Primer on the Rheumatic Diseases

EDITION 12

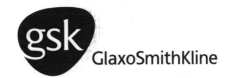

GlaxoSmithKline

*Grateful appreciation is expressed to
GlaxoSmithKline Pharmaceuticals for their support.*

Primer on the Rheumatic Diseases

EDITION 12

JOHN H. KLIPPEL, MD, EDITOR

Leslie J. Crofford, MD, ASSOCIATE EDITOR

John H. Stone, MD, ASSOCIATE EDITOR

Cornelia M. Weyand, MD, ASSOCIATE EDITOR

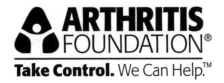

Published by the Arthritis Foundation
1330 West Peachtree Street
Atlanta, Georgia 30309

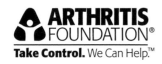

Library of Congress Catalog Card Number: 2001090001
ISBN: 0-912423-29-3

This book is a production of the Arthritis Foundation Publishing Department:
Dennis Bowman, *Senior Vice President, Communications and Health Promotions*
Cindy McDaniel, *Group Vice President, Publishing*
Suzanne Verity, *Associate Vice President, Custom Publishing*
Susan Bernstein, *Director, Book Development and Acquisition*
Susan Siracusa, *Associate Art Director, Publishing*
Elizabeth Compton, *Associate Vice President, Publishing, Production and Operations*
Jamie Lin, *Graphic Designer, Publishing*

Managing Editor: Beth Axtell
Production Designer: Jill Dible
Editorial Contributors: MaryAnne Dunkin, Kim Gochenauer, Rachel Moore, Bruce Tracy

Printed in Canada

CONTRIBUTORS

The following people contributed to the *Primer on the Rheumatic Diseases* by writing or revising chapters and sections for the publication of the twelfth edition. Credits for illustrations are given in figure legends.

Steven B. Abramson, MD
Graciela S. Alarcón, MD, MPH
Ronald J. Anderson, MD
William P. Arend, MD
Frank C. Arnett, MD
Erin L. Arnold, MD
William J. Arnold, MD
John P. Atkinson, MD
Todd Atkinson, MD
W. Timothy Ballard, MD
Thomas Bardin, MD
Karyl S. Barron, MD
Thomas Beardmore, MD
Nicholas Bellamy, MD
Francis Berenbaum, MD, PhD
Clifton O. Bingham, III, MD
Joseph J. Biundo, Jr., MD
Warren D. Blackburn, Jr., MD
David Borenstein, MD
Adele L. Boskey, PhD
Dimitrios T. Boumpas, MD
Laurence A. Bradley, PhD
S. Louis Bridges, Jr., MD, PhD
Joseph A. Buckwalter, MD
Joel Buxbaum, MD
Jill P. Buyon, MD
Leonard H. Calabrese, DO
Kenneth T. Calamia, MD
Leigh F. Callahan, PhD
Grant W. Cannon, MD
Daniel J. Clauw, MD
Philip J. Clements, MD
David R. Cornblath, MD
Leslie J. Crofford, MD
Paul E. DiCorleto, PhD
Jonathan C.W. Edwards, MD
N. Lawrence Edwards, MD
Hani El-Gabalawy, MD
Keith B. Elkon, MD
John M. Esdaile, MD, MPH
Kenneth H. Fye, MD

Allan Gibofsky, MD
Gary S. Gilkeson, MD
Mary B. Goldring, PhD
Duncan A. Gordon, MD
Jörg J. Goronzy, MD
Peter K. Gregersen, MD
Paul B. Halverson, MD
Valee Harisdangkul, MD, PhD
E. Nigel Harris, MD
David B. Hellmann, MD
George Ho, Jr., MD
Marc C. Hochberg, MD, MPH
Gary S. Hoffman, MD
William A. Horton, MD
Robert W. Ike, MD
Gabor G. Illei, MD
Robert D. Inman, MD
Daniel L. Kastner, MD, PhD
Arthur Kavanaugh, MD
Andrew Keat, MD
John Kehrl, MD
Robert P. Kimberly, MD
Warren Knudson, PhD
Klaus E. Kuettner, PhD
Nancy E. Lane, MD
Robert Lash, MD
Thomas J.A. Lehman, MD
Carol B. Lindsley, MD
M. Kathryn Liszewski
Daniel J. Lovell, MD, MPH
Susan Manzi, MD, MPH
Michael Maricic, MD
Manuel Martínez-Lavín, MD
Alfonse T. Masi, MD, DrPH
Eric L. Matteson, MD
Nancy L. McKendree-Smith, PhD
Peter A. Merkel, MD, MPH
Paul Miller, MD
John S. Mort, PhD
Linda Myers, MD
Stanley J. Naides, MD

Michael C. Nevitt, PhD, MPH
Hossein Carlos Nousari, MD
James C. Oates, MD
John J. O'Shea, MD
Kee Duk Park, MD
Stanley R. Pillemer, MD
Robert S. Pinals, MD
David S. Pisetsky, MD, PhD
A. Robin Poole, PhD, DSc
Reed Edwin Pyeritz, MD, PhD
John D. Reveille, MD
Christopher T. Ritchlin, MD
Laura Robbins, DSW
Michael G. Rock, MD
Ann Rosenthal, MD
Lawrence M. Ryan, MD
Kenneth E. Sack, MD
H. Ralph Schumacher, Jr., MD
William W. Scott, Jr., MD
Sean P. Scully, MD, PhD
David D. Sherry, MD
Leonard H. Sigal, MD
Peter A. Simkin, MD
Robert W. Simms, MD
Lee S. Simon, MD
Robert F. Spiera, MD
E. William St.Clair, MD
John H. Stone, MD, MPH
Ioannis O. Tassiulas, MD
Robert A. Terkeltaub, MD
Nelson B. Watts, MD
Cornelia M. Weyand, MD
Barbara White, MD
Fredrick M. Wigley, MD
Ronald L. Wilder, MD, PhD
John B. Winfield, MD
Robert L. Wortmann, MD
Edward H. Yelin, PhD
Steven R. Ytterberg, MD
John B. Zabriskie, MD

TABLE OF CONTENTS

FOREWORD

Publication of this twelfth edition of the *Primer on the Rheumatic Diseases* highlights the Arthritis Foundation's ongoing commitment to the education of health care professionals about arthritis. The *Primer* is recognized as a concise, authoritative, and state of the art summary clinical and scientificwhat physicians and students need to know about the rheumatic diseases. The Foundation hopes that the *Primer* will inspire students in health care professions to dedicate their lives to improving the lives of people with arthritis, and will enable physicians in all fields and in all countries to better understand and improve the care of patients with rheumatic diseases. thus fulfilling the mission of the Arthritis Foundation to better the lives of people with arthritis.

The Arthritis Foundation was founded in 1948 under the name Arthritis and Rheumatism Foundation by an organization of rheumatologists for the purpose of raising funds to support education and research programs. There has been tremendous growth of the Arthritis Foundation over the past half century thanks to the dedication of countless volunteers who remain committed to our mission "to improve lives through leadership in the prevention, control and cure of arthritis and related diseases."

The support of research is a primary goal of the Foundation and critical to our success in achieving the mission. Over the past decade alone, the Foundation's investment in research has exceeded $150 million to fund the work of postdoctoral fellows, new investigators, biomedical and clinical researchers, and health sciences researchers. This year marks the 50th anniversary of the Arthritis Foundation's Postdoctoral Fellowship Program, and we are proud of the role that we have played in supporting the training and career development of researchers and scientists whose work has dramatically improved the lives of people with arthritis.

The effort to improve the quality of life for people with arthritis involves many activities both for people with arthritis and the professionals who care for them. To educate physicians, allied health professionals, and medical students, the Arthritis Foundation offers not only this *Primer*, but the *Bulletin on the Rheumatic Diseases*, videotapes, multimedia resources, and educational symposia.

Through its 150 service points and by means of cooperative agreements with other agencies, the Arthritis Foundation provides programs and services for people with arthritis to help improve the quality of their lives. These programs include exercise classes and videotapes, advocacy programs, self-help courses, and support groups. Educational materials including books, pamphlets, brochures, videotapes, and audiotapes are also available for people with arthritis and their families. The American Juvenile Arthritis Organization, a council of the Arthritis Foundation, provides other materials and programs designed with special attention to the needs of children with arthritis and their parents.

Very importantly, the Arthritis Foundation seeks to increase the awareness of arthritis as a serious health problem. Disability and even mortality from arthritis have profound economic and even more importantly social costs. The Arthritis Foundation is working to convey that message to the public, to health care professionals, and to all levels of government that we must take arthritis much more seriously. The Arthritis Foundation advocates increased funding for research in arthritis and related diseases through the National Institutes of Health and the Centers for Disease Control and Prevention and improved access to medical care for people with arthritis and related diseases.

JOHN H. KLIPPEL, MD
Medical Director
Arthritis Foundation

INTRODUCTION

The *Primer on the Rheumatic Diseases* has always served an important role in the education of students of the rheumatic diseases, including medical students, residents, clinicians, and academics. We are extremely proud to launch the 12th edition of the *Primer*, which comes at a time of great opportunity and optimism that will have a profound impact on the health care of people with arthritis over the next decade. Arthritis is beginning to be taken seriously as an important public health care problem with threats of disability and, in many instances, mortality. We are just beginning to see the results from our investment in research with the introduction of major new drugs that, for many forms of arthritis, have resulted in dramatic improvements in care. Yet these new drugs come with substantial increases in cost, along with specialized expertise and knowledge required for their use. These costs and requirements pose challenges to assure that access to care and new advances in treatment, which will assuredly increase over the next decade, are widely available to all people with arthritis. Finally, we must assure that there are adequate numbers of highly skilled and knowledgeable health care providers to care for people with arthritis.

The *Primer* evolved from several publications of the American Committee for the Control of Rheumatism – What is Rheumatism? in 1928, Rheumatism Primer: Chronic Arthritis in 1932; and Primer on Rheumatism: Chronic Arthritis in 1934 (1). This latter work, generally considered the first edition of the *Primer*, consisted of a 52-page brochure that was prepared for distribution in connection with a scientific exhibit on arthritis at the Annual Convention of the American Medical Association held in Cleveland, Ohio. A revision, the Primer on Arthritis, was published in the *Journal of the American Medical Association* in 1942 (2) as were editions that appeared in 1949 (third), 1953 (fourth), 1959 (fifth), 1964 (sixth), and 1973 (seventh) (3-7). The Arthritis Foundation has published all subsequent editions, which appeared in 1983 (eighth), 1988 (ninth), 1993 (tenth), 1997 (eleventh), as well as the current (twelfth) edition (8-12).

The purpose of this *Primer* remains the same as that of all previous editions – to provide a thorough yet concise description of the current science, diagnosis, clinical consequences, and principles of management of the rheumatic diseases. This edition of the *Primer* has a number of new features that give it a different look. It is noticeably bigger than previous editions as a result of a new, more reader-friendly design. There are many new, first-time Primer authors, each experts in their field and highly respected and capable educators. Chapters on juvenile arthritis, vasculitis, osteoarthritis, and osteoporosis have been expanded to reflect important advances in these fields that have occurred since the previous edition. Finally, the appendices now include a section on herbs and supplements commonly taken by people with rheumatic diseases.

Thanks go to many people who have worked tirelessly for the past two years to make the *Primer* possible. First to the Associate Editors Leslie Crofford, John Stone, and Connie Weyand and their assistants for their help in the planning, organization, editing, and proofing of the chapters – the *Primer* would not have been possible without them. The editorial team wishes to express its sincere thanks to the contributing authors for sharing their expertise, adhering to deadlines, and their understanding and patience in having to deal with the inevitable changes and suggestions offered by the editors. Last but certainly not least, we are all extremely grateful to Beth Axtell and the entire staff at the Arthritis Foundation who coordinated virtually all phases of the *Primer*'s development, rewrote and polished countless chapters to make them readable, and deserve all of the credit for the design of the new *Primer*.

The editors, contributors, and staff of the Arthritis Foundation sincerely hope that it contributes to the education of individuals wanting to learn more about the rheumatic diseases and perhaps to generate new ideas that will provide a better understanding of the causes of rheumatic illness that will lead to improvements in care and eventually ways to prevent and cure arthritis.

JOHN H. KLIPPEL, MD
Editor

1. Benedek TG. A century of American rheumatology. Ann Intern Med 1982;106:304–312.
2. Jordan EP, Bauer W, Boots RH, et al. Primer on arthritis. JAMA 1942;119:1089–1104.
3. McEwen C, Bunim JJ, Freyberg RH, et al. Primer on the rheumatic diseases. JAMA 1949;139 :1068–1076, 1139–1146, 1268–1273.
4. Ragan C, Feldman HA, Clark WS, et al. Primer on the rheumatic diseases. JAMA 1953;152:323–331, 405–414, 522–531.
5. Crain DC, Epstein W, Howell D, et al. Primer on the rheumatic diseases. JAMA 1959;171:1205–1220, 1345–1356, 1680–1691.
6. Decker JL, Bollet AJ, Duff IF, et al. Primer on the rheumatic diseases. JAMA 1964;190:127–140, 425–444, 509–530, 741–751.
7. Rodnan GP, Schumacher HR, Zvaifler NJ. Primer on the rheumatic diseases. JAMA 1973;224:661–812.
8. Rodnan GP, Schumacher HR, Zvaifler NJ. Primer on the Rheumatic Diseases. Atlanta, Arthritis Foundation, 1983.
9. Schumacher HR, Klippel JH, Robinson DR. Primer on the Rheumatic Diseases. Atlanta, Arthritis Foundation, 1988.
10. Schumacher HR, Klippel JH, Koopman WJ. Primer on the Rheumatic Diseases. Atlanta, Arthritis Foundation, 1993.
11. Klippel JH, Weyand CM, Wortmann RL. Primer on the Rheumatic Diseases. Atlanta, Arthritis Foundation, 1997.
12. Klippel JH, Crofford LJ, Stone JH, Weyand CM. Primer on the Rheumatic Diseases. Atlanta, Arthritis Foundation, 2001.

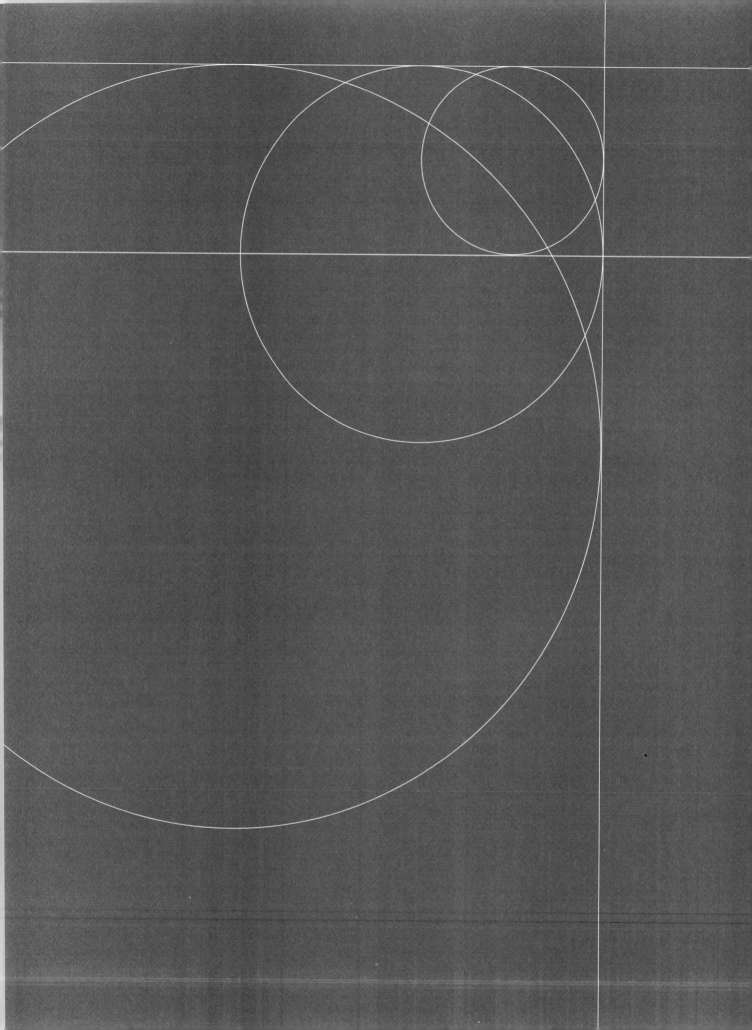

1 THE SOCIAL AND ECONOMIC CONSEQUENCES OF RHEUMATIC DISEASE

Rheumatic diseases, the most prevalent chronic conditions in the United States and a leading cause of disability (1–4), are characterized by chronic pain and progressive physical impairment of joints and soft tissues. They encompass more than 100 diseases and conditions, including osteoarthritis (OA), rheumatoid arthritis (RA), fibromyalgia, systemic lupus erythematosus (SLE), gout, and bursitis. The economic, social, and psychological impact associated with rheumatic diseases is enormous (1,5). Although some of the effects are easily translated into such economic terms as lost wages and medical care costs, many effects, such as pain, reductions in housekeeping activities, or the inability to enjoy leisure activities, are not easily determined. The consequences have a significant impact on individuals with disease, their families, and society. It is important for clinicians and other care providers to understand the burden of rheumatic diseases, so that they may respond to these challenges.

Prevalence and Activity Limitations

Arthritis and rheumatic conditions affected an estimated 43 million Americans in the late 1990s (3,4), and this number is expected to increase to an estimated 60 million by the year 2020 (2). Approximately 21 million people have OA, 3.7 million have fibromyalgia, and 2.1 million have RA (4). Risk factors associated with various forms of arthritis include nonmodifiable and modifiable factors, as well as some demographic factors (2,6–8). Nonmodifiable risk factors are female sex, older age, and genetic predisposition. Modifiable risk factors are obesity, joint injuries, infections, and certain occupations, such as shipyard work, farming, heavy industry, and occupations with repetitive knee bending. The demographic factors associated with the various forms of arthritis include lower levels of formal education and lower income.

Arthritis and rheumatic diseases significantly limit the ability of more than seven million Americans to participate in such daily activities as going to work or school and housekeeping (2). The prevalence of arthritis-related disability, like arthritis prevalence, is also expected to rise. By the year 2020, an estimated 11.6 million individuals will be limited in their ability to perform daily activities.

When the rank and prevalence of chronic conditions causing disability in the United States in 1991–1992 were analyzed, arthritis was the leading cause of disability (Fig. 1-1) (9). Disability was assessed using five measures: 1) ability to perform functional activities; 2) activities of daily living; 3) instrumental activities of daily living; 4) presence of selected impairments; and 5) use of assistive aids. An estimated 42 million persons reported one or more conditions they believed to be associated with their disability. Of those individuals, 17.1% reported arthritis or rheumatism, 13.5% reported back or spine problems, and 11.1% reported heart trouble as being associated with their disability (Fig. 1-1).

Economic Impact

Cost-of-illness studies generally are divided into three categories: direct costs, indirect costs, and intangible costs (10). Direct costs are the costs that accrue when people receive medical care, such as physician visits, hospitalizations, medications, and diagnostic tests. Direct costs also include expenditures for such items as home adaptations and

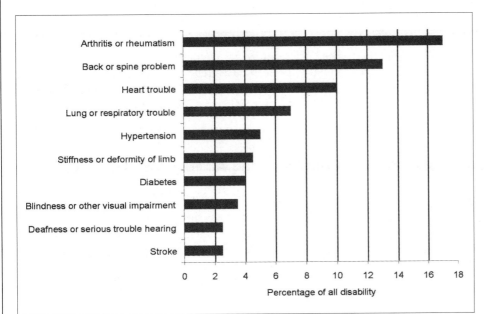

Fig. 1-1. Prevalence of chronic conditions causing disability in the United States in 1991–1992. Data from *Morbidity and Mortality Weekly Report* (9).

transportation to health care providers, but it often is difficult to accurately estimate these expenditures. Indirect costs usually are calculated as costs due to lost wages from a reduction or cessation of work. Intangible costs are the costs of individuals foregoing the activities they and society value. Intangible costs include the costs associated with a decline in functional capacity, increased pain, and reduced quality of life. Most comprehensive studies of the national cost of illness do not include intangible costs, due to the difficulty in assessing all of these costs in population-based studies.

In comprehensive studies of the economic cost of musculoskeletal disease, Rice and colleagues have estimated that the total costs of these conditions are equivalent to 2.5% of the gross national product (GNP) (1). In 1995 dollars, the estimated total economic impact of musculoskeletal conditions on the U. S. economy was $215 billion (Table 1-1) (5). Of that total, direct costs accounted for 41% and indirect costs accounted for 59%. Total costs for arthritis have risen from $65 billion in 1992 dollars to $82.5 billion in 1995 dollars, which represents 38% of the total cost of all musculoskeletal conditions (1,5).

The estimated direct costs of medical care for all forms of arthritis totaled $21.7 billion (Table 1-1). Expenditures for nursing-home care accounted for the largest percentage of direct costs, $12.7 billion (59%) (Fig. 1-2). Hospital inpatient care totaled $3.1 billion, or 14% of direct costs. According to the National Hospital Discharge Survey, patients hospitalized for arthritis account for approximately 2.6 million days of care (5). Administration and physician outpatient costs contribute $1.2 billion and $1.1 billion, respectively (each, approximately 5% of direct costs).

Estimated indirect costs due to arthritis in 1995 dollars were $60.8 billion or 74% of the total costs (Table 1-1) (5). As noted in previous studies of the costs of arthritis, the indirect costs are almost three times greater than the direct costs (1). This estimate would be even larger if the costs attributed to loss of homemaking functions could be determined more easily. Furthermore, older women have lower labor-force participation rates, resulting in lower estimates of economic impact for the current cohort of women.

The costs of rheumatic disease extend far beyond the direct medical care costs and the indirect costs associated with work loss. The intangible costs include pain, psychological distress, changes in family structure, limitations in instrumental and nurturing activities, and changes in appearance resulting from deformity (1,11).

Work Disability and Role Limitations

As reflected in the indirect costs, the capacity of individuals with rheumatic diseases to work is affected significantly (12–15). In fact, rheumatic disease is the leading cause of work loss and the second leading cause of work disability payments (15,16). For two of the most prevalent rheumatic conditions, OA and RA, studies have documented significant work disability (11,16). For example, substantial earnings losses and work disability have been noted in individuals younger than age 65 with asymmetric oligoarthritis, a surrogate for OA (13), and approximately one-half of the people with RA who are working at the onset of disease become work-disabled (15).

Determinants of work disability in individuals with rheumatic disease exist at the societal and individual levels (16). Risk factors on a societal level include economic conditions, attitudinal and architectural barriers, types of jobs available, employer practices, and the characteristics of disability pension plans (16). Individual-level determinants include work autonomy, social factors, and disease factors (14,16).

Rheumatic diseases clearly have negative effects on family-role functioning and the person with the condition (17). Role limitations associated with rheumatic disease include significant reductions in the amount of time individuals spend engaged in such activities as shopping, visiting the bank and supermarket, homemaking, interacting with friends and family, or participating in hobbies (1,17,18). Functional status has been shown to be the most important determinant of household work performance (17).

Psychological Consequences

In addition to the significant economic costs, activity and role limitations, and disability associated with rheumatic disease, the psychological impact of rheumatic disease has been documented in a number of clinical studies (1). The impact has been measured in terms of depression, anxiety, learned helplessness, coping strategies, cognitive changes, and self-efficacy. Most studies note higher levels of psycho-

TABLE 1-1
Direct and Indirect Costs of All Musculoskeletal Conditions and All Forms of Arthritis

Condition	Direct costs	Indirect costs	Total costs
All musculoskeletal conditions	88.7 (41%)	126.3 (59%)	215
All forms of arthritis	21.7 (26%)	60.8 (74%)	82.5

In billions of 1995 dollars. Adapted from Praemer, Furner, Rice (5).

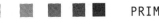

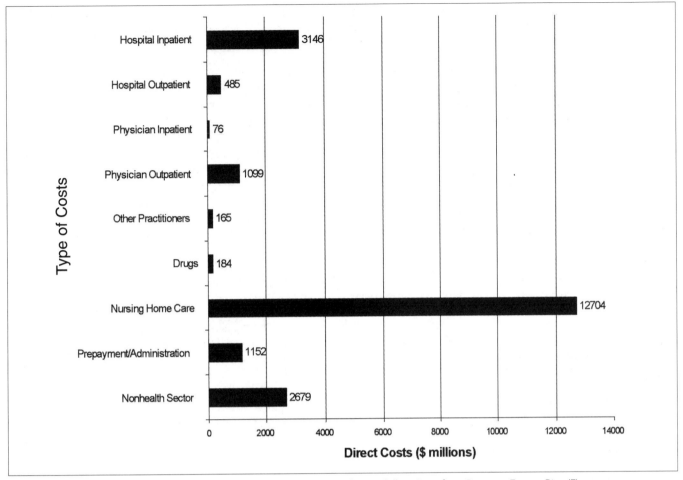

Fig. 1-2. Direct costs of medical care for all forms of arthritis in millions of 1995 dollars. Data from Praemer, Furner, Rice (5).

logical distress in individuals with rheumatic disease than in the general population. The levels of distress reported in people with rheumatic disease are comparable to levels noted in clinical samples of individuals with other chronic conditions (19). Higher levels of psychological distress in individuals with rheumatic disease also have been associated with poorer status on clinical outcome variables and with increased health services utilization (20).

Research into depressive symptoms and disorders has focused on OA, RA, fibromyalgia, and SLE (19). Although depressive symptoms and disorders are more common among clinical samples of individuals with rheumatic disease than in the general population, the majority of individuals with rheumatic disease do not report increased depression. Among persons with RA, the loss of valued activities and the self-perception of the ability to do activities are correlated strongly with psychological status (18).

Conclusions and Policy Implications

Given the high prevalence and significant impact of rheumatic diseases in terms of economic, functional, social, and psychological consequences, these diseases should receive considerable attention from society. The burdens will increase dramatically in the near future due to the aging of the population, underscoring the need for a public health approach. In 1998, a consortium of national organizations produced "The National Arthritis Action Plan: A Public Health Strategy," a comprehensive and ambitious plan for addressing the looming epidemic of arthritis (21). The plan was developed under the leadership of the Centers for Disease Control and Prevention (CDC), the Arthritis Foundation, and the Association of State and Territorial Health Officials. These three organizations were joined by nearly 90 other organizations, including academic institutions, professional societies, government agencies, voluntary health agencies, and others with an interest in arthritis prevention.

The National Arthritis Action Plan is based on the underlying principles that the disability and chronic pain associated with arthritis reduce quality of life and that arthritis can be prevented (21). The plan is based on a growing recognition that public health must shift its emphasis from diseases that kill to diseases that destroy quality of life. In terms of prevention, there is a growing body of evidence that arthritis can be addressed effectively at all three levels of the prevention spectrum – primary, secondary, and tertiary (11). For example, primary prevention of OA is feasible through weight control, exercise, and injury prevention; secondary prevention of RA appears achievable through early diagnosis and aggressive treatment; and tertiary prevention of the negative effects of arthritis can be achieved through self-management classes or increasingly efficacious new therapies (11,21).

The National Arthritis Action Plan outlines a public health strategy with emphasis in three areas: 1) surveillance, epidemiology, and prevention research; 2) communication and education; and 3) programs, policies, and systems (21). Activities in the surveillance and epidemiology area address the need to establish a solid scientific base of knowledge about the prevention of arthritis. The communication and education activities are designed to raise awareness of arthritis as a public health problem and to stimulate creative responses to this problem. The emphasis in the program, policies, and systems area is on developing approaches for systematic change, based on a recognition that arthritis affects individuals in a social context and that this context can be changed in ways that promote health and prevent disease.

The National Arthritis Action Plan follows two historical national efforts to address arthritis. The first was the National Arthritis Act of 1975, which led to the development of Multipurpose Arthritis and Musculoskeletal Disease Centers. The second was the 1986 establishment of an arthritis institute at the National Institutes of Health, the National Institute of Arthritis and Musculoskeletal and Skin Diseases. This third milestone should provide a framework for new partnerships and collaborations to address the important issues and challenges of arthritis. In addition, the incorporation of arthritis-specific objectives in Healthy People 2010 and the launch of the Decade of Bone and Joint Disease in the year 2000 should further enhance society's understanding of the burden of rheumatic disease. Health professionals should familiarize themselves with these public health activities. The success of these approaches will depend on informed participation of health professionals interested in rheumatic diseases.

LEIGH F. CALLAHAN, PhD
EDWARD H. YELIN, PhD

References

1. Yelin E, Callahan LF. The economic cost and social and psychological impact of musculoskeletal conditions. Arthritis Rheum 1995;38:1351–1362.
2. Centers for Disease Control and Prevention. Arthritis prevalence and activity limitations – United States, 1990. MMWR Morb Mortal Wkly Rep 1994;43:433–438.
3. Centers for Disease Control and Prevention. Prevalence and impact of chronic joint symptoms – seven states, 1996. MMWR Morb Mortal Wkly Rep 1998;47:345–351.
4. Lawrence RC, Helmick CG, Arnett FC, et al. Estimates of the prevalence of arthritis and selected musculoskeletal disorders in the United States. Arthritis Rheum 1998;41:778–799.
5. Praemer A, Furner S, Rice D. Musculoskeletal Conditions in the United States. 2nd ed. Rosemont, IL: American Academy of Orthopaedic Surgeons, 1999.
6. Callahan LF, Rao J, Boutaugh M. Arthritis and women's health: prevalence, impact, and prevention. Am J Prev Med 1996;12:401–409.
7. Felson DT, Zhang Y. An update on the epidemiology of knee and hip osteoarthritis with a view to prevention. Arthritis Rheum 1998;41:1343–1355.
8. Felson DT, Hannan MT, Naimark A, et al. Occupational physical demands, knee bending, and knee osteoarthritis: results from the Framingham Study. J Rheumatol 1991;18:1587–1592.
9. Centers for Disease Control and Prevention. Prevalence of disabilities and associated health conditions – United States, 1991–1992. MMWR Morb Mortal Wkly Rep 1994;43:730–739.
10. Hall J, Mooney G. What every doctor should know about economics. Part I. The benefits of costing. Med J Aust 1990;152:29–31.
11. Callahan LF. Impact of rheumatic disease on society. In: Wegener ST, Belza BL, Gall EP (eds). Clinical Care in the Rheumatic Diseases. Atlanta: American College of Rheumatology, 1996; pp 209–213.
12. Yelin E. Arthritis: the cumulative impact of a common chronic condition. Arthritis Rheum 1992;35:489–497.
13. Pincus T, Mitchell JM, Burkhauser RV. Substantial work disability and earnings losses in individuals less than age 65 with osteoarthritis: comparisons with rheumatoid arthritis. J Clin Epidemiol 1989;42:449–457.
14. Yelin EH, Henke CJ, Epstein WV. Work disability among persons with musculoskeletal conditions. Arthritis Rheum 1986;29:1322–1333.
15. Yelin EH. Work disability and rheumatoid arthritis. In: Wolfe F, Pincus T (eds). Rheumatoid Arthritis: Pathogenesis, Assessment, Outcome, and Treatment. New York: Marcel Dekker, 1994; pp 261–271.
16. Allaire SH. Work disability. In: Wegener ST, Belza BL, Gall EP (eds). Clinical Care in the Rheumatic Diseases. Atlanta: American College of Rheumatology, 1996; pp 141–145.
17. Reisine ST. Arthritis and the family. Arthritis Care Res 1995;8:265–271.
18. Katz PP, Yelin EH. Life activities of persons with rheumatoid arthritis with and without depressive symptoms. Arthritis Care Res 1994;7:69–77.
19. DeVellis B. Depression in rheumatological diseases. Bailliere's Clin Rheumatol 1993;7:241–257.
20. Hawley DJ, Wolfe F. Anxiety and depression in patients with rheumatoid arthritis: a prospective study of 400 patients. J Rheumatol 1988;15:932–941.
21. Meenan RF, Callahan LF, Helmick CG. The National Arthritis Action Plan: a public health strategy for a looming epidemic. Arthritis Care Res 1999;12:79–81.

2

THE MUSCULOSKELETAL SYSTEM
A. Joints

Human bones join with each other in a variety of ways to serve the functional requirements of the musculoskeletal system. Foremost among these needs is that of purposeful motion. From the digital dexterity of the accomplished musician to the raw power of the world-class weightlifter, the activities of the human body depend on effective interaction between normal joints and the neuromuscular units that drive them. The same elements interact reflexively to distribute mechanical stresses among the tissues of the joint. Muscles, tendons, ligaments, cartilage, and bone all do their share to ensure smooth function of the human machine. In this role, the supporting elements unite the abutting bones and optimally position the cartilage for low-friction load-bearing.

Classification

Differing designs of human joints usually have been classified according to a scheme based on the histologic features of the union and the range of motion it permits. *Synarthroses*, or "suture lines," are found in the skull where adjoining cranial plates are separated only by thin fibrous tissue as they interlock to prevent detectable motion but provide for orderly growth. When cranial growth ceases, synarthrodial joints have no further role and they close.

In *amphiarthroses*, adjacent bones are bound by flexible fibrocartilage that permits modest motion to occur. In the pubic symphysis and in a portion of the sacroiliac joint, amphiarthroses permit minor rotatory motion of the pelvic bones. Between the vertebral bodies, the intervertebral disc has developed into a more mobile, highly specialized amphiarthrodial articulation.

The third class of joint design, the *diarthroses*, includes the most mobile joints and is by far the most common of the articular design patterns. Because these joints possess a synovial membrane and contain synovial fluid, diarthrodial joints more commonly are referred to as *synovial joints*.

Synovial joints are further subclassified according to shape, i.e., *ball and socket* (hip), *hinge* (interphalangeal), *saddle* (first carpometacarpal), and *plane* (patellofemoral) joints. These widely varying configurations reflect the fact that form parallels function in the design of diarthrodial joints. In every case, a well-lubricated bearing develops from essentially congruent cartilaginous surfaces that slide freely against each other. The direction and the extent of the permitted motion are defined by the shape and size of the opposing surfaces (Fig. 2A-1). Within these limitations, a wide variety of designs permit motion in flexion (bending),

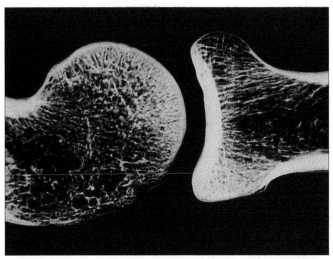

Fig. 2A-1. Radiograph of a 3-mm sagittal slab through an extended elbow joint. The convex distal humerus has a thin subchondral plate and honeycombed underlying trabeculation, whereas the concave, proximal radius has a thick subchondral plate over coarse, vertical trabecular bone. Comparable convex-concave differences are regularly seen in other large human joints. Reprinted with permission from Simkin et al (8).

extension (straightening), abduction (away from the midline), adduction (toward the midline), and rotation. Individual joints thus can act in one (humero-ulnar joint), two (wrist), or even three (shoulder) axes of motion.

Articular Tissues

Articular cartilage comprises the low-friction surface that covers the opposing members of synovial joints. The structure and composition of this unique tissue are described in Chapter 2B.

Synovial joints are surrounded by a capsule that defines the boundary between articular and periarticular tissues. The capsule varies in thickness from an inapparent membrane in some areas to a strong ligamentous band in others. A reinforced capsular plate, for instance, serves as effective prevention against hyperextension of most hinge joints. Over extensor aspects of the same joints, the capsule is a much less consequential structure. Reinforcing the capsule are additional ligaments that sometimes are extracapsular. Further periarticular support is provided by the tendons of muscles acting across the joint. Capsule, ligaments, and tendons are formed primarily from bundles of type I collagen fibers aligned with the axis of tensile stress (1). Tendons and ligaments characteristically include a thin region of fibrocartilage at the entheses, the sites where they attach to bone (2).

The synovial intima comprises the lining tissue (one to three cells deep) that surfaces all intracapsular structures other than the contact areas of cartilage (3). This highly flexible, well-lubricated lining normally is collapsed upon itself and upon articular cartilage to minimize the volume of the joint space it encloses. When opened, most normal human joints reveal moist and tacky synovial and cartilaginous surfaces, but no obvious pool of synovial fluid.

The synovial lining cells reside in a matrix rich in collagen fibrils and proteoglycans. In most areas, the cells do not directly abut each other but are separated by interstitium. Principal cells of the normal synovium come in two forms, type A and type B (Fig. 2A-2). The monocyte-derived type A cell resembles a macrophage in its high content of cytoplasmic organelles, which include lysosomes, smooth-walled vacuoles, and micropinocytotic vesicles. In contrast, the fibroblastic type B cell has fewer organelles and a more extensive endoplasmic reticulum. Other cells sometimes seen in normal synovial tissue include apparent antigen-processing cells with a dendritic configuration, mast cells, and occasional white blood cells.

The synovial lining is supported by a rich bed of fenestrated microvessels (Fig. 2A-3) that, for the most part, lie immediately below the lining cells at the surface of the joint space (4). These vessels are terminal branches of an arterial plexus that supports the capsule and the juxta-articular bone. Synovial tissue also includes a generous complement of lymphatic vessels and nerve fibers. The innervation derives from the nerve roots supplying each of the muscles that cross the joint.

The synovial intima overlies a spectrum of matrices ranging from fibrous capsule through loose areolar connective tissue to organized structures composed mainly of fat. Such "fat pads" serve as flexible, space-occupying structures that help to accommodate the vast changes in geometry imposed by normal articular motion. In other locations, a similar role is played by much more solid fibrocartilaginous structures. The best examples of the latter are found in the knees, where the medial and lateral menisci help preserve alignment and distribute loads (5).

Stress Distribution

In active motion, substantial loading forces cross each normal joint. If these forces exceed the inherent limits of a tissue, the structure will fracture or fail. Normal joints distribute these forces, however, and thus minimize the likelihood of failure in one component. The greatest share of loading energy is taken up within the muscles and tendons crossing each joint. Effective reflexes normally ensure that impact forces are delivered to flexed joints, which bend farther under the acute load in a response of the extensor muscles known as *eccentric contraction*. Most people have experienced the surprise of finding one more step than expected when descending a flight of stairs. The sudden jolt of that moment results from landing on a hip and knee that have not flexed in anticipation of the impact. Appropriate flexion of these joints distributes the stress in time by prolonging the deceleration of landing and in space by loading a larger surface area of each convex joint member as it slides within the embrace of its concave mate.

Loading stress not absorbed by surrounding muscles, tendons, and ligaments impacts directly on the opposing articular cartilage and its underlying trabecular bone. The firm, resilient articular cartilage has viscoelastic properties that allow it to serve as a hydraulic shock absorber analogous to those found in an automobile (6). Despite these desirable characteristics, the cartilage is so thin that the loading energy at contact surfaces is transmitted mainly into bone (7).

Immediately beneath the cartilage is a continuous plate of subchondral bone supported by a complex, fat-filled meshwork of underlying trabeculae. In convex members, such as the femoral and humeral heads, this plate is a thin shell supported by a honeycombed structure of interconnecting bony chambers. In contrast, the opposing concave acetabulum and the glenoid fossa have much thicker subchondral plates supported by a coarser and more open framework of trabecular struts (8). This structural difference in bone is matched by a corresponding difference in the thickness of overlying cartilage. In cartilage, however, the thicker layer is

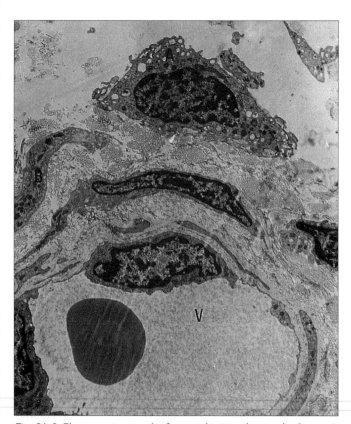

Fig. 2A-2. Electron micrograph of synovial intima showing both type A and type B lining cells within a well-organized synovial matrix. V indicates a superficial synovial vessel. Courtesy of HR Schumacher, MD.

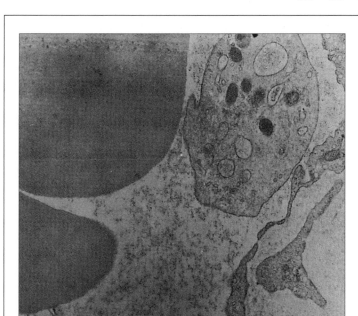

Fig. 2A-3. Higher magnification electron micrograph of a synovial vessel shows red cells and a platelet in the lumen. The endothelium has fenestrations closed by diaphragms. Courtesy of HR Schumacher, MD.

on the convex side, while the thinner layer is concave and tends to have more of a fibrous than hyaline composition. These concave-convex differences in structure provide for stiff concave joint members in opposition to more flexible convex mates. The clinical significance of these structural and functional differences lies in patterns of injury where overwhelming stresses regularly explode the stiff, concave side but do not crush its more flexible, convex opponent. Conversely, raised subchondral pressures in loaded convex bones may play a role in their special vulnerability to ischemic necrosis of bone, or *osteonecrosis* (9).

Stability

A number of factors interact to confer stability while permitting motion in active human joints. First among these factors is the simple shape of the component parts. In the hip, for example, the articular members are configured and positioned so that normal loading enhances the closeness of their fit when weight-bearing drives the femoral head into its acetabular socket.

Ligaments provide a second major stabilizing influence as they guide and align normal joints through their range of motion. An excellent example is the pair of collateral ligaments along each side of interphalangeal joints. These strong, relatively inelastic structures limit articular motion to flexion and extension.

Within the axes of motion, however, more forgiving constraints are required, and this need is met by muscles and tendons. Muscular stabilization is perhaps most obvious in the shoulder, which is the quintessential polyaxial joint. Here, the rotator cuff muscles approximate and stabilize the

articular surfaces, while larger muscles with better leverage provide the power for effective shoulder motion (10).

The synovial fluid contributes significant stabilizing effects as an adhesive seal that freely permits sliding motion between cartilaginous surfaces, but effectively resists distracting forces. This property is most easily demonstrated in small articulations, such as those that occur in the metacarpophalangeal joints. There, the common phenomenon of "knuckle cracking" reflects the fracture of this adhesive bond. Secondary cavitation within the joint space causes a radiologically obvious bubble of gas that requires up to 30 minutes to dissolve before the bond can be re-established and the joint can be "cracked" again (11). This adhesive property depends on the normally thin film of synovial fluid between all intra-articular structures. When this film enlarges as a pathologic effusion, its stabilizing properties are lost.

The intra-articular pressure is about –4 mm Hg in the resting, normal knee, and this pressure falls further when the quadriceps muscle contracts. The difference between atmospheric pressure on overlying tissues and subatmospheric values within the joint helps to hold the joint members together, and thus provides a stabilizing force. In a pathologic effusion, however, the resting pressure is above that of the atmosphere and it rises further when surrounding muscles contract. Thus, reversal of the normal pressure gradient is an additional destabilizing factor in joints with effusions (12).

Lubrication

Synovial joints act as mechanical bearings that facilitate the work of the musculoskeletal machine. As such, normal joints are remarkably effective with coefficients of friction lower than those obtainable with sliding bearings in industrial machines. Furthermore, the constant process of renewal and restoration ensures that living articular tissues have a durability far superior to that of any artificial bearing. It is thus axiomatic that no arthroplastic implant can equal the performance of a normal human joint.

The mechanics of joint lubrication have provided a productive focus of investigation beginning with the unique structure of the bearing surface. Because articular cartilage is elastic, fluid-filled, and backed by a relatively impervious layer of calcified cartilage and bone, load-induced compression of cartilage can be expected to force interstitial fluid to flow laterally within the tissue and to surface through adjacent cartilage. As that area, in turn, becomes load-bearing, it is partially protected by the newly expressed fluid above it. This is a special form of *hydrodynamic lubrication*, so called because the dynamic motion of the bearing areas produces an aqueous layer that separates and thus protects the contact points (6).

Boundary layer lubrication is the second major mechanism considered important in the low-friction characteristics of normal joints. Here, the critical factor is a small glycoprotein called *lubricin*. The lubricating properties of this synovium-derived molecule are highly specific and depend on its ability to provide a slippery coating for the surface of articular cartilage (13).

Another important molecule in articular lubrication is *hyaluronan*, the molecule that makes synovial fluid viscous. It is useful to remember that the term *synovia* was coined to convey the resemblance of joint fluid to highly viscous normal egg white. The viscosity imparted by synovial hyaluronan augments hydrodynamic lubrication as it retards the outflow of load-bearing fluid. Hyaluronan also plays a major role in lubricating a quite different site of surface contact, that of synovium on cartilage. The well-vascularized, well-innervated synovium must sequentially contract and then expand to cover nonloaded cartilage surfaces as each joint moves through its normal range of motion. This process must proceed freely. Were synovial tissue to be pinched, there would be immediate pain, intra-articular bleeding, and inevitable functional compromise. The rarity of these problems testifies to the effectiveness of hyaluronan-mediated synovial lubrication.

Synovial Fluid

In normal human joints, a thin film of synovial fluid covers the surfaces of synovium and cartilage within the joint space. Only in disease does the volume of this fluid increase to produce an effusion that is clinically apparent and may be aspirated easily for study. For this reason, most knowledge of human synovial fluid comes not from normal subjects but from people with joint disease. Because of the clinical frequency, volume, and accessibility of knee effusions, our knowledge is further focused on findings in that joint.

In the synovium, as in all tissues, essential nutrients are delivered and metabolic byproducts are cleared by the bloodstream perfusing the local vasculature. Synovial microvessels contain fenestrations that facilitate diffusion-based exchange between plasma and the surrounding interstitium. Free diffusion provides full equilibration of small solutes between plasma and the immediate interstitial space. Further diffusion, augmented by the convection caused by joint use, extends this equilibration to all other intracapsular spaces, including the synovial fluid and the interstitial fluid of cartilage. Synovial plasma flow and the narrow diffusion path between synovial lining cells provide the principal limitations on exchange rates between plasma and synovial fluid (14).

This process is clinically relevant to the transport of therapeutic agents in inflamed synovial joints. Many investigators have made serial observations of drug concentrations in plasma and synovial fluid after oral or intravenous administration. Predictably, plasma levels exceed those in synovial fluid during the early phases of absorption and distribution. This gradient reverses during the subsequent period of elimination when intrasynovial levels exceed those of plasma. These patterns reflect passive diffusion alone. The delays in equilibration primarily reflect effusion volume, and no therapeutic agent is known to be transported into or selectively retained within the joint space (15).

Metabolic evidence of ischemia provides a second instance when the delivery and removal of small solutes becomes clinically relevant. In normal joints and in most pathologic effusions, essentially full equilibration exists between plasma and synovial fluid. The gradients that drive net delivery of nutrients (glucose and oxygen) or removal of wastes (lactate and carbon dioxide) are too small to be detected. In some cases, however, the synovial microvascular supply is unable to meet local metabolic demand, and significant gradients develop. In these joints, the synovial fluid reveals a low oxygen pressure (P_{O_2}), low glucose, low pH, high lactate, and high carbon dioxide pressure (P_{CO_2}). Such fluids are found regularly in septic arthritis, often in rheumatoid arthritis, and infrequently in other kinds of synovitis. These findings presumably reflect both the increased metabolic demand of hyperplastic tissue and an impaired microvascular response. Consistent with this interpretation is the finding that ischemic rheumatoid joints are colder than are joints containing synovial fluid in full equilibration with plasma (16). Like other peripheral tissues, joints normally have temperatures lower than that of the body's core. The knee, for instance, has a normal intra-articular temperature of 32°C. With acute local inflammation, articular blood flow increases, the temperature approaches 37°C, and the joint feels "hot" to the examining hand. As active rheumatoid synovitis persists, however, microcirculatory compromise may cause the tissues to become ischemic and the temperature to fall.

The clinical implications of local ischemia remain under investigation. Decreased synovial fluid pH, for instance, was found to correlate strongly with radiographic evidence of joint damage in rheumatoid knees (17). Other work has shown that transient increases in intrasynovial pressure may exert a tamponade effect on the synovial vasculature. This finding has led to the suggestion that normal use of swollen joints may create a cycle of ischemia and reperfusion that leads to tissue damage by release of toxic oxygen radicals (18).

Normal articular cartilage has no microvascular supply of its own and, therefore, is conspicuous among the tissues at risk in ischemic joints. In this tissue, the normal process of diffusion is supplemented by the convection induced by cyclic compression and release during joint usage. In immature joints, the same pumping process promotes exchange of small molecules with the well-vascularized interstitial tissue of underlying trabecular bone. In adults, however, this potential route of supply is considered less likely, and all exchange of solutes may occur through synovial fluid. As a result, normal chondrocytes may be farther from their supporting microvasculature than are any other cells in the body. The vulnerability of this extended supply line is clearly shown in synovial ischemia.

The normal proteins of plasma also enter synovial fluid passively. In contrast to small molecules, however, protein concentrations remain substantially less in synovial fluid than in plasma. In aspirates from normal knees, the total protein was only 1.3 g/dl, a value roughly 20% of that in normal plasma (19). Moreover, the distribution of intrasynovial proteins differs from that found in plasma. Large proteins such as immunoglobulin M and α_2-macroglobulin are underrepresented, whereas smaller proteins are present in relatively high concentrations. This pattern reflects transport across the vascular endothelium that becomes progressively more restrictive with increasing molecular size, allowing smaller proteins to enter the joint space at rates proportionately faster than those of large proteins. In contrast, proteins leave synovial fluid through lymphatic vessels, a process that is not selective across the size range of almost all plasma proteins. Thus, in all joints, the continuing, passive transport of plasma proteins involves microvascular delivery, size-dependent transport across the endothelium, and essentially nonselective lymphatic return to plasma. With certain macromolecules, most notably hyaluronan, access to the terminal lymphatics may be restricted, and resultant clearance rates lag behind those of plasma proteins.

The intrasynovial concentration of any protein represents the net contributions of plasma concentration, synovial blood flow, microvascular permeability, and lymphatic removal. In addition, specific proteins may be produced or consumed within the joint space. Thus, lubricin normally is synthesized within synovial cells and released into synovial fluid, where it facilitates boundary layer lubrication of the cartilage-on-cartilage bearing. In disease, additional proteins may be synthesized (e.g., IgG rheumatoid factor in rheumatoid arthritis), released from inflammatory cells (e.g., cytokines or enzymes), or mobilized from articular tissues (e.g., constituents of the cartilage matrix) (20). In contrast, intra-articular proteins may be depleted by local consumption, as are complement components in rheumatoid arthritis.

Synovial fluid protein concentrations vary little between highly inflamed rheumatoid joints and modestly involved osteoarthritic articulations. Microvascular permeability to protein, however, is more than twice as great in rheumatoid arthritis as in osteoarthritis (21). This marked difference in permeability leads to only a minimal increase in protein concentration, because the enhanced ingress of proteins is largely offset by a comparable rise in lymphatic egress. These findings illustrate the fact that synovial microvascular permeability cannot be evaluated from protein concentrations unless the kinetics of delivery or removal are assessed concurrently.

PETER A. SIMKIN, MD

References

1. Amiel D, Frank C, Harwood F, Fronek J, Akeson W. Tendons and ligaments: a morphological and biochemical comparison. J Orthop Res 1984;1:257–265.
2. Benjamin M, Ralphs JR. Fibrocartilage in tendons and ligaments—an adaptation to compressive load. J Anat 1998; 193:481–494.
3. Henderson B, Edwards JCW. The Synovial Lining in Health and Disease. London: Chapman and Hall, 1987.
4. Knight AD, Levick JR. Morphometry of the ultrastructure of the blood-joint barrier in the rabbit knee. Q J Exp Physiol 1984;69:271–288.
5. Messner K, Gao J. The menisci of the knee joint. Anatomical and functional characteristics, and a rationale for clinical treatment. J Anat 1998;193:161–178.
6. Mow VC, Roth V, Armstrong CG. Biomechanics of joint cartilage. In: Frankel VH, Nordin M (eds). Basic Biomechanics of the Skeletal System. Philadelphia: Lea & Febiger, 1980; pp 61–86.
7. Radin EL. Mechanics of joint degeneration. In: Radin EL, Simon SR, Rose RM, Paul IL (eds). Practical Biomechanics for the Orthopedic Surgeon. New York: John Wiley & Sons, 1979.
8. Simkin PA, Graney DO, Feichtner JJ. Roman arches, human joints, and disease: differences between convex and concave sides of joints. Arthritis Rheum 1980;23:1308–1311.
9. Downey DJ, Simkin PA, Taggart R. The effect of compressive loading on intraosseous pressure in the femoral head in vitro. J Bone Joint Surg 1988;70(6):871–877.
10. Jobe CM. Gross anatomy of the shoulder. In: Rockwood CA, Matsen FA (eds). The Shoulder. Philadelphia: WB Saunders, 1990; pp 34–97.
11. Unsworth A, Dowson D, Wright V. "Cracking joints": a bioengineering study of cavitation in the metacarpophalangeal joint. Ann Rheum Dis 1971;30:348–358.
12. Levick JR. Joint pressure-volume studies: their importance, design and interpretation. J Rheumatol 1983;10:353–357.
13. Jay GD, Britt DE, Cha CJ. Lubricin is a product of megakaryocyte stimulating factor gene expression by human synovial fibroblasts. J Rheumatol 2000;27:594–600.
14. Levick JR. Blood flow and mass transport in synovial joints. In: Renkin EM, Michel CC (eds). Handbook of Physiology, Vol. IV. Microcirculation, Part 2. Bethesda, MD: American Physiological Society, 1984; pp 917–947.
15. Simkin PA, Wu MP, Foster DM. Articular pharmacokinetics of protein-bound antirheumatic agents. Clin Pharmacokinet 1993;25:342–350.
16. Wallis WJ, Simkin PA, Nelp WB. Low synovial clearance of iodide provides evidence of hypoperfusion in chronic rheumatoid synovitis. Arthritis Rheum 1985;28:1096–1104.
17. Geborek P, Saxne T, Pettersson H, Wollheim FA. Synovial fluid acidosis correlates with radiological joint destruction in rheumatoid arthritis knee joints. J Rheumatol 1989;16: 468–472.
18. Stevens CR, Williams RB, Farrell AJ, Blake DR. Hypoxia and inflammatory synovitis: observations and speculation. Ann Rheum Dis 1991;50:124–132.
19. Weinberger A, Simkin PA. Plasma proteins in synovial fluids of normal human joints. Semin Arthritis Rheum 1989;19: 66–76.
20. Simkin PA, Bassett JE. Cartilage matrix molecules in serum and synovial fluid. Curr Opin Rheumatol 1995;7:346–351.
21. Wallis WJ, Simkin PA, Nelp WB. Protein traffic in human synovial effusions. Arthritis Rheum 1987;30:57–63.

THE MUSCULOSKELETAL SYSTEM
B. Articular Cartilage

Articular cartilage is a specialized connective tissue that covers the weight-bearing surfaces of articulating (diarthrodial) joints. Its extracellular matrix is composed of an extensive network of collagen fibrils, which confers tensile strength, and an interlocking mesh of proteoglycans, which provides compressive stiffness through its ability to absorb and extrude water. Lubrication by synovial fluid provides frictionless movement of the articulating cartilage surfaces. Chondrocytes, the sole cellular component of adult hyaline articular cartilage, are responsible for synthesizing and maintaining the highly specialized cartilage matrix macromolecules.

Cartilage Structure

The unique structural properties and biochemical components of diarthrodial joints make them extraordinarily durable load-bearing devices (1). The principal role for the cartilage layer is to reduce friction in the joint and absorb the shock associated with locomotion. The articular cartilage is bathed in synovial fluid, a lubricant that serves to some degree as a source of nutrition for chondrocytes. More than 70% of articular cartilage is water. More than 90% of articular cartilage's dry weight consists of two components, type II collagen and the large proteoglycan aggrecan (2,3). However, several "minor" collagens and small proteoglycans also play roles in cartilage matrix organization (4,5). The physical properties of articular cartilage are determined by the unique fibrillar collagen network interspersed with proteoglycan aggregates to bestow tensile strength and resilience. The proteoglycans are associated with large quantities of water, which are bound to the hydrophilic glycosaminoglycan chains. This cartilaginous extracellular matrix, with its tightly bound water, provides a high degree of resistance to deformation by compressive forces. The capacity to resist compressive forces depends on the ability to extrude water as cartilage is compressed. Once the compression is released, the proteoglycans contain sufficient fixed charge to re-absorb water and small solutes into the matrix by osmosis. The articular cartilage then rebounds to its original dimensions.

Normal articular cartilage is white and translucent. It is an avascular tissue nourished by diffusion from the vasculature of the subchondral bone and, to a lesser degree, from the synovial fluid. Cartilage is rather hypocellular, compared with other tissues, because chondrocytes comprise only 1%–2% of the total cartilage volume (6). Despite its thinness (7 mm or less) and apparent homogeneity, mature hyaline articular cartilage is a heterogeneous tissue with four distinct regions: the superficial tangential (or gliding) zone; the middle (or transitional) zone; the deep (or radial) zone; and the calcified cartilage zone, located immediately below the tidemark and above the subchondral bone.

In the superficial zone, the chondrocytes are flattened, and the matrix is composed of thin collagen fibrils in tangential array, associated with a high concentration of the small proteoglycan decorin and a low concentration of aggrecan. The middle zone, comprising 40%–60% of the cartilage weight, consists of rounded chondrocytes surrounded by radial bundles of thick collagen fibrils. In the deep zone, the chondrocytes frequently are grouped in clusters and resemble the hypertrophic chondrocytes of the growth plate. In this region, the collagen bundles are thickest and arranged in a radial fashion. Cell density progressively decreases from the surface to the deep zone, where it is one-half to one-third of the density in the superficial zone. The concentration of collagen relative to proteoglycan also decreases progressively from the superficial to deep zones, and the proportion of proteoglycan increases to 50% of the dry weight in the deep zone. The calcified zone is formed as a result of endochondral ossification and persists as the growth plate is resorbed. The calcified zone serves as an important mechanical buffer between the uncalcified articular cartilage and the subchondral bone.

Cartilage Matrix Composition

The extracellular matrix components synthesized by chondrocytes include highly cross-linked fibrils of triple-helix type II collagen molecules that interact with other collagens, aggrecan, small proteoglycans, and other cartilage-specific and nonspecific matrix proteins (Table 2B-1) (1–3). These organic constituents represent only about 20% of the wet weight (total weight) of cartilage; water and inorganic salts constitute most of the remaining tissue. Water content is 75%–80% of the wet weight in the superficial zone and progressively decreases to 65%–70% with increasing depth. Collagen, primarily type II, accounts for about 15%–25% of the wet weight and about one-half of the dry weight, except in the superficial zone, where it represents most of the dry weight. Proteoglycans, primarily aggrecan, account for up to 10% of the wet weight and about 25% of the dry weight.

The highly cross-linked type II collagen fibrils form a systematically oriented fibrous network that entraps the highly negatively charged proteoglycan aggregates. The importance of these structural proteins may be observed in heritable disorders such as chondrodysplasias, or in transgenic animals where mutations in collagen genes or aggrecan sulfation genes result in cartilage abnormalities (7,8).

The Collagens of Articular Cartilage

Type II collagen fibrils are composed of 300-nm tropocollagen molecules of three identical alpha chains, $[\alpha1(II)]_3$, arranged in a triple helix. These molecules are assembled to form fibrils in a quarter-stagger array that can be observed by electron microscopy (2). The type II procollagen precursor contains nonhelical amino- and carboxyl-terminal propeptides, which are required for correct alignment of the procollagen molecules during fibril assembly and are then removed by specific proteinases. Chondrocalcin, a carboxyl propeptide, remains transiently within the cartilage matrix after cleavage and has been proposed to play a role in mineralization as a calcium-binding protein. The type II collagen in articular cartilage is a product of alternative splicing and lacks the 69-amino acid, cysteine-rich domain of the amino-terminal propeptide encoded by exon 2 in the human type II collagen gene (COL2A1) (Fig. 2B-1) (9). This domain also is found in the amino propeptides of other interstitial collagen types and is speculated to play an inhibitory feedback role in collagen biosynthesis. The type IIA procollagen that contains this domain is expressed during development by interstitial prechondrocytes, but not by fully differentiated chondrocytes.

Although collagen types VI, IX, XI, XII, and XIV are quantitatively minor components, they may have important structural and functional properties (2,10). Types IX and XI are relatively specific to cartilage, whereas types VI, XII, and XIV are distributed widely in other connective tissues. Type VI collagen, which is present in cartilage as microfibrils in very small quantities localized around the chondrocytes, may play a role in cell attachment. Type IX collagen is a proteoglycan and a collagen, as it contains a chondroitin-sulfate–chain attachment site in one of the noncollagen domains. The helical domains of the type IX collagen molecule form covalent cross-links with type II collagen telopeptides and are observed in the electron microscope to "decorate" the surface of the type II collagen fibrils. It has been suggested that type IX collagen functions as a structural intermediate between type II collagen fibers and the proteoglycan aggregates, thereby serving to enhance the mechanical stability of the fibril network and resist the swelling pressure of the entrapped proteoglycans. Destruction of type IX collagen may accelerate cartilage degradation and loss of function. The $\alpha3$ chain of type XI collagen has the same primary sequence as the $\alpha1(II)$ chain, and the heterotrimeric type XI collagen molecule probably is located in the same fibril as type II collagen. The more recently discovered nonfibrillar collagens XII and XIV, which are structurally related to type IX collagen, modulate the packing of collagen fibers in collagen-gel contraction assays in vitro (10). Type X collagen is not present in normal adult articular cartilage, but is expressed transiently in mature hypertrophic chondrocytes during calcification at the growth plate in growing animals and during certain stages of osteoarthritis. Expression of type III and type VI collagens also is induced or increased in osteoarthritic cartilage (11).

The Proteoglycans of Articular Cartilage

Aggrecan consists of a core protein of 225–250 kDa, with covalently attached side chains of glycosaminoglycans (GAGs). These side chains include approximately 100 chondroitin sulfate (CS) chains, 30 keratan sulfate (KS) chains, and shorter N- and O-linked oligosaccharides (1,3,5,12). Link protein, a small glycoprotein, stabilizes the noncovalent linkage between aggrecan and hyaluronic acid (HA; also called hyaluronan) to form the proteoglycan aggregate that may contain as many as 100 aggrecan monomers (Fig. 2B-2). The G1 and G2 N-terminal globular domains of aggrecan and its G3 C-terminal domain have distinct structural properties that function as integral parts of the aggrecan core protein and as cleavage products that accumulate with age or in osteoarthritis. The G1 domain and link protein share sequence homology with the immunoglobulin superfamily. The interaction between these substances and HA may function in cell adhesion and immune recognition. The G2 domain is separated from G1 by a linear interglobular domain and has two proteoglycan tandem repeats, but it does not bind to HA and has no known function. The G3 domain, which contains sequence homologies to epidermal growth factor, lectin, and complement regulatory protein, participates in growth regulation, cell recognition, intracellular trafficking, and the recognition, assembly, and stabilization of the extracellular matrix. Approximately half of the aggrecan molecules in adult cartilage lack the G3 domain, probably due to pro-

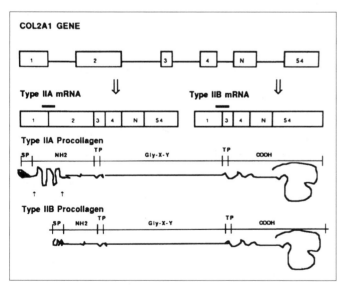

Fig. 2B-1. Diagram of the COL2A1 gene, types IIA and IIB procollagen mRNAs, and types IIA and IIB procollagens. In the COL2A1 gene, exons are indicated as boxes. Bars above the mRNAs indicate oligonucleotide probes specific for types IIA and IIB procollagen mRNAs. In the procollagen molecules: SP, signal peptide; NH2, amino-terminal propeptide; TP, telopeptide; Gly-X-Y, triple helical domain; COOH, carboxy-terminal propeptide; straight lines are triple helical regions; curved lines are globular portions of the protein. In the type IIA procollagen: arrow is the differentially spliced domain. Reproduced with permission from Sandell et al. (9).

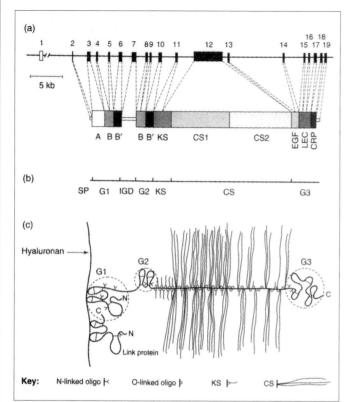

Fig. 2B-2. Schematic representation of aggrecan and its domains aligned with the genomic map of the human gene encoding aggrecan. The coding exons (filled bars), noncoding exon 1 (open bar), and introns (line) are shown in (a) and aligned with domains of the core protein and the aggrecan proteoglycan in (b) and (c), respectively. Interaction of the G1 domain with link protein and hyaluronan is indicated in panel c, as are a few N- and O- linked oligosaccharides. CS, chondroitin sulfate domain; EGF, epidermal growth factor-like domain; IGD, interglobular domain; KS, keratan sulfate domain; LEC, lectin-like domain. Reproduced with permission from Vertel (12).

teolytic cleavage during matrix turnover. Small amounts of other large proteoglycans are found in cartilage, including versican, which forms aggregates with HA, and perlican, which is nonaggregating.

The nonaggregating small proteoglycans are not specific to cartilage but are quite abundant; they are thought to serve important roles in cartilage matrix structure and function (4,5). These leucine-rich repeat (LRR) proteoglycans, including biglycan, decorin, fibromodulin, and lumican, have structurally related core proteins. Biglycan has GAG chains – CS, dermatan sulfate (DS), or both – attached near the N-terminus through two closely spaced serine–glycine dipeptides. Decorin contains only one CS or DS chain. Fibromodulin and lumican contain KS chains linked to the central domain of the core protein and to several sulfated tyrosine residues in the N-terminus. The negatively charged GAG side chains contribute to fixed-charge density of the matrix and, together with the highly anionic tyrosine-sulfation sites, permit multiple-site linkage between adjacent collagen fibrils, thereby stabilizing the

network. Biglycan, decorin, and fibromodulin bind transforming growth factor (TGF)-β, and may thereby modulate growth, remodeling, and repair. Two additional LLR proteoglycans, proline arginine-rich end leucine-rich repeat protein (PRELP) and chondroadherin, may regulate cell-matrix interactions by binding to syndecan and α2β1 integrin, respectively.

Other Matrix and Cell-Surface Proteins

Several other noncollagenous matrix proteins may play important roles in determining cartilage matrix integrity (4). Cartilage oligomeric matrix protein (COMP), a member of the thrombospondin family, is a disulfide-bonded pentameric 550-kDa calcium-binding protein that constitutes approximately 10% of the noncollagenous, nonproteoglycan protein in normal adult cartilage. COMP is localized in the interterritorial matrix of adult articular cartilage, where it may stabilize the collagen network, but it is pericellular in the proliferating region of the growth plate, where it may have a role in cell-matrix interactions. The cartilage matrix protein (or matrilin 1) and matrilin 3 are expressed in cartilage at certain stages of development and are present in tracheal cartilage, but not in mechanically loaded adult articular or intervertebral disc cartilage. The cartilage intermediate layer protein is expressed in the middle to deep zones of articular cartilage as a precursor protein that, when cleaved in conjunction with secretion, also forms the nucleotide pyrophosphohydrolase. The glycoprotein 39 (gp39, or YKL-40) is found only in the superficial zone of normal cartilage. Synthesis or release of these proteins or fragments often is increased in cartilage that is undergoing repair or remodeling. COMP and gp39 have been investigated as markers of cartilage damage in arthritis (13).

Other matrix proteins, including fibronectin and tenascin-c, may mediate cell-matrix interactions in cartilage by binding to cell-surface integrins or other membrane proteins (10). Alternative splicing of fibronectin and tenascin-c mRNAs gives rise to different protein products at different stages of chondrocyte differentiation. Both proteins are increased in osteoarthritic cartilage and thus may serve specific functions in remodeling and repair. Integral membrane proteins found in chondrocytes include the cell-surface proteoglycans CD44 and syndecan 3. CD44 is a receptor for HA and also binds collagen and fibronectin. Syndecan 3 links to the cell surface via glycosyl phosphatidylinositol and binds tenascin-c, growth factors, proteases, inhibitors, and other matrix molecules, through heparan sulfate (HS) side chains on the extracellular domain. Anchorin CII is a 34-kDa integral-membrane protein that binds type II collagen and shares extensive homology with the calcium-binding proteins calpactin and lipocortin.

Chondrocytes

Chondrocytes in adult articular cartilage are terminally differentiated cells that are interspersed in the cartilage matrix in distinct chondrocyte lacunae. The chondrocytes and the surrounding dense extracellular matrix form a functional unit termed a *chondron* (1). Although chondrocytes are biosynthetically active in growing animals, their capacity to replace lost collagen is limited in mature articular cartilage. Only proteoglycans appear to be synthesized continuously. Normally, chondrocytes are in a homeostatic state. In fact, because of their relatively quiescent nature, adult chondrocytes once were thought to be metabolically inactive. However, chondrocytes now are known to be capable of responding to biochemical, structural, and physical stimuli and are able to synthesize various enzymes, enzyme inhibitors, growth factors, and cytokines, as well as all the matrix components described previously (14). Unfortunately, adult chondrocytes have limited repair capacity and may replace damaged or aging articular cartilage with type I collagen-containing fibrotic tissue. Cultured chondrocytes have served as useful models for studying the mechanisms that control synthesis of cartilage matrix proteins (14). Advances in studies of gene expression during development have increased our understanding of cartilage repair mechanisms in the adult (7,15).

Cartilage Matrix Turnover, Degradation, and Repair

In normal adult articular cartilage, turnover of extracellular matrix components is slow compared with turnover in many other connective tissues, and the capacity for repair is limited. The turnover rate of collagen is very slow, except in pericellular sites where there is evidence for ongoing type II collagen cleavage (1). The proteoglycans – particularly the small, sulfated GAG components, which are more susceptible to enzymatic degradation – are resynthesized continuously. With increasing age, human articular cartilage shows increased damage to type II collagen and major changes in the structure and content of the proteoglycan aggregate components. Although the total content of sulfated GAGs does not change significantly with age, notable changes include increased KS associated with decreased CS, decreased size of proteoglycan aggregates, increased amounts of free binding region (G1 or G1 and G2 together with the KS-rich region and proteolytically cleaved link protein), and increased content of HA of shorter chain length.

Pathologic cartilage degradation involves matrix metalloproteinases (MMPs) and other proteinases that are more-or-less specific for cleavage of cartilage collagens and proteoglycans. Degradation results from an imbalance between the active enzymes and their natural inhibitors such as the tissue inhibitors of metalloproteinases (TIMP-1, -2, and -3) (14). The collagenases implicated in type II collagen degradation include collagenases 1, 2, and 3 (MMP-1, -8, -13) and membrane type I (MT1)-MMP (MMP-14). MMP-13 has a major role in cartilage degradation, due to its capacity to degrade type II collagen more effectively than MMP-1. Although MMP-3, MMP-8, and MT1-MMP all have the capacity to degrade aggrecan, there is evidence that degradation at the "aggre-canase" cleavage site is the primary event in chondrocyte-mediated catabolism of aggrecan. The recent cloning and characterization of aggrecanase 1 and 2 as members of the ADAM-TS family of metalloproteinases (ADAM-TS4 and 5) have provided the opportunity to define the precise role of these proteinases in aggrecan degradation and to develop targeted therapies that interfere with aggrecan breakdown. Other proteineases produced by chondrocytes may have roles in degradation of different matrix components or may participate in the proteinase activation cascade. These proteinases include the gelatinases; MMP-2 and -9; the cathepsins B, L, and D; and plasminogen activators.

The failure of cartilage to repair itself once it has begun to degrade is a major public health problem. Current procedures for repairing or transplanting severely damaged articular cartilage do not provide long-term restoration of the normal properties of the cartilage matrix. New therapies involving transplantation of autologous chondrocytes or bone marrow-derived mesenchymal stem cells, with or without biomaterial scaffolds, offer the promise of more effective approaches.

Markers of Cartilage Matrix Degradation and Turnover

With increasing knowledge of the composition of the cartilage matrix, molecular markers in body fluids have been identified for monitoring changes in cartilage metabolism and for assessing joint damage in arthritis (13,16,17). For example, COMP is released in reactive arthritis, and high serum levels in early rheumatoid arthritis can distinguish an aggressive, destructive form of the disease. However, this marker may not be specific for cartilage degradation because COMP also is secreted by synovial cells. Monoclonal antibodies have been developed that recognize products of proteoglycan or collagen degradation (catabolic epitopes) or newly synthesized matrix components (anabolic neo-epitopes), which represent attempts to repair the damaged matrix. For example, different monoclonal antibodies can distinguish subtle biochemical differences in CS or KS chains that result from degraded versus newly synthesized proteoglycans. Such epitopes can be detected in the synovial fluids and sera of people with osteoarthritis and rheumatoid arthritis, and the synovial fluid-to-serum ratio can be useful as a diagnostic indicator. Other antibodies recognize specific aggrecanase or metalloproteinase cleavage sites in the aggrecan core protein (18,19). Similarly, the synthesis of type II collagen can be monitored by measuring serum and synovial-fluid levels of the carboxyl-terminal propeptide, CPII or chondrocalcin, and urinary excretion of hydroxylysyl pyridinoline cross-links may indicate collagen degradation. Specific antibodies that recognize epitopes on denatured type II collagen at the collagenase cleavage site (for example, N-terminus of the three-quarter fragment) are promising diagnostic reagents (20). The use of such assays as research tools has lead to their further development for use in clinical practice.

TABLE 2B-1
Extracellular Matrix Components of Cartilage

Molecule	Structure and size	Function and location
Collagens		
Type II	$[\alpha1(II)]_3$	Tensile strength; major component of collagen fibrils
Type IX	$\alpha1(IX)\ \alpha2(IX)\ \alpha3(IX)$; single CS or DS chain	Regulates fibril size; cross-links to type II collagen
Type XI	$\alpha1(XI)\ \alpha2(XI)\ \alpha3(XI)$	Tensile strength; pericellular within type II fibril
Type VI	$\alpha1(VI)\ \alpha2(VI)\ \alpha3(VI)$	Microfibrils in pericellular space
Type X	$[\alpha1(X)]_3$	Associated with type II collagen in hypertrophic cartilage
Type XII	$[\alpha1(XII)]_3$	Associated with collagen fibrils in perichondrium and articular surface
Type XIV	$[\alpha1(XIV)]_3$	Associated with collagen fibrils throughout articular cartilage
Proteoglycans		
Aggrecan	255-kDa core protein; CS/KS side chains; C-terminal EGF and lectin-like domains	Compressive stiffness through hydration of fixed charge density
Versican	265–370-kDa core protein; CS/DS side chains; C-terminal EGF, C-type lectin, and CRP-like domains	Low levels in articular cartilage throughout life; calcium-binding and selectin-like properties
Perlican	400–467-kDa core protein; HS/CS side chains; no HA-binding	Cell adhesion
Biglycan	38 kDa; LRR core protein with two DS chains (76 kDa)	Contributes fixed charge density and stabilization of collagen network; binds TGF-β
Decorin	36.5 kDa; LRR core protein with one CS or DS side chain (100 kDa)	Same as biglycan
Fibromodulin	58 kDa; containing KS chains in central LRR region and N-terminal tyrosine sulfate domains	Same as biglycan
Lumican	58 kDa; structure similar to fibromodulin	Contributes fixed charge density and stabilization of collagen network
PRELP	58 kDa; LRR core protein; proline- and arginine-rich N-terminal binding domain for heparin and HS	Mediates cell binding through HS sulfate in syndecan
Chondroadherin	LRR core protein without N-terminal extension	Binding to cells via $\alpha2\beta1$ integrin

Molecule	Structure and size	Function and location
Other molecules		
Hyaluronic acid (hyaluronan)	1000–3000 kDa	Retention of aggrecan within matrix
Link protein	38.6 kDa	Stabilizes attachment of aggrecan G1 domain to HA
COMP	550 kDa; five 110-kDa subunits; thrombospondin-like	Interterritorial in articular cartilage; stabilizes collagen network or promotes collagen fibril assembly; calcium binding
Cartilage matrix protein (or matrilin 1)	Three 50-kDa subunits with vWF and EGF domains	Tightly bound to aggrecan in immature cartilage
CILP	92 kDa; N-terminal protein product of gene that also encodes nucleotide pyrophosphohydrolase	Restricted to middle/deep zones of cartilage; increase in early and late OA
Glycoprotein 39 (or YKL-40)	39 kDa; chitinase homology	Marker of cartilage turnover; in superficial zone of cartilage
Fibronectin	Dimer of 220-kDa subunits	Cell attachment and binding to collagen and proteoglycans; increased in OA cartilage
Tenascin-c	Six 200-kDa subunits forming hexabrachion structure	Associated with chondrogenesis; binds syndecan 3
Membrane proteins		
CD44	Integral membrane protein with extracellular HS/CS side chains	Cell-matrix interactions; binds HA
Syndecan-3	N-terminal HS attachment site; cytoplasmic tyrosine residues	Receptor for tenascin-c during cartilage development; cell-matrix interactions
Anchorin CII (or annexin V)	34 kDa; homology to calcium-binding proteins calpactin and lipocortin	Cell-surface attachment to type II collagen; calcium binding
Integrins (α1, 2, 3, 5, 6, 10; β1, 3, 5)	Two noncovalently linked transmembrane glycoproteins (α and β subunits)	Cell-matrix interactions and intracellular signaling

CS, chondroitin sulfate; DS, dermatan sulfate; KS, keratan sulfate; EGF, epidermal growth factor; CRP, complement regulatory protein; HS, heparan sulfate; HA, hyaluronic acid (hyaluronan); LRR, leucine-rich repeat; TGF, transforming growth factor; PRELP = proline- and arginine-rich end leucine-rich repeat protein; COMP, cartilage oligomeric matrix protein; vWF, von Willebrand factor; EGF, epidermal growth factor; CILP, cartilage intermediate layer protein; OA, osteoarthritis.

Conclusion

Articular cartilage is a highly specialized tissue, with a structure and composition more complex than is apparent to the naked eye. Availability of new molecular techniques and reagents has enabled the discovery of structural components that have subtle influences on function. Further understanding of cartilage structure and function will aid in the development of novel therapies for preventing cartilage destruction and promoting cartilage repair.

MARY B. GOLDRING, PhD

References

1. Poole AR. Cartilage in health and disease. In: Koopman WJ (ed). Arthritis and Allied Conditions: A Textbook of Rheumatology. Baltimore: Williams & Wilkins, 1997; pp 255–308.

2. Mayne R. Structure and function of collagen. In: Koopman WJ (ed). Arthritis and Allied Conditions: A Textbook of Rheumatology. Baltimore: Williams & Wilkins, 1997; pp 207–227.

3. Sandy JD, Plaas AHK, Rosenberg L. Structure, function, and metabolism of cartilage proteoglycans. In: Koopman WJ (ed). Arthritis and Allied Conditions: A Textbook of Rheumatology. Baltimore: Williams & Wilkins, 1997; pp 255–308.

4. Heinegard D, Saxne T, Lorenzo P. Noncollagenous proteins: glycoproteins and related molecules. In: Seibel MJ, Robins SP, Bilezekian JP (eds). Dynamics of Bone and Cartilage Metabolism. New York: Academic Press, 1999; pp 59–69.

5. Hardingham T. Proteoglycans and glycoaminoglycans. In: Seibel MJ, Robins SP, Bilezekian JP (eds). Dynamics of Bone and Cartilage Metabolism. New York: Academic Press, 1999; pp 71–81.

6. Stockwell RA, Meachim G. The chondrocytes. In: Freeman MAR (ed). Adult Articular Cartilage. Tunbridge Wells, England: Pitman Medical, 1979; 69–144.

7. Mundlos S, Olsen BR. Heritable diseases of the skeleton. Part II: Molecular insights into skeletal development-matrix components and their homeostasis. FASEB J 1997;11:227–233.

8. Goldring MB. The role of cytokines as inflammatory mediators in osteoarthritis. Lessons from animal models. Connect Tissue Res 1999;40:1–11.

9. Sandell LJ, Morris N, Robbins JR, Goldring MB. Alternatively spliced type II procollagen mRNAs define a distinct population of cells during vertebral development: differential expression of the amino-propeptide. J Cell Biol 1991;114:1307–1319.

10. Olsen BR. Matrix molecules and their ligands. In: Lanza R, Langer R, Chick W (eds). Principles in Tissue Engineering. Austin, TX: R.G. Landes Company, 1997; 47–65.

11. Aigner T, Dudhia J. Phenotypic modulation of chondrocytes as a potential therapeutic target in osteoarthritis: a hypothesis. Ann Rheum Dis 1997;56:287–291.

12. Vertel BM. The ins and outs of aggrecan. Trends Cell Biol 1995;5:458–464.

13. Garnero P, Rousseau JC, Delmas PD. Molecular basis and clinical use of biochemical markers of bone, cartilage and synovium in joint diseases. Arthritis Rheum 2000;43:953–968.

14. Goldring MB. The role of the chondrocyte in osteoarthritis. Arthritis Rheum 2000;43:1916-1926.

15. Mundlos S, Olsen BR. Heritable diseases of the skeleton. Part I: Molecular insights into skeletal development-transcription factors and signaling pathways. FASEB J 1997;11:125–132.

16. Thonar EJ, Lenz ME, Masuda K, Manicourt DH. Body fluid markers of cartilage metabolism. In: Seibel MJ, Robins SP, Bilezekian JP (eds). Dynamics of Bone and Cartilage Metabolism. New York: Academic Press, 1999; pp 453–464.

17. Goldring SR, Goldring MB. Rheumatoid arthritis and other inflammatory joint pathologies. In: Seibel MJ, Robins SP, Bilezekian JP (eds). Dynamics of Bone and Cartilage Metabolism. New York: Academic Press, 1999; pp 623–636.

18. Lark MW, Bayne EK, Flanagan J, et al. Aggrecan degradation in human cartilage. Evidence for both matrix metalloproteinase and aggrecanase activity in normal, osteoarthritic, and rheumatoid joints. J Clin Invest 1997;100:93–106.

19. Hughes CE, Little CB, Buttner FH, Bartnik E, Caterson B. Differential expression of aggrecanase and matrix metalloproteinase activity in chondrocytes isolated from bovine and porcine articular cartilage. J Biol Chem 1998;273:30576–30582.

20. Dahlberg L, Billinghurst RC, Manner P, et al. Selective enhancement of collagenase-mediated cleavage of resident type II collagen in cultured osteoarthritic cartilage and arrest with a synthetic inhibitor that spares collagenase 1 (matrix metalloproteinase 1). Arthritis Rheum 2000;43:673–682.

THE MUSCULOSKELETAL SYSTEM
C. Bone

Bone is a composite tissue consisting of mineral, matrix, cells, and water (Fig. 2C-1). The mineral is an analog of the naturally occurring crystalline calcium phosphate, hydroxyapatite $[Ca_5(PO_4)_3(OH)]$. Compared to geologic apatites, physiologic mineral crystals are very small and imperfect, containing fewer hydroxyl groups and many impurities such as carbonate, fluoride, acid phosphate, magnesium, and citrate. The small size of the bone apatite crystals makes them ideally suited for their function in mineral ion homeostasis, since smaller crystals generally dissolve before larger crystals. Apatite crystals also form in tissues that are not normally calcified, for example, in atherosclerotic plaque, in soft tissues of some people with abnormally high serum calcium or phosphate levels, and in articular cartilage of some people with osteoarthritis (1). These abnormally calcified tissues generally appear distinct from bone because of the larger size of the crystals and the nature of the matrices upon which the crystals are deposited.

Structure and Function

In addition to serving as a source of calcium, magnesium, and phosphate ions, the mineral crystals in bone provide strength and rigidity to the matrix upon which they are deposited. This strength and rigidity provides protection to internal organs and also serves a mechanical function, facilitating mobility. The bone matrix is predominantly type I collagen. The collagen fibrils are arranged in the extracellular matrix in patterns related to the function of the tissue in which they are found. The unique triple helical structure of collagen provides strength and flexibility to most of the connective tissues (2). The mineral crystals add extra rigidity to the collagen fibers. Collagen is stabilized by cross-links formed post-translationally in the extracellular matrix. The nature of these cross-links differs in the mineralized and nonmineralized connective tissues (3). Analyses of serum or urine for the cross-links that stabilize bone collagen, as opposed to skin and tendon collagen, provide useful markers for diseases such as osteoporosis, in which breakdown of the matrix is increased (4). Because the cross-links are formed after the fibrils are assembled in the extracellular matrix, these assays are specific for degradation. In addition to collagen, about 5% of the extracellular matrix of bone is made up of noncollagenous proteins. These proteins play crucial roles in mineral homeostasis, bone metabolism, bone formation, and bone turnover (5–7).

Bone cells govern the metabolism, formation, and turnover of the tissue. Bone has three cell types: osteoblasts, osteocytes, and osteoclasts (Fig. 2C-2). Osteoblasts and osteocytes, both derived from the mesenchymal cell lineage, are closely related, but their functions differ. Osteoblasts synthesize the bone matrix. Osteocytes, enmeshed in the existing bone matrix, convey nutrition throughout bone and are the cells within bone responsible for sensing mechanical signals (8,9). Osteoclasts, multinucleated giant cells of macrophage origin (10), are responsible for removing bone. To accomplish this task, osteoclasts attach to the bone surface and seal off a microenvironment into which they release acid to dissolve the mineral, followed by a series of enzymes that break down the matrix. These enzymes include acid phosphatase, collagenase, cathepsins, and other specialized proteinases (11). In normal bone, the functions of osteoblasts and osteoclasts are coupled such that signals from one affect the other. One of the principal coupling factors between osteoblasts and osteoclasts is osteoprotegerin ligand (OPGL), a factor originally identified as a T-cell activator (TRANCE or RANK-ligand). Osteoprotegerin ligand, produced by osteoblasts (12), binds to a receptor on macrophages or immature osteoclasts and stimulates their maturation.

The distribution of each type of bone cell and the relative activities of these cells varies with type of bone, age, and disease state. Three main hormone groups regulate the activities of bone cells. First, parathyroid hormone (PTH) and 1,25-dihydroxy-vitamin D are responsible for increasing Ca^{+2} levels, and they do so by increasing Ca^{+2} resorption and retention, and by stimulating osteoclasts to remodel bone (via direct effects on osteoblastic synthesis of OPGL).

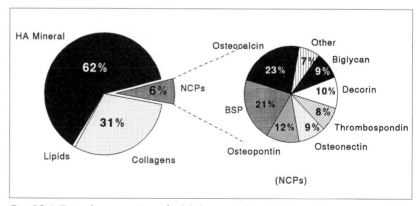

Fig. 2C-1. Typical composition of adult human trabecular bone. Components of the pie chart on the left reflect the weight percent apatite (HA mineral), lipids, collagens, and noncollagenous proteins (NCPs) found in bone. The pie chart on the right shows the relative (weight percent) distribution of the major types of noncollagenous proteins. BSP, bone sialoprotein.

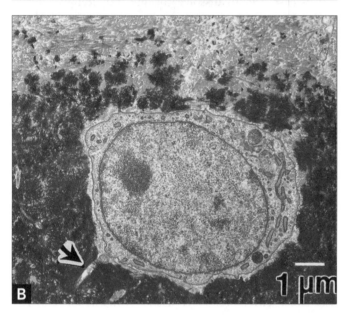

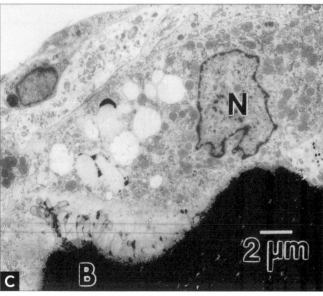

Second, calcitonin is a PTH antagonist that suppresses osteoclast activity. Finally, estrogen and other sex steroids, corticosteroids, and other factors directly affect osteoblasts and the synthesis of the bone matrix.

Bone Formation

It is now recognized that there are key genetic signals (master genes) that regulate bone development (13). These genes include those that determine the shape and orientation of the bone, and those that regulate the function and activity of the bone cells. In general, bone formation occurs through two distinct processes: endochondral ossification, in which bone replaces a cartilage model, and intramembranous ossification, in which bone forms directly. During embryonic development, long bones form by the former process and the bones of the skull by the latter. Fracture healing in the adult recapitulates the events of endochondral ossification.

Endochondral ossification begins when mesenchymal cells differentiate into chondrocytes. This process is modulated by a number of cytokines (14), including Indian hedgehog, parathyroid hormone-related peptide, and the bone morphogenetic proteins. The differentiated chondrocytes produce a cartilage model that matures and is modified to facilitate mineralization, vascular invasion, and replacement by bone.

As they mature, chondrocytes change shape and switch from making collagens found in all cartilage (type II and IX) to producing type X collagen, a form unique to the "hypertrophic" chondrocytes at the interface of cartilage and bone. The precise function of type X collagen is not known; however, defects in its production have been found in several families with various forms of spondyloepiphyseal dysplasias (15). This condition is characterized by extreme curvature of the spine (kyphosis), implying that type X collagen has a role in stabilizing the endochondral structure. Transgenic mice expressing an abnormal type X collagen develop lymphocytopenia in addition to skeletal kyphosis (16), indicating that type X collagen may have some still-undetermined functions in immunoregulation. This is another example of the cross-talk between modulators of the immune system and bone cells, similar to that mediated by OPGL/RANK/TRANCE.

A second alteration occurring in the cartilaginous matrix of the epiphyseal plate as it matures and prepares for calcifi-

Fig. 2C-2. Electron micrographs showing **A**: osteoblasts, **B**: osteocytes, and **C**: osteoclasts in normal rat bone. Note the abundant rough endoplasmic reticulum (arrow) in the osteoblast, a cell actively involved in matrix deposition. The osteocyte, which shows less synthetic activity, is almost entirely engulfed in electron-dense mineral but is connected to other cells by long channels known as canaliculi (arrow). The osteoclast is a larger cell, often with multiple nuclei (N), which attaches to the bone surface (B), and pumps out protons to dissolve mineral. Courtesy of S.B. Doty, Hospital for Special Surgery, New York.

cation is a modification of proteoglycan structure. Several different types of proteoglycans are present in the developing epiphyseal plate and bone (5,17). The large chondroitin sulfate/keratan sulfate molecules (*aggrecan*) associate with hyaluronic acid (*hyaluronan*) to form high-molecular weight, space-filling molecules (*aggregates*) that expand to up to 50 times their volume. The related nonaggregating molecules found in a variety of connective tissues (*versican*) and a unique but related nonaggregating molecule (*epiphycan*) may regulate matrix organization. In addition, a smaller dermatan sulfate-containing molecule with only one glycosaminoglycan chain, called *decorin*, trims the surface of collagen fibrils, as does *biglycan*, a related molecule with two component glycosaminoglycan chains per core protein. Biglycan and decorin also bind growth factors, allowing them to persist in the matrix. Chondroitin sulfate analogs of these dermatan sulfate proteoglycans are found in bone and tendon.

A family of distinct small proteoglycans with leucine-rich core proteins has been identified in cartilage and bone (17). These include fibromodulin, keratocan, lumican, osteoglycin (also called osteoinductive factor), and osteoadherin, in addition to epiphycan and proline arginine-rich end leucine-rich repeat protein. The large cartilage proteoglycans (aggrecan and its aggregates and versican) keep the matrix hydrated and prevent unwanted calcification. The smaller proteoglycans are believed to regulate collagen fibril formation and, because of their ability to bind growth factors, to play a key role in cartilage metabolism signaling. Aggrecan and proteoglycan aggregates in solution are effective inhibitors of mineral crystal growth and formation, a finding that may explain the observation that in severe osteoarthritis, calcification occurs around chondrocytes where the proteoglycans have been degraded.

As the hypertrophic cartilage is modified, mineralization commences. Initial calcification in cartilage occurs in association with both collagen and extracellular membrane-bound bodies known as *matrix vesicles* (Fig. 2C-3). These vesicles are enriched in enzymes that facilitate transport of calcium and phosphate ions into the vesicle and that promote degradation of the matrix around the vesicle. Matrix vesicles thus provide a protected environment in which ions can accumulate and initial mineral deposition can occur in the absence of inhibitors. Mineral crystals break through the vesicles and may fuse with collagen-based mineral as cartilage calcification proceeds (5).

Bone replaces calcified cartilage following vascular invasion. Osteoblasts produce this bone, sequentially elaborating an underlying fibrous network (consisting of fibronectin and vitronectin), type I collagen, and a variety of matrix proteins. Mineral deposition then occurs by processes described below. Once the bone is formed, it remains in a dynamic state, remodeling to provide maximum strength with minimum mass (Wolff's law), allow growth, and provide a source of mineral ion homeostasis. The remodeling processes (formation and resorption) are linked so that factors produced by bone-forming cells (osteoblasts) activate remodeling cells (osteoclasts), and vice versa.

Bone Mineralization

Physiologic mineral deposition is a combination of physicochemical and biochemical processes (5). For mineral crystals to form, the local concentrations of the ions within the crystal must increase to the extent that their ion product exceeds the solubility of the crystal (*supersaturation*). Supersaturation occurs through the actions of cells that pump out these ions and cellular enzymes that modulate their environments in a way that allows ions to be released from proteins in the extracellular matrix. The most extensively studied of these enzymes, alkaline phosphatase, is found on the outer membrane of osteoblasts and chondrocytes and can hydrolyze phosphate esters. Alkaline phosphatase deficiency results in hypophosphatasia, a disease characterized by improper mineral deposition (18). Increasing the supersaturation raises the probability that when these ions collide, they will possess sufficient energy and be in the correct orientation to form the smallest stable version of the crystal, the *nucleus*. The synthesis or exposure of macromolecules that resemble the nucleus in question enhances physiologic nucleation. These macromolecules act as "heterogeneous nucleators." For example, a phosphoprotein, with phosphate groups arranged on its surface in a pattern that matches the phosphate-rich surface of the apatite crystal, could bind Ca^{+2} ions and lead to the formation of an apatite crystal. Once crystal nuclei are formed, they continue to accumulate ions (*crystal growth*) or serve as additional nucleation sites (*secondary nucleation*).

In bone, nucleation starts at many distinct sites in the collagen matrix. However, collagen itself is not an effective nucleator. It is the noncollagenous proteins associated with collagen that provide these nucleation sites (5). Table 2C-1 lists the proteins associated with the bone and cartilage matrix

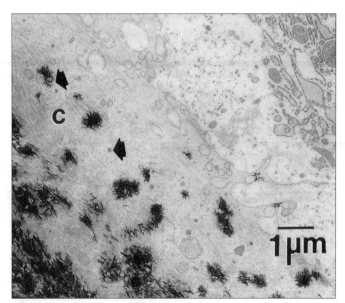

Fig. 2C-3. Electron micrograph illustrating collagen-mediated (c) and matrix vesicle-mediated (arrows) calcification in rat periosteal bone. Courtesy of S.B. Doty, Hospital for Special Surgery, New York.

TABLE 2C-1
Proteins Found in Bone and Cartilage Matrices and Their Effects on Biomineralization

Protein	Tissue expression	In vitro effect on HA formation and growth	Effect of absence on skeleton	Disease where expression is abnormal
Albumin	Liver	Promotes/inhibits	?	?
Aggrecan	Cartilage	Inhibits	Premature growth plate closure	Osteoarthritis
Biglycan	Bone, dentin, skin, cartilage	Promotes/inhibits	Thin cortices; fewer but larger crystals	Absence: Turner's syndrome; excess: Klinefelter's syndrome
Bone proteolipid	Bone, dentin	Promotes	?	?
BSP	Bone, dentin	Promotes/inhibits	No phenotype	?
Decorin	Cartilage, bone, skin	Weak inhibitor	None	?
DMP-1	Dentin, bone	Promotes/inhibits	?	Odontogenesis imperfecta
DSP	Dentin	Weak promoter/ inhibitor	?	Odontogenesis imperfecta
Fetuin (α2-HS-glycoprotein)	Liver, bone	Inhibits	Delayed osteogenesis	?
Immunoglobulin	Liver	No effect	?	?
MGP	Cartilage, smooth muscle cells	Inhibits	Premature death due to tracheal calcification	?
Osteocalcin	Bone, dentin	Inhibits	Increased bone diameter; bone mineral crystals do not mature	Some forms of osteopetrosis
Osteonectin/SPARC	Bone, dentin, cartilage	Promotes/inhibits	Bones thinner and smaller	?
Osteopontin	Bone, dentin, cartilage	Inhibits	Bones thinner; crystals larger	?
TRAMP	Bone	?	?	?
Thrombospondin	Bone, platelets	?	Bones are weaker	?

HA, hyaluronic acid; BSP, bone sialoprotein; DMP-1, dentin matrix protein I; DSP, dentin sialoprotein; MGP, matrix gla protein; SPARC, secreted protein acid-rich and cysteine-containing; TRAMP, tyrosine-rich acidic matrix protein; ?, unknown.

that affect apatite nucleation and growth. Many of these same proteins are involved in regulating cell-matrix interactions, matrix organization, and other bone processes. In terms of mineralization, it is likely that the functions of many of these proteins are redundant, because regulation of biologic mineralization is so important. This redundancy is suggested by animals with null-mutations (knockouts) in which only minor changes in bone phenotype are noted. Proteins that act as apatite nucleators frequently also inhibit apatite crystal growth. This most likely is attributable to the mechanism of action of these proteins: when present in low concentrations, they bind to and stabilize apatite nuclei; when more abundant, they can coat the crystals and inhibit their growth.

There are many examples of human bone disorders linked to defects in specific matrix proteins. Osteogenesis imperfecta or "brittle bone disease" is a heterogeneous set of conditions characterized by fragile bones, and associated in most cases with defects in the type I collagen gene. Alteration in matrix protein synthesis and/or accumulation in association with the collagen fibrils frequently parallel impaired collagen synthesis. The impaired load-bearing properties of bone appear to be attributable to the decrease in collagen content and the inability of the collagen fibrils to form properly. But mineral crystals in these patients and related animal models are also abnormal, being smaller, with altered composition, and often found away from the collagen matrix (19). Turner's syndrome (45 X0) is sometimes associated with abnormal expression of biglycan, a small proteoglycan (20). In mouse models, *osteopetrosis*, the presence of excess bone due to impaired bone remodeling, has been associated with defects in osteocalcin production, osteoprotegerin production, and altered expression of certain cytokines (21). A combination of gene discovery and evaluation of the function of each matrix protein should provide information that links defects in matrix proteins to other musculoskeletal diseases and a unified view of the events surrounding bone formation, mineralization, and remodeling.

ADELE L. BOSKEY, PhD

References

1. Boskey AL, Bullough PG, Vigorita V, Di Carlo E. *Calcium-acidic phospholipid-phosphate complexes in human hydroxyapatite-containing pathologic deposits. Am J Pathol 1988;133:22–29.*
2. Lees S, Hanson D, Page E, Mook HA. *Comparison of dosage-dependent effects of ß-aminopropionitrile, sodium fluoride, and hydrocortisone on selected physical properties of cortical bone. J Bone Miner Res 1994;9:1377–1389.*
3. Knott L, Bailey AJ. *Collagen cross-links in mineralizing tissues: a review of their chemistry, function, and clinical relevance. Bone 1998;22:181–187.*
4. Watts NB. *Clinical utility of biochemical markers of bone remodeling. Clin Chem 1999;45:1359–1368.*
5. Robey PG, Boskey AL. *The biochemistry of bone. In: Marcus R, Feldman D, Kelsey J (eds). Osteoporosis. New York: Academic Press, 1996; pp 95–184.*
6. Sodek KL, Tupy JH, Sodek J, Grynpas MD. *Relationships between bone protein and mineral in developing porcine long bone and calvaria. Bone 2000;26:189–198.*
7. Cowles EA, DeRome ME, Pastizzo G, Brailey LL, Gronowicz GA. *Mineralization and the expression of matrix proteins during in vivo bone development. Calcif Tissue Int 1998;62: 74–82.*
8. Noble BS, Reeve J. *Osteocyte function, osteocyte death and bone fracture resistance. Mol Cell Endocrinol 2000;159:7–13.*
9. Burger EH, Klein-Nulend J. *Mechanotransduction in bone – role of the lacuno-canalicular network. FASEB J 1999;13: S101–S112.*
10. Teitelbaum SL, Abu-Amer Y, Ross FP. *Molecular mechanisms of bone resorption. J Cell Biochem 1995;59:1–10.*
11. Vaananen HK, Zhao H, Mulari M, Halleen JM. *The cell biology of osteoclast function. J Cell Sci 2000;113:377–381.*
12. Lacey DL, Timms E, Tan HL, et al. *Osteoprotegerin ligand is a cytokine that regulates osteoclast differentiation and activation. Cell 1998;93:165–176.*
13. Shapiro IM. *Discovery: Osf2/Cbfa1, a master gene of bone formation. Clin Orthop 1999;2:42–46.*
14. Ferguson CM, Miclau T, Hu D, Alpern E, Helms JA. *Common molecular pathways in skeletal morphogenesis and repair. Ann N Y Acad Sci 1998;857:33–42.*
15. Cremer MA, Rosloniec EF, Kang AH. *The cartilage collagens: a review of their structure, organization, and role in the pathogenesis of experimental arthritis in animals and in human rheumatic disease. J Mol Med 1998;76:275–288.*
16. Jacenko O, LuValle PA, Olsen BR. *Spondylometaphyseal dysplasia in mice carrying a dominant negative mutation in a matrix protein specific for cartilage-to-bone transition. Nature 1993;365:56–61.*
17. Matsushima N, Ohyanagi T, Tanaka T, Kretsinger RH. *Supermotifs and evolution of tandem leucine-rich repeats within the small proteoglycans – biglycan, decorin, lumican, fibromodulin, PRELP, keratocan, osteoadherin, epiphycan, and osteoglycin. Proteins 2000;38:210–225.*
18. Fedde KN, Blair L, Silverstein J, et al. *Alkaline phosphatase knock-out mice recapitulate the metabolic and skeletal defects of infantile hypophosphatasia. J Bone Miner Res 1999;14: 2015–2026.*
19. Boskey AL, Wright TM, Blank RD. *Collagen and bone strength. J Bone Miner Res 1999;14:330–335.*
20. Xu T, Bianco P, Fisher LW, Longenecker G, et al. *Targeted disruption of the biglycan gene leads to an osteoporosis-like phenotype in mice. Nat Genet 1998;20:78–82.*
21. Boyce BF, Hughes DE, Wright KR, Xing L, Dai A. *Recent advances in bone biology provide insight into the pathogenesis of bone diseases. Lab Invest 1999;79:83–94.*

THE MUSCULOSKELETAL SYSTEM
D. Synovium

Synovium is found in many vertebrates, but in different joints in each species. Synovium develops by the splitting apart of adjacent musculoskeletal structures, in contrast to more ancient serosal linings, which form by infolding of extraembryonic spaces (1). In other respects, synovium has similarities to serosa and to a more recent evolutionary development, bone marrow, with which it shares its origin from skeletal blastema. These similarities may help to explain synovium's involvement in autoimmune disease.

Disconnective Tissue

The fluid-filled gap within normal synovial structures rarely is more than 50 μm thick, a smear too thin to see (Fig. 2D-1), rather than the large space often shown in diagrams. The essence of a synovial structure is not so much a cavity as it is a plane of cleavage – a *disconnection*. As such, it allows movement between, rather than within, solid tissues. The main effect of removing synovium is that disconnective surfaces are replaced by adherent connective tissue, resulting in loss of range of movement.

Synovium Is Multilayered

The best account of what synovium really looks like is by Albert Key (2). Synovium often is portrayed as a monolayer of cells, the intima. However, synovium is much more complex, comprising several layers, any of which may appear and disappear as one follows the surface (Fig. 2D-2) (3). The subintimal layers, which confer mobility and packing properties, remain unstudied, and little of interest can be said about their normal structure and function. The subintima cannot be ignored, however, because it forms 95% of what can be felt clinically in synovitis.

The term "synovial membrane" probably refers to a superficial sheet of collagenous tissue that moves readily over underlying ligament or periosteum, which can be found anterior to the femoral condyles, for example. As with many older terms, the definition is vague (see Table 2D-1). Basketworks of ligaments and tendons surround joints and may appear to form a fibrous capsule, but the existence of such a structure is debatable. Synovial fluid is held in place by synovial intima, and synovium is held in place by atmospheric pressure.

Intima

Until the 1960s, there was no good evidence that the cells on the surface of synovium were different from other connective-tissue cells. Electron microscopy studies first showed the superficial cells to be surrounded by a specialized matrix, rich in microfibrils, now known to consist of fibrillins 1 and 2 and collagen VI. Other matrix molecules found in basal laminae are present, including collagen IV, laminin, and chondroitin-6-sulphate-rich proteoglycans, but there is no boundary structure of the sort seen in epithelia or mesothelia (4). The limits of the intima are defined best by the microfibrillar mesh, although the mix of proteins varies from one area to another.

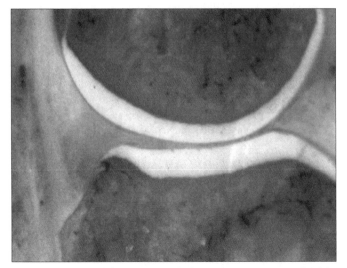

Fig. 2D-1. Normal human interphalangeal joint sectioned while frozen to show true relationships between cartilage and synovium. Synovium forms a tongue of tissue that fills the space between incongruous cartilage surfaces, except for a 50-micron thick film of fluid (just visible as a dark line in this magnified view) so that most of the cartilage is very close to synovial vessels.

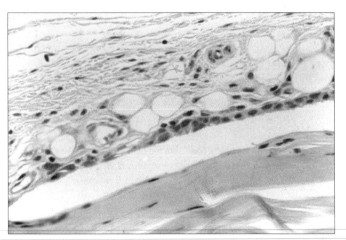

Fig. 2D-2. Section of normal tenosynovium, showing tendon below and synovium above. The synovial surface carries an irregular and incomplete layer of cells. The deeper subintima comprises loose areolar and fatty elements.

Cells embedded in intimal matrix are of two types. In normal tissue, the majority are fibroblasts and the minority are macrophages. This often is reversed in disease. The two types were separated by electron microscopy before the current understanding of cell origins (5). The terms type A (macrophage-like) and type B (fibroblast-like) arose, and for some time it was suggested that these types were two forms of a "synoviocyte" lineage – a term that has been used to mean so many things that it effectively is useless. The type A/B terminology has become obsolete because it has become clear that intimal macrophages are just as much macrophages as are peritoneal or alveolar macrophages. Furthermore, immunochemical markers have shown electron microscopic identification to be unreliable in disease. The terms intimal macrophage and intimal fibroblast are unambiguous (see Table 2D-1).

It is now reasonably certain that synovial intimal macrophages are monocyte-derived (6), and intimal fibroblasts derive locally from embryonic interzone. Both cell types show important specializations within their lineage-specific repertoires. Intimal macrophages express such typical macrophage products as CD14, CD68, and CD163,

but also belong to a subset that express the IgG Fc receptor FcγRIIIa (CD16a) (7). This receptor also is expressed in pericardium, alveoli, bone marrow, salivary glands, and sclera, and on Kuppfer cells. As in serosae, FcγRIIIa is found adsorbed onto intimal fibrillin-1 microfibrils.

Intimal fibroblasts differ from other fibroblasts in their high-level expression of uridine diphosphoglucose dehydrogenase (UDPGD), an enzyme involved in hyaluronan synthesis, vascular cell adhesion molecule 1 (VCAM-1), and complement decay-accelerating factor (DAF) (8–10). All three gene products are strongly expressed by bone marrow stromal cells, although separately on UDPGD$^+$ osteoblastic cells and VCAM-1$^+$DAF$^+$ hemopoietic nurse cells. Synovial and bone marrow stroma both derive from a perichondrial envelope, identifiable early in limb development by staining for the hyaluronan receptor CD44 (Fig. 2D-3) (11). There is a rapidly increasing list of other gene products expressed in both tissues, including chemokines, growth factors, and morphogenetic proteins. The most remarkable recent finding is that lubricin (which lubricates joints) and megakaryocyte stimulating factor come from the same gene (12).

Significant areas of synovial surface do not carry a recognizable intimal cell layer. However, an important property of the whole synovial surface is an absence of interstitial pores >1 µm in diameter, allowing the retention of synovial fluid. This matrix continuity gives rise to two features that distinguish synovial spaces from the ill-defined spaces present between layers of collagen throughout loose connective tissue. Synovium appears to be "folded back" at the margins of the cavity (1). The surface often appears crimped when stretched, although nobody knows exactly what happens to the surface as it stretches and relaxes during movement in vivo.

TABLE 2D-1
Terminology

Components of synovium	Obsolete or ambiguous terms
Intima or lining cell layer:	Synoviocyte
Synovial intimal macrophage	Type A cell
Synovial intimal fibroblast	Type B cell
Intimal matrix	
Superficial capillary plexus	
Subintima:	Synovial membrane
Subintimal macrophage	
Subintimal fibroblast	
Subintimal matrix	
In disease:	
Intimal macrophage recruitment	Synovial hyperplasia
Fibroblast proliferation	Mesenchymal transformation
In vitro:	
Synovial macrophages	
Synovial fibroblasts	

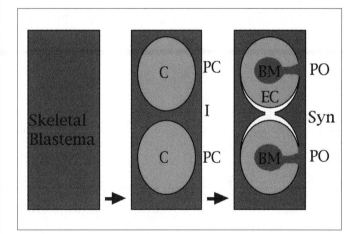

Fig. 2D-3. Development of bone marrow and synovium from a common perichondrial envelope. Within an embryonic skeletal blastemal element, precartilaginous foci (C) form. The surrounding envelope becomes both perichondrium (PC) and, between the elements, interzone (I). Perichondrium invades the cartilage to form bone marrow (BM) stroma and also matures to become periosteum (PO). Interzone detaches from cartilage to form synovium (Syn).

Subintima

Areolar, fatty, and fibrous forms of subintimal connective tissue may look unremarkable, but there are reasons to believe that the stromal cells have the potential to assume the same specialized features as intimal fibroblasts. These tissues may be considered to belong to the same specialized blastemal fibroblast subpopulation. Superficial subintima may form a "membrane" that moves freely over deeper tissues. In other places, it forms surface folds or finger-like villi.

The Superficial Vascular Plexus

Just below the intima is a rich capillary network derived from a plexus of arterioles and venules lying in the subintima, together with lymphatics (13). The capillaries have fenestrations on the side facing the cavity. This network imparts to the synovial surface a high vascular density. The vascular network is associated with nerve fibers, some of which have endings within the intima (14).

Function

Synovium allows disconnection between adjacent moving structures. When disconnection is overtaken by connecting fibrous tissue (as in frozen shoulder), mobility is lost. The detailed mechanical properties of subintima also contribute to mobility. Fatty areas provide isotropic, elastically deformable packing for large spaces between incongruent cartilage surfaces. Areolar areas may stretch, crimp, roll, or slide. Synovial villi, which provide versatile deformability during movement, become more common with age and may compensate for the growing inelasticity and increasingly fibrous character of the subintima. Villi would not be expected to assist molecular exchange, and often are avascular.

Other synovial functions include the provision of nutrition to chondrocytes and the control of synovial-fluid volume and composition.

Chondrocyte Nutrition

Hyaline cartilage has no vasculature. Chondrocytes must obtain glucose and other nutrients from vessels in other tissues. Subchondral bone vessels may contribute, but the diffusion routes are limited. Synovium is the obvious source of nutrients for most cartilage. Articular surfaces are mostly incongruent, with relatively small contact areas. Most of the cartilage surface is effectively in contact with vascular synovium, despite a thin film of fluid between these structures (Fig. 2D-1).

The route of nutrition to areas of cartilage that do not come close to synovium in any position of the joint must be indirect, and may be via adjacent or apposed areas of cartilage, which have better access to synovium (15). It often is assumed that synovial fluid is an important transporter of nutrients, but the volume of fluid is so small that it is unlikely to have much nutrient capacity. The key unanswered question is whether there is ever any real problem in providing adequate nutrition for chondrocytes. Although some chondrocytes are distant from vessels, their minimum metabolic demands may be small. Nasal, intervertebral disc, and costal cartilage survive, cocooned in fibrous tissue. However, chondrocyte starvation, and hypoglycemia in particular, may be a major problem under special circumstances.

Synovial Fluid Volume and Composition

The volume and composition of synovial fluid is determined by the properties of synovial intima and its vasculature. The biophysics are complex and yet appear to be achieved by the simplest of means, the secretion by intimal fibroblasts of the high–molecular-weight polysaccharide known as hyaluronan (16,17). The mechanism appears to be unique, and to have no parallel with glands, glomeruli, or any other fluid-dynamic system.

The water in synovial fluid, like any other interstitial fluid, is a dialysate of plasma. The water is there because the solid elements of the joint do not oppose each other perfectly; if the intervening space were not filled with water, the joint would be under a hard vacuum, and water would filter in. Joint cavities are under only a slight vacuum. The drawback of filling a joint with a pure dialysate of plasma is that during movement, the pumping effect of intermittent tissue compression would squeeze out the water into the lymphatics.

The biologic solution to this is to mix the plasma dialysate with a molecule so enormous that it cannot be squeezed through the collagen VI microfibrillar mesh of the synovial intima. This intimal meshwork is leakier than a basement membrane and allows water, crystalloids, and proteins to pass freely, but obstructs the passage of hyaluronan, which has a molecular mass in the order of 1 million Da. If synovial fluid tries to escape rapidly from the cavity, the hyaluronan "gunks up" the tissue surface, like coffee grounds stopping water percolating through a filter paper. The result is that water can pass in and out of the cavity slowly by diffusion, but cannot be squeezed out. Because the gunking effect of hyaluronan depends on its concentration, the fluid equilibrates at a constant concentration. This means that synovial-fluid volume is determined by the amount of hyaluronan present.

Hyaluronan is not unique to synovium. Muscle cells are surrounded by a film of hyaluronan solution, and dermis is rich in hyaluronan. The fluid dynamics are different in each tissue, but hyaluronan probably plays a role in water retention in many different contexts.

Functions of Synovial Fluid

Maintenance of constant fluid volume by hyaluronan probably has two roles. Preventing formation of a high vacuum in a joint allows synovium to slide, stretch, and crimp without becoming jammed between cartilage surfaces and torn to pieces. Hyaluronan also maintains a fluid film between cartilage surfaces under load, which allows fluid-based (hydrodynamic) lubrication to occur. Hyaluronan maintains the fluid film by using properties related to those involved in preventing fluid leakage. If a very thin film of hyaluronan solution is compressed, water escapes more rapidly than does hyaluronan, with the result that the remaining hyaluronan solution becomes so concentrated, it forms an elastic gel that cannot be squeezed out. This gel maintains its ability to lubricate under high shear stress. When pressure is removed, the elastic hyaluronan gel will recoil and suck back a film of fluid.

The lubricating mechanisms in joints and other tissues still are not understood completely. It is clear that hyaluronan is not itself an important lubricant, but a film-maintaining agent. It has been thought for some time that the true lubricant is lubricin, a glycoprotein (11). However, Hills recently proposed that the common lubricating mechanism for many tissues is a boundary lubrication based on phospholipid, and that lubricin functions as a phospholipid carrier (18).

Synovium as an Immunologic Microenvironment

Intimal macrophages probably have little to do much of the time, and in normal tissue, they are rather sparse. However, synovium has unusually stringent requirements for self-repair. Throughout life, in the face of repeated microtrauma, synovium needs to retain its disconnective properties and suppleness, keep its surface free of large gaps, and maintain a cavity free of debris and pathogenic microorganisms. That synovium uses different strategies than other tissues use to achieve these ends is suggested by the specialized properties of both intimal macrophages and fibroblasts.

The IgG Fc receptor FcγRIIIa is expressed only on a subgroup of tissue macrophages that includes synovial intimal macrophages, serosal macrophages, alveolar macrophages, Kuppfer cells, and macrophages in bone marrow and lymphoid tissue (6). Activation of this receptor by immune complexes generates tumor necrosis factor (TNF) and interleukin 1, which are known to contribute substantially to the clinical spectrum of rheumatoid arthritis. Expression of FcγRIIIa probably is controlled in part by mechanical stress, because in dermis, it is expressed only at the exposed sites where rheumatoid nodules occur.

FcγRIIIa often is expressed at sites rich in the complement regulatory protein DAF, as if the two molecules act in concert. In serosae and synovium, the two molecules are found together, adsorbed on fibrillin-1–based microfibrils. FcγRIIIa probably is the only Fc receptor to generate cytokines in response to small immune complexes of the type that occur early in immune responses (19). This action suggests that the combination of FcγRIIIa and DAF may be used by tissues that require an "early warning system" for responding rapidly to pathogens. Although synovium is embryologically quite unrelated to serosa, it seems that when it developed in evolution, it borrowed this early warning system from the pre-existing tissue linings. At the same time, it may have acquired a susceptibility to involvement in small immune-complex–based autoimmune diseases.

The expression of VCAM-1 by intimal fibroblasts regulates the traffic of white blood cells. Mononuclear leukocytes, but not granulocytes, carry the coligand for VCAM-1, known as α4β1 integrin. The presence of VCAM-1 on intimal cells may arrest mononuclear cells migrating to the surface and prevent them from entering synovial fluid, while allowing granulocytes to pass. This may allow granulocytes to pick up any pathogenic microorganisms in the cavity, but then be reabsorbed into the tissue by intimal macrophages. It also will prevent lymphoid cells from accumulating in the synovial space, where they would be of little value, being unable to control contact-mediated interactions with accessory cells.

There may be another link with serosal linings relating to VCAM-1. In primitive organisms, phagocytes probably arise and function chiefly in serosal cavities. Even in higher vertebrates, early leukocyte precursors arise in splanchnopleural tissue. Leukopoiesis then moves to the liver and on to bone marrow. Stromal cell expression of VCAM-1 is particularly essential for B-lymphocyte development. Thus, stromal cell–leukocyte interactions of the type mediated by VCAM-1 may have arisen in serosal linings and then been taken on by synovium to serve different functions. With the evolution of bone marrow, these interactions again became important for leukopoiesis. The problem for both synovium and bone marrow is that under the influence of such cytokines as TNF, which is produced by its own macrophages in response to immune complexes, the stromal cells express a combination of ligands capable of sustaining the formation of full-blown lymphoid follicles (20); hence, the resemblance of rheumatoid synovium to lymph-node tissue.

Synovium and Cartilage Damage

Synovium plays an important role in disease-driven damage to cartilage. However, the true sequence of events is far from clear. In what conventionally is called osteoarthritis, cartilage fragmentation occurs at load-bearing sites. This fragmentation may be secondary to a wide range of inflammatory or metabolic abnormalities for which the synovial vasculature provides the portal of entry to the joint, although age-related changes in subchondral and periarticular bone structure are thought to be more important in the genesis of primary cartilage fragmentation.

An important possibility remains that, with age, the combination of complete closure of the subchondral plate to diffusion gaps and the loss of synovial vascularity due to fibrosis may lead to chronic chondrocyte ischemia in such joints as the hip. This reopens the issue of the minimum nutrient supply required for chondrocyte survival and whether the critical need is for glucose (for glycolysis), oxygen, or clearance of toxic wastes. Once chondrocytes have died, fragmentation of the matrix probably is inevitable.

Interestingly, chondrocyte death may precede matrix disruption in acute models of osteoarthritis, such as in the Pond-Nuki dog.

In rheumatoid arthritis, cartilage damage occurs particularly at the margins, and there seems little doubt that removal of cartilage matrix is accomplished by such enzymes as metalloproteinases derived from synovial cells. However, therapeutic metalloproteinase inhibition so far has failed to halt the progression of cartilage damage. Again, the maintenance of chondrocyte nutrition may be relevant. Chondrocytes are thought to respire largely by glycolysis. Fluids bathing tissues affected by inflammation in rheumatoid arthritis commonly show very low glucose levels. Thus, chondrocytes may suffer hypoglycemia, rather than ischemia or hypoxia. Samples of cartilage from rheumatoid joints showing cartilage invasion by pannus nearly always show that many of the chondrocytes in the tissue being invaded already are dead.

JONATHAN C.W. EDWARDS, MD

References

1. O'Rahilly R, Gardner E. The embryology of movable joints. In: Sokoloff L (ed). The Joints and Synovial Fluid, Vol 1. New York: Academic Press, 1978; pp 105–176.

2. Key JA. The synovial membrane of joints and bursae. In: Special Cytology, Vol 2. New York: PB Hoeber Inc, 1932; pp 1055–1076.

3. Edwards JCW. Structure of synovial lining. In: Henderson B, Edwards JCW (eds). The Synovial Lining in Health and Disease. London: Chapman & Hall, 1987; pp 31–40.

4. Revell PA, Al-Saffar N, Fish S, Osei D. Extracellular matrix of the synovial intimal cell layer. Ann Rheum Dis 1995;54:404–407.

5. Barland P, Novikoff AB, Hamerman D. Electron microscopy of the human synovial membrane. J Cell Biol 1962;14:207–216.

6. Edwards JCW, Willoughby DA. Demonstration of bone marrow derived cells in synovial lining by means of giant intracellular granules as genetic markers. Ann Rheum Dis 1982;41:177–182.

7. Bhatia A, Blades S, Cambridge G, Edwards JCW. Differential distribution of Fc gamma RIIIa in normal human tissues and colocalization with DAF and fibrillin-1: implications for immunological microenvironments. Immunology 1998;94:56–63.

8. Pitsillides AA, Blake SM. Uridine diphosphoglucose dehydrogenase activity in synovial lining cells in the experimental antigen induced model of rheumatoid arthritis: an indication of synovial lining cell function. Ann Rheum Dis 1992;51:992–995.

9. Morales-Ducret J, Wayner E, Elices MJ, Alvaro-Garcia JM, Zvaifler NJ, Firestein GS. Alpha 4/Beta1 integrin (VLA-4) ligands in arthritis: vascular cell adhesion molecule-1 expression in synovium and on fibroblast-like synoviocytes. J Immunol 1992;149:1424–1431.

10. Medof ME, Walter EI, Rutgers JL, Knowles DM, Nussenzweig V. Identification of the complement decay accelerating factor on epithelium and glandular cells and in body fluids. J Exp Med 1987;165:848–864.

11. Edwards JCW, Wilkinson LS, Jones HM, et al. The formation of human synovial joint cavities: a possible role for hyaluronan and CD44 in altered interzone cohesion. J Anat 1994;185:355–367.

12. Jay GD, Britt DE, Cha CJ. Lubricin is a product of megakaryocyte stimulating factor gene expression by human synovial fibroblasts. J Rheumatol 2000;27:594–600.

13. Davies DV, Edwards DAW. The blood supply of the synovial membrane and intra-articular structures. Ann R Coll Surg 1948;142–156.

14. Mapp PI. Innervation of synovium. Ann Rheum Dis 1995;54:398–403.

15. Edwards JCW. Functions of synovial lining. In: Henderson B, Edwards JCW (eds). The Synovial Lining in Health and Disease. London: Chapman & Hall, 1987; pp 41–74.

16. Simkin PA, Bassett JE, Koh EM. Synovial perfusion in the human knee: a methodologic analysis. Semin Arthritis Rheum 1995;25:56–66.

17. Levick JR, McDonald JN. Fluid movement across synovium in healthy joints: role of synovial fluid macromolecules. Ann Rheum Dis 1995;54:417–423.

18. Hills BA. Boundary lubrication in vivo. Proc Inst Mech Eng H 2000;214:83–94.

19. Abrahams VM, Cambridge G, Edwards JCW. Induction of tumour necrosis factor alpha production by human monocytes: a key role for FcγRIIIa in rheumatoid arthritis. Arthritis Rheum 2000;43:608–611.

20. Edwards JCW, Leigh RD, Cambridge G. Expression of molecules involved in B lymphocyte survival and differentiation by synovial fibroblasts. Clin Exp Immunol 1997;108:407–414.

THE MUSCULOSKELETAL SYSTEM
E. Skeletal Muscle

Skeletal muscle makes up more than 40% of our total body mass. Normal skeletal muscle is composed of multinucleated cells called fibers, grouped anatomically in fascicles, and surrounded by connective tissue called perimysium (1). The space between the muscle fibers (called endomysium) usually is insignificant. Most skeletal muscles are connected to bone by tendons at each end. The parallel arrangements of fascicles between the tendinous ends of muscles allow for an additive force of contraction. Fibers within a fascicle are innervated by different motor neurons. Functionally, muscle fibers are grouped in motor units that consist of a lower motor neuron originating in a spinal cord anterior horn cell and the muscle fibers it innervates (2).

Muscle fibers vary with respect to their metabolism and response to stimuli and may be typed accordingly. A variety of fiber-type classifications have emerged based on different biochemical and physiologic properties (3). For most purposes, fibers are divided among three types. Type 1 fibers, also called slow-twitch fibers, respond to electrical stimulation comparatively slowly, have moderate contractile intensity, and are fatigue-resistant with repeated stimulation. Type 1 cells have greater numbers of mitochondria and higher lipid content. Type 2 fibers, termed fast-twitch fibers, are of two types. Type 2a fibers respond more rapidly than Type 1 fibers and with greater force of contraction, but they fatigue rapidly. These fibers have more glycogen and higher activities of myophosphorylase and myoadenylate deaminase. Type 2b fibers are referred to as "default fibers" because they become more prominent during periods of deconditioning and contract inefficiently (4,5).

Individual human muscles are heterogeneous with regard to fiber type. However, all muscle fibers within a motor unit are of the same type. The characteristics of each fiber type originally are determined during development and are maintained through interaction with the innervating motor neuron. Fiber-type specificity and distribution can be altered by reinnervation with a different type of motor neuron, physical training, or disease processes (6).

Each muscle fiber is an elongated multinucleated cell surrounded by a plasma membrane called the sarcolemma. Fibers contain contractile proteins (actin, troponin, tropomyosin, and myosin) called myofilaments (Fig. 2E-1). The myofilaments are bathed in cytosol, called *sarcoplasm,* and organized within fibrils, which are enveloped by the sarcoplasmic reticulum. Communication between the sarcolemma and sarcoplasmic reticulum is provided through a network of pores and channels known as the *T-tubule system.*

Most of the energy necessary for muscle function is generated in mitochondria. These organelles contain their own DNA, called mitochondrial DNA (7). In contrast to nuclear DNA, mtDNA is circular, maternally derived, and lacks a mechanism for repair. Mitochondria have a limited life span but maintain their numbers by self-replicating through a process similar to binary fission.

Contraction and Relaxation

Muscle contraction requires shortening of fibrils located within muscle fibers (8). Contraction can result from electrical, chemical, or physical stimulation that initiates the

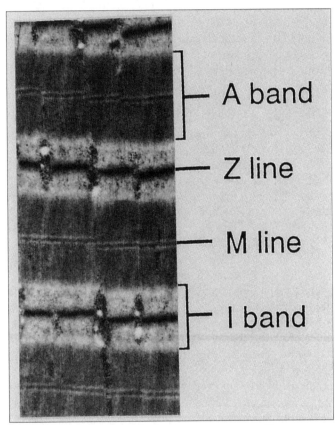

Fig. 2E-1. The varying refractile indices of the myofilaments give skeletal muscle its characteristic ultrastructural cross-striated appearance. The functional contractile unit of the fiber is the sarcomere, defined as the area between two Z lines. Z lines transect the fibrils and connect the actin filaments. The A band is composed of the thick myofilaments (myosin), and the M line is due to the bulges in the middle of the myosin filaments. In cross-section, each myosin filament is surrounded by six actin filaments in a hexagonal pattern. At rest, the I band is the area occupied by the thin filaments (actin, troponin, and tropomyosin) not overlapped by myosin. With contraction, cross-bridges form between actin and myosin; Z lines move toward the M line; and I bands become smaller. Mitochondria (not shown) are located in the I bands on either side of the Z line.

orderly transmission of an action potential along the sarcolemma, through the T-tubule system, and to the sarcoplasmic reticulum. As a result of this stimulation, calcium is released into the sarcoplasm. As calcium concentrations increase within the sarcoplasm, actin is released from an inhibited state, permitting actin-myosin cross-linkage and fibril shortening. Shortening continues until calcium is actively pumped back into the sarcoplasmic reticulum, breaking the cross-linkages and allowing relaxation.

Both contraction and relaxation are active processes that require normal levels of electrolytes and adenosine triphosphate (ATP). Sodium, potassium, calcium, and magnesium are critical to the function of three ATPase proteins that must work effectively for normal fiber contraction and relaxation. Sodium-potassium ATPase activity maintains normal polarity of the sarcolemma. The ATPase that controls actin-myosin cross-linking is magnesium-dependent. A calcium-dependent ATPase pumps calcium from the sarcoplasm into the sarcoplasmic reticulum, permitting relaxation. Phosphorus levels also are critical because phosphorus is the ion that forms the high-energy bonds of ATP, the substrate for the three enzymes.

Energy Metabolism

Energy required for the contraction and relaxation of muscle is derived from the hydrolysis of ATP. Skeletal muscle uses fatty acids and carbohydrates to produce ATP (8–10), with several pathways used to produce energy from each source. The importance of a particular pathway varies with the level of exertion and nutritional status of the individual. Working in concert, these pathways maintain intracellular ATP concentrations at constant levels under most conditions and restore them to normal levels if vigorous activity or hypoxia causes ATP concentrations to fall.

Free fatty acids provide the major source of ATP during fasting intervals, at rest, and for muscle activities of low intensity and long duration. These acids must enter mitochondria to be processed for energy. To enter mitochondria, long-chain fatty acids combine with the carrier molecule carnitine and transfer across the mitochondrial membrane. This process is catalyzed by two enzymes found on the inner membrane, carnitine palmitoyltransferase (CPT) I and CPT II. Once in the mitochondria, fatty acid and carnitine separate. Two carbon fragments of acetyl-CoA are split off the fatty acid by the process of beta-oxidation. The carbon fragments are metabolized sequentially by the tricarboxylic acid cycle and oxidative phosphorylation. By this metabolic route, one molecule of palmitate results in the net gain of 131 molecules of ATP.

Glycogen, the major storage form of carbohydrate, can be metabolized aerobically or anaerobically but provides the primary source of ATP when physical activity is intense or when anaerobic conditions exist. Under such conditions, glycogen is mobilized to form glucose-6-phosphate by the process of glycogenolysis, a process initiated by the activity of myophosphorylase (8,11). Glucose-6-phosphate is metabolized to lactate through the glycolytic pathway.

Under aerobic conditions, this pathway produces pyruvate, which can enter the tricarboxylic acid cycle. The aerobic metabolism of one molecule of glucose nets 38 molecules of ATP, whereas anaerobic processing results in the generation of only two molecules of ATP.

At rest, oxidative metabolism produces excess amounts of ATP, but intracellular levels of ATP remain constant. Creatine phosphokinase (CK) activity plays a pivotal role in maintaining constant intracellular ATP concentrations, functioning to buffer changes in cytosol levels. Creatine phosphokinase catalyzes the reversible transphosphorylation of creatine and adenine nucleotides. At rest, the terminal phosphate of excess ATP is transferred to creatine, forming creatine phosphate and adenosine diphosphate (ADP). The creatine phosphate acts as a reservoir of high-energy phosphates. With muscle activity and ATP hydrolysis, CK catalyzes the transfer of those phosphates to ADP, rapidly restoring ATP levels to normal. Creatine phosphokinase and its products, creatine and creatine phosphate, also serve as a shuttle mechanism for energy transport between mitochondria, where ATP is generated by oxidative metabolism, and the myofilaments, where ATP is consumed in the active processes of muscle contraction and relaxation (12).

The CK-buffering system maintains ATP concentrations at stable levels during exercise until creatine phosphate concentrations are depleted by 50%. If activity continues, ATP concentrations fall and the purine nucleotide cycle begins to play a pivotal role. This cycle tends to occur when anaerobic glycolysis becomes the major route for ATP generation. The first step of the purine nucleotide cycle is conversion of adenosine monophosphate (AMP) to inosine monophosphate (IMP) by myoadenylate deaminase activity, with the generation of ammonia. Both IMP and ammonia stimulate glycolysis. As ATP concentrations fall, IMP concentrations rise stoichiometrically. This process continues until muscle activity decreases and recovery can occur. During recovery, oxidative pathways resume a major functional role. Adenosine monophosphate is regenerated from IMP by a two-step process with the liberation of fumarate (13). Fumarate is converted to malate, which enters mitochondria and participates as an intermediate in the tricarboxylic acid cycle. The higher concentrations of malate thus act to "drive" the cycle, causing efficient regeneration of ATP by oxidative phosphorylation.

ROBERT L. WORTMANN, MD

References

1. Bossen EH. Muscle structure and development. In: Wortmann RL (ed). Diseases of Skeletal Muscle. Philadelphia: Lippincott Williams & Wilkins, 2000; pp 3–9.
2. Landon DN. Skeletal muscle – normal morphology, development and innervation. In: Mastaglia FL, Detchant LW (eds). Skeletal Muscle Pathology, 2nd ed. New York: Churchill Livingstone, 1992; pp 1–94.
3. Kelly AM, Rubinstein NA. The diversity of muscle fiber types

and its origin during development. In: Engel AG, Franzini-Armstrong C (eds). Myology, 2nd ed. New York: McGraw-Hill, 1994; pp 119–133.

4. *Smerdu V, Karsch-Mizrachi I, Campione M, Leinwand L, Schiaffino S. Type IIx myosin heavy chain transcripts are expressed in type IIb fibers of human skeletal muscle. Am J Physiol 1994;267:C1723–C1728.*

5. *Schiaffino S, Reggiani C. Molecular diversity of myofibrillar proteins: gene regulation and functional significance. Physiol Rev 1996;76:371–423.*

6. *Hickey MS, Carey JO, Azevedo JL, et al. Skeletal muscle fiber composition is related to adiposity and in vitro glucose transport rate in humans. Am J Physiol 1995;268:E453–E457.*

7. *Clayton DA: Structure and function of the mitochondrial genome. J Inherit Metab Dis 1992;15:439–447.*

8. *Wortmann RL. Skeletal muscle biology, physiology, and biochemistry. In: Wortmann RL (ed). Diseases of Skeletal Muscle. Philadelphia: Lippincott Williams & Wilkins, 2000; pp 11–22.*

9. *Layzer RB: How muscles use fuel. N Engl J Med 1991;324:411–412.*

10. *Ontko JA. Lipid metabolism in muscle. In: Engel AG, Franzini-Armstrong C (eds). Myology, 2nd ed. New York: McGraw-Hill, 1994; pp 665–682.*

11. *Brown DH: Glycogen metabolism and glycolysis in muscle. In: Engel AG, Franzini-Armstrong C (eds). Myology, 2nd ed. New York: McGraw-Hill, 1994, pp 648–664.*

12. *Erickson-Viitanen S, Geiger P, Yang WC, Bessman SP. The creatine-creatine phosphate shuttle for energy transport-compartmentation of creatine phosphokinase in muscle. Adv Exp Med Biol 1982;151:115–125.*

13. *Aragon JJ, Lowenstein JM. The purine nucleotide cycle. Comparison of the levels of citric acid cycle intermediators with the operation of the purine nucleotide cycle in rat skeletal muscle during exercise and recovery from exercise. Eur J Biochem 1980;110:371–377.*

THE MUSCULOSKELETAL SYSTEM
F. Vascular Endothelium

The entire circulatory system is lined by the vascular endothelium, a continuous membrane that is one cell thick. Originally, the endothelium was viewed simply as a passive permeable barrier, but in recent years, the multifunctional nature of this tissue has been recognized. By virtue of its anatomic location, vascular endothelium provides the interface that defines intra- and extravascular compartments, serves as a selectively permeable barrier, and provides a continuous nonthrombogenic lining for the cardiovascular system.

The endothelial surface covers several thousand square meters. It can function as an immense catalytic surface, a highly selective binding surface, or a relatively nonspecific adsorptive surface. These activities are especially enhanced in the microcirculation, where the ratio of endothelial surface area to blood volume is maximal. Blood vessel walls actively participate in the biochemical reactions of hemostasis (1) and immune response (2). In addition, key surface-related functions of vascular endothelium can be altered dynamically, rendering the endothelial surface an important site of physiologic regulation and pathologic alteration (3–5).

Changes in the structure and function of the endothelium profoundly alter its interactions with the cellular and macromolecular components of circulating blood and underlying tissue. These alterations include enhanced permeability of the endothelium to plasma lipoproteins; oxidative modification of these lipoproteins; increased adhesion of blood leukocytes; and functional imbalances in local pro- and antithrombotic factors, growth stimulators, growth inhibitors, and vasoactive substances. These manifestations, collectively termed endothelial dysfunction, participate in the initiation, progression, and clinical complications of various forms of inflammatory and degenerative diseases. Growth-promoting and promigratory activities for endothelial cells, such as vascular endothelial growth factor (VEGF) family members, are generated at sites of inflammation, leading to aberrant angiogenic responses. In rheumatoid arthritis, these new vessels may play critical roles in the generation and maintenance of the invasive pannus.

Anatomy and Function of Normal Endothelium

The endothelium's location is a key factor in its interactions with cells in the circulating blood and surrounding tissue. Its involvement in the monitoring, integration, and transduction of blood-borne signals makes the endothelium a type of sensory organ. This sensor-transducer function is facilitated by the surfaces of endothelial cells, the clearly definable "apical" or luminal surface facing the blood stream, and the "basal" or abluminal surface in contact with the subendothelial connective tissues. Each surface is outfitted with a distinct complement of functional molecules, including enzymes and receptors.

The endothelium plays a pivotal role in the coagulation and fibrinolytic system (6). Several of the body's natural anticoagulant mechanisms are associated with the endothelium, and their expression levels vary according to the vascular bed (7). These include the heparin-antithrombin mechanism, the protein C-thrombomodulin mechanism, and the tissue plasminogen activator mechanism. Dysfunctional endothelial cells are capable of active prothrombotic behavior, synthesizing such adhesive cofactors for platelets as von

Willebrand factor, fibronectin, and thrombospondin; pro-coagulant components, such as factor V; and an inhibitor of the fibrinolytic pathway, known as plasminogen activator inhibitor-1, which reduces the rate of fibrin breakdown. Thus, the endothelium plays a number of roles, both "pro" and "anti" hemostatic-thrombotic.

Until the discovery of endothelium-derived relaxing factor (EDRF), maintenance of cardiovascular tone was viewed solely as a function of the vascular smooth-muscle cell response to nerve stimulation or circulating hormones. The identification of EDRF as endogenous nitric oxide and recognition of its mechanism of action in vasodilation, cell survival, and gene expression have enhanced greatly our understanding of the regulation of vascular tone (8). A number of endothelial-derived substances balance the vasorelaxor actions of nitric oxide and prostacyclin. These vasoconstrictors include angiotensin II, which is generated at the endothelial surface by angiotensin-converting enzyme; platelet-derived growth factor (PDGF), which is secreted by endothelial cells and acts as an agonist of smooth-muscle contraction; and endothelin 1, a unique vasoconstrictor substance (9).

The vascular endothelial lining produces a variety of cytokines, growth factors, and growth inhibitors that act locally to influence the behavior of adjacent vascular cells and interacting blood elements. This makes the endothelium a special kind of endocrine organ that secretes hormones in a paracrine or autocrine fashion.

The Dysfunctional or Activated Endothelium

Injury to, or activation of, the endothelium may lead to the induction of genes that are suppressed under physiologic conditions and/or the down-regulation of beneficial genes (1–5). As depicted in Fig. 2F-1, specific endothelial cell functions may be directly relevant to chronic inflammatory responses and their clinical sequelae, including the expression of leukocyte-binding sites on the endothelial cell surface; the altered production of paracrine growth factors, chemoattractants, and vasoreactive molecules; the ability to oxidize low-density lipoprotein and respond to oxidized lipids and lipoproteins; the expression of procoagulant activities; and the modulation of plasma-component levels within the surrounding tissue through changes in permeability function. Many factors alter endothelial gene expression during inflammation. Leading candidates include altered hemodynamics, local cytokines or proteases, viral infection, free radicals, and oxidized lipids.

Expression of Leukocyte Adhesion Molecules

The molecular interactions between blood-borne leukocytes and the endothelium play pivotal roles in inflammation. Neutrophils and monocytes produce paracrine growth factors and cytokines, generate cytotoxic factors for neighboring cells, and cause degradation of local connective tissue. The first step in recruiting leukocytes into the subendothelial space is attachment of the cell to the endothelium. Healthy endothelium does not bind leukocytes. However, neutrophils, monocytes, and lymphocytes bind avidly to newly expressed leukocyte adhesion molecules on the endothelial surface in response to such activating agents as interleukin 1, tumor necrosis factor α, lipopolysaccharide, and oxidized lipids (1–5).

The process of leukocyte attachment and diapedesis involves various adhesion molecules and chemokines (10–12). The endothelium and the leukocytes play active roles in the process, which includes an initial rolling or tethering event (selectins), a signaling process (chemokines), a strong attachment step (the immunoglobulin family members), and transendothelial cell migration of the leukocyte. Much has been learned about these processes through the use of genetically engineered mice and various models of inflammation (13,14).

Growth Factor Production by the Activated Endothelium

The activated endothelium is a potential source of growth factor for neighboring smooth-muscle cells and fibroblasts. PDGF, a mitogen implicated in wound healing and atherosclerosis, is expressed

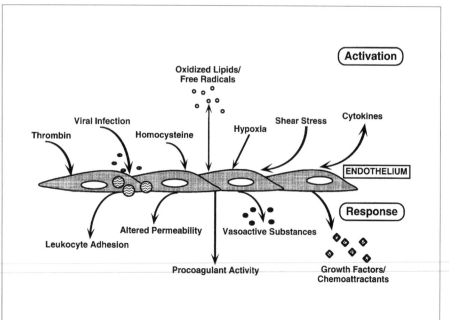

Fig. 2F-1. Generation of a dysfunctional endothelium. A variety of stimulatory or injury-provoking agents have been implicated in the process of endothelial cell activation. Many of the responses of the endothelium are associated with the progression of vascular disease and inflammation (1).

by endothelial cells. Substantial evidence correlates endothelial PDGF expression with vascular dysfunction and disease (15). The most effective natural inducer of PDGF production by endothelial cells is α-thrombin, a protease component of the coagulation system that increases PDGF-gene expression through a unique mechanism (16). The endothelium also is known to produce other growth factors for connective-tissue cells, including insulin-like growth factor 1, basic fibroblast growth factor, and transforming growth factor β (a pleuripotent growth factor/growth inhibitor). These connective-tissue mitogens participate in the fibrosis observed in many inflammatory diseases.

Angiogenic Response of the Activated Endothelium

Recent research has focused on the role of newly formed synovial microvessels in the maintenance of the invasive pannus in rheumatoid arthritis. Members of the VEGF family may be responsible for this angiogenic response at sites of inflammation (17). VEGF induces migration and proliferation of endothelium from existing vessels, and increases the leakiness of new and pre-existing vessels, potentially exacerbating the sequelae of inflammation (18). Inhibition of VEGF through the use of soluble receptors, blocking antibodies, gene therapy, or other approaches may be effective therapeutic strategies for some chronic inflammatory diseases.

PAUL E. DiCORLETO, PhD

References

1. Preissner KT, Nawroth PP, Kanse SM. Vascular protease receptors: integrating haemostasis and endothelial cell functions. J Pathol 2000;190:360–372.
2. Pober JS. Immunobiology of human vascular endothelium. Immunol Res 1999;19:225–232.
3. Mantovani A, Garlanda C, Introna M, Vecchi A. Regulation of endothelial cell function by pro- and anti-inflammatory cytokines. Transplant Proc 1998;30:4239–4243.
4. Drexler H, Horning B. Endothelial dysfunction in human disease. J Mol Cell Cardiol 1999;31:51–60.
5. Gimbrone MA Jr. Endothelial dysfunction, hemodynamic forces, and atherosclerosis. Thromb Haemost 1999;82:722–726.
6. Lijnen HR, Collen D. Endothelium in hemostasis and thrombosis. Prog Cardiovasc Dis 1997;39:343–350.
7. Rosenberg RD, Aird WC. Vascular-bed–specific hemostasis and hypercoagulable states. N Engl J Med 1999;340:1555–1564.
8. Ignarro LJ. Nitric oxide: a unique endogenous signaling molecule in vascular biology. Biosci Rep 1999;19:51–71.
9. Miyauchi T, Masaki T. Pathophysiology of endothelin in the cardiovascular system. Annu Rev Physiol 1999;61:391–415.
10. Kevil CG, Bullard DC. Roles of leukocyte/endothelial cell adhesion molecules in the pathogenesis of vasculitis. Am J Med 1999;106:677–687.
11. Oppenheimer-Marks N, Lipsky PE. Adhesion molecules in rheumatoid arthritis. Springer Semin Immunopathol 1998; 20:95–114.
12. Ebnet K, Vestweber D. Molecular mechanisms that control leukocyte extravasation: the selectins and the chemokines. Histochem Cell Biol 1999;112:1–23.
13. Hynes RO, Wagner DD. Genetic manipulation of vascular adhesion molecules in mice. J Clin Invest 1997;100:S11–S13.
14. Etzioni A, Doerschuk CM, Harlan JM. Of man and mouse: leukocyte and endothelial adhesion molecule deficiencies. Blood 1999;94:3281–3288.
15. DiCorleto PE, Fox P. Growth factor production by endothelial cells. In: Ryan U (ed). Endothelial Cells, Vol. 2. Boca Raton: CRC Press, 1988; pp 51–61.
16. Stenina OI, Poptic EJ, DiCorleto PE. Thrombin activates a Y box-binding protein (DNA-binding protein B) in endothelial cells. J Clin Invest 2000;106:579–587.
17. Ferrara N. Role of vascular endothelial growth factor in the regulation of angiogenesis. Kidney Int 1999;56:794–814.
18. Bates DO, Lodwick D, Williams B. Vascular endothelial growth factor and microvascular permeability. Microcirculation 1999;6:83–96.

THE MUSCULOSKELETAL SYSTEM
G. Peripheral Nerves

Peripheral nerves consist of nerve cell bodies, their peripheral extensions (axons), and Schwann cells, which provide a distinctive axonal covering, the myelin sheath. The axon is a thread-like cylindrical process that varies in length and diameter according to the size and type of neuron. Axons of large diameter (1–22 mm) are myelinated and conduct nerve impulses rapidly due to the advantages conveyed by the myelin sheath. The length of each axon is invested by many Schwann cells, and gaps between these cells, called nodes of Ranvier, allow saltatory conduction of action potentials and rapid transmission of nerve impulses. Axons of small diameter (0.2–2.4 mm) are unmyelinated, but even unmyelinated fibers are ensheathed by Schwann cells (1–3).

Axons are devoid of polyribosomes and rough endoplasmic reticulum, and they depend on the cell body (soma) for sustenance. Anterograde flow of axonal contents from the neuronal soma is essential for maturation, maintenance, and regeneration of the axon. Slow anterograde flow transports proteins and microfilaments; axoplasmic flow of intermediate speed transports mitochondria; and fast axonal flow transports substances contained within vesicles that are needed at the axon terminal during neurotransmission.

Retrograde flow, which allows the periphery to provide feedback to the soma, transports several types of molecules, including materials taken up by endocytosis.

Nerves have a dense external fibrous coat called epineurium, which also fills the space between the nerve fascicles. In turn, each fascicle is surrounded by perineurium, a sleeve formed by layers of flattened epithelial-like cells. Each nerve fiber is surrounded and bound together through endoneurium, which consists of a thin layer of reticular fibers produced by Schwann cells. Although blood vessels are present in all three areas — epineurium, perineurium, and endoneurium — disorders that lead to peripheral nerve damage, such as vasculitis, most frequently involve the epineurial arterioles.

Peripheral nerves are divided according to their function into motor, sensory, and autonomic nervous system fibers. Motor nerve fibers are the axons of lower motor neurons, i.e., of spinal anterior horn cells and motor nerve cells of cranial nerves, that innervate extrafusal and intrafusal striated muscle fibers. The sensory nerves are one of the axons of pseudounipolar sensory neurons in dorsal root or cranial nerve ganglia. Preganglionic sympathetic autonomic nerve cell bodies reside in the intermediolateral gray columns of spinal cord segments T1–L2 (thoracolumbar). Their nerve fibers emerge with ventral roots, enter the sympathetic chain as myelinated white rami, and synapse with sympathetic ganglion cells. These cells give rise to unmyelinated axons, which emerge through gray rami and innervate effector organs such as sweat glands, the smooth muscle of blood vessels, and hair follicles. Preganglionic parasympathetic nerve cell bodies are located in the brainstem (cranial nerves III, VII, IX, and X) and in the S2–S4 segments of the spinal cord (craniosacral). Nerve fibers that release acetylcholine are called cholinergic fibers and include all the preganglionic autonomic fibers and postganglionic parasympathetic fibers that innervate smooth muscle, heart, and exocrine glands.

Sensory fibers may be classified by their size and resultant conduction velocity into A-alpha (30–72 m/s), A-delta (6–36 m/s), and C (0.5–2 m/s) fibers; the former two are myelinated and the latter is unmyelinated. Most peripheral nerves are mixtures of myelinated and unmyelinated fibers. Position and vibration sense are transmitted by large myelinated fibers; touch, by medium-sized myelinated fibers; and pain and temperature, by thinly myelinated (A-delta) or small unmyelinated (C) fibers.

Pathogenic Mechanisms in Peripheral Nerve Diseases

When the primary pathologic process resides in the cell body (neuron), it is called neuronopathy. In motor neuronopathy, the anterior horn cell is affected, and in sensory neuronopathy, the sensory ganglion cell is affected. Pure motor neuronopathies result in weakness and muscle wasting. The most well-known motor neuronopathy is amyotrophic lateral sclerosis (ALS). Sensory neuronopathies usually are

associated with pan-modality sensory losses (large- and small-fiber function) and can be caused by paraneoplastic disorders and Sjögren's syndrome, among others. Impaired neuronal synthesis or axoplasmic transport then causes degeneration of distal axons.

When the primary pathologic process resides in the axon, it is called axonopathy. Most axonopathies start distally, in the longest fibers, with the pathologic process proceeding proximally. This progression results in distal axonal degeneration or "dying back axonopathy," with motor, sensory, and reflex changes greatest in the distal extremities. This is the most common mechanism of neuropathy and may result from literally hundreds of causes. The most common causes are diabetes and such toxins as drugs or alcohol (4).

When the primary pathologic process resides in the Schwann cell or myelin, it is called myelinopathy, or a demyelinating neuropathy. Because of the profound effect on conduction parameters electrophysiologically, demyelinating neuropathy is distinctive and readily recognized by nerve conduction testing. There are two classic forms of demyelinating neuropathy: genetic conditions such as the Charcot-Marie-Tooth diseases, and acquired conditions such as chronic inflammatory demyelinating polyneuropathy (4).

Direct nerve injury results in a range of pathologies depending on the degree of injury to the Schwann cells/myelin sheaths, axons, and supporting elements. Wallerian degeneration describes the process that occurs in the nerve fiber and cell body as a result of anatomic axonal interruption. Distal to the injured site, both the axon and myelin sheath degenerate and their remnants, excluding their connective tissue and perineurial sheaths, are removed by macrophages. The axons just proximal to the injury site also degenerate, but only a short distance. With the degenerative changes, Schwann cells proliferate, giving rise to solid cellular columns that serve as guides to the sprouting axons. Only fibers that find their way in these Schwann-cell columns can be reconnected to the correct target and remyelinated. Axonal interruption induces a series of changes within the cell body called chromatolysis, in which dissolution of Nissl substances leads to a decrease in cytoplasmic basophilia, eccentric positioning of the nucleus, and swelling of the cell body.

Clinical Findings in Peripheral Neuropathies

People with peripheral nerve diseases develop symptoms and signs that depend on the type of nerve fiber involved. With sensory fiber involvement, numbness, paresthesia, pain, dysesthesia, ataxia, and tremor may result. Signs include sensory loss and decreased tendon reflexes. With motor fiber involvement, fasciculations, cramps, and weakness may occur. When autonomic fibers are involved, there may be disturbances in sexual function and bowel or bladder control.

Clinically, peripheral nerve disorders may be categorized into mononeuropathy, multiple mononeuropathy, or polyneuropathy, based on the pattern of involvement. Mononeuropathy, in which a single nerve is involved, usually results from trauma, mechanical compression, or unknown cause. The most well-known mononeuropathy is carpal tunnel syndrome (median neuropathy) at the wrist.

Multiple mononeuropathy is diagnosed when the clinical picture involves multiple individual nerves. A small number of disorders cause the majority of these cases, with vascular etiologies highest on the differential diagnosis. The list includes many forms of vasculitis, sarcoidosis, meningeal carcinomatosis, lymphomatosis, leprosy, hereditary neuropathy with liability to pressure palsies (HNPP), and human immunodeficiency virus infection (5).

Polyneuropathies are diffuse disorders that are most commonly symmetric and involve the distal nerves greater than the proximal (i.e., feet and distal legs before hands). Polyneuropathies may be hereditary or acquired due to metabolic, toxic, infectious, nutritional, and idiopathic causes.

These three categories of neuropathy may be further subclassified by their course (acute, subacute, and chronic), specific type of fiber involved, and electrodiagnostic features. Such subclassification helps narrow the differential diagnosis of peripheral nerve disorders and focuses subsequent evaluations.

Electromyography and Diagnosing Peripheral Nerve Disease

The term electomyography (EMG) includes both nerve conduction studies and needle EMG. Nerve conduction studies provide objective and quantifiable measures of peripheral nerve function including the presence of neuropathy, distribution of nerve involvement, and differentiation between myelinopathy and axonopathy (6). Important parameters in the nerve conduction study are: 1) distal latency; 2) conduction velocity; and 3) evoked response amplitude and duration at each stimulation site. In addition, assessment of proximal portions of peripheral nerves is routinely performed using late responses such as F-wave and H-reflex.

Nerve conduction velocity of motor and sensory fibers is a function of axonal diameter and the degree of myelination. Therefore, reduced conduction velocity can occur by either axonal atrophy or demyelination, but the most striking abnormalities of conduction occur with the latter. Sensory studies are useful in localizing peripheral nerve lesions as either proximal or distal to the dorsal-root ganglia, because standard sensory responses are unaffected by lesions proximal to the dorsal-root ganglia despite the presence of clinical sensory loss.

The main purposes of needle EMG are to differentiate neurogenic processes from myopathic disorders, to separate active denervation from chronic, to categorize myopathies as irritable or nonirritable, and to detect the presence of abnormal discharges.

Routine nerve conduction studies evaluate the function of large myelinated nerve fibers (motor and sensory). Several methods are available to assess small myelinated

and unmyelinated nerve fibers. Quantitative sensory testing is a psychophysiologic test developed to evaluate functions such as heat and cooling thresholds and heat-pain sensation. Quantitation of intraepidermal nerve fiber density by skin punch biopsy is an easy way to assess small fiber pathology objectively.

In practice, differentiating demyelinating and axonal neuropathy is very important. Many of the acquired demyelinating neuropathies are highly treatable if detected early. Myelin injuries can be induced by various causes. Myelin has proteins and lipids that may become immunogenic, and some of the immune-mediated neuropathies are characterized by the binding of circulating antibodies to specialized regions at the nodes of Ranvier, which may lead to damage of adjacent axons. A complement-mediated humoral immune response against the myelin sheath itself also has been delineated. Toxic agents that damage the Schwann cells or their membranes selectively can cause demyelination of peripheral nerves while leaving axons relatively intact.

Demyelination increases membrane capacitance and decreases membrane resistance, which results in current leakage between nodes of Ranvier. If the current becomes low enough, the next node will not depolarize, and conduction will fail (conduction block) in that axon. A few layers of myelin (remyelination) may transform an axon from one with conduction block into one with conduction, albeit with reduced velocity, hence restoring muscle strength. However, when this occurs in sensory fibers that are crucial for tendon reflexes and vibration sense, the asynchronous conduction of nerve volleys may impair these functions, which require synchronous nerve volleys. Patchy demyelination or inhomogenous myelin injury reduces conduction velocity of individual nerve fibers to different extents, resulting in abnormal temporal dispersion. This condition can be detected by examining the actual response waveforms between stimulating sites. At times, these changes may be severe enough to mimic conduction block.

Thus, the primary features of demyelinating neuropathy involve conduction parameters and include prolonged distal, F-wave and H-reflex latencies; reduced conduction velocities; partial motor-conduction block; and abnormal temporal dispersion.

In contrast, axonopathies usually result in loss of nerve fibers with little in the way of conduction abnormalities. Thus, the evoked response amplitudes are reduced, with normal or near-normal distal, F-wave, and H-reflex latencies, and relatively little change in the shape and duration of evoked responses.

In demyelinating neuropathy, rapid recovery of function may result from remyelination that is sufficient to restore conduction. By contrast, in distal axonal degeneration, recovery is slower, often requiring months to years because the axon must first regenerate (1 mm/day) and then reconnect to the target organ.

KEE DUK PARK, MD
DAVID R. CORNBLATH, MD

References

1. Kandel ER, Schwartz JH (eds). *Principles of Neural Science, 2nd edition.* New York: Elsevier, 1985.

2. Junqueira LG, Carneiro J, Kelly RO. *Basic Histology, 9th ed.* Stamford, CT: Appleton & Lange, 1998.

3. Matthews GG. *Cellular Physiology of Nerve and Muscle, 3rd edition.* Malden, MA: Blackwell Science, 1998.

4. Cornblath DR. *The electrophysiology of axonal and demyelinating polyneuropathies. Baillieres Clin Neurol* 1996;5: 107–113.

5. Kim RC, Collins GH. *The neuropathology of rheumatic disease. Hum Pathol* 1981;12:5–15.

6. Mendell JR, Kissel JT, Cornblath DR (eds). *Diagnosis and Management of Peripheral Nerve Disorders.* New York: Oxford University Press, in press.

3 STRUCTURE
A. Collagen and Elastin

Collagen, the major structural protein of the fibrillar component of the extracellular matrix, is the most abundant protein in the body. Defects in the structure of collagen and autoimmunity to collagen have been implicated in many rheumatic diseases, including rheumatoid arthritis, osteoarthritis, scleroderma, spondyloepiphyseal dysplasia, osteogenesis imperfecta, Ehlers-Danlos syndrome, and others. An understanding of the structure and organization of collagen molecules is essential for elucidating the pathophysiology of major rheumatic diseases.

Collagens play a dominant role in maintaining the structural integrity of tissues. Fibrillar collagens, with contributions from elastin and proteoglycans, confer most of the mechanical properties of such diverse connective tissues as tendons, ligaments, cartilage, cornea, and bone. Collagens also are involved in such biologic processes as development, organogenesis, cell attachment, chemotaxis, platelet aggregation, and filtration. By convention, the collagens are defined as extracellular proteins that have a triple-helix conformation in at least a substantial portion of their structure. A unique feature of the biogenesis of collagens is their extensive posttranslational modifications, which are necessary for stabilization of the collagen molecule and maturation of fibrils via lysine-derived covalent cross-links (Table 3A-1).

Structure of Fibrillar Collagens

The fibril-forming collagens, types I, II, III, V, and XI, were the first collagens to be isolated and characterized. They have a highly asymmetric, flexible, rod-like structure, with a diameter of 1.5 nm and a length of 300 nm. Each molecule is composed of three polypeptide chains, called α chains, characterized by a repeating $[Gly-X-Y]_n$ structure, where X and Y residues can be any amino acid, but most commonly are proline and hydroxyproline, respectively. These imino acids constitute 20%–25% of the total amino acid content in most mammalian collagens. The α carbon of the imino acids, unlike other amino acids, is tied up in a ring structure and is not free to rotate. This stereochemical configuration of the imino acids necessitates each α chain to assume a left-handed helical conformation (i.e., minor helix), with a residue repeat distance of 0.291 nm and a relative twist of 110°, a configuration that provides 3.27 residues per turn of the helix and 0.87 nm distance between glycine residues. The positioning of glycine at every third residue is critical; because glycine lacks a bulky side chain, it can occupy the center position along the common axis of the triple helix. As a result, genetic mutations replacing glycine with any other

amino acid are not tolerated because of the space restriction. Interchain hydrogen bonds involving the hydroxyl groups of hydroxyproline stabilize the triple-helix structure.

Under physiologic ionic strength, pH, and temperature, these collagen molecules are not soluble, and they spontaneously aggregate into striated fibrils of the type seen in tissues. The fibril formation occurs by parallel aggregation of the collagen molecules, in which each neighboring row of molecules is displaced along the long axis of the molecule by a distance of 68 nm. Within the same row, there is a gap, or "hole," of approximately 40 nm between the end of one molecule and the beginning of the next. Each triple-helical domain is completely resistant to degradation by nonspecific proteinases.

Classification of Collagens

After fibril-forming collagens were isolated and characterized by the classic techniques of protein chemistry, application of molecular biologic approaches led to the discovery of several additional types of collagen and collagen-like proteins. To date, 19 collagen types have been identified, representing the products of at least 30 genes. It generally is accepted that a protein should be a component of extracellular matrix before it can be classified as a collagen. Thus, certain nonmatrix proteins that contain collagenous domains, such as acetyl cholinesterase and the complement component C1q, have not been classified as collagens, despite having collagen-like domains. Evidence suggests that some of the more recently identified collagens (e.g., type XIII and XVII) may be cell-membrane components, but the question remains whether they should be considered collagens. Because of the complexity of collagens, they have been classified into six different groups (Table 3A-2) based on the characteristics of the polymeric structures they form or the structural features of the collagens themselves.

Fibrillar Collagens

Fibrillar collagens (types I, II, III, V, and XI) are grouped together because they have a tendency to aggregate into characteristic striated fibrils. These collagens are of particular interest to rheumatologists because they are involved prominently in connective-tissue diseases. Defects in type I collagen are associated with osteogenesis imperfecta, which is characterized by brittle bones or skeletal deformities, thin blue sclerae, and abnormal tooth development. Recent data indicates that most people with scleroderma have T-cell sensitivity to type I and/or type III collagens. Type II collagen is

TABLE 3A-1
Collagens

Collagen type	Collagen group	Gene	Chromosome	Tissue
I	Fibrillar	COL 1A1	17q21.3-p22	Bone, cornea, dentin, tendon
		COL 1A2	7q21.3-q22	Dermis, gingiva, heart valve, intestine, large vessel, fibrocartilage
II	Fibrillar	COL 2A1	12q13-q14	Articular cartilage, vitreous humor, fibrocartilage
III	Fibrillar	COL 3A1	2q24.3-q31	Dermis, lung, blood vessels, intestine, uterine wall
IV	Network-forming	COL 4A1	13q34	Endothelial and epithelial basement membranes
		COL 4A2	13q34	
		COL 4A3	2q35-q37	
		COL 4A4	2q35-q37	
		COL 4A5	Xq22	
		COL 4A6	Xq22	
V	Fibrillar	COL 5A1	9q34.2-q34.3	Cornea, placental membrane, large vessel wall, bone, gingiva, heart valves, hyaline cartilage
		COL 5A2	2q34.3-q31	
		COL 5A3		
VI	Bead-forming	COL 6A1	21q22.3	Placenta, aorta, neurofibroma, dermis, nucleus pulposus
		COL 6A2	21q22.3	
		COL 6A3	2q37	
VII	Anchoring-fibril-forming	COL 7A1	3p21	Dermal-epidermal junction, amnionic epithelium
VIII	Network-forming	COL 8A1	3q12-q13.1	Endothelial cell product, Descemet's membrane
		COL 8A2	1p32.3-p34.3	
IX	FACIT	COL 9A1	6q12-q14	Articular cartilage, vitreous humor
		COL 9A2	1p32	
		COL 9A3		
X	Network-forming	COL 10A1	6q21-q22	Hypertrophic cartilage

Collagen type	Collagen group	Gene	Chromosome	Tissue
XI	Fibrillar	COL 11A1 COL 11A2 COL 2A1	1p21 6p21.2 12q13-q14	Articular cartilage, vitreous humor
XII	FACIT	COL 12A1	6	Tendon, skin, peridontal ligament
XIII	Transmembrane	COL 13A1	10q22	Product of fibro-blasts, tendon
XIV	FACIT	COL 14A1		Tendon, skin
XV	Noncollagen collagen	COL 15A1	q21-22	Ubiquitous connective tissues
XVI	FACIT	COL 16A1	1q34-35	Fibroblasts, keratinocytes
XVII	Transmembrane	COL 17A1	10q24.3	Skin, hemidesmosomes
XVIII	Noncollagen collagen	COL 18A1	21q22.3	Many tissues, including liver, kidney, and placenta
XIX	FACIT	COL 19A1	6q12-q14	Rhabdomyosarcoma cells

the major fibrillar collagen of articular cartilage and the vitreous of the eye. Defects in type II collagen result in chondrodysplasias and premature osteoarthritis. Autoimmunity to type II and/or type XI collagen is thought to play a role in rheumatoid arthritis, juvenile rheumatoid arthritis, and polychondritis. Ehlers-Danlos syndrome type IV, which is characterized by loose joints and rupture of bowel and major blood vessels, is associated with mutations that result in abnormal processing of procollagen type III.

The fibrillar collagens are composed of a chains of approximately 95 kDa each and a continuous, uninterrupted triple-helical domain of approximately 300 nm (Fig. 3A-1). These collagen a chains have the repeating $[Gly-X-Y]_n$ structure: 338 triplets (or 1,014 amino-acid residues) in type I chains, and 341 triplets (or 1,023 amino-acid residues) in type III chains. At the NH_2 and COOH termini of each α chain are short, nonhelical sequences of 15–20 residues, referred to as telopeptides. Type I and type III collagens quantitatively are the major collagens in structures requiring great mechanical strength (e.g., bone, tendon, ligament, dermis, and blood vessels), and together they form the striated fibrils. Type I collagen classically is found in a heterotrimeric form, $[\alpha 1(I)_2 \alpha 2(I)]$, although homotrimers of the α1(I) chain have been described. Type II collagen is enriched in hydroxylysine, and is more highly glycosylated than type I collagen. Type III collagen is a homotrimer, $[\alpha 1(III)]_3$, and is found in most tissues along with type I collagen. Type III collagen is characterized by interchain disulfide bonds within the helical domain. Located in most of the same tissues as type I collagen, type V collagen consists of two different a chains, α1(V) and α2(V), and is found

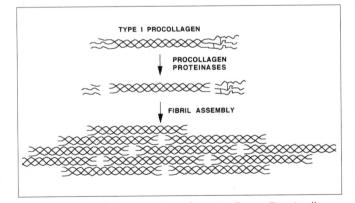

Fig. 3A-1. Extracellular processing of type I collagen. Type I collagen is secreted from the cell with amino- and carboxy-terminal extensions or propeptides. Specific peptidases cleave the propeptides resulting in a marked reduction in solubility. The central, helical region retains short, nonhelical sequences and assembles in a near-quarter stagger fashion into fibrils. The other fibrillar collagens are processed similarly.

TABLE 3A-2
Post-Transcriptional Events and Post-Translational Modification of Collagen

Events	Enzymes and cofactors
Intracellular events	
Proline hydroxylation	Prolyl hydroxlase, ascorbate, iron, α-ketoglutarate
Lysine hydroxylation	Lysyl hydroxylase
Glycosylation of hydroxylysines	Glactosyl transferase and glycosyl transferase
C-terminal disulfide bridge formation and helical assembly	
Secretion	
Extracellular events	
Cleavage of N- and C-termini	Procollagen N-peptidase and C-peptidase
Cross-link formation	Lysyl oxidase, copper
Fibrillogenesis	

either as a heterotrimer of the two a chains or as homotrimers of either chain. Type XI collagen is found in articular cartilage and the ocular vitreous (associated with type II collagen) and consists of heterotrimers of three different chains, α1(XI), α2(XI), and α3(XI). The sequences of the type XI collagen chains strongly resemble those of type V collagen and may play a similar role as type V in influencing fibril size.

FACIT Collagens
Fibril-associated collagens with interrupted triple-helix (FACIT) collagens (i.e., types IX, XII, XIV, XVI, and XIX) contain triple-helical domains with disruptions in the Gly-X-Y sequence, producing interrupted triple helices that vary in number and size. Although FACIT collagens do not form fibrils independently, they are associated with the major fibrils composed of types I, II, and III collagen. Type IX collagen has been studied more extensively than other FACIT collagens, and its importance to rheumatologists is underscored by its location in articular cartilage in association with the striated type II collagen (Fig. 3A-2). Antibodies to type IX collagen have been described in the sera of people with rheumatoid arthritis, suggesting that type IX plays a role in the pathophysiology of the disease. Type IX collagen is a heterotrimer composed of three different chains: α1(IX), α2(IX), and α3(IX). It contains a large noncollagenous (NC) domain at the NH$_2$-terminus of α1(IX), and is further characterized by two short NC segments that interrupt the helix. One of these short NC segments creates a kink in the molecule that is the site of the glycosaminoglycan chain extending from α2(IX). Two collagenous domains associate with the striated fibrils of type II collagen, while the third collagenous domain extends into the interfibrillar space. A large, positively charged NH$_2$-terminal noncollagenous domain (NC4) is presumed to interact with other matrix components. Type XII and type XIV collagens have nearly identical amino-acid sequences, and are associated with type I collagen fibrils in the same way that type IX collagen is associated with type II. These three FACIT collagens are unique in that they all contain a single chondroitin sulfate polysaccharide chain.

Network-Forming Collagens
Types IV, VIII, and X collagens are called network-forming collagens because of their tendency to form three-dimensional networks in tissues (Fig. 3A-3). Type IV collagen, found exclusively in basement membranes, is the best characterized of the group and is of interest to rheumatologists because it contains the putative antigen of Goodpasture's syndrome. In this disease, antibodies to type IV collagen, specifically the NC1 domain of the α3(IV) chain, bind to the glomerular and alveolar basement membranes, causing local immune complexes and autoimmune disease. Alport's syndrome, characterized by hereditary nephritis and deafness, also is associated with abnormalities of type IV collagen and with mutations in the α5(IV) collagen gene.

The foundation for basement membranes is a delicate network formed by the assembly of type IV collagen molecules. Three molecular forms have been identified, the most abundant being the heterotrimer α1(IV)$_2$α2(IV), which is present in all basement membranes. The molecules have a long collagenous domain (400 nm), with multiple interruptions in the triple helix, and they are assembled in a three-dimensional, lattice-like network, with a head-to-head and tail-to-tail arrangement that is created by lysine- and cysteine-derived cross-linkages (Fig. 3A-3). Four amino-terminal domains associate into the proteinase-resistant 7s domain, and the four extending, carboxy-terminal, large noncollagenous (NC1) domains associate tail-to-tail with other type IV collagen tetrads. Side-to-side association of collagen molecules provides a three-dimensional network, which is believed to be important in the filtration function of basement membranes.

Type VIII collagen is a network collagen found in the sheet-like structures of Descemet's membrane. This membrane separates the corneal epithelial cells from the corneal stoma and consists of stacks of collagen lattices. Structurally, type VIII collagen molecules contain a small triple-helical domain and two small globular domains. The other network collagen, type X collagen, is a short-chain homotrimer found in calcifying hypertrophic cartilage and is thought to play a role in endochondral ossification. Type X collagen also is found in osteoarthritic cartilage, specifically at sites of osteophyte formation and surface fibrillation, and around clonal clusters of proliferative cells. It has been speculated that type X collagen weakens osteoarthritic cartilage by altering matrix-molecule interactions.

Anchoring-Fibril-Forming Collagen

Collagen type VII forms anchoring fibrils that stabilize the attachment of basement membranes to the underlying connective tissues. Mutations in the $\alpha1(VII)$ gene result in dystrophic forms of hereditary epidermolysis bullosa. Autoantibodies to type VII collagen can react with anchoring fibrils and produce skin lesions (epidermolysis bullosa

acquisita) in systemic lupus erythematosus. Type VII collagen is distinguished by its extraordinary length, nearly 467 nm, in which all but a very small portion is triple-helical. The molecule extends from the basement membrane to the papillary dermis. It contains a complex, trident-like, carboxy-terminal NC domain with fibrils formed by antiparallel dimerization. The two amino-terminal NC domains associate and are stabilized by cross-link formation.

Other Collagens

Other collagens include the bead-forming collagen type VI, which is widely distributed in cartilage, skin, blood vessels, and other interstitial tissues. Immunolocalization of type VI collagen has identified it as a component of microfibrils in cultured cells. The globular domains of type VI collagen chains, which flank the 336-residue, triple-helical regions, are quite large. Type VI monomers contain three distinct α chains: $\alpha1(VI)$, $\alpha2(VI)$, and $\alpha3(VI)$, with molecular weights of 150, 140, and 300 kDa, respectively. Each chain has regions similar to the type A repeats found in von Willebrand factor. The $\alpha3(VI)$ collagen chain is much longer because it contains 11 repeats of this type A domain. It also has a 73-residue segment analogous to the platelet glycoprotein Ib. This region in the COOH-terminus also is flanked by a type III

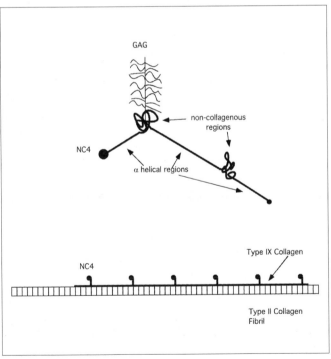

Fig. 3A-2. Type IX collagen and its relation to type II collagen fibrils. The molecular structure of type IX collagen is displayed, showing its characteristic "kink" near the carboxy terminus, a large, C-terminal noncollagenous domain, and a proteoglycan component of the $\alpha2(IX)$ chain at the kink region. This collagen associates with type II collagen fibrils, with the NC4 domain exposed on the fibril surface. Other FACIT collagens (fibril-associated collagens with interrupted triple helix) probably interact with other fibrils in a similar manner.

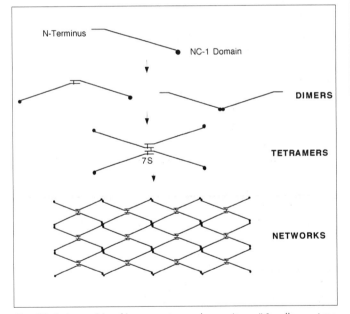

Fig. 3A-3. Assembly of basement membrane (type IV) collagen into networks. The native type IV collagen molecule has multiple interruptions and imperfections in the helical sequences, resulting in flexible regions. Assembly of type IV collagen is by dimerization through "tail-to-tail" interaction between two C-terminal noncollagenous domains (NC-1) and by tetramer-formation through N-terminal interactions. Cross-link formation in the N-terminal region results in a proteinase-resistant region known as 7s collagen. Networks resembling chicken wire then form in a two-dimensional orientation. Side-to-side interactions between molecules and networks result in a three-dimensional network.

repeat of fibronectin and a Kunitz-type proteinase inhibitor. The type III domain suggests a role for type VI collagen in cell adhesion and type I collagen binding.

Transmembrane collagens (i.e., types XIII and XVII) are characterized by a prominent transmembrane domain. Type XIII collagen occurs in many tissues, in varying amounts, depending on the developmental state and specific tissue. The protein of hemidesmosomes, previously referred to as the 180-kDa bullous pemphigoid antigen, now is known to be type XVII collagen.

The remaining collagens (i.e., types XV and XVIII) have not been well-characterized in terms of structure or function and belatedly were found to have short triple-helical collagenous domains. The distribution of type XV and type XVIII varies markedly between tissues. For instance, liver contains type XVIII collagen but no type XV, whereas skin has both.

Collagen Biosynthesis, Post-Translational Modifications, and Processing

Collagen biosynthesis and incorporation into the extracellular matrix occurs via a complex series of intracellular and extracellular events. Certain processes, such as prolyl hydroxylation, are involved in the biosynthesis of all collagens, whereas procollagen processing and cross-link formation are specific to the assembly of fibrillar collagens.

The transcription and translation of collagen mRNA proceeds in a manner similar to the expression of other genes. The precursor collagen chains are synthesized on polyribosomes as prepro-α chains. The hydrophobic leader sequence is removed from the prepro-α chains prior to secretion, and the procollagen molecules, consisting of pro-α chains, are secreted into the extracellular space. The nascent pro-α chains of the major fibrillar collagens are approximately 150,000 kDa, considerably longer than the a chains found in mature collagen fibrils (95,000 kDa). These chains contain NH_2- and COOH-propeptides that largely are nonhelical. Disulfide bonds form between the COOH-terminal nonhelical propeptides of the a chains, which facilitate their folding into a triple helix.

Hydroxylation of proline, which is carried out by prolyl hydroxylase and cofactors, including ascorbate, iron, and α-ketoglutarate, is essential for the stability of the triple helix. Underhydroxylated α chains form unstable helices that denature at the body temperature of 37°C. Prolyl hydroxylase catalyzes the hydroxylation of approximately one-half of the prolyl residues, predominantly at the Y positions, and the molecule folds in its wake. Like proline, several lysine residues are hydroxylated; this process results from the action of lysyl hydroxylase.

Certain hydroxylysines then are glycosylated. The enzyme UDP-galactose:hydroxylysine galactosyltransferase adds a galactose residue to the hydroxyl group of specific hydroxylysine residues. The UDP-glucose:galactosehydrox-

ylysine glucosyltransferase then transfers a glucose residue to some of the hydroxylysine-linked galactose residues. Sequential glycosylation occurs during nascent-chain synthesis and before the formation of triple helices, because the triple-helical collagen cannot act as a substrate for glycosylating enzymes. Glycosylation of specific hydroxylysine that later becomes involved in collagen cross-linking imparts greater stability to the cross-link. These procollagen molecules are transported to the extracellular space, where specific procollagen peptidases cleave the NH_2- and COOH-terminal propeptides to form the native collagen molecule. These proteolytic steps result in a reduction in the solubility of collagen, and the collagen molecules spontaneously assemble into fibrils in a near-quarter stagger fashion.

Once the collagen molecules are assembled into striated fibrils, the fibrils are stabilized by the formation of covalent intermolecular cross-links. Lysyl and hydroxylysyl oxidase catalyze the oxidative deamination of specific lysine or hydroxylysine residues in the NH_2- or COOH-terminal telopeptides to yield aldehyde-containing derivatives, allysine or hydroxyallysine, respectively. Once these reactive aldehydes are formed, they react with the ε-amino group of lysine or hydroxylysine residues on adjacent chains to form cross-links that link collagen chains by covalent bonds. The formation of covalent bonds between the collagen molecules gives the fibrils a much greater tensile strength. Failure to form intermolecular cross-links results in marked fragility of connective tissues.

The metabolic turnover of fibrillar collagen, as measured in a whole animal or in a tissue, is extremely low; the half-life is measured in years. However, in specific physiologic and pathologic situations, such as tissue remodeling and inflammation, a very rapid breakdown and synthesis of collagen must take place. Fibrillar collagens are resistant to the action of general proteases, although they are readily degraded by a wide variety of proteases after the molecules are denatured or the helical structures are disrupted.

Physiologic breakdown of the fibrillar collagens is accomplished by the action of very specific collagenases. Typically, these enzymes cleave the native molecule at a single position within the triple helix (between residues 775 and 776), resulting in a bisection of each a chain into two fragments representing approximately 75% and 25%, respectively, of the intact molecule. The resulting products are unstable and denature spontaneously at body temperature and pH, and the unraveled polypeptides become susceptible to the action of gelatinases and other proteases and are degraded further.

Collagenases are known to be metalloenzymes and belong to a family known as the matrix metalloproteinases. The family consists of at least 28 distinct enzymes, each capable of degrading one or more components of the extracellular matrix. Many of these enzymes are synthesized and secreted as enzymatically inactive proenzymes, which can be converted to active enzymes by proteolytic cleavage of the proenzyme domain. Other family members, the membrane type of matrix metalloproteinases (MT-MMP), function as integral membrane proteins and are activated intra-cellularly. The synthesis of MMPs is induced by many inflammatory cytokines that regulate transcriptional and post-transcriptional mechanisms. Once synthesized, the proteins are secreted constitutively and their extracellular activity is regulated by their activation and by a family of protein inhibitors, referred to as tissue inhibitors of metal-loproteinase (TIMP). Currently there are four distinct TIMP family members (TIMP 1–4). The balance between collagenase and TIMP undoubtedly plays a crucial role in the regulation of collagenolysis.

Regulation of Collagen-Gene Expression

The collagen composition of different tissues in the body reflects the sum of highly coordinated pathways of synthe-sis and degradation elicited in their unique physiologic and pathologic milieus. Expression of various collagen genes is coordinated precisely in the developing embryo, and their aberrant regulation leads to serious disorders, including osteogenesis imperfecta and osteoarthritis. In the adult, col-lagen-gene expression is subject to positive regulation [e.g., transforming growth factor β (TGF-β) and connective-tissue growth factor] as well as negative regulation [e.g., tumor necrosis factor α (TNF-α) and interferon γ] by many cytokines and growth factors elaborated at the sites of postinflammatory tissue repair and regeneration.

Regulation of transcription is the paramount mechanism of collagen-gene expression. However post-transcriptional control of collagen biosynthesis may play a significant role under some conditions. For instance, TGF-β1 can enhance type I collagen-gene expression dramatically by concomi-tantly increasing the rate of transcription and stability of COL1A1 collagen mRNAs. Conversely, interferon γ treat-ment may reduce the stability and translation rate of COL1A1 collagen mRNA. Regulation of collagen biosyn-thesis also may occur during the post-translational modifi-cation and processing steps that precede formation of triple helices by collagen α chains. In fact, feedback mechanisms capable of modulating type I collagen biosynthesis by amino- and carboxy-terminal propeptides have been demonstrated.

The molecular organization and regulation of genes encod-ing α chains of type I collagen may be considered prototypic because these processes have been investigated most exten-sively. The regulatory sequences that potentially dictate the constitutive, tissue-specific, or inducible expression of colla-gen genes are found on both sides of the transcription start site. These sequences may be located in close proximity of the transcription start site or many kilobases (kb) upstream or downstream from it. The promoters of all known COL1A1 and COL1A2 collagen genes contain TATA and CCAAT boxes located at 25–30 and 75–80 bp upstream of the tran-scription start site, respectively. Integrity of TATA and CCAAT boxes is essential for promoter function.

The regulatory motifs located far from the transcription start site are exemplified by an enhancer-like element found between 15 and 17 kb upstream and the 3'-flanking sequences of the COL1A2 and COL1A1 genes of mice, respectively. The first intron of the human COL1A1 gene also contains important regulatory elements.

The regulatory elements of the COL1A1 promoter/ enhancer appear to have a modular organization. The minimal promoter contains two GC-rich motifs capable of binding to Sp1, which appears to be an obligatory tran-scription factor. Other members of the Sp1 family may be involved in the regulation of type I collagen genes. An Sp1-binding motif has been implicated in the enhanced activity of COl1A1 promoter in response to TGF-β1. Reduced bone density and osteoporosis in a subset of humans is associated with a polymorphic Sp1 binding site in the COl1A1 gene.

Elastin and Elastic Fibers

Elastic fibers provide resiliency and elasticity to certain tis-sues, such as large blood vessels, lung, skin, and certain specialized connective tissues of the ocular zonule. There are two components to the elastic fibers: an amorphous element composed mainly of the protein tropoelastin, and

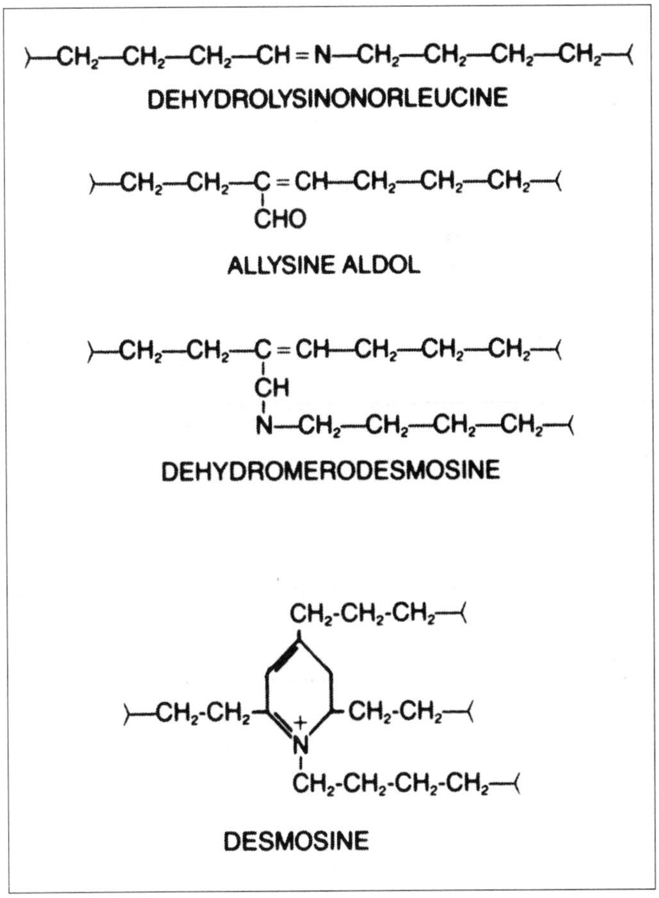

Fig. 3A-4. The structures of cross-links found in elastin. The desmo-sine and isodesmosine represent final products of the lysine-derived cross-links.

a microfibrillar element composed of fibrillin and other proteins. The 360-kDa glycoprotein known as fibrillin, of which there are two known forms, is of interest to rheumatologists. Marfan's syndrome has been associated with mutations in fibrillin 1. Marfan's syndrome includes abnormalities of tissues rich in elastic fibrils, such as ligaments (loose-jointedness), large blood vessels (aortic aneurysms), and ocular zonule (lens subluxation). A gene encoding fibrillin has been linked to congenital contractual arachnodactyly.

Tropoelastin is a single polypeptide with a molecular weight of 72,000 kDa and a unique amino-acid composition. The protein consists of hydrophobic domains composed primarily of glycine, valine, proline, and alanine, alternating with hydrophilic regions rich in lysine residues. The gene encoding for elastin has the hydrophilic domains and hydrophobic regions encoded by different exons.

The lysyl residues of elastin are oxidized enzymatically through the action of lysyl oxidase, a copper-dependent enzyme. These residues form interchain and intrachain cross-links, including desmosine and isodesmosine (Fig. 3A-4). The resulting network of elastic fibers in tissue is resistant to extraction, boiling, and proteolysis by nonspecific proteinases. Specific elastases are required for enzymatic degradation of elastin.

The human gene encoding the elastin protein consists of 34 exons. Alternative splicing appears to occur commonly with transcription, resulting in a variety of species of elastin with unknown roles. The expression of the elastin gene is up-regulated by TGF-β and down-regulated by TNF-α and vitamin D_3.

LINDA MYERS, MD

References

1. Bornstein P. Regulation of expression of the alpha 1 (I) collagen gene: a critical appraisal of the role of the first intron. Matrix Biol 1996;15:3–10.
2. Wang Q, Raghow R. Molecular mechanisms of regulation of type I collagen biosynthesis. Proc Indian Acad Sci (Chem Sci) 1999;111:185–195.
3. Seyer JM, Kang AH. Connective tissues of the subendothelium. In: Loscalzo, Creager, and Dzau (eds). Vascular Medicine. Boston: Little, Brown & Co, 1996; pp 39–67.
4. Goldsmith L (ed). Elastin in Biochemistry and Physiology of Skin, 2nd ed. New York: Oxford University Press, 1991.
5. Perrin S, Foster JA. Developmental regulation of elastin gene expression. Crit Rev Eukaryot Gene Expr 1997;7:1–10.

STRUCTURE
B. Proteoglycans

The proteoglycans are a diverse group of uniquely glycosylated proteins that are ubiquitous in the body and most abundant in the extracellular matrix of connective tissues. Like glycoproteins, proteoglycans often contain both N-linked and O-linked oligosaccharides. However, the addition of one or more sulfated glycosaminoglycan side chains to the protein core distinguishes this group of complex glycoconjugates as proteoglycans. Glycosaminoglycans are linear, anionic polysaccharides with repeating disaccharide units containing a hexosamine residue and usually, but not always, a hexuronic acid residue. Proteoglycans display a broad diversity of structures and sizes well-correlated with their vast array of functions within tissues. One functional property common to all proteoglycans is the capacity to provide a high-density source of fixed negative charges within the extracellular matrix. Within some tissues, such as cartilage, proteoglycans are highly concentrated (to about 100 mg/ml) and compressed within the matrix to approximately 20% of their maximum extended volume (1). This compression of negative charge density, entrapped within a collagen network and not freely mobile, provides the osmotic pressure needed to withstand physiologic loads that can reach 100–200 atm within milliseconds after standing (e.g., in articular cartilage of the lower extremities).

Particular functional attributes of proteoglycans may reside in the glycosaminoglycan structure and/or within the core protein. At present there are at least 20 separate genes that code for proteins and have the capacity to carry one or more glycosaminoglycan side chains (Table 3B-1). Once the nucleic acid sequence of a proteoglycan core-protein gene product has been described and documented, the core proteins often are given functional names, such as aggrecan, decorin, or lumican (2). However, it should be noted that any given proteoglycan found within a tissue may be the product of extensive post-transciptional modifications, including alternative splicing, the use of different start sites of a particular core protein mRNA, variations in glycosaminoglycan type and structure, and selective proteolytic processing (3). Thus, for some proteoglycans no simple nomenclature is adequate, and often a combination nomenclature of named core protein plus glycosaminoglycan type or tissue type of origin often is used (e.g., chondroitin sulfate decorin or corneal decorin).

Glycosaminoglycans

The glycosaminoglycan side chains found on a particular core protein commonly are divided into three basic groups: chondroitins, heparins, and keratan sulfates. The chondroitins contain a linear (i.e., nonbranching), repeating, N-acetylgalactosamine–glucuronic acid, disaccharide structure, commonly sulfated at the 4 or 6 position of the hexosamine residue to yield *chondroitin-4-sulfate* (chondroitin sulfate A) or *chondroitin-6-sulfate* (chondroitin sulfate C). Postsynthesis epimerization of glucuronic acid residues of chondroitin-4-sulfate to iduronic acid yields the glycosaminoglycan called *dermatan sulfate* (chondroitin sulfate B). It should be noted that many of the chondroitin glycosaminoglycans exist as composite polymers containing hybrid regions along the polysaccharide chain of nonsulfated, 4-sulfated, 6-sulfated, or iduronic, acid-containing disaccharides (2).

Although known to exist and to be highly regulated by cells, the specific functions of these composite glycosaminoglycan structures are not completely understood. The length of chondroitin glycosaminoglycan chains varies (see Fig. 3B-1), but seldom is more than 200–250 disaccharide units long. Keratan sulfates generally are shorter glycosaminoglycans (20–40 disaccharide units) that contain repeating galactose, N-acetylglucosamine, disaccharide units that primarily contain sulfate residues at the 6 position of the galactose, the N-acetylglucosamine, or both. The ends of keratan-sulfate chains may be capped by sialic acid residues (2). With such structures, it has been suggested that keratan sulfates represent an evolutionary link between glycoproteins and proteo-

TABLE 3B-1
Summary of Proteoglycan Properties

Proteoglycan	Interacts with	Glycosaminoglycan	Predominant tissue localization
Aggrecan	Hyaluronan	CS/KS	Load-bearing tissues (e.g., cartilage, aorta, disk, tendon)
Versican	Hyaluronan	CS	Ubiquitous, fibrous
Decorin	Collagen I and II	CS or DS	Ubiquitous
Biglycan	Collagen VI	CS or DS	Ubiquitous
Fibromodulin	Collagen I and II	KS	Ubiquitous
Collagen IX	Collagen II	CS	Cartilage
Syndecan-1	Cell membranes	HS/CS	Epithelial cells
Syndecan-2 (fibroglycan)	Cell membranes	HS/CS	Ubiquitous
Syndecan-3 (N-syndecan)	Cell membranes	HS/CS	Ubiquitous
Syndecan-4 (ryudocan or amphiglycan)	Cell membranes	HS/CS	Ubiquitous
Glypican	Cell membranes via glycosylphosphatidylinositol	HS	Ubiquitous
Serglycin	–	Heparin	Mast cells
Perlecan	Basement membranes	HS	Basement membranes, cartilage

Other proteoglycans include agrin, bamican, betaglycan, brevican, CD44, epiphycan, keratocan, lumican, neurocan, osteoadherin, osteoglycin, and thrombomodulin.
CS, chondroitin sulfate; DS, dermatan sulfate; KS, keratan sulfate; HS, heparan sulfate.

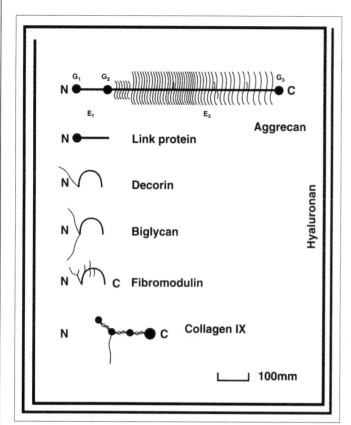

Fig. 3B-1. Structure of some common proteoglycans. Some of the prototypical proteoglycans found in the extracellular matrix of many connective tissues are depicted at approximate scale for each of the molecules at full extension. Note the length of the hyaluronan nearly twice frames the other macromolecules. The structural domains of the aggrecan core protein (G1, G2, G3, E1, and E2) also are depicted. Adapted from an unpublished figure designed by P.J. Roughley.

common tetrasaccharide linkage unit: xylosyl-galactose-galactose-glucuronic acid (2). The linkage region is added to the core protein cotranslationally via interaction of the reducing end of the xylose with the hydroxyl of a serine residue of the core protein. A predominant consensus sequence of serine followed immediately by glycine is required for xylosylation of the core protein. Keratan sulfate has two modes of attachment to core proteins: via a branched hexasaccharide linkage unit O-linked to serine residues or via a branched oligosaccharide linkage unit N-linked to asparagine residues. Keratan sulfate in cartilage generally is attached via O-glycosidic linkages; keratan sulfate of cornea, via N-glycosylamine linkages.

Another member of the family of glycosaminoglycans is the macromolecule *hyaluronan*, or hyaluronic acid (HA). Hyaluronan has a b-linked, repeating, glucuronic acid–N-acetylglucosamine disaccharide structure and thus is similar to the glycosaminoglycans described above. However, HA is not associated with a core protein, is not substituted with sulfate, and exists as a linear, nonbranching polymer about 150 times longer than any other glycosaminoglycan, with molecular mass up to 6×10^6 Da, ~13,700 disaccharide units (Fig. 3B-1). Also, unlike the other glycosaminoglycans, which are synthesized predominately within the Golgi apparatus, HA is synthesized via an HA synthase present within the plasma membrane (4). Thus, it is not surprising that HA is the only glycosaminoglycan synthesized by prokaryotes. Three separate but related mammalian genes have been identified as HA synthases and designated *has*-1, *has*-2 and *has*-3 (4). In some tissues or specific developmental stages, HA functions as an independent glycosaminoglycan. However, in many tissues, HA functions as an integral part or backbone of a tightly bound supramolecular complex, the proteoglycan aggregate.

Proteoglycans That Interact With Hyaluronan

Upon secretion into the extracellular matrix, several proteoglycans self-assemble into larger supramolecular structures by binding to filaments of HA (Fig. 3B-2). All proteoglycans within this group possess at the amino-terminal region a tandem repeat structure or motif within their core protein, called a proteoglycan tandem repeat (PTR). This structure is responsible for the specific, high-affinity binding to the HA filament (5). Included in this PTR family are the proteoglycans *aggrecan*, *versican*, *brevican*, *neurocan*, *CD44*, and *BEHAP*. Aggrecan is by far the most well-documented, and its structure may be used as the prototype for the PTR family. Aggrecan is the predominant proteoglycan of cartilages, representing about 90% of the proteoglycan mass in articular cartilage (1). Human aggrecan contains a protein core (M_r 254 kDa) encoded by 19 exons, with each exon essentially defining a particular protein domain (6). The aggrecan core protein is substituted with two types of glycosaminoglycans (keratan sulfate and chondroitin sulfate), which constitute 90% of the total mass of the macro-

glycans. The heparin glycosaminoglycans exhibit a basic repeating glucuronic acid–N-acetylglucosamine, disaccharide structure; however, the presence of alternating α- and β-glycosidic linkages differentiates heparins from all other glycosaminoglycans, which typically are all β-linkages. This difference is of importance because many enzymes that degrade glycosaminoglycans typically have strict specificities for either α- or β-glycosidic linkages. The basic heparin sequence is subsequently sulfated and modified following polymerization; however, the modifications are more extensive and specific than they are in any other family of glycosaminoglycans. The modifications include unique sulfation patterns of the uronic acid and hexosamine hydroxyl group, N-deacetylation followed by N-sulfation of the hexosamines, and epimerization of particular glucuronic-acid residues to iduronic acid. The degree of modification is sufficient to imbed information and specificity within the polysaccharide structure. Due to historically accepted terminology, the less-modified heparin glycosaminoglycans are called *heparan sulfates* and the more "mature" glycosaminoglycans, *heparins*.

Heparins, as well as chondroitin glycosaminoglycans, are linked via an O-glycosidic bond to a core protein via a molecule (complete aggrecan monomer shown in Fig. 3B-1 = $1-5 \times 10^6$ Da). Aggrecan core proteins can be separated into five functional units: three globular (G_1, G_2, and G_3) and two extended interglobular (E_1 and E_2) domains (Fig. 3B-1). The glycosaminoglycans are clustered primarily in two regions, both within the E_2 domain. The largest (about 260 nm long), called the chondroitin sulfate-rich region, contains all the chondroitin sulfate chains (over 100 chains) and some of the keratan sulfate chains (about 15–25). This distal portion of the E_2 domain is encoded by a single large exon (exon 12). The second glycosaminoglycan attachment region is the keratan sulfate-rich region located in the proximal portion of the E_2 domain near the G_2 domain and before the chondroitin sulfate-rich region. This smaller attachment region is encoded by exon 11 and a small portion of the 5′ end of exon 12 (6).

The carboxy-terminal globular domain (G_3) of the aggrecan core protein, encoded by exons 13–18, exhibits three structural motifs: an epidermal growth factor (EGF)-like domain, a lectin-like domain, and a complement regulatory protein (CRP)-like domain. The presence of the G_3 globular domain is highly variable in mature aggrecan due to alternative splicing and proteolytic processing (7). Only about one-third of the aggrecan molecules isolated from adult cartilage actually contain an intact G_3 domain (1). Many functions related to the homology of these subdomains with other proteins (EGF, hepatic cell-surface lectins, or CRP) have been suggested. Other HA-binding proteoglycans,

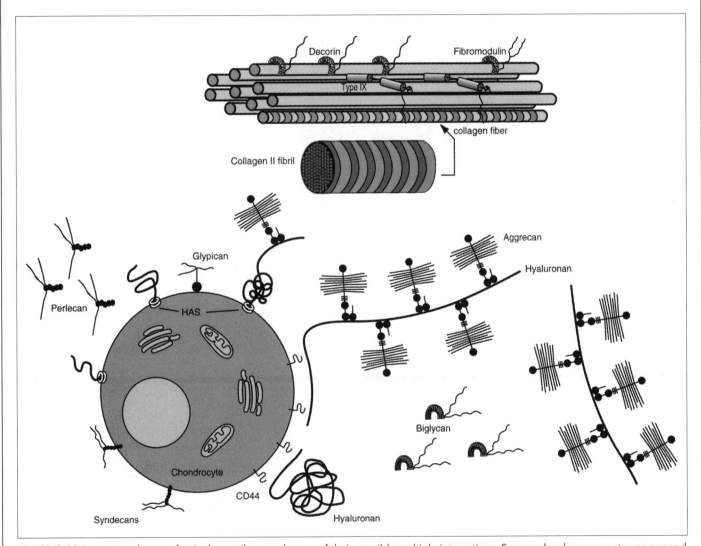

Fig. 3B-2. Major proteoglycans of articular cartilage and some of their possible multiple interactions. Supramolecular aggregates composed of aggrecan and link protein bound to hyaluronan are shown. Some aggregates, especially within the pericellular matrix, are bound to the chondrocyte cell surface via interaction of the central hyaluronan filament with CD44 or newly synthesized hyaluronan still retained by the hyaluronan synthase (HAS). Other aggregates presumably are self-containing within the extensive extracellular matrix. The specific location of biglycan and perlecan is not known but is thought to be predominately within the pericellular matrix. Collagen IX, decorin, and fibromodulin shown decorating the surface of collagen II fibers, illustrate possible proposed interactions. The cell-surface syndecan proteoglycans are depicted with a transmembrane core protein, and glypican is bound to the plasma membrane via a phosphatidylinositol linkage (n). Reproduced with permission from Knudson CB and Knudson W (21).

namely versican, neurocan, and brevican, also contain a G_3 domain similar to aggrecan and have been called *lecticans* (7). Fibulin 1 has been demonstrated as a ligand for the C-type lectin domain of aggrecan and versican (8). Fibulin-1 expression is very low in adult cartilage, but more substantial in growth plate cartilage.

The first globular domain of aggrecan (G_1) at the amino terminal region is responsible for the binding of aggrecan to HA. The G_1 domain has a molecular mass of 38 kDa and is composed of three subdomains that are encoded by exons 3, 4, and 5, respectively (9). Aggrecan molecules bind to HA to form aggregates after they are secreted into the extracellular matrix. These aggregates are stabilized further by an accessory protein called *link protein* (Figs. 3B-1 and 3B-2). Link proteins are not proteoglycans but exhibit a protein motif structure highly homologous to aggrecan G_1: A PTR double loop and a structural motif similar to an immunoglobulin (Ig) fold present on the amino-terminal end of this protein (9). The PTR double loop structure of the G_1 domain and link protein interacts reversibly with five consecutive HA disaccharide repeat units. In addition, aggrecan and link protein interact specifically with each other, forming a ternary complex with HA. Link protein and aggrecan independently exhibit a strong binding affinity for HA in the range of 10^{-9} M. Together, the affinity of the ternary complex essentially is nondissociable. Thus, both HA and link protein are required for the stabilization of the aggregate. Only one link protein molecule is present at each HA-aggrecan linkage site. As many as 200 aggrecan molecules can bind to a single filament of an HA molecule to form supramolecular structures in the range of 5×10^7 to 5×10^8 Da. By electron microscopy, these aggregates are visualized as longer than 8 mm (1).

Little is known about the functions of the G_2 domain of aggrecan. It contains a PTR motif, with considerable homology to the double-loop structure found in the G_1 domain and link protein, yet it does not have the ability to bind to HA or link protein. Unlike the G_1 domain and the link protein, the G_2 does not contain the third Ig-fold loop.

Other members of the PTR family of proteoglycans have core protein structures homologous to aggrecan. Whereas aggrecan is the predominate proteoglycan of cartilage and other load-bearing tissues, *versican* is the predominate PTR proteoglycan common to most other soft connective tissues (e.g., dermis, mesentery, etc). The core protein of versican is similar to that of aggrecan, except it contains only two globular domains, one at each terminal of the protein (analogous to aggrecan G_1 and G_3), and fewer consensus sequences for glycosaminoglycan attachment. Thus, versican, by bearing fewer glycosaminoglycans, may satisfy a space-filling role in tissues but not the role of proteoglycans as a source of high fixed-charge density required to compensate for cyclic loading as in aggrecan-rich tissues (e.g., cartilage). Some of the most recently described members of the PTR family are proteoglycans present within the extracellular matrix of neuronal tissues: *neurocan* and *brevican*. Additional central nervous system PTR proteoglycans, *glial hyaluronan-binding protein* and *hyaluronectin*, have been shown to be related to, or derivatives of, versican. The lymphocyte-homing receptor CD44 is included in the PTR family, even though it contains only one-half of the PTR structural motif (i.e., one loop). CD44 (like *betaglycan* and *thrombomodulin*) is considered a "part-time" proteoglycan because its substitution with glycosaminoglycan is variable, depending on cell type and cell state (3,5). Changes in cellular state also appear to regulate whether CD44 becomes substituted with heparan sulfate or chondroitin sulfate. The role of CD44 as a proteoglycan is not clear. However, on many cells, CD44 serves a more important function (with or without a glycosaminoglycan side chain) as a plasma-membrane intercalated HA receptor (10). For example, on chondrocytes, CD44 serves to anchor a substantial portion of aggrecan molecules within the pericellular matrix, itself tethered to HA (Fig. 3B-2). COS cells transiently transfected with pCD44 gained the capacity to assemble chondrocyte-like pericellular matrices in the presence of added HA and aggrecan. CD44 also participates in the receptor-mediated catabolism of HA.

Proteoglycans That Interact With Collagen

Collagen fibers are a predominant component of all connective tissues, forming a three-dimensional network that bestows, as well as limits, correct tissue shape and integrity. In many tissues, the collagen fibers are complemented by a distinct family of proteoglycans that form tight associations with collagen upon their secretion into the extracellular space. The small proteoglycans *decorin* and *fibromodulin* are the most notable members of this family, called the small leucine-rich proteoglycans (SLRPs) (3,11). Decorin carries predominantly one dermatan sulfate chain located at its amino terminus (except in bone, where the chain is not epimerized and is thus expressed as chondroitin sulfate), whereas fibromodulin carries up to four keratan sulfate chains within the central portion of its protein core (Fig. 3B-1). The lack of dermatan sulfate or chondroitin sulfate substitution by fibromodulin may be due to the presence of several tyrosine sulfate residues at its amino terminal end on the fibromodulin core protein. Both have been shown to bind (or "decorate") the surface of collagen fibers at specific periodic intervals along the fiber. However, the binding sites on the collagen fiber for each of the two proteoglycans are distinct. The horseshoe shape of decorin, biglycan, and fibromodulin (Fig. 3B-2), as well as the overall dimensions of this arch, support a model for its interaction with a single triple helix of collagen (11). The exact function of these proteoglycans is not known. Both have the capacity to inhibit fibrillogenesis in vitro and may therefore regulate collagen fiber diameter. It has been suggested that these proteoglycans maintain proper spacing between collagen fibrils and regulate hydration and movement of molecules within this domain (3). Further, decorin-deficient mice exhibit reduced tensile strength of skin and tendons and irregularities in the collagen fibril diameter (12).

Type IX collagen has a nontriple-helical portion that allows a "kink" in the otherwise linear molecule and extends the noncollagenous region NC4 away from the surface of the fibril (Fig. 3B-2) (1). This conformation would further facilitate interactions with adjacent acidic structures. Interestingly, type IX collagen is itself a proteoglycan often carrying a chondroitin-sulfate chain attached to the NC3 domain of the α(IX) chain. As such, type IX collagen represents another proteoglycan that may participate in controlling collagen fiber diameter. For example, it was shown by immunoelectron microscopy that the collagen fibrils of hyaline cartilage were heterogeneous, with the majority of the thinnest fibrils decorated with type IX collagen, whereas the fibrils of larger diameter were decorated with decorin (13).

The core proteins of decorin and fibromodulin, although the product of separate genes, are highly homologous. The presence of 10 or 11 hydrophobic, adjacent, leucine-rich repeat sequences of 23 or 24 amino acids each, as well as conserved disulfate-bonded loop structures, define these two proteoglycans as members of a common SLRP family (11). Other proteoglycans that belong to this family include *biglycan*, which contains two dermatan-sulfate chains, and the proteoglycans *lumican*, *epiphycan*, *keratocan*, and *osteoadherin* (see Table 3B-1). Although biglycan does not associate with or decorate fiber-forming collagens (e.g., type I or II), it does display affinity for type VI collagen. Mice with a targeted disruption of the biglycan gene appeared normal at birth, but displayed subsequent decreased postnatal skeletal growth. These results indicate that biglycan is a positive regulator of bone formation and bone mass (14). Members of this SLRP family also have shown to bind matrix macromolecules other than collagen, such as fibronectin, and growth factors, such as transforming growth factor β (TGF-β) (15). Thus, these proteoglycans may play a multifaceted role of regulating collagen fiber diameter, cross-linking collagen lattices, cross-linking other matrix components to the collagen network, and serving as an extracellular repository for growth factors.

Cell-Surface Proteoglycans

Although proteoglycans commonly are viewed as components of the extracellular matrix, some proteoglycans are never secreted, and upon synthesis, they remain closely associated with the cellular plasma membrane. The proteoglycans that predominate at the cell surface fall into one of two groups: transmembrane proteoglycans, represented by the *syndecan* family, and *glypican*, a proteoglycan tethered to the cell surface via a glycosylphosphatidylinositol linkage (3,16). These two proteoglycan groups, in different combinations and subtypes, essentially are ubiquitous to all cell types (i.e., not associated selectively with the plasma membranes of connective-tissue cells). For example, it has been demonstrated that human articular chondrocytes express mRNA for syndecan-2, syndecan-4, betaglycan, and glypican, but they express little mRNA for syndecan-1 (17). All members of the syndecan family have homologous core-protein structures that include a C-terminal cytoplasmic domain, a hydrophobic transmembrane domain, and a large N-terminal extracellular domain that bears the glycosaminoglycan chains. Another unique feature of the syndecan core-protein family is the presence of a protease-sensitive site within the proximal portion of the extracellular domain close to the plasma membrane. It has been suggested that the presence of this site allows for rapid regulation of proteoglycan-related functions via proteolytic shedding of the extracellular domain. The syndecan core protein may carry two or more heparan-sulfate chains, alone or in combination with chondroitin sulfate (16). The heparan sulfate typically is located on the distal end of the molecule, and the chondroitin-sulfate chains are localized more centrally along the extracellular domain. The proteoglycan glypican also provides for the regulated expression of heparan-sulfate chains at the cell surface. Glypican core protein is one of several cell-surface proteins that do not exhibit hydrophobic transmembrane domains, but become anchored to the plasma via the covalent linkage to a glycosylphosphotidylinositol attachment site, a process called glypiation (16). As with the syndecans, it is thought that glypican can be shed rapidly via the action of particular phospholipases.

The presence of glycosaminoglycans localized directly on the cell surface provides cells with an exquisite means for controlling the local cell environment. This control may involve all purported functions of glycosaminoglycans, including regulation of local hydration and molecular movement, binding of basic growth factors and cytokines, and binding to other matrix components as well as adjacent cell-surface heparan sulfate receptors. In fact, the binding of other extracellular matrix components (e.g., fibronectin, laminin, or collagen) by cell-surface–associated glycosaminoglycans may serve to classify these proteoglycans as matrix receptors. It is thus not surprising that cell-surface heparan sulfates are found to participate prominently in many cell–cell and cell–matrix interactions. The presence of heparan sulfate proteoglycans on the surface of vasculature-lining endothelial cells may serve to provide other functions specific for heparin/heparan sulfates (e.g., binding to antithrombin III and/or binding to lipoprotein lipase) (16). The more acute anticoagulation properties of the mature mast cell are met by a different heparin-bearing proteoglycan *serglycin*, the core protein of which contains numerous serine/glycine repeats located within the central portion of the molecule (2,3). Although substituted with heparin side chains, serglycin is not a membrane-bound proteoglycan. During resting states, serglycin exists as an intracellular proteoglycan localized within storage granules. Interestingly, other hematopoietic cell types related to mast cells express the same serglycin core protein but substitute the core with chondroitin sulfate rather that heparin chains (3).

In addition to the syndecans and glypican, several other proteoglycans are known to associate with cell surfaces. For many of these proteoglycans, the core proteins are thought to play a major functional role in the molecule. For example, the core protein of *betaglycan* is the type III TGF-β receptor (3). Other cell-surface proteins such as *thrombomodulin*, *transferrin receptor*, and the HA receptor CD44 also may exist as proteoglycans (5). However, in these cases the presence of "part-time" glycosaminoglycan substitution may serve to modulate the intrinsic function of the core protein.

Proteoglycan Metabolism

Under physiologic conditions, cells regulate a dynamic, metabolic steady state, in which anabolism (synthesis of matrix macromolecules) is balanced by catabolism (degradation and loss from the matrix) (1). Different tissues use different methods to maintain this delicate balance. However, the maintenance of proteoglycans within cartilage often provides a useful paradigm because of the relative isolation of the tissue in terms of its metabolism. Cartilage proteoglycans are regulated, for all intents and purposes, solely by the resident chondrocytes. As in all tissues, anabolism in chondrocytes is regulated by cellular responses to biomechanical stimuli as well as a capacity of the cells to "sense" changes in the composition of their extracellular matrix. The mechanism of these two cellular responses is not clear, but likely is mediated via such cell-surface receptors as *anchorin CII* (annexin V), CD44, and/or a variety of integrins (Fig. 3B-2) (1,10). Chondrocytes also are responsive to a variety of cellular mediators, including inflam-

matory mediators [e.g., interleukin (IL)-1α, IL-1β; IL-6, tumor necrosis factor α (TNF-α), and interferon (IFN)-γ], peptide growth factors (e.g., epidermal growth factor, fibroblast growth factors, platelet-derived growth factors, TGF-α, TGF-β, and other members of the TGF-β superfamily, including the bone morphogenic proteins), bacterial lipopolysaccharides, some retinoids, and degraded portions of matrix macromolecules, such as fibronectin fragments (1). These mediators often are bipolar, affecting both anabolism and catabolism. In general, it can be stated that cytokines released by inflammatory cells stimulate cartilage catabolism and inhibit its anabolism, whereas peptide growth factors promote cartilage anabolism and inhibit catabolism (1).

The normal catabolic mechanisms controlled by the chondrocytes are very conservative. Very little is known concerning the turnover of decorin, biglycan, and fibromodulin, the proteoglycans that associate with collagen. As for aggrecan, in vitro explant culture studies of human articular cartilage suggest that 25 days is the average half-life of newly synthesized aggrecan within the tissue (1). It is noteworthy that a comparable half-life (13–25 days) of newly synthesized aggrecan was observed in explant studies on bovine articular cartilage (18). It also was shown that the half-life

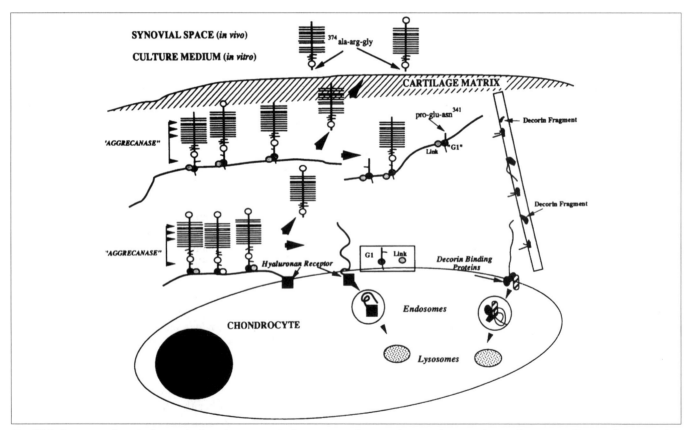

Fig. 3B-3. Summary of catabolic events thought to occur in the turnover of proteoglycan within articular cartilage tissue. Depicted is a postulated scheme for the catabolism of proteoglycans within articular cartilage. Aggrecans, as well as other matrix proteoglycans, are first cleaved at critical sites along their core protein (e.g., between G₁ and G₂ of aggrecan) by matrix metalloproteinases (MMPs). Depicted here is putative action by the MMP termed "aggrecanase" although action by other MMPs has also been postulated. Hyaluronan, possibly still retaining remnants of aggrecan and link protein, is then internalized via interaction with a hyaluronan receptor such as CD44 (10). Courtesy of Drs. A. Plaas and J. Sandy (19); reproduced with permission.

of newly synthesized HA is nearly equivalent to aggrecan, even though the two molecules are believed to be processed via different mechanisms. In general, aggrecan catabolism is thought to occur primarily extracellularly and involve the proteolytic cleavage between the G_1 and G_2 domains of the core protein, resulting in degradation products that are lost rapidly from the cartilage matrix (Fig. 3B-3) (19). The primary proteolytic enzymes responsible for the extracellular cleavage of proteoglycans (as well as other matrix proteins) are the matrix metalloproteases characterized by a bound Zn^{2+} at their active site and a requirement for calcium (1). Extracellular catabolism of HA in cartilage as well as other tissues never has been demonstrated; however, evidence is accumulating to suggest that turnover occurs primarily intracellularly, following endocytosis by HA receptors such as CD44 (10). One unfortunate outcome of cartilage degradation is the exposure of released matrix components, such as aggrecan, to the immune system. Aggrecan and other matrix proteins within healthy cartilage normally are not subjected to immune surveillance, making them potential antigenic determinants upon their release. Thus, molecular fragments of collagen type II and aggrecan are considered potential causal factors in human joint diseases (20).

Summary

Proteoglycans represent a highly complex family of macromolecules. They possess core proteins that undergo extensive post-translational modifications and exhibit structural motifs that not only serve as sites for glycosaminoglycan attachment but allow for specific interactions with other matrix macromolecules, cell membranes, and growth factors. The glycosaminoglycan side chains display a multiplicity of functions, such as supplying a source of fixed, high-density negative charge to the extracellular matrix. Many of these proteoglycans functions still are being elucidated, but given their complexity, proteoglycans have the potential to contribute to both the physiologic functions and the physical properties of all tissues.

WARREN KNUDSON, PhD
KLAUS E. KUETTNER, PhD

References

1. Kuettner KE. Osteoarthritis: cartilage integrity and homeostasis. In: Klippel JH, Dieppe PA, (eds). Rheumatology. St. Louis, MO: Mosby-Year Book Europe Limited, 1994; pp 6.1–6.16.

2. Wight TN, Heinegard DK, Hascall VC. Proteoglycans structure and function. In: Hay ED (ed). Cell Biology of the Extracellular Matrix, 2nd ed. New York: Plenum Press, 1991; pp 45–78.

3. Roughley PJ, Poole AR. Proteoglycans. In: Schumacher HR, Klippel JH, Koopman WJ (eds). Primer on the Rheumatic Diseases, 10th ed. Atlanta: Arthritis Foundation, 1993; pp 23–27.

4. Weigel PH, Hascall VC, Tammi M. Hyaluronan synthases. J Biol Chem 1997;272:13997–14000.

5. Hardingham TE, Fosang AJ. Proteoglycans: many forms and many functions. FASEB J 1992;6:861–870.

6. Valhmu WB, Palmer GD, Rivers PA, et al. Structure of the human aggrecan gene: exon-intron organization and association with the protein domains. Biochem J 1995;309:535–542.

7. Aspberg A, Miura R, Bourdoulous S, et al. The C-type lectin domains of lecticans, a family of aggregating chondroitin sulfate proteoglycans, bind tenascin-R by protein-protein interactions independent of carbohydrate moiety. Proc Natl Acad Sci, USA 1997;94:10116–10121.

8. Aspberg A, Adam S, Kostka G, Timpl R, Heinegard D. Fibulin-1 is a ligand for the C-type lectin domains of aggrecan and versican. J Biol Chem 1999;274:20444–20449.

9. Sandell LJ, Chansky H, Zamparo O, Hering TM. Molecular biology of cartilage proteoglycans and link protein. In: Kuettner KE, Goldberg VM (eds). Osteoarthritic Disorders. Rosemont, IL: American Academy of Orthopaedic Surgeons, 1995; pp 117–130.

10. Knudson W, Knudson CB. Hyaluronan receptor, CD44. http://www.glycoforum.gr.jp/science/hyaluronan/HA10/HA10E.html, 1999.

11. Iozzo RV. The biology of the small leucine-rich proteoglycans. J Biol Chem 1999;274:18843–18846.

12. Danielson KG, Baribault H, Holmes DF, Graham H, Kadler KE, Iozzo RV. Targeted disruption of decorin leads to abnormal collagen fibril morphology and skin fragility. J Cell Biol 1997;136:729–743.

13. Hagg R, Bruckner P, Hedbom E. Cartilage fibrils of mammals are biochemically heterogeneous: differential distribution of decorin and collagen IX. J Cell Biol 1998;142:285–294.

14. Xu T, Bianco P, Fisher LW, et al. Targeted disruption of the biglycan gene leads to an osteoporosis-like phenotype in mice. Nature Gen 1998;20:78–82.

15. Hildebrand A, Romaris M, Rasmussen LM, et al. Interaction of the small interstitial proteoglycans biglycan, decorin and fibromodulin with transforming growth factor β. Biochem J 1994;302:527–534.

16. David G. Integral membrane heparan sulfate proteoglycans. FASEB J 1993;7:1023–1030.

17. Grover J, Roughley PJ. Expression of cell-surface proteoglycan mRNA by human articular chondrocytes. Biochem J 1995;309:963–968.

18. Morales TI, Hascall VC. Correlated metabolism of proteoglycans and hyaluronic acid in bovine cartilage organ cultures. J Biol Chem 1988;263:3632–3638.

19. Plaas AHK, Sandy JD. Proteoglycan anabolism and catabolism in articular cartilage. In: Kuettner KE, Goldberg VM (eds). Osteoarthritic Disorders. Rosemont, IL: American Academy of Orthopaedic Surgeons, 1995; pp 103–116.

20. Glant TT, Mikecz K, Thonar JMA, Kuettner KE. Immune responses to cartilage proteoglycans in inflammatory animal models and human diseases. In: Woessner JF, Howell DS (eds). Joint Cartilage Degradation. New York: Marcel Dekker. 1993; pp 435–473.

21. Knudson CB, Knudson W. Cartilage proteoglycans. Semin Cell Dev Biol 2001;12:69–78.

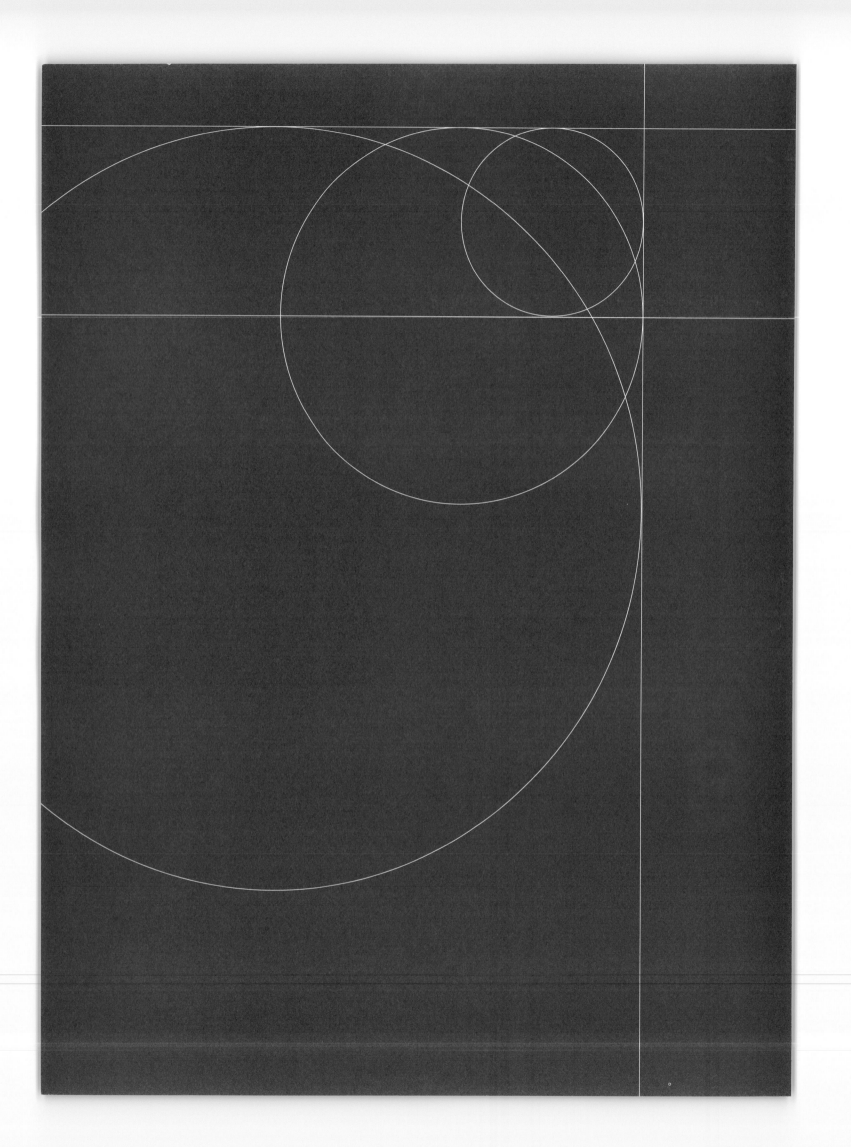

4 MEDIATORS OF INFLAMMATION, TISSUE DESTRUCTION, AND REPAIR
A. Cellular Constituents

Inflammation may be defined as a local tissue reaction to injury initiated by a microbial pathogen, toxin, foreign body, trauma, or malignancy. Activation of endothelial cells and resident cells in tissues results in an influx of circulating granulocytes and monocytes to the area of injury. Released mediators cause increased vasopermeability with a resultant efflux of fluid and plasma proteins with or without a cellular response. We now understand the underlying cells and mediators that are the pathophysiologic causes of the cardinal physical signs of inflammation described by Celsius in the first century: rubor (redness), calor (heat), dolor (pain), and tumor (swelling).

This section will review the major inflammatory cells and their recruitment, activation, products, and interactions that are important in rheumatic diseases. Later sections will review in more detail the soluble mediators these cells release, which include cytokines, proteinases, lipid-derived mediators, nitric oxide, and reactive oxygen species, and will examine the roles of plasma proteins and complement in the initiation and amplification of the inflammatory response.

Neutrophils

Neutrophils, also known as polymorphonuclear leukocytes (PMNs), have a highly condensed, segmented, multilobed nucleus. These cells are terminally differentiated and released from the bone marrow into the circulation in a quiescent state. Their numerous cytoplasmic granules contain preformed mediators sequestered within membrane-bound compartments, preventing cell autolysis. Neutrophils are activated through numerous stimuli including complement components and microbial peptides, and through other cell-surface receptors (Table 4A-1).

Chemotaxis
In most instances, neutrophils must move from the circulation into an inflammatory site. Directed migration, or *chemotaxis*, occurs along a chemical gradient originating from

the target. Neutrophil chemoattractants include bacterial formylated peptides and the activated complement component C5a. Other chemoattractants for PMNs include leukotriene (LT) B_4 (1), and the chemoattractant cytokine (*chemokine*) interleukin (IL)-8 (2). These chemoattractants interact with specific guanosine triphosphate (GTP)-binding protein-linked (G-protein) surface receptors.

Neutrophils express on their surfaces L-selectin (CD62L), which interacts with glycosylated counterligands such as sialyl-Lewis^x expressed on endothelial cells, and glycoproteins, which interact with endothelial cell E- and P-selectins (CD62E and CD62P). These interactions mediate cell-rolling along blood vessels (Fig. 4A-1). An important neutrophil cell-surface receptor is the *integrin* adhesion molecule CD11b/CD18 ($\alpha M\beta 2$, Mac-1), which is responsible for adherence to vascular endothelium and to other neutrophils. The $\beta 2$ integrins containing CD18 bind CD54 (intercellular adhesion molecule [ICAM]-1), the expression

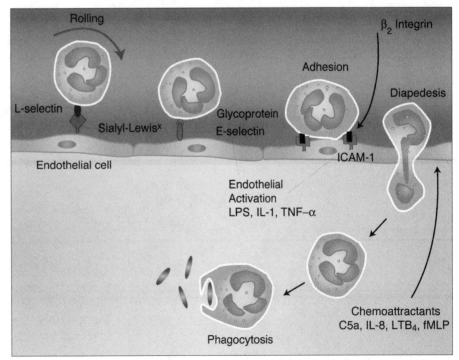

Fig. 4A-1. Neutrophil adhesion and transmigration into tissues. Neutrophils roll along blood vessels tethered by the interactions between L-selectin expressed on the neutrophil and carbohydrate ligands on the endothelial cells. Upon endothelial cell activation, expression of E-selectin and intercellular adhesion molecule (ICAM)-1 is increased. The interaction of neutrophil $\beta 2$ integrins with ICAM-1 leads to a firm adhesion of the cell to the vessel wall. Neutrophils then migrate into the tissues where chemotactic factors target them to the area of injury.

TABLE 4A-1
Major Chemoattractants, Activators, and Products of Inflammatory Cells

Cell	Chemoattractants	Activation
Neutrophil	C5a, LTB$_4$, IL-8, formyl peptides	Opsonized particles, CR1, FcγRI, FcγRII, FcγRIII, GM-CSF
Monocyte/Macrophage	MIP, MCP-1, collagen, fibronectin, TGF-β, PDGF, GM-CSF, M-CSF	Opsonized particles, CR1, FcγRI, FcγRII, FcγRIII, IL-1, IL-3, TNF-α, IFN-γ, LPS, mannose receptor, fibronectin, GM-CSF, M-CSF
Platelet	PAF Collagen	PAF, MBP, fibrinogen, thrombin, CRP, substance P, IgG, FcϵRII, complement components
Mast Cell	SCF	FcϵRI, C3a, C5a, c-kit, IL-1, IL-10, IL-4
Eosinophil	PAF, LTB$_4$, IL-3, GM-CSF, IL-5, eotaxin, RANTES, MCP-2, MCP-3, MCP-4	FcϵRI, FcγRI, FcγRII, FcϵRII, CR1, CR3, C5a

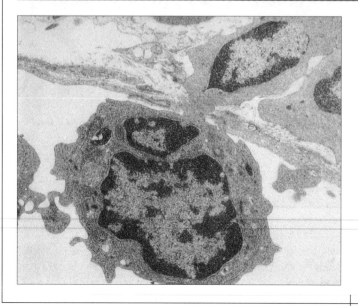

of which is increased on activated endothelial cells. This interaction leads to a tighter leukocyte adhesion followed by cell spreading and crawling. The transmigration of cells across the endothelium, *diapedesis*, is mediated by adhesion of platelet-endothelial cell adhesion molecule-1 (PECAM-1/CD31) on leukocytes interacting with PECAM-1 prominently expressed in the intercellular junctional areas of endothelial cells (Fig. 4A-2). In diseases such as systemic lupus erythematosus (SLE), leukocytoclastic vasculitis, giant cell arteritis, and rheumatoid vasculitis, activation of

Fig. 4A-2. Neutrophil diapedesis. In this electron micrograph, the heavily granulated neutrophil is seen traversing the endothelium. Interactions between the platelet-endothelial cell adhesion molecule-1 (PECAM-1) expressed on neutrophils and in the junctional areas of endothelial cells are important in transmigration.

Granule mediators	Cytokines	Other mediators
1° Azurophilic Lysozyme, myeloperoxidase defensins, collagenase, elastase, gelatinase, proteinase-3, cathepsin-G **2° Specific** Lactoferrin, B12-binding protein **Other granules** PLA_2		LTB_4, PGE_2 PAF O_2^-, free radicals
Lysozyme	IL-1,IL-4, IL-6, IL-10, IL-12, TNFα, IL-8, MIP-1α, MIP1-β, MCP-1, MCP-2, MCP-3, RANTES, TGF-β, PDGF, FGF, GM-CSF	LTB_4, LTC_4, PGE_2, PGI_2, $PGF_{2α}$, PAF, fibronectin, thrombospondin, free radicals, O_2^-, nitric oxide, complement components, coagulation factors
ADP, seratonin, PF-4, vWF, PLA_2, thrombospondin, thromboglobulin	PDGF, FGF, TGF-β, RANTES	PGE, LTC_4, TxA_2, 12-HETE, PAF, coagulation factors, fibrinogen, fibronectin, adenosine
Histamine, tryptase, chymase, carboxypeptidase A, cathepsin-G, heparin, chondroitin sulfate, PLA_2	FGF, TGF-β, PDGF, TNF-α, IL-1, IL-3, IL-4, IL-5, IL-6, IL-8, IL-10, IL-13	LTC_4, PGD_2, PAF
Eosinophil peroxidase, MBP, ECP, EDN, CLC (lysophospholipase)	IL-3, IL-5, GM-CSF, RANTES, MIP-1α, eotaxin, IL-8, TNF-α, IL-1, IL-2, IL-4, IL-6, IL-7, IL-10, IL-16i	LTC_4, PAF, lipoxins

the endothelium is seen with consequent adhesion molecule expression, an event critical to targeting neutrophils to the inflammatory site (3–6).

Phagocytosis

Both neutrophils and monocyte/macrophages are capable of ingesting foreign particles and have been referred to as "professional phagocytes." Phagocytosis is initiated by the attachment or binding of target particles to the cell surface and the subsequent enclosure of the particle within a plasma-membrane pouch. Upon closure, this pouch becomes a cytoplasmic vacuole called a *phagosome*. The membranes of primary or secondary lysosomes fuse with phagosomes to form *phagolysosomes*, which permit entry of lysosomal contents into the phagosome (7). Within this shielded environment, the enzymatic degradation of ingested material occurs, an important aspect of the scavenging function of

neutrophils and macrophages. Phagocytosis thus delivers a microorganism to a sequestered intracellular compartment in which the noxious action of host cytotoxins and degradative enzymes is confined.

Neutrophils and macrophages bind particular plasma immunoglobulins, or antibodies, and certain complement components. These substances are known as *opsonins*, from a Greek word meaning "to prepare food for." The coating of bacteria, cells, other surfaces, and debris with opsonins increases the efficiency with which they undergo phagocytosis. Phagocytes recognize antibody- or complement-coated particles through cell-surface receptors for immunoglobulin and for fragments of the third component of complement, C3b and iC3b. Opsonization of foreign particles is an important component of the innate immune system, permitting the ingestion of a wide variety of particles (8). The stimulus to phagocytosis does not depend on specific recognition of the organism, due to adaptive immune recognition by antibody and T-cell receptors.

Phagocytic cells express receptors for the complement fragment C3b (receptor designated CR1 or CD35) and its inactivated cleavage product iC3b (receptor designated CR3 or CD11b/CD18). Both receptors are important in the clearance of such particles as opsonized bacteria, to which C3b or iC3b are bound, and for the removal of immune complexes that covalently bind C3b and iC3b (9).

Neutrophils, monocytes/macrophages, platelets, B lymphocytes, and natural killer cells all express receptors for immunoglobulin (Ig). Three receptors bind IgG-containing complexes via their Fc fragments: FcγRI (CD64) is the high-affinity receptor for monomeric IgG, whereas FcγRIIa (CD32), and FcγRIII (CD16) are low-affinity receptors that bind multimeric IgG. FcγRI is expressed on neutrophils only after interferon (IFN)-γ stimulation, but is expressed on unstimulated monocytes and macrophages. FcγR polymorphisms that may represent disease susceptibility factors in the development of autoimmunity also affect phagocytic function (10).

Release of Toxic Proteolytic Enzymes

Neutrophils contain four types of morphologically distinct granules, each containing different proteases and other mediators (7,11). When these granule membranes fuse with the plasma membrane through the active process of *exocy-* tosis or *degranulation*, their contents are released into the extracellular microenvironment, where they promote inflammation and tissue damage. The primary azurophilic granules contain microbicidal enzymes including lysozyme, defensins, and myeloperoxidase (MPO), as well as the proteases cathepsin G, proteinase 3, and elastase (which causes destruction of the elastic laminae of blood vessels). The specific or secondary granules contain lactoferrin, gelatinase, and collagenase, which degrade components of the extracellular matrix. Other granules contain gelatinase, lysozyme, and other mediators including bacteriocidal phospholipase A$_2$. Neutrophil degranulation is provoked by soluble stimuli including C5a, IL-8, and immune complexes, and granule release is augmented when neutrophils encounter immune complexes deposited on a surface. The release of lysosomal enzymes from neutrophils contributes to tissue injury in diseases (such as rheumatoid arthritis) characterized by immune-complex deposition on cell surfaces, vascular basement membranes, or articular cartilage (Fig. 4A-3)(12). Neutrophil MPO and proteinase 3 are detected by the antineutrophil cytoplasmic antibodies perinuclear ANCA and cytoplasmic ANCA, respectively. Release of these proteases may be important in vascular injury of several vasculitides (13).

In crystal arthritis, neutrophils are recruited to the synovium in an attempt to eliminate these foreign bodies. Crystals, which cannot be readily digested by the neutrophils,

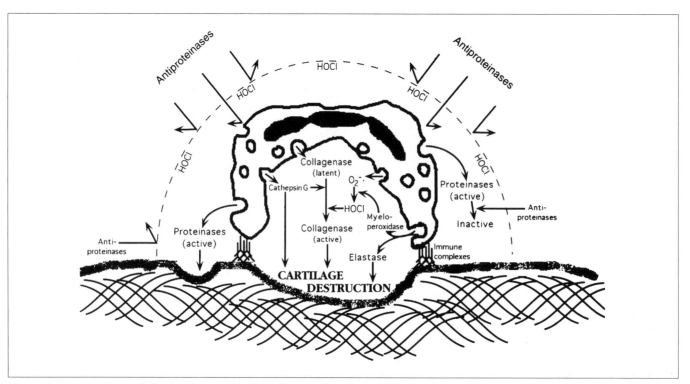

Fig. 4A-3. A model for mechanisms of antiproteinase defense and cartilage destruction by neutrophils in rheumatoid arthritis. Fc receptors of neutrophils engage immune complexes associated with or embedded in articular cartilage. Neutrophil activation following Fc receptor engagement results in the release of latent and active proteinases and the products of NAPDH oxidase into the space between the neutrophil and cartilage. Here the proteases are protected from degradation by antiproteinases, thus facilitating the breakdown of collagen and proteoglycans. Proteinases released into the adjacent synovial fluid may be inactivated by antiproteinases or may be protected from inactivation by neutrophil-derived hypochlorous acid (HOCl).

cause a breach in cellular structure integrity, with subsequent release of toxic proteases into the extracellular environment and resultant signs and symptoms of inflammation.

Production of Toxic Oxygen Radicals

Phagocytic cells, when activated, consume molecular oxygen. Most of this oxygen is transformed directly into superoxide anion radicals (O_2^-), causing tissue injury and irreversible modification of macromolecules. Other toxic oxygen metabolites produced by neutrophils are generated through the MPO-hydrogen peroxide-halide system (7). Myeloperoxidase, present in azurophilic granules, catalyzes the reaction of hydrogen peroxide with a halide, such as chloride, to form hypohalous acids (e.g., hypochlorous acid). These compounds are capable of killing a variety of microorganisms and are cytotoxic to host cells (Table 4A-2).

Macrophages

Macrophages are important in the inflammatory response, as phagocytic cells and as effector cells producing many mediators (Table 4A-1). Tissue macrophages, which may have life spans measured in years, develop from circulating bone marrow-derived monocytes. Monocytes are recruited into tissues from the circulation in response to such chemotactic factors as formylated bacterial proteins, C5a, and the C-C chemokines, which include RANTES, macrophage inflammatory protein (MIP)-1α, MIP-1β, and monocyte chemoattractant protein (MCP)-1 (2). Monocyte chemoattractants also include two growth and differentiation factors, transforming growth factor (TGF)-β and platelet-derived growth factor (PDGF), as well as extracellular matrix components. As with neutrophil recruitment, β1 and β2 integrins on the surface of monocytes engage the endothelial cells ICAM-1 and vascular cell adhesion molecule (VCAM)-1 (CD106) to facilitate adhesion and transmigra-

tion into tissues. Monocytes differentiate within a few hours into tissue macrophages under the influence of locally produced cytokines including IL-1, IL-3, tumor necrosis factor (TNF)-α, and IFN-γ, and growth factors including the macrophage and granulocyte-macrophage colony stimulating factors (M-CSF and GM-CSF). Interactions with extracellular matrix proteins including fibronectin, collagen, and laminin through β1 and β3 integrins further influence macrophage differentiation and maturation (14).

Similar to neutrophils, receptors are present on macrophages for FcγRI, FcγRII, and FcγRIII, and CR1 and CR3 are also expressed, allowing the recognition of opsonized particles with subsequent phagocytosis. Macrophages additionally possess the mannose receptor that recognizes glycoproteins on microbial cell surfaces, permitting their phagocytosis.

Release of Inflammatory Mediators and Proteases

Macrophages may be activated by cytokines, immune complexes, endotoxin, and complement components. A large number of substances are produced by macrophages, ranging from free radicals such as superoxide anion to large macromolecules such as fibronectin (Table 4A-1) (15). Some products are actively secreted in response to inflammatory stimuli, whereas others are released constitutively. Stimulated macrophages produce coagulation factors of both the intrinsic and extrinsic pathways, procoagulant tissue factor, prothrombin activator, and plasmin inhibitors. Monocytes isolated from people with rheumatic disease have increased procoagulant activity, which may contribute to the deposition of fibrin at inflammatory sites and is implicated in the formation of crescents in glomerulonephritis. Like neutrophils, macrophages release proteases, including collagenase and elastase and the bactericidal lysozyme. Macrophages also are the source of many of the proteins of both the alternative and classical complement cascades.

TABLE 4A-2
Potential Effects of Reactive Oxygen Intermediates

On cells
Killing of microbes (viruses, bacteria, fungi, protozoa)
Injury of tumor cells
Stimulation of secretion by platelets, mast cells, endothelial cells, glomerular cells
Mutagenesis of bacteria and mammalian cells
Tumor promotion and carcinogenesis

On extracellular products
Generation of chemotactic lipids from arachidonate
Activation of leukocyte collagenase and gelatinase
Inactivation of chemotactic leukotriennes, chemotactic peptides, α-1-antiprotease, met-enkephalin, leukocyte hydrolases, and bacterial toxins

Production of Cytokines

Macrophages secrete a variety of cytokines that regulate immune function and inflammation as well as participate in wound healing and repair. Macrophages produce the cytokines IL-1 and TNF-α, which not only have overlapping functions, but are also capable of inducing each others' release (15). Interleukin 1, an endogenous pyrogen, is a major macrophage product with proinflammatory effects on many cells. Interleukin 6 activates lymphocytes and induces the synthesis of acute phase reactants by hepatocytes. Interleukin 12 release stimulates IFN-γ and the induction of T helper (Th)1-type lymphocyte response. Macrophages also release the Th2 cytokine IL-4, a stimulus of antibody production, and the predominantly anti-inflammatory IL-10. Macrophages are a source of chemokines including the neutrophil attractant IL-8, as well as others including MCP-1, MCP-2, MCP-3, RANTES, MIP-1α, and MIP-1β, which act on monocytes but not neutrophils and have additional activities toward basophil, eosinophils, and T lymphocytes (2). The growth factors TGF-β, GM-CSF, PDGF, and basic fibroblast growth factor lead to further monocyte activation and recruitment, as well as fibroblast activation and angiogenesis. For more on cytokines, see Chapter 4B.

Production of Arachidonic Acid-Derived Mediators

Macrophages are significant sources of the eicosanoid lipid mediators of inflammation derived from arachidonic acid (AA). Phospholipase (PL)A_2 enzymes liberate free AA and lyso-phospholipids from cell-membrane phospholipids (16). Different cell-associated and secreted PLA_2 may release AA for the generation of distinct eicosanoid end-products and may themselves represent proinflammatory mediators acting through cell-surface receptors. Arachidonic acid is metabolized either via constitutive and inducible cyclooxygenases (COX, prostaglandin endoperoxide synthase) to generate prostaglandins (PG) and thromboxanes (TX)(17) or via lipoxygenases to generate leukotrienes and lipoxins. Lysophospholipids generated by PLA_2 are important as precursors of the mediator platelet-activating factor (PAF).

Macrophages have both COX-1 and inducible COX-2. The primary prostanoid product of macrophages is PGE_2, which vasodilates, increases vascular permeability, and activates osteoclastic bone resorption. These cells also are sources of PGF_2-α, the vasodilator prostacyclin, and TXA_2. Macrophages are sources of LTB_4, lesser amounts of LTC_4-, and PAF, which is important in the regulation of platelet function but is also a potent neutrophil chemotaxin. For more on AA-derived mediators, see Chapter 4E.

Nitric Oxide as a Modulator of Inflammation

Macrophages also are sources of the reactive intermediate nitric oxide. Although originally identified as endothelium-derived relaxation factor, nitric oxide is a product of multiple cells with diverse biologic functions (18). Exposure of macrophages to such cytokines as IL-1β and IFN-γ markedly increases their nitric oxide production. Activities of nitric oxide that may contribute to the inflammatory response include vasodilation and reaction with superoxide anion to form toxic peroxynitrite compounds. In humans, the production of nitric oxide by synovial macrophages and articular chondrocytes has been demonstrated in both rheumatoid arthritis and osteoarthritis, as well as in the endothelium of people with SLE (19,20). For more on nitric oxide, see Chapter 4E.

Platelets

Platelets are derived from marrow megakaryocytes and function in hemostasis, wound healing, and cellular responses to injury. Platelets are also inflammatory effector cells. Both PAF and collagen fragments cause platelet chemotaxis to areas of endothelial activation or injury, and products released after activation recruit other cells and contribute to the amplification of the inflammatory reaction (Table 4A-1) (21,22).

Normal platelet adhesion to extracellular matrix proteins requires von Willebrand factor (vWF), which binds to the platelet glycoprotein Ib/IX and serves as a molecular bridge between platelets and subendothelial collagen. Platelets may be activated through their receptors for IgG, IgE, PAF, C-reactive protein, and substance P, and through many activated complement components. With activation, platelets release granular contents that promote clotting and further platelet aggregation. A variety of protein- and lipid-derived mediators have chemotactic, proliferative, thrombogenic, and proteolytic activity. Stimuli that activate platelet adhesion and degranulation also trigger the release of AA from the membrane via PLA_2, initiating the synthesis of TXA_2 via COX-1 and the lipoxygenase product 12-hydroxytetraenoic acid (12-HETE), which is metabolized to lipoxins.

Products released from platelet granules also promote the local inflammatory reaction (21,22). Dense granules contain adenosine diphosphate (ADP), an important platelet agonist that activates platelet fibrinogen-binding sites of the $\beta3$ integrin glycoprotein IIb/IIIa, and serotonin, a potent vasoconstrictor that activates neutrophils and endothelial cells. The alpha granules contain platelet factor 4 and beta-thromboglobulin, which activate both mononuclear and polymorphonuclear leukocytes and are also the source of PDGF and TGF-β, both of which stimulate proliferation of smooth-muscle cells and fibroblasts and are important in angiogenesis and tissue repair. Additional platelet granule products include thrombospondin, which promotes neutrophil adhesion, the coagulation factors V and VIII, vWF, fibrinogen, and fibronectin.

Mast Cells

The tissue-based mast cell, a primary effector cell of IgE-mediated immediate-type hypersensitivity reactions, may contribute to the inflammatory response in many rheumatic diseases. This long-lived cell commonly is positioned at the interface of the external environment and often along blood vessels. Mast cells are derived from a pluripotent bone marrow progenitor that diverges early in development from other leukocytes. The cytokine c-*kit* (or stem cell factor) is the major cytokine influencing mast cell chemotaxis and development. Like the macrophage, mast cells in different sites demonstrate heterogeneity and may undergo phenotypic changes in response to local cytokines, growth factors, and cellular and matrix interactions (23,24). The mast cell is a large cell with a single, usually indented nucleus containing numerous secretory granules; however, mast cells may be difficult to detect with routine fixation and staining, and often require specific techniques for identification (25).

The major stimulus to mast cell activation is IgE through its high-affinity receptor FcɛRI. Hoewever, mast cells also respond to C3a, C5a, neuropeptides, many cytokines, and eosinophil-derived cationic proteins (Table 4A-1). Mast cell activation results in the rapid exocytosis of secretory granules and eicosanoid generation, followed by the later generation of eicosanoids and the production of numerous cytokines and growth factors. Interactions with extracellular matrix proteins through integrins augments mast cell degranulation. The mast cell secretory granule contains abundant proteoglycans including heparin and chondroitin sulfate. The mast cell proteases – tryptase, chymase, and carboxypeptidase – may cause tissue injury and activate proenzymes such as matrix metalloproteinases. Mast cells also contain the vasodilatory and vasopermeability-inducing histamine and are an important source of LTC_4 and PGD_2, as well as PAF and PLA_2. Mast cell cytokines are of Th1 and Th2 type with a significant amount of TNF-α, IL-4, IL-5, and IL-6. Fibroblast growth factor, TGF-β, and tryptase made by mast cells are important in fibroblast activation, reflected in a potential role in fibrotic reactions and scleroderma. Mast cell-specific products also are found in synovial fluid, and increased numbers of activated mast cells have been identified in the synovium of people with arthritis (25). Mast cells are important effector cells in the pathogenesis of urticaria and urticarial vasculitis, both of which are associated with autoimmunity.

Eosinophils

Eosinophils are important inflammatory effector cells (26). More commonly associated with allergic diseases and parasitic infection, eosinophils contribute to the inflammatory reaction of several rheumatic diseases. Eosinophilic granulocytes have bilobed nuclei that are easily identified by their granules containing cationic proteins; these granules are stained with acidic dyes including eosin. Mature eosinophils are released from the bone marrow, where IL-5 is an important growth, differentiation, and survival factor. They circulate in the peripheral blood and are recruited to tissues by LTB_4, PAF, and chemokines including eotaxin,

RANTES, MCP-2, MCP-3, and MCP-4. The interaction between the very late antigen (VLA)-4 (α4β1 or CD49d/CD29) integrin on eosinophils with VCAM-1 on endothelial cells is important for migration into inflammatory sites. Eosinophils are activated through numerous cell-surface receptors, including the low-affinity receptors for IgG, FcγRII, and FcγRIII; the high- and low-affinity receptors for IgE, FcɛRI, and FcɛRII; and the IgA receptor. The complement receptors CR1 and CR3, and the C5a receptor also are expressed (Table 4A-1). The granules of eosinophils contain major basic protein and eosinophil cationic protein, both of which are toxic to helminths and which activate neutrophils and mast cells. The eosinophil peroxidase generates hypobromous acid, a toxin to parasites and a contributor to tissue injury. The eosinophil is also a source of numerous cytokines, chemokines, and growth factors, as well as the lipid-derived mediators LTC_4, lipoxins, and PAF. In rheumatic diseases, eosinophils contribute to vascular injury in Churg-Strauss syndrome and hypersensitivity vasculitides. There is also a role for eosinophils in some fibrotic diseases including eosinophilic fasciitis and the eosinophilia myalgia syndrome, caused by contaminated L-tryptophan.

CLIFTON O. BINGHAM, III, MD
STEVEN B. ABRAMSON, MD

References

1. Serhan CN, Prescott SM. *The scent of a phagocyte: advances on leukotriene B_4 receptors. J Exp Med* 2000;192:F5–F8.
2. Luster AD. *Chemokines – chemotactic cytokines that mediate inflammation. N Engl J Med* 1998;338:436–445.
3. Belmont HM, Abramson SB, Lie JT. *Pathology and pathogenesis of vascular injury in systemic lupus erythematosus. Interactions of inflammatory cells and activated endothelium. Arthritis Rheum* 1996;39:9–22.
4. Cid MC, Cebrian M, Font C, et al. *Cell adhesion molecules in the development of inflammatory infiltrates in giant cell arteritis: inflammation-induced angiogenesis as the preferential site of leukocyte-endothelial cell interactions. Arthritis Rheum* 2000;43:184–194.
5. Verschueren PC. Voskuyl AE, Smeets TJ, Zwinderman KH, Breedveld FC, Tak PP. *Increased cellularity and expression of adhesion molecules in muscle biopsy specimens from patients with rheumatoid arthritis with clinical suspicion of vasculitis, but negative routine histology. Ann Rheum Dis* 2000;59:598–606.
6. Cronstein BN, Weissmann G. *The adhesion molecules of inflammation. Arthritis Rheum* 1993;36:147–157.
7. Hampton MB, Kettle AJ, Winterbourn CC. *Inside the neutrophil phagosome: oxidants, myeloperoxidase, and bacterial killing. Blood* 1998;92:3007–3017.
8. Medzhitov R, Janeway C. *Innate Immunity. N Engl J Med* 2000;343:338–344.
9. Schifferli JA, Ng YC, Peters DK. *The role of complement and its receptor in the elimination of immune complexes. N Eng J Med* 1986;315:488–495.

10. Salmon JE, Edberg JC, Brogle NL, Kimberly RP. Allelic polymorphisms of human Fc gamma receptor IIA and Fc gamma receptor IIIB. Independent mechanisms for differences in human phagocyte function. J Clin Invest 1992;89:1274–1281.

11. Borregaard N, Cowland JB. Granules of the human neutrophilic polymorphonuclear leukocyte. Blood 1997;89: 3503–3521.

12. Pillinger MH, Abramson SB. The neutrophil in rheumatoid arthritis. Rheum Dis Clin North Am 1995;21:691–714.

13. Harper L, Savage CO. Pathogenesis of ANCA-associated systemic vasculitis. J Pathol 2000;190:349–359.

14. Thomas R, Wong R, Lipsky PE. Monocytes and Macrophages. In: Kelley WN, Harris ED, Ruddy S, Sledge CB (eds.). Textbook of Rheumatology, 5th ed. Philadelphia: W.B. Saunders, 1997; pp 128–145.

15. Nathan CF. Secretory products of macrophages. J Clin Invest 1987;79:319–326.

16. Bingham CO III, Austen KF. Phospholipase A_2 enzymes in eicosanoid generation. Proc Assoc Am Physicians 1999;111: 516–524.

17. Crofford LJ, Lipsky PE, Brooks P, Abramson SB, Simon LS, Van de Putte LBA. Basic biology and clinical application of specific cyclooxygenase-2 inhibitors. Arthritis Rheum 2000;43:4–13.

18. Clancy RM, Abramson SB. Nitric oxide: a novel mediator of inflammation. Proc Soc Exp Biol Med 1995;210:93–101.

19. Belmont HM, Levartovsky D, Goel A, et al. Increased nitric oxide production accompanied by the up-regulation of inducible nitric oxide synthase in vascular endothelium from patients with systemic lupus erythematosus. Arthritis Rheum 1997;40:1810–1816.

20. Amin AR, Abramson SB. The role of nitric oxide in articular cartilage breakdown in osteoarthritis. Curr Opin Rheumatol 1998;10:263–268.

21. Ginsberg MH. Role of platelets in inflammation and rheumatic disease. Adv Inflamm Res 1986;2:53–71.

22. Marcus AJ. Platelets: their role in hemostasis, thrombosis, and inflammation. In: Gallin JI, Snyderman R (eds). Inflammation: Basic Principles and Clinical Correlates, 3rd ed. Philadelphia: Lippincott Williams and Wilkins, 1999; pp 77–95.

23. McNeil HP, Gotis-Graham I. Human mast cell subsets – distinct functions in inflammation? Inflamm Res 2000;49:3–7.

24. Bingham CO III, Austen KF. Mast cell responses in the development of asthma. J Allergy Clin Immunol 2000;105: S527–S534.

25. Church MK, Levi-Schaffer F. The human mast cell. J Allergy Clin Immunol 1997;99:155–160.

26. Weller PF. Human eosinophils. J Allergy Clin Immunol 1997; 100:283–287.

MEDIATORS OF INFLAMMATION, TISSUE DESTRUCTION, AND REPAIR
B. Growth Factors and Cytokines

Cytokines are small molecular-weight proteins that mediate communication between cells. The generic term "cytokine" includes colony-stimulating factors, growth factors, interleukins, and interferons. The terminology of these molecules is confusing because it is largely historically based rather than functionally based. For example, some interleukins primarily serve to regulate cell growth and differentiation, whereas some growth factors have other major properties.

Cytokines carry out their functions largely in the immediate pericellular environment, either in an autocrine fashion, influencing the same cell that produced the cytokine, or in a paracrine fashion, influencing adjacent cells. Cytokines bind to specific plasma-membrane receptors on target cells. Subsequent activation of secondary messenger pathways or other intracellular mechanisms leads to alterations in transcription and production of proteins.

Cytokines are involved as mediator molecules in normal biologic processes. These physiologic functions include growth and differentiation of hematopoietic, lymphoid, and mesenchymal cells, as well as orchestration of host defense mechanisms. Multiple cytokines operate as a network in a redundant, overlapping, and synergistic manner. However, the cytokine network is largely self-regulating, and pathophysiologic consequences may result from the unregulated

action or inappropriate production of particular cytokines.

This chapter's review of cytokines uses arbitrary groupings based on primary functions. These categorizations include colony-stimulating factors, growth and differentiation factors, immunoregulatory cytokines, and proinflammatory cytokines (Table 4B-1). This chapter also emphasizes the relevance of each cytokine to the function of lymphoid and inflammatory cells, particularly its possible role in rheumatic diseases. The self-regulatory nature of the cytokine network also is discussed, in a review of mechanisms that inhibit the effects of cytokines.

Colony-Stimulating Factors

Colony-stimulating factors (CSFs) and related molecules function primarily as hematopoietic growth factors (1). However, this group of cytokines also demonstrates profound effects on mature lymphocytes, neutrophils, monocytes, and macrophages. It is in these latter effects that CSFs may play significant roles in rheumatic diseases.

Granulocyte-macrophage CSF (GM-CSF) and interleukin (IL)-3 potentiate the growth of numerous early bone marrow precursor cells, whereas erythropoietin influences only erythroid precursor cells. Each of these factors is preceded in its

TABLE 4B-1
Functional Classification of Cytokines

Colony-stimulating factors (CSFs)
  GM-CSF (granulocyte-macrophage CSF)
  G-CSF (granulocyte CSF)
  M-CSF (macrophage CSF or CSF-1)
  IL-3 (interleukin 3)
  Erythropoietin

Growth and differentiation factors
  PDGF (platelet-derived growth factor)
  EGF (epidermal growth factor)
  FGF (fibroblast growth factor)
  TGF-β (transforming growth factor β)
  ODF (osteoclast differentiation factor)

Immunoregulatory cytokines
  IFN-γ (interferon γ)
  IL-2, 4, 5, 7, and 9–18

Proinflammatory cytokines
  TNF-α (tumor necrosis factor α)
  IL-1, 6, and 8

Anti-inflammatory cytokines and growth and differentiation factor inhibitors
  IL-1Ra (interleukin-1 receptor antagonist)
  IL-4, 10, and 13
  OPG (osteoprotegerin)

the presence of GM-CSF produce more IL-1 receptor antagonist (IL-1Ra), possibly leading to an inhibition of IL-1 effects. These properties of GM-CSF illustrate an essential principle of cytokine biology: A single cytokine may exhibit activating and suppressing effects simultaneously.

The possible role of GM-CSF in rheumatic diseases is illustrated best by rheumatoid arthritis (RA). This is the only human disease in which both GM-CSF protein and mRNA are known to be localized in the damaged tissue. GM-CSF also is present in RA synovial fluids. The enhanced expression of class II MHC molecules observed on macrophages from RA synovial tissue may be secondary to the effects of GM-CSF.

Interleukin 1 and tumor necrosis factor α (TNF-α) stimulate monocytes, fibroblasts, and endothelial cells to produce more GM-CSF. Some investigators believe that chronic inflammation and tissue destruction in some people with RA may result from a cytokine-mediated self-perpetuating cycle without a significant component of continuous T-cell activation.

Growth and Differentiation Factors

A number of cytokines exhibit as their major property a growth enhancement of specific cell types. These cytokines include platelet-derived growth factor (PDGF), epidermal growth factor (EGF), fibroblast growth factor (FGF), and transforming growth factor β (TGF-β). Other cytokines, such as the CSFs and many of the interleukins, also promote growth.

PDGF primarily is a product of platelets but also is produced by macrophages, endothelial cells, and other cells. There are three different forms of PDGF and two different PDGF receptors. The biologic properties exhibited by PDGF vary with the form synthesized by a particular cell and the predominant receptor expressed on a target cell. EGF is found throughout the body and is a potent angiogenic factor, as is FGF. Two main forms of FGF exist, but many structural variants have been described. Both EGF and FGF induce the growth and proliferation of a variety of mesenchymal and epithelial cells, and FGF also may stimulate osteoclasts in the rheumatoid synovium.

The marked proliferation of synovial fibroblasts that occurs in RA synovium probably is secondary to the effects of PDGF, EGF, and FGF. Tissue fibrosis present in other diseases, such as scleroderma, may also be due in part to PDGF, EGF, and FGF. The greatly enhanced growth of new capillaries that characterizes synovitis in RA likely is a result of multiple factors, including FGF, IL-8, TNF-α, and vascular endothelial growth factor (VEGF). These growth factors are all present in synovial fluids of people with RA and are produced by synovial macrophages.

The importance of angiogenesis in the pathophysiology of rheumatoid synovitis has been reviewed (2). Both angiogenic inducers and inhibitors are present in the joint fluid and tissue, with the balance between the two sets of factors deter-

actions by other stem-cell growth and differentiation factors. The effects of GM-CSF and IL-3 are enhanced by the presence of IL-1 and IL-6. In contrast, granulocyte CSF (G-CSF) influences the growth and function of mature neutrophils, and macrophage CSF (M-CSF) serves the same role for monocytes and macrophages. GM-CSF, G-CSF, and M-CSF are produced by monocytes, fibroblasts, and endothelial cells; in addition, GM-CSF is produced by T lymphocytes.

In addition to its effects as a growth factor, GM-CSF influences the function of mature cells of the granulocytic and monocytic lineages. GM-CSF primes neutrophils, eosinophils, and basophils to respond to triggering agents with enhanced chemotaxis, oxygen radical production, and phagocytosis. GM-CSF also enhances eosinophil cytotoxicity and stimulates basophil release of histamine. These multiple effects of GM-CSF serve to heighten the inflammatory response in acute rheumatic diseases.

GM-CSF also influences diverse functions of monocytes and macrophages, leading to an enhanced ability of these cells to present antigen and induce an immune response. These functions include increased expression of membrane-bound IL-1a and of class II molecules of the major histocompatibility complex (MHC). Monocytes differentiated in mining whether new capillary growth will predominate. Compared with cells from controls, peripheral blood monocytes from RA patients produce greatly enhanced amounts of VEGF in response to TNF-α stimulation, and synovial lining macrophages in this disease contain large amounts of VEGF mRNA. In fact, when IL-1 and TNF-α in rheumatoid synovial membrane cultures were neutralized with IL-1Ra and a monoclonal antibody to TNF-α, VEGF release was reduced by approximately 50%. The administration of angiogenesis inhibitors effectively reduced inflammation and tissue destruction in two animal models of arthritis.

The last and most important growth factor to be discussed, TGF-β, has both potent proinflammatory and anti-inflammatory effects (Table 4B-2) (3). TGF-β exhibits many biologic properties, but its most important effects in rheumatic diseases include recruitment of monocytes into tissues, dampening of lymphocyte and macrophage functions, and stimulation of tissue fibrosis. More than any other cytokine, TGF-β exemplifies the apparent paradox of simultaneously enhancing inflammatory responses and promoting repair. In general, TGF-β is stimulatory toward resting or immature cells and when confined to local environments, but is inhibitory toward differentiated cells and when present systemically.

TGF-β is the major member of a family of molecules that may serve important roles in embryogenesis of mesenchymal tissues. Many cells in the adult contain mRNA for TGF-β, but macrophages and platelets are the main sources of protein. TGF-β is released in a latent form and must be activated in tissues, presumably by proteases.

The presence of other cytokines in a particular tissue may influence whether TGF-β enhances or inhibits growth and differentiation in fibroblasts. For example, TGF-β and EGF together may suppress the growth of particular types of fibroblasts, whereas the combination of TGF-β and PDGF stimulates their growth. The enhancing effects of TGF-β on cell growth may be mediated by inducing PDGF production. TGF-β induces production of collagen and fibronectin in fibroblasts; however, interferon gamma (IFN-γ) and TNF-α both oppose this effect on collagen synthesis. In the presence of PDGF, EGF, or FGF, TGF-β inhibits fibroblast production of collagenase and other neutral proteases, while enhancing production of inhibitors of these enzymes.

TGF-β is thought to be responsible, at least in part, for tissue fibrosis in a variety of human diseases, including scleroderma, pulmonary fibrosis, and chronic glomerulonephritis. Infiltrating monocytes in skin and organ lesions of scleroderma contain TGF-β mRNA. TGF-β protein has been found in skin lesions adjacent to fibroblasts and areas of fibrosis. The observation that IFN-γ inhibits TGF-β–induced collagen production by fibroblasts in vitro led to clinical trials of IFN-γ in people with scleroderma. Unfortunately, no clear clinical benefit of IFN-γ administration was observed in established dermal fibrosis in this disease.

TGF-β exhibits potent effects on monocytes and lymphocytes. TGF-β is the strongest known chemotactic agent for monocytes. In addition, TGF-β enhances expression of Fc receptor III on these cells but may block production of cytokines. It may promote inflammation; injection of TGF-β into rat joints leads to an influx of monocytes, with swelling, redness, and eventual hyperplasia of synovial fibroblasts. However, the net effects of TGF-β on macrophage function are suppressive and include a decrease in human leukocyte antigen (HLA)-DR expression and a deactivation of H_2O_2 production. Overall, TGF-β is thought to call monocytes into an acutely inflamed tissue, contribute to fibroblast proliferation, and then promote fibrosis.

TGF-β exhibits immunosuppressive effects on B cells, T cells, and natural killer (NK) cells. TGF-β inhibits IL-1–induced T-cell proliferation, B-cell growth, and immunoglobulin (Ig) production after stimulation by IL-

TABLE 4B-2
Roles of TGF-β in Human Inflammatory Diseases

Proinflammatory effects of TGF-β
Locally stimulates resting or immature monocytes, lymphocytes, and chondrocytes
Recruits monocytes into inflammatory tissues
Enhances cell growth primarily through induction of PDGF production
Stimulates collagen production by fibroblasts, with subsequent tissue fibrosis
May be involved in inducing fibrosis in scleroderma and interstitial lung disease
Stimulates angiogenesis

Anti-inflammatory effects of TGF-β
Inhibitory towards differentiated cells and when present systemically
Leads to a decrease in monocyte HLA-DR expression and in H_2O_2 production
Inhibits B-cell and T-cell growth and proliferation and is generally immunosuppressive
Blocks NK-cell activation induced by IFN-γ
Inhibits IFN-γ–induced collagen production in fibroblasts

TGF, transforming growth factor; PDGF, platelet-derived growth factor; HLA-DR, human leukocyte antigen-DR; NK, natural killer; IFN, interferon.

2 and IL-4. IFN-γ–induced NK-cell function is opposed by TGF-β. The immunosuppression that occurs in streptococcal cell-wall–induced arthritis in rats is thought to be secondary to TGF-β, and a similar situation may exist in the joints of people with RA.

Bone resorption in RA may be secondary to the effects of osteoclasts under the influence of osteoclast differentiation factor (ODF) (4). ODF may be synthesized by synovial fibroblasts and T cells, and it acts with M-CSF to induce differentiation of synovial monocytes into osteoclasts. A specific inhibitor of ODF has been described, osteoprotegerin (OPG), which binds to both soluble and membrane ODF to prevent interaction with cell-surface receptors on osteoclast precursors. Treatment of animal models of arthritis with OPG prevents cartilage and bone destruction but does not reduce inflammation. The balance between ODF and OPG in the rheumatoid synovium may influence the relative degree of bone erosion. These exciting new findings establish a foundation for novel therapeutic approaches to inhibit the effects of osteoclasts, not only in RA but also in osteoporosis.

Thus, growth and differentiation factors may be primarily responsible for fibroblast proliferation, angiogenesis, and bone resorption in many human chronic inflammatory diseases. In addition, TGF-β may be involved in enhancing acute inflammatory events. It should be emphasized that these net biologic effects are secondary to multiple cytokines acting in both synergistic and opposing fashions, and the state of differentiation of potential target cells for growth factors influences the resultant biologic response.

Immunoregulatory Cytokines

Interleukins 2, 4, 5, 7, 9, 10, and 11 and IFN-γ are produced by T-cell subsets during an immune response, and they exert effects primarily on that response. In addition, IL-4, IL-10, and IFN-γ exhibit important effects on monocytes and macrophages. Other recently described immunoregulatory cytokines include interleukins 12–18.

T helper (Th) cells are divided into two subsets: Th1 cells produce IFN-γ, IL-2, TNF-α, and IL-1; Th2 cells secrete IL-4, IL-5, and IL-10. In part, these cytokines function to regulate differentiation of T-cell subsets. Th1-cell differentiation is enhanced by IFN-γ and IL-12, the latter of which is produced primarily by macrophages and NK cells. However, Th1-cell differentiation is suppressed by IL-4 and IL-10. In contrast, Th2-cell differentiation is enhanced by IL-4 and inhibited by IFN-γ and IL-12.

Macrophage presentation of processed antigen in complex with a class II MHC molecule stimulates IL-2 production by CD4$^+$ helper T cells. Interleukin 2 then binds to a specific two-chain receptor on target cells in the immediate microenvironment. Interleukin 2 induces a clonal expansion of T cells, enhances B-cell growth, augments NK-cell function, and activates macrophages.

Interleukin 2 production originally was thought to be deficient in people with such autoimmune diseases as RA

and systemic lupus erythematosus (SLE). However, these observations may represent an in vitro artifact, and IL-2 production actually may be excessive in these diseases in vivo. The administration of monoclonal antibodies to the IL-2 receptor ameliorates collagen-induced arthritis (CIA) and lupus in mice. This observation argues for the probable importance of IL-2–driven T-cell responses in the counterpart human diseases of RA and SLE.

Soluble IL-2 receptors are found in the circulation of many people with autoimmune, chronic inflammatory, or neoplastic diseases. These receptors probably are released by activated T cells, and their circulating levels correlate with clinical disease activity in some diseases, including SLE. However, these molecules do not inhibit IL-2 in vivo and their presence in circulation merely reflects T-cell activation.

Like Th2 cells, mast cells produce IL-4 (5). Interleukin 4 exerts a major influence on B cells by enhancing IgG$_1$ and IgE production, inducing the expression of Fc receptors for IgE, and stimulating the expression of class II MHC molecules. Interleukin 4 exhibits stimulatory and suppressive effects on mononuclear phagocytes, again illustrating the principle that a single cytokine may produce mixed or opposing consequences. Interleukin 4 enhances the ability of these cells to present antigen by inducing the expression of class II MHC molecules. Paradoxically, IL-4 directly inhibits monocyte production of IL-1, IL-6, and TNF-α at the level of transcription; these effects of IL-4 potentially are quite anti-inflammatory.

Interleukin 10 and IL-13 function similarly to IL-4 in suppressing monocyte function, although IL-13 is present only in low amounts in the rheumatoid synovium (6,7). Further anti-inflammatory effects of IL-4, IL-10, and IL-13 include the induction of IL-1Ra production. Interleukin 4 also inhibits the production of tissue-degrading neutral metalloproteinases by rheumatoid synovial cells in vitro. Administration of IL-4, either by recombinant-protein injection or gene therapy, is markedly inhibitory to cartilage and bone destruction in CIA in mice (8). IL-4–induced signal transduction molecules are up-regulated in the rheumatoid synovium, although IL-4 protein is present only in small amounts (9). Thus, IL-4 may be exerting anti-inflammatory effects in this tissue, but the cytokine balance remains in favor of the proinflammatory cytokines such as IL-1 and TNF-α.

Interleukins 5, 7, 9, 11, 14, 15, and 16 function primarily as growth and differentiation factors. Interleukin 5 is produced by T cells and enhances the immune response through effects on T and B cells. IL-5 increases IL-2 receptor expression on these cells and promotes antibody secretion by B cells. In addition, IL-5 is the most active known cytokine on eosinophils, inducing chemotaxis, enhancing growth, and stimulating superoxide production. Interleukin 14 is a potent growth factor for B cells.

Interleukins 7, 9, 11, 15, and 16 are primarily growth factors for T lymphocytes. IL-7 and IL-11 are synthesized by bone marrow stromal cells and exhibit additional effects on B cells and hematopoietic cells. Interleukin 7 is a requisite factor for IL-1–induced thymocyte proliferation. These cytokines influence the function of other cells in addition to T lymphocytes. Interleukin 9 induces proliferation of mast cells; IL-11 synergizes with IL-3 stimulation of megakaryocytes; IL-11, like IL-1 and IL-6, induces the hepatic synthesis of acute-phase proteins; and IL-11 enhances antigen-specific B-cell responses. IL-15 shares biologic properties with IL-2 and is present in high concentrations in RA joints, where it may be responsible for attracting and activating T cells. IL-16 is a chemoattractant for CD4+ T cells.

Unlike IL-2, most immunoregulatory cytokines have not been directly incriminated in pathophysiologic events in rheumatic diseases. However, these cytokines are involved indirectly through their effects on T lymphocytes and other cells. Endogenous IL-4 and IL-5 may play a role in asthma, and endogenous IL-4, IL-10, and IL-13 may dampen synovitis in RA.

Interleukin 17 is a recently characterized cytokine that exhibits biologic functions relevant to joint diseases (Table 4B-3). IL-17 is produced by activated memory CD4+ T cells, and this protein and mRNA are found in large amounts in rheumatoid synovium (10). IL-17 exhibits many proinflammatory effects, including induction of IL-1 and TNF-α production by human macrophages, stimulation of metalloproteinase (MMP)-1 and MMP-9 production by synovial cells, enhancement of nitric oxide production by cartilage, and stimulation of osteoclast differentiation. A single injection of IL-17 into the knees of normal rabbits led to proteoglycan degradation, similar to the effects of IL-1. Inhibition of the production or effects of IL-17 is a potential therapeutic strategy in RA.

Interleukin 18 is another new cytokine that may be important in human disease, particularly in RA as an inducer of the chronic Th1 response present in the synovium (Table 4B-3) (11). The combination of IL-18 with IL-12 or IL-15 induces IFN-γ production in Th1 and NK cells. However, IL-18 exhibits other proinflammatory effects, such as enhancement of GM-CSF, IL-1, and TNF-α production by synovial-lining macrophages. Elevated levels of IL-18 protein and mRNA are present in the rheumatoid synovium, with production by macrophages, chondrocytes, and osteoblasts. A natural inhibitor of IL-18, the IL-18 binding protein, recently has been described and currently is being examined for effects in animal models of arthritis.

IFN-γ is produced simultaneously with IL-2 by antigen-stimulated T cells. A major function of IFN-γ is to enhance antigen presentation by stimulating the expression of MHC class I and II molecules on macrophages, endothelial cells, fibroblasts, and other more tissue-specific cells. IFN-γ also is a potent activator of macrophages, cytotoxic T cells, and NK cells. In addition, IFN-γ stimulates antibody production by B cells but, paradoxically, opposes the effects of IL-4 on these cells. This paradox is an example of self-regulation of the cytokine network through opposing effects.

IFN-γ may be relevant to many human autoimmune diseases, particularly SLE and RA. In SLE, the poor production of IFN-γ by T cells in vitro and the weak response to IFN-γ may reflect cells exhausted by intense IFN-γ effects in vivo, similar to IL-2. In RA, IFN-γ could antagonize the stimulatory effects of TNF-α on many functions of synovial fibroblasts. IFN-γ production probably is deficient in the

TABLE 4B-3
Roles of Interleukins 17 and 18 in Inflammatory Joint Disease

Interleukin 17
Produced by activated memory CD4+ T cells
Protein and mRNA present in high levels in the rheumatoid synovium
Stimulates IL-1 and TNF-α production in human monocytes and macrophages
Induces MMP production by synovial fibroblasts
Enhances nitric oxide production by chondrocytes
Decreases chondrocyte proliferation and proteoglycan synthesis
Stimulates osteoclast differentiation into bone-resorbing cells

Interleukin 18
Produced by macrophages, keratinocytes, chondrocytes, fibroblasts, and osteoblasts
Production stimulated by IL-1 and TNF-α
Protein and mRNA present in high levels in the rheumatoid synovium
Stimulates IFN-γ production by Th1 and NK cells, in combination with IL-12 and IL-15, to promote a Th1 phenotype
Induces GM-CSF, IL-1, and TNF-α production by synovial macrophages
Stimulates nitric oxide production by synovial cells
Relative effects in vivo may be counteracted by IL-18 binding protein, a naturally occurring inhibitor

IL, interleukin; TNF, tumor necrosis factor; MMP, metalloproteinase; IFN, interferon; Th, T helper; NK, natural killer; GM-CSF, granulocyte-macrophage colony-stimulating factor.

rheumatoid synovium, predisposing to unregulated TNF-α effects. However, the therapeutic administration of IFN-γ in RA patients appears to offer only modest benefit.

IL-10 is overproduced in SLE, RA, and Sjögren's syndrome and may be involved in some of the pathophysiologic events in these diseases. IL-10 may be involved in enhancing autoantibody production and in inhibiting T-cell function in people with SLE. First- and second-degree relatives of people with SLE demonstrate markedly increased IL-10 production by peripheral B cells and monocytes, in comparison with controls, further implicating excess IL-10 as one predisposing factor in this disease (12). Anti-IL-10 treatment prevents and ameliorates murine models of SLE and appears to have beneficial effects in people with SLE (13).

Thus, the immunoregulatory cytokines may be important in rheumatic disease for their effects on immune cells and macrophages. The possibility of manipulating this group of cytokines for therapeutic advantage has yet to be completely explored.

Proinflammatory Cytokines

The last group of cytokines to be discussed includes TNF-α and interleukins 1, 6, and 8. The functions of these molecules in normal physiology remain unclear, but an understanding of their possible role as inadvertent mediators of inflammation and tissue necrosis continues to grow. TNF-α and IL-1 usually are produced together and may act separately or together in different diseases. The roles of IL-1 and TNF-α in RA have assumed increasing importance with the successful development of therapeutic agents that inhibit their effects (14–16).

TNF-α and TNF-β are related molecules that share the same receptors on the plasma membranes of target cells. TNF-α structurally resembles a transmembrane molecule, and 1%–2% of TNF-α produced resides in the plasma membrane. TNF-α is produced by monocytes, macrophages, lymphocytes, and a variety of transformed cell lines. TNF-α production is stimulated by endotoxin, viruses, and other cytokines. TNF-α receptors p55 and p75 are present on a variety of target cells, and the extracellular portions of these receptors can be cleaved, probably by proteases, releasing soluble receptors. Endogenously produced soluble TNF receptors may function as regulators of extracellular TNF-α effects.

TNF-α exhibits many biologic properties that may be relevant to rheumatic diseases. Along with IL-1, TNF-a induces collagenase and prostaglandin E_2 (PGE_2) production in synovial fibroblasts. TNF-α is present in RA synovial tissues and may be an important inducer of IL-1 in this disease. TNF-α also may induce muscle breakdown and has been associated with the cachexia of congestive heart failure and other chronic diseases. In addition, TNF-α may play pathophysiologic roles in sepsis syndrome and in acute respiratory distress syndrome.

The IL-1 family has at least three known members: two proinflammatory agonists, IL-1α and IL-1β, and a specific naturally occurring inhibitor, IL-1Ra. The two agonists bind to the same receptors and generally produce the same biologic responses, whereas IL-1Ra competitively inhibits receptor binding of IL-1 (14). IL-1α and IL-1β primarily are products of monocytes and macrophages but may also may be produced by endothelial cells, epithelial cells, fibroblasts, activated T cells, and numerous other cells. In humans, IL-1β is the major extracellular product, whereas IL-1α remains primarily membrane-bound.

Two different IL-1 receptors exist. Type I receptors are present on T cells, endothelial cells, and fibroblasts, and type II receptors predominate on B cells, monocytes, and neutrophils (14). Only type I IL-1 receptors are functionally active, whereas type II IL-1 receptors are not capable of inducing intracellular signals. Target cells are exquisitely sensitive to small concentrations of IL-1; occupancy of only 1%–2% of available type I IL-1 receptors stimulates a cell to display complete biologic responses. The expression of type I IL-1 receptors can be down-regulated by TGF-β, partially explaining the immunosuppressive properties of this cytokine.

IL-1 exhibits systemic and local biologic effects in acute and chronic inflammatory disease. Some systemic effects of IL-1 include fever, muscle breakdown and, like IL-6 and IL-11, induction of acute-phase proteins in the liver. The local effects of IL-1 are important in the pathophysiology of joint disease in RA (15). Early in this disease process, IL-1 may enhance expression of adhesion molecules on endothelial cells and induce chemotaxis of neutrophils, monocytes, and lymphocytes into the synovium. Furthermore, IL-1 may contribute to tissue destruction in the rheumatoid joint by inducing PGE_2 and collagenase production by synovial fibroblasts and by chondrocytes present in the articular cartilage. IL-1 may exert similar effects on fibroblasts in other immune and inflammatory diseases, producing tissue damage in lungs, kidneys, or other organs.

IL-6 and IL-8 also play important roles in acute inflammatory diseases. IL-6 is produced in many cells, including synovial cells stimulated by IL-1 or TNF-α. The major functions of IL-6 probably are to induce hepatic synthesis of acute-phase proteins and to enhance Ig synthesis by B cells (17). High levels of IL-6 are present in inflammatory synovial fluids, and IL-6 is present in fibroblasts found in the synovium of RA patients. However, in RA, IL-6 does not induce collagenase and PGE_2 production by synovial fibroblasts and actually may enhance synthesis of a collagenase inhibitor. Interleukin 6 may be primarily responsible for the hypergammaglobulinemia that characterizes many chronic inflammatory diseases.

Interleukin 8 is one member of a family of chemotactic peptides (18). TNF-α and IL-1 stimulate IL-8 production by monocytes, macrophages, endothelial cells, fibroblasts, and other cells. IL-8 is an extremely potent chemotactic factor for neutrophils and may be responsible for attracting these cells into the joint in RA, gout, and other forms of inflammatory arthritis. In addition, IL-8 enhances other neutrophil properties, including expression of adhesion molecules, generation of oxygen radicals, and release of lysosomal enzymes. Thus,

IL-8 may contribute to rheumatic diseases by calling neu-trophils into sites of acute inflammation and by activating these cells into an enhanced destructive profile. Other chemokines may be involved in the migration of monocytes into inflamed joints, such as macrophage inflammatory pro-tein-1α and monocyte chemoattractant protein 1.

Regulation of Cytokine Effects

As emphasized throughout this chapter, the cytokine net-work functions in a self-regulatory fashion. Five different mechanisms regulate the actions of cytokines: specific receptor antagonists, soluble cytokine receptors, antibodies to cytokines, opposing actions of different cytokines, and protein binding of cytokines. Cytokine-inhibiting therapeu-tic agents would appear to have an important effect in RA (Table 4B-4).

A specific receptor antagonist of IL-1 originally was described in the supernatants of monocytes cultured on adherent IgG and in the urine of febrile patients (19). IL-1Ra is related structurally to IL-1 and binds to both types of human IL-1 receptors on a variety of target cells without inducing discernable biologic responses. IL-1Ra represents the first known naturally occurring molecule that functions as a specific receptor antagonist.

A secreted form of IL-1Ra is produced by monocytes, macrophages, and neutrophils. An intracellular variant of IL-1Ra (icIL-1Ra), which lacks the structural characteristics that lead to secretion, is produced by keratinocytes and other epithelial cells. Additional forms of icIL-1Ra have been described in macrophages, neutrophils, and other cells; it remains unknown whether these molecules perform unique functions inside cells. Alveolar and synovial macrophages secrete little IL-1β, but synthesize large

TABLE 4B-4
Inhibition of Cytokine Effects in RA

Agents with demonstrated clinical responses
IL-1Ra (anakinra)
Soluble TNF receptors (etanercept)
Monoclonal antibody to TNF-α (infliximab)

Possible future directions
Combination of IL-1Ra and a TNF inhibitor
Administer anti-inflammatory cytokines such as IL-4,
   IL-10, or IL-13

Block effects of additional inflammatory cytokines
Monoclonal antibody to IL-6, IL-8, or IL-12
Receptor antagonists to IL-8, IL-12, or IL-17
Soluble receptor to IL-15
Specific binding protein to IL-18

IL-1Ra, interleukin-1 receptor antagonist; TNF, tumor necrosis factor.

amounts of IL-1Ra, particularly under the influence of GM-CSF. Thus, IL-1Ra is a major product of tissue macrophages and may offer significant antagonism to IL-1 in the pericel-lular microenvironment of inflammatory tissues.

IL-1Ra has been extensively evaluated in vitro and in vivo, and this molecule blocks the inflammatory effects of IL-1 in every system evaluated. Most importantly, IL-1Ra does not affect normal T- or B-cell responses in vitro or in vivo, suggesting that IL-1 is not required for these responses. IL-1Ra has shown beneficial effects in many animal and in vitro models of human disease, including RA, septic shock, graft-versus-host disease, inflammatory bowel disease, chronic myelogenous leukemia, diabetes mellitus, and asth-ma. However, very high concentrations of IL-1Ra are required to block the effects of IL-1 in vivo, and IL-1Ra was found ineffective for treating people with sepsis syndrome.

Clinical trials in people with RA indicate that the daily subcutaneous administration of recombinant human IL-1Ra is clinically efficacious and safe. In a six-month trial, 43% of patients experienced a 20% American College of Rheumatology (ACR) response to IL-1Ra administration, compared with 27% in the placebo group (20). Furthermore, treatment with IL-1Ra for six or 12 months reduced radio-logic evidence of progression of both joint-space narrowing and bone erosion (21). IL-1Ra also has been delivered suc-cessfully by gene therapy in early feasibility trials in RA. A clinical trial in RA examining the simultaneous administra-tion of agents to inhibit both IL-1 and TNF-α is in progress.

Soluble cytokine receptors offer another possible mecha-nism to inhibit the cytokine network in vivo by binding cytokines in solution and blocking their interaction with tar-get cells. A truncated form of the type I IL-1 receptor was genetically engineered, but it was not effective as a thera-peutic agent in RA. Both types of TNF receptors occur in soluble forms and may be effective in blocking TNF effects in vitro and in vivo. Other soluble cytokine receptors have been described, but their in vivo relevance remains unclear.

A therapeutic agent containing the extracellular portion of the p75 TNF receptor coupled to the Fc portion of human IgG1, called etanercept, has proved effective and safe in RA. After six months of twice-weekly subcutaneous injections of this soluble TNF receptor, 20% ACR responses were observed in 59% of treated patients, compared with 11% in controls receiving placebo injections (22). Furthermore, in patients poorly responsive to methotrexate alone, ACR 20% responses were observed in 71% of patients receiving a combination of etanercept and methotrexate for six months, compared with 27% of patients treated with methotrexate alone (23).

Antibodies to many cytokines have been described in the serum of normal individuals, including antibodies to IL-1α (but not IL-1β), TNF-α, and IL-6. These antibodies appear to block the biologic effects of some cytokines, but their in vivo relevance has not been established. A chimeric murine/human monoclonal antibody to TNF-α, called infliximab, has been shown to be quite effective in the treat-ment of RA. This agent was administered by intravenous infusion every one or two months. In people treated with both infliximab and methotrexate for 30 weeks, 50% experienced a 20% ACR response, compared with 20% receiving methotrexate and placebo (24).

Inhibition of TNF in RA also led to a decrease in radiologic progression of the disease after six to 12 months of treatment. Other forms of arthritis responding to anti-TNF therapy include juvenile rheumatoid arthritis (25), psoriatic arthritis (26), and ankylosing spondylitis (27). TNF inhibitors should not be administered to patients with active or latent infections, and the long-term risk of developing malignancies is not known. Up to 15% of patients receiving anti-TNF agents have developed antinuclear antibodies, with a few patients exhibiting a reversible clinical SLE syndrome.

Numerous examples have been given throughout this chapter of the opposing action of different cytokines. TGF-β has some opposing effects to IL-1 and TNF-α, whereas some effects of TGF-β are opposed by IFN-γ and TNF-α. IL-4 and IL-10 block monocyte production of IL-1, TNF-α, IL-6, and other cytokines. Whether these opposing biologic effects of cytokines can be used to treat human diseases has not been determined. Multiple cytokines bind to α2-macroglobulin in circulation; however, many of these cytokines retain partial or full biologic activities. Thus, protein binding of cytokines as a mechanism to inhibit the effects of cytokines in vivo has not been proved.

Conclusion

The field of cytokine biology is in its infancy. New cytokines continue to be discovered, and existing cytokines are found to possess previously unrecognized biologic properties. Cytokines do not exist solely to cause human diseases; rather, they are mediators of normal cellular events. Particular cytokines may cause unwanted consequences in human disease because they are produced in excess or because their effects are unregulated. Interference with the effects of IL-1 or TNF-α has proved efficacious in subsets of people with RA, and anti–IL-10 therapy may be effective in some people with SLE. Additional anticytokine therapies are under development for these and other rheumatic diseases (Table 4B-4).

WILLIAM P. AREND, MD

References

1. Lieschke GJ, Burgess AW. Granulocyte colony-stimulating factor and granulocyte-macrophage colony-stimulating factor. N Engl J Med 1992;327:28–35, 99–106.
2. Koch AE. Angiogenesis. Implications for rheumatoid arthritis. Arthritis Rheum 1998;41:951–962.
3. Blobe GC, Scheimann WP, Lodish HF. Mechanisms of disease: Role of transforming growth factor β in human disease. N Engl J Med 2000;342:1350–1358.
4. Gravallese EM, Goldring SR. Cellular mechanisms and the role of cytokines in bone erosions in rheumatoid arthritis. Arthritis Rheum 2000;43:2143-2151.
5. Paul WE. Interleukin-4: a prototypic immunoregulatory lymphokine. Blood 1991;77:1859–1870.
6. Mosmann TR. Properties and functions of interleukin-10. Adv Immunol 1994;56:1–26.
7. Woods JM, Haines GK, Shah MR, Rayan G, Koch AE. Low-level production of interleukin-13 in synovial fluid and tissue from patients with arthritis. Clin Immunol Immunopathol 1997;85:210–220.
8. Lubberts E, Joosten LAB, Chabaud M, et al. IL-4 gene therapy for collagen arthritis suppresses synovial IL-17 and osteoprotegerin ligand and prevents bone erosion. J Clin Invest 2000;105:1697–1710.
9. Muller-Ladner U, Judex M, Ballhorn W, et al. Activation of the IL-4 STAT pathway in rheumatoid synovium. J Immunol 2000;164:3894–3901.
10. Chabaud M, Durand JM, Buchs N, et al. Human interleukin-17: A T cell-derived proinflammatory cytokine produced by rheumatoid synovium. Arthritis Rheum 1999;42:963–970.
11. Gracie JA, Forsey RJ, Chan WL, et al. A proinflammatory role for IL-18 in rheumatoid arthritis. J Clin Invest 1999;104:1393–1401.
12. Llorente L, Richaud-Patin Y, Couderc J, et al. Dysregulation of interleukin-10 production in relatives of patients with systemic lupus erythematosus. Arthritis Rheum 1997;40:1429–1435.
13. Llorente L, Richaud-Patin Y, Garcia-Padilla C, et al. Clinical and biologic effects of anti-interleukin-10 monoclonal antibody administration in systemic lupus erythematosus. Arthritis Rheum 2000;43:1790–1800.
14. Dinarello C. Biologic basis for interleukin-1 in disease. Blood 1996;87:2095–2147.
15. Arend WP, Dayer JM. Inhibition of the production and effects of interleukin-1 and tumor necrosis factor a in rheumatoid arthritis. Arthritis Rheum 1995;38:151–160.
16. Feldmann M, Elliott MJ, Woody JN, Maini RN. Anti-tumor necrosis factor-α therapy of rheumatoid arthritis. Adv Immunol 1997;64:283–350.
17. Papanicolaou DA, Wilder RL, Manolagas SC, Chrousos GP. The pathophysiologic roles of interleukin-6 in human disease. Ann Intern Med 1998;128:127–137.
18. Luster AD. Chemokines – chemotactic cytokines that mediate inflammation. N Engl J Med 1998;338:436–445.
19. Arend WP, Malyak M, Guthridge CJ, Gabay C. Interleukin-1 receptor antagonist: role in biology. Annu Rev Immunol 1998;16:27–55.
20. Bresnihan B, Alvaro-Gracia JM, Cobby M, et al. Treatment of rheumatoid arthritis with recombinant human interleukin-1 receptor antagonist. Arthritis Rheum 1998;41:2196–2204.
21. Jiang Y, Genant HK, Watt I, et al. A multicenter, double-blind, dose-ranging, randomized, placebo-controlled study of recombinant human interleukin-1 receptor antagonist in patients with rheumatoid arthritis: radiologic progression and correlation of Genant and Larsen scores. Arthritis Rheum 2000;43:1001–1009.
22. Moreland LW, Schiff MH, Baumgartner SW, et al. Etanercept therapy in rheumatoid arthritis. A randomized, controlled trial. Ann Intern Med 1999;130:478–486.
23. Weinblatt ME, Kremer JM, Bankhurst AD, et al. A trial of etanercept, a recombinant tumor necrosis factor receptor: Fc

fusion protein, in patients with rheumatoid arthritis receiving methotrexate. N Engl J Med 1999;340:253–259.

24. *Maini R, St Clair EW, Breedveld F, et al. Infliximab (chimeric anti-tumour necrosis factor α monoclonal antibody) versus placebo in rheumatoid arthritis patients receiving concomitant methotrexate: a randomised phase III trial. Lancet 1999;354:1932–1939.*

25. *Lovell DJ, Giannini EH, Reiff A, et al. Etanercept in children with polyarticular juvenile rheumatoid arthritis. N Engl J Med 2000;342:763–769.*

26. *Mease PJ, Goffe BS, Metz J, VanderStoep A, Finck B, Burge DJ. Etanercept in the treatment of psoriatic arthritis and psoriasis: a randomised trial. Lancet 2000;356:385–390.*

27. *Brandt J, Haibel H, Cornely D, et al. Successful treatment of active ankylosing spondylitis with the anti-tumor necrosis factor α monoclonal antibody infliximab. Arthritis Rheum 2000; 43:1346–1352.*

MEDIATORS OF INFLAMMATION, TISSUE DESTRUCTION, AND REPAIR
C. The Complement System

The complement system, discovered more than 100 years ago as a bactericidal (lytic) substance, provides an innate defense against microbes and a "complement" to humoral immunity (see references 1–3 for in-depth reviews). It accomplishes this task by depositing on a target and promoting the inflammatory response. The early reaction sequences behave as biologic cascades in which, by limited proteolysis, one component activates the next, producing a rapid and robust amplification of the system. Because of their capacity to injure tissue, nearly one-half of complement proteins function as regulators or inhibitors (4,5).

In the setting of autoantibodies, complement components unwittingly serve as "inappropriately" guided missiles. Many rheumatic diseases are mediated by immune complexes (ICs). The complement system is critical to the normal handling of ICs, but it also can produce inflammation and tissue damage if ICs lodge in inappropriate locations, such as the joints or kidneys. Deficiencies of the activating components predispose the host to infections (6) and, surprisingly, autoimmune diseases, especially systemic lupus erythematosus (SLE) (7). Complement measurements facilitate the diagnosis and management of lupus and related rheumatic diseases. Further, the system's genetic deficiencies provide intriguing clues relative to the etiology of autoimmune syndromes. These issues, plus complement's putative role in clearance of apoptotic cells and tissue injured by ischemia-reperfusion, have led to a renaissance in the study of complement and its role in innate and adaptive immunity.

Complement Discovery and Function

An ancestral version of the complement system emerged more than 600 million years ago as a host defense system, predating adaptive immunity. Complement systems similar to that of mammals have been found in birds, reptiles, amphibians, fish, sharks, and ascidians. Complement was first identified in the 1890s as a heat-labile fraction of serum that assists (complements) a heat-stable fraction (antibody) to produce bacterial lysis. In the 1950s, a second pathway of complement activation was discovered; the alternative pathway, which provides natural (innate) immunity, can identify and destroy foreign elements *without the need for antibody*. The lectin pathway, characterized more recently, is similar to the activation scheme of

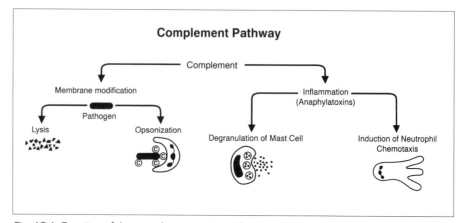

Fig. 4C-1. Function of the complement system. The most important function of complement is to alter the membrane of a pathogen by coating its surface with clusters of complement components (the phenomenon of opsonization). These complements, in turn, facilitate interactions with complement receptors and, in some cases, such as with certain Gram-negative bacteria and viruses, induce lysis. The second function of complement is to promote the inflammatory response. The complement fragments C3a and C5a (called anaphylatoxins) activate many cell types, such as mast cells, to release their contents and phagocytic cells to migrate to an inflammatory site (chemotaxis).

the classical pathway, except that it is triggered when a plasma protein with a lectin (sugar)-binding domain attaches to a carbohydrate moiety (such as mannose on the surface of a pathogen).

The complement system consists of plasma and membrane proteins. Plasma proteins are synthesized primarily in the liver but also locally by monocytes, macrophages, fibroblasts, and many types of epithelial cells. Membrane proteins are receptors with limited tissue distribution (mostly present on peripheral blood cells) and widely expressed regulatory proteins.

Following activation, the complement system functions in two major ways: it modifies membranes and promotes inflammation (Fig. 4C-1).

Membrane Modification

Activated complement components deposit in large amounts on microbes and ICs. For example, several million activation fragments can attach in clusters to a bacterial surface in less than five minutes. The most critical function of these deposited complement proteins is to *opsonize* or coat the target. These opsonic fragments are ligands for complement receptors on peripheral blood cells and tissue macrophages. This interaction, known as immune adherence, often is followed by phagocytosis of the opsonized IC. Such processing leads to elimination of the particle or IC. Additionally, the membranes of some microorganisms can be disrupted by the terminal complement components, resulting in lysis.

Promotion of Inflammation by Cell Activation

During complement activation, mediators are released to elicit a *local* inflammatory reaction. These fragments (C4a, C3a, and C5a) are called *anaphylatoxins* because, in excessive amounts, they may induce a reaction resembling anaphylaxis. By binding to their receptors at the site of complement activation, the anaphylatoxins trigger release of mediators (such as histamine) and cause smooth-muscle contraction. C5a and C3a also are chemotactic factors for phagocytic cells and eosinophils, respectively.

Nomenclature

The complement system is divided into three branches: the originally discovered classical pathway (CP), the antibody-independent alternative pathway (AP), and the recently described lectin pathway (LP). These pathways all lead to C3 activation and proceed to a common lytic pathway called the *membrane attack complex* (MAC). Nomenclature is as follows: the CP proteins are identified by numbers (C1, C2, C3, and C4,) and the AP proteins by capital letters (factors B, D, and P). The MAC consists of C5, C6, C7, C8, and C9. Upon proteolytic activation, a smaller fragment may be liberated and is designated by a lowercase "a," as in C3a. The larger fragment often attaches to a target and is noted with a "b," as in C3b. Limited proteolytic cleavage produces further breakdown

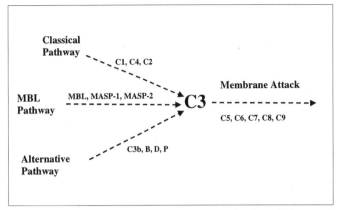

Fig. 4C-2. Pathways of complement activation. The three pathways of complement activation are shown, each leading to generation of activated C3 complex. The classical pathway is triggered by antibody interacting with antigen, and the lectin pathway is activated by a lectin binding to a sugar. The alternative pathway turns over continuously and becomes engaged only in the setting of a foreign material. Not shown are the anaphylatoxins, C3a, C4a, and C5a, that are liberated into the surrounding milieu. Modified with permission from Cooper NR. Inflammation: Basic Principles and Clinical Correlates, 3rd edition. Philadelphia: Lippincott Williams & Wilkins, 1999.

products designated by lowercase letters, such as when C3b is cleaved to iC3b, and then iC3b is in turn cleaved to C3c and C3dg.

Classical Pathway

Initiation

The CP is activated primarily by an interaction between C1 and immune complexes (see Fig. 4C-2). C1 is a large multicomponent protein consisting of a single molecule of C1q (bearing six globular "heads") and a serine-protease tetramer C1s-C1r-C1s-C1r. When at least two of the globular regions of C1q attach to the Fc portion of antibody, the CP is initiated. Immunoglobulin (Ig) M and IgG subclasses 1, 2, and 3 activate the CP, but IgA, IgD, IgE, and IgG_4 do not. C-reactive protein is an acute-phase reactant that can activate the CP upon binding to its ligand.

Enzyme Activation

After C1 binds to antibody, the C1r subcomponent undergoes an autoactivation cleavage process and then cleaves C1s. C1s, in turn, cleaves C4 and C2. Large cleavage fragments derived from C4 (C4b) and C2 (C2a, an exception to the rule that only smaller fragments are designated with an "a") assemble on the target surface and on antibody, forming the C3 convertase, or C3-cleaving enzyme, C4b2a. C4 possesses a thioester that, upon activation by cleavage of C4 to C4b, allows C4b to covalently attach via ester or amide linkages. C3 also possesses this structural feature and usually binds to a substrate via an ester linkage. It is this remarkable mechanism that enables complement components to transfer from plasma to a target.

Amplification

Each activated C1 generates many C4b and C2a fragments. Most deposited C4bs serve as opsonins, but some engage a C2a to form a C3 convertase. Each C3 convertase can rapidly generate many activated C3 molecules. In a study quantitating CP-mediated activation by an antibody to a membrane antigen of nucleated cells (8), 2.4×10^6 C4 molecules and 0.67×10^6 C2a molecules subsequently attached. Within five minutes, 2.1×10^7 molecules of C3b were deposited, and approximately 1×10^6 MACs were formed in the same time period. Concomitantly, anaphylatoxins C4a, C3a, and C5a were generated, equal to the number of C4b, C3b, and C5b fragments formed.

Attack

Most C3bs that deposit on targets serve as opsonins. A smaller percentage covalently binds to C4b in the C4b2a enzymatic complex (C3 convertase) to generate a C5 convertase, C4b2a3b. C5 is the substrate for this trimeric enzyme complex. Generation of C5b leads to the formation of the MAC (C5b + C6 + C7 + C8 + multiple C9s). This assembly of the MAC occurs through protein–protein interactions (i.e., no proteolysis is involved after the step of C5 cleavage).

Lectin Pathway

Lectins are carbohydrate-binding proteins (9). They initially were described as proteins capable of agglutinating red blood cells, and they have been found to be important players in innate immunity and rheumatic diseases. In particular, mannan-binding lectin (MBL) is a serum protein that preferentially binds to repeating mannoses on pathogens. MBL resembles C1q in that it is an oligomer with a terminal collagenous domain on one end and a globular domain on the other. The main difference is that the carboxyl-terminus of MBL possesses a carbohydrate-recognition domain, whereas C1q has an immunoglobulin-binding domain. Like C1q, MBL engagement with a sugar leads to the activation of serine proteases similar to C1r and C1s, called MASP-1 and MASP-2, which also cleave C2 and C4. MBL deficiency is associated with recurrent infections early in life, and accumulating evidence suggests that this deficient state is a predisposing factor for SLE and rheumatoid arthritis and a disease severity indicator (9–12).

Alternative Pathway

The AP does not require antibody. Instead, a small amount of auto-activated C3 continuously turns over (so-called "C3 tickover") such that, if it encounters a foreign surface, it binds to the microbe and serves as the nidus for engagement of the AP. Although this is an apparent shotgun approach to host defense, it nonetheless provides an important surveillance or sentry-like role in the nonimmune host. Amplification rapidly occurs in the presence of foreign material but is blocked on host tissue by endogenous regulators.

Target-bound C3b binds factor B. The latter undergoes proteolytic cleavage mediated by a plasma serine protease factor D to produce the fragments Bb and Ba. The alternative pathway C3 convertase thus formed, C3bBb, is stabilized by properdin. As the stabilized convertase cleaves more C3 to C3b, a feedback loop (i.e., auto-amplification) is set in motion, resulting in the deposition of large amounts of C3b on a microbe (Fig. 4C-3). The AP also engages the MAC. In this case, the C5 convertase (C3bBbC3bP) cleaves C5 to C5b, and C5b initiates assembly of the MAC. A second major activity of the AP is to amplify, via the feedback loop, C3b deposition on a target. The initial C3b may be deposited by the CP, LP, or spontaneous tickover.

Complement Receptors

The complement system exerts many of its effects through its receptors (Table 4C-1). The ligands are generated during the activation process. For example, the vasomodulatory and chemotactic effects of C3a and C5a are due to interaction with their respective receptors. The opsonic fragments C4b and C3b mediate clearance of ICs and bacteria through complement receptors. Degradation of C3b by regulators leads to formation of iC3b and then C3dg, which in turn interact with additional complement receptors.

Complement receptor (CR) 1 plays an important role in IC clearance. CR1 on erythrocytes binds C3b/C4b-coated ICs for processing and transport to the liver and spleen. In these organs, the ICs are transferred from the erythrocyte to tissue macrophages, allowing the erythrocyte to return to the circulation for another round of clearance. CR1 on granulocytes and monocytes promotes IC adherence and

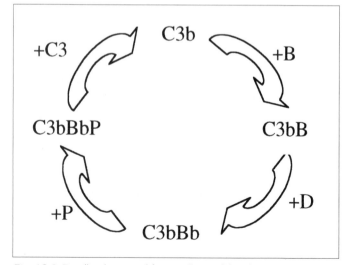

Fig. 4C-3. Feedback or amplification loop of the alternative pathway. If C3b is deposited by the alternative pathway (the classical or lectin pathways), it can engage the components shown above to generate more C3b. C3bBbP is the physiologic C3 convertase of the alternative pathway. The net effect of such amplification is rapid and massive deposition of C3b and convertases on the target. Not shown are the liberated fragments Ba and C3a.

TABLE 4C-1
Complement Receptors for C3 and C4

Name	Primary ligand	Location	Function
CR1	C3b/C4b	Peripheral blood cells, FDC	Immune adherence, phagocytosis, antigen localization
CR2	C3dg/C3d	B lymphocytes, FDC	Coreceptor for B-cell signaling; antigen localization
CR3/CR4	iC3b	Myeloid lineage	Phagocytosis, adherence

The CD numbers are CR1, CD35; CR2, CD21; CR3, CD11b/CD18; CR4, CD11c/CD18.
FDC, follicular-dendritic cells.

phagocytosis, whereas CR1 on B lymphocytes, tissue macrophages, and follicular-dendritic cells facilitates trapping and processing of ICs in lymphoid organs. CR2 is expressed on B lymphocytes and follicular-dendritic cells where it facilitates antigen localization and is a coreceptor for activation of the B cell antigen receptor (13). Coating of an antigen with several C3d fragments may enhance immunogenicity of the antigen up to 10,000-fold (14).

Control of the Complement System

Unregulated, the complement system would fire to exhaustion, a point well-illustrated by inborn errors of several regulatory proteins. Checks and balances occur at each of the major steps in the pathways (4,5). This regulation is designed to prevent excessive activation on one target, fluid-phase activation (i.e., no target), and activation on self (i.e., wrong target) but does not interfere with appropriate activation. In the early phase of the CP, C1 inhibitor prevents excessive fluid-phase C1 activation. The C3 and C5 convertases are regulated by a family of proteins that include the membrane proteins decay-accelerating factor (CD55) and membrane cofactor protein (CD46), and the serum inhibitors C4b-binding protein and factor H. These proteins function in two ways: by disassembling the convertases (decay-accelerating activity) and/or by facilitating proteolytic inactivation of C4b or C3b. The latter occurs in collaboration with the plasma serine protease factor I and is called cofactor activity. The MAC also is regulated by both a serum and a cell-anchored protein. CD59 is a glycolipid anchored protein that binds C8 and C9 to prevent proper MAC insertion, while the plasma protein vitronectin (S-protein) binds to and thereby inactivates the fluid-phase MAC. As a result of these regulators, complement attack is focused on foreign surfaces (which usually lack complement regulators)

and is held in check on host cells and in body fluids. Interestingly, a number of microorganisms have "captured" complement regulators or have evolved proteins that inhibit the system (virulence factors). However, the activation of the CP by antibody is so efficient that the inhibitors, in general, have modest effects on limiting damage by complement-fixing autoantibodies.

Complement and Rheumatic Disease

Complement is a double-edged sword in rheumatic diseases. It is needed for proper handling of ICs, but it also mediates tissue damage, especially in the setting of autoantibodies and excessive ICs. Deficiencies of any one of the early components of the CP represent a single gene defect that leads to autoimmunity, especially SLE (7,15).

Immune Complex Diseases
The pathophysiology of many inflammatory diseases involves the synthesis of autoantibodies and the presence of excessive quantities of IC. For example, if the host synthesizes an antibody reacting with a self-antigen on an erythrocyte, antibody will bind to the autoantigen and activate the complement cascade. Just as the complement system can destroy a microbe, it may lyse an erythrocyte, phagocytose a platelet, or disrupt a basement membrane. If ICs lodge in blood vessel walls of tissues, they may activate complement to produce synovitis, vasculitis, dermatitis, and glomerulonephritis.

Complement Deficiency
Inherited deficiencies of complement components predispose to bacterial infections (expected) or autoimmunity (unexpected), especially SLE (see Table 4C-2). Deficiencies are inherited as autosomal codominant (recessive) traits, except those of C1 inhibitor (autosomal dominant), and properdin and factor D (X-linked). Approximately 90% of

C1q-deficient individuals, 80% of C4-deficient individuals, and 40% of C2-deficient individuals present with lupus (7,16). The clinical illness tends to be more severe in C1q and C4 deficiency than in C2 deficiency. Early age of onset, prominent cutaneous manifestations, and presence of anti-Ro antibodies are features suggestive of a complement deficiency. C1r- or C1s-deficient patients also present with SLE.

Acquired complement deficiency results from accelerated consumption, as is the case for SLE, where CP activation is observed in >50% of people with SLE. Generally, the more active the disease, the more likely complement levels will be low, because consumption outstrips synthesis. Low complement values are a poor prognostic factor in SLE and correlate with anti-DNA antibodies and nephritis. Complement deposition in tissue, especially in the kidney glomerulus as detected by immunofluorescence, assists in the diagnosis and classification of lupus nephritis. Antibodies to C1q occur in 15%–30% of people with SLE, but their contribution to disease pathogenesis is not well understood. On certain genetic backgrounds, C1q-knockout mice develop a lupus syndrome with glomerulonephritis and antinuclear antibodies (ANA) (15,16). C4- or C2-knockout mice develop ANAs but no clinical disease (16).

TABLE 4C-2
Inherited Complement Deficiencies

Components	Major associated illness
C1, C4, or C2	SLE[a]
C3	Pyogenic infections
C5-9	*Neisseria* infections
D, B or Properdin	*Neisseria meningitides*
C1 Inhibitor	Hereditary angioedema
Factor H or I	Pyogenic infections (secondary deficiency of C3)

[a] More than 90% of C1q-deficient and more than 80% of C4-deficient individuals develop systemic lupus erythematosus (SLE); (7,15). Nearly 50% of C2-deficient individuals have lupus or a related rheumatic syndrome. C1r- or C1s-deficient patients also present with lupus. Further, partial deficiency of C4 also predisposes to SLE (7). C4 is synthesized as two proteins, called C4A and C4B, that are more than 99% homologous. C4 genes (two for C4A and two for C4B) are tandemly arranged on chromosome 6 in the major histocompatibility locus. The C4A deficiency in SLE is usually found as part of a human leukocyte antigen haplotype containing B8 and DR3. About 10%–15% of Caucasian SLE patients are homozygous for C4A deficiency.

"C3 nephritic factor" is an autoantibody against the alternative pathway C3 convertase. The autoantibody stabilizes the convertase to the point that excessive C3 cleavage and a secondary deficiency of C3 results. Most patients with C3 nephritic factor are children, who may present with glomerulonephritis, partial lipodystrophy, or frequent infections with encapsulated bacteria.

Complement Measurement

Complement can be assessed by functional or antigenic assays (Table 4C-3). The most commonly used functional measurement in clinical practice is the total hemolytic complement assay (THC, CH_{50}). The THC is based on the ability of the test serum to lyse sheep erythrocytes optimally sensitized with rabbit antibody. All nine components of the classical pathway (i.e., C1–C9) are required for a normal THC. A THC of 200 means that, at a dilution of 1:200, the test serum lysed 50% of the antibody-coated sheep erythrocytes. THC is a useful screening tool for detecting a homozygous deficiency of a complement component because a total deficiency of any one of the C1–C8 components will produce a zero THC. Deficiency of C9 will give a low but detectable THC.

Assays for C3 and C4 are widely available and usually are measured by nephelometric-based immunoassays. They are useful in the initial diagnosis of lupus and related syndromes and for following the course of patients who present with low levels while undergoing treatment. Table 4C-3 provides examples of serum-complement test results and their interpretation in rheumatic diseases.

Tests for the detection of activation fragments (such as C3a and C5a), neoantigens, and fragments of activation proteins (C3d, C4d, Bb) have become more available. Their clinical utility relates to the fact that they are dynamic activation parameters and thus reflect ongoing turnover of the system. These tests are not affected by partial inherited deficiencies or alterations in the synthetic rate, but they are more costly, not widely available, and not necessary in most clinical situations.

Therapeutic Implications of Complement

Study of the complement system has undergone a renaissance over the past decade. Much of this revival relates to: 1) the discovery and characterization of the regulatory and receptor proteins (4,5); 2) the development of inhibitors for experimental and clinical use (17,18); 3) strong association of deficiency states with autoimmunity (especially the recognition that C1q, C4, or C2 deficiency are single-gene defects that reproducibly lead to SLE in the human population, independent of background genetic influences) (7,15); 4) greater appreciation of the importance of the innate immune system in instructing the adaptive immune response (9,14,15,19); and 5) availability of knockout mice to analyze more precisely the role of complement in the normal immune response and in autoim-

TABLE 4C-3
Interpretation of the Results of Complement Determinations

THC (units/ml)	C4 (mg/dl)	C3 (mg/DL)	Interpretation
150–200	16–40	100–180	Normal range
250	40	200	Acute-phase response
100	10	80	CP activation
100	30	50	AP activation
<10 or 0	30	140	Inherited deficiency or in vitro activation[a]
50	<8	100	Partial C4 deficiency or fluid-phase activation[b]

THC, total hemolytic complement or CH_{50}; CP, classical pathway; AP, alternative pathway.

[a] In vitro activation is more common than an inherited deficiency state. The lack of activity (<10 THC) in the setting of normal C4 and C3 antigenic levels suggests: 1) an improperly handled sample; 2) cold activation (such as by cryoglobulins) following collection of the sample; or 3) homozygous component deficiency (most commonly C2 with a lupus presentation or, if a *Neisserial* infection, of an AP or membrane-attack-complex component).

[b] Because THC is detectable, this cannot be a complete deficiency of C4. A partial C4 deficiency, such as of C4A, could give this result. Some types of immune complexes or a deficiency of the C1-inhibitor (hereditary angioedema) also would give this pattern. Measurement of C2 would be helpful – a low value suggests activation, whereas a normal value suggests an inherited, partial C4 deficiency. Also, C4A and C4B alleles can be assessed by commercial laboratories.

munity (15,16). Of much potential interest and importance, especially for the treatment of rheumatic diseases, would be the development of complement inhibitors for clinical use. Currently, two such compounds, a monoclonal antibody to C5 and a solubilized version of CR1, are in clinical trials (17,18). Both are effective in attenuating tissue destruction and inflammatory responses in animal models, where considerable evidence already has pointed to a role for complement (e.g., Arthus reaction, serum sickness, and SLE). Complement inhibition also reduced infarct size in experimental models of myocardial infarction and tissue damage in many other types of ischemia-reperfusion injury. A role for complement in clearing apoptotic cells also is likely (20). These remarkable results suggest that the complement system is a major participant for removing necrotic and injured tissue. Although these two recombinantly produced inhibitors are not commercially available, they are undergoing phase II and phase III trials. These and other approaches eventually will spawn a complement inhibitor for clinical use.

Summary

The complement system provides natural immunity against microbes and "complements" the antibody-mediated system. It opsonizes targets and promotes the inflammatory process. In rheumatic disease states (especially those with

autoantibodies and excessive IC formation), complement contributes to tissue destruction, but it also is critical to the proper handling of ICs and to preventing autoimmunity, as evidenced by the development of SLE in most people with C1q or C4 deficiency. The development of inhibitors of the complement system for use in rheumatic diseases is much anticipated.

JOHN P. ATKINSON, MD
M. KATHRYN LISZEWSKI

References

1. Volanakis JE, Frank MM. *The Human Complement System in Health and Disease.* New York: Marcel Dekker, 1998.
2. Morgan BP. *Complement: Clinical Aspects and Relevance to Disease.* London: Harcourt Brace Jovanovich, 1990.
3. Whaley K, Loos M, Weiler JM. *Immunology and Medicine: Complement in Health and Disease,* 2nd ed. Boston: Kluwer Academic Publishers, 1993.
4. Morgan BP, Harris CL. *Complement Regulatory Proteins.* San Diego: Harcourt Brace & Company, 1999.
5. Liszewski MK, Farries TC, Lublin DM, Rooney IA, Atkinson JP. Control of the complement system. *Adv Immunol* 1996; 61:201–283.
6. Figueroa JE, Densen P. Infectious diseases associated with complement deficiencies. *Clin Microbiol Rev* 1991;4:359–395.

7. Bala Subramanian V, Liszewski MK, Atkinson JP. The complement system and autoimmunity. In: Lahita R, Chiorazzi N, Reeves W (eds). Textbook of the Autoimmune Diseases. Philadelphia: Lippincott-Raven, 2000; pp 117–135.

8. Ollert MW, Kadlec JV, David K, Petrella EC, Bredehorst R, Vogel CW. Antibody-mediated complement activation on nucleated cells. A quantitative analysis of the individual reaction steps. J Immunol 1994;153:2213–2221.

9. Turner MW. Mannose-binding lectin: the pluripotent molecule of the innate immune system. Immunol Today 1996;17:532–540.

10. Graudal NA, Madsen HO, Tarp U, et al. The association of variant mannose-binding lectin genotypes with radiographic outcome in rheumatoid arthritis. Arthritis Rheum 2000;43:515–521.

11. Garred P, Madsen HO, Halberg P, et al. Mannose-binding lectin polymorphisms and susceptibility to infection in systemic lupus erythematosus. Arthritis Rheum 1999;42:2145–2152.

12. Ip WK, Lau YL, Chan SY, et al. Mannose-binding lectin and rheumatoid arthritis in Southern Chinese. Arthritis Rheum 2000;43:1679–1687.

13. Nielsen CH, Rischer EM, Leslie RGQ. The role of complement in the acquired immune response. Immunology 2000;100:4–12.

14. Dempsey PW, Allison ME, Akkaraju S, Goodnow CC, Fearon DT. C3d of complement as a molecular adjuvant: bridging innate and acquired immunity. Science 1996;271:348–350.

15. Walport MJ, Davies KA, Morley BJ, Blotto M. Complement deficiency and autoimmunity. Annals NY Acad Sci 1997;815:267–281.

16. Holers VM. Phenotypes of complement knockouts. Immunopharmacology 2000;49:125–131.

17. Klickstein LB, Moore Jr FD, Atkinson JP. Therapeutic inhibition of complement activation with emphasis on drugs in clinical trials. In: Austen KF, Burakoff SJ, Strom TB, Rosen FS (eds). Therapeutic Immunology. Malden, MA: Blackwell Science, 2000.

18. Lambris JD, Holers VM. Therapeutic Interventions in the Complement System. Totowa, NJ: Humana Press, 1999.

19. Carroll MC. A protective role for innate immunity in autoimmune disease. Clin Immunol 2000;95:S30–S38.

20. Vaishnaw AK, McNally JD, Elkon KB. Apoptosis in the rheumatic diseases. Arthritis Rheum 1997;40:1917–1927.

MEDIATORS OF INFLAMMATION, TISSUE DESTRUCTION, AND REPAIR
D. Proteases and Their Inhibitors

The diarthrodial joint is composed of several different connective tissue types: cartilage, bone, synovium, ligament, tendon, and joint capsule. Turnover of extracellular matrix in these tissues occurs in the course of normal remodeling. Degradation of these components also is an important aspect of arthritis pathology, particularly in articular cartilage and subchondral bone, where destruction leads to pain and loss of joint function. The principal molecules of extracellular matrices are the fibrillar collagens (types I, II, and III), other less-abundant nonfibrillar collagens, and various proteoglycans and glycoproteins. In cartilage, the large aggregating proteoglycan aggrecan forms complexes with hyaluronan and link protein, giving this tissue its water-binding ability. Type II collagen fibrils provide a structural framework. Fibrillar collagens are resistant to attack by tissue proteases. Excessive cleavage of fibrillar collagens by specific collagenases represents an irreversible step in joint destruction.

Degradative Mechanisms

There are three major degradative mechanisms for the turnover of extracellular matrix molecules. First, the carbohydrate components of proteoglycans and glycoproteins are susceptible to attack by glycosidases. There is, however, little evidence for the extracellular action of such enzymes; rather, the glycosaminoglycans and carbohydrate portion of glycoproteins appear to be degraded by a broad array of lysosomal enzymes only after endocytosis. Important exceptions are the recently characterized heparanases, which degrade the glycosaminoglycan part of heparan-sulfate proteoglycans in the extracellular milieu. In addition, the mechanism for the turnover of hyaluronate, which is present at high levels in cartilage, synovial fluid, and many other tissues, is not clear and may involve extracellular hyaluronidases.

A second, and more general, destructive mechanism for proteins and carbohydrates is free-radical attack. There is good evidence for the presence of reactive oxygen species (ROS) in the joint, particularly under inflammatory conditions. In addition, due to their longevity, many components of the extracellular matrix present in cartilage and the intervertebral disc undergo various radical-mediated changes as they accumulate with age.

Overall, however, extracellular glycosidases and the ROS appear to be of minor importance in joint destruction relative to the action of the third mechanism: proteolytic enzymes (also referred to as proteases, proteinases, or peptidases). Proteases cleave peptide bonds with various degrees of sequence selectivity or, in some cases, sequence specificity. However, the ability of a protease to cleave its substrate is limited by the accessibility of the appropriate

TABLE 4D-1
Classification of Proteases

Protease class	Catalytic group	Archetype	Relevant proteases
Serine	–OH	Chymotrypsin Subtilisin	Cathepsin G Prohormone convertases
Threonine	–OH	Proteasome	Proteasome
Aspartic	$COO^-/COOH$	Pepsin	Cathepsin D
Cysteine	S^-	Papain	Cathepsins B, C, K, L, S Caspases
Metalloprotease	Zn^{2+}	Thermolysin	MMPs, ADAMs, ADAMTSs

MMPs, matrix metalloproteases; ADAMs, a disintegrin and a metalloprotease; ADAMTSs, a disintegrin and a metalloprotease with thrombospondin motifs

peptide bonds, so that surface loops and unfolded areas of the protein substrates are the locations most susceptible to cleavage. There are two approaches that a protease can take for the degradation of a protein substrate. The peptide chains can be "trimmed" from either end by the action of proteases called exopeptidases, or they can be cleaved internally by endopeptidase action. The majority of proteases considered to be of major importance in joint destruction are endopeptidases because their action leads to the immediate loss of function of most proteins.

Proteases and Their Classification

A vast number of proteases have been described, especially as a result of cDNA cloning and the Human Genome Project. These enzymes are widespread and essential for most aspects of normal life. In some cases, a clear function has been attributed to a particular protease, as demonstrated by the consequences of natural or experimental gene deletion. In many other instances, results suggest there is considerable redundancy in the protease repertoire so that individuals can adapt to the loss of some enzymes under normal conditions. Since the 1960s, proteases have been classified into four major groups based on the nature of their catalytic centers, which are provided by specific amino-acid residues (serine, aspartic acid, or cysteine) present in the protease structure or by a chelated metal ion (usually zinc) (Table 4D-1). It has become clear that, in several cases, the same mechanistic approach has developed several times through convergent evolution, so that very different protein frameworks have been adapted for the same type of chemistry. This finding has important consequences in terms of natural protease inhibitors that function by complementing the particular three-dimensional structures of different protease types. The protease universe has been

reviewed exhaustively (1) and is catalogued continuously on the MEROPS database (http://www.merops.ac.uk/).

Serine Proteases

Serine proteases, in which the catalytic group is a hydroxyl moiety, represent the most abundant class. These enzymes are active at neutral pH and are best exemplified by the proteases of the digestive system (trypsin, chymotrypsin, etc.). In contrast, elastase and cathepsin G, the polymorphonuclear leukocyte (PMN) proteases, are extremely destructive enzymes secreted by these cells. Other effector cells, such as mast cells and cytotoxic lymphocytes, contain various granzymes, which also are serine proteases. Plasmin, the plasma protease found in synovial fluid, is known to be an activator of inactive protease precursors.

The protease classification scheme has been refined to include the proteasome, a cytoplasmic multi-subunit assembly responsible for the turnover of such cytoplasmic proteins as transcription factor NF-κB and its inhibitor I-κB, which are prominent mediators of inflammation. Proteasomes also participate in the processing of antigens for presentation through the class I pathway. The proteasome is composed of protease subunits where the catalytic hydroxyl is provided by a threonine residue.

Aspartic Proteases

Aspartic proteases represent the second mechanistic class. Due to their low pH optima, they are not thought to play a major role in extracellular proteolysis, but the major lysosomal protease cathepsin D represents an important mediator of intracellular proteolysis. Discovery of a membrane-bound aspartic protease that has an acid pH optimum in vitro, yet is responsible for cleavage at the cell surface of the Alzheimer disease amyloid precursor protein, points to other possible roles for members of this protease class.

Cysteine Proteases

Cysteine proteases can be divided into two structurally unrelated subclasses. First, a large family of caspase proteases is present in the cytoplasm. Many of these enzymes are mediators of the proteolytic events associated with programmed cell death (apoptosis), whereas caspase 1, also known as ICE (interleukin 1 converting enzyme), is responsible for the activation of the precursor of interleukin 1 (IL-1). Caspases cleave at specific sites in their target substrates. All cleavages occur following an aspartic acid residue, but the nature of other residues upstream of this site and the site's overall accessibility also contribute to actual cleavage susceptibility. This specificity underlies the caspase terminology (cysteine protease, with specificity for aspartic acid, plus "ase," meaning enzyme).

The second group of 11 human cysteine proteases is found mainly in the lysosome and is generically termed cathepsins (although, for historical reasons, some serine and aspartic proteases also have this designation). These enzymes are responsible for intracellular protein degradation in the lysosome and play an important role in antigen processing for presentation through the class II pathway. Extracellular roles have been proposed for members of this family, such as cathepsins B and L. Of particular importance is the recently characterized cysteine protease cathepsin K, which is the principal protease of the osteoclast and is responsible for the degradation of the organic component of bone matrix. Cathepsin K also is one of the few proteases that can degrade native fibrillar collagen efficiently (2).

Metalloproteases

The final protease class consists of several families of metalloproteases, which appear to be the most important mediators of extracellular matrix degradation (Fig. 4D-1). These enzymes depend on the presence of a zinc ion bound to their active site for their catalytic activity. They are active at neutral pH, and are either secreted in the extracellular matrix or are anchored at the cell surface. Members of this class of enzymes can be divided into three families, the matrix metalloproteases (MMPs), the ADAMs (a disintegrin and a metalloprotease), and the ADAMTS (a disintegrin and a metalloprotease with thrombospondin motifs).

It has been known for many years that MMPs are responsible for the degradation of collagen and other matrix molecules. More than 20 members of this family have been described, including four true collagenases (MMP-1, -8, -13, and -14) (3). Although most of the proteases discussed previously consist solely of a dedicated proteolytic unit, the MMPs are examples of multidomain proteases in which additional protein modules are present. These proteases can contribute to substrate binding or to localization of the enzyme with other components of the extracellular matrix or at the cell surface. In the case of the collagenases, the C-terminal domain, called the hemopexin domain due to its sequence homology, is responsible for binding the enzyme to triple-helical collagen. By an unclear mechanism, cooperation between the hemopexin module and the catalytic domain when binding to the collagen substrate allows the individual chains to become accessible for cleavage. Other members of the MMP family have different

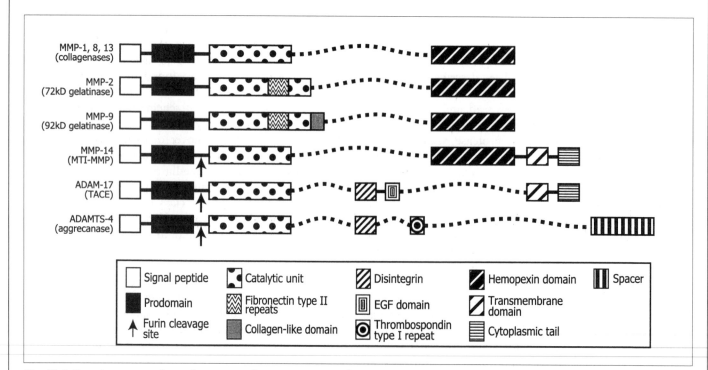

Fig. 4D-1. Domain structure of metalloproteases. Representative metalloproteases are illustrated as assemblies of their constituent modules. The domains are arranged in groups and aligned to show maximum homology. Solid lines indicate linker regions between domains. Dotted lines also indicate linker regions, but these lines have been extended to facilitate grouping of the different modules, and are not drawn to scale.

substrate selectivities; for example, the gelatinases (MMP-2 and MMP-9) contain additional fibronectin type II repeats that aid in binding their substrate, denatured collagen. Another variant of the MMPs are the membrane-type MMPs (MT-MMPs), which are localized to the plasma membrane though a C-terminal transmembrane domain, allowing restricted protease activity.

The ADAMs family members are multidomain proteases. They are membrane-localized and contain a disintegrin domain in addition to the catalytic unit. The disintegrin domain has the ability to bind to cell-surface integrins, allowing it to disrupt interactions between the cell and the extracellular matrix. Of particular interest is ADAM-17, also called TACE (tumor necrosis factor alpha converting enzyme), which processes the cell-surface form of tumor necrosis factor α (TNF-α) to the soluble cytokine.

The ADAMTS family is related to the ADAMs, but they lack a membrane-spanning domain and contain one or more thrombospondin type I motifs, which assist with substrate binding to glycosaminoglycans, for example (4). Of particular importance with respect to cartilage pathology are ADAMTS-4 and ADAMTS-5 (also called aggrecanases), which are the principal mediators of aggrecan degradation. These proteases cleave this proteoglycan following glutamic-acid residues at five unique sites in the aggrecan core protein.

Specific examples of proteases involved in extracellular matrix degradation are given in Table 4D-2.

Protease Activation

Proteases are synthesized as inactive proenzymes that are processed to their functional forms by two proteolytic mechanisms. In the case of the cathepsin cysteine proteases, autoprocessing results in the removal of the inhibitory proregion. In contrast, metalloproteases are activated through propeptide cleavage by a processing protease. For example, the prohormone convertase furin, a Golgi-resident serine protease, cleaves at specific processing sites in MMP-11, MMP-14, and the aggrecanases. Since furin-mediated cleavage occurs intracellularly, active enzyme is secreted from the cell or delivered to the plasma membrane. In the case of other MMPs, the propiece is removed by the action of other active MMPs or serine proteases. Thus, pro-MMP-13 can be activated by MMP-2, MMP-3, MMP-14, or plasmin. It remains unclear which proteases are involved naturally in the activation of most of these enzymes. Observations made in MMP-14 and MMP-3 null mice suggest that these proteases are involved in the activation of pro-MMP-13 in bone and skin (MMP-14) and in cartilage (MMP-3) (5,6).

The proregion of the MMPs interacts with the active-site zinc ion through a cysteine residue in the propeptide. Artificial activation of the pro-MMPs can be achieved by the so-called "cysteine-switch" mechanism, whereby this interaction is disrupted by organomercurial aminophenylmercuric acetate (APMA) (7). APMA activation commonly is used for in vitro studies of these enzymes.

Regulation of Metalloprotease Activity

Growth Factors, Hormones, Cytokines, and Matrix Molecules

Although some metalloproteases are produced constitutively, the synthesis of the majority of these enzymes is modulated by the presence of extracellular signaling molecules. IL-1 and TNF-α, singly or, more potently, in combination, and IL-1 in combination with fibroblast growth factor 2 (FGF-2) or oncostatin M can produce potent up-regulation of MMP expression. Interferon g, insulin-like growth factor-1 (IGF-1), and transforming growth factor β (TGF-β) can arrest/suppress MMP expression and negate the stimulatory effects of IL-1. TGF-β also can suppress IL-1 receptor expression, whereas FGF-2 up-regulates these receptors.

Matrix molecules and their degradation products also differentially regulate MMP expression in fibroblasts and chondrocytes. For example, type I collagen and fibronectin, or fragments derived from these molecules, can suppress or activate MMP-1 expression. These effects of the intact molecule or its degradation products are mediated by different cell-surface integrin receptors. The sites of proteolysis may determine whether matrix degradation products enhance or suppress MMP expression.

Cellular responses to these stimuli are mediated through binding to specific cell-surface receptors that initiate a series of intracellular signaling cascades, the final result of which is increased production of active transcription factors.

Gene Expression
The first point of control for protease production is at the transcription level. This is understood particularly well in the case of the MMPs. The activator protein-1 (AP-1) binding site is present within the promoter region of all of the MMPs except MMP-2 (gelatinase A). Fos and Jun are transcription factors that form a heterodimeric complex that binds to this regulatory DNA sequence. TNF-α, for example, induces a prolonged increase of Jun and Fos production, leading to MMP expression.

The AP-1 site also plays a dominant role in the suppression of MMP gene expression induced by TGF-β and glucocorticoids. TGF-β inhibits MMP-3 expression through an upstream sequence in the promoter described as the TGF-β inhibitory element. This sequence binds a nuclear protein complex containing Fos. Induction of Fos expression is required for this inhibition.

Other specific transcription factors may be involved in gene regulation of MMPs. For example, Cbfa1 (a runt family member) regulates MMP-13 expression in hypertrophic chondrocytes. Its absence in null mice can lead to a lack of MMP-13 expression.

Protease Inhibitors
To control unwanted proteolysis, natural protease inhibitors for most protease types are present in cells and

TABLE 4D-2
Proteolysis of Extracellular Matrix: Representative Proteases

Proteinase	Substrates	Comments	Natural inhibitor
Metalloproteases			
Collagenases: MMP-1 (collagenase 1) MMP-8 (collagenase 2) MMP-13 (collgenase 3)	Fibrillar collagens	Require hemopexin domain for binding to collagen and cleavage of triple helix.	TIMPs
Stromelysins: MMP-3 (stromelysin 1) MMP-11 (stromelysin 3)	Procollagenases (MMP-3), aggrecan (MMP-3)	MMP-11 has furin activation cleavage site – probably MMP activator.	TIMPs
Gelatinases: MMP-2 MMP-9	Denatured collagens General proteinases	Controversial as to whether MMP-2, -9 are collagenases. MMP-9 is involved in angiogenesis.	TIMPs
Macrophage elastase: MMP-12	Elastin	Absence results in emphysema.	TIMPs
Membrane type MMPs: MMP-14 (MT1-MMP)	Pro-MMP-13	Required for angiogenesis and bone development. Has furin cleavage site.	TIMPs
Matrilysin MMP-7	Proenzymes, fibronectin, and other matrix proteins	Mainly in epithelial cells and monocytes. Lacks a hemopexin domain	TIMPs
Adamalysins/Aggrecanases ADAM-17 (TNF-α-converting enzyme, TACE)	Pro-TNF-α	TACE releases TNF-α from cell surface.	TIMP-3
ADAMTS-4 (aggrecanase 1) ADAMTS-5 (or -11) (aggrecanase 2) ADAMTS-1 (aggrecanase 3)	Aggrecan	ADAMTS proteinases have a furin activation/cleavage site. Thrombospondin domain binds to glycosaminoglycan and increases activity.	TIMP-3
Serine Proteases			
Plasminogen/Plasmin	Plasmin cleaves fibrin and activates pro-MMPs	Activation by PA and kallikrein generates plasmin.	Protease nexins, α_1-antiplasmin
Plasminogen activators (PA) Tissue type (tPA)	Plasminogen	Plasmin generation	Plasminogen activator inhibitors 1 and 2
Urokinase type (uPA)	Plasminogen	Plasmin generation	Protease nexin

Proteinase	Substrates	Comments	Natural inhibitor
Kallikrein	Activates proplasminogen, uPA and procollagenase; factor XII	Chemotactic for neutrophils and activates them.	C1 inhibitor and α_2 –macroglobulin
Polymorph Elastase	Elastin, fibrillar collagen and other matrix proteins	Neutrophil specific	α_1-proteinase inhibitor (α_1-antitrypsin)
Cathepsin G	TIMP, elastin, collagens	Neutrophil specific	α_1-antichymotrypsin α_1-proteinase inhibitor
Mast cell tryptase	Broad substrate activity	Mast cell specific	Resistant to most natural serine proteinase inhibitors
Granzymes A, B, M	Broad specificity	Lymphocyte specific. Involved in T-cell mediated killing.	Endogenous serpins, protease nexin
Cysteine Proteases			
Cathepsin B	Broad specificity	Broad distribution	Cystatins
Cathepsin K	Type I collagen	Osteoclastic bone resorption. Active at neutral pH.	Cystatins
Cathepsin L	Elastin/other substrates	Monocytes/macrophages	Cystatins
Cathepsin S	Elastin, collagen	Active at neutral pH.	Cystatins
Caspase-1 (ICE)	Pro-IL-1	Key enzyme in IL-1 generation	
Caspase-3	Regulatory molecules in homeostasis and cell repair	Required for apoptosis.	Inhibitor of apoptosis (IAPs)

MMP, matrix metalloprotease; TIMPs, tissue inhibitors of metalloproteases; MT, membrane type; ADAM, a disintegrin and a metalloprotease; TNF, tumor necrosis factor; TACE, TNF-α converting enzyme; ADAMTS, a disintegrin and a metalloprotease with thrombospondin motifs; IL, interleukin.

tissues. The large cystatin families control the cathepsin cysteine proteases, and many families of inhibitors are present for the different serine proteases. Of particular importance are the plasma proteins α_1-antitrypsin and α_1-antichymotrypsin, which are present in synovial fluid and neutralize soluble elastase and cathepsin G released from PMNs. The four members of the tissue inhibitors of metalloproteases (TIMPs) represent the principle regulators of proteolysis in connective tissues (8). These are two-domain proteins consisting of an inhibitory domain that binds to the active site of the metalloprotease, and a second domain that has alternate binding specificities. In addition to acting as inhibitors of metalloproteases, some TIMPs are involved in the activation of MMPs. The activation of pro-MMP-2 requires a trimolecular interaction at the cell membrane between TIMP-2, MT1-MMP (MMP-14), and pro-MMP-2. Here, TIMP-2 links the MMP-14 and pro-MMP-2 through its first and second domains, allowing a second molecule of MMP-14 to cleave and activate the pro-MMP-2.

While the TIMPs show little selectivity in their affinity for the different MMPs, TIMP-3 is unique in its ability to inhibit ADAM-17 (TACE) and the aggrecanases (ADAMTS-4 and ADAMTS-5). TIMP-3 also binds to glycosaminoglycans in the extracellular matrix, which presumably serves to retain it in higher concentrations.

Mechanisms of Fibrillar Collagen Cleavage

Collagens essentially are triple-helix molecules with small nonhelical telopeptide domains at each end. Although the collagen helix generally is resistant to proteolysis, the telopeptides are susceptible to the action of proteases, such as elastase, cathepsin G, and stromelysin 1 (MMP-3). To allow turnover of the collagen fibrils, a region located three-quarters of the distance along the molecule allows the triple helix to relax enough for collagenases to bind and cleave all three chains at this site. The primary cleavage site is at Gly^{775}-Ile in the α1(I) chain and at Gly^{775}-Leu in the α2(I) chain of type I collagen. Cleavage of the three α1(II) chains of type II collagen occurs at the corresponding Gly-Ile bond, and in type III at the corresponding Gly-Leu bond. These cleavages produce characteristic TC^A and TC^B or $^3/_4$ and $^1/_4$ fragments. Cleavage can be demonstrated immunologically in situ, and the types I and II products are present in both healthy and diseased tissues and can be detected in body fluids. There are four collagenases that can produce this cleavage, namely MMP-1, -8, -13, and -14 or collagenases 1, 2, 3, and 4, respectively. Although there have been reports that the gelatinases MMP-2 and MMP-9 can act as collagenases, this theory is controversial for human type II collagen. MMP-13 is the most effective collagenase for digesting type II collagen, whereas MMP-1 cleaves type III collagen more effectively than it cleaves type II. MMP-8 (a PMN product) can digest both types I and III collagens, but not type II, when it is in the form of a native fibril. Following cleavage of the triple helix, the α chains denature (unwind) and become susceptible to further digestion by collagenases and other proteases, such as stromelysin-1 (MMP-3) and the gelatinases (MMP-2 and MMP-9).

Cathepsin K can be considered a collagenase. In bone, this osteoclast product cleaves the carboxy terminal telopeptide, leading to the release of a telopeptide fragment and its accompanying intermolecular cross-links. It also is able to cleave the triple-helix region at multiple sites. Cathepsin K functions optimally under the acidic conditions found in the osteoclast ruffled border, where bone resorption occurs.

Sequence of Events During the Degradation of Extracellular Matrix

When pathology is initiated, not all proteases act at once on all the molecules of the extracellular matrix. Studies of the proteolysis of collagen and proteoglycans, in vitro and in vivo, have revealed that aggrecan is cleaved rapidly following induction of proteolysis by molecules that induce joint inflammation, such as TNF-α and IL-1. This process involves aggrecanase(s) of the ADAMTS family, and later involves MMPs. Cleavage of collagen II also is observed in the same sites that aggrecanases cleave aggrecan (6).

The in vitro use of cartilage explants has permitted a clearer understanding of the temporal sequence of specific proteolytic events and has demonstrated that collagenase-mediated cleavage of type II collagen is secondary to aggrecan cleav-

age (Fig. 4D-2). In nasal cartilages, this delay is a few days, and up to one week in mature articular cartilages (9). Delayed activation of proenzymes is one causative factor. Induction of cartilage degradation by IL-1 in explant cultures results first in aggrecan cleavage by aggrecanases, accompanied by removal of the NC4 (noncollagenous) domain of the α1(IX) chain that projects from the collagen fibril surface. This action is followed by the loss of the COL2 (collagenous) domain of the α1(IX) chain, which abuts the type II collagen fibril, and simultaneous cleavage of type II collagen by collagenases. In vivo, type XI collagen degradation is observed early, together with cleavage of type II collagen, following induction of experimental joint inflammation (10). Decorin also is present on the surface of the collagen fibril in articular cartilage, particularly at the articular surface and in pericellular sites. Surprisingly, decorin and other leucine-rich fibril-associated proteoglycans, such as biglycan and lumican, are very resistant to proteolysis and may be lost only after the type II collagen is digested. In contrast, another molecule in this family, fibromodulin, is susceptible to early cleavage. In advanced osteoarthritis (OA), this fibril damage is accompanied by loss of decorin and biglycan close to and at the articular surface, where excessive collagen cleavage develops (11). These molecules that resist cleavage may protect the fibril against proteolysis.

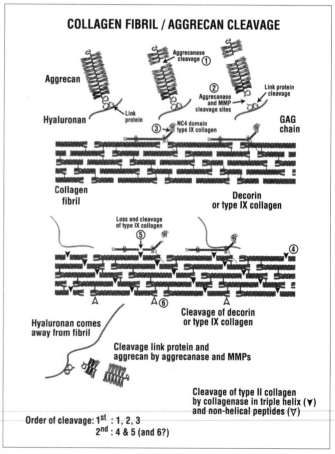

Fig. 4D-2. Steps in matrix cleavage in cartilage undergoing stimulated degradation in culture.

In established arthritis, cleavage of aggrecan and type II collagen usually are seen at the same sites. In established human OA and rheumatoid arthritis (RA), there is clear evidence for cleavage of aggrecan by both aggrecanase(s) and MMPs (12). Wherever aggrecan is lost, type II collagen is badly damaged. The organization of these molecules is very much related, in that aggrecan is localized within the collagen fibril network. When the fibrils are lost, there is no effective way of retaining macromolecular aggregates of aggrecan, leading to permanent and irreparable damage to the articular cartilage.

Articular Cartilage Resorption in Arthritis

Cells of the musculoskeletal and immune systems are capable of producing a wide range of proteases. A variety of metallo, cysteine, and serine proteases are produced by synovial cells, chondrocytes, skin fibroblasts, keratinocytes, osteoblasts, osteoclasts, macrophages/monocytes, PMNs, and lympho-

cytes (Fig. 4D-3). However, some proteases are restricted to a particular cell type as befits the functional requirements. For example, osteoclasts use cathepsin K as a major protease in bone resorption. Chondrocytes of hypertrophic lineage, which rapidly resorb and calcify their extracellular matrix in skeletal growth and repair, do not produce MMP-1 (collagenase 1), the major collagenase produced by other cell types, but rather produce MMP-13 (collagenase 3), which is capable of rapid cleavage of the fibrils of type II collagen found in cartilage. Macrophage metalloelastase (MMP-12) and the PMN collagenase (MMP-8) also are examples of proteases in which expression is tightly restricted.

In arthritis, many MMPs and other proteases are up-regulated (13). The principal intra-articular sources are chondrocytes, PMNs, and synovial cells in RA, and chondrocytes in OA. In RA, neutrophils concentrate in large numbers in inflamed joints, releasing neutrophil elastase, cathepsin G, and MMP-1. Together, this broad spectrum of proteases can degrade many protein substrates, including collagen. However, there currently is no convincing evidence for a primary role of neutrophil proteases in the cleavage of type II collagen in cartilage, although these proteases may play a role in the degradation of aggrecan at the articular surface. Experimental studies have revealed that cartilage degradation is dependent upon adherence of these cells to articular surfaces and the activation of Fc receptors.

In both RA and OA, articular cartilage is progressively destroyed, with proteolysis appearing centered around the chondrocyte, as revealed by analyses of type II collagen degradation. Collagenases and other MMPs involved in this proteolysis are detected in those same locations. However, the diseases clearly are distinguishable with regard to the sites in cartilage where degradation takes place. In RA, cleavage of aggrecan by metalloproteases occurs at the articular surface and is accompanied by a loss of metachromatic staining with such dyes as toluidine blue. Denaturation of type II collagen is observed throughout the

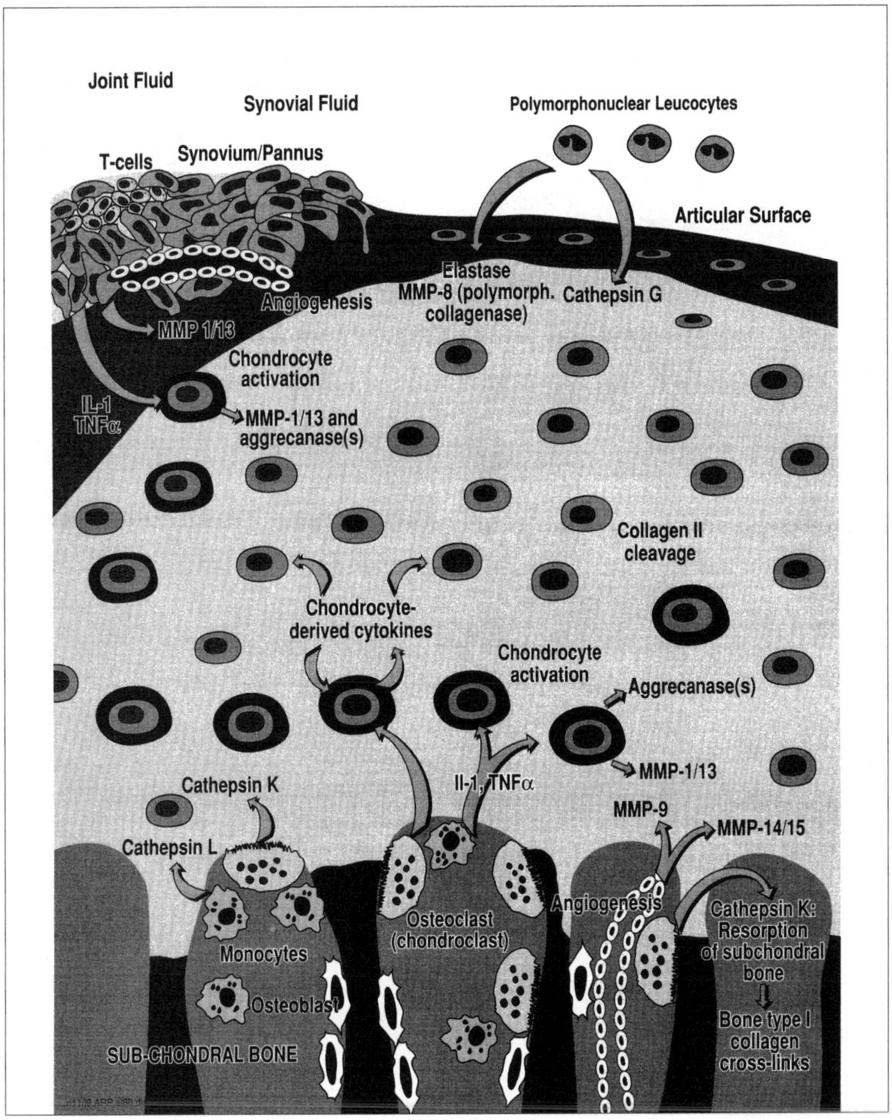

Fig. 4D-3. Summary of the sources of proteases and cytokines in cells from different tissues in the inflamed joint. Articular cartilage is depicted with the underlying subchondral bone and invading synovium to the left. Dark regions in the cartilage indicate areas where type II collagen degradation is observed immunohistochemically.

cartilage, but tends to be more intense around chondrocytes adjacent to pannus, and interestingly, also adjacent to subchondral bone (11). Collagenase-mediated cleavage of collagen is prominent around chondrocytes in the same areas. The concentration of damaged collagen around chondrocytes suggests that these cells generate or activate collagenases in response to signals, such as IL-1 and TNF-α, from adjacent inflammatory cells in pannus and bone.

The picture of cartilage in OA is different. Both in aging and in the development of OA, the loss of aggrecan and type II collagen due to cleavage usually starts at, and close to, the articular surface around chondrocytes. The loss extends progressively into the underlying middle and deep zones, with increased degeneration of the cartilage. Cleavage of collagen is accompanied by the loss of aggrecan and collagen fibril-associated proteoglycans, such as decorin. Biglycan also is lost from the more superficial sites (13). The resorption process in OA ordinarily does not appear to be driven by inflammation, as it is in RA. Instead, it is likely that a chronic cycle of degeneration occurs when the chondrocytes respond to changes in the extracellular matrix and to abnormal loading by increased proteolysis.

Angiogenesis and Cell Migration

Proteases play a pivotal role in the formation of new vessels and in capillary invasion, a requirement for synovial hyperplasia. MMP-9 is concentrated in sites of angiogenesis; in its absence, angiogenesis is suppressed. A role for MMP-14 in angiogenesis was revealed by MMP-14 null mice, which exhibit a delay in the formation of the secondary center of ossification as a result of impaired vascular invasion. Yet, the primary center of ossification is unaffected. This finding also points to site-specific differences in the roles of these proteases in angiogenesis.

Endothelial cells involved in angiogenesis do not require the plasminogen activator (PA) system to invade fibrin gels, because cells isolated from PA-deficient or plasminogen-deficient mice successfully vascularize fibrin gels. This is because MMP-14 (MT1-MMP) expressed on the cell surface permits invasion. Type I collagen-rich tissues also can be invaded, provided MT1-MMP or MT2-MMP (MMP-15) is expressed. Other migrating cells also use such proteases as collagenases for detachment from fibrillar collagen substrates to allow locomotion.

Proteases in Normal Physiology, and Their Regulation in Arthritis

It is clear that proteases play a critical role in normal homeostasis, so they cannot be inhibited excessively with impunity (14). Protease activity is very carefully regulated at a variety of levels, ranging from receptor-mediated activation of specific cells to transcriptional and translational regulation and the controlled secretion, activation, and inhibition of protease. In pathology, these controls may be lost at one or more levels. The excessive generalized inhibi-

tion of proteases could therefore induce pathology, and this action has been observed in clinical trials of MMP inhibitors developed for the treatment of joint damage in arthritis. Such unfavorable outcomes may have led to the premature abandonment of potentially valuable preclinical and clinical programs.

Sometimes an experimental genetic deletion of a specific protease results in a pathology that is not dissimilar to the side effects seen in clinical studies. The intra-articular cellular proliferation observed in rats treated with some MMP inhibitors, which are prone to inhibition of MMP-14 along with the intended target MMP, is not unlike the intra-articular pathology observed in the MMP-14 null mouse (5). This similarity may well indicate the inhibition of MMP-14, which clearly plays a key regulatory role in the proliferation of these cells.

There is evidence for a role of collagenases (such as MMP-13, MMP-1), other MMPs (such as stromelysin 1) and the ADAMTS proteases (aggrecanases) in the damage done to articular cartilage macromolecules in arthritis. There also is evidence for a role of proteases in inflammation, angiogenesis, and cell recruitment. In the future, we must regulate the activities of these proteases in a more enlightened manner to provide therapeutic benefit while minimizing interference with normal protease physiology.

JOHN S. MORT, PhD
A. ROBIN POOLE, PhD, DSc

References

1. Barrett AJ, Rawlings ND, Woessner JF. Handbook of proteolytic enzymes. San Diego: Academic Press, 1998.
2. Chapman HA, Riese RJ, Shi GP. Emerging roles for cysteine proteases in human biology. Annu Rev Physiol 1997;59: 63–88.
3. Nagase H, Woessner JF. Matrix metalloproteinases. J Biol Chem 1999;274:21491–21494.
4. Kaushal GP, Shah SV. The new kids on the block: ADAMTSs, potentially multifunctional metalloproteinases of the ADAM family. J Clin Invest 2000;105:1335–1337.
5. Holmbeck K, Bianco P, Caterina J, et al. MT1-MMP-deficient mice develop dwarfism, osteopenia, arthritis, and connective tissue disease due to inadequate collagen turnover. Cell 1999; 99:81–92.
6. van Meurs J, van Lent P, Stoop R, et al. Cleavage of aggrecan at the Asn^{341}-Phe^{342} site coincides with the initiation of collagen damage in murine antigen-induced arthritis: a pivotal role for stromelysin 1 in matrix metalloproteinase activity. Arthritis Rheum 1999;42:2074–2084.
7. Springman EB, Angleton EL, Birkedal-Hansen H, Van Wart HE. Multiple modes of activation of latent human fibroblast collagenase: evidence for the role of a Cys73 active-site zinc complex in latency and a "cysteine switch" mechanism for activation. Proc Natl Acad Sci USA 1990;87:364–368.
8. Brew K, Dinakarpandian D, Nagase H. Tissue inhibitors of metalloproteinases: evolution, structure and function. Biochim Biophys Acta 2000;1477:267–283.

9. Dahlberg L, Billinghurst RC, Manner P, et al. Selective enhancement of collagenase-mediated cleavage of resident type II collagen in cultured osteoarthritic cartilage and arrest with a synthetic inhibitor that spares collagenase 1 (matrix metalloproteinase 1). Arthritis Rheum 2000;43:673–682.

10. Kojima T, Mwale F, Yasuda T, Girard C, Poole AR, Laverty S. Early degradation of type IX and type II collagen with the onset of experimental inflammatory arthritis. Arthritis Rheum 2001;44:120–127.

11. Poole AR, Alini M, Hollander AP. Cartilage biology and cartilage destruction. In: Henderson B, Edwards JCW, Pettipher ER (eds). Mechanisms and models in rheumatoid arthritis, New York: Academic Press, 1995; pp 163–204.

12. Lark MW, Bayne EK, Flanagan J, et al. Aggrecan degradation in human cartilage. Evidence for both matrix metalloproteinase and aggrecanase activity in normal, osteoarthritic, and rheumatoid joints. J Clin Invest 1997;100:93–106.

13. Poole AR. Cartilage in health and disease. In: Koopman WJ (ed). Arthritis and Allied Conditions, Baltimore: Lippincott, Williams & Wilkins, 2001; pp 226–284

14. Vincenti PM, Clark IM, Brinckerhoff CE. Using inhibitors of metalloproteinases to treat arthritis. Easier said than done? Arthritis Rheum 1994;37:1115–1126.

MEDIATORS OF INFLAMMATION, TISSUE DESTRUCTION, AND REPAIR
E. Arachidonic Acid Derivatives, Reactive Oxygen Species, and Other Mediators

A number of inflammatory mediators modulate the immune response. Cytokines, chemokines, and surface receptor ligands are discussed in detail in other sections of this chapter. Prostaglandins, leukotrienes, kinins, thromboxanes, isoprostanes, nitric oxide, and reactive oxygen species are important mediators of localized inflammation. In addition to their common role in inflammation, some of these molecules are linked by common derivation from arachidonic acid (i.e., prostaglandins, lipoxins, and leukotrienes) or by linkage in signals necessary for their production (prostaglandins, reactive oxygen species, and nitric oxide).

Prostaglandins

Prostaglandins initially were identified by the ability of prostatic secretions to stimulate uterine contraction. The active component of prostatic secretions was found to be lipid-based, and subsequently, similar compounds with diverse activities were isolated from a variety of tissues.

Prostanoids encompass lipid mediators, such as prostaglandins, thromboxanes, and isoprostanes, that are derived from arachidonic acid (AA) or arachidonyl-containing lipids. Prostaglandins are derived predominantly from AA stored as phosphatidylinositol and phosphatidylcholine in the cellular membrane of all cells (1). Arachidonic acid is released from membrane phospholipids primarily via the enzyme phospholipase A_2; phospholipase C_2 also may release AA from the cell membrane (Fig. 4E-1). Phospholipase A_2 has a natural inhibitor, lipomodulin, whose expression is stimulated by glucocorticoids. Release of AA is a key rate-determining step of prostaglandin synthesis. Once released, AA can be oxidized directly or con-

verted via a number of biochemical pathways to prostaglandins, thromboxanes, or leukotrienes. Tissue type, enzyme concentrations, and cytokine milieu, among other factors, determine the metabolic pathway to which available AA is directed.

Prostaglandins (PGs) derived from AA are produced through a series of biosynthetic pathways. The initial enzyme is cyclooxygenase (COX), which also is called prostaglandin endoperoxide synthase, or prostaglandin H synthase (PGHS). Two different cyclooxygenases have been identified: COX-1 (PGHS-1) and COX-2 (PGHS-2). COX-1 and COX-2 are derived from two genes, on different chromosomes, that share significant similarities in sequence and structure (2). COX-1 is expressed constitutively, suggesting that PGs produced by this enzyme play a homeostatic role that is particularly important in gastric mucosal protection, renal hemodynamics, and platelet thrombogenesis. COX-1 messenger RNA is relatively long-lived and stable, allowing long-term and rapid transcription.

In contrast, COX-2 is induced in but not limited to fibroblasts, endothelial cells, and macrophages by cytokines, mitogens, and tumor promoters. COX-2 expression is induced in physiologic and pathologic settings, such as in the human kidney during salt restriction (3,4), in and around atherosclerotic plaques (5), in the degenerative brain lesions of Alzheimer disease (6), and in many malignant neoplasms (7). In neoplasms, COX-2 plays a pathologic role, inhibiting apoptosis and increasing proliferation (7). In atherosclerosis, COX-2 may play both protective and pathologic roles (5).

Cyclooxygenases catalyze two sequential reactions. During the first, oxygen is incorporated into AA, and ring closure occurs, yielding the first unstable prostaglandin structure PGG_2 (Fig. 4E-1). The second reaction involves reduction of PGG_2 to PGH_2. Both of these reactions require heme as a cofactor. The reduction step can be accelerated for COX-2 by the presence of lipid hydroperoxides or peroxynitrite (see the nitric oxide section in this chapter), which are formed by inflammatory cells, such as polymorphonuclear leukocytes (PMNs) and macrophages. PGH_2 then is converted by various isomerases to the biologically active PGs: PGD_2, PGI_2, PGE_2, and PGF_{2a}.

Two isoforms of PGE_2 synthase have been isolated and cloned (8,9). A cytoplasmic, constitutively expressed PGE_2 synthase isoform is linked functionally with COX-1; the other isoform is membrane-associated, inducible, and linked functionally with COX-2, suggesting that the latter plays a role in inflammation (8,9). Thromboxane (TX) A_2 also is produced via isomerization of PGH_2. Which PG is produced depends on tissue type, as tissues produce different isomerases. Prostaglandins can act in an autocrine, paracrine, or endocrine manner. They are relatively short-lived as active compounds, being converted rapidly to biologically inactive or other biologically active derivatives that are excreted in the kidney or further modified to form other derivatives.

The biologic effect of PGs depends on their interactions with their receptors and the relative amounts of the types of prostaglandins produced. Eight surface receptors for PGs are known; each is a member of the family of receptors characterized by seven membrane-spanning domains that interact with G proteins for intracellular signal transduction. Four different PGE_2 receptors (EP_1, EP_2, EP_3, and EP_4), one PGD_2 (DP), one PGI_2 (IP), one PGF_{2a} (IF), and one TXA_2 (TP) receptor have been isolated. All of these receptors are expressed on smooth muscle, although the type of receptor expressed varies in different organs. Stimulation of EP_2, EP_4, IP, and DP leads to smooth-muscle relaxation by raising intracellular cAMP (cyclic 3′, 5′-adenosine monophosphate). Stimulation of EP_1, FP, and TP initiates smooth-muscle contraction by increasing signaling via the inositol triphosphate/diacylglycerol pathway, and stimulation of EP_3 induces the same vasoconstrictive effect by reducing cAMP (10).

Two receptors expressed on platelets have opposing actions: IP inhibits platelet aggregation, whereas TP induces platelet aggregation. EP_2, which is expressed on PMNs and lymphocytes, modulates many of the prostaglandin effects in immunity. $EP_{(1-4)}$, FP, and TP are expressed in the kidney. EP_1 appears to have a role in renal sodium transport, whereas EP_2 and EP_4 (expressed in the glomerulus) appear to play a role in reducing blood pressure. A confounding factor is that most receptors can be stimulated by most PGs; the receptors differ merely in their relative affinity for each individual PG. Thus, if PGI_2 is present in large amounts in a tissue with PGE_2 receptors, a PGE_2-like response will

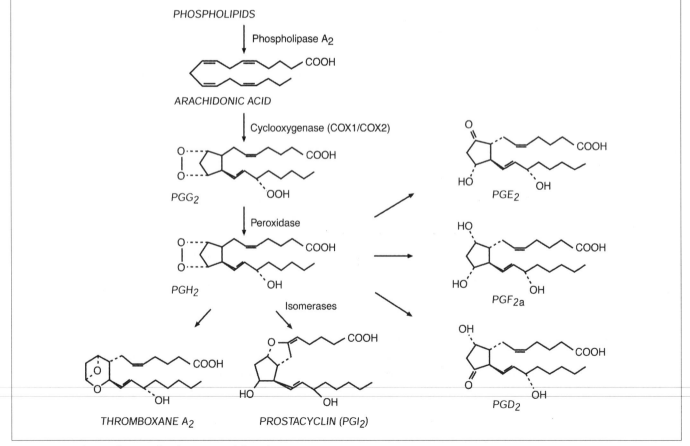

Fig. 4E-1. Synthesis of prostaglandins (PG) and thromboxane A_2.

occur. The controls of receptor production currently are being delineated.

Overall, PGE_2 and PGI_2 have proinflammatory effects, leading to vasodilation and increased vascular permeability. IP knockout mice have impaired inflammatory and pain responses [11]. PGE_2 also induces T-cell migration and production of metalloproteinases and plays a role in the febrile response via the EP_3 receptor [10,11]. However, not all effects of PGE_2 are proinflammatory. Both EP_2 and EP_4 are expressed on macrophages, which themselves make large amounts of PGE_2 in response to inflammatory stimuli. EP_2 is induced in macrophages by inflammatory stimuli, and EP_4 appears to be expressed constitutively. Stimulation of these receptors inhibits cytokine release, suggesting the receptors act in a negative feedback fashion in macrophages. PGE_2 also inhibits T-cell responses in vitro and blocks B-cell maturation. Recent data suggest that PGs and TXs play key roles in thymic T-cell development and selection. PGE_2 appears to protect a developing T cell from negative selection. EP_4 knockout mice do not undergo inflammatory osteoclast bone resorption, suggesting a role for PGs in inflammatory bone erosions. EP_1 knockout mice fail to develop carcinogen-induced colon cancer [11]. These results highlight the therapeutic potential for specific receptor antagonists in inflammatory and malignant diseases.

PGJ_2 is formed by dehydration of PGD_2. A "PGJ_2 synthase" has not been isolated, making it difficult to study the regulation and localization of PGJ_2 production. The importance of PGJ_2 during an in vivo inflammatory response is unclear, but PGJ_2 and its metabolites (15-deoxy and 15-deoxy D12,14 PGJ_2) have anti-inflammatory properties that appear to act, in part, via stimulation of the nuclear receptor known as peroxisome proliferator-activated receptor-gamma (PPARγ). Currently marketed diabetes drugs of the thiazolidinedione class (rosiglitazone and pioglitazone) are PPARγ agonists. Animal studies of thiazolidinediones indicate that these drugs are successful for the treatment of experimental arthritis [12], colitis [13], and insulinitis [14]. Pharmacologic doses of 15-deoxy D12,14 PGJ_2 have been used successfully to treat adjuvant-induced arthritis in rats [12]. PPARγ ligands, such as PGJ_2, its metabolites, and the thiazolidinediones, offer a novel avenue for the treatment of inflammatory diseases and are being researched.

Thromboxane

As described earlier, TXA_2 is derived from AA through the same biosynthetic pathways as the PGs, with the initial steps catalyzed by the COXs. Subsequently, TX synthase converts PGH_2 to TXA_2 (Fig. 4E-1). TXA_2 differs from the PGs in having a six-carbon primary ring rather than the five-member ring that characterizes prostaglandins.

The TXA_2 receptor (TP) is found in the kidney, on epithelial cells, on platelets, and on smooth muscles of the arterial system, venous system, and pulmonary airways. Stimulation of TP results in smooth-muscle contraction, platelet aggregation, increased intestinal secretion, and increased glomerular filtration.

TXA_2 has been shown to be a key mediator in inflammatory renal disease and asthma [15]. Levels of TX are elevated in murine lupus models. High levels of TXA_2 in the kidney result in intense vasoconstriction, platelet aggregation, mesangial cell contraction, and increased production of extracellular matrix, which lead to decreased renal function. Blocking TXA_2 synthesis results in short- and long-term improvement in renal function and survival in lupus mice. Disease is not totally inhibited, however, as mice in which TXA_2 synthesis is blocked eventually develop renal disease. Thus, TXA_2 plays a role, but is not the sole inflammatory mediator, in lupus nephritis. However, antagonism of the TP in murine lupus nephritis results in significant reductions in proteinuria and glomerular damage/cellular infiltration [16,17]. Any differential effect of TP antagonism versus TXA_2 synthase inhibition may be due to the ability of other prostanoids (such as PGH_2 or the isoprostane 8-isoPGF_{2a}) to act as TP agonists and thus act as inducers of lupus nephritis.

TXA_2 and leukotrienes are important in asthma. Healthy individuals who inhale preparations containing TXA_2 develop bronchoconstriction and increased airway secretions. Metabolites of TXA_2 (TXB_2) are increased in the blood, urine, and bronchoalveolar lavage fluids of people with asthma. Agents that block TXA_2 production or the TXA_2 receptor are effective for treating bronchoconstriction in humans and animals. Indeed, blocking TXA_2 alone is effective therapy, even when leukotriene levels remain high. It is very likely that inhibitors of TXA_2 will quickly become part of the treatment regimen for asthma. Other uses for TXA_2 inhibitors remain to be defined.

The role of TXA_2 as a vasoconstrictor may be important in the development of Raynaud's phenomenon in systemic sclerosis (SSc). Compared with controls, subjects with SSc have elevated levels of a renally excreted systemic TXA_2 metabolite. In addition, when these SSc subjects are exposed to a cold stimulus that induces Raynaud's phenomenon, levels of this metabolite are increased further [18].

TXA_2 appears to be important in thymic development because it induces cell death in developing thymocytes, indicating a role in negative selection. PGE_2 inhibits TXA_2-induced cell death. Production of eicosanoids by thymic epithelial cells and expression of eicosanoid receptors by developing thymocytes appear to be important in positive and negative selection of T cells and the resultant T-cell repertoire.

Leukotrienes

Like PGs, leukotrienes (LTs) are produced primarily from AA that is released by phospholipase A_2 from phospholipids in the cellular membrane [19]. Specific cellular signals lead to translocation of the phospholipase–AA complex to the nuclear membrane. The same signals cause the enzyme 5-lipoxygenase (5-LO) to migrate from the cytoplasm to the

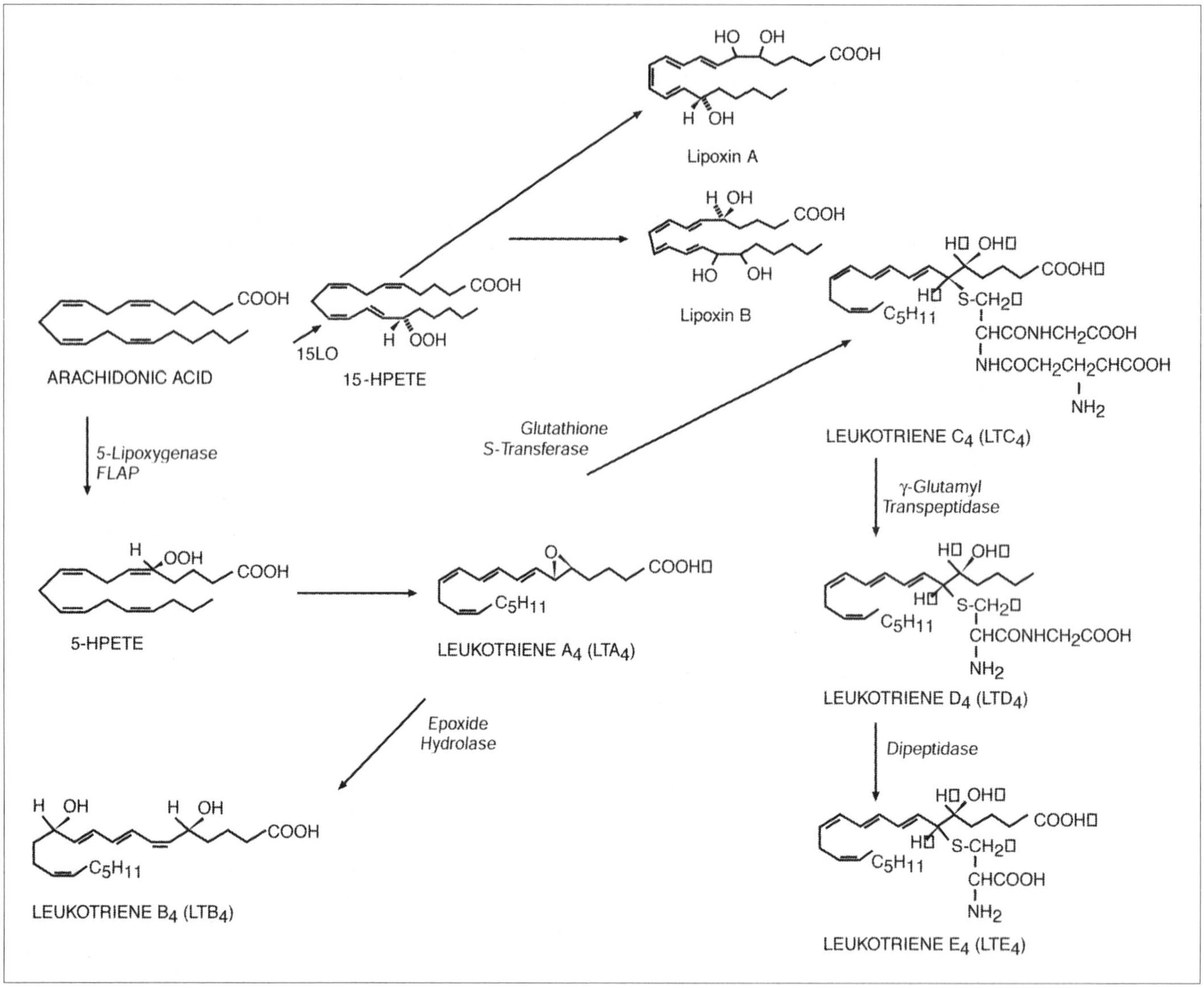

Fig. 4E-2. Synthesis of leukotrienes.

nuclear membrane (Fig. 4E-2). A protein called 5-lipoxygenase–activating protein (FLAP) facilitates the transfer of AA from phospholipase A_2 to 5-LO. In the test tube, 5-LO alone can convert AA to LTs; in the cell, however, FLAP is necessary for the series of reactions that convert AA to LTs.

Arachidonic acid is converted by 5-LO to 5-hydroperoxyeicosa-tetranoic acid (5-HPETE) by a dioxygenase reaction. 5-HPETE subsequently is transformed to LTA_4 via dehydrase activity. LTA_4 then enters divergent pathways: LTA_4 hydrolase converts LTA_4 to LTB_4 by the addition of H_2O; or LTC_4 synthetase, with the addition of a glutathione, transforms LTA_4 to LTC_4. By the action of gamma-glutamyl transferase, LTC_4 is converted to LTD_4, and removal of the terminal glycine by dipeptidase produces LTE_4. LTC_4, LTD_4, and LTE_4 commonly are referred to as the cysteinyl or *peptide leukotrienes*; they make up the majority of biologic activity in SRS-A (the slow-reacting substance of anaphylaxis).

The cysteinyl LTs have significant biologic effects, including constriction of respiratory, gastrointestinal, and vascular smooth muscle. Other actions include increasing vascular permeability, constricting mesangial cells, stimulating bronchial mucus secretion, inhibiting ciliary function, and enhancing mucosal edema. These agents also enhance the responsiveness of the airway to other bronchoconstrictors. The primary action of LTB_4, a noncysteinyl LT, is to accentuate PMN function. It is a potent chemoattractant for PMNs and results in degranulation and release of reactive oxygen species and proteolytic enzymes. LTB_4 also has effects on lymphocytes, enhancing the effects of gamma interferon on classical cellular activation pathways, inhibiting apoptosis of thymic T cells, and inducing differentiation of resting B cells. LTB_4 also enhances proliferation and synthetic responses of B cells.

Receptors for LTs are of the seven-domain transmembrane motif with signaling through G proteins. Specific receptors for LTB_4 and the cysteinyl LTs have been isolated, and they are located at the sites where these compounds are active. LTB$_4$ receptors are found primarily on PMNs and lymphocytes, whereas LTC$_4$ receptors are found in respiratory, gastrointestinal, and vascular epithelia. Disruption of the gene for the LTB$_4$ receptor prevented inflammatory responses in the ear and peritoneum following injection of inflammatory mediators, indicating a critical role for LTB$_4$ in acute inflammation. Recently, two receptors for the cysteinyl leukotrienes were cloned, expressed, and knocked out in animal models. These receptor studies provided important confirmation of the biologic activity of the cysteinyl LTs, and indicated the receptors as a new therapeutic target for inhibiting cysteinyl LT activity. Indeed, a new class of available pharmacologic agents (including montelukast and zafirlukast) for asthma treatment targets the cysteinyl LT receptors. Other uses of these drugs may develop with better understanding of the function of the cysteinyl LTs and their receptors.

Therapeutic trials of LT inhibitors in other diseases have not been as promising. Trials in psoriasis, rheumatoid arthritis (RA), and inflammatory bowel disease produced minimal, if any, improvement. In some of these trials, inhibition of 5-LO activity was incomplete, suggesting that more effective 5-LO inhibition subsequently may prove useful in these diseases. Other studies have demonstrated profound effects of LT on nitric oxide production, reactive oxygen species production, tumor growth, tumor regression, cognition, and central pain perception. These effects of LTs have obvious clinical applications, but their clinical significance has yet to be defined.

Lipoxins

Lipoxins (LXs) are a group of compounds related to LTs in that they are derived from AA through lipoxygenase activity (20). The lipoxygenases 12-LO and 15-LO are involved in lipoxin formation, producing 12- or 15-HPETE. Through a series of reactions, the lipoxins LXA$_4$ and LXB$_4$ are formed. These molecules primarily are vasodilatory and immunomodulatory. Elevated levels of LXs are found in inflammatory lesions, including some forms of inflammatory arthritis and glomerulonephritis. Lipoxins are produced primarily by PMNs and platelets. A lack of specific inhibitors of LX formation limits the understanding of their true biologic functions in normal immunity or in autoimmune diseases.

Kinins

Kinins are a group of proteins activated in a sequence similar to the coagulation cascade. Tissue and plasma prekallikreins are cleaved via trauma, immunologic signals, or plasmin, which produces activated kallikrein. Plasma kallikrein then acts on high-molecular weight kininogen to produce bradykinin, a biologically active nonpeptide. Tissue kallikrein cleaves low-molecular weight kininogen to release kallidin, which has many of the same properties of bradykinin (Fig. 4E-3). The ability to produce kinins is ubiquitous throughout body tissues. Specific receptors for bradykinin have been isolated, and these receptors vary in their tissue localization (21).

The kinins have a wide spectrum of biologic activities. They stimulate smooth-muscle contraction and bronchospasm, increase vascular permeability, mediate pain and vasodilation, and induce hypotension. At an inflammatory site, kinins enhance the release of phospholipids, freeing AA for the production of PGs and LTs. Kinins also stimulate the production of platelet-activating factor. Thus, kinins act as proinflammatory agents and are present in increased concentrations in the rheumatoid joint. Specific inhibitors of bradykinin have been developed that block the development of inflammation in animal models, including induced rodent models of RA. Such agents, given systemically or locally, may be beneficial in treating inflammatory lesions.

Dipeptidases are natural inhibitors of bradykinin. One, kininase II, is identical to angiotensin-converting enzyme (ACE). ACE inhibitors block the function of kinase II. In clinical situations where bradykinin is overproduced, ACE inhibitors may accentuate the clinical syndrome by blocking the metabolic breakdown of bradykinin.

Coagulation System

The coagulation system is intricately involved in inflammation. Fibrin is a prominent component of any inflammatory reaction, indicating that activation of the coagulation system is integral to the immune response. Components of the coagulation system and the fibrinolytic system can become proinflammatory by their activation of other factors. Hageman factor is able to activate the kinin system. Certain fibrin split products are potent chemoattractants for PMNs. Plasmin is capable of cleaving the complement component C3. Fibrin stimulates interleukin (IL)-1 and IL-8 production by macrophages. Thus, the coagulation system can be an active component of the inflammatory reaction (22).

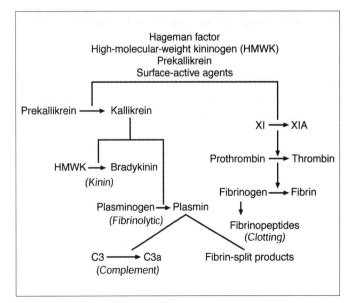

Fig. 4E-3. Kinins and the coagulation system.

Much of the damage done by inflammation is secondary to the scarring and fibrosis that follow an acute inflammatory response. Fibrin plays a key role in the early component of this scarring. Certain inflammatory diseases in animals have been treated successfully with heparin, but it is not clear if therapeutic benefits are secondary to anticoagulation or other effects of heparin. There are no convincing data to date that anticoagulation is useful for treating inflammatory diseases in humans.

Vasoactive Amines

Some low-molecular weight amines have potent inflammatory effects. The role of histamine in the allergic response is well-known. Histamine is stored in mast-cell granules and released by activating signals, such as immunoglobulin (Ig) E binding to antigen. Histamine then binds to cellular receptors, resulting in the clinical effects of vasodilation, increased vascular permeability, bronchoconstriction, and increased mucus production.

Serotonin is noted for its role in depression, but it also plays a role in inflammation. Outside the central nervous system, it is stored primarily in dense body granules of platelets. Serotonin causes vasoconstriction and increased vascular permeability. Blocking serotonin can cause fibrotic changes, as exemplified by the infrequent side effect of retroperitoneal fibrosis by the drug methysergide maleate (Sansert), which is used to treat severe vascular headaches.

Another amine with biologic activity is adenosine, notable as an agent for blocking tachyarrhythmias. Accumulation of adenosine and its resulting toxic effects on lymphocytes are the proximate cause of combined immunodeficiency due to adenosine deaminase deficiency. Adenosine has been known for many years to have anti-inflammatory effects at the site of its release, and evidence suggests that the effects of methotrexate may be mediated by adenosine (23). In therapeutic doses, methotrexate promotes accumulation of the compound 5-aminoimidazole-4-carboxamide ribonucleotide (AICAR), which enhances local release of adenosine. The addition of adenosine deaminase breaks down adenosine and abrogates the anti-inflammatory actions of methotrexate. Adenosine also may abrogate inflammatory responses by blocking AA release, limiting PG and LT production. Other methods of increasing local adenosine release may be of use in the treatment of inflammatory diseases.

Nitric Oxide

The important role of nitric oxide (NO) in health and disease has been the subject of intensive investigation. Interest in NO began when it was identified as the endothelial-derived relaxation factor. Subsequently, NO was shown to play a key role in cell-mediated immunity and also to serve as a neurotransmitter.

Nitric oxide is derived from the amino acid arginine through the activity of the enzyme NO synthase (NOS) (Fig. 4E-4). There are at least three forms of NOS derived from three separate genes. Two forms of NOS (endothelial and neuronal) are expressed constitutively and are dependent on calcium and calmodulin. Both forms produce the NO that is responsible for maintaining vascular tone and neurotransmission. In the vascular system, NO is a potent vasodilator and is the active moiety of sodium nitroprusside and nitroglycerin (24).

The third NOS gene produces an inducible form called iNOS, which primarily is found in immune cells, most notably macrophages and macrophage-derived cells. In addition, iNOS is present in endothelial cells, some neuronal cells, PMNs, lymphocytes, and natural killer cells. Nitric oxide produced by immune cells participates in killing intracellular pathogens and certain tumors. A key role of NO in autoimmunity was demonstrated in animal models of arthritis, diabetes, multiple sclerosis, and systemic lupus erythematosus. Blocking the production of NO with such arginine analogs as N-monomethyl arginine (NMMA) prevented or treated autoimmune disease in these animals (25).

The role of NO in human disease is not as clear as it is in murine disease. Unlike macrophages from rodents, human macrophages cannot be stimulated to produce NO by immune activators, such as cytokines or endotoxin. Recent studies provide evidence that NO is overproduced in human autoimmune diseases. Elevated serum levels of NO metabolites are present in patients with RA, ulcerative colitis, and systemic lupus erythematosus (26). Peripheral blood monocytes and synovial cells from people with RA demonstrate increased levels of iNOS, compared with measurements from controls.

Nitric oxide can cause direct tissue injury by interfering with the function of enzymes in the respiratory burst chain. It also can interact with superoxide to form peroxynitrite, a highly toxic compound that can nitrate tyrosine residues

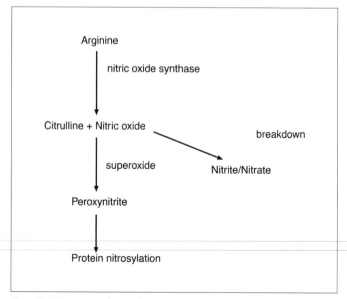

Fig. 4E-4. Nitric oxide synthesis and metabolism

and oxidize cysteine, tryptophan, and tyrosine residues in proteins, altering their function (27). Inducible NOS activity directly affects prostanoid synthesis. Peroxynitrite, an indirect iNOS product, increases COX-2 activity by acting as a substrate for its peroxidase activity (28). Peroxynitrite directly oxidizes arachidonyl-containing lipids to form isoprostanes, and experiments with iNOS-knockout mice indicate that up to 50% of basal 8-isoPGF$_{2a}$ levels in mice is iNOS-derived (29). In addition to these direct actions on tissues, NO apparently has other functions in immunity. It blocks apoptosis of B lymphocytes, participates in maintaining viral latency, and alters the ratio of T-helper (Th)1 to Th2 cells.

Reactive Oxygen Species

Because oxygen possesses two unpaired electrons, it is converted easily to reactive and toxic species by the simple addition or subtraction of electrons. The addition of one electron to oxygen forms the superoxide radical O_2^-, whereas subtracting the two electrons via superoxide dismutase (SOD) forms hydrogen peroxide H_2O_2. Another reduction product of oxygen is the hydroxyl radical OH, formed by the reaction of hydrogen peroxide with iron (Fenton reaction).

Oxygen radicals appear to be important in the ability of PMNs to kill bacteria and other pathogens. Indeed, a defect in the generation of superoxide by PMNs is the underlying pathogenesis of chronic granulomatous disease. Confirmation of this point has been derived from knockout mice in which a subunit of cytochrome b oxidase was inactivated. PMNs from these mice could not produce superoxide, and the mice were susceptible to staphylococcal and fungal infections.

Increased levels of reactive oxygen species have been found in autoimmune diseases, including animal models of disease and human disease (30). Similar to NO, the role of reactive oxygen species in inflammatory diseases has been the focus of increased investigation. Reactive oxygen species can induce apoptosis and tissue damage and/or regulate immune responses. Use of superoxide knockout mice and SOD knockout mice may provide insight into the role of oxygen radicals in disease. Agents that prevent oxygen radical production or quench radicals after they are produced are being studied as treatments for inflammatory diseases (31).

JAMES C. OATES, MD
GARY S. GILKESON, MD

References

1. O'Neill C. The biochemistry of prostaglandins: a primer. Aust N Z J Obstet Gynaecol 1994;34:332–337.

2. Goetzl EJ, An S, Smith WL. Specificity of expression and effects of eicosanoid mediators in normal physiology and human diseases. FASEB J 1995;9:1051–1058.

3. Komhoff M, Grone HJ, Klein T, Seyberth HW, Nusing RM. Localization of cyclooxygenase-1 and -2 in adult and fetal human kidney: implication for renal function. Am J Physiol 1997;272:F460–F468.

4. Harding P, Carretero OA, Beierwaltes WH. Chronic cyclooxygenase-2 inhibition blunts low sodium-stimulated renin without changing renal haemodynamics. J Hypertens 2000;18:1107–1113.

5. Schonbeck U, Sukhova GK, Graber P, Coulter S, Libby P. Augmented expression of cyclooxygenase-2 in human atherosclerotic lesions. Am J Pathol 1999;155:1281–1291.

6. Ho L, Pieroni C, Winger D, Purohit DP, Aisen PS, Pasinetti GM. Regional distribution of cyclooxygenase-2 in the hippocampal formation in Alzheimer's disease. J Neurosci Res 1999;57:295–303.

7. Fosslien E. Molecular pathology of cyclooxygenase-2 in neoplasia. Ann Clin Lab Sci 2000;30:3–21.

8. Tanioki T, Nakatani Y, Sammyo N, Murakami M, Kudo I. Molecular identification of cytosolic prostaglandin E$_2$ synthase that is functionally coupled with cyclooxygenase-1 in immediate prostaglandin E$_2$ biosynthesis. J Biol Chem 2000; 42:32775–32782.

9. Murakami M, Naraba H, Tanioka T, et al. Regulation of prostaglandin E$_2$ biosynthesis by inducible membrane-associated prostaglandin E$_2$ synthase that acts in concert with cyclooxygenase-2. J Biol Chem 2000;42:32783–32792.

10. Breyer MD, Breyer RM. Prostaglandin receptors: their role in regulating renal function. Curr Opin Nephrol Hypertens 2000;9:23–29.

11. Sugimoto Y, Narumiya S, Ichikawa A. Distribution and function of prostanoid receptors: studies from knockout mice [Review]. Prog Lipid Res 2000;39:289–314.

12. Kawahito Y, Motoharu K, Yasunori T, et al. 15-deoxy-D^{12,14}-PGJ2 induces synoviocyte apoptosis and suppresses adjuvant-induced arthritis in rats. J Clin Invest 2000;106: 189–197.

13. Su CG, Wen X, Bailey ST, et al. A novel therapy for colitis utilizing PPAR-gamma ligands to inhibit the epithelial inflammatory response. J Clin Invest 1999;104:383–389.

14. Takamura T, Ando H, Nagai Y, Yamashita H, Nohara E, Kobayashi K. Pioglitazone prevents mice from multiple low-dose streptozotocin-induced insulitis and diabetes. Diabetes Res Clin Pract 1999;44:107–114.

15. Obata T, Yamashita N, Nakagawa T. Leukotriene and thromboxane antagonists. Clin Rev Allergy 1994;12:79–93.

16. Salvati P, Lamberti E, Ferrario R, et al. Long-term thromboxane-synthase inhibition prolongs survival in murine lupus nephritis. Kidney Int 1995;47:1168–1175.

17. Spurney RF, Fan PY, Ruiz P, Sanfilippo F, Pisetsky DS, Coffman TM. Thromboxane receptor blockade reduces renal injury in murine lupus nephritis. Kidney Int 1992;41: 973–982.

18. Reilly IA, Roy L, Fitzgerald GA. Biosynthesis of thromboxane in patients with systemic sclerosis and Raynaud's phenomenon. Br Med J Clin Res Ed 1986;292:1037–1039.

19. Harris RR, Carter GW, Bell RL, Moore JL, Brooks DW. Clinical activity of leukotriene inhibitors. Int J Immunopharmacol 1995;17:147–156.

20. Serhan CN. Lipoxin biosynthesis and its impact in inflammatory and vascular events. Biochim Biophys Acta 1994;1212: 1–25.

21. Sharma JN, Buchanan WW. Pathogenic responses of bradykinin system in chronic inflammatory rheumatoid disease. Exp Toxicol Pathol 1994;46:421–433.

22. Cotran RS, Kumar V, Robbins SL. Inflammation and repair. In: Cotran RS, Kumar V, Robbins SL (eds). Robbins Pathologic Basis of Disease, 4th ed. Philadelphia: WB Saunders, 1989; pp 29–86.

23. Cronstein BN, Naime D, Ostad E. The antiinflammatory mechanism of methotrexate. Increased adenosine release at inflamed sites diminishes leukocyte accumulation in an in vivo model of inflammation. J Clin Invest 1993;92:2675–2682.

24. Nathan C. Nitric oxide as a secretory product of mammalian cells. FASEB J 1992;6:3051–3064.

25. Weinberg JB, Granger DL, Pisetsky DS, et al. The role of nitric oxide in the pathogenesis of spontaneous murine autoimmune disease: increased nitric oxide production and nitric oxide synthase expression in MRL-lpr/lpr mice, and reduction of spontaneous glomerulonephritis and arthritis by orally administered NG-monomethyl-L-arginine. J Exp Med 1994;179:651–660.

26. Godkin AJ, De Belder AJ, Villa L, et al. Expression of nitric oxide synthase in ulcerative colitis. Eur J Clin Invest 1996;26: 867–872.

27. Lincoln J, Hoyle CHV, Burnstock G. Nitric oxide in health and disease. In: Lucy JA (ed). Biomedical Research Topics. Vol. 1. New York: Cambridge University Press, 1997.

28. Landino LM, Crews BC, Timmons MD, Morrow JD, Marnett LJ. Peroxynitrite, the coupling product of nitric oxide and superoxide, activates prostaglandin biosynthesis. Proc Natl Acad Sci USA 1996;93:15069–15074.

29. Marnett LJ, Wright TL, Crews BC, Tannenbaum ST, Morrow JD. Regulation of prostaglandin biosynthesis by nitric oxide is revealed by targeted deletion of inducible nitric oxide synthase. J Biol Chem 2000;275:13427–13430.

30. Greenwald RA. Oxygen radicals, inflammation, and arthritis: pathophysiological considerations and implications for treatment. Semin Arthritis Rheum 1991;20:219–240.

31. Bauerova K, Bezek A. Role of reactive oxygen and nitrogen species in etiopathogenesis of rheumatoid arthritis. Gen Physiol Biophys 1999;18:15–20.

5 IMMUNITY
A. Molecular and Cellular Basis of Immunity

The immune system, a coordinated response of highly anti-gen-specific cells with nonspecific inflammatory cells and soluble factors, evolved to protect the body from infectious microorganisms. Although these responses generally provide a highly effective system, they can go awry, resulting in immune-mediated disease. This chapter briefly reviews the cardinal features of the immune system, including antigen recognition, diversity, specificity, tolerance, and memory. Also discussed are the mechanisms and molecules that underlie these features and how they relate to the pathogenesis of immune-mediated diseases. Despite the gaps in our understanding of the pathogenesis of rheumatic diseases, there are numerous examples (albeit for the most part in animal models) in which mutation of a single gene leads to immunologic disease. Perhaps the surprise is that so many different genetic lesions can lead to autoimmune disease.

Overview of the Immune System

The immune response typically is divided into innate and adaptive responses, but it is very clear that both arms work in concert for host defense and both contribute to immune-mediated disease. The innate immune response consists of such barriers as skin and mucosa, phagocytic cells of the myelomonocytic lineage, and serum constituents, such as complement (1). The cells that contribute to adaptive immunity include T and B lymphocytes. In contrast to T and B cells, the natural killer (NK) cells that form a third lymphocyte subset lack specific antigen receptors (2). Rather, NK cells recognize and kill virus-infected cells and tumors that lack major histocompatibility class (MHC) I molecules. Natural killer cells are included in the innate immune system, but they also regulate adaptive immunity by the production of cytokines. Antigen-presenting cells (APC), like macrophages, are key constituents of both adaptive and innate immunity; these cells have direct host-defense activity, but also promote T-cell responses. Another major subset of APC is dendritic cells (DC), which serve key functions in regulating the immune response (3,4).

The adaptive immune response is further divided into humoral and cell-mediated immunity. Humoral immunity principally consists of the B-cell and immunoglobulin (Ig) response, whereas cell-mediated immunity refers to the T-cell and APC-dependent response. Although useful concep-tually, the division of the immune response between innate versus adaptive immunity and humoral versus cellular immunity is somewhat arbitrary. Not only do T cells (cell-mediated immunity) regulate immunoglobulin production

by B cells (humoral immunity), but T cells (adaptive immu-nity) also secrete cytokines that recruit inflammatory cells of the myelomonocytic lineage (innate immunity). It is par-ticularly relevant to understand this coordination of responses in considering the pathogenesis and treatment of immunologic diseases.

Lymphocytes and mononuclear phagocytes are derived from hematopoietic stem cells. Embryonically, stem cells arise from the fetal yolk sac and populate the bone marrow, spleen, and liver. In the adult, bone marrow is the predom-inant source of lymphocytic and myelomonocytic progeni-tor cells. Lymphoid organs include the thymus, spleen, lymph nodes, and Peyer's patches. Immature T cells develop into mature T lymphocytes in the thymus, and B cells devel-op within the bone marrow. The spleen, lymph nodes, and Peyer's patches in the intestine are sites where B-cell differ-entiation occurs and T and B cells engage antigen. Antigen presentation to T cells occurs here, as do B-cell–T-cell inter-actions. The spleen, the major site where lymphocytes encounter blood-borne antigen, clears the circulation of senescent red blood cells and foreign substances. Lymph-borne antigen is encountered in the lymph nodes.

The ability of immune system cells to function depends on their ability to localize within specific tissues and to interact with each other in a coordinated fashion. During normal homeostasis and inflammation, chemokines and their cognate receptors provide a flexible code for immune-cell trafficking (5,6). Varying levels of chemokine receptor expression, responsiveness, and production contribute to the complex migration patterns of immune cells. Not sur-prisingly, chemokine receptors are exploited by several pathogens. For example, during infection with the human immunodeficiency virus, HIV gains entry into permissive cells by using several different chemokine receptors, CCR5 and CXCR4 being the best-known.

Antigens, Antigen-Presenting Cells, and MHC Molecules

A fundamentally important concept in immunology is that of antigenicity. Simply speaking, an antigen is a substance that generates an immune response. What does this mean mechanistically? Lymphocytes recognize antigen by virtue of clonally specific antigen receptors. These receptors are immunoglobulin-like molecules located in the plasma mem-branes of T cells and B cells. Although T and B cells use a similar strategy to produce these extraordinary receptors, they "see" antigen very differently. B cells recognize soluble peptides, proteins, nucleic acids, polysaccharides, lipids, and small synthetic molecules. These antigens bind directly to the B-cell antigen receptor (BCR), a membrane-associated form of immunoglobulin. Consequently, B cells have no need for antigen-presenting cells (Fig. 5A-1).

In contrast, T cells need antigen to be presented – that is, the T-cell antigen receptor (TCR) recognizes peptide fragments only when they are bound to MHC molecules. There are two types of MHC molecules, class I and class II. The three-dimensional structure of both classes creates a cleft, or groove, in which peptides are bound and can be recognized by T cells. MHC molecules, therefore, are antigen-presenting molecules for T cells (7,8). The association of peptides with MHC molecules is determined by primary and secondary structures of these molecules. Each MHC molecule binds a single peptide, but the pool of MHC molecules produced can bind an array of peptides. Thus, MHC molecules are important determinants in controlling the immune response to protein antigens. The association of autoimmune disease with specific HLA alleles is well-documented and makes sense, given the critical role of MHC molecules in antigen presentation. The types of antigens that each class bind are quite distinct (Fig 5A-2).

The primary function of MHC class I molecules is to present endogenous peptides. Class I molecules are expressed on nearly all cells and consist of two subunits. The α chain of class I proteins, encoded by genes within the HLA locus (HLA-A, -B, and -C), associates with a non– MHC-encoded protein, β2-microglobulin. Class I molecules bind fragments of proteins that are degraded within the cell, including peptides derived from pathogens, such as viruses, as well as normal cellular proteins. Cytosolic proteins are degraded in the proteasome and transferred to the endoplasmic reticulum by peptide transporter molecules, which also are encoded within the MHC locus. There the MHC class I molecules are synthesized and assembled. The nascent MHC molecules associate with peptides and translocate to the plasma membrane, where they can be recognized by T cells. Class I molecules bind peptides that are nine to 11 amino acids in length. The T-cell accessory molecule, CD8, binds to class I molecules in a region distinct from the TCR; thus, *CD8-expressing T cells are class I-restricted*. Because of their ability to bind MHC, the CD8 and CD4 molecules are called coreceptors. When CD8 T cells are activated, they become cytotoxic T lymphocytes, which are important in controlling viral infections by destroying virally infected cells.

The primary function of class II molecules is to present exogenous peptides. Class II molecules are composed of two chains that are products of different MHC genes (HLA-DR, -DQ, and -DP). A limited array of cells, including B cells, macrophages, DC, activated T cells, and activated endothelial cells, express class II molecules. Bone marrow-derived DCs, which are present in lymph nodes and the spleen, are extremely efficient APCs.

Antigen processing by class II-expressing APCs occurs in three steps: extracellular antigens are ingested, internalized, and proteolyzed. MHC class II molecules are synthesized and assembled, but they are prevented from binding endogenous peptide antigens because the class II complex associates with a molecule called the invariant chain. In the appropriate intracellular compartment, however, the invariant chain is cleaved and removed by the action of proteases and HLA-DM. This action allows processed, extracellularly derived antigen to bind to class II molecules, enabling the presentation of these antigens to T cells. Class II molecules bind peptides that range from 10 to 30 amino acids in length. The CD4 molecule binds MHC class II molecules, and therefore, *CD4-expressing or helper T cells are class II-restricted*. Helper T cells, which account for about 60% of all T cells, are key immunoregulatory cells that control cellular and humoral immune responses.

Although most T cells recognize peptides, γδ T cells, a subset representing about 5% of peripheral blood T cells, can recognize nonpeptide antigen, such as prenyl pyrophosphate derivatives of mycobacteria. Lipid antigens also can be presented to T cells by the MHC-related CD1 family of molecules (9).

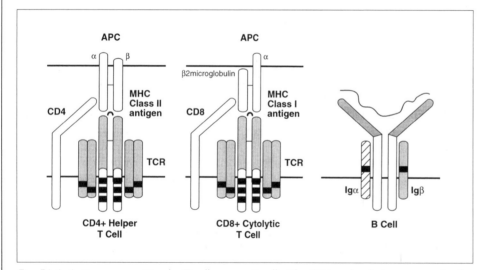

Fig. 5A-1. Antigen recognition by T cells versus B cells. The CD4 molecule is a coreceptor for major histocompatibility complex (MHC) class II molecules. CD4 or helper T cells recognize processed peptide antigen presented by class II molecules, which are expressed only on specialized cells. The CD8 molecule is a coreceptor for class I molecules, so CD8 T cells recognize peptide antigens presented by cells expressing class I molecules, which are present on most cells. In contrast, γδ T cells do not express either CD4 or CD8 and, unlike αβ T cells, can recognize nonpeptide antigens. B cells recognize many different types of soluble antigens in their native state and do not require antigen presentation. The black boxes indicate immune tyrosine-based activation (ITAM) motifs.

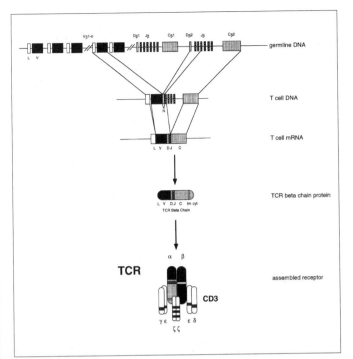

Fig. 5A-2. Processes that generate a T-cell receptor (TCR). DNA is in the germline configuration in T cell precursors. During T-cell development in the thymus, the TCR gene segments rearrange in a specific order, bringing variable (V), diversity (D), joining (J), and constant (C) segments into proximity to generate functional receptor genes. Random nucleotide additions (N) are inserted by terminal deoxytransferase. The β locus has 75 V, two D, 10 or 12 J, and two C segments. The α gene has 50 V, 70 J, and one C segments. The δ gene, which is embedded within the α gene, has four V, two D, three J, and one C segments, whereas the γ locus has eight V, five J, and two C segments. After DNA rearrangement, messenger RNA is produced and spliced to form the mature RNA. After transcription, the receptor subunit associates with another subunit that also is the product of a gene rearrangement plus invariant chains. This process occurs in the endoplasmic reticulum, and the receptor complex is transported to the cell surface.

Recognition of Antigen by T Cells

The TCR complex is composed of both antigen-recognition and signal-transducing subunits. Four TCR genes encode the subunits responsible for antigen recognition: α, β, γ, and δ. The TCR genes are members of the Ig gene superfamily and are similar in other respects to Ig genes. TCR genes undergo DNA rearrangement of variable (V), diversity (D), joining (J), and constant (C) region segments (Fig. 5A-3). This recombination of gene segments is generated by the action of a number of enzymes, including the recombinase-activating genes RAG-1 and RAG-2. The rearranged gene is then transcribed and translated to produce a protein subunit. Two of these subunits combine to form the two types of heterodimeric receptors, αβ and γδ receptors, which function as the antigen-recognition unit; the majority of T cells in peripheral blood, lymph nodes, and spleen express αβ receptors.

V-region gene segments are highly polymorphic, and recombinant assembly of the different V, D, and J segments further increases their diversity. Even greater diversity occurs with the insertion of random nucleotides at the junctions by the enzyme terminal deoxytransferase. An individual has the genetic capacity of producing a vast number of T-cell clones with specific antigen receptors – potentially, about 10^{16} αβ T-cell receptors.

TCR genes show allelic exclusion; that is, if one chromosome undergoes rearrangement and produces a functional receptor chain, the genes on the other chromosome are prevented from rearranging. Hence, each T-cell clone expresses only one antigen receptor, and antigen-specific T cells develop in unimmunized or naive individuals independent of exposure to antigen. Subsequent antigen exposure leads to clonal selection or expansion of lymphocytes with the appropriate antigen receptors. Clonal selection improves the efficiency of the immune response and produces immunologic memory.

TCR αβ or γδ subunits provide an elegant solution to the problem of antigen recognition, but these subunits do not transmit activation signals. Instead, the antigen-recognizing subunits associate with signaling subunits called invariant chains because they are not polymorphic. The invariant subunits include the CD3 family of molecules (γ, δ, ε) and the ζ chain, which can exist as a homodimer (ζ–ζ) or a heterodimer (ζ–η), the η chain being an alternatively spliced form of ζ. The stoichiometry of the TCR most likely is TCRαβ/CD3γδε₂ζ₂.

TCR Signal Transduction

In response to recognition of foreign antigen by the antigen-recognition subunits, the first known biochemical event is phosphorylation of the invariant chains on tyrosine residues by protein tyrosine kinases (PTK) (Fig. 5A-4) (10). Upon recognition of antigen–MHC complex, Lck (a PTK that binds CD4 and CD8 molecules) is brought into the TCR complex, where it phosphorylates the invariant chains. A protein tyrosine phosphatase, CD45, is critical for TCR signaling. The phosphorylated sites on the γ, δ, ε, and ζ subunits of CD3 are called ITAMs (immune tyrosine-based activation motifs) and consist of 17 amino acids with a duplicated sequence: tyrosine-X-X-leucine (X denotes any amino acid). ITAMs are present in receptors other than the TCR, including the B-cell and Fc receptors (11), and are docking sites for proteins with SH2 (Src homology 2) domains that bind phosphotyrosine. A second PTK, Zap-70 (zeta-associated protein of 70 kDa) binds the TCR ITAMs via its SH2 domain. Along with members of a third PTK family (e.g., Itk), Zap-70 activation leads to phosphorylation of the adapter protein LAT (linker of activated T cells). Phosphorylated LAT binds other proteins that have SH2 domains, including adapters like Grb2, Gads, and SLP-76, which effect the activation of several pathways, including the cascade of serine–threonine kinases activated by Ras. In addition, phospholipase C (PLC)γ is activated and catalyzes cleavage of phosphatidylinositol bisphosphate (PIP₂) to pro-

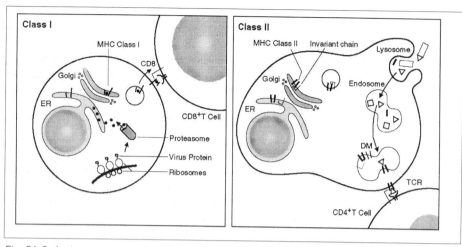

Fig. 5A-3. Antigen presentation: Endogenous antigens are presented by major histocompatibility complex (MHC) class I molecules to CD8+ T cells, whereas exogenous antigens are presented by MHC class II molecules to CD4+ T cells.

duce diacylglycerol and inositol trisphosphate; the former intermediate activates protein kinase C, and the latter releases intracellular calcium. Elevation of calcium in the cell activates calcineurin, which dephosphorylates NFAT (nuclear factor of activated T cells), allowing the translocation of this transcription factor to the nucleus; this step is blocked by the immunosuppressive drugs cyclosporine and FK506 (12). Transcription factors like NFAT, NFκB, Fos, and Jun are key molecules regulated by receptor-derived signals that modulate the expression of genes encoding cytokines, receptors, and other proteins.

It should be noted that in addition to ITAMs, some lymphocyte receptors have motifs called ITIMs (immunoreceptor tyrosine-based inhibitory motif) that can recruit phosphatases and thus attenuate signaling. The NK inhibitory receptors function in this manner (2).

Costimulation

Occupancy of the T-cell receptor alone does not lead to T-cell activation; perturbation of other surface molecules is necessary to provide a full activation signal (Fig. 5A-4). Receptors that provide these additional signals include costimulatory molecules, such as CD28 (13), and adhesion molecules (CD11a/CD18, CD2, and others). TCR stimulation in the absence of a CD28-mediated signal can lead to a state of anergy, or unresponsiveness. Interestingly, interference of CD28 signaling in murine lupus ameliorates autoimmune disease in mice. The counter-receptors for CD28 are B7-1 and B7-2, which are expressed on APC. In addition, a molecule related to CD28, CTLA-4, also binds B7-1 and B7-2. Unlike CD28, which provides costimulatory signals, CTLA-4 functions to down-regulate the immune response. This is illustrated by CTLA-4 knockout mice, which develop lethal lymphoproliferative disease. Several new members of this family of receptors and counter-receptors include B7-1, B7-2, B-7RP.1, B7-H3, PDL-1, PDL-2, CD28, CTLA-4, ICOS, and PD-1. It appears that these

molecules play important sequential roles in regulatory T-cell function and tolerance (14).

Costimulation works in both directions, activating APCs as well as lymphocytes. An example of this is CD40 (on APCs and B cells) and CD40 ligand (on activated T cells). Occupancy of CD40 activates APC to produce such cytokines as IL-12. Mutation of CD40 ligand (CD40L) is the basis of the primary immunodeficiency X-linked hyper-IgM syndrome, and interference with the CD40–CD40-ligand interaction is being studied as a means of treating autoimmune disorders. Increasingly, it is recognized that APC and their trafficking are critical factors in determining antigenicity and the character of the immune response (1,4,15,16). Indeed, it is thought that the mechanism through which adjuvants increase the antigenicity of vaccines is their ability to activate APC. APCs exposed to pathogens or "dangerous" stimuli are thought to be more efficient in inducing antigenicity. Alternatively, the amount of antigen and the time in which it is transported to lymphoid tissue are thought to be factors in immune reactivity.

T-cell Development

Precursor T cells originate in the bone marrow from stem cells, which are progenitors of other hematopoietic cells. These cells migrate to the thymus, where they begin differentiation. The most immature cells lack CD4 and CD8, and are called double-negative cells; these cells do not express a mature TCR but do express the pre-T receptor. These cells mature to cells expressing TCR and both CD4 and CD8; such cells are called double-positive (DP) thymocytes. DP thymocytes mature to become single-positive (SP) thymocytes, which express either CD4 or CD8, as well as TCR. Of considerable interest is that the vast majority of T cells entering the thymus die there. To survive, T cells must have produced TCRs that recognize self-MHC molecules, a process called positive selection. Cells lacking an appropriate receptor undergo "death by neglect." Some TCRs recognize self-MHC molecules and self-peptides with high affinity, and these potentially autoreactive clones are eliminated (negative selection or clonal deletion). Positive and negative selection occur at the DP and SP stages of T-cell development. This mechanism is believed to achieve tolerance to self, which is termed central tolerance. Much of the T-cell death that occurs in the thymus is due to programmed cell death (apoptosis). There are additional mechanisms for achieving tolerance outside the thymus and this process is referred to as peripheral tolerance.

Immunoglobulins and B Cells

Immunoglobulin molecules, inserted into the membrane of a B lymphocyte, are responsible for the ability of B cells to recognize antigen (Fig. 5A-1). In addition, Ig secreted by terminally differentiated B lymphocytes, called plasma cells, assists in the clearance of pathogenic organisms. Ig molecules are composed of two types of polypeptides, light and heavy chains. There are two Ig light (L) chain classes (isotypes), κ and λ, and nine distinct Ig heavy (H) chain isotypes (Table 5A-1). The H chain isotypes correspond with the five different classes of immunoglobulins – γ, α, μ, δ, and ε for IgG, IgA, IgM, IgD, and IgE, respectively – and the subclasses of IgG (γ1, γ2, γ3, and γ4) and IgA (α1 and α2). For example, an IgG1 molecule contains two identical γ1 chains and two identical L chains (either κ or λ) bound together by noncovalent and disulfide bonds. In contrast, most IgM and many IgA molecules are higher order multimers of H and L chains that are interconnected via interdisulfide bonds and a unique protein called a J chain. IgA often functions at epithelial surfaces and, when secreted through the epithelium, is associated with a secretory fragment.

Each H and L chain has a variable and a constant region. Many of the effector functions of Ig, such as binding to complement and Fc receptors, depend on the constant region of H chain isotype, while the antigen-binding capability of Ig resides in the variable regions of both the H and L chains. Each developing B cell has the genetic potential for assembling an antigen-receptor complex of a unique specificity, and the vast sum of the specificities is called the

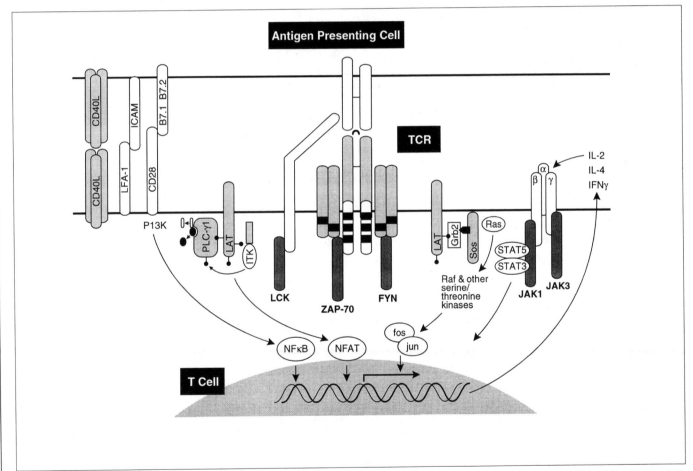

Fig. 5A-4. T-cell activation. Upon encountering foreign antigen in association with the major histocompatibility complex (MHC), CD4 or CD8 is brought into proximity of the T-cell receptor (TCR) complex with the protein tyrosine kinase Lck, which phosphorylates the TCR invariant subunits on immune tyrosine-based activation motif (ITAM) sites (shown as black boxes on the receptor subunits). The site formed can be bound by the SH2-containing kinase, Zap-70, which phosphorylates adapter molecules like LAT and SLP-76. This action propagates signaling by the recruitment of enzymes like PLCγ, which in turn activate serine/threonine kinases and elevate intracellular calcium ($Ca2^+$) levels. These signals regulate the function of transcription factors, such as nuclear factor of activated T cells (NFAT), NFκB, Fos, and Jun. These factors, in turn, regulate the expression of T-cell activation genes, such as interleukin 2 (IL-2) and the IL-2Rα subunit. IL-2 is secreted and activates T cells through its receptor, which interacts with the tyrosine kinases JAK1 and JAK3. These kinases then activate STATs, a class of transcription factors. Also shown are adhesion molecules (ICAM and LFA-1 [CD11a/CD18]) and important costimulatory molecule CD28. IP3 and PIP_2 are phosphorylated derivatives of a phospholipid component of the plasma membrane and PI3K is a lipid kinase. Other abbreviations are diacylglycerol (DG) and protein kinase C (PKC).

TABLE 5A-1
Human Immunoglobulin Classes (Heavy Chain Isotypes)

	IgM	IgD	IgG1	IgG2	IgG3	IgG4	IgA1	IgA2	IgE
H chain	μ	δ	γ1	γ2	γ3	γ4	α1	α2	ε
Molecular weight (kDa)	900	180	150	150	150	150	160–350	160–350	190
Serum concentration (mg%)	100	3	900	300	100	50	300	50	0.001
Complement fixation by classical pathway	+++	–	++	+	+++	–	–	–	–
Placental transfer	–	–	+	+	+	+	–	–	–
Plasma half life (days)	5	3	21	20	7	21	6	6	2
$(H_2L_2)_n$, n=	5	1	1	1	1	1	1,2	1,2	1
Number of domains per heavy chain	5	5	4	4	4	4	4	4	5
Carbohydrate (%)	12	12	3	3	3	3	9	9	12

B-cell repertoire. Similar to the T-cell repertoire, the B-cell repertoire is diversified by using different V genes, imprecise joining of different D and J segments, and diversification of N segments (nucleotide insertions). In addition, the B-cell repertoire is capable of somatic hypermutation.

B-Cell Development

B-cell lymphopoiesis begins in the fetal liver and later switches to the bone marrow. While conventional B cells (B2) are generated continuously in the adult bone marrow, B1 (formerly called CD5) B cells predominantly are produced early in ontogeny. Two major events occur in B-cell development: the rearrangement and expression of Ig genes (17). All the H chain genes are on chromosome 14. Their successful rearrangement requires the joining of a J_H segment, a D_H segment, and a V_H region (Fig. 5A-5). B-cell precursors first assemble $D_H J_H$ rearrangements, and after V_H is successfully joined to $D_H J_H$, H-chain rearrangements cease. B-cell precursors that have not initiated Ig rearrangement or that include only DJ rearrangements are called pro-B cells. Precursors that have rearranged, transcribed, and translated an H chain are called pre-B cells. The translated μ chains in pre-B cells are intracellular, with the exception of small amounts found on the plasma membrane in conjunction with surrogate L chain (derived from the λ5 and V pre-β gene products). Together, the H chain and the surrogate L chain form the pre-B-cell receptor complex. This complex signals the pre-B cells to proliferate and to rearrange one of its L chains. The κ and λ loci are on chromosomes 2 and 22, respectively. Their rearrangement requires a VJ joint. Once a B-cell precursor successfully rearranges an H and L gene, the process stops, and the cell expresses surface Ig; it then is termed an immature B cell. Many precursor cells fail to make successful rearrangements or to express a func-

tional pre–B-cell receptor, and these precursor cells die in situ via apoptosis.

The protein RAG-2 is required for rearrangement of the Ig and TCR loci. The lack of RAG-2 results in the absence of mature lymphocytes. In general, any mutation that impairs H-chain rearrangement or expression will block B-cell development (18). In addition, the cytokine IL-7, the kinase Syk, the cell-survival gene bcl-x, and the transcription factors E2A, EBF, and BSAP have critical roles in B-cell development, as does Bruton's tyrosine kinase (BTK) gene. Mutations in the BTK gene cause Bruton's X-linked agammaglobulinemia, a disease characterized by impaired B-cell development (19). B-cell development also is impaired in mice that lack the chemokine SDF-1 or its cognate receptor CXCR4 (20).

B-Cell Activation

Once a B-cell precursor expresses surface Ig, it can respond to exogenous and self-antigens. However, the binding of antigens to the BCR on immature B cells does not trigger cellular activation, but rather, a cellular response leading to self-tolerance. Multivalent self-antigens, such as double-stranded DNA, induce programmed cell death, whereas oligovalent self-antigens render immature B cells refractory to further stimulation. Such a cell may escape anergy by rearranging another L-chain Ig gene, changing its BCR specificity, and losing its self-reactivity, a process called receptor editing.

Mature B cells with non–self-reactive BCRs enter secondary lymphoid tissues, such as spleen or lymph nodes, where they may encounter foreign antigens. B-cell antigens are divided broadly into thymus-dependent (TD) and thymus-independent (TI) antigens. TD antigens are largely soluble protein antigens that require MHC class II-restricted T-cell help for antibody production, whereas TI antigens do not require such help. TI antigens often are multivalent and poorly degraded in vivo; bacterial polysaccharides are examples of these antigens. In general, TI responses generate poor immunologic memory, induce minimal germinal-center formation, and trigger IgG2 secretion (21). The B cells responding to TI antigens have a distinct phenotype and localize in the marginal zone of the spleen. Dependence on these splenic B cells for responses to TI antigens may account for the poor responses to polysaccharide antigens seen in splenectomized individuals and in infants (the marginal zone B cells do not mature until about two years of age). Coupling polysaccharides to a carrier protein produces an effective infant vaccine, because the conjugate triggers a TD response.

The BCR has a dual role: 1) it binds and internalizes antigen for processing into peptides that assemble with class II molecules for presentation to CD4 T cells; and 2) it activates the antigen-recognizing B cell (22). The signal-transducing capability of the BCR lies not with surface Ig, but with two associated transmembrane proteins: Ig-α and Ig-β. Similar to the TCR-associated molecules, their intracellular domains contain ITAM motifs. Ig-α/Ig-β heterodimers couple the BCR to the Src-related kinases Lyn, Blk, and Fyn, and the Zap-70-related tyrosine kinase Syk. The B-cell transmembrane proteins CD19 and CD22 modulate BCR signaling. CD19 enhances and CD22 impairs B-cell activation through the BCR. Although the ligands for CD19 and CD22 are unknown, their intracellular portions associate with tyrosine kinases. In Lyn-deficient mice,

defective B-cell clonal expansion and terminal differentiation occur, as does a failure to eliminate autoreactive B cells. The Syk- and the Src-related kinases phosphorylate other downstream effectors, activating the B cell and increasing the membrane levels of the T-cell costimulatory ligands B7-1 and B7-2, which are needed for B-cell and T-cell collaboration.

B-Cell Differentiation

Exposure to a TD antigen triggers two pathways of B-cell differentiation: the extrafollicular pathway, which leads to early antibody production, and the germinal-center pathway, which leads to germinal-center formation, immunologic memory, and generation of plasma-cell precursors (23,24). In the spleen, antigen-activated B cells migrate to T-cell–rich zones in the periarteriolar lymphoid sheath searching for T-cell help. Failure to find this help likely results in anergy, but successful B-cell–T-cell collaboration produces short-lived oligoclonal proliferative foci (each derived from several B cells). Many of the B cells in these foci secrete IgM and undergo isotype switching, a DNA-splicing event that exchanges the H-chain constant regions of an Ig gene, while the VDJ gene segments remain the same. By this mechanism, IgM antibodies of a given antigen specificity can be converted to IgG, IgA, or IgE. These events depend on direct costimulatory signals, CD40 and CD40L interactions, and such cytokines as TGF-β, IL-2, IL-4, IL-6, and IL-10. Antibody affinity also may be altered by the introduction of mutations in variable gene segments, a process known as somatic mutation.

Some B cells migrate from these proliferative foci to primary follicles and enter the germinal-center pathway. Within a primary follicle, an oligoclonal expansion of B cells forms the dark zone. Eventually, these cells migrate into a region called the light zone, where they interact with helper T cells and follicular dendritic cells that have trapped and localized antigen on their surfaces. Here, B cells that possess high-affinity BCRs are selected to survive, whereas those that do not possess this affinity die. B cells in which somatic mutations generated an autoreactive BCR also are eliminated. Rescue signals induce the survival genes *bcl-x* and *bcl-2*, resulting in the persistence of the selected cells. B7-1, CD19, CD40 on B cells, and CD40L on activated T cells, have critical roles in germinal-center formation. Individuals with the X-linked hyper IgM syndrome do not express functional CD40L following T-cell activation, which underscores the importance of CD40L. Consequently,

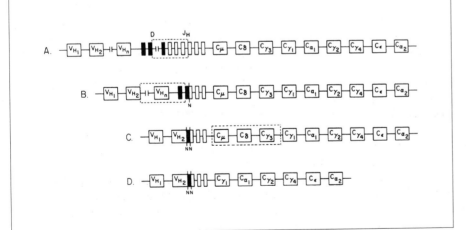

Fig. 5A-5. Genetic organization and rearrangement of immunoglobulin heavy chain genes. Shown is a simplified version of the portion of chromosome 14 containing the immunoglobulin heavy chain variable region and constant region genes. A: Genomic organization found in all cells except committed B cells. B: Initial rearrangement produces the D-J joining, which results from deletion of the DNA enclosed in the dashed box in A. The junction between D and J regions includes additional random nucleotides constituting an N region. C: The next step in rearrangement is V-D-J joining, which results from the deletion of the DNA enclosed in the dashed box in B. A B cell expressing the rearrangement gene shown in C might express IgM with the V_{H2} variable region. D: Such a B cell could then undergo an isotype switch by deleting the DNA shown in the dashed box in C to express IgGl with the same V_{H2} variable region.

B cells do not form germinal centers, and their Ig genes are unable to undergo class switching. CD40 and CD40L are members of the tumor necrosis factor α (TNF-α) family.

Passage through the germinal center leads to the formation of memory B cells or plasma-cell precursors; few antibody-secreting cells remain within the germinal center. Cytokines and CD40L influence this decision; IL-2, IL-10, and IL-6 promote differentiation into plasma cells, whereas CD40–CD40L interactions promote memory-cell formation and inhibit plasma-cell generation. Cytokines also contribute to isotype switching. IL-4 enhances switching to IgE and IgG4; IL-10 to IgG1, IgG3, and IgA; and transforming growth factor β (TGF-β) to IgA.

Plasma cells secrete large amounts of Ig, but they are short-lived cells that need constant replenishment to sustain high antibody levels. Plasma cells lose their membrane Ig and many of the markers that identify B cells, although they express high levels of CD38. Memory B cells are long-lived cells that contain somatically mutated V genes and are morphologically distinct from naive B cells. They can be restimulated to rapidly generate a secondary antibody response. Together, the extrafollicular and germinal-center pathways of B-cell differentiation lead to a coordinated humoral response that provides the very rapid production of low-affinity antibodies, the subsequent production of high-affinity antibodies, and the potential for a rapid amnestic response.

The migration of B cells into splenic follicles and lymph node follicles requires a chemokine called B-lymphocyte chemoattractant (BLC/BCA1) and its receptor, CXCR5. The development of most lymph nodes and Peyer's patches requires this chemokine/receptor pair (5,6). In addition, BLC expression by follicular stromal cells is defective in TNF- and lymphotoxin-deficient mice. This defect explains the lack of normal B-cell follicles in the spleen of these mice.

Immunoregulation and Cytokines

The ability of the immune system to mount a response is regulated at many levels. MHC and TCR molecules determine which antigens will be recognized. Other factors that influence the immune response include the nature of antigen, the route of exposure, and the quantity of antigen. Co-administration of an adjuvant increases the immunogenicity of a substance because adjuvants activate antigen-presenting cells and other components of the innate immune system. Another major immunoregulatory mechanism is the production of a large number of cytokines by lymphoid and nonlymphoid cells; many of the cytokines that mediate innate immunity and inflammation are of great importance in the pathogenesis of rheumatic disease. For example, IL-1 and TNF-α are major mediators of inflammation and tissue injury; interfering with the action of TNF-α is one strategy for treating rheumatoid arthritis (25). Of note, mutations of the TNF receptor in humans result in a periodic fever syndrome called TRAPs (TNF receptor-associated periodic syndrome) (26). Other cytokines are critically important in hematopoiesis, and several are widely used clinically (e.g., erythropoietin and granulocyte colony-stimulating factor). However, only those cytokines with important immunoregulatory activities will be reviewed here.

T-Helper Cells

CD4 or helper T cells differentiate to one of two phenotypes (27,28): T-helper 1 (Th1) and T-helper 2 (Th2) cells. Th1 cells produce lymphotoxin α and interferon (IFN)-γ, promoting a cell-mediated response. IFN-γ activates macrophages, enhances their ability to kill microorganisms, up-regulates class II expression, and suppresses Th2 responses. IL-12 is a key inducer of Th1 differentiation and is produced by B cells and monocytes in response to pathogenic organisms. It also enhances T- and NK-cell cytolytic activity and induces IFN-γ secretion.

In contrast, Th2 cells produce IL-4, IL-5, IL-9, and IL-10, promoting humoral or allergic responses. IL-4 is a major regulator of allergic responses. It inhibits macrophage activation, blocks the effects of IFN-γ, is a growth factor for mast cells, and is required for class switching of B cells to produce IgE. IL-4 also greatly influences Th2 differentiation of naive helper T cells. IL-5 promotes the growth, differentiation, and activation of eosinophils, and IL-9 supports growth of T cells and bone marrow-derived mast-cell precursors. In contradistinction to IFN-γ, IL-10 inhibits macrophage antigen presentation and decreases expression of class II molecules. The importance of IL-10 as an endogenous inhibitor of cell-mediated immunity is underscored by the finding that IL-10 knockout mice develop autoimmune disease.

Precisely how Th1 versus Th2 differentiation occurs is not fully understood, but cytokines, especially IL-12 and IL-4, clearly are important in the outcome; mice and humans with mutations of these cytokines or their receptors have the expected impaired responses and host-defense deficits. Transcription factors, such as GATA-3, c-Maf, NFAT, and T-Bet, regulate Th differentiation, as do dendritic cells (27).

Interleukin 2, an autocrine T-cell growth factor, is important in determining the magnitude of T-cell and NK-cell responses. Interestingly, mice that lack IL-2 do not have immunodeficiency, but rather, they display autoimmunity and lymphoproliferation. This condition is thought to be to due to impaired apoptosis. IL-15 has similar effects, as it binds the β and γ subunits of IL-2R. However, IL-15 is produced by nonlymphoid cells and is important for NK and memory cell development; it appears to be of importance in immunologically mediated diseases as well.

Many, but not all, cytokines bind to receptors that are members of the hematopoietic cytokine receptor superfamily. A family of cytoplasmic PTKs known as Janus kinases (JAKs) is particularly important for signaling by these receptors. JAKs bind to cytokine receptors, become activated following cytokine binding, and phosphorylate the receptor (29). Different JAKs are activated by different cytokines. The importance of this family is supported by the demonstration that patients who lack JAK3 are immunodeficient. JAK3 binds to the cytokine subunit γχ, which is a component of the receptors for IL-2, IL-4, IL-7, IL-9, and IL-15, all of which activate JAK3. Deficiency of either γχ or JAK3 leads to the same phenotype of severe combined immunodeficiency.

An important class of substrate for the JAKs is the STAT (signal transducers and activators of transcription) family of transcription factors. Having SH2 domains, STATs bind the phosphorylated cytokine receptor, become phosphorylated by the JAKs, and then translocate to the nucleus where they regulate gene expression. Different cytokine receptors recruit and activate different members of the STAT family. The importance of STAT molecules in the immune response is underscored by the generation of STAT knockout mice. Mice deficient in STAT4, which is activated by IL-12, have impaired Th1 differentiation; mice deficient in STAT6, which is activated by IL-4, have impaired Th2 responses. STAT1 and STAT2 knockouts show impaired IFN responses.

Turning Off the Immune Response

An essential feature of immune responses is that they are self-limited. A number of mechanisms serve to attenuate immune responses. As discussed, ITIM-containing receptors inhibit signaling by recruiting protein tyrosine phosphatases, which counteract PTK. Moth-eaten mice have deficiency of SHP1 (SH-2 that contains phosphatase 1) and suffer from severe immunologic disease. CTLA-r recruits tyrosine phosphatases; accordingly, CTLA-4–deficient mice develop a fatal lymphoproliferative disorder. Like IL-10, TGF-β1 is an important cytokine that suppresses immune responses. TGF-β1 knockout mice die of overwhelming immunologic disease, associated with autoantibodies (30), that is characterized by lymphoid and mononuclear infiltration of the heart, lung, and other tissues. SOCS (suppressor of cytokine signaling) proteins are a family of cytokine-induced inhibitors that attenuate signaling, and absence of SOCS-1 in mice causes lethal immunologic disease.

Another important mechanism that dampens the immune response is mediated by the Fas molecule, which induces T cells to undergo apoptosis. The importance of this molecule is illustrated by the discovery of *Fas* gene mutations, in both mice and humans, that cause severe lymphoproliferative disease associated with autoimmunity, which in humans is called autoimmune lymphoproliferative syndrome (31). FAS-dependent apoptosis is one mechanism of achieving peripheral tolerance.

The Immune Response to Pathogenic Organisms

Different types of infectious organisms elicit different types of immune responses. Even though these mechanisms evolved to protect the host, tissue injury and disease can occur as a consequence of host response. It is well-established that, through a variety of immunologic and inflammatory mechanisms, some rheumatic diseases are triggered by infectious agents.

A major host response to such endotoxins as lipopolysaccharide, produced by Gram-negative bacteria, is the production of such cytokines as TNF by macrophages, vascular endothelium, and other cells. A severe consequence of this response is septic shock. *Staphylococci*, in contrast, produce enterotoxins that are the most potent natural T-cell mitogens. The enterotoxins bind TCR variable regions (Vβ) and class II molecules, activating T cells, which can result in toxic shock syndrome characterized by fever, exfoliative skin disease, disseminated intravascular coagulation, and cardiovascular shock.

The immune response to extracellular bacteria largely is humoral. Toxins are neutralized by antibody, and organisms are lysed by complement or opsonized with antibody and complement and then phagocytosed. An exaggerated response can lead to disease in the host, such as poststreptococcal glomerulonephritis, in which the profuse production and deposition of antigen–antibody (immune) complexes lead to kidney damage.

Cell-mediated immunity is the primary defense against intracellular pathogens like *Mycobacteria*. When antigen-specific T cells recognize foreign peptides presented by APCs, the T cells proliferate and secrete cytokines that activate endothelial cells, resulting in the recruitment and activation of other leukocytes. Monocytes are recruited, differentiate to macrophages, and kill the microorganisms. With chronic stimulation, however, macrophages fuse together and generate multinucleate giant cells that can participate in granuloma formation. Fibrin also is deposited, causing tissue induration. This response is called delayed-type hypersensitivity (DTH). The immune response then may subside, without permanent damage to the host tissue, although this is not always the case. Cell-mediated immunity to such intracellular organisms as *M. tuberculosis* can cause significant tissue destruction and fibrosis. Granulomatous diseases, such as sarcoidosis and Wegener's granulomatosis, may be due to a cell-mediated response to an unknown organism.

Immunity to viruses is mediated by IFN α and β (innate immunity) and the production of specific antibodies (adaptive immunity). Immune-complex disease can occur as a consequence of viral infection (e.g., hepatitis B infection and arteritis). CD8 T cells that recognize viral peptides in association with class I molecules mediate the cellular response to virus. These T cells can destroy virally infected cells, a process called cell-mediated cytotoxicity. In addition, NK cells lyse virally infected cells.

The Th2 response, characterized by production of IL-4 and IL-5 and subsequent eosinophilia, is key to the immune response to parasitic infestations. The importance of this response is demonstrated by IL-4 knockout mice, which rapidly succumb to certain parasitic infestations.

Self–Nonself Recognition, Tolerance, Autoimmunity, and Pathogenesis of Immune-Mediated Disease

A fundamental aspect of the immune response is that dangerous foreign antigens are recognized, but the host generally does not attack its own tissues, an unresponsive state called tolerance. Exactly how the immune system makes this distinction is poorly understood. Accordingly, the mechanisms that control tolerance are incompletely defined.

Historically, it was proposed that self–nonself recognition occurred through clonal selection, i.e., self-reactive clones of B cells and T cells are deleted during development. However, because development of T cells in the thymus cannot occur without some degree of self-recognition, in a sense, self-reactive lymphocytes are generated constantly. Still, a major function of the thymus is to delete potentially pathogenic T-cell clones with high avidity for self-antigens (central tolerance). Peripheral tolerance is achieved by anergy, Fas-mediated deletion of activated cells, and other immune homeostatic mechanisms. In terms of disease pathogenesis, there are more examples in which failure of immune homeostasis causes autoimmune disease (both natural and experimental) than alterations in self–nonself recognition.

Another paradigm that relates to tolerance is that immune response is mounted against "dangerous" stimuli (15). In other words, pathogenic organisms, in addition to being recognized as foreign to cells of adaptive immune response, provoke inflammatory responses through innate immune responses, enhancing antigenicity (1,15). By inference, autoimmune responses are proposed to be initiated in a similar manner in the context of inflammation. Immune reactivity also is thought to be regulated by the timing and amount of antigen delivery to organized lymphoid tissue by APCs, especially DC; at the extremes, antigen is either ignored or tolergenic (16).

Although the pathogenesis of rheumatic diseases is not fully understood, immune-mediated diseases have been characterized based on their predominant immunopathologic lesion. While this classification can be useful, it is equally important to bear in mind that 1) the components of the immune system are interdependent; and 2) similar immunopathologic abnormalities may arise by different mechanisms.

Diseases Caused by Antibodies

Immediate hypersensitivity (type I hypersensitivity) is due to the production of IgE that binds to Fc receptors on mast cells and basophils. Antigen cross-linking of receptor-bound IgE triggers the release of histamine and the production of proinflammatory lipid mediators and cytokines. The inflammatory component (late-phase response) is clinically important in such diseases as asthma. Allergic rhinitis and anaphylaxis are other examples of immediate hypersensitivity disease.

Antibodies against circulating or fixed cells (type II hypersensitivity) are involved in the pathogenesis of a variety of diseases, including autoimmune hemolytic anemia, autoimmune thrombocytopenia, Goodpasture's syndrome, pemphigus, pemphigoid, pernicious anemia, myasthenia gravis, and Graves' disease. Pathogenic antibodies cause tissue damage by a variety of mechanisms, including lysis by complement and phagocytosis of opsonized cells. In addition, inflammatory cells are recruited to tissues by antibody deposition and complement activation. Antibodies also bind to receptors and alter cellular function without damaging the cells. Antibodies can be present but not involved in disease pathogenesis, which likely is the case in rheumatoid arthritis.

In immune-complex disease (type III hypersensitivity), antibody and antigen form complexes that activate complement. These complexes normally are cleared by macrophages in the spleen and elsewhere. However, immune complexes may be deposited in other organs and tissues, such as the kidney, skin, and serosal surfaces. A number of factors influence immune-complex deposition, including physicochemical properties, anatomic site of deposition, local tissue response (e.g., local production of cytokines), and the host's ability to clear the complexes. Examples of immune-complex disease include systemic lupus erythematosus, polyarteritis nodosa, and poststreptococcal glomerulonephritis.

Considerable evidence supports a role for B cells and their production of autoantibodies in the pathogenesis of rheumatoid arthritis and systemic lupus erythematosus. The molecule BLys, which stimulates B cells to become plasma cells (32), has been found to be elevated in the serum of both groups of patients. Furthermore, a preliminary study indicates that the depletion of B cells may provide an effective alternative treatment for people with rheumatoid arthritis.

Diseases Caused by T Cells

In a number of animal models and human diseases, T cells have a pathogenic role. The mechanisms of T-cell–mediated tissue injury include delayed-type hypersensitivity (DTH) and direct lysis by cytolytic (CD8) T cells. Contact dermatitis is a typical DTH process. T cells also play a role in the pathogenesis of insulin-dependent diabetes mellitus, experimental allergic encephalomyelitis (a mouse model for multiple sclerosis), myasthenia gravis, and Graves' disease.

Although it is useful to classify diseases according to B- or T-cell involvement, there is a great deal of overlap. For example, B-cell antibody production (the mediator of types I, II, and III hypersensitivity) is regulated to a great extent by T cells. Thus, T cells may have a major pathogenic role in these diseases. In addition, increasing information about the function of chemokines in regulating leukocyte migration and function helps explain how various lineages are recruited to sites of inflammation (33).

Summary

The human immune response is composed of highly antigen-specific cells that work in concert with cells involved in innate immunity. Ordinarily, this orchestrated process efficiently rids the host of pathogenic organisms, but not always. Because the immune response is the result of the recruitment and activation of a variety of cells through an array of cytokines, immunologic disease can occur as a consequence of dysregulation at many different steps. Indeed, mutations of many diverse genes have been documented to result in immunologic disease. Immune-mediated tissue injury also can occur as a byproduct of the normal response. The molecular basis for the common autoimmune diseases in humans probably is heterogenous – that is, a variety of mutations or polymorphisms in an array of separate genes could contribute to disease susceptibility. Although this probability makes the study of the pathogenesis of rheumatic diseases extraordinarily complex, it also provides many distinct avenues for therapeutic intervention.

JOHN J. O'SHEA, MD
JOHN KEHRL, MD

References

1. Medzhitov R, Janeway C Jr. Innate immunity. N Engl J Med 2000;343:338-344.
2. Ravetch JV, Lanier LL. Immune inhibitory receptors. Science 2000;290:84–89.
3. Banchereau J, Briere F, Caux C, et al. Immunobiology of dendritic cells. Annu Rev Immunol 2000;18:767–811.
4. Moser M, Murphy KM. Dendritic cell regulation of TH1-TH2 development. Nature Immunology 2000;1:199–205.
5. Sallusto F, Mackay CR, Lanzavecchia A. The role of chemokine receptors in primary, effector, and memory immune responses. Annu Rev Immunol 2000;18:593–620.
6. Ansel KM, Ngo VN, Hyman PL, et al. A chemokine-driven positive feedback loop organizes lymphoid follicles. Nature 2000;406:309–314.
7. Abbas AK, Lichtman AH, Pober JS (eds): Cellular and Molecular Immunology, 4th ed. Philadelphia: WB Saunders, 2000.
8. Klein J, Sato A. The HLA system. First of two parts. N Engl J Med 2000;343:702–709.
9. Park SH, Bendelac A. CD1-restricted T-cell responses and microbial infection. Nature 2000;406:788–792.
10. Zhang W, Samelson LE. The role of membrane-associated adaptors in T cell receptor signaling. Semin Immunol 2000;12:35–41.
11. Benschop RJ, Cambier JC. B cell development: signal transduction by antigen receptors and their surrogates. Curr Opin Immunol 1999;11:143–151.
12. Bierer BE. Mechanisms of action of immunosuppressive agents: cyclosporin A, FK506, and rapamycin. Proc Assoc Am Physicians 1995;107:28–40.
13. Slavik JM, Hutchcroft JE, Bierer BE. CD28/CTLA-4 and CD80/CD86 families: signaling and function. Immunol Res 1999;19:1–24.
14. Coyle AJ, Gutierrez-Ramos JC. The expanding B7 superfamily: increasing complexity in costimulatory signals regulating T call function. Nat Immunol 2001;2:203-209.
15. Matzinger P. An innate sense of danger. Semin Immunol 1998;10:399–415.
16. Zinkernagel RM. Localization dose and time of antigens determine immune reactivity. Semin Immunol 2000;21:63–71.
17. Max EE. Immunoglobulins: molecular genetics in fundamental immunology. In: Paul WE (ed). Fundamental Immunology, 4th ed. New York: Raven Press, 1999.
18. Loffert D, Schaal S, Ehlich A, et al. Early B-cell development in the mouse: insights from mutations introduced by gene targeting. Immunol Rev 1994;137:135–153.
19. Puck JM. Molecular and genetic basis of X-linked immunodeficiency disorders. J Clin Immunol 1994;14:81–89.
20. Ma Q, Jones D, Springer TA. The chemokine receptor CXCR4 is required for the retention of B lineage and granulocytic precursors within the bone marrow microenvironment. Immunity 1999;10:463-471.
21. Mond JJ, Lees A, Snapper CM. T cell-independent antigens type 2. Annu Rev Immunol 1995;13:655–692.
22. Gold MR, DeFranco AL. Biochemistry of B lymphocyte activation. Adv Immunol 1994;55:221–295.
23. MacLennan IC. Germinal centers. Ann Rev Immunol 1994;12:117–139.
24. Banchereau J, Briere F, Liu YJ, Rousset F. Molecular control of B lymphocyte growth and differentiation. Stem Cells 1994;12:278–288.
25. Feldmann M, Brennan FM, Elliott MJ, Williams RO, Maini RN. TNF alpha is an effective therapeutic target for rheumatoid arthritis. Ann N Y Acad Sci 1995;766:272–278.
26. Galon J, Aksentijevich I, McDermott MF, O'Shea JJ, Kastner DL. TNFRSF1A mutations and autoinflammatory syndromes. Curr Opin Immunol 2000;12:479–486.
27. Glimcher LH, Murphy KM. Lineage commitment in the immune system: the T helper lymphocyte grows up. Genes Dev 2000;14:1693–1711.
28. Romagnani S. T-cell subsets (Th1 versus Th2). Ann Allergy Asthma Immunol 2000;85:9–18.
29. Leonard WJ, O'Shea JJ. Jaks and STATs: biological implications. Annu Rev Immunol 1998;16:293–322.
30. Letterio JJ, Roberts AB. Regulation of immune responses by TGF-beta. Annu Rev Immunol 1998;16:137–161.
31. Fisher GH, Rosenberg FJ, Straus SE, et al. Dominant interfering Fas gene mutations impair apoptosis in a human autoimmune lymphoproliferative syndrome. Cell 1995;81:935–946.
32. Moore PA, Belvedere O, Orr A, et al. BLyS: member of the tumor necrosis factor family and B lymphocyte stimulator. Science 1999;285:260–263.
33. Mackay CR. Chemokines: immunology's high impact factors. Nat Immunol 2001;2:95-101.

IMMUNITY
B. Neuroendocrine Influences

The neuroendocrine and immune systems are mediated by a large number of shared signal molecules and regulated receptors (1). For example, the neuroendocrine system produces cytokines, particularly interleukin 1 (IL-1) and IL-6. Analogously, various immune cells produce typical neuroendocrine products, such as proopiomelanocortin (POMC), corticotropin (ACTH), corticotropin-releasing hormone (CRH), and growth hormone (GH), which act locally and systemically to exert diverse effects on many tissues (1,2).

Interactions between the neuroendocrine and immune systems of whole organisms are profoundly complex, poorly defined, and not clearly understood. This section reviews the better-understood aspects of neuroendocrine–immune interactions that may apply to rheumatic and autoimmune diseases. Human studies are emphasized because of their more direct relevance to clinical circumstances (3). In vitro and animal models are reviewed for their role in interpreting biologic mechanisms.

The Hypothalamic–Pituitary–Adrenal Axis

Cortisol is the most important hormone of the hypothalamic–pituitary–adrenal (HPA) axis. It influences immune reactions by inhibiting most aspects of the immune response (4,5). In turn, the immune system participates in a regulatory loop with the cortisol–HPA axis. Deficiencies or interruption of this neuroendocrine–immune (NEI) regulatory loop may result in increased susceptibility to, or severity of, autoimmune inflammatory disease (3,4).

The HPA axis is activated by a wide variety of physical and psychological stressors, as well as products of an upregulated immune system that potently increase HPA axis function by stimulating CRH production. Hypothalamic CRH stimulates release of ACTH from the anterior pituitary, which results in increased production of cortisol by the adrenal cortex. Optimally, the HPA axis response to cytokine stimulation serves to modulate acute-phase inflammatory reactions, including immunologic and microvascular changes (4–7).

Cytokine Stimulation

A number of immune and inflammatory mediators, particularly IL-1, stimulate HPA hormone synthesis and secretion. Interleukin 1 stimulates the hypothalamus to secrete CRH and arginine vasopressin (AVP), an adjunctive ACTH secretagogue (4–7). The precise mechanisms behind these actions are not understood (8,9).

Interleukin 6 is a potent stimulus for HPA axis activation at the level of the hypothalamus (10). However, IL-6 directly stimulates release of ACTH by the pituitary, and synergizes with ACTH to increase production of cortisol by adrenocortical cells (8). Adrenal cells also synthesize IL-6 after stimulation by IL-1 or ACTH (7). Tumor necrosis factor α (TNF-α) acutely stimulates HPA axis activation, whereas IL-2 and interferon γ (IFN-γ) promote a more delayed HPA axis activation (9).

Modulation of Immune and Inflammatory Processes

Corticosteroids inhibit immune and inflammatory responses at multiple steps, including neutrophil and monocyte migration, antigen presentation, lymphocyte proliferation and differentiation, cytokine production by monocytes and certain lymphocyte subtypes, synthesis of eicosanoids and other lipid mediators, and production of nitric oxide (NO) and metalloproteinases (7,9). Corticosteroids also regulate thymocyte maturation and differentiation. Thymocytes are more sensitive to the effects of corticosteroids than mature T cells and undergo apoptosis after exposure to corticosteroids. A number of stressors can cause thymocyte apoptosis by inducing physiologically increased plasma corticosteroid levels (9).

Data support the contention that endogenous corticosteroids are involved in modulating the activation, expansion, and clonal deletion of peripheral T cells in vivo, thereby contributing to long-term modeling of the immune system (11). Corticosteroids regulate development of T-helper (Th) subtypes, shifting responses from Th1 to Th2. They also suppress production of the Th1 cytokines IL-2 and IFN-γ, but not such Th2 cytokines as IL-4. This differential effect on Th1 and Th2 cytokine balance may be important in the control of immune responses, because Th2 cells inhibit the Th1 subset and may function as suppressor cells in autoimmune disease (8,9).

The HPA Axis in Human Autoimmune Disease

The discovery of the anti-inflammatory properties of corticosteroids and the dramatic clinical response of people with rheumatoid arthritis (RA) to corticosteroids led to the hypothesis that RA develops as a consequence of adrenal insufficiency (12). Increasingly, data from humans suggest that dysregulation of the HPA axis may contribute to certain rheumatic diseases (13). Premenopausal RA patients show relatively subnormal serum cortisol responsiveness to adrenal stimulation by either ACTH or insulin hypoglycemia, compared with controls (14). Also, elevated serum levels of IL-6 fail to cause sustained hypercortisolism in early, untreated RA, suggesting relative adrenal hyporesponsiveness (15).

Impaired HPA Axis Activation and Autoimmune Inflammatory Disease

The concept that impaired NEI counterregulatory activity might increase susceptibility to, or affect severity of, autoimmune inflammatory diseases is bolstered by observations in experimental animals (Table 5B-1). Lewis rats, unlike Fischer rats, are susceptible to a wide range of experimentally induced autoimmune inflammatory diseases that include models for RA and multiple sclerosis. These rats differ markedly in the severity of their inflammatory responses to nonspecific irritants, possibly because they display dramatically different HPA axis responses to inflammatory stimuli (7,16,17). Lewis rats exhibit blunted CRH, ACTH, and cortisol secretion in response to many types of stressors, including IL-1, whereas Fischer rats robustly increase these HPA axis hormones. Because small, supplemental, physiologic doses of corticosteroids profoundly suppress the severity of inflammation in Lewis rats, and administration of a glucocorticoid-receptor antagonist leads to severe inflammatory disease in Fisher rats, the HPA axis is believed to play a critical role in determining disease severity.

Inbred mouse strains, including MRL lpr/lpr and NZB/NZW F_1, that develop systemic autoimmune disease resembling systemic lupus erythematosus (SLE) exhibit blunted IL-1–stimulated corticosterone levels (9). In the nonobese diabetic (NOD) mouse strain, both T and B lymphocytes display extended survival, and thymocytes are relatively resistant to corticosteroid-induced apoptosis (7).

OS chickens are an inbred strain that develop spontaneous autoimmune thyroiditis, clinically similar to Hashimoto's thyroiditis. OS chickens have decreased free corticosterone levels primarily due to increased levels of cortisol-binding globulin. They also have blunted corticosterone response to IL-1, similar to the Lewis rat (9). University of California at Davis Line 200 (UCD-200) chickens spontaneously develop systemic inflammatory disease and fibrosis similar to scleroderma. This strain displays markedly increased ACTH production and normal levels of corticosterone in response to administration of cytokine-containing conditioned media. These corticosterone levels are blunted in relation to ACTH levels, indicating adrenal hyporesponsiveness (9).

Prolactin and Growth Hormone

Prolactin (PRL) and GH are immunostimulatory pituitary hormones produced by pituitary and immune cells. Hypophysectomy leads to profound immunodeficiency and thymic hypoplasia, which can be reversed by PRL or GH, but not other pituitary hormones (18). Most data suggest that GH promotes thymocyte proliferation, whereas PRL promotes proliferation and differentiation of antigen-specific T cells (19). Bromocriptine, a drug that inhibits pituitary release of PRL, selectively reduces lymphocyte reactivity in rats. Prolactin stimulates the expression of IL-2 receptors and enhances the IL-2–induced proliferative response of T lymphocytes. Both GH and PRL have cell-surface receptors structurally homologous to the receptor for IL-6 and other cytokines, and these hormone receptors are present on lymphocytes (18,19).

It has been suggested that PRL levels modulate expression of autoimmune disease. Some people with SLE or other autoimmune diseases show elevated PRL levels, and bromocriptine has been shown to ameliorate some types of experimental autoimmune diseases in animals. However, because estrogens can stimulate PRL levels, the independent effects of these hormones need to be critically analyzed in human and animal models of disease (18).

The Hypothalamic–Pituitary–Gonadal Axis

A striking female preponderance characterizes many autoimmune diseases, and estrogens activate humoral immunity (20). Estrogens appear to play an important role in the pathogenesis of SLE. The disease often begins at the time of menarche or in younger menstruating women, and some patients experience exacerbations of symptoms during specific phases of the menstrual cycle or with pregnancy. Furthermore, oral contraceptives or estrogen replacement

TABLE 5B-1
HPA Axis Defects in Animal Models of Autoimmune Disease

Strain	Disease model	HPA axis defect
Lewis rat	RA, multiple sclerosis	Blunted CRH to IL-1 and other stressors
NZB/NZW F_1	SLE	Blunted IL-1–stimulated corticosterone
MRL lpr/lpr	SLE	Blunted IL-1–stimulated corticosterone
NOD	Diabetes mellitus	Thymocyte resistance to corticosteroid-induced apoptosis
OS chicken	Hashimoto's thyroiditis	Decreased free corticosterone; blunted corticosterone response to IL-1
UCD-200 chicken	Scleroderma	Adrenal hyporesponsiveness to increased ACTH

RA, rheumatoid arthritis; HPA, hypothalamic–pituitary–adrenal; CRH, corticotropin-releasing hormone; IL, interleukin; SLE, systemic lupus erythematosus; ACTH, adrenocorticotropic hormone.
Modified from Wick et al. (9) with permission.

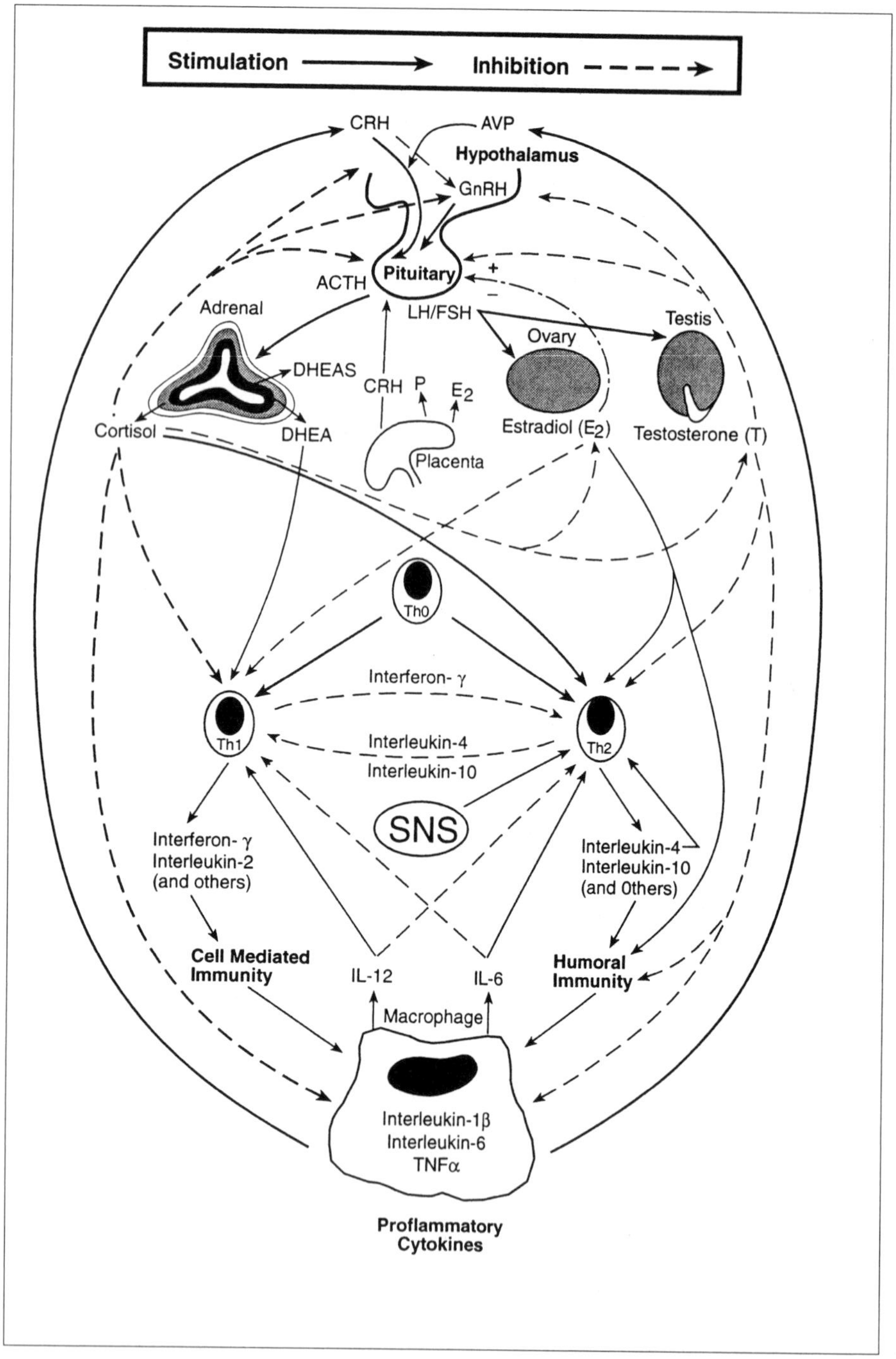

Fig. 5B-1. Reciprocal regulations and modeling of the neuroendocrine and immune systems. The neuroendocrine and immune systems are modulated bidirectionally and may be modeled over the long term by homeostatic control mechanisms. The acute-phase response of active inflammation generates such proinflammatory cytokines as interleukin (IL)-1β, IL-6, and tumor necrosis factor (TNF)-α, which stimulate the hypothalamic–pituitary–adrenal (HPA) axis to increase cortisol production. In turn, cortisol modulated inflammatory responsiveness by diverse mechanisms and favors a T-helper 2 (Th2) humoral response over a Th1 cell-mediated response. The major sex hormones, including estradiol (E_2) and testosterone (T), also modulate immune responsiveness and contribute to gender dimorphism. In physiologic concentration, E_2 tends to enhance humoral immunity and favors a Th2 cytokine pattern, but T tends to be immunosuppressive. Dehydroepiandrosterone (DHEA) may favor Th1 immune responsiveness and progesterone (P) favors Th2 function, as does activation of the sympathetic nervous system (SNS).

Placental corticotropin-releasing hormone (CRH) stimulates the HPA axis to increase cortisol and adrenal androgen production. In turn, hypothalamic CRH decreases, due to cortisol–HPA negative feedback. During pregnancy, adrenal cortical function and hormonal production increases, and the gland may hypertrophy. Postpartum, placental CRH is lost and the adrenal gland my become understimulated, but hypothalamic production of CRH still is decreased. Physiologic variations in CRH and HPA-axis function during pregnancy and during the postpartum period may contribute to the notable changes in onset risks and clinical activity of RA.

therapy may exacerbate SLE, and patients may have disease remission at menopause (7,20). Additionally, men and women with SLE may have imbalances of sex steroid metabolism. However, sex hormones are not likely to be the underlying cause of this disease, but rather modulators, possibly through immunoregulatory effects (20). Klinefelter's syndrome, a condition associated with the XXY genotype and abnormal sexual development, also has been associated with SLE, but it is difficult to quantitate the degree of concurrence.

The risk of RA increases significantly in pubertal girls and premenopausal women, compared with the risk for male cohorts (11). However, unlike in SLE, estrogens and androgens do not appear to be major factors in this increase. Pregnancy is a protective factor for risk of developing RA, and patients usually experience amelioration of disease activity during gestation. The ameliorating effects of pregnancy on RA, but not on SLE or ankylosing spondylitis, are not well understood (11,21,22). Low serum total testosterone levels have been reported in male RA patients with active disease (21), and exogenous testosterone therapy over six months showed favorable clinical and immunologic changes in a small series of cases (23). Combined low serum levels of cortisol (<140 nmol/l) and testosterone (<10 nmol/l) have been found to predict the long-term development of RA in a small proportion of men (11). Such observations suggest that sex steroids contribute to the expression of autoimmune diseases, but the effects are limited and variable, depending on specific immune mechanisms of disease (3,13,24).

Sex Steroid Influences on the Immune Response

Sexual dimorphism occurs in immune responses, and may, in part, underlie the differential expression of autoimmune diseases in males and females (20,25). Estrogens may influence immune responses indirectly through their ability to stimulate prolactin (18). However, direct sex steroid effects probably are operative (7,20,25,26). Estrogen receptors are present in lymphoid and thymic tissue, and androgen receptors are present in thymic epithelial cells. Both estrogen and testosterone appear to alter thymocyte development; castration leads to thymic enlargement, and estrogen and testosterone decrease thymic mass (25). Estrogen stimulates hyperreactivity in humoral immune responses, whereas testosterone appears to depress humoral immunity. For example, females display increased immunoglobulin concentrations and greater primary and secondary antibody responses to certain infectious agents. Estrogen treatment of castrated males reproduces hyperactive humoral immune responses similar to that of females. Sex steroid hormone effects on cellular immune processes are less clear (25,26). Cell-mediated immune responses also seem to be more active in women than in men, except during pregnancy. Female sex hormone effects on cellular immunity may be indirect, although estrogens appear to suppress at least some T-cell–dependent immune responses. Complex steroid hormone and immunological counterregulatory interactions are summarized in Fig. 5B-1.

Sex Steroids in Animal Models of Autoimmune Disease

The role of sex steroids has been investigated intensively in the NZB/NZW F_1 mice, a model for SLE (7,18,20). In these mice, renal disease and autoantibody production progress more rapidly in females than in males. Although castration or androgen therapy decreases disease activity in females, castration or estrogen therapy increases disease activity in males. Data using the autoimmune-prone MRL +/+ mice demonstrate that estrogens selectively enhance such B-cell–mediated humoral immune responses as immunoglobulin levels, autoantibody production, and immune-complex glomerulonephritis, but T-cell–mediated immune responses are diminished by estrogens (7). Animal models of RA demonstrate differences in sexual dimorphism depending upon the species and model (7).

Dehydroepiandrosterone

The adrenal androgens dehydroepiandrosterone (DHEA) and DHEA sulfate (DHEAS) are synthesized under the control of ACTH and other ill-defined factors (5,21). DHEAS is the predominant circulating adrenal androgen, having the highest concentration in healthy, young, nonpregnant persons. The presence of DHEA sulfatase in lymphoid tissues allows conversion of DHEAS to the more metabolically active DHEA (7). Levels of DHEAS vary greatly over life cycles and decline with age, which contrasts with typically stable cortisol levels. Levels of DHEAS are lower in pubertal juvenile RA (27) and premenopausal RA (21) patients not treated with corticosteroids than in controls, and levels are inversely correlated with disease severity (7). Premenopausal women, but neither postmenopausal women nor men, show decreased serum DHEAS levels many years prior to the development of RA (11). Low adrenal androgen levels currently are interpreted to be a marker for relative adrenal cortical (i.e., glucocorticoid) insufficiency, which is suspected to be a potential risk factor for an earlier onset age of RA in women (11,27).

Therapeutic use of DHEA in women with SLE in controlled trials has resulted in modestly favorable clinical and immunological effects (20); the same results have not been achieved for people with RA (24). Mechanisms of these effects are unknown, but potentially are contributed by DHEA enhancement of IL-2 synthesis by helper T cells, as described in mice (28), or by conversion of this precursor hormone to sex steroids (5,11,25,26,29).

Summary

Reciprocal regulation of the neuroendocrine and immune systems is profoundly complex. Dysfunctions of these systems, in conjunction with perturbations of the microvascular endothelial compartments, are believed to contribute to the physiopathogenetic processes operating in RA and some other systemic, rheumatic, and autoimmune diseases (3). Elucidation of specific mechanisms will require integrated basic and controlled clinical experimental research directed toward understanding these complex systems.

ALFONSE T. MASI, MD, DrPH
LESLIE J. CROFFORD, MD

References

1. Blalock JE. Proopiomelanocortin and the immune-neuroendocrine connection. Ann N Y Acad Sci 1999;885:161–172.

2. Weigent DA, Blalock JE. Associations between the neuroendocrine and immune systems. J Leukoc Biol 1995;58:137–150.

3. Masi AT, Bijlsma JW, Chikanza IC, Cutolo M (eds). Neuroendocrine mechanisms in rheumatic diseases. Rheum Dis Clin North Am 2000;26:693-1042.

4. Chrousos GP. The hypothalamic-pituitary-adrenal axis and immune-mediated inflammation. N Engl J Med 1995;332: 1351–1362.

5. Orth DN, Kovacs WJ. The adrenal cortex. In: Wilson JD, Foster DW, Kronenberg HM, Larsen PR (eds). Williams Textbook of Endocrinology, 9th ed. Philadelphia: WB Saunders, 1998; pp 517–664.

6. Reichlin S. Neuroendocrinology. In: Wilson JD, Foster DW, Kronenberg HM, Larsen PR (eds). Williams Textbook of Endocrinology, 9th ed. Philadelphia: WB Saunders, 1998; pp 165–248.

7. Wilder RL. Neuroendocrine-immune system interactions and autoimmunity. Annu Rev Immunol 1995;13:307–338.

8. Busbridge NJ, Grossman AB. Stress and the single cytokine: interleukin modulation of the pituitary-adrenal axis. Mol Cell Endocrinol 1991;82:C209–214.

9. Wick G, Hu Y, Schwarz S, Kroemer G. Immunoendocrine communication via the hypothalamo-pituitary-adrenal axis in autoimmune diseases. Endocr Rev 1993;14:539–563.

10. Mastorakos G, Weber JS, Magiakou MA, Gunn H, Chrousos GP. Hypothalamic-pituitary-adrenal axis activation and stimulation of systemic vasopressin secretion by recombinant interleukin-6 in humans: potential implications for the syndrome of inappropriate vasopressin secretion. J Clin Endocrinol Metab 1994;79:934–939.

11. Masi AT. Hormonal and immunological risk factors for the development of rheumatoid arthritis: an integrative physiopathogenetic perspective. In: Masi AT, Bijlsma JW, Chikanza IC, Cutolo M (eds). Neuroendocrine mechanisms in rheumatic diseases. Rheum Dis Clin North Am 2000;26:775-803.

12. Hench PS, Kendall EC, Slocumb CH, Polley HF. The effect of a hormone of the adrenal cortex (17-hydroxy-11-dehydrocorticosterone: compound E) and of pituitary adrenocorticotropic hormone on rheumatoid arthritis. Mayo Clin Proc 1949;24: 181–197.

13. Masi AT. Neuroendocrine immune mechanisms in rheumatic diseases: an overview and future implications. In: Masi AT, Bijlsma JW, Chikanza IC, Cutolo M (eds). Neuroendocrine mechanisms in rheumatic diseases. Rheum Dis Clin North Am 2000;26:1003–1017.

14. Masi AT, Aldag JC, Chatterton RT, Adams RF, Kitabchi AE. Adrenal androgen and glucocorticoid dissociation in premenopausal rheumatoid arthritis: a significant correlate or precursor to onset? Z Rheumatol 2000;59:54–61

15. Crofford LJ, Kalogeras KT, Mastorakos G, et al. Circadian relationships between interleukin (IL)-6 and hypothalamic-pituitary-adrenocortical axis hormones: failure of IL-6 to cause hypercortisolism in patients with early untreated rheumatoid arthritis. J Clin Endocrinol Metab 1997;82: 1279–1283.

16. Sternberg EM, Hill JM, Chrousos GP, et al. Inflammatory mediator-induced hypothalamic-pituitary-adrenal axis activation is defective in streptococcal cell wall arthritis-susceptible Lewis rats. Proc Natl Acad Sci USA 1989;86:2374–2378.

17. Sternberg EM, Young WS III, Bernardini R, et al. A central nervous system defect in biosynthesis of corticotropin-releasing hormone is associated with susceptibility to streptococcal cell wall-induced arthritis in Lewis rats. Proc Natl Acad Sci USA 1989;86:4771–4775.

18. Walker SE, Jacobson JD. Roles of prolactin and gonadotropin releasing hormone in rheumatic disease. In: Masi AT, Bijlsma JW, Chikanza IC, Cutolo M (eds). Neuroendocrine mechanisms in rheumatic diseases. Rheum Dis Clin North Am 2000;26:713–736.

19. Goetzl EJ, Sreedharan SP. Mediators of communication and adaptation in the neuroendocrine and immune systems. FASEB J 1992;6:2646–2652.

20. Lahita RG. Sex hormones and systemic lupus erythematosus. In: Masi AT, Bijlsma JW, Chikanza IC, Cutolo M (eds). Neuroendocrine mechanisms in rheumatic diseases. Rheum Dis Clin North Am 2000;26:951-968.

21. Masi AT, Feigenbaum SL, Chatterton RT. Hormonal and pregnancy relationships to rheumatoid arthritis: convergent effects with immunologic and microvascular systems. Semin Arthritis Rheum 1995;25:1-27.

22. Olsen NJ, Kovacs WJ. Hormones, pregnancy and rheumatoid arthritis. J Gender-Specific Med (in press).

23. Cutolo M, Balleari E, Giusti M, Intra E, Accardo S. Androgen replacement therapy in male patients with rheumatoid arthritis. Arthritis Rheum 1991;34:1–5.

24. Gooren LJ, Giltay EJ, van Schaardenburg D, Dijkmans BA. Gonadal and adrenal sex steroids in ankylosing spondylitis. In: Masi AT, Bijlsma JW, Chikanza IC, Cutolo M (eds). Neuroendocrine mechanisms in rheumatic diseases. Rheum Dis Clin North Am 2000;26:969–987.

25. Olsen NJ, Kovacs WJ. Gonadal steroids and immunity. Endocr Rev 1996;17:369–384.

26. Cutolo M, Wilder RL. Different roles for androgens and estrogens in the susceptibility to autoimmune rheumatic diseases. In: Masi AT, Bijlsma JW, Chikanza IC, Cutolo M (eds). Neuroendocrine mechanisms in rheumatic diseases. Rheum Dis Clin North Am 2000;26:825–839.

27. Khalkhali-Ellis Z, Moore TL, Hendrix MJ. Reduced levels of testosterone and dehydroepiandrosterone sulphate in the serum and synovial fluid of juvenile rheumatoid arthritis patients correlates with disease severity. Clin Exp Rheumatol 1998;16:753–756.

28. Suzuki T, Suzuki N, Daynes RA, Engleman EG. Dehydroepiandrosterone enhances IL-2 production and cytotoxic effector function of human T cells. Clin Immunol Immunopathol 1991;61:202-211.

29. Cutolo M. Sex hormone adjuvant therapy in rheumatoid arthritis. In: Masi AT, Bijlsma JW, Chikanza IC, Cutolo M (eds). Neuroendocrine mechanisms in rheumatic diseases. Rheum Dis Clin North Am 2000;26:881–895.

IMMUNITY
C. Autoimmunity: Self Versus Nonself

The immune system is composed of innate, early-response elements (macrophages, neutrophils, natural killer [NK] cells, and mast cells) and later-acting, adaptive components (predominantly lymphocytes) that have exquisite specificity. Immune responses are capable not only of killing foreign organisms that invade the host, but of killing the host itself – as may occur in septic shock or certain autoimmune disorders. The fundamental task of the immune system is to protect the individual from infectious organisms (nonself) without serious injury to self.

Any molecule capable of eliciting an immune response is a potential immunogen. Humans are exposed constantly to large doses of potential immunogens at epithelial surfaces (e.g., skin, lung, and gastrointestinal tract) not only from foreign organisms, but also through the constant turnover of host cells, especially within the immune system itself. The concept of immunologic tolerance was evoked to explain the immune system's robust response to almost any foreign substance, compared with its failure to react against self molecules. Tolerance must, of necessity, apply to both the innate and adaptive immune responses. Tolerance of the innate immune response is an evolutionary process; over time, best-fit receptors have been selected that link binding to foreign molecules with a proinflammatory response. On the other hand, tolerance of the adaptive immune response largely is a somatic process; lymphocyte receptors and the thresholds for activation are selected during the lifetime of an individual.

To be able to recognize the universe of foreign antigens, T- and B-lymphocyte antigen receptors (TCR and BCR, respectively) are generated randomly. The consequence of this strategy is that lymphocytes with reactivity against self antigens also are produced and, if the host is to survive, must be eliminated or held in check. Lymphocyte tolerance is a multistep process. The initial "education" of lymphocytes is achieved in central organs (the thymus and bone marrow), but the regulation of all cells belonging to the peripheral immune system (within the blood, spleen, lymph nodes, and mucosal immune system) requires constant and diverse strategies to avoid autoimmunity. These strategies can be classified as central or peripheral tolerance.

Central Tolerance

Billions of lymphocyte progenitor cells are produced by the bone marrow daily, and many of these cells die due to faulty rearrangement of their antigen receptor genes. For cells that undergo productive rearrangement of their antigen receptors in the bone marrow or thymus, the receptor is forced to engage the environment as a test for self-reactivity. Cells that bind to antigen with high affinity at this stage of maturation are deleted by a programmed cell death pathway associated with apoptosis (see Fig. 5C-1). Many of the principles that control tolerance of immature cells are similar between T and B cells, but there are some important differences.

T Cells
T-cell maturation in the thymus is conveniently monitored by the display of the coreceptors CD4 and CD8, as well as the TCR and signaling complex

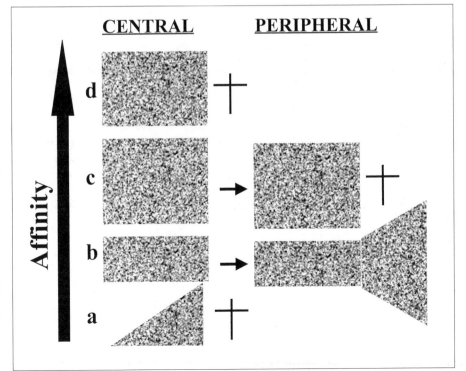

Fig. 5C-1. The affinity of antigen receptor binding determines the fate of lymphocytes in central lymphoid organs and sets the threshold for activation in the periphery. Lymphocytes with no (a) or very high (d) affinity of binding die by apoptosis. Lymphocytes with intermediate affinity (b and c) survive but, within this population, cells with the highest affinity (c) have their signaling tuned down so they are nonresponsive to antigen (anergic) in the periphery. A small proportion (b) of the original number of surviving cells selected in the thymus (T cells) or bone marrow (B cells) can be activated in the periphery, provided the cells receive additional activation signals (see Figs. 5C-2 and 5C-3).

CENTRAL   PERIPHERAL

Affinity

d

c

b

a

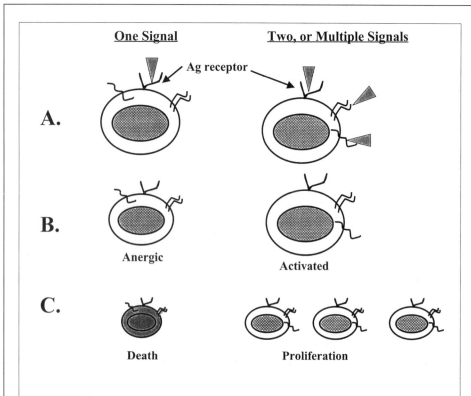

Fig. 5C-2. Costimulation usually is required for efficient activation of lymphocytes. In the left panel, a lymphocyte binds to an antigen but does not receive additional signals (A). Because the threshold is set such that this binding to self antigen is insufficient for full activation (see Fig. 5C-1), the cell is rendered anergic (B) and dies (C). In the right panel, a lymphocyte binds to antigen and receives additional signals through costimulatory molecules or cytokines (see text for details and differences between T and B cells). The cell becomes activated (B) and proliferates (C, clonal expansion).

CD3. Pre-T cells entering the cortex of the thymus initially do not express any of these phenotypic markers. As they mature, they express CD4 and CD8 (double-positive), and the TCR/CD3 complex, and they enter the corticomedullary junction. Through the random nature of TCR generation, some of the T cells will engage antigens – major histocompatibility complex (MHC) alone or MHC containing a peptide – and some will not. T cells die if they do not receive any signals through their TCR, and T cells that engage antigen with high affinity are deleted (negative selection). T cells that engage antigen with low affinity are positively selected and mature into either CD4 or CD8 (single-positive) T cells in the thymic medulla. These cells then seed into the periphery to perform their protective function. Kinetic studies in animals suggest that only about 5% of all thymocytes survive the selection process and mature into single-positive T cells (1).

B Cells

In humans, B cells develop from progenitors within the bone marrow. The stages of B-cell ontogeny from pro-B to pre-B to early B to mature B cell are marked by phenotypic changes, the most important of which is expression of the BCR for antigen on the cell surface at the early B-cell stage of development. Analogous to T-cell ontogeny, large numbers of cells die through faulty rearrangement of receptors in the pro- to pre–B-cell transition (2).

In early B cells, the BCR is a transmembrane form of immunoglobulin M (sIgM). As in the case of cortical thymocytes that express TCR, high-affinity interaction with antigen leads to cell death. Unlike the TCR, the BCR binds to epitopes on soluble antigens and does not require presentation by MHC molecules. Because IgM is pentavalent, antigens that cross-link sIgM most efficiently (e.g., cell-membrane antigens) usually are highly efficient at negative selection. Some self-reactive B cells avoid death by switching their light chain expression so as to avoid self-reactivity, a process called receptor editing. Experiments with transgenic mice suggest that B cells that bind to antigen with low affinity or those that encounter oligovalent antigens unable to cross-link sIgM become anergized. Anergy refers to functional inactivation of the lymphocyte so that re-exposure of the cell to the antigen in the periphery will result in a failure to produce antibodies. Fully mature B cells express surface IgD as well as IgM through alternative splicing of the pre-mRNA for IgM. Each B cell, therefore, expresses sIgM and sIgD with the same immunoglobulin variable region but different constant regions. Compared with T cells, a higher proportion of immature B cells seed to the periphery where additional self-reactive cells are eliminated.

Key Points

Immature lymphoid cells in the central lymphoid organs cannot distinguish self from foreign antigens, as shown by the ready ability of animals to be rendered tolerant to foreign antigens by systemic immunization during the neonatal period. Because almost all antigens encountered in the thymus or bone marrow in neonates would be expected to derive from self antigens, autoreactive cells that bind to these antigens with moderate-to-high affinity are tolerized (deleted or inactivated).

The avidity or relative affinity of the antigen receptor for antigen is key to determining the fate of immature lymphocytes.

Signaling thresholds are established so that cells emerging from central lymphoid organs have higher thresholds for activation, compared with immature cells within the thymus or bone marrow.

Peripheral Tolerance

Lymphocytes in the thymus and bone marrow are exposed to antigens derived from fixed and circulating cells, as well as from serum components. Tolerance to these self components is induced readily by the mechanisms described previously, but cannot be complete. A number of self antigens expressed in low concentrations at specialized sites in the body are unlikely to be present in the thymus or bone marrow. In addition, "new" antigens are expressed during different periods in life. Finally, lymphocytes *require very low-affinity binding* to self antigens to remain viable in the periphery. These constraints require that the host be capable of employing a number of additional strategies to avoid autoimmunity. These strategies include minimizing the opportunity for an immune response to self, active suppression of immune responses to self (with additional specialized mechanisms at "privileged sites"), and mechanisms to actively terminate immune responses. The decision of the immune cells to ignore, suppress, or attack is not left to lymphocytes alone. "Pattern recognition" of self and foreign molecules is a critical function of phagocytes that links innate immunity to the adaptive immune response.

Clonal Encounters with Self and Induction of Anergy

In the thymus, T cells are exposed continuously to antigens on stromal cells and other professional antigen-presenting cells. In contrast, the cells in nonlymphoid organs throughout the body are not directly in contact with lymphocytes under normal conditions, and the probability of a low-affinity, self-reactive cell encountering a specific self antigen is small. There are several sites within the body where even a minor degree of immune activation can cause immense damage in very short time. These sites include the brain, eye, and gonads. In the brain, the limited permeability of the blood–brain barrier, minimal lymphoid drainage, paucity of dendritic cells, and absent or low expression of MHC molecules on neurons also minimize the opportunity for inflammation.

In some cases, a lymphocyte clone will encounter self antigen. In the absence of additional signals, however, the lymphocyte will be rendered anergic (Fig. 5C-2).

Immune Deviation and Immune Suppression

Powerful mechanisms operate to prevent immune activation and inflammation at certain anatomic sites. The largest exposure of the host to a diverse array of foreign antigens occurs by ingestion of food and microorganisms. Although enzymes in the gut break down most proteins, numerous studies in animals have shown that this process is incomplete. Experiments performed more than 50 years ago demonstrated that ingestion of an antigen, prior to immunization by a systemic route, was capable of abrogating the immune response to that specific antigen. Although a number of different mechanisms may be responsible, the most important appears to be a phenomenon referred to as immune deviation, i.e., preferential production of transforming growth factor (TGF)-β and T-helper 2 (Th2) cytokines (3). Immune deviation may also be responsible for the neonatal tolerance discussed previously.

Multiple mechanisms contribute to immune privilege in the brain, eye, and testis. In the anterior chamber of the eye, constitutive production of the cytokine TGF-β suppresses immune responses. In addition, Fas ligand (FasL), a molecule that induces apoptosis of immune cells, is expressed constitutively in the eye and testis. If activated cells manage to enter these sites, FasL induces apoptosis of the cells, leading to their rapid phagocytosis and suppression of inflammation (see below).

Other mechanisms of immune suppression exerted by select subpopulations of CD4, CD8, or NK cells may play a role in the maintenance of tolerance, but these mechanisms are not yet well defined.

Discrimination Between Self and Foreign

The peripheral immune system is exposed constantly to potential immunogens comprising foreign microorganisms and dead and dying host cells. How does the immune system distinguish between these potential immunogens? A key role is played by phagocytes expressing pattern-recognition receptors that show relative specificity for such molecules as lipids or carbohydrates. For example, bacterial lipopolysaccharides interact with macrophage receptors that initiate the release of molecules (reactive oxygen and nitrogen intermediates) directly injurious to bacteria and initiate the release of proinflammatory cytokines, such as interleukin (IL)-1 and tumor necrosis factor (TNF). These proinflammatory cytokines link the innate and adaptive immune responses by directly enhancing activation of lymphocytes and by inducing the high level of expression of the key B7 costimulatory molecules on the macrophage. B7 binds to CD28 on T cells, providing the critical second signal required to overcome the high activation threshold of mature lymphocytes (Figs. 5C-2 and 5C-3). Fully activated T cells release interferon γ (IFN-γ), which feeds back on the macrophage to enhance antigen presentation, providing a positive feedback loop (Fig. 5C-3). Some bacterial products, such as superantigens, are able to induce T-cell activation without a need for costimulatory molecules.

A strikingly different immune response occurs when phagocytes encounter dying host cells during normal cell turnover. The dying cells undergo numerous changes to their surface membranes, including translocation of phosphatidyl serine to the outer layer of the membrane. These molecules are recognized by different pattern-recognition receptors, and they trigger the release of the immunosuppressive cytokine TGF-β. The active induction of an anti-inflammatory response following phagocytosis of normal apoptotic cells provides a potent mechanism to prevent immune responses to self (Fig. 5C-3).

It should be noted that, for most antigens, B cells also require more than one signal for full activation. This signal may be provided by engagement of C3d by the coreceptor

CR2/CD19 on B cells, by activated T cells through CD40 ligand, and/or by such cytokines as IL-4 (4–6).

Termination of the Immune Response

As discussed, during the inflammatory immune response, antigen-presenting cells (macrophages, dendritic cells, and B cells) express high levels of costimulatory products that promote lymphocyte activation. Due to the constant processing of self proteins, self antigens are efficiently presented together with these costimulatory molecules. The coincidence of self-antigen presentation and lymphocyte activation provides a fertile opportunity for self-reactivity and, indeed, low titers of autoantibodies frequently are expressed transiently during infections and other forms of tissue injury (7).

To ensure termination of immune responses and to limit the opportunity for lymphocyte reactivity to host antigens, activated cells are eliminated by several mechanisms (Fig. 5C-4). Destruction of the microorganism by the immune system will reduce stimulation of inflammatory cytokines and chemokines, preventing further recruitment and activation of immune cells. Autoregulatory circuits come into play. A second receptor for the B7 molecules is CTLA-4, a protein that is expressed only on activated T cells and has a much higher affinity for binding to B7 than does CD28. In contrast to CD28, engagement of CTLA-4 results in T-cell inhibition and down-modulation of the immune response. Cytokine withdrawal causes apoptosis of some previously stimulated cells, but lymphocyte-mediated induction of activation-induced cell death (AICD) occurs predominantly through the Fas (APO-1/CD95) and TNF receptors, both members of the nerve growth factor receptor family (8).

The Fas receptor is expressed at low levels on resting T and B lymphocytes, as well as on macrophages. When these cells are activated by antigens, certain ligands, and/or cytokines (e.g., IFN-γ), Fas expression is up-regulated and the Fas signal transduction pathway is facilitated. Because the FasL is expressed predominantly on activated CD4+ Th1 and CD8+ T cells, these T-cell subsets are major regu-

lators of AICD through this pathway. FasL-bearing cells are able to induce apoptosis of other activated T cells, B cells, and macrophages. The Fas pathway plays a key role in terminating the immune response, as illustrated by the development of a systemic autoimmunity, similar to systemic lupus erythematosus (SLE), in mice and humans with mutations in the Fas or FasL. The receptors for TNF-α are expressed ubiquitously, but TNF-α appears to induce apoptosis predominantly of activated CD8+ T cells.

Unlike T cells, activated B cells are subjected to a third round of selection in germinal centers located within the spleen and lymph nodes. Here, B cells that have been triggered by antigen undergo somatic hypermutation and are positively selected (high-affinity clones) or die by apoptosis (low-affinity clones). Because mutations are generated randomly in the variable regions of the immunoglobulin heavy and light chains, it is likely that autoreactive cells also are generated by this mechanism. It is not yet certain how autoreactive B cells are eliminated in this microenvironment, but elimination most likely involves Fas.

Apoptosis

Apoptosis is the form of cell death seen during normal physiologic processes, such as tissue remodeling during embryogenesis and metamorphosis, but it also can be observed in certain pathologic situations, such as cancers. The term was first applied to the morphologic appearance of these dying cells, as depicted by electron microscopy. In contrast to necrotic cells, apoptotic cells are shrunken, have condensed nuclei, and undergo dissolution by blebbing.

Apoptosis is of particular relevance to immunology because most cell death that occurs in the induction and maintenance of tolerance occurs by apoptosis. As in the case of cells dying during embryogenesis, lymphocytes and cells of the myeloid series probably die by a programmed pathway during normal cell turnover, unless they are recruited into the immune response. It is relevant to note that cytotoxic T cells, NK cells, and antibody-dependent cytotoxic cells are, themselves, inducers of apoptosis

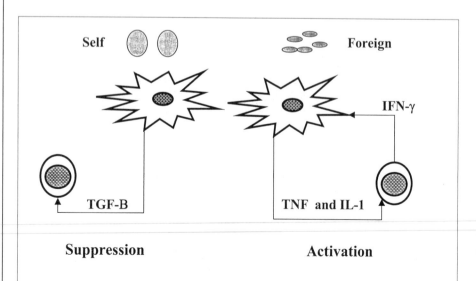

Fig. 5C-3. Self–nonself discrimination occurs at the level of the phagocyte. During normal cell turnover, apoptotic cells are removed rapidly by macrophages and induce the expression of cytokines, such as TGF-β, that suppress lymphocyte responses (left panel). In contrast, uptake of most foreign organisms induces the expression of cytokines, such as TNF and IL-1, that activate lymphocytes and/or induce costimulation (see Fig. 5C-2). When T cells are activated, they produce IFN-γ, which feeds back on the macrophage to enhance antigen presentation.

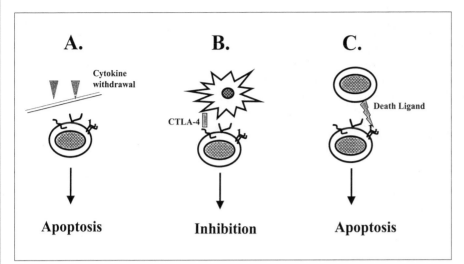

Fig. 5C-4. Termination of the immune response. During inflammation, activated lymphocytes are eliminated by cytokine withdrawal (**A**), inhibitory counter-receptors such as CTLA-4 (**B**) and by active induction of death through death receptors such as Fas (**C**). Failure of these mechanisms results in persistence of inflammation with increased opportunity for reactivity to self (autoimmunity).

in their corresponding targets. The resulting apoptotic bodies are phagocytosed by surrounding cells and rapidly degraded in lysozymes.

An important difference between programmed (apoptotic) versus accidental/toxic (necrotic) death is that programmed cell death results in the ordered fragmentation of the cell. As discussed above, phagocytosis of apoptotic bodies by neighboring cells and/or professional phagocytes does not cause activation of the engulfing cell and, in many instances, promotes an anti-inflammatory response. Although cell death by apoptosis takes hours, removal of apoptotic fragments is so rapid that apoptotic cells rarely are seen, even in such tissues as the thymus, where up to 95% of cells undergo apoptosis.

The mechanisms that identify, remove, and degrade apoptotic cells are not well-understood. Initial studies suggested that a lectin–sugar interaction might be responsible for clearance of apoptotic thymocytes. More recently, a number of receptors and potential ligands involved in the clearance of apoptotic fragments have been reported.

Autoimmunity: Models and Mechanisms

Given the sophisticated and overlapping mechanisms to avoid autoimmunity, how do autoimmune diseases occur? While in no case have the etiology and pathogenesis of human systemic autoimmune diseases been resolved, a number of important clues are available from both human and mouse studies.

Autoimmunity by Immunization

In several mouse models of autoimmunity, tolerance can be overcome by immunization with antigen in the pres-

ence of an adjuvant. For example, myelin basic protein has been effective in the case of experimental allergic encephalomyelitis, and collagen in the case of collagen-induced arthritis. These models illustrate a number of important points.

Potentially autoreactive T cells exist in healthy people. Several scenarios could explain how immunization with a foreign antigen leads to autoimmunity. The immunogen may share sequence similarity with self antigen; this obviously is the case when mice are immunized with chick collagen and develop autoimmunity against mouse collagen. In this case, the immune response is at first focused on the immunogen, but then cross-reacts with self antigen (molecular mimicry).

Although loss of tolerance often is initiated with foreign antigen, many of these diseases can be induced with self antigen in the presence of a powerful adjuvant, such as Freund's complete, that contains *Mycobacteria*. This adjuvant markedly facilitates the immune response by inducing cytokines such as TNF and IFN-γ, resulting in enhanced antigen presentation and up-regulation of costimulatory molecules. Self antigens therefore are presented in a proinflammatory context.

Autoimmunity is strain-dependent, suggesting that peptide binding to MHC dictates susceptibility to disease and/or that T-cell autoreactivity might be explained by failure of certain peptide-specific T cells to be tolerized.

Infection and Initiation of Autoimmunity

Certain diseases considered autoimmune in nature (such as reactive arthritis) unequivocally are initiated by exposure to bacteria, such as *Salmonella*, *Shigella*, and *Yersinia*. Although the mechanisms of inflammation are unclear, the association between HLA-B27 and these diseases suggests the possibility that bacterial peptide antigens presented by MHC class I induce immune responses that cross-react between host and bacterial products. In the setting of costimulation, a powerful immune response ensues. This may be another example of molecular mimicry.

Apart from serving as targets of the immune response, infectious organisms can manipulate the immune response. Viruses have been shown to induce polyclonal B-cell activation, interfere with the complement cascade, modify cytokine expression and receptor function, and inhibit MHC class I expression. A number of viruses subvert the regulation of cell survival and death. Mammalian DNA viruses synthesize proteins that inhibit cell death, including a Bcl-2 homologue, BHRF (Epstein-Barr virus), and the E1B 19-kDa protein (adenovirus). Disruption of apoptotic pathways predisposes to autoimmunity.

Cryptic Epitopes

During central tolerance, T lymphocytes that react with high affinity to peptide antigens are deleted. In most situations, only a very limited number of peptides derived from each protein are presented to T cells. In fact, usually one peptide is "dominant." This dominance is explained by the highly ordered degradation, transport, and binding of peptides to the MHC molecules. This being the case, tolerance will only be induced to the dominant, and perhaps subdominant, epitopes. Several studies have suggested that tolerance to a protein antigen may be broken if a new, "cryptic" peptide is presented to peripheral T cells. Presentation of this cryptic peptide may occur through a variety of mechanisms – binding of either an antibody or a foreign protein may alter the processing or intracellular transport of the protein. If this process occurs in an inflammatory setting (presence of costimulatory molecules), a vigorous immune response to self could occur.

Defined Mutations Predisposing to Autoimmunity

Loss-of-function mutations of the early complement components (particularly C1q, C2, and C4) predispose to SLE in humans. Although the mechanisms remain controversial, recent studies suggest that early complement deficiencies lead to defective clearance of apoptotic cells and/or interfere with the activation threshold of B lymphocytes.

The targeted deletions of a number of gene products involved in T- or B-lymphocyte signal transduction cause systemic autoimmunity in mice. The common feature of these knockouts is that the activation threshold of lymphocytes is reduced (lesser requirement for costimulation), resulting in increased activation of the cells in the peripheral immune system.

Mice with spontaneous mutations of the Fas receptor or its ligand develop massive lymphadenopathy and lupus-like autoimmunity. It is interesting to note the highly variable expression of lupus in terms of disease severity, organ involvement, and autoantibody production in these strains as well as other normal strains onto which the *lpr* mutation has been crossed. This variability stresses the importance of background genes in the expression of mutations affecting the same receptor/ligand pair. Although Fas mutations have been reported in a small number of humans, Fas expression and function appear to be normal in most people with SLE. However, failure of apoptosis in the peripheral immune system allows for the persistence of activated lymphocytes and some antigen-presenting cells. Targeted deletion of several other molecules that regulate apoptosis of lymphocytes have also been reported to lead to systemic autoimmunity (9).

KEITH B. ELKON, MD

References

1. Amsen D, Kruisbeek AM. *Thymocyte selection: not by TCR alone. Immunol Rev 1998;165:209–229.*

2. Goodnow CC. *Balancing immunity and tolerance: deleting and tuning lymphocyte repertoires. Proc Natl Acad Sci USA 1996;93:2264–2271.*

3. Weiner HL, Friedman A, Miller A, et al. *Oral tolerance: immunologic mechanisms and treatment of animal and human organ-specific autoimmune diseases by oral administration of autoantigens. Ann Rev Immunol 1994;12:809.*

4. Bretscher P, Cohn M. *A theory of self-nonself discrimination. Science 1970;169:1042–1049.*

5. Janeway CA Jr. *The immune system evolved to discriminate infectious nonself from noninfectious self. Immunol Today 1992;13:11–16.*

6. Matzinger P. *Tolerance, danger, and the extended family. Ann Rev Immunol 1994;12:991–1045.*

7. Van Parijs L, Abbas AK. *Homeostasis and self-tolerance in the immune system: turning lymphocytes off. Science 1998;280:243–248.*

8. Ashkenazi A, Dixit VM. *Death receptors: signaling and modulation. Science 1998;281:1305–1308.*

9. Elkon KB. *Immunologic tolerance and apoptosis. In: Rich RR, Fleisher TA, Kotzin B, Shearer W, Schroeder HW (eds). Clinical Immunology. 2nd ed. London: Harcourt International, 2001.*

6 GENETICS

Inherited traits account for much of the variation between individuals. This phenotypic diversity extends to differences in immune responsiveness and explains, for example, why some individuals respond poorly to immunization against hepatitis B, but others mount a vigorous antibody response (1). The primary genes that determine immune-response patterns are located within the major histocompatibility complex (MHC) on chromosome 6; they encode the human leukocyte antigens (HLA), which often are referred to as HLA molecules. The MHC is of great interest to rheumatologists because this region encodes HLA genes that are associated with a variety of autoimmune diseases. These genetic associations provide an important paradigm for approaching the larger question of genetic susceptibility to rheumatic disorders.

Traditionally, a chapter about genetics in rheumatic disease would have focused almost exclusively on the MHC. However, it has become apparent that numerous genes outside the MHC contribute to autoimmune and inflammatory disorders. Advances in this area include identification of the genes underlying several periodic fever syndromes, such as familial Mediterranean fever and tumor necrosis factor (TNF) receptor-associated periodic syndrome (2,3). In the latter case, gene identification has led to improved clinical management through manipulation of the TNF cytokine pathway (3).

The more common rheumatic diseases, such as rheumatoid arthritis (RA) and systemic lupus erythematosus (SLE), present enormous challenges in identifying genes outside the MHC. Students of rheumatic diseases need to have some understanding of the basic approaches used to detect and describe the relationship of genes to clinical phenotypes. This chapter provides a conceptual framework for an informed interpretation and incorporation of findings into both research and clinical practice.

Probability, Not Certainty

Most of the common rheumatic diseases, including autoimmune diseases, result from the interaction of genetic and nongenetic factors. Over time, this interaction may lead to the clinical expression of disease. Nongenetic factors may include environmental exposures, such as infection, and stochastic factors, which are random events that occur from early fetal life into adulthood (4). These etiologic factors combine to produce clinical disease and the variable manifestations and degrees of severity commonly observed. Because of the complexity of these interactions, a simple one-to-one correlation between genes and disease is not observed, and predicting disease outcomes for individual patients will remain difficult.

It is possible to assign weight to the role of a particular factor in susceptibility to, or risk for, a specific disease or clinical manifestation. In the case of genetic factors, the goal is to identify particular genetic variants, or *alleles*, that confer risk for disease. (Table 6-1 contains a glossary of genetic terms.). In the simplest formulation, an allele confers increased risk when the conditional probability of disease (D) in a population (P) is greater over a lifetime in the presence of particular allele (A) than it would be in the absence of the allele. This concept can be expressed as:

$$P(D \mid A) > P(D \mid \text{not } A)$$

The ratio of these two probabilities can be estimated in various ways. Modern approaches to genetics and epidemiology allow us to quantify these effects and ultimately identify genes that confer disease risk, even when many other factors may contribute "noise" and obscure the underlying genetic component.

Knowing a Disease Has a Genetic Component

Although researchers sometimes discover a particular gene that associates with disease, it usually is the occurrence of disease in families that suggests a genetic component. For most autoimmune diseases, however, aggregation in families is rather modest; in most cases, a person with RA or SLE will not have a close relative with the same illness. Therefore, it is necessary to study carefully the prevalence of disease among populations of individuals with different degrees of genetic relatedness. The most useful types of populations for these comparisons are genetically identical individuals (monozygotic twins), individuals who share approximately 50% of their genes in common (dizygotic twins and siblings), and unrelated individuals in the population. For the group of unrelated individuals, the overall degree of genetic similarity (at polymorphic loci) is relatively low, with approximately a 0.1% difference over the entire genome (4). Note that a 0.1% difference over the entire human genome of 3.2×10^9 base pairs implies at least three million base-pair differences between any two unrelated individuals; in fact, this figure may be an underestimate.

For monozygotic (MZ) twins, concordance rates for most autoimmune disease are between 15% and 30% (4). The fact

TABLE 6-1
Glossary of Genetic Terms

Alleles:	Alternative forms or variants of a gene at a particular locus.
Haplotype:	A group of alleles located at adjacent or closely linked loci on the same chromosome that usually are inherited as a unit.
Heterozygote:	An individual who inherits two different alleles at a given locus on two homologous chromosomes.
Linkage disequilibrium:	The preferential association, in a population, of two alleles or mutations, more frequently than predicted by chance. Linkage disequilibrium is detected statistically, and except in unusual circumstances, generally implies that the two alleles lie very close to one another in the genome.
Linkage:	The coinheritance, within a family, of two (nonallelic) genes or loci that lie close to one another in the genome. This phenomenon forms the basis of linkage analysis, in which the coinheritance of a marker locus is examined in relation to a disease locus within families.
Polymorphism:	The degree of allelic variation at a locus, within a population. Specific criteria differ, but a locus is said to be polymorphic if the most frequent allele does not occur in more than 98% of the population. Occasionally, the term polymorphism is used in the same way as "allele" to refer to a particular genetic variant.

that these concordance rates are substantially less than 100% indicates that nongenetic factors play a role. However, if one compares this MZ-twin concordance rate with the concordance rate among dizygotic (DZ) twins or siblings (who share half of their alleles in common), the rate drops to approximately 2%–5%. This fact indicates that complete sharing of genetic background with an affected individual substantially increases one's risk for disease. (In this case, we are assuming that shared environmental factors are approximately equivalent among MZ and DZ twin pairs).

To get a sense of the overall genetic risk, we need to compare these rates to the prevalence of disease in a genetically unrelated population (i.e., the background population prevalence). Depending on the autoimmune disease, background population prevalences range from 0.1% to 1%. These values can be used to calculate two ratios, the relative risk to siblings (λ_S) and the relative risk to MZ twins (λ_{MZ}):

$$\lambda_S = \frac{\text{Disease prevalence in siblings of affected individuals}}{\text{Disease prevalence in general population}}$$

$$\lambda_{MZ} = \frac{\text{Disease prevalence in co-twins of affected individuals}}{\text{Disease prevalence in general population}}$$

The values of these two ratios for various autoimmune disorders are given in Table 6-2 (5). Compared with the general population, an individual who has an identical twin or sibling with one of these disorders clearly is at substantially increased risk for the disease. It is likely that

genetic factors are largely responsible for this increased risk, although these risk ratios also account for environmental factors that may be preferentially shared among family members. HLA-linked genes probably account for 50% or less of this risk in most cases.

The MHC – Assigning Genetic Risk

Since the mid-1970s, research in the genetics of rheumatic disease has focused primarily on the MHC, which is known to encode the HLAs directly involved in antigen presentation to the immune system. The MHC also illustrates many of the concepts and complexities involved in assigning genetic risk to specific alleles, and it emphasizes the importance of combining genetics with biology when assigning such risk.

TABLE 6-2
Relative Risks of Autoimmune Disease in Siblings (λ_S) and Monozygotic Twins (λ_{MZ})

Disease	λ_S	λ_{MZ}
Rheumatoid arthritis	2–17	12–60
Multiple sclerosis	20	250
Type I diabetes	15	60
Systemic lupus erythematosus	20	250
Ankylosing spondylitis	54	500

Data in part from Vyse and Todd (5).

The Function of HLA Molecules

The major function of HLA molecules is to present peptide antigen fragments for recognition by T cells. As discussed in other chapters, T-cell recognition of foreign antigen requires antigen-presenting cells to process and present antigen on their surface, in physical association with HLA molecules. This process, called *antigen presentation*, is a highly complex and regulated cellular activity. The end result is that antigenic peptides are bound within the peptide-binding cleft of the HLA molecule, and it is this complex that is recognized by T cells through a specific interaction with their T-cell receptor molecules (6).

Different HLA alleles have different binding affinities for particular sets of antigenic peptides, which enables them to determine which antigens may be presented to T cells in a given individual. T cells undergo a process of education during thymic development, so that mature T cells generally interact successfully only with HLA molecules from the same individual from whom the T cells were derived. This phenomenon is known as *MHC-restricted T-cell recognition*, and is due to the fact that HLA molecules exhibit a high degree of structural (genetic) polymorphism.

Organization of the Human MHC

A bewildering array of genes and alleles is encoded within the MHC gene cluster. A highly simplified map of the MHC is shown in Fig. 6-1. The entire 3.4 million base-pair region has been sequenced, and the actual number of genes far exceeds what is shown in Fig. 6-1 (7). Indeed, the MHC is an exceedingly gene-rich region, containing more than 200 loci and at least 128 functional genes, of which approximately 40% appear to be primarily involved in immune

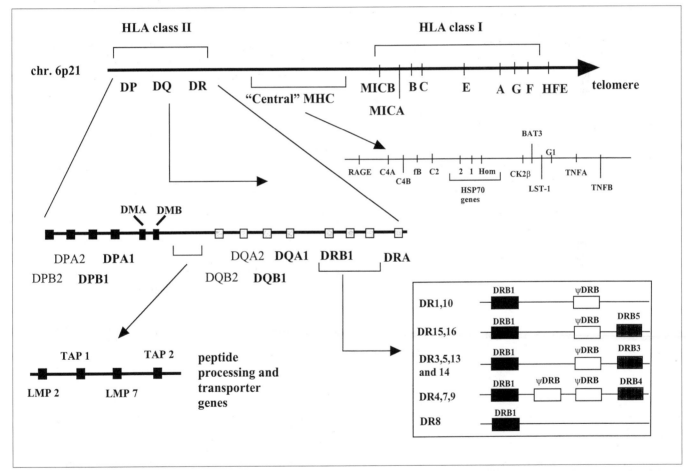

Fig. 6-1. Map of the human major histocompatibility complex (MHC). The human leukocyte antigen (HLA) class I and class II molecules are encoded in distinct regions of the MHC, located approximately 1 million base pairs apart. In between are encoded complement components (C4A, C4B, C2 and factor B), tumor necrosis factors (TNF)-α and -β, and the heat shock protein Hsp70. The HLA class II region contains three subregions, DR, DQ, and DP. Each of these subregions contains a variable number of α- and β-chain genes. HLA class II loci with known functional protein products are labeled in bold. In the case of DR, different numbers of DRB genes are present in different haplotypes, and the most common are shown in the boxed inset. (The DR3, 5, and 6 group includes haplotypes carrying the DR11, 12, 13 and 14 allelic families; most of these carry a functional DRB3 gene). The DQ and DP subregions each contain one pair of functional α- and β-chain genes. A number of genes involved in antigen processing and presentation (TAP, LMP genes) by class I molecules are situated between the DP and DQ subregions. The DMA and DMB genes encoded in this region are required for normal antigen presentation by HLA class II molecules. A more detailed map and references to these genes can be found in supplementary materials for reference 5 at www.nature.com.

function (7). For a more detailed map of the region, see http://www.nature.com (7).

The MHC can be broadly divided into the class I and class II regions, which contain the "central" MHC between them. The central MHC contains many genes, including genes for several complement components (C4A, C4B, C2) and TNF-α and -β. The class I region contains the standard class I genes (HLA-A, -B and -C) and several genes with similar structure. In the class II region, there are several subregions, referred to as HLA-DR, -DQ, and -DP. Each of these subregions contains its own cluster of genes. For example, in the HLA-DR subregion, there is one gene (DRA) encoding the DR alpha chain. This gene is notable because it generally is not polymorphic. The DR beta chains are encoded by several genes (DRB1, DRB2, DRB3, etc.), the number of which varies according to the particular haplotype. All haplotypes contain a DRB1 gene; the DRB1 locus generally is the most variable within the DR subregion.

The complexity of the MHC is evident from the large number of genes and the many alleles of these genes found in human populations. This property is referred to as *polymorphism*. Many of the HLA loci exhibit extraordinarily high levels of polymorphism. For example, more than 100 different alleles have been described for the HLA-B locus and for the DRB1 locus. A full list of these alleles, their sequences, and explanations of nomenclature can be found at http://www.ebi.ac.uk/imgt/hla/allele.html.

This high level of diversity in HLA genes is thought to be a result of selective pressure during evolution. It is presumed that the wide array of HLA molecules available to present antigen confers a survival advantage against infectious organisms or other environmental challenges.

Association Studies and the Concept of Relative Risk

The association of HLA with disease provides a classic example of how to develop evidence that a particular allele confers risk for disease, namely that [P (D | A) > P (D | not A)], as discussed previously. One could measure these probabilities directly by conducting a *cohort study*, in which a large number of subjects carrying (or not carrying) allele A are followed over a lifetime and observed for disease. Although this approach is impractical, the results could be presented as shown in Table 6-3A, and used to calculate the relative risk (RR) as follows:

$$RR = a/(a + b) \div c/(c + d)$$

The RR is a measure of how much more (or less) likely a person is to develop the disease (over a lifetime) if that person inherits allele A. If the disease is uncommon (i.e., if a and c are small), the RR can be estimated from $(a \times d) \div (c \times b)$, also known as the cross product of Table 6-3A.

A more practical approach is to perform a *case control study*, in which the test and control populations are selected based on whether or not they have disease. The frequency of the allele is then measured in each group. The

TABLE 6-3
Association Analyses

A. Cohort study groups	Disease	No disease
Exposed	a	b
Not exposed	c	d

B. Case control study groups	Exposed	Not exposed
Disease	a	b
No disease	c	d

a, b, c, d = number of individuals in each category.

results are tabulated as shown in Table 6-3B. If the disease is rare, as is the case for the major rheumatic diseases, an estimate of the RR, also known as the *odds ratio*, can be calculated by using the cross product $(a \times d) \div (c \times b)$ from Table 6-3B.

The vast majority of data showing the association between HLA alleles and autoimmune disease have been generated using a case control study design. In general, the estimated RRs are less than 10, with the exception of HLA-B27 and the spondyloarthropathies, where the RR values approach 100 for ankylosing spondylitis (8). Even when HLA analysis is based on particular amino acid sequences, such as the association of the "shared epitope" on HLA-DR4 with RA, the overall risk calculations still are rather modest (4).

Case Control Studies and the Concept of Linkage Disequilibrium

Although the positive association (RR > 1) between an allelic polymorphism and a disease seems to suggest that the allele is directly involved with the disease's pathogenesis, this conclusion cannot be made without establishing that the association is statistically significant, and that cases and controls are properly matched for ethnicity and other factors. Beyond these considerations, it is critical to understand that most positive associations do *not* reflect causation by the allele associated with disease. Genetic polymorphisms occur at particular locations on chromosomes and are surrounded by many other polymorphisms in the genome. These "neighborhoods" of alleles tend to cluster together on haplotypes in human populations, a phenomenon known in population genetics as *linkage disequilibrium*. This term refers to the fact that alleles located very near to one another (less than 200,000 base pairs apart) are found together in the same individual more often than would be expected by chance.

For example, hemochromatosis is an iron metabolism disorder that is caused by mutations in the HFE gene on chromosome 6, quite near the MHC (9). A typical class I allele within the MHC, HLA-A3, is present in approximately 25% of the Caucasian population. Because HLA-A3 has nothing to do with the cause of hemochromatosis, one might also expect that only 25% of people with this disease would carry HLA-A3. However, it has been observed frequently in Caucasian populations that 70% or more of people with hemochromatosis carry HLA-A3. This phenomenon occurs because HLA-A3 is in linkage disequilibrium with common mutations in the HFE gene. The estimated RR for HLA-A3 and hemochromatosis is in the range of 10, yet HLA-A3 has nothing whatsoever to do with the pathogenesis of hemochromatosis. Many, indeed most, genetic associations likely are due to linkage disequilibrium between the test allele and the disease alleles; the actual genes responsible for the association are located elsewhere in the genetic neighborhood. Using case control methods, it is nearly impossible to prove definitively that a particular allele is the "cause" of the association, without using other experimental methods to show the mechanism underlying the association.

Almost all current data supporting a role for HLA in autoimmune diseases are derived from associations detected by case control studies. As the hemochromatosis example shows, this data alone does not prove that HLA alleles actually cause or are directly involved in disease mechanism. The fact that MHC genes are known to directly control immune-response patterns in experimental animals makes such a conclusion compelling, and this conclusion is supported by the wealth of ancillary data on the molecular basis of immune recognition. Nevertheless, the fact that the exact mechanisms underlying HLA associations with disease are not defined precisely provides a caution for students and a challenge for researchers. Ultimately, basic biologic research, not genetics, will resolve this issue.

Going Beyond the MHC

The study of association and linkage disequilibrium is useful only when there is some previous evidence that a gene of interest lies near to the chromosomal region under investigation, as is the case with the HLA region. Genes outside the HLA are important, but information about their location in the genome may be unavailable. One approach is to make an intelligent guess and select a "candidate" gene, such as a cytokine gene, to examine for polymorphisms. If polymorphisms are found, a case control design may be used to search for an association with the disease. The obvious disadvantage of this approach is the possibility of error when selecting a candidate gene – after all, there are at least 30,000 genes to choose from in the genome.

An alternative approach is to develop evidence that a particular location in the genome contains a disease gene, and then pursue association studies, using the more limited selection of genes in that region. The usual methods for doing this are based on a phenomenon known as *linkage*. A full discussion of linkage methods is beyond the scope of this chapter, and can be found elsewhere (10). However, it

is useful to contrast gene mapping by linkage with mapping by linkage disequilibrium. As discussed, studies based on linkage disequilibrium are focused on the *association* of particular *alleles* in *populations* of (usually) unrelated subjects. In contrast, linkage methods are focused on the *coinheritance* of disease with a *genetic marker*, regardless of the particular allele, within families.

Classic linkage analysis has been used to confirm HLA involvement in ankylosing spondylitis (11) and in some studies of SLE (12). However, for the major rheumatic diseases, the most widely utilized method of analysis based on linkage is known as the affected sibling pair (ASP) method. Consider the family shown in Fig. 6-2 in which there are two siblings, each exhibiting the same disease or phenotype. In these types of families, the affected siblings within each family are highly likely, although not certain, to be carriers of the same disease alleles. This conclusion assumes that the genes involved are not so heterogeneous and so common in the population that affected siblings might have developed the same disease by inheriting different susceptibility genes.

In the family shown, both siblings have inherited identical alleles at marker locus X. In this case, there is only a 25% probability of this happening by chance. For example, given the fact that the first-born sibling (#1) inherited genotype 1,3, sibling #2 could have inherited one of four genotypes (1,3; 2,3; 1,4; or 2,4) with equal probability. By similar reasoning, there is a 50% probability that these two siblings will share only one allele, and a 25% chance that they will share nothing in common at this marker locus. If, however, the marker locus X is located very near to a disease gene, affected siblings would be expected to

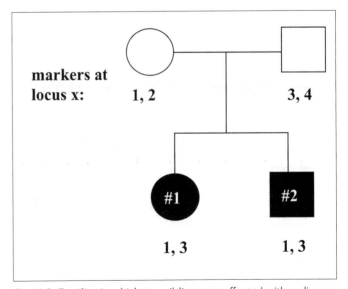

markers at
locus x: 1, 2   3, 4

#1   #2

1, 3   1, 3

Fig. 6-2. Families in which two siblings are affected with a disease can be useful for detecting genetic linkage using the affected sibling pair (ASP) method. The segregation of alleles 1, 2, 3, and 4 are shown for a generic marker "X" for parents and affected siblings. The first-born (#1) and second-born (#2) are indicated to aid discussion (see text).

share marker alleles more frequently than predicted by mendelian segregation ratios. Examining large numbers of affected sibling pairs helps develop statistical evidence that this is the case for a given test marker locus using a χ^2 analysis, with the null hypothesis being that there is no increased sharing of alleles at the marker locus. This is the essence of ASP analysis (13).

Searching the Genome for Non-MHC Genes

By using ASP analysis and other linkage methods, it has become apparent that many genes outside the MHC contribute to rheumatic/autoimmune disorders. Although none of these genes have been identified definitively, it is likely that they will be identified in the near future. Perhaps the most compelling candidate is SLE, in which a gene, or genes, on chromosome 1 clearly are important, both in human and murine lupus (14,15). Genome-wide searches in ankylosing spondylitis (16) and rheumatoid arthritis (17,18) also are beginning to reveal chromosomal regions of interest. There is a developing impression that multiple genes in complex and overlapping patterns, including genes within the MHC, are involved in these disorders. Presumably, this involvement reflects an overlapping set of molecular pathways that underlie the pathogenesis of autoimmune diseases.

PETER K. GREGERSEN, MD

References

1. Egea E, Iglesias A, Salazar M, et al. The cellular basis for lack of antibody responses to Hepatitis B vaccine in humans. J Exp Med 1991;173:531–538.
2. Samuels J, Aksentijevich I, Torosyan Y, et al. Familial Mediterranean fever at the millennium. Clinical spectrum, ancient mutations, and a survey of 100 American referrals to the National Institutes of Health. Medicine (Baltimore) 1998; 77:268–297.
3. Galon J, Aksentijevich I, McDermott MF, O'Shea JJ, Kastner DL. TNFRSF1A mutations and autoinflammatory syndromes. Curr Opin Immunol 2000;12:479–486.
4. Gregersen PK. Genetics of rheumatoid arthritis: confronting complexity. Arthritis Res 1999;1:37-44. Available at: http://arthritis-research.com/26oct99/ar0101r04.
5. Vyse TJ, Todd JA. Genetic analysis of autoimmune disease. Cell 1996;85:311-8.
6. Bjorkman PJ, Saper MA, Samraoui B, et al. Structure of the human class I histocompatibility antigen, HLA-A2. Nature 1987;329:506-512.
7. The MHC sequencing consortium. Complete sequence and gene map of a human major histocompatibility complex. Nature 1999;401:921–923.
8. Khan MA. HLA-B27 and its subtypes in world populations. Curr Opin Rheumatol 1995;7:263-269.
9. Feder JN, Penny DM, Irrinki A, et al. The hemochromatosis gene product complexes with the transferrin receptor and lowers its affinity for ligand binding. Proc Natl Acad Sci USA 1998;95:1472–1477.
10. Ott J. Analysis of Human Genetic Linkage. 2nd ed. Baltimore: Johns Hopkins Univ Press, 1991.
11. Rubin LA, Amos CI, Wade JA, et al. Investigating the genetic basis for ankylosing spondylitis. Arthritis Rheum 1994;37: 1212-1220.
12. Moser KL, Neas BR, Salmon JE, et al. Genome scan of human systemic lupus erythematosus: evidence for linkage on chromosome 1q in African-American pedigrees. Proc Natl Acad Sci USA 1998;95:14869–14874.
13. Risch N. Linkage strategies for genetically complex traits. II. The power of affected relative pairs. Am J Hum Genet 1990; 46:229–241.
14. Harley JB, Moser KL, Gaffney PM, Behrens TW. The genetics of human systemic lupus erythematosus. Curr Opin Immunol 1998;10:690–696.
15. Criswell LA, Amos CI. Update on genetic risk factors for systemic lupus erythematosus and rheumatoid arthritis. Curr Opin Rheumatol 2000;12:85–90.
16. Brown MA, Pile KD, Kennedy LG, et al. A genome-wide screen for susceptibility loci in ankylosing spondylitis. Arthritis Rheum 1998;41:588–595.
17. Cornelis F, Faure S, Martinez M, et al. New susceptibility locus for rheumatoid arthritis suggested by a genome-wide linkage study. Proc Natl Acad Sci USA 1998;95:10746-10760.
18. Jawaheer D, Seldin MF, Amos CI, et al. A genomewide screen in multiplex rheumatoid arthritis families suggests genetic overlap with other autoimmune diseases. Am J Hum Genet 2001;68:927-936.

7 EVALUATION OF THE PATIENT
A. History and Physical Examination

Musculoskeletal complaints are among the most common problems in clinical medicine. Physicians must be able to conduct an evaluation that identifies the presence of pathology or dysfunction in musculoskeletal structures.

Rheumatologic History

A thoughtful, detailed history plays a critical role in determining the nature of the complaint and helps focus the clinical evaluation (1). The history should be structured to answer specific questions:

- Is the problem regional or generalized, symmetric or asymmetric, peripheral or central? Is it an acute, subacute, or chronic problem? Is it progressive?
- Do the symptoms suggest inflammation or damage to musculoskeletal structures?
- Is there evidence of a systemic process? Are there associated extra-articular features?
- Has there been functional loss and disability?
- Is there a family history of a similar or related problem?

Location and Symmetry

The location of a musculoskeletal problem often is the most important clue to identifying the specific cause. Musculoskeletal problems can be categorized broadly as regional or generalized, although there often is considerable overlap between these two categories. Regional syndromes typically affect a single joint or periarticular structure, or an entire extremity or body region. A regional pain syndrome can be on a referred basis, in which the painful area is unrelated to the actual source of the disorder.

Specific arthropathies have a predilection for involving specific joint areas (2). Involvement of the wrists and the proximal small joints of the hands and feet is an important feature of rheumatoid arthritis (RA). In contrast, psoriatic arthritis (PsA) often involves the distal joints of the hands and feet. An acutely painful and swollen great toe most likely is caused by a gouty attack.

Symmetry is an important aspect of articular patterns of involvement. For example, RA tends to involve joint groups symmetrically, whereas the seronegative spondyloarthropathies tend to be asymmetrical.

Onset and Chronology

The mode of onset and evolution of musculoskeletal symptoms can help establish a diagnosis. For most chronic arthropathies, such as RA, onset typically is subacute, occurring over weeks to months rather than hours to days. Attacks

of gout and septic arthritis, however, have an acute onset, reaching a crescendo within hours. The pain of fibromyalgia often is reported as being present for years with episodic exacerbations. A temporally associated traumatic event or a history of repetitive use of a joint can provide good clues to diagnosing a regional musculoskeletal syndrome.

Inflammation and Weakness

Articular pain and swelling can be inflammatory or noninflammatory. When intra-articular inflammation is present, the process involves the synovial membrane and is called synovitis. Swelling usually is due to accumulation of fluid in the articular cavity. Pain and swelling associated with synovitis often occur at rest, whereas in disorders such as osteoarthritis (OA), symptoms become more evident with joint use. When synovitis is present, the patient may also complain of difficulty moving the joints after a period of immobility, a symptom referred to as stiffness. In inflammatory disorders, such as RA, this stiffness is most evident in the early morning. The duration of morning stiffness is a semi-quantitative measure of the degree of articular inflammation, typically established by asking the patient, "How long does it take you before you are moving as well as you are going to move for the day?" Complaints of limited joint motion, deformity, and joint instability usually are caused by damage to articular and periarticular structures. Patients should be questioned carefully to establish the circumstances around which these symptoms began, and the type of movements that aggravate them.

People with musculoskeletal pathology often complain of muscle weakness. This feeling of weakness may be associated with pain, stiffness, and in some cases, paresthesia or other neurologic symptoms. Generalized weakness may be in response to pain from articular or periarticular inflammation, as in the case of RA and polymyalgia rheumatica. Alternatively, a primary neuropathic or myopathic process may cause weakness. In the case of myopathies, weakness typically is symmetrical and involves proximal muscles most severely. In the case of neuropathies, the distal musculature is affected more commonly.

Systemic and Extra-Articular Features

Constitutional symptoms of fatigue, weight loss, anorexia, and low-grade fever may be associated with any systemic inflammatory process, and their presence is an important diagnostic clue. Systemic rheumatic diseases commonly are associated with specific nonarticular features that are of value in diagnosis. For example, a history of recent genitourinary symptoms in association with lower-extremity asymmetric oligoarthritis is highly suggestive of reactive arthritis, whereas this same articular pattern in association with recurrent abdominal pain and bloody diarrhea is more suggestive of the arthropathy of inflammatory bowel disease. It is thus important that the clinician perform a complete review of systems and question the patient regarding such symptoms as rashes or skin changes, photosensitivity, Raynaud's phenomenon, mouth ulcers, and dryness in the eyes and mouth.

Functional Losses

Questions regarding functional loss are essential for understanding the impact of a musculoskeletal disorder and developing a management plan. Questions should span the spectrum of activities, from simple activities of daily living, such as dressing and grooming, to more physically demanding activities, such as sports. In some cases, the functional loss may be quite severe, impairing such basic activities as stair climbing and gripping, while in others it may be subtle, detectable only as a reduction in strenuous activities, such as jogging.

Family History

A number of rheumatic diseases have a strong genetic basis. Some disorders, such as ankylosing spondylitis (AS), are much more common in human leukocyte antigen (HLA)-B27–positive families than in the general population. Questions about family history should not be restricted to ascertaining whether other family members have a similar "arthritis," but should be as complete as possible regarding autoimmune diseases, many of which (e.g., RA, thyroid disease, and diabetes) tend to cluster in families.

Principles of Rheumatologic Examination

Evaluation of musculoskeletal complaints involves examination of the joints and their soft-tissue support structures, the bony skeleton, and the muscle groups that move the skeletal structures (3). Joints, bones, and muscles may be directly accessible, as in the extremities, or they may be inaccessible to direct examination, as in the case of the spine and hip joints.

The cardinal signs of articular inflammation are joint-line tenderness; pain on motion, particularly at the extremes of the range of motion; and intra-articular swelling or effusion. In acute inflammation, such as that caused by septic arthritis, the joint usually is red and hot to the touch. These findings often are not present in more chronic articular inflammation, such as that found in RA.

Joint motion should be tested both by having the patient move the joint to its extremes (active range of motion) and by having the examiner move the joint through its range (passive range of motion). Loss of range of motion is seen with acute articular inflammation and with chronic arthritis and damage. In acute synovitis, loss of range of motion

usually is reversible, and is associated with pain at the extremes of the range of motion. When irreversible articular damage is present, such as in advanced RA and OA, the loss of range of motion has a more "fixed" quality to it, and may not be associated with pain on movement.

Deformity caused by loss of alignment is a consequence of destructive arthropathies, such as RA. The damage commonly is associated with loosening of the soft-tissue support structures surrounding the joints. In some cases, the joint may not exhibit any obvious deformity, but may be unstable when put through its range of motion or when it is stressed mechanically.

A key part of the musculoskeletal evaluation involves examination of the ligaments, tendons, menisci, and muscles. These structures may be the primary source of the pathology, or may be involved secondary to the articular pathology. Examination of individual muscle groups requires a basic knowledge of the origin and insertion of each muscle, and the primary joint that is moved by the muscle. Atrophy and weakness of the muscles surrounding a joint are important indicators of chronic articular pathology.

A Screening Musculoskeletal Exam

The GALS (gait, arms, leg, spine) system has been devised to rapidly screen for musculoskeletal disease (4). Initially, the patient is asked three basic questions: 1) Have you any pain or stiffness in your muscles, joints, or back? 2) Can you dress yourself completely without any difficulty? and 3) Can you walk up and down stairs without any difficulty? Depending on the answers, further questioning should explore specific areas of concern.

The examiner then systematically inspects the patient's gait, arms, legs, and spine, first with the patient standing still, and then with the patient responding to instructions (Table 7A-1). Abnormalities detected on this screening are followed with a more detailed regional or generalized musculoskeletal examination.

Examination of Specific Joint Areas

The Hand and Wrist

A number of generalized arthropathies have distinctive patterns of hand involvement, and the recognition of these patterns is highly valuable diagnostically. Examination of the hands should be initiated with the patient sitting comfortably, hands open and the palms facing down. In this position, the examiner can inspect the alignment of the digits relative to the wrist and forearm. Atrophy of the intrinsic muscles of the hands can be readily apparent as a hollowing out of the spaces between the metacarpals. The nails should be inspected for evidence of onycholysis or pitting suggestive of psoriasis. Redness and telangiectasia of the nail-fold capillaries can be detected on close inspection, and often is indicative of a connective-tissue disease, such as systemic lupus erythematosus, scleroderma, or dermatomyositis. Tightening of the skin around the digits,

TABLE 7A-1
Main Features of the GALS Screening Inspection

Position/activity	Normal findings
Gait	Symmetry, smoothness of movement Normal stride length Normal heel strike, stance, toe-off, swing through Able to turn quickly
Inspection from behind	Straight spine Normal, symmetric paraspinal muscles Normal shoulder and gluteal muscle bulk Level iliac crests No popliteal cysts No popliteal swelling No hindfoot swelling/deformity
Inspection from the side	Normal cervical and lumbar lordosis Normal thoracic kyphosis
"Touch your toes"	Normal lumbar spine (and hip) flexion
Inspection from the front Arms "Place your hands behind your head (elbows out)"	Normal glenohumeral, sternoclavicular, and acromioclavicular joint movement
"Place your hands by your side (elbows straight)"	Full elbow extension
"Place your hands in front (palms down)"	No wrist/finger swelling or deformity Able to fully extend fingers
"Turn your hands over"	Normal supination/pronation Normal palms
"Make a fist"	Normal grip power
"Place the tip of each finger on the tip of the thumb"	Normal fine precision, pinch
Legs	Normal quadricep bulk/symmetry No knee swelling or deformity No forefoot/midfoot deformity Normal arches No abnormal callous formation
Spine "Place your ear on your shoulder"	Normal cervical lateral flexion

Modified from Doherty et al. (4), with permission.

or sclerodactyly, is typical of scleroderma and usually is visible and palpable. The pulp of the digits should be examined for the presence of digital ulcers, also seen most commonly in scleroderma.

Articular swelling of the distal interphalangeal (DIP) and proximal interphalangeal (PIP) joints may signify bony osteophytes, as in the case of Heberden's and Bouchard's nodes in the DIP and PIP joints, respectively, or it may indicate an intra-articular effusion associated with synovitis in the joint. Palpation will help differentiate these conditions. Swelling and redness of an entire digit, termed dactylitis, is highly suggestive of a spondyloarthropathy, such as psoriatic arthritis or reactive arthritis.

Swelling of the metacarpophalangeal (MCP) joints can be seen as a fullness in the valleys normally found between the knuckles (heads of the metacarpal bones). In cases of RA where the MCP synovitis has been long-standing, this swelling often is associated with ulnar subluxation of the extensor tendons, resulting in the ulnar drift of the digits typical of this diagnosis. Swelling on the dorsum of the wrist can result from synovitis of the wrist or tenosynovitis of the extensor tendons. Getting patients to gently wiggle the fingers helps differentiate these two findings because swelling tends to move with the tendons if it is a result of tenosynovitis. Inspection of the palmar aspect of the hands is important for identifying atrophy of the thenar or hypothenar eminences, which can result from disuse due to articular involvement of the wrist or, in the case of the thenar eminence, carpal tunnel syndrome.

Global function of the hand should be evaluated by asking the patient to make a fist, and then fully extend and spread out the digits. Pincer function of the thumb and fingers should be tested. Grip strength can be estimated by having the patient squeeze two of the examiner's fingers. Individual hand joints should be palpated to determine the presence of joint-line tenderness and effusion, the most important indicators of synovitis. The technique for palpating the DIP and PIP joints is similar. The thumb and index finger of one hand palpates in the vertical plane, while the thumb and index finger of the other hand palpates in the horizontal plane (Fig. 7A-1). Alternating gentle pressure between the two planes will displace small amounts of syn-

ovial fluid back and forth, allowing the examiner to detect effusions in these small joints. Tenderness suggestive of synovitis also can be elicited by this technique. The technique for palpating the MCP joints is somewhat modified because of the inability to directly palpate these joints from the horizontal plane. The thumbs are used to palpate the dorsolateral aspects of the joint, while the index fingers palpate the palmar aspect.

Palpation of the wrist involves a technique similar to that used for the MCPs. Using thumbs, the examiner palpates the dorsum of the joint, while the index fingers palpate the volar aspect (Fig. 7A-2). Synovial thickening and tenderness suggestive of wrist joint synovitis usually can be palpated on the dorsum of the joint. Particular attention should be paid to swelling and tenderness in the area just distal to the ulnar styloid, where the extensor and flexor carpi ulnaris tendons are directly palpable. This area is involved very commonly in early RA. Pain and tenderness confined to the radial aspect of the wrist are due most commonly to OA of the first carpometacarpal joint or to DeQuervain's tenosynovitis.

The Elbow

Flexion and extension of the forearm occur exclusively at the elbow joint and involve hinge articulation between the proximal ulna and distal humerus. When examining the elbow, it is necessary to identify the olecranon process, the medial and lateral epicondyles of the humerus, and the radial head. A triangular recess is formed in the lateral aspect of the joint between the olecranon process, the lateral epicondyle, and the radial head. This recess is the point where the synovial cavity of the elbow is most accessible to inspection and palpation.

Examination of the elbow should be undertaken with the patient sitting comfortably, and the entire arm well-supported to eliminate muscle tension. Initially, the joint should be inspected while the forearm is flexed to 90°. Particular attention should be paid to the lateral recess described previously. Obvious bulging in this area is highly suggestive of an effusion and synovitis. In contrast, swelling directly over the olecranon process is more suggestive of olecranon bursitis. Any process that causes true synovitis of the elbow typically is associated with a reduction in the range of motion of the joint, both in flexion-extension and in supination-pronation. Having the patient extend the forearm as much as possible will detect the presence of a flexion contracture, an almost invariant feature of elbow synovitis. With this maneuver, the bulge in the lateral recess tends to enlarge, becoming more tense, due to the reduction in the internal dimension of the elbow in the position of extension.

The synovial cavity and joint line are best palpated for swelling and tenderness in the area of the lateral recess. This also is the site where arthrocentesis of the elbow is performed. It should be noted that pain in the lateral aspect of the elbow is a common clinical problem, and usually is due to lateral epicondylitis, or tennis elbow, rather than elbow-joint pathology. Tenderness directly palpable over the lateral epicondyle is suggestive of this diagnosis.

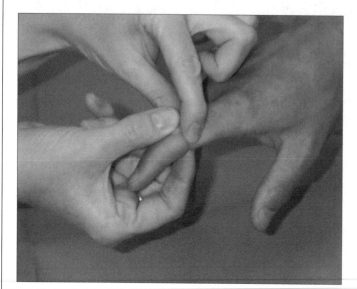

Fig. 7A-1. Technique for examining the small joints of the hands and feet. The thumb and index finger of the examiner's hands are used to gently move small amounts of intra-articular fluid back and forth, and to elicit evidence of joint-line tenderness.

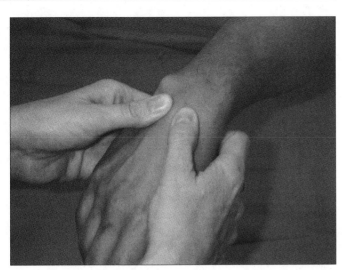

Fig. 7A-2. Using thumbs, the examiner palpates the dorsum of the wrist joint for tenderness and swelling. The wrist should be examined in slight flexion to allow the joint line of the radiocarpal, intercarpal, and carpometacarpal joints to be palpated optimally.

The Shoulder

Proper examination of the shoulder should begin with appropriate visual examination of the entire shoulder girdle area, from the front and the back. Comparison should be made with the contralateral shoulder. Any asymmetry between the two sides should be noted. For example, patients with rotator cuff tears often hold the affected shoulder higher than the other side. A prominent bump in the area of the acromioclavicular joint often is associated with osteophytes resulting from OA. Atrophy of the shoulder girdle musculature is an important sign of chronic glenohumeral joint pathology, as occurs in RA. This condition is most evident as squaring of the shoulder, due to deltoid atrophy, and scooping out of the upper scapular area, due to supraspinatus atrophy. Effusions in the shoulder joint are visible anteriorly just medial to the area of the bicipital groove and, if large enough, also are evident laterally below the acromion. It should be noted that large amounts of fluid can accumulate in the glenohumeral joint space without much visible evidence. This phenomenon is due to considerable redundancy in the joint capsule.

After the shoulder area is inspected in the resting position, the patient is asked to demonstrate active range of motion of the arms in several planes. Flexion is observed by having the patient lift the outstretched arms from the side directly in front, to the highest point above the head. Abduction is observed as the patient moves the outstretched arms from the side in the lateral plane until the palms meet overhead. Active internal rotation is observed by having the patient reach behind the back and attempt to touch the highest point possible on the scapula. External rotation is tested by having the patient attempt to touch the back of the head with the palm of the hand while extending the flexed elbow. Internal and external rotation of the shoulder are movements that are particularly sensitive to glenohumeral pathology.

Palpation should include the entire shoulder girdle, the cervical spine, and the thoracic wall. The cervical musculature is palpated for spasm. The costochondral joints, sternal joints, and ribs are palpated for tenderness and swelling. The sternoclavicular joint is palpated, then the fingers are "walked" laterally over the clavicle to the acromioclavicular joint, which is palpated for tenderness and swelling. Immediately below the acromioclavicular joint, the coracoid process should be identified. The short head of the biceps inserts on this process. The long head of the biceps can be palpated lateral to this process in the bicipital groove. The anterior aspect of the glenohumeral joint can be palpated between the coracoid process and the long head of the biceps, and it follows the contour on the rounded anterior aspect of the humeral head. Shoulder synovitis can be palpated in this area as joint-line tenderness and/or boggy effusion.

Passive range of shoulder motion then is evaluated. The most informative parts of this evaluation are internal/external rotation and abduction. When testing these movements, it is very important to immobilize the scapula to prevent rotation at the scapulothoracic area. In this way, glenohumeral motion can be isolated and appropriately evaluated. One effective technique to achieve this immobilization is to press down firmly on the top of the shoulder with the palm of one hand, while the other hand moves the arm through the range of motion (Fig. 7A-3). Internal/external rotation should be tested with the arm by the patient's side and with the arm abducted to 90°.

Some special maneuvers are useful in detecting specific clinical syndromes in the shoulder. Forced supination of the hand with the elbow flexed at 90° will cause pain in the area of the long head of the biceps in people with bicipital tendinitis. Supraspinatus tendinitis can be detected by having the patient position the outstretched arm at 90° of abduction while maximally internally rotating the glenohumeral joint such that the thumb is pointing downward. The examiner then asks the patient to resist attempts to push down the arm. In patients with supraspinatus tendinitis, the maneuver will be associated with pain, and may result in the patient suddenly dropping the arm.

The Hip

Pain resulting from hip arthritis typically is experienced in the groin or, less commonly, the buttock. It tends to radiate down the anteromedial aspect of the thigh, occasionally to the knee. Pain in the lateral trochanteric area most often is indicative of bursitis involving the trochanteric bursa.

Because the hip joint cannot be examined directly, the examiner needs to observe important diagnostic clues from the patient's gait, buttock and thigh musculature, and the hip joint's active and passive range of motion. The patient with true hip disease often walks with a "coxalgic" gait, quickly swinging the pelvis forward on the affected side to avoid weight-bearing on the affected hip. If hip arthritis is prolonged and severe, the buttock musculature tends to atrophy, as does the thigh musculature. In severe cases, the abductor muscles are unable to hold the pelvis

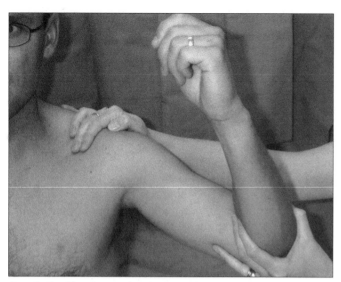

Fig. 7A-3. Glenohumeral joint motion is best examined with the elbow flexed to 90° and the upper arm partially abducted. Internal and external rotation of the shoulder then are examined in this position. Care should be taken to immobilize the scapula by using a technique such as the one shown.

in a horizontal position when the patient is asked to stand on only the leg with the affected hip. This position forms the basis of the Trendelenburg test, where the patient's pelvis tends to sag on the contralateral side when the patient is asked to support the entire body weight on the affected leg.

Hip range of motion is tested by having the patient actively flex, extend, abduct, and adduct the leg. With the patient supine, passive range of motion initially should be screened by "log rolling" the entire extended leg. The leg then is flexed maximally to assess completeness of this motion. With the knee flexed to 90° and the hip flexed to 90°, internal and external rotation of the hip are tested. Care should be taken that the hip movements are isolated, and that the patient's pelvis is not rotating to compensate for lost range of motion. Pain and loss of motion on internal rotation are particularly sensitive indicators of hip pathology. Flexion contracture of the hip tends to accompany severe, long-standing hip arthritis.

The Sacroiliac Joint

Palpation of the sacroiliac (SI) joint is undertaken with the patient lying flat on the abdomen. With the palm of the examiner's hand held around the iliac crest, the thumb tends to fall directly over the joint, which extends down below the dimples in the posterior pelvic area. To elicit tenderness in the SI joint, direct pressure is applied with the thumb in this area. In addition to direct palpation, other maneuvers help establish the presence of sacroiliitis. Direct pressure over the sacrum will produce pain in an inflamed SI joint. Gaenslen's maneuver is performed by having the patient hyperextend the leg over the edge of the examining table, thereby stressing the ipsilateral SI joint.

The Spine

The spine should be examined initially with the patient standing and the entire spine visible. The normal curvature of the spine, lumbar lordosis, thoracic kyphosis, and cervical lordosis should be evaluated by observing the patient from the back and the side, and noting any loss or accentuation of these curves. If scoliosis is noted when the patient is standing, the patient should be asked to bend forward and flex the spine. This movement helps in the evaluation of the scoliosis. True scoliosis will be present irrespective of the state of spinal flexion, but a functional scoliosis due to leg-length discrepancy tends to decrease with spinal flexion. The level of the iliac crests relative to the spine also should be evaluated by observing the patient from the back, with the examiner sitting approximately at eye level with the iliac crests. A tilted pelvis can be due to compensation for primary scoliosis in the spine or, alternatively, due to a leg-length discrepancy.

The range of motion of the entire spine should be examined in segments. The lumbar spine is assessed by having the patient attempt to touch the toes and then extend the back. Lateral flexion is assessed by having the patient reach the fingertips as far as possible down the lateral aspect of the leg. Lateral rotation, which involves both the lumbar and thoracic spine, is tested by having the patient turn the upper body while the examiner holds the pelvis stable. Pathology involving the anterior parts of the spinal column, such as intervertebral disc disease, generally will be aggravated by flexion, whereas pathology involving the posterior structures, as is seen with facet-joint arthritis, will be aggravated by extension and lateral flexion of the spine.

The Schöber test is performed to specifically assess movement in the lumbar spine. With the patient standing, a distance of 10 cm is measured up the lumbar spine from the lumbosacral junction at the level of the sacral dimples. Marks are placed at both ends of this 10-cm segment. The patient then is asked to flex forward as far as possible, attempting to touch the toes. With this motion, the marks identifying this 10-cm segment normally expand to 15 cm or more, indicative of distraction between the vertebrae. If the lumbar spine is fused, such as in ankylosing spondylitis, the increase in the length of the segment with flexion will be diminished.

Patients presenting with symptoms suggestive of a lumbar radiculopathy, such as pain and paresthesia shooting down the leg, need to undergo an examination of the lumbosacral area and a detailed neurologic examination of the leg. Maneuvers that put traction on the lumbar spinal roots are used to provide further evidence of a radiculopathy. The most commonly used of these maneuvers is the straight leg raising test, in which the patient lies supine and the examiner raises the leg, knee fully extended. A positive test requires that the patient experience pain and paresthesia shooting down the leg to the foot.

Thoracic motion should be examined by measuring chest expansion at the level of the nipples. Ankylosing spondylitis can markedly reduce chest expansion from the

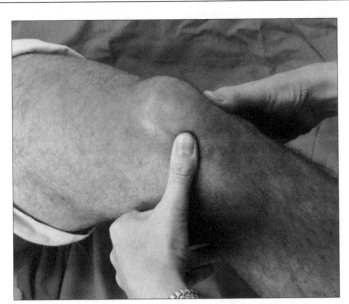

Fig. 7A-4. The joint line of the knee is palpated on the medial and lateral aspects for tenderness suggestive of synovitis. Stability of the cruciate ligaments also can be assessed in this position. Using the bulge sign or patellar tap sign, with the joint fully extended, an effusion can be detected in the knee.

normal 5–6 cm. Cervical range of motion should be tested with the patient upright and while lying down. The head is flexed, extended, laterally flexed (patient attempts to touch the ear to the shoulder) and laterally rotated (patient attempts to touch the chin to the shoulder). It should be noted that pain in the neck often radiates down the arm, up the occiput, or down to the scapular area. The pain may be aggravated by particular parts of the range of motion.

The Knee

Examination of the knee starts with inspection from both the front and the back, with the patient standing. From the front, areas above and below the knee should be inspected first. Atrophy of the quadriceps usually indicates chronic knee pathology. Swelling in the knee may be severe enough to compromise the venous return from the lower legs and cause pedal and tibial edema. Swelling due to synovial-fluid accumulation or synovial infiltration and thickening is most readily apparent in the suprapatellar bursa. When a large effusion is present, it can cause bulging of the lateral and medial compartments of the knee. Inspection of the knee from the back with the patient standing is the best way to evaluate the alignment of the femur relative to the tibia. Varus deformities, which cause a bow-legged appearance, result most commonly from OA preferentially involving the medial compartment. Valgus deformities, which cause a knock-kneed appearance, are more commonly associated with RA. Posterior inspection also is important for detecting popliteal or Baker's cysts, which can be large enough to track down the calf.

After the patient is inspected in the standing position, the knee is evaluated with the patient supine and the joint

fully extended. Flexion contractures should be noted. With the knee in partial flexion, the medial and lateral joint line are palpated for tenderness (Fig. 7A-4).

Synovial fluid in the knee is an important diagnostic clue. Large amounts of fluid cause distention of the joint in the suprapatellar area and in the medial and lateral compartments. The fluid can be confirmed by using the palm of one hand to firmly push the swelling in the suprapatellar area into the main compartment of the knee. While maintaining pressure over the suprapatellar area, the examiner's other hand is used to move the fluid back and forth, between the medial and lateral compartments of the knee; alternatively, the examiner may perform the patellar tap by pushing the patella up and down against the femoral condyles. Small amounts of fluid in the knee may be detected with the bulge sign. The medial aspect of the knee is stroked from the inferior aspect towards the suprapatellar area to move the fluid into the lateral compartment. The lateral aspect of the knee then is stroked in a similar manner, while the medial compartment is observed for the return of the fluid bulge.

To test the medial and collateral ligaments, varus and valgus stresses are applied gently to the joint while the examiner firmly supports the joint with one hand. The cruciate ligaments are tested using the drawer sign, in which anteroposterior stress is placed on the upper tibia with the knee in flexion; instability of the ligaments will result in the tibia moving back and forth relative to the femur, much as a drawer would if pushed back and forth.

The Ankle and Hindfoot

The ankle and hindfoot should be examined as a unit, because arthropathies often involve several structures in this area concurrently. Valgus deformities of the ankle and hindfoot can best be seen by inspecting the area from

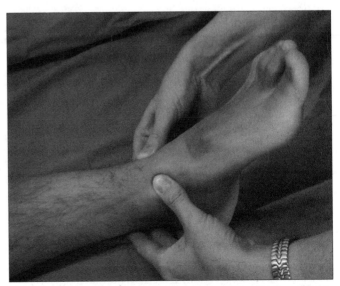

Fig. 7A-5. Palpation for tenderness and swelling in the ankle is undertaken medial and lateral to the extensor tendons on the anterior part of the joint below the malleoli.

behind, with the patient standing. Swelling in the ankle area eliminates the normal contours associated with the malleoli.

The joint line of the ankle is palpated anteriorly (Fig. 7A-5). Boggy swelling and tenderness in this area are typical of ankle synovitis. Tenderness and swelling posteriorly, at the insertion of the Achilles tendon, usually indicates enthesitis, although it also can result from bursitis of the retrocalcaneal bursa. Tenderness in the heel can indicate plantar fasciitis, another enthesitis associated with spondyloarthropathies.

The ankle and hindfoot unit should be put through the range of motion, isolating parts of the range associated with specific joints. The ankle proper, or tibiotalar joint, is capable only of dorsi and plantar flexion. Pain and limitation in this part of the range is associated with ankle synovitis. The subtalar joint, which separates the talus from the calcaneus, can be tested by rocking the calcaneus from side to side, while holding the talus stable.

The Midfoot and Forefoot

Observation of the standing patient may reveal abnormalities in the longitudinal arch and the anterior part of the foot. Pes planus (flat foot, collapsed arch) or pes cavus (high arch) will be most evident with the patient standing. Hallux valgus deformities, which cause bunions, are some of the most commonly observed problems in the joints.

Swelling of the metatarsophalangeal (MTP) joints causes a visible spreading of the toes, referred to as the daylight sign. Direct pressure over each of the MTP joints will confirm the presence of tenderness and swelling. In cases of advanced RA, subluxation of the MTP joint results in a hammertoe deformity, which can cause skin breakdown on the dorsum of the toes, due to constant rubbing against footwear. Inflammation of the interphalangeal joints of the toes is more common with spondyloarthropathies. In some cases, the entire digit becomes swollen and inflamed, a process termed dactylitis and referred to as sausage digit. Examining the plantar aspect of the forefoot is important to identify areas of callus formation. Calluses tend to occur in conjunction with subluxation of the MTP joint, where the metatarsal head can be directly palpated subcutaneously.

HANI EL-GABALAWY, MD

References

1. *Dieppe PA, Sergent JS. History. In: Klippel JH, Dieppe PA (eds). Rheumatology. 2nd ed. London: Mosby, 1998; pp 2:1.1–2:1.6.*
2. *Hubscher O. Pattern recognition in arthritis. In: Klippel JH, Dieppe PA (eds). Rheumatology. 2nd ed. London: Mosby, 1998; pp 2:3.1–2:3.6.*
3. *Grahame R. Examination of the patients. In: Klippel JH, Dieppe PA (eds). Rheumatology. 2nd ed. London: Mosby, 1998; pp 2:2.1–2:2.16.*
4. *Doherty M, Dacre J, Dieppe P, Snaith M. The GALS locomotor screen. Ann Rheum Dis 1992;51:1165–1169.*

EVALUATION OF THE PATIENT
B. Health Status Questionnaires

Qualitative and quantitative patient assessments are essential for effective treatment and clinical research. Standardized measurements form the basis of descriptive, predictive (including diagnostic), and evaluative activities (1). Health status questionnaires (HSQs) play a quintessential role in data acquisition. From a clinical standpoint, health status measurements: 1) describe the health status of an individual or a group of patients; 2) predict future health outcomes from information regarding current health status; 3) evaluate the efficacy, effectiveness, and safety of therapy in an individual patient or a group of patients; 4) communicate the health status of an individual to other professionals or lay people in compensation or litigation environments; and 5) dissect operational problems in health care systems, for purposes of total quality management, forecasting, and facilitation of health care policy planning.

Since the work of such early pioneers as Taylor, Steinbrocker, and Keele (2), there has been a progressive evolution in the sophistication of HSQs and in the scope and depth of measurements acquired through them. Terminology has developed to describe the different components of the measurement process (Table 7B-1). Data no longer are spoken of as being "hard" or "soft," but are characterized according to their points of origin and the clinimetric properties of the instruments used to collect data. Indeed, health status questionnaires are referred to as instruments and valid tools of measurement, placing them on an equal standing with technical and electromechanical devices.

There are two levels at which a clinician may encounter these instruments, as originator or user. Originators are the research scientists who develop measuring instruments and who determine their clinimetric properties. Originators often are the best sources of information, particularly regarding the application and utility of new instruments. In contrast, users often are practitioners using a technique, maybe for the first time, to address clinical problems of a descriptive, predictive, or evaluative nature.

Fundamentals of Clinical Measurement

Clinical measures can be subdivided into observer-dependent and observer-independent. Observer-dependent methods include interviewer-scored HSQs, examination-based physical findings, and observed physical performance tests using technical instruments. Interviewer-scored HSQs require proper training of the interviewers to achieve standardization and impartiality. Observer-independent measures are based on self-administered patient questionnaires. Such measures are free of observer bias, relatively inexpensive, and generally convenient and undemanding for the patient.

Paradigms and Constructs

The impact of disease can be subdivided into components called dimensions or domains. The paradigm of the five Ds (death, discomfort, disability, dollar costs, and drug or other iatrogenic effects) has been popularized by Fries (3). Along similar lines, the World Health Organization (WHO) has developed a functional classification system based on impairment, activity, and participation (4). These constructs attempt to capture the multidimensional nature of health and disease. Health-related quality of life (HRQOL) exists within the larger domain of quality of life, which encompasses issues related to human rights, nutritional adequacy, and education. HRQOL is determined by factors affecting its component domains. These factors may include pain, physical function, social function, emotional function, impairment, handicap, coping, helplessness, fatigue, well-being, cost of illness, and adverse effects of treatment and work loss. HRQOL measurement uses purpose-built multi-dimensional questionnaires that provide specific data on several key domains, or utility-based measures that generate a value between zero (death) and one (complete health) to characterize the HRQOL of specific health states.

In addition to generic HRQOL measures, there are HSQs designed for general-purpose or disease-specific applications in different musculoskeletal conditions (Table 7B-2). Measurement batteries containing both generic HRQOL and disease-specific instruments can be extremely powerful in dissecting the dimensionality of treatment response.

In assessing the adequacy and appropriateness of specific techniques, four primary and six secondary criteria should be considered. The primary criteria, similar to those described by the Outcome Measures in Rheumatology Clinical Trials (OMERACT) group, are referred to in the literature as the OMERACT filter (5). The OMERACT filter encompasses issues of validity, sensitivity to change (reliability plus responsiveness), and feasibility (practicality). The issues of validity, reliability, and responsiveness are critical to an understanding of the measurement literature.

Validity

Validity gauges the extent to which an instrument specifically measures the phenomenon of interest (Fig. 7B-1) (6). Validity and reliability are separate clinimetric issues; it does not follow that because a measure is reliable, it also is valid (or vice versa). Validity is concerned with sources of nonrandom error (i.e., systematic error or bias), and reliability is concerned with sources of random error, also known as noise. It should be noted that validity is not a fixed property, but is assessed in relation to a specific purpose and particular patient population. Instruments rarely are transferable directly from one patient population to another without reassessment of their psychometric properties. When selecting an outcome measure, it is important to know how the instrument was validated, in what populations of patients, and for what purpose (i.e., research or clinical practice). From a clinimetric standpoint, there are four basic types of validity: face, content, construct, and criterion.

Face Validity

A measure has face validity if experts judge that it measures at least part of the defined phenomenon. For many measurement procedures, this aspect is self-evident. In the case of some functional status measures, however, the extent to which the measurement taps into physical, social, or emotional aspects of functioning may not be obvious.

Content Validity

Content validity is a measure of comprehensiveness, which is the extent to which the measure encompasses all relevant aspects of the defined attribute. An instrument can have face validity but fail to capture the dimension of interest in its entirety. The issue of importance can be decided either by patients, who rate the importance of their symptoms, or by clinical assessors, who base their decisions on perceptions of patient symptoms.

Construct Validity

Construct validity is of two types: convergent and discriminant (6). Both are tested by demonstrating relationships between measurement scores and a theoretical manifestation of the disease, which typically is a construct or consequence of an attribute.

Convergent construct validity testing is based on the statistical correlation between scores on a single health component, as measured by two different instruments. If the correlation coefficient is positive and appreciably above zero, the new measure is said to have convergent construct validity.

In contrast, discriminant construct validity testing compares correlation coefficients between scores on the same health component, as measured by two different instruments (e.g., separate measures of physical function), and between scores on that health component and each of several other health components (e.g., measures of social and emotional function). A measure has discriminant construct validity if the proposed measure correlates better with a second measure (e.g., the other measure of physical function), accepted as being more closely related to the construct, than it does with a third, more distantly related measure (e.g., psychosocial function).

TABLE 7B-1
Glossary of Terms

Aggregated multidimensional index (AMI): A measure in which scores on several different aspects of health are combined and expressed as a single number.

Ceiling effect: An attribute of an outcome measure that limits its ability to detect deterioration in patients who score at the upper (i.e., more symptomatic) end of the scale (i.e., patients who have severe disease, pain, disability, etc.).

Clinical judgement analysis: A statistical method that identifies those clinical, laboratory, and patient data on which specific clinical decisions are based.

Disease-specific measures: Measures that are designed to quantify outcome related to specific diseases or disease groups. These measures enable problems related to particular diseases to be identified and evaluated.

Floor effect: An attribute of an outcome measure that limits its ability to detect improvement in patients who score at the lower (i.e., less symptomatic) end of the scale (i.e., patients who have mild disease, little pain, disability, etc.).

Generic measures: Outcome measures that are designed to quantify outcome in all disease groups (and sometimes in the healthy population). These enable outcomes such as quality of life or general health status to be compared across different diseases. For this reason, generic measures are used in some economic (cost-utility) analyses.

Health-related quality of life (HRQOL): A concept that some aspects of QOL are specific to health and can be measured using one or more health status questionnaires. There are different conceptual approaches to measurement, some based on utility theory, others not.

Health status questionnaire (HSQ): An interviewer-administered or self-administered questionnaire that probes one or more aspects of health/disease.

Index: A measure that uses more than one probe to evaluate health status.

Individualized measures: Outcome measures (usually questionnaires) that elicit each individual patient's priorities, problems, limitations in activities or participation, quality of life, and so on. This outcome is achieved by using a standardized prompt or question but allowing free response answers.

Likert scales: Adjectival scales with five, seven, or more categories and a neutral midpoint, which often are used to measure attitudes (e.g., strongly agree, agree, unsure, disagree, strongly disagree).

Measurement error: Problems and limitations in measurement that affect its accuracy. **Random** error relates to individual variability in measurement (e.g., patients completing a pain visual analog scale may not place the line in exactly the same place on repeated measurements, even when pain levels have not altered). **Systematic** error is a property of **bias** rather than measurement error. Forms of bias that can affect outcome measurement include bias related to the completion of questionnaires (halo and social desirability effects), item bias (background variables, such as age and gender, influence the response to certain items on questionnaires), mood effects, and the sample population (e.g., inpatient and outpatient populations).

Criterion Validity
Criterion validity is assessed by comparing a new measurement technique to either an independent criterion or standard (concurrent validity) or a future standard (predictive validity), using tests of statistical significance. Criterion validity is an estimate of the extent to which a measure agrees with a "gold standard" (i.e., an external criterion of the phenomenon being measured). The major problem in criterion validity testing is the paucity of gold standards.

Reliability
Reliability is the degree to which the instrument is free from random error (Fig. 7B-1), and is the amount of the score that is attributable to "signal" rather than "noise" (1). In this respect, reliability is an essential attribute because it is important to establish that changes in the score obtained from the instrument reflect real change in the attribute being measured and are not simply the result of problems within the instrument itself. Consistency, reproducibility, repeatability, and agreement are synonyms for reliability (6). As with validity, the reliability of an instrument is context- and population-specific. For example, the reliability requirements are more stringent for an individual than for a group of patients.

Reliability of an HSQ refers to the degree to which the measurement produced can be replicated. This may be assessed either from the result of different measurements performed at the same time, or from the same measurements

Patient-centered outcomes: A term used to refer to outcomes that are related to the patient, rather than the biological disease process, and which include such symptoms as pain and fatigue, disability, quality of life, and so on. Such measures reflect the subjective experience of disease.

Reliability: The extent to which repeated measures of the same static phenomenon yield the same results.

Responsiveness: The ability of a measure to detect even minimally important clinical changes. Also called sensitivity.

Shared clinical decision-making: A process of decision-making in which the patient and clinician are equal partners, and decisions are based on evidence and patient priorities and preferences.

Standardized measures: Structured questionnaires that ask each respondent the same questions and force them to select from the same set of responses. Standardized questionnaires are favored in epidemiologic studies and clinical trials because data is easy to manipulate statistically and such measures facilitate comparisons between groups of patients.

Type I Error: The detection of a statistically significant difference when, in truth, none exists.

Type II Error: The failure to detect a statistically significant difference when, in truth, one exists.

Segregated multidimensional index (SMI): A measure in which separate scores are generated for different dimensions of health.

Utility-based measures: Assessment of the value or preference that patients attach to their health, requiring patients to combine the positive and negative aspects of a health state or intervention into one single value. Methods for eliciting utilities include rating scales, standard gamble, and time trade-off.

Validity (Face): Whether the instrument measures what is intended.

Validity (Construct): Whether predicted relationships are observed to hold true.

Validity (Content): Whether the instrument captures the dimensionality of the problem.

Validity (Criterion): Whether instrument scores agree with those of a gold standard.

Visual analog scale (VAS): A horizontal or vertical line, usually 100 mm long, with anchors at each end used to represent a continuum of the attribute being measured (e.g., pain).

Weighting: Transformation of scores from health status questionnaires, using a variety of techniques, to represent the relative importance of the domains measured. If no system of weighting is applied, equal weights are assumed.

performed at different times. With interviewer-administered HSQs, individuals should be "measured" by several observers at the same time to test interobserver variability. With self-administered HSQs, it may be necessary to have individuals complete the same measure on more than one occasion to assess intrarater variability. When evaluating several items within an HSQ, the average interitem correlation can be used as a measure of internal consistency.

Responsiveness (Sensitivity to Change)

The primary goal of outcome assessment is to detect clinically important change in some aspect of a condition (1). To detect change, a measurement technique needs to be targeted to aspects of the disease amenable to change; use scaling methods that allow detection of change; and be applied at a point in time when change might occur. Validity and reliability are important aspects of measurement techniques, but the capacity to detect change is the quintessential requirement of a successful outcome measure. An assessment technique may fail to record any clinical improvement for a number of reasons: the patient lacked response potential, there was poor compliance with the treatment program, the treatment was ineffective, the outcome measure employed was insensitive, or a Type II error occurred due to inadequate sample size. One of the inherent problems in measuring outcomes in chronic musculoskeletal conditions is that an absence of deterioration (i.e., no change) may be clinically important.

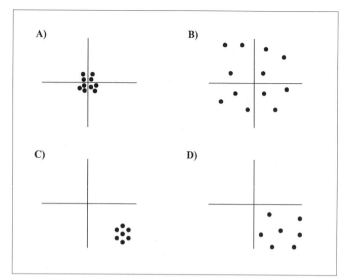

Fig. 7B-1. Schematic representation of systematic error (bias) and random error (noise) shows a comparison of measurements that are A) valid and reliable; B) valid but unreliable; C) reliable but invalid; and D) unreliable and invalid. The center of the target represents the true value, and the black circles (•) represent the measured values of a single static phenomenon.

Scaling

Several different types of scales are used in scoring health status (Fig. 7B-2) (1). The most popular are adjectival (Likert) scales and visual analog (VA) scales. Adjectival scales are ordinal-level scales in which categories are hierarchically ordered, but the interval between adjacent categories may not be equal. Adjectival scales often use three, five, or seven categories, and are suitable for assessing current health status as well as changes in health status. Individual categories usually are assigned numbers, and the data often are treated as interval-level data using parametric or nonparametric statistical methods.

Much has been written about the length, orientation, and segmentation of VA scales. The simplest form, and that which is used most often, is a 100-mm horizontal line with small vertical markers at either end, beside which are placed terminal descriptors, such as "none" (left-hand end) and "extreme" (right-hand end). Between 0% and 4% of patients are reported to have difficulty understanding the VA concept, but the scale may be slightly more sensitive to change than comparable Likert scales. Other types of scales used in musculoskeletal clinical metrology include numerical rating scales, continuous chromatic analogs, and faces scales. Comparative studies in rheumatoid arthritis (RA) and osteoarthritis (OA) have shown that all such scales are responsive, and there is no evidence that scales that are more complex outperform simpler scales (7,8). The idea that patients should be shown their prior score when completing a new blank scale is controversial, but comparative studies of "blind versus informed" presentation have not demonstrated any systematic differences in the scores obtained (1).

Weighting and Aggregation

Health status questionnaires can be divided into those that collect information on multiple dimensions and create subscale scores on each separate dimension (segregated multidimensional indices), and those that collect information on multiple dimensions and combine the information into a single or aggregate score (aggregated multidimensional indices). Methods used to create the total score for aggregated multidimensional indices may not correspond to the relative importance of the component subscales and may be influenced by differing scale lengths of the components. Comparative studies suggest that this phenomenon may distort data interpretation (1).

Specific Measures

Three types of studies can be recognized in the literature: validation studies, which evaluate the clinimetric properties of a single measure; comparative studies, in which the relative performance of two or more measures is assessed; and application studies, in which instruments have been used to address specific clinical questions. Each type contributes useful information for readers interested in particular measurement procedures, and standard or specialty texts can provide a comprehensive review of instruments (1). For convenience, the major HSQs are identified in Table 7B-2.

Clinical Assessment

Health status questionnaires are used to assess pain, physical function, and patient and physician global assessments.

Pain

Pain is an entirely subjective sensation known only to the sufferer. Much has been written on the validity of various approaches to pain measurement. Pain measures may be simple or complex (9), and may score pain severity as a single entity to give a global score, or probe each of several pain situations to provide a composite score. The various approaches all seem to be responsive. As noted earlier, Likert and VA scales frequently are used for pain assessment.

Physical Function

Unlike measurement tools for pain, physical function scales almost always use multiple probes to address several different aspects of everyday living. Geography, topography, culture, and climate may all be relevant to the item inventory. Likert and VA scales frequently are used to assess physical function.

Global Assessments

Global assessments are general impressions made by the patient or physician regarding either a particular aspect of the disease or the condition overall. The exact mental processes used to sort through arrays of sometimes complex symptoms, assign weights to individual symptoms, and aggregate the information into a single score is poorly understood. There is no international agreement on a standard wording for the global question or a preferred response scale. Nevertheless, global measures have face validity to clinicians, appear to be responsive, and in clinical trials, have low sample size requirements.

HRQOL

Although not claiming disease-specificity, HRQOL measures provide an opportunity to probe quality of life in broad terms and conduct comparative analyses between very diverse conditions, such as arthritis and cardiovascular disease. HRQOL measures may differ conceptually, and users should be aware of the differences. In general, HRQOL measures are less responsive than arthritis-specific measures, but capture elements of health beyond the scope of the latter. As a result, HRQOL and disease-specific measures often are used in combination.

Health Economic Assessment

Health economic assessments generally take one of four forms: cost-minimization, cost-benefit, cost-effectiveness, or cost-utility. Cost-minimization studies concern the costs of alternatives with similar outcomes. In cost-benefit analyses, both costs and benefits are valued in monetary terms. Cost-effectiveness studies value costs in monetary terms but measure outcomes in health terms, often using disease-specific HSQs, and express the results in such terms as cost per unit improvement in health. Finally, cost-utility studies value costs in monetary terms, but value outcome using generic utility-based HSQs, and express the results in such terms as cost per quality-adjusted life-year (Cost/QALY) gained (10).

Disease-Specific Issues

Consensus-building in outcome measurement has been led by the OMERACT group and carried forward by major national and international agencies and organizations, such as the American College of Rheumatology (ACR) and the Osteoarthritis Research Society International (OARSI). HSQs play a key role in the measurement of musculoskeletal symptoms in each of the core sets and responder criteria described in the following paragraphs.

Rheumatoid Arthritis

Consensus on core set measures for RA was established at OMERACT I and ratified by the ACR. The ACR clinical core set measures are pain, function, number of tender joints, number of swollen joints, patient global assessment, physician global assessment, and for studies longer than one year in duration, imaging (11). Based on this core set of clinical measures, the ACR has proposed responder criteria (12). The ACR 20 criteria are as follows: 20% or more improvement in the number of both tender and swollen joint counts, and 20% or more improvement in three or more of the remaining five ACR core set measures (pain, function, patient global assessment, physician global assessment, and an acute-phase reactant) (12). Similar criteria based on higher thresholds of 50% (ACR 50) and 70% (ACR 70) improvement sometimes are reported in the literature.

Osteoarthritis

Consensus on core set measures for OA (namely pain, physical function, patient global assessment, and imaging in studies lasting one year or more) was established at OMERACT III and ratified by the OARSI (13). Based on these core set clinical measures, the OARSI has proposed two sets of class-specific responder criteria, requiring minimal percentage improvements and accompanying absolute improvements, as defined by normalized units (NU) (14). These response criteria are more complex than those for RA. They attempt to address simultaneously issues of class-specificity (e.g., oral NSAIDs versus intra-articular therapy), joint specificity (e.g., hip versus knee), differences in the pharmacodynamic profile of different interventions, minimum clinically important effects in patients with low baseline values, and optimal separation of active versus placebo responders.

For example, two proposals outline criteria for use of oral NSAID-class drugs in knee OA. Proposal A recommends a 45% (and 20 NU) or greater improvement in pain, or two or more of the following conditions: a 15% (and 10 NU) or greater improvement in pain; a 30% (and 15 NU) or greater improvement in function; and a 35% (and 10 NU) or greater improvement in patient global assessment. Proposal B suggests a 50% (and 20 NU) or greater improvement in pain, and a 60% (and 20 NU) or greater improvement in function, or two or more of the following conditions: a 30% (and 15 NU) or greater improvement in pain; a 20% (and 25 NU) or greater improvement in function; and a 25% (and 10 NU) or greater improvement in patient global assessment (14).

Ankylosing Spondylitis

The Bath ankylosing spondylitis (AS) series of clinical and radiographic measures represent a significant clinimetric development. Progress toward core set measures for AS was made at OMERACT IV. Different core sets pertain to

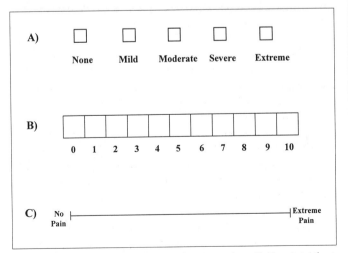

Fig. 7B-2. Three different types of pain scales: A) 5-point Likert (adjectival) scale; B) 11-point numerical rating scale; and C) visual analog scale.

TABLE 7B-2
Categorization and Reference Sources for Key Health Status Questionnaires

General Measures

Health Related Quality of Life
- EuroQol: Hurst NP, Jobanputra P, Hunter M, Lambert M, Lochhead A, Brown H. Validity of Euroqol – a generic health status instrument – in patients with rheumatoid arthritis. Economic and Health Outcomes Research Group. Br J Rheumatol 1994;33:655–662.
- HUI: Feeny D, Furlong W, Barr RD, Torrance GW, Rosenbaum P, Weitzman S. A comprehensive multiattribute system for classifying the health status of survivors of childhood cancer. J Clin Oncol 1992;10:923–928.
- NHP: Hunt SM, McKenna SP, McEwen J, Williams J, Papp E. The Nottingham Health Profile: subjective health status and medical consultations. Soc Sci Med [A] 1981;15:221–229.
- Quality of Well-Being Scale: Kaplan RM, Bush JW, Berry CC. Health status: types of validity and the Index of Well-Being. Health Serv Res 1976;11:478–507.
- SF-36: Ware JE, Sherbourne CD. The MOS 36-item short-form health survey (SF-36). I. Conceptual framework and item selection. Med Care 1992;30:473–483.
- Sickness Impact Profile: Bergner M, Bobbitt RA, Carter WB, Gilson BS. The Sickness Impact Profile: development and final revision of a health status measure. Med Care 1981;19:787–805.
- Standard Gamble: Torrance GW. Social preferences for health states: an empirical evaluation of three measurement techniques. Socioecon Plann Sci 1976;10:129–136.
- Time Trade-Off: Torrance GW. Measurement of health state utilities for economic appraisal. J Health Econ 1986;5:1–30.

General Arthritis Measures
- Arthritis Impact Measurement Scales (AIMS): Meenan RF, Gertman PM, Mason JH. Measuring health status in arthritis. The arthritis impact measurement scales. Arthritis Rheum 1980;23:146–152.
- Arthritis Impact Measurement Scales (AIMS2): Meenan RF, Mason JH, Anderson JJ, Guccione AA, Kazis LE. AIMS2. The content and properties of a revised and expanded Arthritis Impact Measurement Scales Health Status Questionnaire. Arthritis Rheum 1992;35:1–10.
- Clinical Health Assessment Questionnaire (CLINHAQ): Wolfe F. A brief clinical health status instrument: CLINHAQ. Arthritis Rheum 1989;32:S99.
- Health Assessment Questionnaire (HAQ): Fries JF, Spitz P, Kraines RG, Holman HR. Measurement of patient outcome in arthritis. Arthritis Rheum 1980;23:137–145.

Condition-Specific Measures

Osteoarthritis
- Australian/Canadian Hand Index (AUSCAN): Arthritis Rheum 1997;40(9 Suppl):S110.
- Dreiser Algofunctional Index: Dreiser RL, Maheu E, Guillou GB, Caspard H, Grouin JM. Validation of an algofunctional index for osteoarthritis of the hand. Rev Rhum Engl. Ed 1995;62(Suppl 1):43S–53S.
- Indices of Clinical Severity (Lequesne): Lequesne M. Indices of severity and disease activity for osteoarthritis. Semin Arthritis Rheum 1991;20(Suppl 2):48–54.
- Western Ontario and McMaster Universities (WOMAC) Osteoarthritis Index: Bellamy N, Buchanan WW, Goldsmith CH, Campbell J, Stitt. Validation study of WOMAC: a health status instrument for measuring clinically important patient relevant outcomes to antirheumatic drug therapy in patients with osteoarthritis of the hip or knee. J Rheumatol 1988;15:1833–1840.
- Radiographic Assessment: Atlas of individual features in osteoarthritis. Altman RD, Hochberg M, Murphy WA, Wolfe F, Lequesne M. Atlas of individual radiographic features in osteoarthritis. Osteoarthritis Cartilage 1995;3(Suppl A):3–70.

Rheumatoid Arthritis
- McMaster Toronto Arthritis Patient Preference Disability Questionnaire (MACTAR): Tugwell P, Bombardier C, Buchanan WW, Goldsmith CH, Grace E, Hanna B. The MACTAR Patient Preference Disability Questionnaire—an individualized functional priority approach for assessing improvement in physical disability in clinical trials in rheumatoid arthritis. J Rheumatol 1987;14:446–451.
- Rapid Assessment of Disease Activity in Rheumatology (RADAR): Mason JH, Anderson JJ, Meenan RF, Haralson KM, Lewis-Stevens D, Kaine JL. The rapid assessment of disease activity in rheumatology (RADAR) questionnaire. Validity and sensitivity to change of a patient self-report measure of joint count and clinical status. Arthritis Rheum 1992;35:156–162.
- Imaging; Larsen Score, Sharp Score: van der Heijde DM. Plain X-rays in rheumatoid arthritis: overview of scoring methods, their reliability and applicability. Baillieres Clin Rheumatol 1996;10:435–453.

Ankylosing Spondylitis
- Bath Ankylosing Spondylitis Indices: Calin A. The Dunlop-Dottridge Lecture. Ankylosing spondylitis: defining disease status and the relationship between radiology, metrology, disease activity, function, and outcome. J Rheumatol 1995;22:740–744.

- Dougados Functional Index: Dougados M, Gueguen A, Nakache JP, Nguyen M, Mery C, Amor B. Evaluation of a functional index and an articular index in ankylosing spondylitis. J Rheumatol 1988;15:302–307.
  Dutch AS Index: Creemers MC, Van't Hof MA, Franssen MJ, Van de Putte LB, Gribnau FW, Van Riel PL. A Dutch version of the functional index for ankylosing spondylitis: development and validation in a long-term study. Br J Rheumatol 1994;33:842–846.
- HAQ-S: Daltroy LH, Larson MG, Roberts NW, Liang MH. A modification of the Health Assessment Questionnaire for the spondyloarthropathies. J Rheumatol 1990;17:946–950.

Fibromyalgia
- Fibromyalgia Impact Questionnaire (FIQ): Burckhardt CS, Clark SR, Bennett RM. The fibromyalgia impact questionnaire: development and validation. J Rheumatol 1991;18:728–733.

Low Back Pain
- Low Back Pain Scale: Leavitt F, Garron DC, Whisler WW, Sheinkop MB. Affective and sensory dimensions of back pain. Pain 1978;4:273–281.
- Million Instrument: Million R, Hall W, Nilsen KH, Baker RD, Jayson MI. Assessment of the progress of the back-pain patient 1981 Volvo Award in Clinical Science. Spine 1982;7:204–212.
- Oswestry Low Back Pain Disability Questionnaire: Fairbank JC, Couper J, Davies JB, O'Brien JP. The Oswestry low back pain disability questionnaire. Physiotherapy 1980;66:271–273.
- Roland & Morris Scale: Roland M, Morris R. A study of the natural history of back pain. Part I: development of a reliable and sensitive measure of disability in low-back pain. Spine 1983;8:141–144.

Systemic Lupus Erythematosus
- British Isles Lupus Assessment Group's Index (BILAG): Symmons DP, Coppock JS, Bacon PA, Bresnihan B, Isenberg DA, Maddison P, et al. Development and assessment of a computerized index of clinical disease activity in systemic lupus erythematosus. Members of the British Isles Lupus Assessment Group (BILAG). Q J Med 1988;69:927–937.
- Systemic Lupus Activity Measure (SLAM): Liang MH, Socher SA, Larson MG, Schur PH. Reliability and validity of six systems for the clinical assessment of disease activity in systemic lupus erythematosus. Arthritis Rheum 1989;32:1107–1118.

- Systemic Lupus Erythematosus Disease Activity Index (SLEDAI): Bombardier C, Gladman DD, Urowitz MB, Caron D, Chang CH. Derivation of the SLEDAI. A disease activity index for lupus patients. The Committee on Prognosis Studies in SLE. Arthritis Rheum 1992;35:630–640.

Handicap
- Disease Repercussion Profile (DRP): Carr AJ. Margaret Holroyd Prize Essay. A patient-centred approach to evaluation and treatment in rheumatoid arthritis: the development of a clinical tool to measure patient-perceived handicap. Br J Rheumatol 1996;35:921–932.

Fatigue
- Multidimensional Assessment of Fatigue: Belza BL, Henke CJ, Yelin EH, Epstein WV, Gilliss CL. Correlates of fatigue in older adults with rheumatoid arthritis. Nurs Res 1993;42:93–99.
- Piper Fatigue Scale: Piper BF. Piper fatigue scale available for clinical testing. Oncol Nurs Forum 1990;17:661–662.

Coping
- Coping with Rheumatic Stressors (CORS): van Lankveld W, van't Pad Bosch P, van de Putte L, Naring G, van der Staak C. Disease-specific stressors in rheumatoid arthritis: coping and well-being. Br J Rheumatol 1994;33:1067–1073.
- Coping Strategies Questionnaire: Rosenstiel AK, Keefe FJ. The use of coping strategies in chronic low back pain patients: relationship to patient characteristics and current adjustment. Pain 1983;17:33–44.
- London Coping with RA Questionnaire: Newman S, Fitzpatrick R, Lamb R, Shipley M. Patterns of coping in rheumatoid arthritis. Psychol Health 1990;4:187–200.
- Self Efficacy Scale: Lorig K, Chastain RL, Ung E, Shoor S, Holman HR. Development and evaluation of a scale to measure perceived self-efficacy in people with arthritis. Arthritis Rheum 1989;32:37–44.

Helplessness
- Arthritis Helplessness Index: Stein MJ, Wallston KA, Nicassio PM. Factor structure of the Arthritis Helplessness Index. J Rheumatol 1988;15:427–432.
- Rheumatology Attitudes Index: Callahan LF, Brooks RH, Pincus T. Further analysis of learned helplessness in rheumatoid arthritis using a "Rheumatology Attitudes Index." J Rheumatol 1988;15:418–426.

different clinical environments (15). The clinical core set for symptom-modifying and disease-modifying studies includes pain, function, patient global assessment, stiffness, spinal mobility, and related to spinal mobility, peripheral-joint and enthesis assessments. Responder criteria have not been established for AS clinical trials.

Other Conditions

Progress has been described in RA, OA, and AS, and other working groups are developing similar initiatives for other musculoskeletal conditions. Instruments exist to assess such conditions as fibromyalgia and low back pain (Table 7B-2). One of the more difficult challenges has been the development of multidimensional outcome measures for the connective-tissue diseases. Although their multiorgan involvement creates numerous problems in clinical measurement, several indices suitable for assessing patients with systemic lupus erythematosus, systemic sclerosis, and Wegener's granulomatosis have emerged.

Future Perspective

Over the last half century, musculoskeletal clinical metrology has evolved (1). Although many obstacles encountered in early studies have been overcome, much remains to be achieved. Three areas in particular deserve special attention: globalization, electronic data capture, and measurement in clinical practice.

Globalization

Opportunities to accelerate the speed at which clinical trials can be completed and to address regulatory issues in different jurisdictions have facilitated the globalization of several popular HSQs. Standard procedures require forward and backward translations by one or more teams of fluent bilingual translators, followed by on-site linguistic and cultural validation in a reference group in the target country. Target populations include, for example, the many English-speaking, French-speaking, Spanish-speaking, and German-speaking populations. Precise phraseology may differ slightly between countries sharing a common language, reflecting variability in word usage and comprehension. Transcultural adaptation of instruments is progressing rapidly, using standard operating procedures in some cases, and being performed ad hoc in others. The majority of indices reported in the literature have their geographic origins in multicultural societies in North America and Europe, necessitating a structured and comprehensive linguistic validation for application in other areas of the world.

Electronic Data Capture

Traditionally, HSQs are completed on paper in the clinic or hospital and the data later is entered into a database for analysis. There has been considerable interest in recent years in accelerating the data-capture process. One approach uses telephone interviews to capture data without patients leaving their own homes, a process that provides data comparable to that acquired from the same patients in a clinic setting (16). Similarly, direct data entry can be achieved using mouse-driven cursor and touch-screen technology, alternatives that appear valid, convenient, and rapid. Based on these technologies, hand-held computers, and scannable or Internet forms, significant additional progress is likely.

Quantitative Measurement in Clinical Practice

In contrast to what is found in clinical research, structured, standardized, quantitative, state-of-the-art health-status measurement occurs infrequently in rheumatology outpatient practice (17,18). Practitioners indicate that they require instruments that are valid, reliable, and responsive, but also fast, brief, and easy to score. The problem can be partitioned into instruments and systems. Some instruments are inherently short, but short forms of longer and more complex measures also exist. Major hurdles to using HSQs in routine clinical care include staff time and costs involved in supervising the completion of questionnaires, scoring forms, inputting data, and outputting results in a format usable by health care providers and intelligible to patients. In general, these activities receive little priority and no financial support from health care systems. In addition, some types of assessment, such as performing joint counts, require professional expertise and are time-consuming. However, with the advent of electronic data capture, user-friendly, touch-screen technology provides an opportunity to collect HSQ data without significant staff involvement (19). Additional work is required on such instruments and systems. Clinicians also want to know whether routine monitoring with HSQs can have a favorable impact on the long-term outcome of individual patients. Comparative studies on the effectiveness, cost-effectiveness, and cost-utility of quantitative measurement are needed to establish the marginal costs and benefits prior to widespread promotion.

NICHOLAS BELLAMY, MD

References

1. Bellamy N. Musculoskeletal Clinical Metrology. Dordrecht, the Netherlands: Kluwer Academic Publishers, 1993.
2. Bellamy N, Buchanan WW. Clinical outcome measurement. In: Dieppe P, Schumacher HR Jr, Wollheim FA (eds). Classic Papers in Rheumatology. London: Martin Dunitz, 2001 (in press).
3. Fries JF, Bellamy N. Introduction. In: Bellamy N (ed). Prognosis in the Rheumatic Diseases. Dordrecht, the Netherlands: Kluwer Academic Publishers, 1991; pp 1–10.
4. World Health Organization. International Classification of Impairments, Activities and Participation (ICIDH-2). Geneva: World Health Organization, 1998.
5. Boers M, Brooks P, Strand CV, Tugwell P. The OMERACT filter for Outcome Measures in Rheumatology. J Rheumatol 1998;25:198–199.

6. Carmines EG, Zeller RA. *Reliability and Validity Assessment.* Beverly Hills, CA: Sage Publications, 1979; pp 5–71.
7. Bellamy N, Campbell J, Syrotuik J. Comparative study of self-rating pain scales in osteoarthritis patients. *Current Med Res Opin* 1999;15:113–119.
8. Bellamy N, Campbell J, Syrotuik J. Comparative study of self-rating pain scales in rheumatoid arthritis patients. *Current Med Res Opin* 1999;15:121–127.
9. Melzack R. The McGill Pain Questionnaire: major properties and scoring methods. *Pain* 1975;1:277–299.
10. Drummond MF, O'Brien B, Stoddart GL, Torrance GW. *Methods for the Economic Evaluation of Health Care Programmes,* 2nd ed. Oxford: Oxford University Press, 1997.
11. Felson DT, Anderson JJ, Boers M, et al. The American College of Rheumatology preliminary core set of disease activity measures for rheumatoid arthritis clinical trials. *Arthritis Rheum* 1993;36:729–740.
12. Felson DT, Anderson JJ, Boers M, et al. The American College of Rheumatology preliminary definition of improvement in rheumatoid arthritis. *Arthritis Rheum* 1995;38:727-735.
13. Altman R, Brandt K, Hochberg M, et al. Design and conduct of clinical trials in patients with osteoarthritis: recommendations from a task force of the Osteoarthritis Research Society. *Osteoarthritis Cartilage* 1996;4:217–243.
14. Dougados M, LeClaire P, van der Heijde D, Bloch DA, Bellamy N, Altman RD. Response criteria for clinical trials on osteoarthritis of the knee and hip: a report of the Osteoarthritis Research Society International Standing Committee for Clinical Trials response criteria initiative. *Osteoarthritis Cartilage* 2000;8:395-403.
15. Van der Heijde D, Calin A, Dougados M Khan MA, van der Linden S, Bellamy N. Selection of instruments in the core set for DC-ART, SMARD, physical therapy and clinical record keeping in ankylosing spondylitis. Progress Report of the ASAS Working Group. *J Rheumatol* 1999;26:951–954.
16. Bellamy N, Campbell J, Hill J, Goodman A, Band P. Validation of telephone-administration of the WOMAC osteoarthritis index. 14th European League Against Rheumatism Congress. June 6-11 1999. Glasgow, UK. *Ann Rheum Dis* 1999:P1079.
17. Bellamy N, Kaloni S, Pope J, Coulter K, Campbell J. Qualitative rheumatology: a survey of outcome measurement procedures in routine rheumatology outpatient practice in Canada. *J Rheumatol* 1998;25:852–858.
18. Bellamy N, Muirden KD, Brooks PM, Barraclough D,Tellus MM, Campbell J. Quantitative rheumatology: a survey of outcome measurement procedures in routine rheumatology outpatient practice in Australia. *J Rheumatol* 1999;26:1593–1599.
19. Wolfe F, Pincus T. Data collection in the clinic. *Rheum Dis Clin North Am* 1995;21:321–358.

EVALUATION OF THE PATIENT
C. Laboratory Assessment

Rapid advances in medical technology have provided a plethora of diagnostic tests and procedures for the practicing physician. This phenomenon is particularly evident in rheumatology, where laboratory results sometimes define a disease. Unfortunately, such results confuse as often as they clarify clinical reasoning. However, a broad knowledge of the methodology and interpretation of relevant laboratory tests enables the clinician to use these tests appropriately to confirm diagnoses, follow the activity of disease, and monitor toxicity of drugs.

Screening

A screening test helps determine which patients *might* have a given disease. Such a test should be highly sensitive, i.e., almost always give positive results when the suspected disease is present. Thus, one might regard sensitivity as the likelihood that a test will show positive results in people with the disease. If negative, a test with high sensitivity virtually excludes the disease in question. An example is the test for antinuclear antibody (ANA), autoantibodies that occur in more than 95% of people with systemic lupus erythematosus (SLE). When negative, this sensitive test virtually eliminates SLE as a diagnostic possibility. Yet, because ANAs occur in so many other diseases, as well as in

healthy people, a positive result does not confirm the diagnosis of SLE.

Diagnosis

Using the laboratory to confirm diagnoses requires an understanding of the terms specificity and predictive value. A highly specific laboratory test nearly always is negative in the *absence* of a particular disease. Tests with high specificity are rare in rheumatic diseases, but a few do exist. In SLE, for example, antibodies to native (double-stranded) DNA are less common than ANAs, but they seldom occur in other diseases (i.e., the false-positive rate is low). Therefore, when present, they help solidify the diagnosis.

The positive predictive value of a test refers to the likelihood that a patient for whom test results are positive has that particular disease. The usefulness of a high positive predictive value in making a diagnosis depends on the *prevalence* of the suspected disease in a given population. Even tests that are highly specific for a given disease, but which occasionally give positive results in people without the disease, will give a large number of false-positive results when the suspected disease is rare. For example, clinicians commonly use human leukocyte antigen (HLA)-B27 to confirm ("predict") the diagnosis of ankylosing spondylitis

(AS). In many cases, however, the results of such a test could be misleading. Although 90% of people with this disease are HLA-B27 positive, 8% of normal individuals also carry this antigen. Because only one of every 1000 whites living in the United States has AS, fewer than 1% of randomly chosen individuals who test positive for HLA-B27 would be true positives. If, however, after taking a careful history and performing a thorough physical examination, the clinician is "on the fence" (i.e., believes that there is a 50% chance that the patient has AS), a positive test for HLA-B27 tips the scales in favor of the diagnosis. In the situation described, the prevalence of AS in this clinician's population has risen from 1 in 1000 to 1 in 2, and the likelihood of a false-positive test drops dramatically. Likewise, a negative test in this setting helps exclude the disease.

Follow-Up

Laboratory tests can help monitor the activity of an illness, but the results of such tests are meaningful only when they correlate with clinical findings. Thus, a fall in serum complement levels or a rise in titers of anti-DNA antibody does not necessarily predict a flare of SLE. Similarly, an elevated erythrocyte sedimentation rate (ESR) by itself does not signal the need to treat an *asymptomatic* patient with polymyalgia rheumatica.

Periodic routine laboratory tests, such as complete blood counts, serum creatinine levels, liver function studies, and urinalyses are required to monitor for toxicities associated with nonsteroidal anti-inflammatory drugs and immunosuppressive agents. The frequency of such tests must be individualized according to the specific medication and individual risk factors.

Laboratory Tests Commonly Used in the Rheumatic Diseases

Erythrocyte Sedimentation Rate (ESR)

Asymmetric plasma proteins (e.g., fibrinogen, immunoglobulins), formed in abundance during the acute-phase response, interact with the red blood cell (RBC) membrane, causing the cells to stick together in stacks (*rouleaux*) (1). Because these stacked RBCs are heavier than individual RBCs, they fall (*sediment*) rapidly to the bottom of a column of blood.

Method (Westergren)

Blood diluted with sodium citrate is transferred into a tube (2.5-mm internal diameter, 200-mm height) and allowed to stand vertically. After one hour, the distance (mm) between the top of the plasma column and the top of the sedimented RBCs is the ESR. The normal values in most laboratories (up to 15 mm/h for women and up to 10 mm/h for men) do not take into account the increase in these values that occurs with aging. To calculate the upper limit for a man, divide the age by two; for a woman, add 10 to the age and divide by two (2).

Interpretation

An elevated ESR usually indicates the presence of an inflammatory process – infectious, immunologic, or neoplastic. At best, however, the ESR is a crude guide to the severity of inflammation. The ESR ordinarily increases with anemia, renal failure, and pregnancy, and it decreases with changes in RBC morphology, hypofibrinogenemia, cryoglobulinemia, and congestive heart failure (3).

C-Reactive Protein (CRP)

CRP derives its name from its ability to react with and precipitate the somatic C-polysaccharide of the pneumococcus. The protein is synthesized in the liver promptly after tissue injury. Plasma levels of CRP increase as early as four to six hours after such injury, peak in 24–72 hours, and return to normal within a week (4).

Method

The availability of specific antibodies to CRP allows quantification of this protein by a variety of methods. One such method is nephelometry, which consists of adding constant amounts of purified, optically clear antiserum to varying amounts of antigen (e.g., CRP), placing the reactants in a high-intensity light beam, and measuring the degree of light scatter in a photoelectric cell (5). The resultant optical density correlates with the concentration of antigen. Normal levels of CRP are <1.0 mg/dl.

Interpretation

Synthesis of CRP depends on a sufficient concentration of inflammatory mediators reaching the liver. Therefore, a normal level of CRP does not necessarily indicate absence of inflammation. Because the CRP level changes rapidly after tissue injury, this test is a more timely indicator of disease activity than is the ESR, which changes slowly in response to inflammation (6).

Rheumatoid Factor (RF)

Rheumatoid factor is an immunoglobulin (Ig) that binds to the constant (Fc) portion of IgG. Although several immunoglobulin isotypes – IgG, IgA, and IgM – may demonstrate RF activity, the IgM isotype is detected most easily in the serum.

Method

The latex fixation test uses IgG-coated latex particles to detect the pentameric IgM RF, which binds to and agglutinates the coated particles. A positive titer is >1/20. Nephelometry can detect all three Ig isotypes and likely will replace the more subjective and labor-intensive latex fixation test. A positive result by this method is ≥20 IU.

Interpretation

Approximately 1%–2% of healthy people have detectable serum RF (7). Although a few patients with various chronic inflammatory conditions (autoimmune, infectious, and neoplastic) also have detectable serum RF (8), at least 75%

of people with rheumatoid arthritis do. High serum levels correlate with the severity of joint damage and the degree of morbidity.

Antinuclear Antibody (ANA)

Antinuclear antibodies are autoantibodies that react with a variety of nuclear antigens, including nucleic acids, histones, and components of the centromere.

Method

Cells from a human tumor cell line are placed on a slide and coated with serial dilutions of the patient's serum. Using fluorescein-labeled anti-human IgG to detect the bound autoantibodies, the technician reports the pattern of staining (Table 7C-1) and the last dilution (i.e., titer) that shows staining. A positive titer is >1/40.

Interpretation

ANAs are sensitive markers for SLE, occurring in >95% of people with this disease. However, these antibodies also occur in up to 5% of healthy people, especially women, and in a variety of inflammatory and other autoimmune diseases (9,10). Consequently, the specificity of this test is low. In addition, determining the titer and pattern of the ANA is highly subjective, reducing the test's reliability.

Specific Autoantibodies

Immunoassay techniques allow the detection of autoantibodies against a variety of cellular antigens (11). Many of these autoantibodies (Table 7C-2) correlate with specific rheumatic diseases and, in some instances, predict disease severity.

Antineutrophil Cytoplasmic Antibody (ANCA) Assay

ANCAs are autoantibodies directed against primary granule components of neutrophils and monocytes. Two distinct staining patterns – cytoplasmic (c-ANCA) and perinuclear (p-ANCA) – correspond to antibodies against the antigens serine protease-3 (PR3) and myeloperoxidase (MPO), respectively (12). Antibodies directed against other granule components (e.g., lactoferrin, elastase, and cathepsin G) may give positive ANCA tests by immunofluorescence.

Method

An indirect immunofluorescence assay uses the patient's serum, layered on a substrate of ethanol-fixed human neutrophils, to determine the pattern and titer of ANCA. An antigen-specific enzyme-linked immunosorbent assay (ELISA) identifies autoantibodies to the more specific antigens, PR3 and MPO.

The p-ANCA staining pattern is an artifact of ethanol fixation, which induces positively charged cytoplasmic granules to rearrange around the negatively charged nuclear membrane. However, antinuclear antibodies may cause a similar staining pattern. Using formalin-fixed neutrophils avoids this potential confusion. When formalin-fixed neutrophils are used, serum containing a true p-ANCA displays diffuse cytoplasmic staining, whereas an ANA-containing serum sample will continue to display perinuclear staining.

Interpretation

ANCAs, per se, are limited in their diagnostic usefulness. The c-ANCA staining pattern (and antibodies to PR3) correlates best with active, widespread Wegener's granulomatosis (WG), and less so with upper airway-restricted (limited) WG. However, these antibodies also occur in other immunologic, infectious, and drug-induced diseases (12).

The ANCAs causing the perinuclear pattern are most commonly directed against MPO, but they also may be directed against other cellular antigens (e.g., elastase, cathepsin G, lactoferrin, lysozyme). Antibodies to MPO are characteristic of microscopic polyangiitis – a small-vessel vasculitis that is not associated with granulomatous inflammation – but they also accompany other forms of vasculitis, inflammatory bowel disease, numerous autoimmune and infectious diseases, and use of various medications (12,13).

Complement

The complement system comprises at least 30 interacting, circulating blood proteins that serve as mediators and

TABLE 7C-1
Antinuclear Antibody Patterns

Pattern	Nuclear antigen	Clinical association
Homogeneous	Histone/DNA	SLE, drug effect
Speckled	Saline-ENAs	MCTD, SLE, Sjögren's syndrome, poly/dermatomyositis
	Other	Various autoimmune diseases, infection, neoplasia
Nucleolar	RNA-associated antigens	Scleroderma
Peripheral (Rim)	DNA	SLE
Centromere	Centromere	Limited scleroderma (e.g., CREST syndrome)

SLE, systemic lupus erythematosus; ENAs, extractable nuclear antigens; MCTD, mixed connective tissue disease; CREST, calcinosis, Raynaud's phenomenon, esophageal dysmotility, sclerodactyly, telangiectasia.

TABLE 7C-2
Autoantibodies in Rheumatic Diseases[a]

Type	Description	Clinical association
Anti-dsDNA	Antibodies to double-stranded DNA; greater specificity than those to single-stranded DNA	High specificity for SLE; occasionally appears in other illnesses and in normal people
Anti-histone	Most assays do not differentiate the antibodies to the five major types of histones	SLE, drug-induced lupus, other autoimmune diseases
Anti-ENA	Typical assays test for antibodies to two extractable nuclear antigens: Sm (Smith)[b] RNP (ribonucleoprotein)	High specificity for SLE MCTD, SLE
Anti-SS-A/Ro	Ribonucleoproteins	SLE (especially subacute cutaneous lupus), neonatal lupus, Sjögren's syndrome
Anti-SS-B/La	Ribonucleoproteins	Sjögren's syndrome, SLE, neonatal lupus
Anti-centromere	Antibodies to the centromere/kinetochore region of the chromosome	Limited scleroderma (i.e., CREST syndrome)
Anti-Scl 70	Antibody to DNA topoisomerase I	Diffuse scleroderma
Anti-Jo-1	Antibody to transfer RNA synthetase	Poly/dermatomyositis; especially in patients with interstitial lung disease, Raynaud's phenomenon, cracked skin on hands ("mechanic's hands"), arthritis, and resistance to treatment
Anti-PM-Scl	Antibodies to a nucleolar granular component	Polymyositis/scleroderma overlap syndrome
Anti-Mi-2	Antibodies to a nucleolar antigen of unknown function	Dermatomyositis

[a] For detailed information, consult references 9 and 10.
[b] Designations of autoantibodies are typically the first two letters of the last name of the patient in whom they were discovered. In this case: Smith.

amplifiers of inflammatory responses. Two pathways in this system, called *classic* (C1 – C4 – C2) and *alternative* (factors B, D, and properdin), lead to cleavage of the third component of complement (C3). In turn, C3 activates the terminal components: the so-called *membrane attack complex* (C5–C9). In addition to inducing lysis of antibody-coated cells and promoting chemotaxis and anaphylaxis, the complement system increases vascular permeability and participates in the clearance of immune complexes (14).

Method
The total hemolytic complement assay (CH50) evaluates the functional integrity of the classical complement pathway by determining the dilution of serum required to lyse 50% of antibody-coated RBCs. The reciprocal of this dilu-

tion is reported in U/mL; normal values depend on the reference ranges of the laboratory. Immunoassay techniques and nephelometry measure individual components of the complement system (e.g., C3, C4).

Interpretation
Decreased levels of serum complement often reflect increased utilization of the system during active, immune-complex mediated diseases, such as SLE. Similar changes may occur in nonrheumatic diseases, such as subacute bacterial endocarditis and post-streptococcal glomerulonephritis (15,16). Persistently low or absent CH50 suggests an inherited deficiency of a complement component. Deficiencies of C1, C2, C3, or C4 increase susceptibility to SLE (14). In contrast, deficiencies of terminal complement

components are associated with an increased risk of *Neisserial* infections. Several complement components are acute-phase reactants, and their serum levels may rise during active inflammation in diseases not mediated by immune complexes.

Cryoglobulins

Cryoglobulins are immunoglobulins that precipitate when serum is incubated at <4°C. As currently classified, cryoglobulins are of three types: type I consists solely of a monoclonal protein (paraprotein), most frequently IgM; type II consists of a mixture of a monoclonal Ig, typically IgM, directed against polyclonal IgG; and type III consists of a mixture of polyclonal Ig, usually IgM and IgG (17,18).

Method

Blood is collected in a warm syringe and maintained at 37°C (body temperature) until coagulation has occurred and the serum has been centrifuged. The serum is maintained at 0°–4°C and then centrifuged. The "cryocrit" is reported in the same manner as the hematocrit. An alternative is to quantify the proteins that remain at the bottom of the tube after centrifugation. Unfortunately, results will differ depending on how the laboratory handles the precipitate (18). Techniques such as immunoelectrophoresis, immunofixation, or immunoblotting can determine the isotype and clonality of the cryoglobulin.

Interpretation

Type I cryoglobulins usually reflect a lymphoproliferative disease. Type II and III cryoglobulins accompany chronic hepatitis C infection, often in association with a systemic vasculitis (17). These latter types sometimes accompany a variety of infectious and autoimmune diseases, as well as lymphoid malignancies. When cryoglobulins precipitate, they may fix early components of the complement system, causing "spurious" hypocomplementemia (19), particularly of the C4 component.

KENNETH E. SACK, MD

References

1. Zlonis M. The mystique of the erythrocyte sedimentation rate. A reappraisal of one of the oldest laboratory tests still in use. Clin Lab Med 1993;13:787–800.

2. Miller A, Green M, Robinson D. Simple rule for calculating normal erythrocyte sedimentation rate. BMJ 1983;286:266.

3. Harber HL, Leavy JA, Kessler PD, et al. The erythrocyte sedimentation rate in congestive heart failure. N Engl J Med 1991;324:353–358.

4. Kushner I. Acute phase response. Clin Aspects Autoimmunity 1989;3:20–30.

5. Stites DP, Rodgers C, Folds JD, et al. Clinical laboratory methods for detection of antigens and antibodies. In: Stites DP, Terr AE, Parslow TG (eds). Medical Immunology. Stanford, CT: Appleton & Lange, 1997; pp 211–253.

6. Gabay C, Kushner I. Acute-phase proteins and other systemic responses to inflammation. N Engl J Med 1999;340:448–454.

7. Cathcart ES, O'Sullivan JB. Rheumatoid arthritis in a New England town. A prevalence study in Sudbury, Massachusetts. N Engl J Med 1970;282:421–424.

8. Sibley J. Laboratory tests. Rheum Dis Clin North Am 1995; 21:407–428.

9. von Muhlen CA, Tan EM. Autoantibodies in the diagnosis of systemic rheumatic diseases. Semin Arthritis Rheum 1995;24: 323–358.

10. Hansen KE, Arnason J, Bridges AJ. Autoantibodies and common viral illnesses. Semin Arthritis Rheum 1998;27:263–271.

11. Saitta MR, Keene JD. Molecular biology of nuclear autoantigens. Rheum Dis Clin North Am 1992;18:283–310.

12. Hoffman GS, Specks U. Antineutrophil cytoplasmic antibodies. Arthritis Rheum 1998;41:1521–1537.

13. Ahmed AEE, Aziz DC. Antineutrophil cytoplasmic antibodies. An update on clinical utility. J Clin Rheumatol 1999;5: 151-156.

14. Ratnoff WD. Inherited deficiencies of complement in rheumatic diseases. Rheum Dis Clin North Am 1996;22:75–94.

15. Bush TM, Shlotzhauer TL, Grove W. Serum complements. Inappropriate use in patients with suspected rheumatic disease. Arch Intern Med 1993;163:2363–2366.

16. Fleisher TA, Tomar RH. Introduction to diagnostic laboratory immunology. JAMA 1997;278:1823–1834.

17. Agnello V, Romain PL. Mixed cryoglobulinemia secondary to hepatitis C virus infection. Rheum Dis Clin North Am 1996; 22:1–21.

18. Trendelenburg M, Schifferli JA. Cryoglobulins are not essential. Ann Rheum Dis 1998;57:3–5.

19. Schwartz B. Abdominal pain, purpura, and death in an elderly woman. Am J Med 1985;78:839–849.

EVALUATION OF THE PATIENT
D. Arthrocentesis, Synovial Fluid Analysis, and Synovial Biopsy

Despite the development of increasingly sophisticated serologic tests and imaging techniques, synovial fluid (SF) analysis remains one of the most important diagnostic tools in rheumatology (1). Normal SF lubricates the joint and, along with blood vessels in subchondral bone, supplies nutrients to the avascular articular cartilage. The majority of SF constituents diffuse through the synovium from the subsynovial vasculature, although certain important proteins, such as hyaluronic acid and lubricin, are synthesized in and secreted from synoviocytes. Plasma proteins not found in SF include prothrombin, fibrinogen, factor V, factor VII, antithrombin, large globulins, and a few complement components(2).

Synovial fluid protein concentrations reflect the interplay between plasma concentration, synovial blood flow, endothelial cell permeability, and lymphatic drainage. There are few cells in normal SF. In arthritis, infiltrating inflammatory cells produce additional proteins and release activated cytokines into SF. In addition, the relative ischemia of the microvasculature caused by increased intra-articular pressure due to increased SF alters the diffusion process that supplies synovial nutrients (3). Offending pathologic substances, including microorganisms or abnormal crystals, may be present. Analyzing SF from people with arthritis may yield information invaluable in making the diagnosis, determining the prognosis, and choosing the appropriate therapy (4).

Arthrocentesis

Indications

An acute, inflammatory, monarticular arthritis should be considered either infectious or crystal-induced until proven otherwise. Arthrocentesis with adequate SF analysis is the only way to identify infection or crystal-induced disease unequivocally. Because acute bacterial infections can lead rapidly to joint and bone destruction, arthrocentesis must be done immediately when there is any suspicion of infection. If preliminary analysis of the SF is consistent with infection – i.e., the white blood cell (WBC) count is markedly elevated but no crystals are identified – antibiotic therapy should be initiated pending the definitive culture results. SF analysis can establish the presence of crystal-induced arthritis and enable the clinician to identify the specific form of crystal-induced disease. If a polarized microscope is used, the sensitivity of this test for identifying a crystal-induced arthropathy is 80%–90% (4). Trauma sometimes can result in an acute monarticular arthropathy. Analysis of joint fluid is the only way to distinguish post-traumatic hemarthrosis from post-traumatic arthritis with bland SF.

Arthrocentesis also can be useful in evaluating chronic or polyarticular arthropathies. SF analysis enables the clinician to differentiate inflammatory and noninflammatory arthritides, and often is essential in distinguishing rheumatoid disease from chronic microcrystalline diseases, such as polyarticular gout or calcium pyrophosphate dihydrate deposition disease. Although chronic mycobacterial or fungal infections sometimes can be identified in SF, synovial biopsy frequently is necessary to distinguish indolent infections from other unusual chronic inflammatory processes, such as pigmented villonodular synovitis. Because people with chronic inflammatory arthropathies such as rheumatoid arthritis (RA) have an increased susceptibility to infection, acute monarticular arthritis in a patient whose disease is otherwise well-controlled is an indication for a diagnostic arthrocentesis.

The cellular and humoral components of inflammatory SF can damage articular and periarticular tissues (5). Therefore, arthrocentesis can be therapeutic. The activated enzymes in septic SF are highly destructive to cartilage, so repeated arthrocentesis may be necessary to remove purulent material (6). If purulent SF reaccumulates despite repeated arthrocenteses, surgical arthroscopy and drain placement should be performed to ensure adequate drainage of an infected joint. Blood in a joint can lead quickly to adhesions that inhibit joint mobility. Therefore, therapeutic arthrocentesis is indicated in any patient with a hemarthrosis. Drainage of as much SF as possible from a noninfected, inflamed joint will decrease intra-articular pressure and remove inflammatory cells and activated enzymes, decreasing the likelihood of articular damage (7) and increasing the efficacy of intra-articular corticosteroids.

Techniques

Infections caused by arthrocentesis are very rare. However, the consequences of a joint infection are so significant that it is prudent to take a few precautionary steps to minimize the likelihood of a post-arthrocentesis infection. Betadine or povidine should be applied to the aspiration site and allowed to dry. Alcohol should then be used to swab the area to prevent an iodine burn. Although it is wise to wear gloves during any procedure involving exposure to potentially infected body fluids, the routine use of *sterile* gloves is not necessary. However, sterile gloves should be used if the clinician has to manually palpate the target anatomy after antiseptic preparation of the arthrocentesis site.

Local anesthesia with 1% lidocaine without epinephrine significantly reduces discomfort associated with the procedure. One-quarter to one cc of lidocaine usually is sufficient, depending on the joint being anesthetized. A 25- or

27-gauge needle should be used to infiltrate the skin, subcutaneous tissue, and pericapsular tissue. Larger caliber needles are more uncomfortable and can lead to local trauma. Although many clinicians apply ethyl chloride to the skin before injecting the anesthetic, others believe this practice is cumbersome and results in no clinically significant additional anesthesia.

After the periarticular tissues have been anesthetized, a 20- or 22-gauge needle can be used to aspirate small- to medium-sized joints. An 18- or 19-gauge needle should be used for aspirating large joints, if there is a suspicion of infection or intra-articular blood, or if there is a likelihood of viscous or loculated fluid. Small syringes are easier to use but need to be changed frequently when aspirating large joints with copious amounts of SF. When using a large syringe to aspirate a significant amount of fluid, be sure to break the suction in the syringe before use and draw back slowly, as too much negative pressure can suck synovial tissue into the needle and prevent an adequate joint aspiration. It is often helpful to use a Kelly clamp to stabilize the hub of the needle while replacing a full syringe.

Typical landmarks often are obscured around a swollen joint. Therefore, after a thorough physical examination and before anesthetizing the skin, it is often helpful to mark the approach with a ballpoint pen. If landmarks still are obscure, use sterile gloves to maintain a clean field while using palpation to identify an aspiration site in the target joint. Many joints, such as the knee, ankle, and shoulder, are amenable to a medial or lateral approach. It usually is prudent to attempt aspiration where joint fluid is most obvious. Unlike injection, aspiration is best done when a joint is in a position of maximum intra-articular pressure.

For example, injection of the knee is best done with the joint flexed to 90° while the patient is seated at an examining table and the foot is dangling. This position allows gravity to open the joint and offers easy access to the intra-articular space from either side of the infrapatellar tendon. However, because such flexion decreases intra-articular pressure, decreasing the likelihood of a successful aspiration, aspirate the knee with the patient supine and the joint in full extension. Aspiration of *any* joint should be done only when the patient is sitting or lying down, to decrease the chance of injury in the event of a vasovagal reaction. Although most joints can be aspirated without radiologic assistance, some joints, such as the hips, sacroiliac joints, or zygoapophyseal joints, require aspiration by interventional radiologists under computed tomography guidance. Table 7D-1 lists suggestions for optimal anatomic approaches to aspirating specific joints. Aspirations should not be done through areas of infection, ulceration, or tumor, or through obvious vascular structures.

Efforts should be made to minimize trauma to the target joint. If corticosteroids are to be injected after aspiration is complete, the drug should be prepared in a separate syringe ahead of time, so that the aspirating needle already in the joint can be used for the injection. If difficulties arise during the procedure, the needle should not be manipulated aggressively because of the risk of damaging the cartilage, capsule, or periarticular supporting structures. If bone is encountered, withdraw the needle a little and reattempt aspiration. If no SF can be aspirated, try to analyze and correct the problem without undue manipulation. The needle may be outside the joint space, blocked by synovium or SF debris, or the wrong size for the SF's viscosity.

TABLE 7D-1
Anatomic Approach to Aspiration

Joint	Position of the joint	Direction of the approach
Knee	Extended	Medial or lateral under the patella
Shoulder	Neutral adduction External rotation	Anterior: inferolateral to coracoid Posterior: under the acromion
Ankle	Plantar flexion	Medial or lateral: anterior to the medial or lateral malleolus
Subtalar	Dorsiflexion to 90°	Inferior to tip of lateral malleolus
Wrist	Midposition	Dorsal into radiocarpal joint
First carpometacarpal	Thumb abducted and flexed	Proximal to base of the metacarpal
Metacarpophalangeal and interphalangeal	Finger slightly flexed	Just under extensor mechanism Dorsomedial or dorsolateral
Metatarsophalangeal and interphalangeal	Toes slightly flexed	Dorsomedial or dorsolateral
Elbow	Flexed to 90°	Just under the lateral epicondyle

Synovial Fluid Analysis

Gross Examination

Certain characteristics of SF provide the clinician with valuable clues as to the nature of an arthropathy. Normal SF is colorless and clear. The yellow color characteristic of SF from people with arthritis is due to xanthochromia, which reflects the breakdown of heme from blood cells that leak into the joint space from diseased synovium. Gross, fresh bleeding due to trauma or to any number of pathologic processes will result in red or bloody SF. Clarity reflects the density of particulate matter in SF. Generally, it is the number of WBCs that determines the opacity of inflammatory SF (8). Synovial fluid from people with degenerative joint disease is clear, whereas the SF of mild rheumatoid arthritis or systemic lupus erythematosus (SLE) may be translucent, and SF from a septic joint will be opaque. Other materials that can opacify SF include lipids, crystals (such as calcium pyrophosphate dihydrate, monosodium urate, or hydroxyapatite), and debris that accumulates in destructive forms of arthritis (such as severe rheumatoid arthritis or Charcot's arthropathy). Normal joint fluid is viscous due to the presence of hyaluronan. Enzymes present in inflammatory arthropathies digest hyaluronic acid, resulting in a decrease in fluid viscosity. When a single drop of SF is expressed from a syringe, a "tail" or "string" of fluid should stretch approximately 10 cm before surface tension is broken. The more inflammatory the arthropathy, the higher the number of inflammatory cells and the greater the release of activated enzymes that lead to breakdown of hyaluronan. The "string" formed by inflammatory SF may be only 5 cm or less. Extremely viscous fluid with a very long "string" is suggestive of hypothyroidism (9). One can also determine the integrity of hyaluronic acid by placing a few drops of SF into 2% acetic acid. In normal SF, a stable clump of hyaluronate-protein complex ("mucin") will form. In inflammatory fluid, the clump will fragment easily, reflecting the loss of integrity of hyaluronan. Although of historical interest, the mucin clot test rarely is performed, because the integrity of hyaluronic acid is basically a reflection of the WBC count.

Cell Count

The WBC count and differential are among the most valuable diagnostic characteristics of SF. Cell counts can be done manually using normal or 0.3% saline as a diluent. However, modern automated counters are convenient and give reliable results if the SF is anticoagulated with sodium heparin or ethylenediaminetetraacetic acid (EDTA). Normal fluid contains fewer than 200 cells/mm^3, whereas SF from noninflammatory arthropathies may have WBC counts of up to 2000 cells/mm^3 (9). Noninfectious inflammatory arthropathies have WBC counts that vary widely and range from 2000 to 100,000 cells/mm^3 (10). Although the autoimmune arthropathies generally present with WBC counts of 2000 to 30,000 cells/mm^3, in patients with rheumatoid arthritis, cell counts of 50,000 or more are not unusual. People with crystal-induced arthritis, such as acute gout, usually have WBC counts of greater than 30,000 cells/mm^3, and counts of 50,000 to 75,000 are common. The closer the WBC count approaches 100,000 cells/mm^3, the greater the likelihood of a septic arthritis. Although a rare patient with crystal-induced arthropathy, rheumatoid arthritis, or even a seronegative arthropathy may have a WBC count of greater than 100,000, such patients generally should be treated for joint infection until microbiologic data exclude the possibility of an infectious process.

Unfortunately, a WBC count of less than 100,000 cells/mm^3, or even the presence of another form of arthritis, does not preclude the possibility of infection. People with chronic inflammatory arthritides, such as RA, SLE, or psoriatic arthritis, have an increased risk of joint sepsis because of the structural joint damage caused by chronic inflammation and the immunosuppressive effects of many of the drugs used to treat those diseases. In addition, many disease-modifying agents, such as methotrexate, cyclosporine, leflunomide, azathioprine, cyclophosphamide, or other cytotoxic agents, can blunt the WBC response to infection and spuriously lower the WBC count in SF. Indolent infections, such as tuberculosis or fungal infection, may not generate WBC counts of greater than 50,000 cells/mm^3 in the SF.

The differential WBC count can provide valuable information (11). SF from a septic joint will contain greater than 95% polymorphonuclear leukocytes (PMNs). Most forms of inflammatory arthritis also reveal a preponderance of PMNs. Frequently, more than 90% of the WBC in the SF from people with crystal-induced arthropathy or RA will be granulocytes. On the other hand, the differential WBC count of noninflammatory SF characteristically reveals less than 50% granulocytes.

Examination of a wet preparation can reveal valuable information regarding the cellular and crystalline content of SF. The wet preparation is best done on SF applied directly from the syringe to a slide, but SF anticoagulated with sodium heparin or EDTA also can be used. "Ragocytes," which are PMNs with refractile inclusions containing immune complexes and complement, can be observed on wet-preparation examination of SF from people with RA. SF from people with SLE may contain LE cells. Cytologic examination may reveal malignant cells in the SF of patients with synovial metastases. The "Reiter's cell" is a macrophage that has ingested a PMN. Although originally described in Reiter's syndrome, Reiter's cells may be seen in any inflammatory process characterized by synovial proliferation and granulocyte chemotaxis.

Blood

The presence of blood in a joint usually is the result of acute trauma. If arthrocentesis reveals a hemarthrosis, the bloody SF should be evacuated to prevent synovial adhesions that can decrease range of motion of the injured joint. Hemarthrosis sometimes is seen in Charcot's arthropathy because of chronic trauma to the affected joint. In the absence of a history of trauma, bloody SF could represent a traumatic aspiration. The blood seen in a traumatic aspiration is not homogenous throughout the sample and usually appears only after the clinician encounters difficulty during the procedure.

If the procedure was not traumatic, the presence of bloody SF should alert the clinician to several possibilities. Recurrent hemarthrosis is common in people with severe coagulation disorders such as hemophilia, von Willebrand's disease, and platelet disorders, and in patients on anticoagulant therapy. The SF from people with pigmented villonodular synovitis virtually always is hemorrhagic or xanthochromic. In fact, the pigmentation derives from hemosiderin accumulated from recurrent hemorrhage. The SF from patients with tuberculous arthritis often is hemorrhagic, as is the SF from joints with local or metastatic tumors. Patients with congenital, metabolic, or hematologic disorders, such as Ehlers-Danlos syndrome, pseudoxanthoma elasticum, sickle cell disease, or scurvy, also may develop hemarthrosis.

Crystals

Although crystals can be identified in SF that is a few days old, optimal examinations for crystals are performed on wet preparations of SF soon after aspiration (12). If the SF is to be anticoagulated before examination, only sodium heparin and EDTA are acceptable; lithium heparin and calcium oxalate are both associated with the formation of birefringent crystals, which confound the fluid examination. In addition, a clean slide and cover slip should be used, because talc, dust, or other debris may mimic crystalline materials.

Although monosodium urate crystals can be seen with ordinary light microscopy (13), an adequate crystal examination requires a polarized light microscope with a red compensator (14). The lower polarizing plate (the polarizer), inserted between the light source and the study material, blocks all light waves except those that vibrate in a single direction. The second polarizing plate (the analyzer) is positioned between the study material and the observer and oriented 90° from the polarizer. No light passes through to the observer, who sees only a dark field through the microscope. Birefringent study material will bend light waves that have passed through the polarizer, so they can pass through the analyzer to the observer, who now sees a white object on a dark field. If a first-order red compensator is placed between the polarizer and the analyzer, the field becomes red and a birefringent crystal becomes yellow or blue, depending on its identity and orientation to the direction of the slow-vibration axis of the red compensator.

Light passing through a birefringent crystal is refracted into two waves, a "fast" and a "slow" wave, with vibration axes perpendicular to each other. The fast-wave vibration of monosodium urate is oriented along the long axis of the crystal. When a monosodium urate crystal is parallel to the slow-wave axis marked on the red compensator, a color-subtraction interference pattern of fast and slow vibration occurs, resulting in a yellow color. A crystal that is yellow when parallel to the slow axis of the red compensator is, by convention, considered to be negatively birefringent. If the slow wave of vibration is parallel to the long pole of the crystal when this pole is oriented parallel to the slow axis of the red compensator, an addition pattern of slow-plus-slow vibration will result in a blue color. By convention, a crystal that is blue when the long pole is parallel to the slow vibration of the red compensator, such as a calcium pyrophosphate dihydrate crystal, is considered to be positively birefringent. Birefringence can be "strong," meaning the birefringent crystal is bright and easy to see, or "weak," meaning the birefringent crystal is muted and difficult to see.

Crystals can be identified by a combination of shape and birefringence characteristics. Monosodium urate crystals generally are needle-shaped and have strongly negative birefringence, whereas calcium pyrophosphate dihydrate crystals are short and rhomboid, and show weakly positive birefringence. Other, less common types of crystals may be encountered. Calcium oxalate crystals, which can be seen in chronic renal failure, are rod- or tetrahedron-shaped and positively birefringent. Cholesterol crystals are flat and box-like, tend to stack up, and often have notched corners. Spherules with birefringence in the shape of a Maltese cross are not uncommon and generally represent lipid. However, it has been suggested that some forms of urate or apatite may take this shape (15,16). Hydroxyapatite usually is difficult to recognize in SF, partly because it is not birefringent. However, sometimes it forms clumps large enough to be seen when stained with alizarin red S.

The presence of intracellular crystals is virtually diagnostic of a crystal-induced arthropathy. However, a superimposed infection must be excluded even if a crystal is identified. In addition, a patient may have more than one crystal-induced disorder. For example, up to 15% of patients with gout also have calcium pyrophosphate dihydrate deposition disease. It is important to make that determination, because it will affect therapy. A patient with chronic gout might require only ongoing hypouricemic therapy (and perhaps prophylactic colchicine). In contrast, a patient with both gout and calcium pyrophosphate dihydrate deposition disease may require continued nonsteroidal anti-inflammatory therapy in addition to ongoing hypouricemic therapy.

Attempts to aspirate inflammatory joints are not always successful. For instance, aspiration of an inflamed first metatarsophalangeal joint is difficult. However, if the clinician keeps negative pressure on the syringe as the needle is withdrawn from articular or periarticular tissues, there is almost always enough interstitial fluid in the needle to allow adequate polarized-light examination for crystals. Simply remove the needle from the syringe, fill the syringe with air, reattach the needle, and use the air to blow the fluid onto a slide. This is a particularly valuable technique when looking for monosodium urate crystals in podagra.

Culture

An inflammatory monarticular arthritis should be considered infectious until proven otherwise. In most bacterial infections, Gram stain and culture and sensitivity yield valuable diagnostic information and are crucial components of analysis. Generally, SF need only be collected in a sterile culture tube and transported to the laboratory for routine analysis. Unfortunately, some important infectious agents are difficult to culture, so negative Gram stains and cultures do not preclude an infection. For example, SF cultures are negative in more than two-thirds of people with gonococcal arthritis, even if chocolate agar is used as the culture medium. In addition, tuberculosis often is difficult to culture from SF, and special techniques and culture media are required for anaerobic or fungal pathogens. Sometimes mycobacterial (17) or fungal (18) infections can be detected only on synovial biopsy material. Because bacterial infections can lead rapidly to joint destruction, early antibiotic therapy is essential. Antibiotic therapy should be initiated based on the results of WBC count, WBC differential, and Gram stain, and adjusted later, depending on the results of culture and sensitivity.

Chemistry

Although glucose and protein levels are often measured in SF, neither of these measurements provides information beyond that derived from cell counts with differential, examination for crystals, Gram stain, and culture (19). Measurement of glucose and protein levels are no longer recommended.

Classes of SF

There are four classes of SF, defined by differences in gross examination, total WBC count, WBC differential, the presence or absence of blood, and results of Gram stain and culture (Table 7D-2). Class I (noninflammatory) SF is clear, yellow, and viscous. The WBC count is less than 2000, with a predominance of mononuclear cells. Class I SF is typical of osteoarthritis or post-traumatic arthropathy (Table 7D-3). Class II (inflammatory) fluid is yellow, translucent or opaque, and of low viscosity. The total WBC count generally ranges

from 2,000 to 75,000, although cell counts of up to 100,000 sometimes are seen. Greater than 50% of the cells are PMNs. All of the autoimmune, seronegative, and crystal-induced arthropathies tend to have Class II SF, as do infectious diseases of low virulence, such as the postviral arthropathies, fungal and mycobacterial infections, and Lyme arthritis. Class III (septic) SF, associated with bacterial infections, is yellow to white in color, opaque, and of low viscosity. WBC counts generally are greater than 100,000, but counts as low as 50,000 are not uncommon. Gram stain and culture generally reveal bacterial organisms, except in the case of gonococcal arthritis, which typically is culture-negative. Polymorphonuclear leukocytes make up more than 95% of the cells. Class IV SF is hemorrhagic and characteristic of post-traumatic effusions, hemorrhagic diatheses, pigmented villonodular synovitis, metastatic joint disease, and tuberculous arthritis. It must be emphasized that the SF characteristics of arthritic conditions can be extremely variable and may change with therapy. Therefore, this categorization of SF is meant only as a general guide to aid in the diagnosis of arthritis.

Synovial Biopsy

Arthroscopy has greatly facilitated the clinician's ability to obtain synovial tissue for analysis. At one time, synovial tissue could be obtained only by open arthrotomy or blind needle biopsy (20). Advances in the technology of arthroscopy have led to the development of small, flexible instruments that allow direct visualization and biopsy of synovium (21). In certain clinical settings, synovial biopsy can add significant diagnostic information.

The granulomatous diseases frequently are difficult to diagnose by SF analysis alone. SF acid-fast smears and cultures are negative in a significant number of people with tuberculosis. The diagnosis of tuberculous arthritis is often based on histologic demonstration of caseating granulomata

TABLE 7D-2
Classes of Synovial Fluid

	Class I (noninflammatory)	Class II (inflammatory)	Class III (septic)	Class IV (hemorrhagic)
Color	Clear/yellow	Yellow/white	Yellow/white	Red
Clarity	Transparent	Translucent/opaque	Opaque	Opaque
Viscosity	High	Variable	Low	Not applicable
Mucin clot	Firm	Variable	Friable	Not applicable
WBC count	<2000	2000–100,000	>100,000	Not applicable
Differential	<25% PMNs	>50% PMNs	>95% PMNs	Not applicable
Culture	Negative	Negative	Positive	Variable

PMN, polymorphonuclear leukocytes.

TABLE 7D-3
Diagnosis by Synovial Class

Class I	Class II	Class III	Class IV
Osteoarthritis	Rheumatoid arthritis	Bacterial arthritis	Trauma
Traumatic arthritis	Systemic lupus erythematosus		Pigmented villonodular synovitis
Osteonecrosis	Poly/dermatomyositis		Tuberculosis
Charcot's arthropathy	Scleroderma		Tumor
	Systemic necrotizing vasculitides		Coagulopathy
	Polychondritis		Charcot's arthropathy
	Gout		
	CPPD deposition disease		
	Hydroxyapatite deposition		
	Juvenile rheumatoid arthritis		
	Seronegative spondyloarthropathies		
	Psoriatic arthritis		
	Reactive arthritis		
	Chronic inflammatory bowel disease		
	Hypogammaglobulinemia		
	Sarcoidosis		
	Rheumatic fever		
	Indolent/low virulence infections (viral, mycobacterial, fungal, Whipple's disease, Lyme arthritis)		

and acid-fast stain or culture evidence of *Mycobacterium tuberculosis* in synovial tissue. Atypical mycobacterial and fungal arthropathies can be indolent, inflammatory, oligoarticular infections that cannot be diagnosed without obtaining synovial tissue for histologic and microbiologic analysis (18). In patients without pulmonary involvement, the diagnosis of sarcoid arthropathy may rest on the demonstration of noncaseating granulomata in synovial tissue.

Malignant infiltrations of the synovium can be seen in synovial sarcomas, lymphomas, metastatic disease, and leukemias. The diagnosis of synovial osteochondromatosis can be made based on the presence of foci of osteometaplasia or chondrometaplasia on synovial biopsy. Sometimes cytologic examination of SF will reveal the presence of a malignancy. However, the diagnosis of a malignant arthropathy is based generally upon histologic demonstration of malignant cells in synovial tissue. Therefore, synovial biopsy is indicated if there is a suspicion of articular malignancy.

The diagnosis of some infiltrative processes depends on the histologic or microbiologic evaluation of synovial biopsy material. A diagnosis of amyloid arthropathy can be made if apple-green birefringence is observed in Congo-red–stained synovial biopsy material examined under polarized light. Hemochromatosis is characterized by the deposition of golden-brown hemosiderin in synovial lining cells. Hydroxyapatite deposits in synovial tissue appear as clumps of material that stain with alizarin red S and have a typical appearance on electron micrography. The synovium

of people with multicentric reticulohistiocytosis is filled with multinucleated giant cells and histiocytes with a granular ground-glass appearance. The SF from patients with ochronosis has a ground-pepper appearance due to pigmented debris. The synovial biopsy from these patients contains shards of ochronotic pigment that is diagnostic. In Whipple's disease, foamy macrophages containing periodic acid-Schiff (PAS)-positive material can be seen on synovial biopsy. Pigmented villonodular synovitis is defined by the presence of giant cells, foamy cells, and hemosiderin deposits in synovial tissue.

The ease of direct biopsy of target tissues that has resulted from advances in arthroscopic techniques has not changed the clinical indications for synovial biopsy. Biopsy should be done only if the diagnosis cannot be made using traditional, less-invasive procedures.

KENNETH H. FYE, MD

References

1. *ACR Ad Hoc Committee on Clinical Guidelines. Guidelines for the initial evaluation of the adult patient with acute musculoskeletal symptoms. Arthritis Rheum 1996;39:1–8.*
2. *Gatter RA, Schumacher HR, Jr. A Practical Handbook of Joint Fluid Analysis, 2nd ed. Philadelphia: Lea & Febiger, 1991.*
3. *Gaffney K, Williams RB, Jolliffe VA, Blake DR. Intra-articular pressure changes in rheumatoid and normal peripheral joints. Ann Rheum Dis 1995;54:670-673.*

4. Shmerling RH. Synovial fluid analysis. A critical reappraisal. Rheum Dis Clin North Amer 1994;20:503-512.

5. Chapman PT, Yarwood H, Harrison AA, et al. Endothelial activation in monosodium urate monohydrate crystal-induced inflammation. Arthritis Rheum 1997;40:955-965.

6. Sack KE. Joint aspiration and injection: a how-to guide. J Musculoskel Med 1999;16:419-427.

7. James MJ, Cleland LG, Rofe AM, Leslie AL. Intraarticular pressure and the relationship between synovial perfusion and metabolic demand. J Rheumatol 1990;17:521-527.

8. Gatter RA. A Practical Handbook of Joint Fluid Analysis. Philadelphia: Lea & Febiger, 1984.

9. Dorwart BB, Schumacher HR. Joint effusions, chondrocalcinosis and other rheumatic manifestations in hypothyroidism. A clinicopathologic study. Am J Med 1975;59:780-790.

10. Krey PR, Bailen DA. Synovial fluid leukocytosis. A study of extremes. Am J Med 1979;67:436-442.

11. Shmerling RH, Delbanco TL, Tosteson AN, Trentham DE. Synovial fluid tests. What should be ordered? JAMA 1990; 264:1009-1014.

12. Kerolus G, Clayburne G, Schumacher HR. Is it mandatory to examine synovial fluids promptly after arthrocentesis? Arthritis Rheum 1989;32:271-278.

13. Gordon C, Swan A, Dieppe P. Detection of crystals in synovial fluids by light microscopy: sensitivity and reliability. Ann Rheum Dis 1989;48:737-742.

14. Gatter RA. Use of the compensated polarizing microscope. In: William Kelley (ed). Clinics in Rheumatic Diseases, Vol 3. London: WB Saunders, 1977.

15. McCarty DJ, Halverson PB, Carrera GF, Brewer BJ, Kozin F. "Milwaukee shoulder" – association of microspheroids containing hydroxyapatite crystals, active collagenase, and neutral protease with rotator cuff defects. Arthritis Rheum 1981; 24:464-473.

16. Beaudet F, de Medicis R, Magny P, Lussier A. Acute apatite podagra with negatively birefringent spherulites in the synovial fluid. J Rheumatol 1993;20:1975-1978.

17. Garrido G, Gomez-Reino JJ, Fernandez-Dapica P, Palenque E, Prieto S. A review of peripheral tuberculous arthritis. Semin Arthritis Rheum 1988;18:142-149.

18. Cuellar ML, Silveira LH, Citera G, Cabrera GE, Valle R. Other fungal arthritides. Rheum Dis Clin North Am 1993;19:439-455.

19. Wheeler AP, Graham BS. Pseudogout presenting with low synovial fluid glucose: identification of crystals by gram stain. Am J Med Sci 1985;289:68-69.

20. Schumacher HR, Kulka JP. Needle biopsy of the synovial membrane – experience with the Parker-Pearson technic. N Eng J Med 286:416-419, 1972.

21. Halbrecht JL, Jackson DW. Office arthroscopy: a diagnostic alternative. Arthroscopy 1992;8:320-326.

EVALUATION OF THE PATIENT
E. Arthroscopy

Arthroscopy is a procedure that permits visualization of superficial intra-articular structures (1). The knee is the joint most frequently examined arthroscopically; however, arthroscopes have been used for nearly all joints, including temporomandibular, interphalangeal, and spinal facet joints. Regardless of the joint examined, the procedure has diagnostic, therapeutic, and research indications.

Cartilage surfaces are examined most effectively by direct arthroscopic visualization, which is considerably superior to plain radiographs and even magnetic resonance imaging, particularly with regard to the area of surface viewed (2,3) (Fig. 7E-1). Mechanical abnormalities, including meniscal tears, cruciate lesions, cartilage fractures, osteochondritis dissecans, and loose bodies are visualized readily by arthroscopy. Furthermore, visually directed biopsy can be performed easily and is of considerable use in the person with an undefined arthritis. Visually directed biopsy is superior to blind biopsy because it allows clinicians to sample several areas of abnormal synovium, and because lesions are patchy (Fig. 7E-2). Material obtained from directed biopsies may lead to the diagnosis of indolent infection (tuberculosis or fungi), metabolic abnormalities (ochronosis, hemochromatosis), or neoplasia (pigmented villonodular synovitis, metastatic cancer). Coupled with newer laboratory testing, synovial biopsies may reveal evidence of infection with organisms responsible for reactive arthritis or Lyme disease.

Therapeutically, arthroscopic interventions largely have replaced open arthrotomies for many indications. Repair of symptomatic meniscal lesions and cruciate ligaments are common examples. Although synovial plicae are seen frequently in normal knees, removal of an inflamed plica occasionally alleviates symptoms in arthritis. In patients with rheumatoid arthritis or other forms of inflammatory arthritis, synovectomy may lead to symptomatic improvement, although its role in modifying the disease process remains unclear. Symptoms of osteoarthritis also improve after arthroscopy and joint lavage; however, the mechanism of this improvement has not been elucidated, and the process does not likely result in functional improvement (4). Debridement of abnormal cartilage is performed occasionally, but it is not clear whether this procedure is more effective than lavage. Septic arthritis that has not responded to antibiotics and closed needle drainage can be treated successfully via arthroscopic drainage.

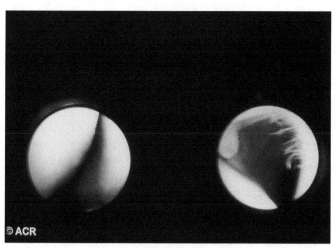

Fig. 7E-1. Osteoarthritis: knees (arthroscopic views). Left: This arthroscopic view shows early loss of articular cartilage of the femoral condyle. Right: There is fibrillation of the patellar cartilage. Reprinted from Clinical Slide Collection on the Rheumatic Diseases, with permission of the American College of Rheumatology.

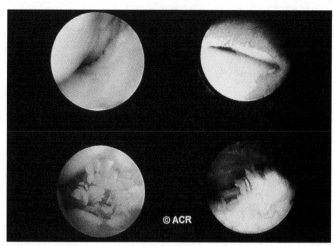

Fig. 7E-2. Rheumatoid arthritis: synovitis, knees (arthroscopic view). Upper left: This arthroscopic view demonstrates normal articular surfaces and medial meniscus. Upper right: An example of early rheumatoid arthritis shows the characteristic hyperemic proliferative synovium with normal cartilage. Lower right: A more advanced hyperemic and villous synovium is seen in the suprapatellar pouch. Lower left: Edematous hypertrophied villi are characteristic of more advanced rheumatoid arthritis. Reprinted from Clinical Slide Collection on the Rheumatic Diseases, with permission of the American College of Rheumatology.

Joints other than the knee have been subject to arthroscopic therapeutic interventions. Oral surgeons have used arthroscopy to debride and repair the temporomandibular joint. Shoulders, ankles, elbows, and wrists also can be investigated and debrided arthroscopically. Rotator cuff lesions or lesions of the glenoid labrum can be repaired (with or without acromioplasty) with an arthroscope. Even hips have been entered, using extended arthroscopes.

Arthroscopic equipment has been used in treating other musculoskeletal disorders. For example, in carpal tunnel release, the joint itself is not entered, but arthroscopic equipment produces results equivalent to an open procedure and is less invasive.

The arthroscope has developed into an indispensable research tool. Direct visualization and grading of cartilage and synovium has been accomplished on multiple occasions during therapeutic trials (5,6). Arthroscopic sampling of synovium for ex vivo investigation is a useful mechanism for evaluating therapeutic interventions. Arthroscopically directed biopsies may give a better view of the degree of synovial inflammation than blind biopsies (7) and may detect lesions prior to the development of symptoms (8).

In general, arthroscopic evaluation is well tolerated. Infection rates are well under 1%, presumably due to the high volume of fluid used for lavage. Effusions are common, particularly in people who have had therapeutic procedures, but they generally subside without further intervention. Stasis, particularly in conjunction with tourniquets, may lead to venous thrombosis. Other neurovascular or ligamental complications are infrequent and usually are due to extensive tourniquet time or vigorous stress on the joint. Improvements in the instruments have made breakage within the joint rare.

Arthroscopic equipment has continued to evolve. Glass lens systems are the standard and provide excellent visualization, but their size and flexibility are somewhat limiting. Recently, systems have been developed using fiber-optic technology, allowing extraordinary flexibility. Using fiber-optic technology, arthroscopes with diameters of less than 1 mm have been developed. As might be expected, the field of view of these instruments is smaller than with the larger glass lens systems and visual quality is not as high. However, joints can be visualized easily with only local anesthesia. As this technology improves, visual quality, and perhaps, field of view will improve.

WARREN D. BLACKBURN, Jr., MD

References

1. Halbrecht JL, Jackson DW. Office arthroscopy: a diagnostic alternative. Arthroscopy 1992;8:320–326.
2. Fife RS, Brandt KD, Braunstein EM, et al. Relationship between arthroscopic evidence of cartilage damage and radiographic evidence of joint space narrowing in early osteoarthritis of the knee. Arthritis Rheum 1991;34:377–382.
3. Blackburn WD Jr, Bernreuter WK, Rominger M, Loose L. Arthroscopic evaluation of knee articular cartilage: a comparison with plain radiographs and magnetic resonance imaging. J Rheumatol 1994;21:675–679.
4. Ravaud P, Moulinier L, Giraudeau B, et al. Effects of joint lavage and steroid injection in patients with osteoarthritis of the knee: results of a multicenter, randomized controlled trial. Arthritis Rheum 1999;42:475–482.

5. Ike R, O'Rourke KS. Compartment-directed physical examination of the knee can predict articular cartilage abnormalities
   disclosed by needle arthroscopy. Arthritis Rheum 1995;38:
   917–925.
6. Blackburn WD Jr, Chivers S, Bernreuter W. Cartilage imaging
   in osteoarthritis. Semin Arthritis Rheum 1996;25:273–281.
7. Youssef PP, Kraan M, Breedveld F, et al. Quantitative microscopic analysis of inflammation in rheumatoid arthritis synovial membrane samples selected by arthroscopy compared
   with samples obtained blindly by needle biopsy. Arthritis
   Rheum 1998;41:663–669.
8. Kraan M, Versendaal H, Jonker M, et al. Asymptomatic synovitis precedes clinically manifest arthritis. Arthritis Rheum
   1998;41:1481–1488.

EVALUATION OF THE PATIENT
F. Imaging Techniques

Imaging techniques may aid in making diagnoses, permit objective assessments of disease severity and response to treatment, and promote new understanding of disease processes. Imaging modalities important in rheumatology include plain radiography, digital radiography, conventional tomography, computed tomography (CT), magnetic resonance imaging (MRI), ultrasound, radionuclide imaging, arthrography, bone densitometry, and angiography. A basic knowledge of the merits and limitations of these techniques is essential in selecting the most appropriate and cost-effective method. This chapter reviews the basic imaging techniques with regard to spatial and contrast resolution (which determine the degree to which individual structures are visualized), radiation dose to the patient, availability, interpretational expertise required, and specific uses in assessing musculoskeletal signs and symptoms.

Conventional Radiography

The conventional radiographic examination is the starting point for most imaging evaluations in the rheumatic disorders, even when other studies such as MRI are expected to follow. The cost is low and spatial resolution is very high, permitting good visualization of trabecular detail and tiny bone erosions. When necessary, resolution can be enhanced further by magnification techniques and film-screen combinations optimized for detail. However, contrast resolution is poor, compared with CT and MRI. This limitation is especially noticeable when trying to evaluate soft tissues. Although plain radiography is a useful tool for assessing the effect of a soft-tissue mass on nearby bone and for detecting calcification within soft tissue, other techniques should be employed if optimal soft-tissue imaging is required.

Examination of peripheral structures, such as the hands and feet, delivers a low radiation dose to the patient, and serial studies can be performed without concern about excessive radiation exposure. However, studies of central structures, such as the lumbar spine and thick areas of the body, expose patients to high radiation doses. Close proximity to the gonads and to bone marrow increases the potential detrimental effects on the patient. Whenever possible, the pelvic region of pregnant or potentially pregnant women should not be exposed to x-rays, and radiation to children should be min-

imized stringently. When such studies are necessary in these patients, radiation physicists can calculate the minimum radiation dose required for the imaging study. These same basic principles apply to all other x-ray imaging techniques.

Conventional radiography is widely available and convenient. Moreover, a vast fund of knowledge about plain radiographic findings in various rheumatic diseases is available (Figs. 7F-1–7F-3).

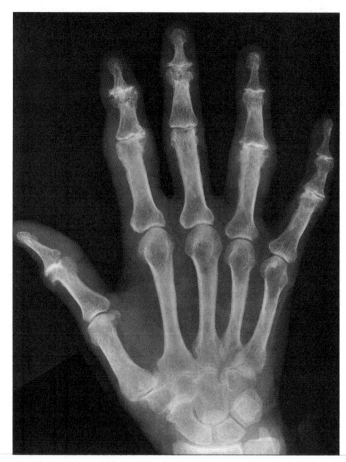

Fig. 7F-1. Typical radiographic findings in osteoarthritis of the hand, showing asymmetric joint narrowing with osteophyte formation. The distal interphalangeal joints, proximal interphalangeal joints, and first carpometacarpal joint are most commonly involved.

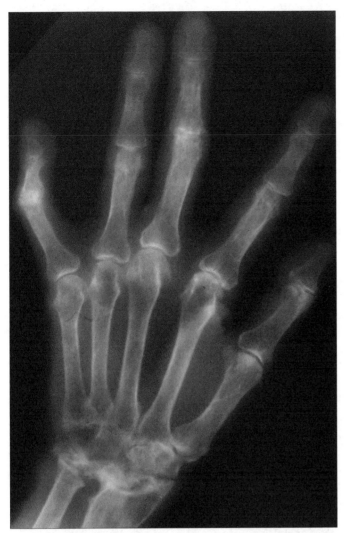

Fig. 7F-2. Rheumatoid arthritis of the hand, showing osteoporosis and severe erosive changes of distal radioulnar, wrist, and intercarpal joints. Some alignment abnormalities of the fingers are present.

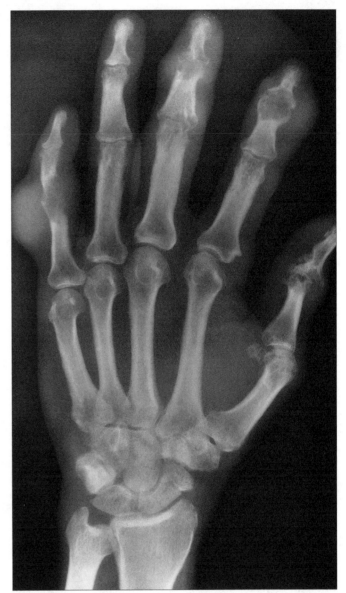

Fig. 7F-3. Advanced changes of gout in the hand. Note soft-tissue masses due to tophi and the large, sharply defined bone erosions, some not immediately at the joint. Scattered distribution of changes is typical.

Digital Radiography

Computed radiography (CR) is a recent innovation for obtaining images that look like conventional radiographs (1). Instead of x-ray film, CR uses a photosensitive phosphor plate to create a digital image, rather than the analog image of conventional radiography. At present, CR images are somewhat higher in cost and lower in resolution than conventional radiographs. However, the resolution is adequate for many routine joint evaluations and can be improved by magnification. The radiation dose is approximately the same as for conventional radiography.

Direct radiography (DR) is another recently developed technique whereby digital images are created at the time of x-ray exposure. The advantages of digital images (whether digitized conventional radiographs, CR, or DR) include the ability to manipulate images electronically and to display images simultaneously in several locations. Image manipulation permits technically excellent final images to be

obtained under adverse circumstances. For this reason, CR currently is popular in emergency departments and intensive care units, locations where it often is difficult to obtain optimal radiographic exposures. The ability to manipulate digital data also could be useful to researchers wishing to make automated measurements on radiographs and to clinicians wishing to send images via the Internet.

The resolution of CR can be improved, and conventional high-resolution radiographs can be converted into digital format. Computed tomography (CT), magnetic resonance imaging (MRI), and ultrasound images are acquired in digital form, and all have a similar transport and manipulation capability. Digital images appear to be the future of imaging, once rapid transmission, cost-effective storage, and easy retrieval become common. Another advantage of this technology is the elimination of the "lost" radiograph, a major waste of time and money.

Conventional Tomography

Conventional tomography is a technique in which the film and x-ray source are moved during radiographic exposure in such a manner that one plane through the structure of interest remains in focus on the resultant radiograph. Conventional tomography and computed tomography are especially useful in areas of complex anatomy and where overlying structures obscure the anatomy.

Tomography is similar in cost to CT. Resolution of bone structures is slightly better than for CT, but visualization of soft tissues is much poorer. Sometimes the primary imaging plane for conventional tomography is especially advantageous for demonstrating pathologic features, such as a fracture or other abnormality of the odontoid process of C2 or pseudoarthrosis in a spinal fusion. Where available, conventional tomography is still useful in limited circumstances, but CT generally has replaced this technique. The radiation dose associated with a conventional tomogram is higher than that of an equivalent CT study.

Computed Tomography

Although relatively expensive, CT is less costly than MRI. The spatial resolution is better than with MRI, but inferior to that of conventional radiography. CT demonstrates soft-tissue abnormalities far better than does conventional radiography, but not as well as MRI. CT is widely available, and many physicians are expert in its interpretation.

Computed tomography is an excellent technique for evaluating degenerative disc disease of the spine and possi-

ble disc herniations in older patients, in whom radiation dose is less critical than in young patients. CT myelography and CT with intravenous contrast enhancement are used to evaluate disc disease and other spinal diseases. Bony impingement on the spinal canal and neural foramina is evaluated more effectively than by MRI. High-quality MRI, if available, is preferred as the second study for investigating disc disease (following plain radiography), but CT is a good alternative and may be useful in circumstances where additional information about osteophytes is important. Elsewhere in the musculoskeletal system, CT is useful for evaluating structures in areas of complex anatomy where overlying structures obscure the view on conventional radiographs. Examples include tarsal coalitions not visible on plain radiographs (2) (Fig. 7F-4); sacroiliitis, especially that of infectious origin (Fig. 7F-5); and articular collapse of the femoral head following osteonecrosis, indicating the need for joint replacement rather than a core procedure. The sternoclavicular joint, which is notoriously difficult to see on conventional radiography, is quite visible with CT.

The radiation dose from CT is relatively high, compared with a single plain radiograph of the same region, but the radiation dose is comparable when several conventional radiographic views of the same area are required.

If the correct initial data are obtained by appropriately adjusting the location and thickness of the slices, images from CT can be reconstructed satisfactorily in almost any plane. Three-dimensional images can be obtained, which may aid in evaluating abnormalities of the pelvis and other areas of complex anatomy. In spiral CT, the data for many images is acquired during a single breath-hold, which pro-

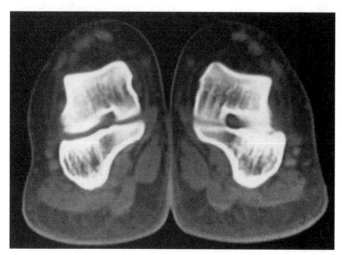

Fig. 7F-4. Middle-aged woman with rigid flat foot and suspected tarsal coalition. Plain radiographs of the left foot did not demonstrate the coalition. Computed tomography scan shows the talocalcaneal coalition on the left, between the sustentaculum of the calcaneus and the talus above.

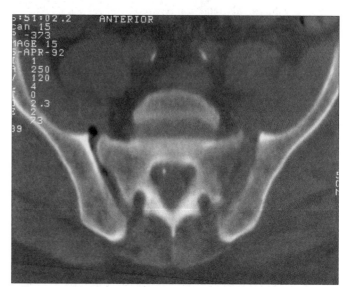

Fig. 7F-5. A 67-year-old man with diabetes and left hip pain. Plain radiographs demonstrated no abnormalities. Computed tomography scan shows marked erosion and widening of the left sacroiliac joint. Blood cultures were positive for *Escherichia coli*, and surgical drainage was performed. Note the "vacuum cleft" in the right sacroiliac joint, a common degenerative phenomenon in middle-aged and older persons.

duces better images of joints affected by respiratory motion, such as the shoulder.

Because a number of rheumatologic disorders are associated with pulmonary abnormalities, it is appropriate to note that high-resolution CT of the lung may reveal details of disease not seen on thicker CT slices of the thorax. The demonstration of "ground glass" infiltrates connotes an active process that may respond to treatment (3).

Magnetic Resonance Imaging

MRI has brought huge advances to musculoskeletal imaging because of its ability to image soft-tissue structures not visible on conventional radiographs. The technique derives structural information from the density of protons in tissue and the relationship of these protons to their immediate surroundings. It is a complex technique that involves changing the strength and timing of magnetic-field gradients, as well as altering radiofrequency pulses and sampling the emitted energy. By altering these factors appropriately, varying amounts of T1 and T2 weighting are imparted to the images to highlight different types of tissue and metabolic states. Altering these parameters can produce radically different images of the same anatomic site. However, because CT images map the density of electrons in tissue, as conventional radiographs do, they may be intuitively easier to grasp than are MR images.

MRI is more expensive than most other imaging studies, largely because of the cost of equipment and the time required to perform the studies. In the future, more attention probably will be given to tailored, limited imaging sequences, which could lower the cost. Newer, faster imaging sequences continue to be developed, which may reduce the time and cost of MRI, as well as provide dynamic studies of joint motion.

MRI is free of the hazards of ionizing radiation, a major advantage in examining central portions of the body where x-ray studies require the highest radiation doses. It has several small hazards of its own, however (4). The strong magnetic field can move such metal objects as surgically implanted vascular clips and foreign bodies in the eyes, cause pacemaker malfunction, heat metal objects if wire loops are within the magnetic field (and produce burns), and draw metal objects into the magnet. Metallic objects in the vicinity of the magnetic field can compromise the quality of MRI images, so operators must screen patients and visitors carefully. Patients suffering from claustrophobia may be unable to tolerate the procedure, a problem also incurred to a lesser degree with CT. More open configurations for the magnet are available to circumvent this problem, but the quality of images produced by these devices varies. On rare occasions, a patient may experience an unfavorable reaction to gadolinium-containing contrast agents used in some MRI studies. Finally, hearing protection should be provided for the patient because application of gradient fields is noisy.

MRI is widely available, and expertise in its interpretation is growing rapidly. However, techniques vary considerably from one imaging center to another, and unfamiliar imaging sequences may be difficult to interpret.

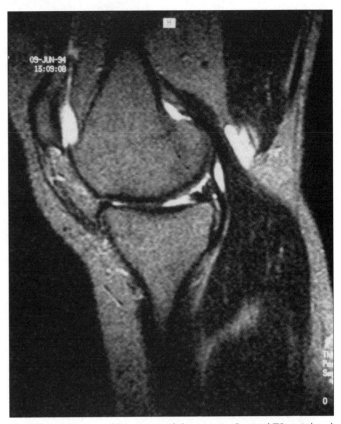

Fig. 7F-6. A 47-year-old woman with knee pain. Sagittal T2-weighted magnetic resonance image shows a high-signal joint effusion, a small popliteal cyst, and multiple tears of the posterior horn of the medial meniscus, which normally has a smooth, triangular configuration.

Spatial resolution using the latest MRI equipment rivals that of CT, and contrast resolution in soft tissues is superior to that obtained by any other modality. Soft-tissue joint structures, such as the menisci and cruciate ligaments of the knee, are demonstrated clearly by MRI (Fig. 7F-6). The synovium can be imaged, especially using gadolinium. Joint effusions, popliteal cysts, ganglion cysts, meniscal cysts, and bursitis are clearly imaged (Fig. 7F-7), and the integrity of tendons can be assessed (5). MRI is becoming increasingly popular for evaluating intercarpal ligaments and the triangular fibrocartilage (6).

Calcifications in soft tissues emit low signal and are not seen as well as in x-ray images. It was supposed initially that bone, which also emits low signal, might pose a problem, but because of the high-signal bone marrow, MRI is extremely sensitive to subtle bony abnormalities. In fact, microfractures due to trauma or stress – often referred to as bone bruises – essentially were unknown before MRI. Recognizing the presence of such microfractures is quite important. For example, much of the pain accompanying some acute meniscal tears may be caused by associated bone bruises. When the bruise heals, the pain disappears, despite the persistent meniscal tear. This finding could have important implications for therapy, and it helps explain why MRI studies of the knee in older people often reveal

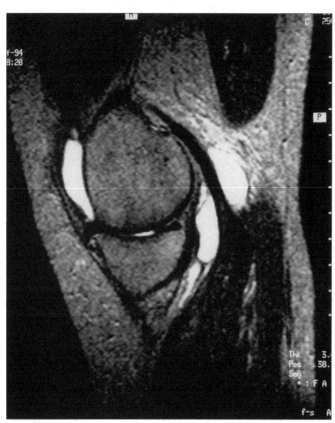

Fig. 7F-7. A 44-year-old woman with knee pain and swelling. Sagittal T2-weighted magnetic resonance image shows joint effusion and a popliteal cyst.

asymptomatic meniscal tears. The pattern of bone bruises also is closely related to ligamentous injuries.

Although plain radiography is the initial method of evaluation in cases of suspected disc herniation, MRI also produces an excellent study of the spine and its contents. (Fig. 7F-8). MRI may be preferred for young patients, because it does not employ ionizing radiation.

MRI is the study of choice for diagnosing osteonecrosis (Fig 7F-9), which can mimic other causes of joint pain, especially in the hip. MRI can detect osteonecrosis early in the course of disease, when plain radiographs show no abnormalities.

MRI also is the best method for evaluating the extent of soft-tissue and bone neoplasms, and generally has replaced CT in this role (7). Plain radiographs still are the mainstay for diagnosing bone neoplasms, but CT may identify characteristic matrix calcifications that are helpful in diagnosing this type of neoplasm.

MRI is sensitive to the presence of bone infection because of alterations in the marrow signal (8). It is a good choice for evaluating a localized area of suspected osteomyelitis, although radionuclide bone scan is preferred for assessing a multifocal hematogenous process. Small studies have shown variable results for MRI in diagnosing osteomyelitis of the foot in people with diabetes and in differentiating osteomyelitis from neuropathic arthropathy,

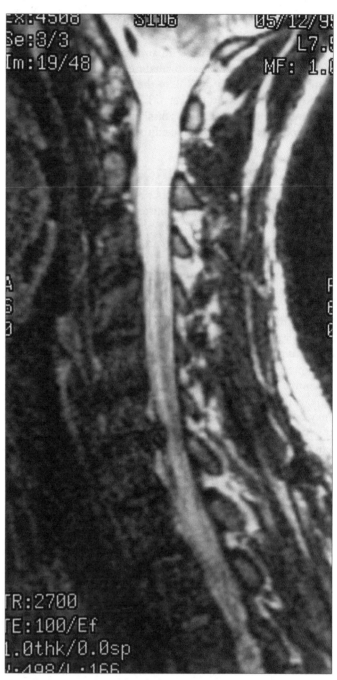

Fig. 7F-8. A 29-year-old radiology resident experienced sudden neck pain and loss of left arm strength during weight lifting. Sagittal T2-weighted magnetic resonance image demonstrates a herniated disc at C6-C7 on the left side.

which is very difficult with other imaging techniques. MRI can also identify soft-tissue abscesses.

Muscle abnormalities such as tears and contusions can be identified on MRI. The activity of different muscles during joint motion can be studied by noting signal changes that occur with muscle activity. MRI is the study of choice for evaluating osteochondritis dissecans when information is needed about whether or not a bone fragment is attached.

Alterations in joint cartilage are visible on MRI. Although direct observation with arthroscopy is more sensitive to small superficial changes, refinements are being made in MRI that improve the images (9). Certainly MRI provides a useful noninvasive research technique; however, the detection of small abnormalities is useful clinically only if it alters therapy. Medical therapy usually is employed until a joint requires replacement, a need that can be diagnosed with plain radiographs.

In certain circumstances, MRI is cost-effective as the primary method of investigating suspected internal derangement of the knee. Arthroscopy proves unnecessary in a large percentage of such cases (10).

Scintigraphic Techniques

Scintigraphy following intravenous administration of agents such as 99m technetium methylene diphosphonate (^{99m}Tc MDP) for bone scans, ^{99m}Tc sulphur colloid for bone marrow scans, 67 gallium citrate (^{67}Ga citrate), and leukocytes labeled with 111 indium (^{111}In-labeled WBCs) are useful for evaluating a variety of musculoskeletal disorders. These studies are similar in cost to CT and deliver a radiation dose similar to a CT scan of the abdomen. Scintigraphy is quite sensitive for detecting many disease processes, and has the advantage of imaging the entire body at once. The technique is nonspecific, however, because a number of processes may cause radionuclide accumulation. When areas of increased uptake are detected, additional studies such as radiography often are necessary to further define the type of abnormality. In clinical situations where the presence of skeletal disease is uncertain, a bone scan can be useful in excluding disease. These studies are available at major medical centers.

The most commonly used radionuclide, ^{99m}Tc MDP, accumulates in areas of bone formation, calcium deposition, and high blood flow. ^{99m}TC sulphur colloid localizes in the reticuloendothelial system (liver, spleen, and bone marrow). ^{67}Gallium citrate accumulates in inflammatory and certain neoplastic processes, and ^{111}In-labeled WBCs localize in inflammatory sites, especially in acute inflammatory processes.

The ^{99m}Tc MDP triple-phase bone scan is the study most widely used for early detection of osteomyelitis (11). Images are obtained in the early vascular phase (during bolus injection of the radionuclide), intermediate blood-pool phase (five minutes postinjection), and late bone phase (three hours postinjection). A fourth phase (24 hours postinjection) can be added to accentuate areas of increased bone uptake, during which time soft-tissue background is decreased, although delayed imaging is not widely used because of its inconvenience. If necessary, the specificity of scanning can be increased by also using ^{67}Ga citrate or ^{111}In-labeled WBCs. The ^{111}In-labeled WBC scan is especially useful when osteomyelitis is suspected to be superimposed on a healing fracture or surgical incision, since uptake of ^{99m}Tc MDP is increased at these sites even in the absence of infection. ^{111}In-labeled WBC scans also may be useful in

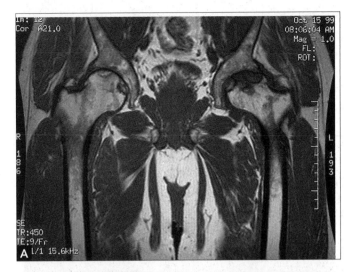
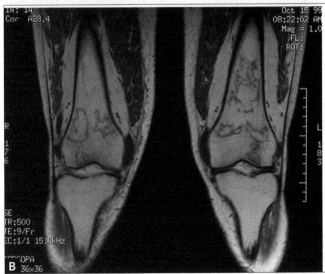

Fig. 7F-9. Magnetic resonance images of hips and knees of a 39-year-old male treated with corticosteroids for severe sarcoid pulmonary sarcoidosis. A: T1-weighted image of hips demonstrates large focus of necrosis in left femoral head and a smaller area in right femoral head. Note collapse of articular surface on left. B: T1-weighted image of knees shows the low-signal, serpiginous margins of multiple infarcts in the distal femurs. Multiple sets of knee radiographics were entirely negative.

diagnosing osteomyelitis of the foot in people with diabetes. In suspected osteomyelitis of the hematopoietic bone marrow, the combination of ^{99m}Tc MDP and ^{111}In-labeled WBC appears to be an effective diagnostic technique. Spatial localization of bone scans can be improved with single-photon emission computed tomography (SPECT), and radiographs of scan-positive areas can be used to increase specificity.

Joints affected by inflammatory or degenerative arthritis show increased uptake and can map the extent of disease in a single examination. This feature has not proved generally useful, but it can help in certain instances. For example, in a patient with inflammatory arthritis and widespread changes on radiographs, scintigraphy may help locate areas of active

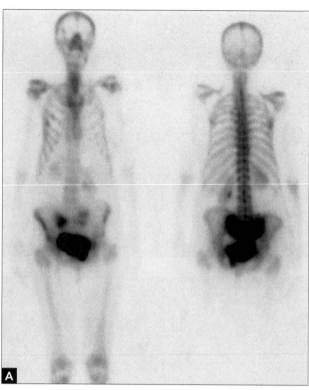

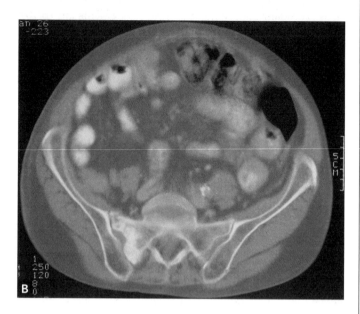

Fig. 7F-10. **A:** An 82-year-old woman with a history of breast cancer and recent onset of lower back pain. Metastases were suspected. ^{99m}Tc methylene diphosphonate bone scan shows increased uptake in the sacrum and right pubic ramus, which are typical of insufficiency fractures. **B:** Computed tomography scan adds specificity to the diagnosis by demonstrating the linear nature of the healing fracture in the sacrum adjacent to the right sacroiliac joint.

inflammation. Bone scans are a reasonable alternative for early detection of osteonecrosis if MRI is not available. Bone scans also can detect stress injuries such as shin splints, tendon avulsions, insufficiency fractures, and stress fractures, which sometimes mimic arthritic complaints (Fig. 7F-10).

Ultrasound

Ultrasound provides unique information by creating images based on the location of acoustic interfaces in tissue. It is relatively inexpensive, widely available, and free of the hazards of ionizing radiation. Spatial resolution is similar to CT and MRI, but the resolution depends on the transducer and is limited by the depth of tissue being studied; resolution is much higher for superficial structures.

One limitation of ultrasound is that it is not always possible for one investigator to reproduce the results of another. Furthermore, because ultrasound has no cross-sectional orientation, it may be difficult for individuals who were not present during the study to interpret the images later.

In some centers ultrasound has proved accurate in detecting rotator cuff tears. It also is excellent for assessing fluid collections, such as joint effusions, popliteal cysts, and ganglion cysts, and it therefore can be used to guide aspiration of fluid in joints and elsewhere. Superficially located tendons, such as the Achilles tendon and patellar tendon, can be studied for tears.

Ultrasound is excellent for differentiating thrombophlebitis from pseudothrombophlebitis. With real-time compression ultrasonography, venous thrombosis and popliteal cysts can be identified (12).

Ultrasound has shown promise in evaluating osteoporosis (13). Sound transmission through bone provides some information about the microtrabecular structure, which relates to bone strength, but cannot be assessed directly with radiographic techniques. This information may prove to be complementary to information provided by bone mineral density studies in evaluating a patient's fracture risk. Ultrasound also has been used to assess the surface properties of cartilage (14).

Arthrography

Arthrography involves injecting a contrast agent into the joint and following with radiography. In conventional arthrography, the joint cavity is filled with an iodine-containing contrast medium and, sometimes, air. The cost is less than that of CT or MRI, and the procedure can be performed wherever fluoroscopy is available. The possibility of introducing bacteria into a joint or encountering reactions to the local anesthetic or contrast medium must be considered, but these complications are very rare.

One of the major reasons for developing arthrography was to examine structures within the joint, such as the

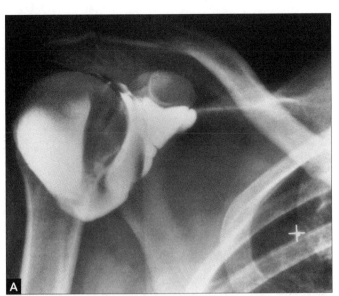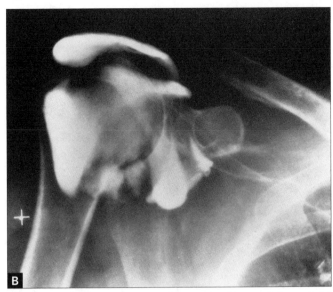

Fig. 7F-11. **A:** Single-contrast arthrogram of a normal shoulder. **B:** Single-contrast shoulder arthrogram of a 66-year-old man with a painful shoulder and history of a past injury. Contrast media fills not only the shoulder joint (as in Fig. 11A) but has filled the subdeltoid-subacromial bursa superiorly, a finding diagnostic of full-thickness rotator cuff tear.

menisci of the knee, which were not visible on conventional radiographs. Now these structures can be imaged noninvasively by MRI. However, certain important roles remain for arthrography.

Conventional arthrography, using iodine-containing contrast medium, either alone or combined with air, accurately detects full-thickness rotator cuff tears (Fig. 7F-11).

Computed tomography scanning can be added to the air-contrast arthrogram (CT arthrography), providing an excellent study of the glenoid labrum that is comparable to, or perhaps better than, MRI (15).

Knee arthrography can confirm the diagnosis of a popliteal cyst and permit injection of corticosteroids at the same time. It is an excellent substitute for evaluating the menisci in patients who are claustrophobic or whose size precludes MRI examination (Fig. 7F-12).

Wrist arthrography is excellent for evaluating the integrity of the triangular fibrocartilage, ligaments between the scaphoid and lunate, and ligaments between the lunate and triquetrum (16). Many clinicians prefer arthrography to MRI in this situation.

MRI arthrography is performed by distending the shoulder joint with a dilute solution of gadolinium-containing contrast medium. This technique has been studied widely and probably increases accuracy of diagnosis of glenoid and acetabular labral tears and rotator cuff tears (17).

Imaging-Guided Aspiration and Injection

Examination of joint fluid often plays an important part in the diagnosis of such arthritic conditions as septic arthritis, gout, and pseudogout. In most instances, the rheumatologist obtains fluid by using external landmarks for needle placement. In more difficult cases, aspiration using imaging

Fig. 7F-12. A 40-year-old woman, too large to fit in the magnetic resonance imaging scanner, was suspected of having a popliteal cyst. Double contrast arthrogram demonstrated a popliteal cyst and also a torn medial meniscus.

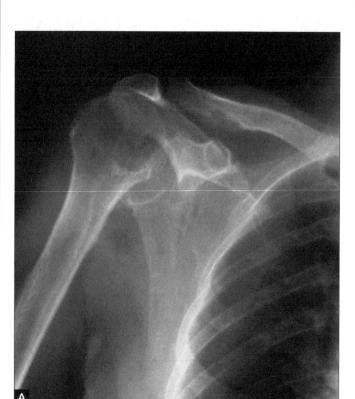

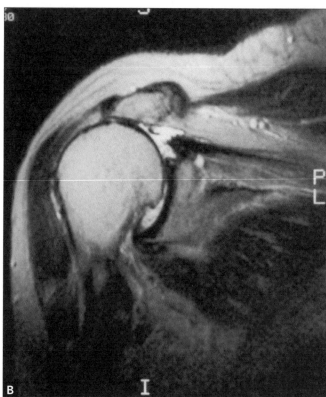

Fig. 7F-13. **A:** An 80-year-old woman with weakness and pain in the right shoulder. Radiograph shows superior subluxation of the humeral head and markedly decreased space between humeral head and acromion. **B:** Oblique-coronal T2-weighted magnetic resonance image (MRI) shows similar decreased distance between the acromion and humeral head, as well as a complete rotator cuff tear and retraction of the supraspinatus muscle and remaining tendon. MRI findings could have been predicted from the plain radiograph and the clinical history.

guidance may prove useful. The source of the specimen can be documented by contrast injection and radiography.

Using imaging guidance to be certain of needle tip position, injection of specific joints with local anesthetic can prove whether or not the joint is responsible for the patient's pain. The injection of corticosteroids for longer-term relief can be similarly directed for greater precision in administration.

Bone Densitometry

Bone densitometry is used primarily for evaluating osteoporosis. Two precise, accurate, and widely available techniques are dual-energy x-ray absorptiometry (DEXA) and quantitative computed tomography (QCT) (18).

DEXA scans with a narrow x-ray beam that alternates energy (kilovoltage peak). A sensitive receptor detects the fraction of the x-ray beam that traverses the body at each point along the scan path. Because the absorption characteristics of bone and soft tissue vary at different x-ray

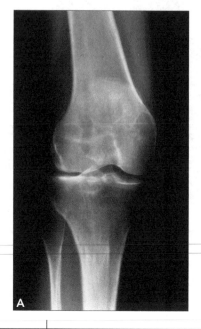

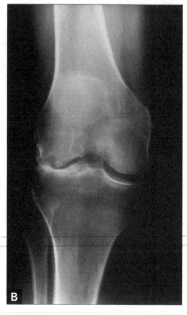

Fig. 7F-14. **A:** A 60-year-old woman with knee pain. Standing anteroposterior radiograph shows what appears to be minimal narrowing of the cartilage of the lateral compartment of the knee joint. **B:** Standing posteroanterior flexed view of the same knee shows severe cartilage loss with bone-on-bone contact in the lateral compartment. This view frequently shows cartilage loss not seen on the anteroposterior standing view.

energies, the amount of radiation absorbed by bone can be calculated. Using this calculation, the amount of bone in the path of the x-ray beam at any point along the scan is determined.

DEXA is relatively inexpensive and delivers very little radiation to the patient. It is thus a good choice for studies that must be repeated. Any part of the body can be studied, and standard values are available for lumbar spine and proximal femur, the most widely studied areas.

QCT scans several lumbar vertebrae while simultaneously scanning a phantom containing different concentrations of bone-equivalent material. A standard curve is constructed from the concentration values versus CT attenuation, and bone density at any location scanned is determined from the standard curve. The cost of this study is moderate and the radiation dose fairly low, although not as low as that for DEXA. One purported advantage of this technique is that it allows evaluation of cancellous bone in the middle of the vertebrae because it does not measure overlying cortical bone and posterior elements of the vertebrae. The cancellous bone has tremendous surface area and is more rapidly affected during bone loss than is cortical bone.

Angiography

Angiography is useful in the primary diagnosis of rheumatologic disorders with vascular components. In polyarteritis nodosa, for example, angiography can demonstrate the existence of multiple small aneurysms of medium-sized visceral arteries. Angiography is an expensive and invasive procedure that should be used only in specific limited circumstances when other modalities will not provide the required diagnostic information.

Imaging Decisions

Almost all imaging should begin with plain radiography, which frequently is the only procedure required. If additional diagnostic information is needed to make clinical decisions, MRI often is the second imaging study conducted. In many cases, MRI findings must be correlated with plain films because MRI does not demonstrate calcifications or subtle cortical abnormalities.

Recent MRI studies demonstrate that many individuals have anatomic abnormalities unrelated to symptoms (19). Therefore, imaging findings must be correlated with clinical presentation. Imaging studies should not be obtained unless they have the potential to answer clinically significant questions.

In many cases simple, low-cost imaging may provide all the information necessary to make clinical decisions. If a plain radiograph of the shoulder shows upward subluxation of the humeral head and erosion of the inferior aspect of the acromion, the clinician can be quite certain that the rotator cuff is torn and atrophic without obtaining an MRI study (Fig. 7F-13). Standing anteroposterior and standing flexed posteroanterior radiographs of the knees cannot show the minimal erosions that are visible on MRI, but abnormalities are seen when the cartilage is gone (Fig. 7F-14). This condition is the end point for failed medical treatment of arthritis and indicates that it is time to consider joint replacement.

It is critically important for the clinician to work closely with the radiologist to decide exactly what information is needed from an imaging study, and then to select the technique that will supply that information. MRI provides such a wealth of information about so many structures that an exhaustive MRI study may be appropriate in a very puzzling joint condition. In other instances, a tailored, abbreviated MRI or a simpler imaging procedure may provide the specific diagnostic information in less time for less money.

WILLIAM W. SCOTT, Jr., MD

References

1. Murphey MD. Computed radiography in musculoskeletal imaging. Semin Roentgenol 1997;32(1):64–76.
2. Wechsler RJ, Karasick D, Schweitzer ME. Computed tomography of talocalcaneal coalition: imaging techniques. Skeletal Radiol 1992;21:353–358.
3. Lee JS, Im JG, Ahn JM, Kim YM, Han MC. Fibrosing alveolitis: prognostic implication of ground-glass attenuation at high-resolution CT. Radiology 1992;184:451–454.
4. Kanal E, Shellock FG, Talagala L. Safety considerations in MR imaging. Radiology 1990;176:593–606.
5. Schweitzer ME, Caccese R, Karasick D, Wapner KL, Mitchell DG. Posterior tibial tendon tears: utility of secondary signs for MR imaging diagnosis. Radiology 1993;188:655–659.
6. Schweitzer ME, Brahme SK, Hodler J, et al. Chronic wrist pain: spin-echo and short tau inversion recovery MR imaging and conventional and MR arthrography. Radiology 1992;182: 205–211.
7. Kransdorf MJ, Jelinek JS, Moser RP Jr. Imaging of soft tissue tumors. Radiol Clin North Am 1993;31:359–372.
8. Erdman WA, Tamburro F, Jayson HT, Weatherall PT, Ferry KB, Peshock RM. Osteomyelitis: characteristics and pitfalls of diagnosis with MR imaging. Radiology 1991;180:533–539.
9. McCauley TR, Disler DG. MR imaging of articular cartilage. Radiology 1998;209:629–640.
10. Ruwe PA, Wright J, Randall RL, Lynch JK, Jokl P, McCarthy S. Can MR imaging effectively replace diagnostic arthroscopy? Radiology 1992;183:335–339.
11. Schauwecker DS. The scintigraphic diagnosis of osteomyelitis. AJR Am J Roentgenol 1992;158:9–18.
12. Heijboer H, Buller HR, Lensing AWA, Turpie AGG, Colly LP, ten Cate JW. A comparison of real-time compression ultrasonography with impedance plethysmography for the diagnosis of deep-vein thrombosis in symptomatic outpatients. N Engl J Med 1993;329:1365–1369.
13. Herd RJM, Blake GM, Ramalingam R, Miller CG, Ryan PJ, Fogelman I. Measurements of postmenopausal bone loss with a new contact ultrasound system. Calcif Tissue Int 1993;53: 153–157.

14. Adler RS, Dedrick DK, Laing TJ, et al. *Quantitative assessment of cartilage surface roughness in osteoarthritis using high frequency ultrasound. Ultrasound Med Biol* 1992;18:51–58.

15. Stiles RG, Otte MT. *Imaging of the shoulder. Radiology* 1993;188:603–613.

16. Metz VM, Mann FA, Gilula LA. *Three-compartment wrist arthrography: correlation of pain site with location of uni- and bidirectional communications. AJR Am J Roentgenol* 1993;160:819–822.

17. Palmer WE, Brown JH, Rosenthal DI. *Labral-ligamentous complex of the shoulder: evaluation with MR arthrography. Radiology* 1994;190:645–651.

18. Guglielmi G, Grimston SK, Fischer KC, Pacifici R. *Osteoporosis: diagnosis with lateral and posteroanterior dual x-ray absorptiometry compared with quantitative CT. Radiology* 1994;192:845–850.

19. Jensen MC, Brant-Zawadzki MN, Obuchowski N, Modic MT, Malkasian D, Ross JS. *Magnetic resonance imaging of the lumbar spine in people without back pain. N Engl J Med* 1994;331:69–73.

8 MUSCULOSKELETAL SIGNS AND SYMPTOMS
A. Monarticular Joint Disease

Pain or swelling of a single joint merits prompt evaluation to identify people in need of urgent and aggressive care (1). Although there are many minor and easily managed causes of monarthritis, infectious arthritis with its risk of prolonged morbidity (and even mortality, if untreated) requires that this more serious problem always be considered.

The underlying causes of monarthritis are divided into two groups: inflammatory diseases (Table 8A-1) and mechanical or infiltrative disorders (Table 8A-2). Triage into one of these categories is the first step in the differential diagnosis of monarthritis.

Diagnosis
History
It is important to determine the course and duration of symptoms, although patients frequently have difficulty establishing the exact time of onset and the rate of evolution. Acute problems or sudden onset of monarthritis often require immediate evaluation and therapy. The course of symptoms may provide critical information. Bacterial infection tends to increase in severity until treated. Viral monarthritis often resolves spontaneously. Osteoarthritic symptoms wax and wane with physical activity. Morning stiffness lasting more than an hour suggests inflammatory disease.

A history of previous episodes provides support for a crystalline or other noninfectious cause. Patients with established rheumatoid arthritis (RA) who develop a dramatic monarthritis out of proportion to involvement of other joints should always be evaluated for septic arthritis or superimposed crystal-associated disease (2). Antecedent joint disease or surgery should raise the clinician's concern about infection. For patients with a prosthesis in the involved joint, loosening of the implant should be investigated.

Monarticular arthritis occasionally is the first symptom of polyarticular disease, such as reactive arthritis, inflammatory bowel disease, psoriatic arthritis, or – rarely – RA. A history of fever, chills, tick bites, sexual risk factors, intravenous drug use, and travel outside the country can contribute clues to infectious causes. Such symptoms as rash, diarrhea, urethritis, or uveitis might suggest reactive arthritis. Weight loss can suggest malignancy or other serious systemic disease.

A history of trauma suggests fracture or an internal derangement, but minor trauma also can precipitate acute gout or psoriatic arthritis, or can introduce infection. Occupations involving repetitive use of the joint favor osteoarthritis. Concurrent illnesses and medication use also may provide important clues; in addition, they can affect test results and influence the choice or outcome of therapy.

TABLE 8A-1
Some Inflammatory Causes of Monarthritis

Crystal-induced arthritis
  Monosodium urate (gout)
  Calcium pyrophosphate dihydrate
  Apatite
  Calcium Oxalate
  Liquid lipid microspherules

Infectious arthritis
  Bacteria
  Fungi
  Lyme disease or disease due to other spirochetes
  Mycobacteria
  Virus (HIV, other)

Systemic diseases presenting with monarticular involvement
  Psoriatic arthritis
  Reactive arthritis
  Rheumatoid arthritis
  Systemic lupus erythematosus

TABLE 8A-2
Some Noninflammatory Causes of Monarthritis

Amyloidosis
Osteonecrosis
Benign tumor
  Osteochondroma
  Osteoid osteoma
  Pigmented villonodular synovitis
Fracture
Hemarthrosis
Internal derangement
Malignancy
Osteoarthritis

Because some monarticular diseases are inherited, a thorough family history can be helpful.

Physical Examination

The clinician must first distinguish arthritis, which involves the articular space, from problems in periarticular areas, such as bursitis, tendinitis, or cellulitis. In arthritis, the swelling and tenderness tend to surround the joint. Even in relatively noninflammatory conditions, such as osteoarthritis of the knee, the joint can be warm and tensely swollen. If full normal joint motion is retained, true arthritis is unlikely. Painful limitation of motion in all planes usually indicates joint involvement. Pain limited to one movement or tenderness on only one side of the joint suggests a periarticular problem.

In any patient with acute monarthritis, it is important to look for extra-articular signs that might provide clues to specific causes. For example, mouth ulcers may occur in Behçet's disease, reactive arthritis, and systemic lupus erythematosus (SLE). Small patches of psoriasis may be found in the anal crease or behind the ears. The keratoderma blennorrhagicum of reactive arthritis can be subtle and often affects only the feet. Erythema nodosum may occur in sarcoidosis and inflammatory bowel disease. A heart murmur might suggest bacterial endocarditis.

Synovial Fluid Analysis

Arthrocentesis should be performed in almost every person with monarthritis, and it is obligatory if infection is suspected. Virtually all the important information from synovial fluid analysis is obtained through the gross examination, total leukocyte and differential counts, cultures, Gram staining, and examination of a wet preparation for crystals and other microscopic abnormalities (3). All these studies can be performed with only 1–2 mL of fluid. Even a few drops may be adequate for culture, Gram staining, and wet preparations. Cloudy synovial fluid is likely to be caused by inflammatory arthritis and is confirmed by a leukocyte count.

Normally, synovial fluid contains fewer than 180 white blood cells per mm^3, most of which are mononuclear cells. The fluid is considered to be "noninflammatory" if it contains fewer than 2000 cells/mm^3, although most samples of synovial fluid from people with osteoarthritis contain fewer than 500 cells/mm^3. Synovial fluid with a count of more than 2000 leukocytes/mm^3 indicates a definite inflammatory process. In general, the leukocyte count and the suspicion of infection should rise at the same rate – the higher the count, the greater the suspicion. Effusions with more than 100,000 leukocytes/mm^3 are considered septic until proved otherwise. However, leukocyte counts vary widely in sterile and septic inflammatory arthritis. Synovial fluid should be cultured if there is any suggestion of infection. Special stains and cultures for mycobacteria and fungi sometimes are appropriate.

Careful examination for crystals in synovial fluid can establish a diagnosis early and avoid unnecessary hospital admissions for treatment of suspected infectious arthritis. A tentative diagnosis can be made by standard light microscopy. Monosodium urate crystals are needle-shaped, and calcium pyrophosphate dihydrate (CPPD) crystals usually are rods, squares, or rhomboids. Polarized light examination can confirm the nature of these crystals. Individual apatite crystals, which cause acute monarthritis or periarthritis, are visible only on electron microscopy. However, masses of these crystals look like shiny, nonbirefringent clumps that resemble cell debris. Special stains, such as alizarin red S, can confirm that these clumps are masses of calcium crystals.

The presence of crystals does not exclude infection, however, especially since antecedent joint disease such as gout may increase the likelihood of septic arthritis. Large fat droplets in synovial fluid suggest a bone fracture involving the marrow space. Small lipid droplets may indicate fracture or pancreatic fat necrosis. Coulter counters sometimes misread these small droplets as leukocytes, providing false elevations of synovial fluid cell counts.

Laboratory Tests

Synovial fluid may give negative cultures in some infectious arthritis. This is especially true for gonococcal arthritis, as only about 25% of patients have positive synovial fluid cultures. For this reason, cultures and Gram stains of blood, skin lesions or ulcers, cervical or urethral swabs, urine, or any other possible source of microorganisms should be ordered when infectious arthritis is suspected. For chronic monarthritis, include cultures for mycobacteria and fungi. Tests for human immunodeficiency virus (HIV) and Lyme antibodies also may be appropriate. However, no single serologic test can establish the cause of any arthritis. For example, rheumatoid factor can be positive in many diseases besides RA, including sarcoidosis and subacute bacterial endocarditis. Similarly, an elevated serum uric acid does not mean a patient has gout, and conversely, normal levels can be seen during the acute phase of gouty arthritis.

Radiographs

Radiologic findings typically are unremarkable in most people with acute inflammatory arthritis, other than showing soft-tissue swelling. However, x-ray studies can help exclude some causes and can provide a useful baseline for future comparisons. Radiographs of the involved joint may show fractures, tumors, or signs of antecedent chronic disease such as osteoarthritis. Chondrocalcinosis in the involved joint suggests, but does not prove, that the arthritis is caused by CPPD crystals. Magnetic resonance imaging is most useful in the identification of meniscal tears and ligament damage (4).

Synovial Biopsy

Needle biopsy of the synovial membrane or a biopsy obtained during arthroscopy may be critical in patients with monarthropathy that remains undiagnosed (5). A culture of synovial tissue may be more informative than a synovial fluid culture in certain settings, such as when mycobacterial or infiltrative diseases are suspected, or when no fluid is available for culture. Biopsies can identify infiltrative diseases, such as amyloidosis, sarcoidosis, pigmented vollonodular synovitis, or tumor. The polymerase chain reaction and immunoelectron microscopy may help identify DNA sequences from *Borrelia burgdorferi*, *Neisseria gonorrhoeae*, chlamydia, and ureaplasma (6).

Initial Treatment

Management decisions often must be made before all test results are available. For instance, a patient with synovial fluid indicating a highly inflammatory process, a negative Gram stain, and no obvious cause or source of infection might require antibiotic coverage while testing proceeds. It is important, however, to obtain several cultures before treatment.

Suspected crystal-induced arthritis in a patient whose course is uncomplicated can be treated with doses of nonsteroidal anti-inflammatory drugs (NSAIDs) near the upper limit of each agent's recommended range, with the dosage tapered as the inflammation subsides. Oral or intravenous colchicine may be effective in some cases of gout. Systemic or intra-articular corticosteroids also are effective in gout and pseudogout. NSAIDs are an acceptable symptomatic treatment in other unexplained inflammatory arthritis. Acetaminophen may be used during the evaluation of noninflammatory arthritis. However, because NSAIDs and acetaminophen can interrupt fever patterns and delay diagnosis, propoxyphene or codeine might be preferred in some instances. Acutely swollen joints can safely be rested, but should not be casted unless a fracture is proved.

Specific Types of Monarthritis

Infection

Between 80% and 90% of nongonoccocal bacterial infections are monarticular. Most joint infections develop from hematogenous spread. The discovery of a primary site of infection can be an important clue to the infectious agent involved. By far the most common agents are Gram-positive aerobes (approximately 80%), with *Staphylococcus aureus* accounting for 60% (7). Gram-negative bacteria account for 18% of infections, and anaerobes are increasingly common causes, as a result of parenteral drug use and the rising number of immunocompromised hosts. Anaerobic infections also are more common in patients who have extremity wounds or gastrointestinal cancers.

N. gonorrhoeae probably still is the most common cause of septic arthritis. It often is preceded by a migratory tendinitis or arthritis. Mycobacterial infection may cause monarthritis or may involve several joints. The disease is more likely to be chronic, but acute mycobacterial arthritis has been reported and may even cause podagra (8). Atypical mycobacterial infections can involve the synovium and should be considered in the differential diagnosis, especially in immunocompromised hosts and in patients whose joints have been injected frequently with corticosteroids.

Fungal arthritis usually is indolent, but cases of acute monarthritis due to blastomycosis or *Candida* species have been reported. Acute monarthritis associated with herpes simplex virus, Coxsackie B, HIV, parvovirus, and other viruses also has been described (9,10).

Symptoms of joint involvement in Lyme disease range from intermittent arthralgias to chronic monarthritis (most often in the knee) to oligoarthritis. Monarthritis also can be caused by other spirochetes, such as *Treponema pallidum*.

Crystal-Induced Arthritis

Gout, which is caused by monosodium urate crystals, is the most common type of inflammatory monarthritis. Typically, gout involves the first metatarsophalangeal (MTP) joint, ankle, midfoot, or knee. However, acute attacks of gout can occur in any joint. Later attacks may be monarticular or polyarticular. Accompanying fever, although less common with monarticular than with polyarticular gout, can mimic infection.

CPPD crystals can cause monarthritis that is clinically indistinguishable from gout and often is called pseudogout. Pseudogout is most common in the knee and wrist, but it has been reported in a variety of other joints, including the first MTP joint. Among other crystals known to cause acute monarthritis are apatites, calcium oxalate, and liquid lipid crystals. Apatites also have been emphasized recently as a cause of gout-like podagra.

Osteoarthritis, Osteonecrosis, Trauma, and Foreign-Body Reactions

Although osteoarthritis primarily is a chronic and slowly progressive disease, it may present with suddenly worsening pain and swelling in a single joint. New pain in the knee often is due to an effusion as a result of overuse or minor trauma. Spontaneous osteonecrosis, especially of the knee, is seen in elderly patients and can lead to pain in a single joint with or without effusion (11). Trauma to a joint leading to internal derangement, hemarthrosis, or fracture also can lead to monarticular disease. Penetrating injuries from thorns, wood fragments, or other foreign materials can cause monarthritis (12).

Hemarthrosis

The most common causes of hemarthrosis, or bleeding into a joint, are clotting abnormalities due to anticoagulant therapy or such congenital disorders as hemophilia. Hemarthrosis also can result from scurvy. Fracture of the joint should always be considered in people with hemarthrosis, especially if the synovial fluid is bloody and contains fat.

Systemic Rheumatic Diseases and Monarthritis of Undetermined Cause

Many systemic diseases may present as acute monarticular arthritis, but this possibility is decidedly uncommon and should not be emphasized in the differential diagnosis. Rheumatoid arthritis, SLE, arthritis of inflammatory bowel disease, psoriatic arthritis, Behçet's disease, and reactive arthritis can begin as acute monarthritis. Other causes include sarcoidosis, serum sickness, hepatitis, hyperlipidemias, and malignancies. Persistence in evaluating patients for underlying systemic diseases can lead to an early diagnosis of systemic disease.

In a substantial number of patients with synovial fluid findings indicative of inflammatory arthritis, the cause cannot be determined. Many of these patients have transient monarthritis with no recurrences (13) and can be treated purely symptomatically. Some such patients have recently been shown to harbor parvovirus B19 in synovium, adding support to a viral cause for some otherwise unexplained monarthritis (14). Guidelines for the initial evaluation of patients with acute musculoskeletal symptoms have been published and include aspects of evaluation of monarthropathy (15) (see Appendix I).

H. RALPH SCHUMACHER, Jr., MD

References

1. Baker DG, Schumacher HR. Acute monarthritis. N Engl J Med 1993;329:1013–1020.
2. Van Linthoudt D, Schumacher HR. Acute monosynovitis or oligoarthritis in patients with quiescent rheumatoid arthritis. J Clin Rheumatol 1995;1:46–53.
3. Gatter RA, Schumacher HR. Joint aspiration: indications and technique. In: Gatter RA, Schumacher HR (eds). A Practical Handbook of Synovial Fluid Analysis, 2nd edition. Philadelphia: Lea & Febiger, 1991; pp 14–23.
4. Weissman BN, Hussain S. Magnetic resonance imaging of the knee. Rheum Dis Clin North Am 1991;17:637–668.
5. Schumacher HR, Kulka JP. Needle biopsy of the synovial membrane – experience with the Parker-Pearson technic. N Engl J Med 1972;286:416–419.
6. Branigan PJ, Gerard HC, Hudson AP, Schumacher HR, Pando J. Comparison of synovial tissue and synovial fluid as the source of nucleic acids for detection of Chlamydia trachomatis by polymerase chain reaction. Arthritis Rheum 1996;39:1740–1746.
7. Goldenberg DL, Reed JI. Bacterial arthritis. N Engl J Med 1985;312:764–771.
8. Boulware DW, Lopez M, Gum OB. Tuberculous podagra. J Rheumatol 1985;12:1022–1024.
9. Rivier G, Gerster JC, Terrier P, Cheseaux JJ. Parvovirus B19 associated monarthritis in a 5-year-old boy. J Rheumatol 1995;22:766–777.
10. Nussinovitch M, Harel L, Varsano I. Arthritis after mumps and measles vaccination. Arch Dis Child 1995;72:348–349.
11. Lotke PA, Ecker ML. Osteonecrosis of the knee. Orthop Clin North Am 1985;16:797–808.
12. Olenginski TP, Bush DC, Harrington TM. Plant thorn synovitis: an uncommon cause of monarthritis. Semin Arthritis Rheum 1991;21:40–46.
13. Devlin J, Gough A, Huissoon A, Perkins P, Jubb R, Emery P. The outcome of knee synovitis in early arthritis provides guidelines for management. Clin Rheumatol 2000;19:82–85.
14. Stahl HD, Seidl B, Hubner B, et al. High incidence of parvovirus B19 DNA in synovial tissue of patients with undifferentiated mono- and oligoarthritis. Clin Rheumatol 2000;19:281–286.
15. American College of Rheumatology Ad Hoc Committee on Clinical Guidelines. Guidelines for the initial evaluation of the adult patient with acute musculoskeletal symptoms. Arthritis Rheum 1996;39:1–8.

MUSCULOSKELETAL SIGNS AND SYMPTOMS
B. Polyarticular Joint Disease

A thorough history and physical examination are the most important diagnostic tools in the evaluation of polyarticular joint complaints (1–4). Potentially useful information includes preceding illnesses or trauma, prior episodes of joint pain, and a family history of arthritis or back pain. The pattern and evolution of joint involvement may offer clues. Are large or small joints affected? Is the arthritis limited to just a few joints? Is it symmetrical? Does it involve several joints simultaneously, or does it appear in an additive or migratory fashion? In the additive pattern, new joint involvement occurs at intervals, but symptoms persist once the joint is involved; with migratory arthritis, the duration of involvement for each joint is only a few days. What is the pattern of pain? In osteoarthritis (OA), pain is aggravated by use and weight-bearing and is relieved by rest. In inflammatory arthritis, particularly rheumatoid arthritis (RA), symptoms are aggravated by immobility. Is there evidence of systemic disease or other organ involvement?

On physical examination, the presence of soft-tissue swelling and effusion should be noted. These signs usually point toward an inflammatory synovitis, even when redness, warmth, and marked tenderness are absent. However, swelling and effusion also may occur in noninflammatory arthritis. If the joints appear normal in patients with widespread pain, nonarticular causes should be considered (e.g., fibromyalgia, polymyalgia rheumatica, bone disease, neuropathy). Because joint pain sometimes is the initial manifestation of systemic illnesses, a complete physical examination is appropriate for all patients with polyarthritis. Particular attention should be given to examining the skin for rashes, subcutaneous nodules, and other lesions associated with rheumatic diseases. The musculoskeletal examination should include the spine and muscles, as well as the joints.

Laboratory studies include standard hematologic and biochemical tests; nonspecific indicators of inflammation or dysproteinemia, such as erythrocyte sedimentation rate;

TABLE 8B-1
Classification of Polyarticular Joint Disease

Inflammatory
Crystal-induced arthritis
Infectious arthritis
  Bacterial
    Gonococcal and meningococcal
    Lyme disease
    Bacterial endocarditis
  Viral
  Other infections
Postinfectious or reactive arthritis
  Enteric infection
  Urogenital infection
  Rheumatic fever
Other seronegative spondyloarthropathies
  Ankylosing spondylitis
  Psoriatic arthritis
  Inflammatory bowel disease
Rheumatoid arthritis
Inflammatory osteoarthritis
Systemic rheumatic illnesses
  Systemic lupus erythematosus
  Systemic vasculitis
  Systemic sclerosis
  Polymyositis/dermatomyositis
  Still's disease
  Behçet's disease
  Relapsing polychondritis
Other systemic illnesses
  Sarcoidosis
  Palindromic rheumatism
  Familial Mediterranean fever
  Malignancy
  Hyperlipoproteinemias
  Whipple's disease

Noninflammatory
Osteoarthritis
  Metabolic/Endocrine
  Hemochromatosis
  Acromegaly
  Ochronosis
Hematologic
  Amyloidosis
  Leukemia
  Hemophilia
  Sickle cell disease
Hypertrophic pulmonary osteoarthropathy

antibody tests for exposure to pathogens (e.g., group A streptococci, parvovirus B19, *Borrelia burgdorferi*); and autoantibodies that may be associated with a single condition or limited group of illnesses.

If the diagnosis is uncertain after history, physical examination, and results of standard laboratory tests are evaluated, synovial fluid should always be examined if it is readily obtainable. Synovial fluid analysis must be done immediately on patients who are febrile or acutely ill. The analysis may be diagnostic in patients with bacterial infections or crystal-induced synovitis. In other conditions, it may permit the examiner to classify the arthritis as either inflammatory or noninflammatory.

Imaging studies may yield valuable information in people with chondrocalcinosis caused by calcium pyrophosphate dihydrate deposition (CPPD) disease, with back pain typical of sacroiliac joint involvement, or erosions typical of RA. However, most imaging studies and many laboratory tests are expensive and should not be ordered routinely, nor should imaging include all involved joints. The physician should first outline the differential diagnosis and estimate the likelihood that a test or study will distinguish between the leading diagnoses or alter the treatment plan.

Biopsy of the synovium or other tissue may be necessary to confirm or establish a diagnosis of a rare disease, such as Whipple's disease, vasculitis, mycobacterial arthritis, or fungal infections.

Classification of Polyarticular Joint Disease

There are two main categories of polyarticular joint disease: inflammatory and noninflammatory. Both groups include conditions with great etiologic and clinical diversity (Table 8B-1). The presence of abnormal findings in another organ system often is valuable in the diagnosis of polyarthropathy, because many of the possible causes involve multiple systems (Table 8B-2).

Polyarticular arthritis also can be grouped by mode of presentation (acute, subacute, chronic), occurrence in different age groups, pattern of joint involvement, or immunogenetic associations. However, not all patients fit the expected profile, and atypical presentations do occur. For example, the onset of RA typically is insidious or subacute and involves multiple small and some large joints, but occasionally its onset is acute and joint involvement is monarticular or oligoarticular. Middle-aged women are affected most often, but RA can occur at any age and also can affect men. The following discussions focus on the most typical presentations of disorders that can cause polyarticular arthritis.

Acute Inflammatory Polyarthritis

People with acute inflammatory polyarthritis frequently have a high- or low-grade fever (Table 8B-2). *Rheumatic fever* is the prototype in this group. Children typically are affected with migratory arthritis that involves several joints simultaneously but persists in each joint for only a few days. In adults, the arthritis often is additive and of longer duration. Carditis may not be evident initially. Streptococcal pharyngitis preceding the symptoms commonly is asymptomatic, but serologic evidence should be sought in all people with acute polyarthritis and fever. Fever usually fluctuates without returning to a normal temperature for a week or more, but characteristically in children, fever and arthritis respond dramatically to high-dose aspirin therapy. Rheumatic fever in

TABLE 8B-2
Systemic and Organ Involvement Associated With Polyarthropathy

Disorder	Organ Involvement				
	Fever	Lungs	Eye	GI System	Heart
Amyloidosis	–	–		X	X
Bacterial arthritis	X	–	–	–	–
Bacterial endocarditis	X	–	–	–	X
Behçet's disease	–		X	–	
Crystal-induced arthritis	X	–	–	–	–
Erythema nodosum	X	–	X	–	–
Familial Mediterranean fever	X	X	–	X	–
Hemochromatosis	–	–	–	–	X
Hypertrophic pulmonary osteoarthropathy	–	X	–	–	–
Inflammatory bowel disease	X	–	X	X	–
Intestinal bypass surgery	–	–	X	X	X
Juvenile chronic arthritis	–	–	X	–	X
Leukemia	X	–	X	–	–
Lyme disease	X	–	–	–	X
Polymyositis/dermatomyositis	–	X	–	–	X
Reactive arthritis	X	–	X	X	–
Relapsing polychondritis	X	X	X	–	X
Rheumatic fever	X	X	–	–	X
Rheumatoid arthritis	–	X	X	–	X
Sarcoidosis	X	X	X		X
Seronegative spondyloarthropathy	–	–	X	X	X
Sjögren's syndrome	–	X	X	–	–
Still's disease	X	X	X	–	X
Systemic lupus erythematosus	X	X	X	X	X
Systemic sclerosis	–	X	–	X	X
Systemic vasculitis	X	X	X	X	X
Viral arthritis	X	–	–	–	–
Whipple's disease	X	X	X	X	X

young children is less likely to present with arthritis; in these cases, aspirin should be used with caution because of the increased risk of Reye's syndrome.

Septic arthritis generally affects a single joint, but about 20% of adults with this condition have two or more large joints involved. Risk factors for polyarthritis include immunosuppression, intravenous drug use, and preexisting joint disease, particularly RA.

Gonococcal and *meningococcal arthritis* frequently are polyarticular and may present with a migratory pattern. Typical vesiculopustular skin lesions on an erythematous base provide an important diagnostic clue in gonococcemia. Tenosynovitis frequently is found in the wrist and ankle extensor tendon sheaths. Synovial fluid usually is sterile in polyarticular neisserial infection, but blood cultures may be diagnostic.

In early *Lyme disease,* dissemination of *B. burgdorferi* often is manifested by fever and migratory arthralgia, with little or no joint swelling. A persistent oligoarticular arthritis may appear months later.

Bacterial endocarditis may present with fever, back pain, and arthralgia. A minority of patients have large-joint oligoarticular arthritis, usually with sterile synovial fluid cultures. Endocarditis should be suspected in people with a heart murmur and fever, and confirmed by blood cultures.

Mycobacterial or fungal arthritis usually is monarticular, but occasionally an indolent oligoarthritis occurs.

Acute polyarthritis may be a sequel to *parvovirus B19* and *rubella* infection, especially in young women. Although self-limited, viral arthropathies resemble acute RA, with morning stiffness, symmetric involvement of the hands and wrists, and occasionally a positive test for rheumatoid factor. The typical viral exanthem may be absent, but the diagnosis should be suspected in patients exposed to one of these viruses and can be confirmed serologically. A similar arthritis may precede the symptoms of *hepatitis B* viral infection and often is accompanied by an urticarial rash. *Hepatitis C* viral infection may be associated with a more chronic polyarthritis, cutaneous vasculitis, and cryoglobulinemia.

Several types of arthropathy may occur in people with *human immunodeficiency virus (HIV)* infection, including acute episodic oligoarthritis and persistent polyarthritis. HIV-induced arthropathies may be related directly to viral infection or to secondary septic or reactive arthritis.

Crystal-induced arthritis is generally monarticular, but it may present as acute oligoarticular arthritis, often with fever. Typically the joints are warm and erythematous, and swelling extends to the soft tissue well beyond the joint. With both crystal-induced and septic arthritis in large joints of the lower extremity, the patient may be unable to bear weight or may walk with a pronounced limp. Gouty arthritis usually affects the feet, especially the first metatarsophalangeal (MTP) joint, and tophi may be present. In older women with OA, gout sometimes presents with acute inflammation in a Heberden's node. Demonstration of crystals in synovial fluid confirms the diagnosis. Radiographs showing chondrocalcinosis support the diagnosis of CPPD disease.

Palindromic rheumatism and *familial Mediterranean fever (FMF)* cause recurrent attacks of acute synovitis or periarticular inflammation, usually in one or two joints, with long symptom-free intervals between attacks. In FMF there usually is a family history of similar attacks starting in childhood; pleuritis and abdominal pain also may occur. Episodic arthritis and periarthritis also have been described in some types of hyperlipoproteinemia.

Relapsing seronegative symmetrical synovitis with pitting edema (RS3PE syndrome) is associated with marked joint stiffness and symmetric polysynovitis involving especially the hands and feet (5). The onset typically is abrupt, and profound pitting edema of the hands may lead to carpal tunnel syndrome. Large-joint involvement also may occur, but like most periodic syndromes, it is not associated with joint destruction. The incidence of RS3PE is unknown; it typically is seen in patients over the age of 60 and is more common in men (5,6).

Acute leukemia in children may cause recurrent acute episodes of arthralgia, arthritis, and bone pain.

Acute *sarcoid arthritis* usually is accompanied by fever, erythema nodosum, and hilar adenopathy. Marked periarticular swelling and erythema in both ankles should suggest sarcoid arthritis.

Subacute and Chronic Inflammatory Polyarthritis

Rheumatoid arthritis, the most prominent member of this group, varies in its presentation. Some patients have a symmetric polyarthritis that usually affects small joints, such as metacarpophalangeal and proximal interphalangeal joints of the fingers. Other patients have an additive pattern with a monarticular or oligoarticular onset. Symptoms are worse upon awakening (morning stiffness) or after periods of inactivity. In the early stages, joint tenderness and swelling are the main physical findings, but later, limitation of motion and joint deformity develop. Although subcutaneous nodules develop in fewer than half of people with RA, their presence may support the diagnosis. About two-thirds to three-fourths of people with RA test positive for rheumatoid factor, including almost all patients with nodules.

Seronegative RA may be difficult to distinguish from some varieties of *seronegative spondyloarthropathy*. This clinically heterogeneous group of disorders includes ankylosing spondylitis, psoriatic arthritis, and reactive arthritis. The spine and sacroiliac joints are frequently involved, and isolated dactylitis (sausage digit) and enthesopathy (pain at sites of tendon or ligament attachment to bone) are common findings. Disease susceptibility often is genetically determined.

Ankylosing spondylitis may present with peripheral joint symptoms, but the axial joints (hips and shoulders especially) are more likely to be affected than in early RA, and low back pain usually is present. As in RA, pain and stiffness are prominent after inactivity and improve after movement.

Psoriatic arthritis has several variants, but it typically is oligoarticular at onset and may evolve into a polyarthritis indistinguishable from RA, particularly if the appearance of skin lesions is delayed. Prominent involvement of the distal interphalangeal joints and pitting of the nails support the diagnosis of psoriatic arthritis.

Reactive arthritis may develop following certain enteric or genitourinary infections, particularly in HLA-B27 positive individuals, as a postinfectious, sterile, lower-extremity oligoarthritis. Large-joint oligoarthritis also may occur in active *inflammatory bowel disease,* and usually remits when the bowel inflammation is suppressed. In many patients, large effusions, particularly in the knees, are accompanied by little or no pain.

In *juvenile chronic polyarthritis* and *Still's disease,* polyarthritis is accompanied by systemic signs that resemble an infectious illness, with high spiking fever, neutrophilic leukocytosis, and evanescent macular rash. Many patients also have lymphadenopathy, splenomegaly, and pericarditis. Synovitis may be absent or intermittent initially, but a persistent polyarthritis resembling RA develops in most patients. Still's disease may occur in adults as well as children.

Whipple's disease is a chronic infection that may cause enteritis and oligoarticular or migratory arthritis. Multiple organ involvement may suggest the diagnosis; confirmation is by biopsy of intestinal mucosa or lymph nodes. Intermittent polyarthritis has been described in morbidly obese patients following *intestinal bypass surgery.* Joint symptoms often are accompanied by a variety of skin lesions.

Polyarthritis is a common mode of presentation in *systemic lupus erythematosus (SLE),* and differentiation from RA may be difficult if nonarticular manifestations of SLE have not yet appeared. Symptoms vary and may be migratory or intermittent. Morning stiffness generally is not as prominent as in RA. Although hand deformities may develop, they are not accompanied by articular erosions on radiographs. *Drug-induced lupus* presents with a symmetric polyarthritis and frequently with systemic manifestations, including low-grade fever and serositis. Many drugs can provoke this reaction, but procainamide is the most common causative agent.

Polyarthritis may occur in other systemic rheumatic illnesses, at presentation and later in the disease course, and the presence of extra-articular manifestations can help distinguish these conditions from RA. For example, Raynaud's phenomenon and skin thickening usually are found in *systemic sclerosis* and *mixed connective tissue disease. Polymyositis* and *dermatomyositis* are accompanied by proximal muscle weakness. People with *systemic vasculitis* have characteristic skin lesions, neuropathy, and visceral involvement. *Polymyalgia rheumatica* presents with diffuse pain and morning stiffness, but usually, joint pain is most prominent in the axial areas (hips and shoulders), joint swelling is absent, small effusions in the knees are minimally symptomatic, and cell counts are lower than in RA.

In *Behçet's disease,* recurrent oral and genital ulcerations often are accompanied by skin, eye, and neurologic manifestations. About half of these patients have arthritis at some time during the course of the disease. *Relapsing polychondritis* presents with extra-articular manifestations, including inflammation and destruction of cartilaginous tissue in the nose, ears, and upper airway. Recurrent oligoarticular arthritis is a frequent early or late finding.

Noninflammatory Polyarthropathy

Osteoarthritis is characterized by progressive attrition of articular cartilage and new bone formation at the margins of the joint. Typically, pain is aggravated by weight-bearing and motion, and is relieved by rest. In more advanced disease, particularly in OA of the hip, there may be nocturnal pain. Pain usually is much less severe in nonweight-bearing joints. On examination, bony enlargement may be detected (such as Heberden's and Bouchard's nodes), and crepitus confirms the presence of articular cartilage roughening. Although less prominent than in inflammatory arthritis, synovial effusions may occur, especially in the knees. However, the fluid does not show inflammatory changes. Joint involvement in OA usually is focal rather than generalized; joints frequently involved include the hips and knees, and the acromioclavicular, first MTP, first carpometacarpal, and interphalangeal joints. Patients with hand involvement often have a strong family history of OA.

Erosive inflammatory OA of the distal and proximal finger joints causes more pain, tenderness, and soft-tissue swelling than does ordinary OA. Patients with this variant also experience more rapid loss of motion and bone erosion, culminating in bony ankylosis. The intermittent signs of inflammation may resemble RA, but erosive inflammatory OA is limited to the fingers.

Primary generalized OA is caused by several conditions, some of which may have a genetic basis. The arthritis involves many joints, and often begins at an earlier age than is typical of OA. Several metabolic disorders, including hereditary *CPPD disease,* can cause premature OA. Patients with this disorder also may have episodes of acute crystal-induced inflammation (pseudogout). *Acromegaly* causes cartilage overgrowth initially, but arthropathy seen in the later stages resembles generalized OA. In *ochronosis,* the enzyme that metabolizes homogentisic acid is absent, and polymers of this acid, a tyrosine derivative, are deposited in cartilage. The cartilage takes on a gray or black discoloration, a pigmentation that also may be detected in the ears and sclerae.

Polyarthropathy is common in early stages of *hemochromatosis* and typically involves the hands, particularly the metacarpophalangeal joints. This pattern resembles RA rather than OA, and the presence of mild soft-tissue swelling may suggest an inflammatory arthritis. However, examination of the synovial membrane reveals iron deposition rather than inflammatory cells. Elevated iron saturation or ferritin levels support the diagnosis.

Other systemic illnesses may cause noninflammatory arthropathy. *Amyloidosis* due to AL amyloid deposition may be a primary disease or secondary to multiple myeloma.

Most patients have prominent renal involvement and evidence that other organs are affected. Arthritis due to amyloid deposits in and around the joints is the main symptom only in a minority of patients. Shoulder swelling may be impressive (shoulder-pad sign), and hand swelling and deformity may resemble patterns seen in RA. Monoclonal immunoglobulins or light chains usually are found in the serum or urine. Patients receiving hemodialysis may have amyloid deposits derived from β_2-microglobulin in articular tissues, resulting in chronic arthritis and carpal tunnel syndrome.

Hypertrophic pulmonary osteoarthropathy is a syndrome that may be caused by many thoracic or abdominal disorders, but carcinoma of the lung is the most common. The main features are clubbing of the fingers, osteoarticular pain, and radiographic evidence of periosteal new bone formation. Some patients have symmetric joint swelling, warmth, and effusions, suggesting the possibility of RA, but synovial fluid analysis fails to confirm inflammation.

Hemophilia causes recurrent episodes of pain and swelling due to intra-articular and periarticular hemorrhage. The attacks start in childhood and usually affect only one or two joints at a time. In the absence of factor VIII replacement therapy, a deforming polyarthritis may develop. *Sickle cell disease*, which also begins in childhood, often involves bones and joints; monarticular or oligoarticular joint swelling is an occasional finding.

Epidemiology of Polyarthritis

A patient's age, gender, and race may provide helpful clues in the differential diagnosis of polyarthritis. Young women are the likeliest group to have gonococcal arthritis, parvoviral and rubella arthritis, and SLE. Young men are more likely to develop ankylosing spondylitis, reactive arthritis, and human immunodeficiency virus-related arthritis. Rheumatoid arthritis and OA of the fingers are seen most frequently in middle-aged women, whereas gout, hemochromatosis, and polyarteritis nodosum are more common in middle-aged men. Elderly patients are more likely to have generalized OA, CPPD disease, and polymyalgia rheumatica. African Americans have a high prevalence of SLE, sarcoidosis, and arthritis due to sickle cell disease, and a decreased prevalence of ankylosing spondylitis and polymyalgia rheumatica. In some regions, infectious or postinfectious illnesses are endemic, such as Lyme disease in southern New England, the midAtlantic states, the upper Midwest, and northern California, and rheumatic fever in various South American and Asian nations. Geographic location and race may be closely intertwined. Behçet's disease occurs much more frequently in Japan and the Eastern Mediterranean than in other parts of the world.

ROBERT S. PINALS, MD

References

1. Pinals RS. Polyarthritis and fever. N Engl J Med 1994;330: 769–774.
2. Hübscher O. Pattern recognition in arthritis. In Klippel JH, Dieppe PA (eds). Rheumatology. 2nd edition. London: Mosby, 1998; pp 3.1–3.6.
3. Sergent JS. Polyarticular arthritis. In: Ruddy S, Harris ED, Sledge CB (eds). Kelley's Textbook of Rheumatology, 6th edition. Philadelphia: WB Saunders, 2000; pp 379–385.
4. McCarty DJ. Differential diagnosis of arthritis: analysis of signs and symptoms. In: Koopman WJ (ed). Arthritis and Allied Conditions, 13th edition. Baltimore: Williams & Wilkins, 1997; pp 35–46.
5. McCarty DJ, O'Duffy JD, Pearson L, Hunter JB. Remitting seronegative symmetrical synovitis with pitting edema. RS3PE syndrome. JAMA 1985;254:2763–2767.
6. Bridges AJ, Hickman PL. RS3PE syndrome and polymyalgia rheumatica: distinguishing features. J Rheumatol 1991;18: 1764–1765.

MUSCULOSKELETAL SIGNS AND SYMPTOMS
C. Disorders of the Low Back and Neck

Low back and neck pain are second only to the common cold as the most common affliction of mankind. Approximately 10%–20% of the US population has back or neck pain each year (1). Low back pain is the fifth most common reason for visiting a physician, according to a US National Ambulatory Care Survey (2).

The symptom of axial skeleton pain is associated with a wide variety of mechanical and medical disorders (3,4; Table 8C-1). Mechanical disorders of the axial skeleton are caused by overuse (muscle strain), trauma, or physical deformity of an anatomic structure (herniated intervertebral disc). Medical disorders that cause spine pain are associated with constitutional symptoms, disease in other organ systems, and inflammatory or infiltrative disease of the axial skeleton. As many as 90% of people with low back or neck pain have a mechanical reason for their discomfort. Characteristically, mechanical disorders are exacerbated by certain physical activities and are relieved by others, and most of these disorders resolve over a short period of time. More than 50% of all patients will improve after one week, and up to 90% are better at eight weeks. However, a recurrence of spinal pain occurs in up to 75% of people over the next year. Back pain will persist for one year and longer in 10% of the spinal pain population (5).

TABLE 8C-1
Disorders Affecting the Low Back and/or Neck

Mechanical
- Muscle strain
- Herniated intervertebral disc
- Osteoarthritis
- Spinal stenosis
- Spinal stenosis with myelopathy[a]
- Spondylolysis/spondylolisthesis[b]
- Adult scoliosis[b]
- Whiplash[a]

Rheumatologic
- Ankylosing spondylitis
- Reactive arthritis
- Psoriatic arthritis
- Enteropathic arthritis
- Rheumatoid arthritis[a]
- Diffuse idiopathic skeletal hyperostosis
- Vertebral osteochondritis[b]
- Polymyalgia rheumatica
- Fibromyalgia
- Behçet's disease[b]
- Whipple's disease[b]
- Hidradenitis suppurativa[b]
- Osteitis condensans ilii[b]

Endocrinologic/Metabolic
- Osteoporosis[b]
- Osteomalacia[b]
- Parathyroid disease[b]
- Microcrystalline disease
- Ochronosis[b]
- Fluorosis[b]
- Heritable genetic disorders

Neurologic/Psychiatric
- Neuropathic arthropathy[b]
- Neuropathies
  - Tumors
  - Vasculitis
  - Compression
- Psychogenic rheumatism
- Depression
- Malingering

Miscellaneous
- Paget's disease
- Vertebral sarcoidosis
- Subacute bacterial endocarditis[b]
- Retroperitoneal fibrosis[b]

Infectious
- Vertebral osteomyelitis
- Meningitis[a]
- Discitis
- Pyogenic sacroiliitis[b]
- Herpes zoster
- Lyme disease

Neoplastic/Infiltrative
- Benign tumors
  - Osteoid osteoma[a]
  - Osteoblastoma
  - Osteochondroma
  - Giant cell tumor
  - Aneurysmal bone cyst
  - Hemangioma
  - Eosinophilic granuloma
  - Gaucher's disease[b]
  - Sacroiliac lipoma[b]

Malignant tumors
- Skeletal metastases
- Multiple myeloma
- Chondrosarcoma
- Chordoma
- Lymphoma[b]
- Intraspinal lesions
- Metastases
- Meningioma
- Vascular malformations
- Gliomas
- Syringomyelia[a]

Hematologic
- Hemoglobinopathies[b]
- Myelofibrosis[b]
- Mastocytosis[b]

Referred Pain
- Vascular
  - Abdominal aorta[b]
  - Carotid[a]
  - Thoracic aorta[a]
- Gastrointestinal
  - Pancreas
  - Gallbladder
  - Intestine
  - Esophagus[a]

Genitourinary[b]
- Kidney
- Ureter
- Bladder
- Uterus
- Ovary
- Prostate

[a] neck predominant
[b] low back predominant
Modified from references 3 and 4, with permission of W.B. Saunders.

Initial Evaluation

In the initial evaluation of patients with spinal pain, the physician must separate individuals with mechanical disorders from those with systemic illnesses. The patient's symptoms and physical signs help differentiate mechanical from systemic causes of axial pain. The initial diagnostic evaluation includes a history and physical examination with complete evaluation of the musculoskeletal system, including palpation of the axial skeleton and assessment of range of motion and alignment of the spine. Neurologic examination to detect evidence of spinal cord, spinal root, or peripheral nerve dysfunction is essential. In most patients, radiographic and laboratory tests are not necessary. Plain radiographs and erythrocyte sedimentation rate (ESR) are most informative in patients who are 50 years or older, who have a previous history of cancer, or who have constitutional symptoms (6).

The initial evaluation should eliminate the presence of cauda equina syndrome and cervical myelopathy, which are rare conditions that require emergency interventions. *Cauda equina compression* is characterized by low back pain, bilateral motor weakness of the lower extremities, bilateral sciatica, saddle anesthesia, and bladder or bowel incontinence. The common causes of cauda equina compression include central herniation of an intervertebral disc, epidural abscess or hematoma, or tumor masses. In the cervical spine, myelopathy with long tract signs (e.g., spasticity, clonus, positive Babinski's sign, incontinence) indicate compression of the spinal cord. The common causes of myelopathy include disc herniation and osteophytic overgrowth. If cauda equina syndrome or cervical myelopathy is suspected, radiographic evaluation is mandatory. Magnetic resonance imaging (MRI) is the most sensitive radiographic technique for visualizing the spine. If the clinician's suspicion is confirmed, surgical decompression of the compromised neural elements is indicated (7).

Systemic Disorders

The majority of people with spinal pain and systemic illnesses can be identified by the presence of one or more of the following: fever or weight loss; pain with recumbency; prolonged morning stiffness; localized bone pain; or visceral pain.

Fever and Weight Loss

In people with a history of fever or weight loss, spinal pain frequently is caused by an infection or tumor (8). Vertebral osteomyelitis causes pain that is slowly progressive, may be either intermittent or constant, is present at rest, and is exacerbated by motion. Tumor pain progresses more rapidly. Plain radiographs generally are not helpful unless more than 30% of the bone calcium has been lost in the area of the lesion. Bone scintigraphy is a sensitive but nonspecific test for bone lesions. Areas of bony involvement and soft-tissue extension are identified best by computed tomography (CT) or MRI, respectively.

Pain with Recumbency

Tumors, benign or malignant, of the spinal column or spinal cord are the prime concern in patients with nocturnal pain or with recumbency (9). Compression of neural elements by expanding masses and associated inflammation accounts for the pain. Physical examination demonstrates localized tenderness, and if the spinal cord or roots are compressed, neurologic dysfunction. MRI is the most sensitive method to detect bony abnormalities, spinal cord or root compromise, and soft-tissue extension of neoplastic lesions.

Morning Stiffness

Morning stiffness lasting an hour or less is a common symptom of mechanical spinal disorders. In contrast, morning stiffness of the lumbar or cervical spine lasting several hours is a common symptom of seronegative spondyloarthropathy. Bilateral sacroiliac pain is associated with ankylosing spondylitis and enteropathic arthritis, whereas reactive arthritis and psoriatic spondylitis may have unilateral sacroiliac pain, or spondylitis without sacroiliitis. Women with spondyloarthropathy may have neck pain and stiffness with minimal low back pain. On physical examination, these patients demonstrate stiffness in all planes of spinal motion. Plain radiographs of the lumbosacral spine are helpful for identifying early changes, loss of lumbar lordosis, joint erosions in the lower one-third of the sacroiliac joints, and squaring of vertebral bodies. More costly radiographic tests are not necessary to identify skeletal abnormalities in people with spondylitis.

Localized Bone Pain

Spinal pain localized to the midline over osseous structures is associated with disorders that fracture or expand bone. Any systemic process that increases mineral loss from bone (osteoporosis), causes bone necrosis (hemoglobinopathy), or replaces bone cells with inflammatory or neoplastic cells (multiple myeloma) weakens vertebral bone to the point that fractures may occur spontaneously or with minimal trauma. Patients with acute fractures experience sudden onset of pain. Bone pain may be the initial manifestation of the underlying disorder. On physical examination, palpation of the affected area produces pain. Plain radiographs may reveal alterations but do not show microfractures. Scintigraphy can detect increased bone activity soon after a fracture occurs, and a CT scan may identify the abnormality. However, locating the lesion is not sufficient to define the specific cause of the bony changes. Laboratory tests including ESR, serum chemistries, and complete blood count are most helpful in differentiating between metabolic and neoplastic disorders that cause localized bone pain.

Visceral Pain

Abnormalities in organs that share segmental innervation with part of the axial skeleton can cause referred back pain. Viscerogenic pain may arise as a result of vascular, gastrointestinal, or genitourinary disorders. The duration and sequence of back pain follows the periodicity of the diseased organ. Colicky pain is associated with spasm in a hollow structure, such as the ureter, colon, or gallbladder. Throbbing pain occurs with vascular lesions. Exertional pain that radiates into the left arm in a C7 distribution may be associated with angina and coronary artery disease. Back pain that coincides with a woman's menstrual cycle may be related to endometriosis.

Physical examination of the abdomen may reveal tenderness over the diseased organ. Laboratory tests are useful to document the presence of an abnormality in the genitourinary (hematuria) or gastrointestinal (amylase) systems. Radiographic tests are helpful for diagnosing some visceral disorders. For example, a CT of the aorta can show abdominal aneurysm and a barium swallow test can reveal esophageal diverticulum.

Mechanical Disorders of the Lumbosacral Spine

Mechanical disorders are the most common causes of low back pain. They include muscle strain, herniated nucleus pulposus, osteoarthritis, spinal stenosis, spondylolisthesis, and adult scoliosis. The clinical characteristics of these disorders are listed in Table 8C-2.

TABLE 8C-2
Mechanical Low Back Pain

	Back strain	Herniated nucleus pulposus	Osteoarthritis	Spinal stenosis	Spondylolisthesis	Adult scoliosis
Age at onset (years)	20–40	30–50	>50	>60	20–30	20–40
Pain pattern						
Location	Back	Back/leg	Back	Leg	Back	Back
Onset	Acute	Acute	Insidious	Insidious	Insidious	Insidious
Upright	I	D	I	I	I	I
Sitting	D	I	D	D	D	D
Bending	I	I	D	D	I	I
SLR	–	+	–	+(exertion)	–	–
Plain x-ray	–	–	+	+	+	+
CT/myelo	–	+	+/–	+	+	–
MR	–	+	+/–	+	+/–	+/–

I, Increase; D, decrease; SLR, straight leg raising; CT, computed tomography; MR, magnetic resonance

Back Strain

Back strain is preceded by some traumatic event that can range from coughing or sneezing to lifting an object heavier than can be supported by the muscles and ligaments of the lumbosacral spine (10). The typical history of muscle strain is acute back pain that radiates up the ipsilateral paraspinous muscles, across the lumbar area, and sometimes caudally to the buttocks without radiation to the thigh. Physical examination reveals limited range of motion in the lumbar area, with paraspinous muscle contraction. No neurologic abnormalities are present.

The Agency for Health Care Policy and Research published an evidence-based review of the effective therapies for acute low back pain in 1994 (11; Table 8C-3). Therapy that combines controlled physical activity with NSAIDs and muscle relaxants can help resolve acute low back pain (12).

Lumbar Disc Herniation

Intervertebral disc herniation causes nerve impingement and inflammation that results in radicular pain (sciatica). Herniation occurs with sudden movement, and frequently is associated with heavy lifting. Sciatica is exacerbated by activities that increase intradiscal pressure, such as sitting, bending, or Valsalva's maneuver. On physical examination, any movement that creates tension in the affected nerve, such as the straight-leg raising test, elicits radicular pain. Neurologic examination may reveal sensory deficit, asymmetry of reflexes, or motor weakness corresponding to the damaged spinal nerve root and degree of impingement (Table 8C-4). An MRI is the best technique to identify the location of disc herniation and nerve impingement, but is significant only when correlated with clinical symptoms

TABLE 8C-3
AHCPR Guidelines for Treatment of Acute Low Back Pain

Patient Education
Natural history of rapid recovery and recurrence
Safe and effective methods of symptom control
Activity modifications
Limit recurrences
Special investigations required with systemic disorders suspected
Risks of common diagnostic tests
Treatment recommendations for persistent symptoms

Medications
Acetaminophen
NSAIDs: decision based on comorbidities, toxicities, cost, patient preferences

Physical treatments
Spinal manipulation in the first month in the absence of radiculopathy (efficacy short term)

Activity Modification
Bed rest no more than four days
Gradual return to normal activities
Low-stress aerobic exercise

(13). Large disc fragments that enhance with gadolinium during MRI examination are more likely to resorb spontaneously without the need for surgical excision (14). Electromyography (EMG) and nerve conduction tests may document abnormal nerve function after impingement has been present for eight weeks or longer.

Therapy for disc herniation includes controlled physical activity, NSAIDs, and epidural corticosteroid injection. For most patients, radicular pain resolves in a 12-week period. Only 5% or fewer of patients with a herniated disc require surgical decompression.

Lumbosacral Spondylosis

Osteoarthritis of the lumbosacral spine may cause localized low back pain. The disorder may progress, causing increased narrowing of the spinal canal that results in spinal stenosis and compression of neural elements (lumbosacral spondylosis). The clinical manifestation of spinal stenosis is neurogenic claudication. As the intervertebral disc degenerates, intersegmental instability and approximation of the vertebral bodies shift the compressive forces across the zygapophyseal joints. The transition of these facet joints from nonweight-bearing to weight-bearing joints leads to zygapophyseal osteoarthritis. As a result, patients develop lumbar pain that increases at the end of the day and radiates across the low back. Physical examination reveals that pain worsens with extension of the spine, and no neurologic deficits are present. Pain radiates into the posterior thigh and is exacerbated by ipsilateral bending to the side with the osteoarthritic joints (facet syndrome). Oblique views of the lumbar spine demonstrate facet joint narrowing, periarticular sclerosis, and osteophytes. These findings have significance only with clinical correlation with historical and physical factors (15).

Lumbar Spinal Stenosis

Spinal stenosis is secondary to the growth of osteophytes, redundancy of the ligamentum flavum, and posterior bulging of the intervertebral discs. Lumbar stenosis may be located in the center of the canal, the lateral recess, or the intervertebral foramen, and may occur at single or multiple levels. The pattern of radiation depends on the location of nerve compression (16). With central canal stenosis, pain in one or both legs occurs with walking. Unlike vascular claudication, leg pain appears after walking variable distances. Individuals with vascular claudication must stop walking to gain relief of pain, whereas those with neurogenic claudication must sit or flex forward, which increases room in the spinal canal and restores blood flow to the spinal roots to decrease pain.

Lateral stenosis causes unilateral leg pain with standing. Stenosis of the intervertebral foramen causes leg pain that is persistent, regardless of the patient's position. The physical examination may be unrevealing unless the patient exercises to the point of developing symptoms. Sensory, motor, and reflex examination during the episode of pain reveals

TABLE 8C-4
Radicular Symptoms and Signs

	Pain distribution	Sensory loss	Motor loss	Reflex loss
Lumbar				
4	Anterior thigh to medial leg	Medial leg to medial malleolus	Anterior tibialis	Patellar
5	Lateral leg to dorsum of foot	Lateral leg to dorsum of foot	Extensor hallucis longus	(Posterior tibial)
S1	Lateral foot	Lateral foot, sole	Peroneus longus and brevis	Achilles
Cervical				
5	Neck to outer shoulder, arm	Shoulder	Deltoid	Biceps, supinator
6	Outer arm to thumb, index fingers	Thumb, index fingers	Biceps, wrist extensors	Biceps, supinator
7	Outer arm to middle fingers	Index, middle fingers	Triceps	Triceps
8	Inner arm to ring, little fingers	Ring, little fingers	Hand muscles	None

abnormal function that reverses when the pain disappears. Motor weakness is present in one-third of patients, and one-half have reflex abnormalities. Plain radiographs of the lumbar spine may demonstrate degenerative disc disease with zygapophyseal joint narrowing, even in patients who are asymptomatic. Thus radiographic alterations are significant only if the patient has corresponding symptoms. A CT scan can identify the presence of zygapophyseal joint disease, trefoil configuration of the spinal canal, and reduced dimensions of the canal. An MRI can document the location of neural compression (Fig. 8C-1).

Prescribing NSAIDs and teaching patients appropriate spinal biomechanics are the initial therapies for osteoarthritis and spinal stenosis. Facet joint injections should be considered when conservative medical therapy does not provide enough relief. People with spinal stenosis may benefit

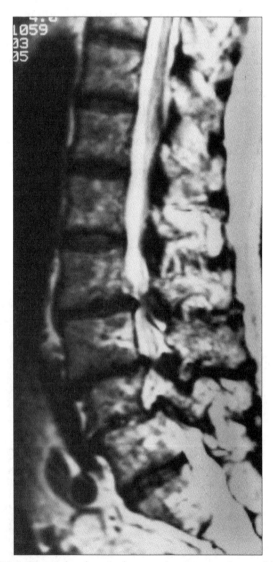

Fig. 8C-1. T2-weighted sagittal magnetic resonance image (MRI) of the lumbar spine. This 82-year-old man had neurogenic claudication in the right leg after walking one block. MRI reveals severe degenerative disc disease with spinal stenosis at multiple levels in the lower lumbar spine.

from epidural corticosteroid injections given every two to three months. Surgical decompression is reserved for patients who are totally incapacitated by pain. Most people with spinal stenosis do not require surgery. In patients of any age who have no serious comorbid illness, the first decompression operation for spinal stenosis has the greatest chance for an excellent outcome (17).

Spondylolisthesis

Spondylolisthesis is the anterior displacement of a vertebral body in relation to the underlying vertebra. Spondylolisthesis usually is secondary to degeneration of intervertebral discs and reorientation of the plane of motion of the zygapophyseal joints. The process also may occur as a developmental abnormality with separation of the pars interarticularis (spondylolysis) (18). People with spondylolisthesis complain of low back pain that is exacerbated with standing and is relieved with rest. Individuals with severe subluxation also have leg pain. Physical examination reveals increased lordosis with a "step off." The neurologic examination reveals no abnormality. Plain radiographs are adequate to demonstrate the lytic lesions in the pars interarticularis, and lateral x-rays demonstrate the degree of subluxation (Fig. 8C-2). An MRI can detect the entrapment and direct impingement of spinal nerve roots associated with this disorder.

Treatment of spondylolisthesis includes flexion strengthening exercises, NSAIDs, and orthopedic corsets. Fusion surgery is useful for patients with greater than grade II slippage and persistent symptoms of neural compression.

Scoliosis

Scoliosis, a lateral curvature of the spine in excess of 10°, most commonly begins to develop in adolescent girls (19). In the lumbar spine, a curve greater than 40° generally leads to a constant rate of progression of 1° per year. Patients complain of increasing back pain that is relieved with bed rest. Neurologic examination reveals findings of nerve compression in more severely affected patients. Plain radiographs allow the clinician to measure the degree of scoliosis by Cobb's method.

In people with scoliosis of 40° or less, exercises, braces, and NSAIDs are effective in reducing pain and maintaining function. Surgical fusion and placement of Harrington rods are reserved for patients with progressive scoliosis who are at increased risk for pulmonary compromise (20).

Mechanical Disorders of the Cervical Spine

Mechanical disorders of the cervical spine are less common than lumbar spine disorders, tend to be less disabling, and result in fewer physician consultations (Table 8C-4).

Neck Strain

Neck strain causes pain in the middle or lower part of the posterior aspect of the neck. The area of pain may be uni-

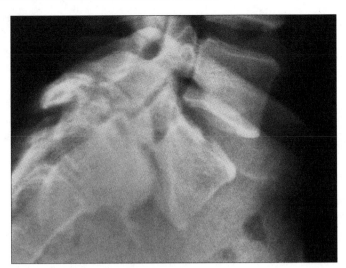

Fig. 8C-2. Lateral spot view of the lumbosacral spine. A grade II spondylolisthesis is seen, with 50% slippage of the vertebral body.

lateral or bilateral and may cover a diffuse area. Pain may radiate toward the head and shoulder, sparing the arms. Neck strain, which rarely is associated with a specific trauma, typically is triggered by sleeping in an awkward position, turning the head rapidly, or sneezing. Physical examination reveals local tenderness in the paracervical muscles, with decreased range of motion and loss of cervical lordosis (21). Muscles most commonly affected include the sternocleidomastoid and the trapezius. No abnormalities are found on shoulder or neurologic examination, laboratory tests, or radiographic studies.

Treatment of neck strain includes controlled physical activity, limited use of cervical orthoses, NSAIDs, and muscle relaxants. Injections of anesthetic and corticosteroid are helpful to decrease local muscle pain, and isometric exercises should be prescribed to maintain strength in the neck. Modifications in the body mechanics while the patient is at work may help prevent recurrences.

Cervical Disc Herniation

Intervertebral disc herniation in the cervical spine causes radicular pain (brachialgia) that radiates from the shoulder to the forearm to the hand (22). The pain may be so severe that the use of the arm is limited. Neck pain is minimal or absent. Cervical herniation occurs with sudden exertion and frequently is associated with heavy lifting. Physical examination reveals increased radicular pain with any maneuver that narrows the intervertebral foramen and places tension on the affected nerve. Spurling's sign (compression, extension, and lateral flexion of the cervical spine) causes radicular pain. Neurologic examination may reveal sensory deficit, reflex asymmetry, or motor weakness corresponding to the damaged spinal nerve root and degree of impingement (Table 8C-3). An MRI is the best tool to identify the location of disc herniation and nerve impingement. An EMG and nerve conduction tests may document abnormal nerve function.

Therapy includes controlled physical activity, cervical orthoses, NSAIDs, and cervical traction. The pain typically subsides within three months; only 20% or fewer of patients require surgical decompression.

Cervical Spondylosis

Osteoarthritis of the cervical spine produces a clinical syndrome similar to that in the lumbosacral spine. As the disc degenerates and the articular structures are brought closer together, the cervical spine becomes unstable. Increased instability results in osteophyte formation in the uncovertebral and zygapophyseal joints, and local synovial inflammation (cervical spondylosis). Neck pain is diffuse and may radiate to the shoulders, suboccipital areas, interscapular muscles, or anterior chest. Involvement of the sympathetic nervous system may cause blurred vision, vertigo, or tinnitus. Physical examination of most patients reveals little, other than midline tenderness. Plain radiographs of the cervical spine are adequate to show the intervertebral narrowing and facet joint sclerosis (Fig. 8C-3). The presence of abnormalities is not necessarily associated with clinical symptoms. For example, an MRI study of individuals 40 years of age or older found more than one-half had degenerative cervical discs (23).

Conservative therapy is effective for cervical spondylosis. NSAIDs and local injections may diminish neck and referred pain. The appropriate amount of immobilization is controversial, however. The use of cervical orthoses may increase neck stiffness and pain. Patient education should stress the importance of balancing the need to restrict neck movement with a cervical collar and to maintain neck flexibility with range-of-motion exercises. Most people with cervical spondylosis have a relapsing course, with recurrent exacerbations of acute neck pain.

Myelopathy

The most serious sequelae of cervical spondylosis is myelopathy. This disorder occurs as a consequence of spinal cord compression by osteophytes, ligamentum flavum, or intervertebral disc (spinal stenosis). Cervical spondylotic myelopathy is the most common cause of spinal cord dysfunction in individuals older than 55 years (24). With disc degeneration, osteophytes develop posteriorly and project into the spinal canal, compressing the cord and its vascular supply. Symptoms may occur with or without movement. The size of the spinal canal is the important static component. Stenosis is associated with an anteroposterior diameter of 10 mm or less. Dynamic stenosis, which is secondary to instability, causes compression of the spinal cord with flexion or extension of the neck. Protruding structures that are located anterior to the spinal cord can compress the posterior and lateral columns. Compression of the anterior spinal artery in the lower cervical spine is another mechanism of spinal cord injury (25). Neck pain is mentioned by only one-third of people with myelopathy.

Clinical symptoms include a history of peculiar sensations in the hands, associated with weakness and uncoordi-

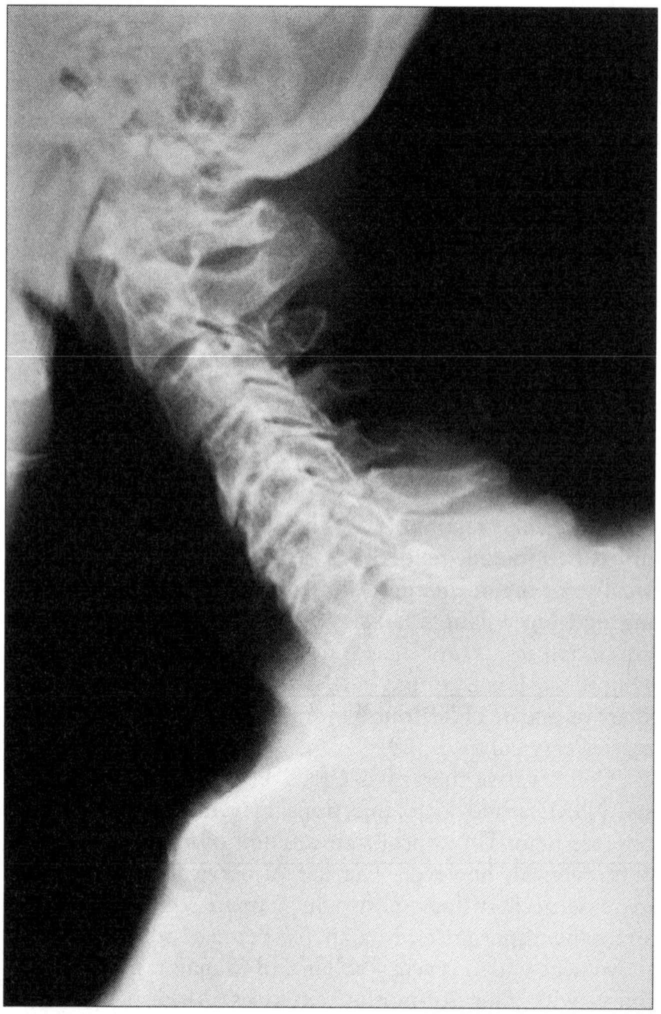

Fig. 8C-3. Lateral view of the cervical spine. This 85-year-old man had localized neck pain with limited cervical rotation. This radiograph reveals diffuse intervertebral disc-space narrowing, with anterior osteophytes characteristic of cervical spondylosis.

nation. In the lower extremities, this disorder can cause gait disturbances, spasticity, leg weakness, and spontaneous leg movements. Older patients may describe leg stiffness, foot shuffling, and a fear of falling. Incontinence is a late manifestation. Physical examination reveals weakness of the appendages in association with spasticity and fasciculations. Sensory deficits include decreased dermatomal sensation and loss of proprioception. Hyperreflexia, clonus, and positive Babinski's sign are present in the lower extremities. Plain radiographs reveal advanced degenerative disease with narrowed disc spaces, osteophytes, facet joint sclerosis and cervical instability. An MRI is the most useful method to detect the extent of spinal cord compression and the effects of compression on the integrity of the cord. Combined CT-myelogram imaging is useful for distinguishing protruding discs from osteophytes.

Although some patients improve with conservative therapy, progressive myelopathy requires surgery to prevent further cord compression and vascular compromise. Surgical intervention works best before severe neurologic deficits are present.

Whiplash

Cervical hyperextension injuries of the neck are associated with rear-collision motor vehicle accidents. Impact from the rear causes acceleration-deceleration injury to the soft-tissue structures in the neck. Paracervical muscles (sternocleidomastoid, longus coli) are stretched or torn, and the sympathetic ganglia may be damaged, resulting in Horner's syndrome (ptosis, meiosis, anhydrosis), nausea, or dizziness. Cervical intervertebral disc injuries may occur.

The symptoms of stiffness and pain with motion are first noticed 12–24 hours after the accident. Headache is a common complaint. Patients may have difficulty swallowing or chewing, and may have paresthesias in the arms. Physical examination reveals decreased range of neck

TABLE 8C-5
Mechanical Neck Pain

	Neck strain	Herniated nucleus pulposus	Osteoarthritis	Myelopathy	Whiplash
Age at onset (years)	20–40	30–50	>50	>60	30–40
Pain pattern					
Location	Neck	Neck/arm	Neck	Arm/leg	Neck
Onset	Acute	Acute	Insidious	Insidious	Acute
Flexion	I	I	D	D	I
Extension	D	I/D	I	I	I
Plain x-ray	–	–	+	+	–
CT/myelo	–	+	+/–	+	–
MR	–	+	+/–	+	–

motion and persistent paracervical muscle contraction. Neurologic examination is unremarkable, and radiographs do not show soft-tissue abnormalities other than loss of cervical lordosis.

Treatment of whiplash includes the use of cervical collars for minimal periods of time (26). Mild analgesics, NSAIDs, and muscle relaxants are prescribed to encourage motion of the neck. Most patients improve after about four weeks of therapy. Patients with persistent symptoms for greater than six months rarely experience significant improvement. The mechanism of chronic pain in whiplash patients remains to be determined (27).

DAVID BORENSTEIN, MD

References

1. *Frymoyer JW, Pope MH, Costanza MC, Rosen JC, Goggin JE, Wilder DG. Epidemiologic studies of low-back pain. Spine 1980;5:419–423.*

2. *Hart LG, Deyo RA, Cherkin DC. Physician office visits for low back pain. Frequency, clinical evaluation, and treatment patterns from a U.S. national survey. Spine 1955;20:11–19.*

3. *Borenstein DG, Wiesel SW, Boden SD. Low Back Pain: Medical Diagnosis and Comprehensive Management, 2nd edition. Philadelphia: W.B. Saunders, 1995.*

4. *Borenstein DG, Wiesel SW, Boden SD. Neck Pain: Medical Diagnosis and Comprehensive Management. Philadelphia: W.B. Saunders, 1996.*

5. *van den Hoogen HJM, Koes BW, Deville W, van Eijk JTM, Bouter LM. The prognosis of low back pain in general practice. Spine 1997;22:1515–1521.*

6. *Deyo RA, Rainville J, Kent DL. What can the history and physical examination tell us about low back pain? JAMA 1992;268:760–765.*

7. *Shapiro S. Medical realities of cauda equina syndrome secondary to lumbar disc herniation. Spine 2000;25:348–351.*

8. *Zimmermann B, Lally EV. Infectious disease of the spine. Semin Spine Surg 1995;7:177–186.*

9. *Nicholas JJ, Christy WC. Spinal pain made worse by recumbency: a clue to spinal cord tumors. Arch Phys Med Rehabil 1986;67:598–600.*

10. *Cooper RG. Understanding paraspinal muscle dysfunction in low back pain: a way forward? Ann Rheum Dis 1993;52: 413–415.*

11. *Agency for Health Care Policy and Research. Acute low back problems in adults, clinical practice guideline. Rockville, MD: Agency for Health Care Policy and Research, 1994: Publication no. 95-0642.*

12. *Cherkin DC, Wheeler KJ, Barlow W, Deyo RA. Medication use for low back pain in primary care. Spine 1998;23:607–614.*

13. *Jensen M, Brant-Zawadzki M, Obuchowski N, Modic MT, Malkasian D, Ross JS. Magnetic resonance imaging of the lumbar spine in people without back pain. N Engl J Med 1994;331:69–73.*

14. *Komori H, Okawa A, Haro H, Muneta T, Yamamoto H, Shinomiya K. Contrast-enhanced magnetic resonance imaging in conservative management of lumbar disc herniation. Spine 1998;23:67–73.*

15. *Boden SD. The use of radiographic imaging studies in the evaluation of patients who have degenerative disorders of the lumbar spine. J Bone Joint Surg Am 1996;78:114–124.*

16. *Moreland LW, Lopez-Mendez A, Alarcon GS. Spinal stenosis: a comprehensive review of the literature. Semin Arthritis Rheum 1989;19:127–149.*

17. *Airaksinen O, Herno A, Turunen V, Saari T, Suomlainen O. Surgical outcome of 438 patients treated surgically for lumbar spinal stenosis. Spine 1997;22:2278–2282.*

18. *Fredrickson BE, Baker D, McHolick WJ, Yuan HA, Lubicky JP. The natural history of spondylolysis and spondylolisthesis. J Bone Joint Surg Am 1984;66:699–707.*

19. *Perennou D, Marcelli C, Herisson C, Simon L. Adult lumbar scoliosis: Epidemiologic aspects in a low-back pain population. Spine 1994;19:123–128.*

20. *Rizzi PE, Winter RB, Lonstein JE, Denis F, Perra JH. Adult spinal deformity and respiratory failure. Surgical results in 35 patients. Spine 1997;22:2517–2531.*

21. *Helliwell PS, Evans PF, Wright V. The straight cervical spine: does it indicate muscle spasm? J Bone Joint Surg Br 1994;76: 103–106.*

22. *Rechtine GR, Bolesta MJ. Cervical radiculopathy. Semin Spine Surg 1999;11:363–372.*

23. *Lehto IJ, Tertti MO, Komu ME, Paajanen HE, Tuominen J, Kormano MJ. Age-related MRI changes at 0.1 T in cervical discs in asymptomatic subjects. Neuroradiology 1994;36:49–53.*

24. *Bernhardt M, Hynes RA, Blume HW, White AA III. Cervical spondylotic myelopathy. J Bone Joint Surg Am 1993;75: 119–128.*

25. *Fehlings MG, Skaf G. A review of the pathophysiology of cervical spondylotic myelopathy with insights for potential novel mechanisms drawn from traumatic spinal cord injury. Spine 1998;24:2730–2737.*

26. *Spitzer WO, Skovron ML, Salmi LR, et al. Scientific monograph of the Quebec Task Force on whiplash-associated disorders: redefining "whiplash" and its management. Spine 1995;20:1S–73S.*

27. *Freeman MD, Croft AC, Rossignol AM, Weaver DS, Reiser M. A review and methodologic critique of the literature refuting whiplash syndrome. Spine 1999;24:86–96.*

MUSCULOSKELETAL SIGNS AND SYMPTOMS
D. Regional Rheumatic Pain Syndromes

Regional rheumatic pain syndromes present challenges to the clinician because of their prevalence, complexity, and lack of diagnostic laboratory tests, but success in the diagnosis and treatment of these disorders is most gratifying. The conditions discussed in this chapter include disorders involving muscles, tendons, entheses, joints, cartilage, ligaments, fascia, bone, and nerve. A working knowledge of regional anatomy and an approach that uses a regional differential diagnosis will help in obtaining a specific diagnosis (1).

A precise history is needed to identify the conditions present; more than one syndrome can occur concomitantly. A complete neuromusculoskeletal examination should be performed, emphasizing careful palpation, passive range of motion (ROM), active ROM, and sometimes, active ROM with resistance. Some guidelines for the management of these conditions are provided in Table 8D-1.

Causative Factors

Many syndromes of the neuromusculoskeletal system are the result of injury from a specific activity or event, ranging from one episode to repetitive overuse, especially when abnormal body position or mechanics is present. Tendons become less flexible with aging, heightening their susceptibility to injury. Due to aging and with disuse atrophy, the muscles become weaker and exhibit less endurance and bulk, resulting in a decreased ability of the muscle to absorb mechanical forces. Consequently, such forces are transmitted to joints, tendons, ligaments, and entheses. A musculotendinous unit shortened from lack of stretching is more prone to injury. In addition, genetic predisposition to certain regional syndromes results from variations in anatomy and abnormal biomechanics. Systemic inflammatory diseases may have local manifestations that are characteristic. Unfortunately, causative factors often are not identified.

General Management Concepts
Drug Therapy
Oral medications, including nonsteroidal anti-inflammatory drugs (NSAIDs) and analgesics, play a role in the management of regional musculoskeletal disorders. The NSAIDs help reduce inflammation and pain. For additional pain relief, such analgesics as acetaminophen can be added. Tricyclic antidepressants, such as amitriptyline, also may be useful in chronic pain syndromes, particularly in neurogenic or myofascial pain.

Rather than relying on oral medications alone, comprehensive management of these regional syndromes is essential. The causative aspects should be evaluated, and activity modification should be advised as needed. Local injections and physical therapy also are useful components of treatment.

Intralesional Injections

After making a specific diagnosis of a regional rheumatic pain syndrome, local injection with lidocaine, corticosteroids, or both often is beneficial (2). In fact, the immediate pain relief from a properly directed injection into a tendon sheath, bursa, enthesis, or nerve area may validate the diagnosis. Injections with corticosteroid preparations into areas of nonspecific muscle tenderness should be discouraged.

Basic principles of intralesional injections include aseptic technique and use of small needles (a 25-gauge 5/8" or 1 1/2", or a 22-gauge 1 1/2"). The use of separate syringes for lidocaine and corticosteroid avoids mixing the two substances and permits infiltration of lidocaine, beginning intracutaneously with a small wheal and continuing to the site of the lesion. This method makes the injection relatively painless. When the needle reaches the desired site, the syringe is changed, but the needle is left in place, and the corticosteroid is injected. This technique helps avoid possible sub-

TABLE 8D-1
Guidelines for Management of Regional Rheumatic Pain Syndromes

1. Exclude systemic disease and infection by appropriate methods. Diagnostic aspiration is mandatory in suspected septic bursitis. Gram stain and culture of bursal fluid provide prompt diagnosis of a septic bursitis.

2. Teach the patient to recognize and avoid aggravating factors that cause recurrences.

3. Instruct the patient in self-help therapy, including the daily performance of mobilizing exercises.

4. Provide an explanation of the cause of pain, thus alleviating concern for a crippling disease. When the regional rheumatic pain syndrome overlies another rheumatic problem, the clinician must explain the contribution each disorder plays in the symptom complex and then help the patient deal with each one.

5. Provide relief from pain with safe analgesics, counterirritants (heat, ice, vapocoolant sprays), and if appropriate, intralesional injection of a local anesthetic or anesthetic with depository corticosteroid agent.

6. Provide the patient with an idea of the duration of therapy necessary to restore order to the musculoskeletal system

7. Symptomatic relief often corroborates the diagnosis.

cutaneous and skin atrophy secondary to corticosteroid use. When injecting a tendon sheath, the needle should be directed as parallel as possible to the tendon fibers, not into the tendon itself. Using a more water-soluble corticosteroid preparation, such as a betamethasone phosphate and betamethasone acetate combination, may lessen the possibility of corticosteroid-induced tendon weakness or post-injection flare.

Physical Therapy

The goals of therapeutic exercise are to increase flexibility by stretching, improve muscle strength by resistive exercises, and augment muscle endurance by repetition. The physician should become knowledgeable about exercise prescriptions for the various conditions (3). For example, older women tend to have tight calf muscles, which predispose to calf cramps, Achilles tendon problems, or other ankle and foot disorders. Tight quadriceps, hamstring, and iliopsoas muscles are related to problems in the low back, hip, and knee regions. Exercises to stretch these muscles can be taught by the physician. Instruction can be given in the office for quadriceps strengthening, especially by straight-leg raising from the sitting position, and for pelvic tilt exercise (4).

Heat or cold modalities provide pain relief and muscle relaxation, and they serve as a prelude to an exercise regimen. These modalities are of doubtful benefit when used alone over extended periods.

Disorders of the Shoulder Region

Shoulder pain is one of the most common musculoskeletal complaints in people over the age of 40. In younger people, athletic injuries are a frequent source of such pain. The shoulder itself is a remarkable ball-and-socket joint, which allows for considerable motion. This mobility, however, is accompanied by some instability, from which shoulder problems can result. Many shoulder conditions have similar precipitating factors and symptoms, and multiple lesions involving different structures around the joint may be present. Understanding the anatomy is important to diagnosis and management (see Chapter 2).

The glenohumeral, acromioclavicular, sternoclavicular, and scapulothoracic joints work synchronously to achieve most shoulder motions. Important shoulder ligaments include the acromioclavicular, capsular, coracoacromial, coracoclavicular (trapezoid and conoid), coracohumeral, sternoclavicular, and glenohumeral ligaments. The subacromial bursa, which is inferior to the acromion, is contiguous to the subdeltoid bursa and covers the humeral head. Overlying the bursa is the deltoid muscle. The rotator cuff, composed of the tendons of the supraspinatus, infraspinatus, teres minor, and subscapularis muscles, attaches at the humeral tuberosities. The rotator cuff provides internal and external rotation of the shoulder. It also fixes the humeral head in the glenoid fossa during abduction to counteract the pull of the deltoid, which tends to displace the humeral head from the glenoid. The mechanism whereby the deltoid

muscle and the downward-acting short rotators combine to produce abduction is called *force-couple*. After 30° of abduction, a constant 1:2 ratio exists between movement of the scapular articulation and the glenohumeral joint, with a combined movement known as *scapulohumeral rhythm*.

Pain may be referred to the shoulder from the cervical region due to cervical spondylosis; from the thorax due to a Pancoast tumor; from the abdomen area secondary to lesions in the liver, spleen, or gallbladder; or from the diaphragm.

Rotator Cuff Tendinitis

Rotator cuff tendinitis, or impingement syndrome, is the most common cause of shoulder pain. Tendinitis (and not bursitis) is the primary cause of pain, but secondary involvement of the subacromial bursa occurs in some cases. The condition may be acute or chronic and may or may not be associated with calcific deposits within the tendon. The key finding is pain in the rotator cuff on active abduction, especially between 60° and 120°, and sometimes when lowering the arm. In more severe cases, however, pain may begin on initial abduction and continue throughout the ROM. In acute tendinitis, pain comes on more abruptly and may be excruciating. Such cases tend to occur in younger patients and are more likely to have calcific deposits in the supraspinatus tendon insertion (Fig. 8D-1). The deposits are best seen on radiographs in external rotation, appearing round or oval and several centimeters in length. These deposits may resolve spontaneously over

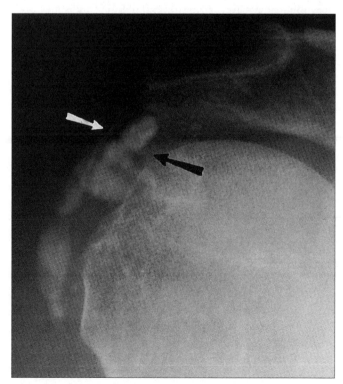

Fig. 8D-1. Right shoulder of a 44-year-old man, illustrating massive calcareous deposits in the supraspinatus tendon (white arrow) and subdeltoid bursa (black arrow).

time. A true subacromial bursitis also may result from the rupture of calcific material into the bursa.

Chronic rotator cuff tendinitis typically presents as an ache in the shoulder, usually over the lateral deltoid, and occurs with various movements, especially on abduction and internal rotation. Other symptoms include difficulty in dressing oneself and night pain due to difficulty in positioning the shoulders. Tenderness on palpation and some loss of motion may be evident on examination. The initial movement to detect rotator cuff tendinitis is to determine whether pain is present on active abduction of the arm in the horizontal position. Passive abduction then is carried out. Usually less pain is present on passive abduction than active abduction. Conversely, pain may be increased on active abduction against resistance. The impingement sign nearly always is positive. This maneuver is performed by the examiner using one hand to raise the patient's arm in forced flexion while the other hand prevents scapular rotation (5). A positive sign occurs if pain develops at or before 180° of forward flexion. Another useful test to confirm rotator cuff disease is the *impingement test*, performed by injecting 2–4 mL of 2% lidocaine into the subacromial bursa. Pain relief on abduction following the injection denotes a positive impingement test. The same test can be used in another way to determine whether apparent shoulder weakness is due to pain; once the injection eliminates the pain, the arm is retested for weakness. If the weakness still is present, the result is considered positive.

The causes of rotator cuff tendinitis are multifactorial, but relative overuse, especially from overhead activity causing impingement of the rotator cuff, commonly is implicated. Compression of the rotator cuff occurs by the edge and undersurface of the anterior third of the acromion above, and the coracohumeral ligament by the humeral head below. Age-related factors include degeneration and decreases in vascularity of the cuff tendons as well as reduction of muscle strength. Osteophytes on the inferior portion of the acromioclavicular joint or acute trauma to the shoulder region contribute to tendinitis development. Finally, inflammatory processes, such as rheumatoid arthritis (RA), cause rotator cuff tendinitis, independent of impingement.

Treatment consists of rest and such modalities as hot packs, cold applications, or ultrasound with specific ROM exercises as soon as tolerated. NSAIDs often are beneficial; however, the most frequent treatment is injection of a depot corticosteroid into the subacromial bursa, the floor of which is contiguous with the rotator cuff (6).

Rotator Cuff Tear

Acute rotator cuff tears after trauma are easily recognized. The trauma may be superimposed on an already attenuated, and possibly partially torn, cuff. In cuff rupture resulting from trauma (especially falls), fractures of the humeral head and dislocation of the shoulder joint should be considered. Conversely, when a humeral fracture is the presenting problem, a tear of the rotator cuff may be present, but unrecognized. However, at least one-half of patients with tears recall no trauma. In such cases, degeneration of the rotator cuff occurs gradually, eventually resulting in a complete tear. Rotator cuff tears are classified as small (1 cm or less), medium (1 – 3 cm), large (3 – 5 cm), or massive (>5 cm) (7). Shoulder pain, weakness on abduction, and loss of motion occur in varying degrees, ranging from severe pain and mild weakness to no pain and marked weakness. A positive drop-arm sign, with inability to actively maintain 90° of passive shoulder abduction, may be present in large or massive tears. Surgical repair is indicated in younger patients.

Less easily diagnosed are the smaller, chronic, full-thickness tears of the rotator cuff and partial, incomplete or non–full-thickness tears. Pain on abduction, night pain, weakness, loss of abduction, and tenderness on palpation can be present in these types of tears. A small complete tear, however, can exist despite fairly good abduction. Tears of the rotator cuff may occur as a result of chronic RA inflammation, and they often present with cystic swelling around the shoulder.

The definitive diagnosis of a ruptured rotator cuff is established by an abnormal arthrogram showing a communication between the glenohumeral joint and the subacromial bursa. In a partial tear, in which an intact layer of rotator cuff tissue still separates the joint space from the subacromial bursa, a small, ulcer-like crater is seen on the arthrogram. Diagnostic ultrasonography or magnetic resonance imaging (MRI) can identify rotator cuff tears (8). At most centers, MRI has become the most expeditious imaging technique to diagnose tears. Small, complete tears and incomplete tears of the rotator cuff are treated conservatively with rest, physical therapy, and NSAIDs. Although their role has not yet been established by careful studies, subacromial injections of a corticosteroid may relieve pain.

Bicipital Tendinitis

Bicipital tendinitis is manifested by pain, most often in the anterior region of the shoulder, but occasionally more diffuse. The pain may be acute, usually is chronic, and is related to impingement of the biceps tendon by the acromion. Tenosynovitis of the long head of the biceps is present, and the tendon may be frayed and fibrotic. Palpation over the bicipital groove reveals localized tenderness. The patient's response should be compared with palpation of the opposite side, as the bicipital tendon typically shows some degree of tenderness. Pain may be reproduced over the bicipital tendon by supination of the forearm against resistance (Yergason's sign), shoulder flexion against resistance (Speed's test), or by extension of the shoulder. Bicipital tendinitis and rotator cuff tendinitis may occur at the same time. Treatment of bicipital tendinitis consists of rest, hot packs, ultrasound, and as pain subsides, passive followed by active ROM exercises. NSAIDs may be helpful, and occasionally, a small quantity of corticosteroid carefully injected into or around the tendon sheath may be beneficial.

Subluxation of the bicipital tendon is manifested as pain, with the shoulder going out and then popping back in. Tenderness may be present over the bicipital tendon, and a snap over the tendon may be noted in the shoulder when the arm is passively abducted to 90° and then moved from internal to external rotation and back. Rupture of the biceps tendon occurs at the superior edge of the bicipital groove. Full rupture of the long head of the tendon produces a characteristic bulbous enlargement of the lateral half of the muscle belly. Generally, these two latter conditions of the biceps tendon are treated conservatively.

Adhesive Capsulitis

Known also as *frozen shoulder* or *pericapsulitis*, adhesive capsulitis is associated with generalized pain and tenderness, and accompanied by severe loss of active and passive motion in all planes. It is rare before age 40 and may be secondary to any type of shoulder problem. Muscle atrophy may occur early in the course. Every stiff and painful shoulder, however, is not necessarily adhesive capsulitis. Inflammatory arthritis and diabetes may cause adhesive capsulitis. Additional factors, such as immobility, low pain threshold, depression, neglect, or improper initial treatment, also favor the development of a frozen shoulder. Many cases, however, are idiopathic. The joint capsule adheres to the anatomic neck, and the axillary fold binds to itself, causing restricted motion. The capsule becomes thickened and contracted.

Arthrography helps confirm this diagnosis by showing decreased shoulder joint capsule volume, loss of the normal axillary pouch, and often, the absence of dye in the biceps tendon sheath. The joint may accept as little as 0.5–3.0 mL of dye, whereas a normal shoulder joint has a capacity of 28–35 mL. A frozen shoulder is treated most effectively with a comprehensive program involving NSAIDs, corticosteroid injections into the glenohumeral joint and the subacromial bursa, and physical therapy (9). Initial physical therapy consists of ice packs, ultrasound, transcutaneous electrical nerve stimulation, and gentle ROM exercises, beginning with pendulum exercises and wall-climbing with the fingers. Active ROM and strengthening exercises conclude the rehabilitation process, which typically requires months. Manipulation under anesthesia may be needed in rare refractory cases.

Suprascapular Neuropathy

The suprascapular nerve, which innervates the supraspinatus and infraspinatus muscles, may be damaged by trauma, overactivity of the shoulder, or a fracture of the scapula. The nerve may be compressed at the suprascapular notch. The condition is marked by weakness on abduction and external rotation. In chronic cases, atrophy of the supraspinatus and infraspinatus muscles may be seen. Electrodiagnostic studies help confirm the diagnosis. Treatment generally consists of physical therapy and may include a local corticosteroid injection into the area of the suprascapular notch. In some chronic cases, surgical decompression is needed.

Long Thoracic Nerve Paralysis

Injury to the long thoracic nerve produces weakness of the serratus anterior muscle, resulting in a winged scapula. Pain may be felt along the base of the neck and downward over the scapula and deltoid region, along with fatigue on elevation of the arm. The winging of the scapula becomes apparent when the patient pushes against a wall with outstretched arms. Trauma and diabetes seem to be common causes of this disorder, but it often is idiopathic and usually self-limited.

Brachial Plexopathy

Brachial plexopathy presents with a deep, sharp shoulder pain of rapid onset, which is exacerbated by abduction and rotation, followed by weakness of the shoulder girdle. An electromyogram helps confirm this diagnosis by demonstrating positive sharp waves and fibrillations in the involved muscles. Recovery may take from one month to several years. Brachial plexopathy can result from trauma, tumor, radiation, post-vaccination neuritis, diabetes, infection, or median sternotomy done for cardiac surgery. Idiopathic cases also occur.

Thoracic Outlet Syndrome

Thoracic outlet syndrome includes a constellation of symptoms, resulting from compression of the neurovascular bundle where the brachial plexus and subclavian artery and vein exit beneath the clavicle and subclavius muscle. The neurovascular bundle is bordered below by the first rib, anteriorly by the scalenus anterior muscle, and posteriorly by the scalenus medius muscle. The clinical picture depends on which component is compressed – neural, vascular, or both. Neurologic symptoms predominate in most patients. Pain, paresthesia, and numbness are the principal symptoms, radiating from the neck and shoulder down to the arm and hand, especially involving the fourth and fifth digits. Activity worsens symptoms. Weakness and atrophy of intrinsic muscles are late findings. Vascular symptoms consist of discoloration, temperature change, pain on use, and Raynaud's phenomenon.

The differential diagnosis is large, and the diagnosis is partly one of exclusion. Incidence is greater in men than in women. Inquiries about the relationship of symptoms to activities are essential, because shoulder abduction may initiate or worsen symptoms. A careful neurologic examination and evaluation for arterial and venous insufficiency and postural abnormalities should be conducted. The Adson test, in which the patient holds a deep breath, extends the neck, and then turns the chin toward the side being examined, is positive when the radial pulse becomes extremely weak or disappears. Many normal people have this finding, but if the maneuver reproduces the patient's symptoms, it is more significant. With the hyperabduction maneuver, the radial pulse is monitored when the patient raises an arm above the head. A reduction in the radial pulse strength may indicate arterial compression. Again, this test may be positive in normal individuals. Chest radiography may exclude a cervical rib, an elongated transverse process of C7, healing fractures, and exostoses. Because of the difficulty in measuring nerve conduction velocity of the involved nerves, results of these tests are somewhat inconsistent, but in capable hands, they furnish additional supporting information. Somatosensory evoked potentials also have been used successfully. An angiogram or venogram can be obtained in cases of suspected arterial or venous compression.

In general, management of thoracic outlet syndrome is conservative. Good posture is emphasized. Stretching of the scalene and pectoral muscles, together with scapula mobilization and strengthening of the shoulder girdle musculature is beneficial. A local anesthetic injection into the scalene anticus muscle may be helpful if a trigger point is present. In resistant or severe cases of thoracic outlet syndrome, the first rib and the scalene muscle may be resected.

Disorders of the Elbow Region

Olecranon Bursitis
The subcutaneous olecranon bursa frequently is involved with bursitis, usually secondary to chronic, low-grade trauma or a systemic inflammatory condition, such as RA or gout. The bursa characteristically is swollen and tender on pressure, but pain may be minimal and ROM usually is preserved. Aspiration may yield clear or blood-tinged fluid with a low viscosity, or grossly hemorrhagic fluid. Aspiration alone and protection from trauma generally are sufficient to resolve the condition. A small dose of corticosteroid may be injected, but there is a possibility of secondary infection, skin atrophy, or chronic local pain that apparently results from subclinical skin atrophy (10).

Inflammatory olecranon bursitis may be due to gout, RA, or calcium pyrophosphate deposition disease. Olecranon bursitis has been seen in uremic patients undergoing hemodialysis. With septic olecranon bursitis, localized erythema is the major clue. Heat, pain, and a positive culture frequently are present. The condition is treated by aspiration, drainage, and the administration of appropriate antibiotics. Surgical excision occasionally is needed.

Lateral Epicondylitis
Lateral epicondylitis, or tennis elbow, is a common condition in those who overuse their arms. Localized tenderness directly over or slightly anterior to the lateral epicondyle is the hallmark of this disorder. Pain may occur during handshakes, lifting a briefcase, or similar activities. Probably fewer than 10% of patients actually acquire lateral epicondylitis through playing tennis; job and recreational activities, including gardening and other athletics, are the usual causes. Pathologically, the condition consists of degeneration of the common extensor tendon, particularly the extensor carpi radialis brevis tendon. Tendon tears may be the cause of chronic cases.

Treatment is aimed at altering activities and preventing overuse of the forearm musculature. Ice packs, heat, and NSAIDs are of some benefit. A forearm brace also can be used. A local corticosteroid injection with a 25-gauge needle over the lateral epicondyle often produces satisfactory initial relief. Isometric strengthening is important as the initial part of a rehabilitation program.

Evaluation of chronic cases should include radiography to check for calcification, exostosis, or other bony abnormalities. Entrapment of the radial nerve at the elbow can cause discomfort and a vague aching at that site. Forced forearm supination against resistance aggravates symptoms of a neural entrapment more than those of lateral epicondylitis, in which resisted wrist extension aggravates the pain.

Medial Epicondylitis
Medial epicondylitis, or golfer's elbow, which mainly involves the flexor carpi radialis, is less common and less disabling than lateral epicondylitis. Local pain and tenderness over the medial epicondyle are present, and resistance to wrist flexion exacerbates the pain. Alteration of activities and use of NSAIDs usually alleviate the problem, although a local corticosteroid injection occasionally is required.

Tendinitis of Musculotendinous Insertion of Biceps
Tendinitis of the distal insertion of the biceps (lacertus fibrosus) may cause dull pain throughout the antecubital fossa of the elbow (11). Palpation confirms the source of pain, and mild swelling may be present. Heat, NSAIDs, rest, and occasionally, a local injection of corticosteroids generally are beneficial in this self-limited condition.

Ulnar Nerve Entrapment
Entrapment of the ulnar nerve at the elbow produces numbness and paresthesia of the little finger and the adjacent side of the fourth digit, as well as aching of the medial aspect of the elbow. Hand clumsiness can be present. Tenderness may be elicited when the ulnar nerve groove, located on the posteroinferior surface of the medial epicondyle, is compressed. The little finger may have decreased sensation and weakness on abduction and flexion. Elevating the hand by resting the forearm on the head for one minute may produce paresthesia. In long-standing cases, atrophy and weakness of the ulnar intrinsic muscles of the hand occur. A positive Tinel's sign, elicited by tapping the nerve at the elbow, often is present. Similar symptoms may result from subluxation of the nerve.

Ulnar nerve entrapment has many causes, including external compression from occupation, compression during anesthesia, trauma, prolonged bed rest, fractures, and inflammatory arthritis. A nerve conduction test that demonstrates slowing of ulnar nerve motor and sensory conduction and prolonged proximal latency aids in the diagnosis. Avoiding pressure on the elbow and repetitive elbow flexion may be all that is necessary for improvement, but in severe, persistent cases, surgical correction is needed.

Disorders of the Wrist and Hand

Ganglion

A ganglion is a cystic swelling arising from a joint or tendon sheath that occurs most commonly over the dorsum of the wrist. It is lined with synovium and contains thick, jelly-like fluid. Ganglia generally are of unknown cause but may develop secondary to trauma or prolonged wrist extension. Usually, the only symptom is swelling, but occasionally, a large ganglion produces discomfort on wrist extension. Treatment, if indicated, consists of aspiration of the fluid, with or without injection of corticosteroid. Use of a splint may help prevent recurrence. In severe cases, the whole ganglion may be removed surgically.

de Quervain's Tenosynovitis

De Quervain's tenosynovitis may result from repetitive activity that involves pinching with the thumb while moving the wrist. It has been reported to occur in new mothers as a complication of pregnancy. In the past, it was thought to be caused by repetitive diapering using safety pins, but it also may be a result of injury to the wrist area caused by lifting the baby. The symptoms are pain, tenderness, and occasionally, swelling over the radial styloid. Pathologic findings include inflammation and narrowing of the tendon sheath around the abductor pollicis longus and extensor pollicis brevis. A positive Finkelstein test result usually is seen: pain increases when the thumb is folded across the palm, and the fingers are flexed over the thumb, as the examiner passively deviates the wrist toward the ulnar side. This test, however, also may be positive in osteoarthritis (OA) of the first carpometacarpal joint. Treatment involves splinting, local corticosteroid injection, and NSAIDs as indicated (12). Rarely, surgical removal of inflamed tenosynovium is needed.

Tenosynovitis of the Wrist

Tenosynovitis occurs in other flexor and extensor tendons of the wrist in addition to those involved in de Quervain's tenosynovitis (13). The individual tendons on the extensor side that may be vulnerable are the extensor pollicis longus, extensor indicis proprius, extensor digiti minimi, and extensor carpi ulnaris; on the flexor side, the flexor carpi radialis, flexor carpi ulnaris, flexor digitorum superficialis, and flexor digitorum profundus are susceptible.

The findings vary depending on which tendon is involved. Localized pain and tenderness usually are present, and there sometimes is swelling. Pain on resisted movement often is seen. The tenosynovitis may be misinterpreted as arthritis of the wrist.

This problem may be due to repetitive use, a traumatic episode, or inflammatory arthritis, or it may be idiopathic. Treatment consists of avoiding overuse, splinting, and NSAIDs. A local corticosteroid injection into the tendon sheath, avoiding direct injection into the tendon itself, usually is beneficial.

Pronator Teres Syndrome

The pronator teres syndrome, an uncommon condition, may be difficult to diagnose because some features are similar to carpal tunnel syndrome. In this case, however, the median nerve is compressed at the level of the pronator teres muscle. The patient may complain of aching in the volar aspect of the forearm, numbness in the thumb and index finger, weakness on gripping with the thumb, and writer's cramp. The most specific finding is tenderness of the proximal part of the pronator teres, which may be aggravated by resistive pronation of the forearm. The pronator compression often produces paresthesia after 30 seconds or less. In some patients, a positive Tinel's sign is found at the proximal edge of the pronator teres. Unlike carpal tunnel syndrome, nocturnal awakening and numbness in the morning are absent. Pronator teres syndrome is thought to result from overuse by repetitive grasping or pronation, trauma, or a space-occupying lesion.

Electrodiagnostic studies often fail to localize the lesion, but may reveal signs of denervation of the forearm muscles supplied by the median nerve, but sparing the pronator teres. If the condition does not improve with alteration of activities and with time, exploratory surgery may be undertaken to exclude fibrous or tendinous bands, or a hypertrophied pronator muscle may be found.

Anterior Interosseous Nerve Syndrome

Compression of the anterior interosseous nerve near its bifurcation from the median nerve produces weakness of the flexor pollicis longus, flexor digitorum profundus, and pronator quadratus muscles. Sensation is not affected, but a person with this syndrome cannot form an "O" with the thumb and index finger, because motion is lost in the interphalangeal (IP) joint of the thumb and the distal interphalangeal (DIP) joint of the index finger. Electromyography may confirm the diagnosis. Repetitive overuse, trauma, and fibrous bands are the principal causes of this syndrome. Protection from trauma usually results in improvement; if not, surgical exploration may be indicated.

Radial Nerve Palsy

The most common type of radial nerve palsy is the spiral groove syndrome, or bridegroom palsy, in which the radial nerve is compressed against the humerus. The most prominent feature is a wrist-drop with flexion of the metacarpophalangeal (MCP) joints and adduction of the thumb. Anesthesia in the web space and hypesthesia from the dorsal aspect of the forearm to the thumb, index, and middle fingers may be present. If the radial nerve is compressed more proximally through improper use of crutches or prolonged leaning of the arm over the back of a chair ("Saturday night palsy"), weakness of the triceps and brachioradialis muscles may occur. Compression injuries generally heal over a period of weeks. Splinting the wrist during this recovery time prevents overstretching of the paralyzed muscles and ligaments. Electrodiagnostic studies are helpful in determining the specific point of compression.

Posterior Interosseous Nerve Syndrome

The posterior interosseous nerve, a branch of the radial nerve, primarily is a motor nerve, so sensory disturbances are rare. Posterior interosseous nerve entrapment in the radial tunnel produces discomfort in the proximal lateral portion of the forearm. The fingers cannot be extended at the MCP joints. Occupational or recreational repetitive activity, with forceful supination, wrist extension, or radial deviation against resistance may contribute to this syndrome. Direct trauma and such nontraumatic conditions as ganglion cysts also have been implicated. In RA, this syndrome is caused by synovial compression of the nerve and, therefore, must be distinguished from a ruptured extensor tendon (14).

Superficial Radial Neuropathy (Cheiralgia Paresthetica)

A lesion of the radial nerve is more common than once thought and causes such symptoms as a burning or shooting pain and, sometimes, numbness and tingling over the dorsoradial aspect of the wrist, thumb, and index fingers. Hyperpronation and ulnar wrist flexion may be provocative. Decreased pinprick sensation and a positive Tinel's sign may be elicited. Electrodiagnostic studies are helpful in the diagnosis.

Tight wrist restraints from handcuffs or watchbands are well-known causes. Trauma to the area, repetitive wrist motion, diabetes, ganglion cyst, venipuncture, and local surgical procedures are other possible etiologies. The neuropathy may resolve with time. Treatment consists of splinting, NSAIDs, local corticosteroid injection, or surgical neurolysis in some cases.

Carpal Tunnel Syndrome

Carpal tunnel syndrome is the most common cause of paresthesias and numbness in the hands. At the wrist, the median nerve and flexor tendons pass through a tunnel with rigid walls that are bound dorsally and on the sides by the carpal bones, and on the volar aspect by the transverse carpal ligament (Fig. 8D-2). Any process encroaching on this tunnel compresses the median nerve, which innervates the thenar muscles (for flexion, opposition, abduction), the radial lumbricales, and the skin of the radial side of the palm, thumb, second and third fingers, and the radial half of the fourth finger.

Symptoms are variable, but episodes of burning pain or tingling in the hand are common, usually occur at night, and are relieved by vigorous shaking or movement of the hand. Some patients experience only numbness, without much pain. Numbness may occur with such activities as driving or holding a newspaper or book. Patients may have the sensation of hand swelling, when in fact, no swelling is visible. Occasionally, the pain spreads above the wrist into the forearm or, rarely, above the elbow and up the arm. Bilateral disease is common.

A positive Tinel's sign or Phalen's sign may be present. Phalen's test is performed by holding the wrist flexed at 90° for one minute. Loss of sensation may be demonstrated in the index finger, middle finger, or radial side of the fourth finger. Weakness and atrophy of the muscles of the thenar eminence appear gradually in chronic cases. The diagnosis can be confirmed by demonstrating prolonged distal latency during electrodiagnostic studies.

A variety of disorders may cause carpal tunnel syndrome, including edema from pregnancy or trauma, osteophytes, ganglia related to tenosynovial sheaths, lipomata, and anomalous muscles, tendons, and blood vessels that compress the median nerve. Carpal tunnel syndrome has been observed in various infections, including tuberculosis, histoplasmosis, sporotrichosis, coccidioidomycosis, and rubella. Rheumatoid arthritis, gout, pseudogout, and other inflammatory diseases of the wrist can cause compression of the median nerve. Amyloid deposits of the primary type or in association with multiple myeloma can occur at this site, and carpal tunnel syndrome may be the initial manifestation of the disease. The syndrome has been reported to occur in myxedema and acromegaly. In many cases, however, no obvious cause can be found or a nonspecific tenosynovitis is evident. Many idiopathic cases may be due to occupational stress.

In mild cases, splinting the wrist in a neutral position may relieve symptoms (15). Local injections of corticosteroids into the carpal tunnel area, using a 25-gauge needle, are helpful for nonspecific or inflammatory tenosynovitis. The benefit may be only temporary, depending on the degree of compression and the reversibility of the neural injury. When conservative treatment fails, surgical decompression of the tunnel by release of the transverse carpal ligament and removal of tissue compressing the median nerve often is beneficial. Even with surgery, however, symptoms may recur.

Ulnar Nerve Entrapment at the Wrist

The ulnar nerve can become entrapped at the wrist proximal to Guyon's canal, in the canal itself, or distal to it (16). Guyon's canal is bounded roughly medially by the pisiform bone, laterally by the hook of the hamate, superiorly by the volar carpal ligament (pisohamate ligament), and inferiorly

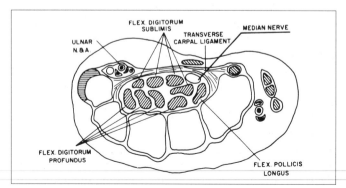

Fig. 8D-2. Cross section of wrist, illustrating the position of the transverse carpal ligament (flexor retinaculum) and the structures occupying the osseous-fibrous carpal tunnel.

by the transverse carpal ligament. Because the ulnar nerve bifurcates into the superficial (sensory) and deep (motor) branches upon entering Guyon's canal, the clinical presentation may vary, with only sensory, only motor, or both sensory and motor findings.

The complete clinical picture includes pain, numbness, paresthesias of the hypothenar area, clumsiness, difficulty using the thumb in a pinching movement, and a weak handgrip. Pressure over the ulnar nerve at the hook of the hamate may cause tingling or pain. Atrophy of the hypothenar and intrinsic muscles can occur. Clawing of ring and little fingers may be seen, resulting from weakness of the third and fourth lumbricales. Loss of sensation occurs over the hypothenar area.

If the superficial branch alone is involved, only numbness, pain, and loss of sensation occur. Entrapment of the deep branch produces only motor weakness. The sites of motor weakness depend on the exact location of nerve compression. For example, if the compression is distal to the superficial branch, but proximal to the branch of the hypothenar muscles, these muscles and the intrinsics may be spared, causing weakness and atrophy of only the adductor pollicis, deep head of the flexor pollicis brevis, and first dorsal interosseous muscles. The causes of ulnar neuropathy at the wrist include trauma, ganglia, bicycling, inflammatory arthritis, flexor carpi ulnaris hypertrophy, fractures, neuroma, lipomata, and diabetes.

The diagnosis is assisted by electrodiagnostic studies, indicating a prolonged distal latency of the ulnar nerve at the wrist and denervation of the ulnar innervated muscles. Treatment includes rest from offending activities, splinting, or a local corticosteroid injection; however, surgical exploration and decompression may be necessary.

Volar Flexor Tenosynovitis
Inflammation of the tendon sheaths of the flexor digitorum superficialis and flexor digitorum profundus tendons in the palm is extremely common, but often unrecognized. Pain in the palm is felt on finger flexion, but in some cases, the pain may radiate to the proximal interphalangeal (PIP) and MCP joints on the dorsal side, misleading the examiner. The diagnosis is made by palpation and identification of localized tenderness and swelling of the volar tendon sheaths. The middle and index fingers are involved most commonly, but the ring and little fingers also can be affected. Often, a nodule composed of fibrous tissue can be palpated in the palm just proximal to the MCP joint on the volar side. The nodule interferes with normal tendon gliding and can cause a triggering or locking, which may be intermittent and may produce an uncomfortable sensation. Similar involvement can occur at the flexor tendon of the thumb. Volar tenosynovitis may be part of inflammatory conditions, such as RA, psoriatic arthritis, or apatite crystal deposition disease. It frequently is seen in conjunction with OA of the hands. The most common cause is overuse trauma of the hands from gripping, with increased traction on the flexor tendons. Injection of a long-acting cortico-

steroid into the tendon sheath usually relieves the problem (17), although surgery on the tendon sheath may be needed in unremitting cases.

Infection of the tendon sheaths in the hand requires drainage and antibiotics. People with drug addictions or diabetes may be at increased risk for such infections. Atypical mycobacterium or fungal infections also cause a chronic tenosynovitis in the hands. *Mycobacterium marinum*, found in infected fish, barnacles, fish tanks, and swimming pools, is a common culprit (18).

Dupuytren's Contracture
In Dupuytren's contracture, a thickening and shortening of the palmar fascia occurs. In established cases, the diagnosis is obvious due to typical thick, cord-like superficial fibrous tissue felt in the palm and causing a contracture, usually of the ring finger. The fifth, third, and second fingers are involved in decreasing order of frequency. Initially, a mildly tender fibrous nodule in the volar fascia of the palm may be the only finding, leading to a confusion with volar flexor tenosynovitis. Dimpling or puckering of the skin over the involved fascia helps identify early Dupuytren's contractures. The initial nodules probably result from a contraction of proliferative myofibroblasts. The tendon and tendon sheaths are not implicated, but the dermis frequently is involved, resulting in fixation to the fascia. Progression of the disease varies, ranging from little or no change over many years to rapid progression and complete flexion contracture of one or more digits.

The cause of this condition is unknown, but a hereditary predisposition appears to be present. Some patients also have associated plantar fasciitis, knuckle pads, and fibrosis in the shaft of the penis (Peyronie's disease). Dupuytren's contracture is about five times more frequent in men, occurs predominantly in whites, and is more common in Europe. Incidence increases gradually with age. Associations exist between Dupuytren's contracture and chronic alcoholism, epilepsy, and diabetes.

Treatment depends entirely on the severity of the findings. Heat, stretching, ultrasound, and intralesional injection of corticosteroids may be helpful in early stages. When actual contractures occur, surgical intervention may be desirable. Limited fasciectomy is effective in most instances, but more radical procedures, including digital amputation, may be necessary. Palmar fasciotomy is a useful and more benign procedure, but if the disease remains active, recurrence is likely.

Disorders of the Hip Region
Trochanteric Bursitis
Although common, trochanteric bursitis frequently goes undiagnosed. It occurs predominantly in middle-aged to elderly people, and somewhat more often in women than in men. The main symptom is aching over the trochanteric area and lateral thigh. Patients usually complain of a "hip problem." Walking, various movements, and lying on the

involved side may intensify the pain. Onset may be acute but more often is gradual, with symptoms lasting for months. In chronic cases, the patient may struggle to locate or describe the pain, and the physician may fail to note the symptoms or interpret them correctly. Occasionally, the pain may mimic a radiculopathy, radiating down the lateral aspect of the thigh. In a few cases, the pain is so severe that the patient cannot walk and complains of diffuse pain of the entire thigh.

The best way to diagnose trochanteric bursitis is to palpate the trochanteric area and elicit point tenderness. In addition to specific pain on deep pressure over the greater trochanter, other tender points may be noted throughout the lateral aspect of the thigh muscle. Pain may worsen with external rotation and abduction against resistance. Although bursitis generally is considered the principal problem, the condition actually may arise from the insertions of the gluteus maximus and gluteus medius tendons. Local trauma and degeneration play a role in the pathogenesis. In some cases, calcification of the trochanteric bursa is seen. Conditions that may contribute to trochanteric bursitis by adding stress to the area include OA of the hip or lumbar spine, leg-length discrepancy, and scoliosis.

Treatment consists of local injection of depot corticosteroid using a 22-gauge needle. Sometimes a 3.5" needle is needed to ensure that the bursal area is reached (19). Nonsteroidal anti-inflammatory drugs, weight loss, and strengthening and stretching of the gluteus medius muscle and iliotibial band help in overall management.

Iliopsoas (Iliopectineal) Bursitis
The iliopsoas bursa lies behind the iliopsoas muscle, anterior to the hip joint and lateral to the femoral vessels. It communicates with the hip in 15% of iliopsoas bursitis cases. When the bursa is involved, groin and anterior thigh pain are present. This pain becomes worse on passive hyperextension of the hip and sometimes on flexion, especially with resistance. Tenderness is palpable over the involved bursa. The patient may hold the hip in flexion and external rotation to eliminate pain and may limp to prevent hyperextension. The diagnosis is more apparent if a cystic mass, which is present in about 30% of cases, is seen; however, other causes of cystic swelling in the femoral area must be excluded. A bursal mass may cause femoral venous obstruction or femoral nerve compression. As with most bursitis, acute or recurrent trauma and such inflammatory conditions as RA may be a cause. The diagnosis is confirmed by plain radiography and injection of a contrast medium into the bursa, or by computed tomography or MRI. Iliopsoas bursitis generally responds to conservative treatment, including corticosteroid injections. With recurrent involvement, excision of the bursa may be necessary.

Ischial (Ischiogluteal) Bursitis
Ischial bursitis is caused by trauma or prolonged sitting on hard surfaces as evidenced by the name, *weaver's bottom*. Pain often is exquisite when sitting or lying down. Because the ischiogluteal bursa is located superficial to the ischial tuberosity and separates the gluteus maximus from the tuberosity, the pain may radiate down the back of the thigh. Point tenderness over the ischial tuberosity is present. Use of cushions and local injection of a corticosteroid are helpful.

Piriformis Syndrome
Piriformis syndrome is not well-recognized and not completely understood, even though it was first described in 1928 (20). The main symptom is pain over the buttocks, often radiating down the back of the leg, as in sciatica. A limp may be noted on the involved side. Women are affected more often, and trauma plays a major role. Diagnosis is aided by tenderness of the piriformis muscle on rectal or vaginal examination. Pain is evident on internal rotation of hips against resistance. Pain and weakness also have been noted on resisted abduction and external rotation. A carefully performed local injection of lidocaine and corticosteroid into the piriformis muscle may help.

Meralgia Paresthetica
The lateral femoral cutaneous nerve (L2–L3) innervates the anterolateral aspect of the thigh and is a sensory nerve. Compression of the nerve causes a characteristic intermittent burning pain, associated with hypesthesia and sometimes with numbness of the anterolateral thigh. Extension and abduction of the thigh or prolonged standing and walking may make symptoms worse, whereas sitting may relieve the pain. Touch and pinprick sensation over the anterolateral thigh may be decreased. Pain can be elicited by pressing on the inguinal ligament just medial to the anterior superior iliac spine. This syndrome is seen more commonly in people who have diabetes, are pregnant, or are obese. Direct trauma, compression from a corset, or a leg-length discrepancy may be factors. Nerve conduction velocity studies help confirm the diagnosis. Weight loss, heel correction, and time generally alleviate the problem. Because entrapment of the nerve often occurs just medial to the anterior superior iliac spine, a local injection of a corticosteroid at that site may help.

Disorders of the Knee Region
Popliteal Cysts
Popliteal cysts, also known as *Baker's cysts*, are not uncommon, and the clinician should be well aware of the possibility of dissection or rupture. A cystic swelling with mild or no discomfort may be the only initial finding. With further distention of the cyst, however, a greater awareness and discomfort is experienced, particularly on full flexion or extension. The cyst is best seen when the patient is standing and is examined from behind. Any knee disease having a synovial effusion can be complicated by a popliteal cyst. A naturally occurring communication may exist between the knee joint and the semimembranosus-gastrocnemius bursa, which is located beneath the medial head of the gastrocnemius muscle. A one-way, valve-like mechanism between the joint

and the bursa is activated by pressure from the knee effusion. An autopsy series has shown that about 40% of the population have a knee-joint–bursa communication.

Popliteal cysts are most common secondary to RA, OA, or internal derangements of the knee. There are a few reported cases secondary to gout and Reiter's syndrome. A syndrome mimicking thrombophlebitis may occur, resulting from cyst dissection into the calf or actual rupture of the cyst. Findings include diffuse swelling of the calf, pain, and sometimes erythema and edema of the ankle. An arthrogram of the knee will confirm both the cyst and the possible dissection or rupture. Ultrasound is used increasingly to make a diagnosis and monitor the course. History of a knee effusion often is a clue that a dissected Baker's cyst is the cause of the patient's swollen leg. If necessary, a venogram can exclude the possibility of concomitant thrombophlebitis. A cyst related to an inflammatory arthritis is treated by injecting a depot corticosteroid into the knee joint and possibly into the cyst itself, which usually resolves the problem. If the cyst results from OA or an internal derangement of the knee, surgical repair of the underlying joint lesion usually is necessary to prevent recurrence of the cyst.

Anserine Bursitis

Seen predominantly in overweight, middle-aged to elderly women, with obese legs and OA of the knees, anserine bursitis produces pain and tenderness over the medial aspect of the knee, about 2" below the joint margin. Pain is worsened by climbing stairs. The pes anserinus (Latin for "goose foot") is composed of the conjoined tendons of the sartorius, gracilis, and semitendinosus muscles. The bursa extends between the tendons and the tibial collateral ligament. The diagnosis is made by eliciting exquisite tenderness over the bursa and by relieving pain with a local lidocaine injection. The treatment is rest, stretching of the adductor and quadriceps muscles, and a corticosteroid injection into the bursa.

Anserine bursitis often is overlooked, as it frequently occurs concomitantly with OA of the knee, which when present, is the assumed cause of pain; however, in some cases of dual involvement, anserine bursitis is the principal source of pain.

Prepatellar Bursitis

Manifested as a swelling superficial to the kneecap, prepatellar bursitis results from trauma, such as frequent kneeling, leading to the name "housemaid's knee." The prepatellar bursa lies anterior to the lower half of the patella and the upper half of the patellar ligament. The pain generally is slight, unless pressure is applied directly over the bursa. The infrapatellar bursa, which lies between the patellar ligament and the tibia, also is subject to trauma and swelling. Chronic prepatellar bursitis can be treated by protecting the knee from the irritating trauma.

Septic prepatellar bursitis should be considered when swelling is noted in this area. Generally, erythema, heat, and increased tenderness and pain are present. When obtained, the history may include trauma to the knee, with puncture or abrasion of the skin overlying the bursa. The bursal fluid should be aspirated and cultured, and treatment with appropriate antibiotics should be instituted if infection is demonstrated.

Medial Plica Syndrome

A plica is a synovial fold in the knee joint, and infrapatellar, suprapatellar, and medial plicae have been identified. The medial plica can sometimes cause knee symptoms (21). Patella pain may be the predominant complaint, and snapping or clicking of the knee, a sense of instability, and possible pseudolocking of the knee may be seen. The plica become symptomatic through any traumatic or inflammatory event in the knee. Diagnosis and treatment are made by arthroscopy, in which a thickened, inflamed, and occasionally fibrotic medial patella plica, leading to a bowstring process, is seen.

Popliteal Tendinitis

Pain in the posterolateral aspect of the knee may occur secondary to tendinitis of the popliteal tendons (hamstring and popliteus). With the knee flexed at 90°, tenderness on palpation may be found. Straight-leg raising, with or without palpation, may cause pain. Running downhill increases the strain on the popliteus and can lead to tendinitis. Rest and conservative treatment are indicated; occasionally a corticosteroid injection may be beneficial.

Pellegrini–Stieda Syndrome

Pellegrini–Stieda syndrome, which generally occurs in men, is thought to result from trauma, and is followed by an asymptomatic period. Later, the symptomatic stage of medial knee pain and progressive restriction of knee movement coincides with the beginning of calcification of the medial collateral ligament, typically appearing as an elongated, amorphous shadow on radiograph (22). The pain is self-limited, and improvement usually occurs within several months.

Patellar Tendinitis

Patellar tendinitis, or jumper's knee, is seen predominantly in athletes engaging in repetitive running, jumping, or kicking activities. Pain and tenderness are present over the patellar tendon. Treatment consists of rest, NSAIDs, ice, knee bracing, and stretching and strengthening of the quadriceps and hamstring muscles. Corticosteroid injections usually are contraindicated, due to the risk of tendon rupture. In some chronic cases, surgery is needed.

Rupture of Quadriceps Tendon and Infrapatellar Tendon

When the tendons around the patella rupture, the quadriceps tendon is involved about 50% of the time; otherwise, the infrapatellar tendon is involved. Quadriceps tendon rupture generally is caused by sudden, violent contractions of the quadriceps muscle when the knee is flexed. A hemarthrosis of the knee joint may follow. Rupture of the infrapatellar tendon has been associated with a specific episode of trauma, repetitive trauma from sporting activities, and systemic diseases. People with chronic renal failure, RA, hyperparathyroidism, or gout, as well as people with systemic lupus erythematosus taking corticosteroids, have been reported to have spontaneous ruptures of the quadriceps tendon. The patient experiences a sudden, sharp pain and cannot extend the leg. Radiographs may show a high-riding patella. The tendon generally is found to be degenerated, and surgical repair is necessary.

Peroneal Nerve Palsy

In peroneal nerve palsy, a painless foot drop with a steppage gait usually is evident. Pain sensation may be decreased slightly along the lower lateral aspect of the leg and the dorsum of the foot. Direct trauma, fracture of the lower portion of the femur or upper portion of the tibia, compression of the nerve over the head of the fibula, and stretch injuries are causes of this palsy. Generally, the common peroneal nerve is compressed, affecting the muscles innervated by the superficial peroneal nerve (which supplies the everters) and the deep peroneal nerve (which supplies the dorsiflexors of the foot and toes). Nerve conduction studies are helpful in demonstrating decreases in conduction velocities. Treatment consists of removing the source of compression, if there is one, and use of an ankle-foot orthosis if necessary. Occasionally, surgical exploration is needed. Systemic vasculitides, such as polyarteritis nodosa, frequently cause peroneal neuropathies; evidence of multiple nerve dysfunction (mononeuritis multiplex) often is manifest on nerve conduction velocity studies.

Patellofemoral Pain Syndrome

This syndrome consists of pain and crepitus in the patellar region (23). Stiffness occurs after prolonged sitting and is alleviated by activity; overactivity involving knee flexion, particularly under loaded conditions such as stair climbing (or stair descent), aggravates the pain. On examination, pain occurs when the patella is compressed against the femoral condyle or when the patella is displaced laterally. Joint effusions are uncommon and usually are small. The symptoms of patellofemoral pain syndrome often are bilateral and occur in a young age group. This syndrome may be caused by a variety of patellar problems such as patella alta, abnormal quadriceps angle, and trauma. The term *chondromalacia patellae* has been used for this syndrome, but patellofemoral pain syndrome is preferred by many. Treatment consists of analgesics, NSAIDs, ice, rest, and avoidance of knee overuse. Isometric strengthening exercises for the quadriceps muscles are beneficial. In some patients, however, surgical realignment may be an option.

Disorders of the Ankle and Foot

Achilles Tendinitis

Usually resulting from trauma, athletic overactivity, or improperly fitting shoes with a stiff heel counter, Achilles tendinitis also can be caused by inflammatory conditions, such as ankylosing spondylitis, Reiter's syndrome, gout, RA, and calcium pyrophosphate dihydrate crystal deposition disease. Pain, swelling, and tenderness occur over the Achilles tendon at its attachment and in the area proximal to the attachment. Crepitus on motion and pain on dorsiflexion may be present. Management includes NSAIDs, rest, shoe corrections, heel lift, gentle stretching, and sometimes, a splint with slight plantar flexion. Because the Achilles tendon is vulnerable to rupture when involved with tendinitis, treatment with a corticosteroid injection could worsen this condition.

Retrocalcaneal Bursitis

The retrocalcaneus bursa is located between the posterior surface of the Achilles tendon and the calcaneus. The bursa's anterior wall is fibrocartilage where it attaches to the calcaneus, whereas its posterior wall blends with the epitenon of the Achilles tendon. Manifestations of bursitis include pain at the back of the heel, tenderness of the area anterior to the Achilles tendon, and pain on dorsiflexion. Local swelling is present, with bulging on the medial and lateral aspects of the tendon. Retrocalcaneal bursitis, also called sub-Achilles bursitis, may coexist with Achilles tendinitis; distinguishing the two sometimes is difficult. This condition may be secondary to RA, spondylitis, Reiter's syndrome, gout, or trauma. Treatment consists of NSAIDs, rest, and a local injection of a corticosteroid carefully directed into the bursa.

Subcutaneous Achilles Bursitis

A subcutaneous bursa superficial to the Achilles tendon may become swollen in the absence of systemic disease. Sometimes called pump-bumps, this bursitis is seen predominantly in women and results from pressure of shoes, although it also can result from bony exostoses. Other than relief from shoe pressure, no treatment is indicated.

Plantar Fasciitis (Subcalcaneal Pain Syndrome)

Plantar fasciitis, which is seen primarily in persons between 40 and 60 years of age, is characterized by pain in the plantar area of the heel. The onset may be gradual or may follow some trauma or overuse from an athletic activity, prolonged walking, using improper shoes, or striking the heel with some force. Plantar fasciitis may be idiopathic; it also is likely to be present in younger patients with spondyloarthritis. The pain characteristically occurs in the morning upon arising, and is most severe for the first few steps. After an initial improvement, the pain may worsen later in the day, especially after prolonged standing or walking. The pain is burning, aching, and occasionally lancinating. Palpation typically reveals tenderness anteromedially on the medial calcaneal tubercle at the origin of the plantar fascia.

Treatment includes relative rest with a reduction in stressful activities, NSAIDs, use of heel-pad or heel-cup orthoses, arch support, and stretching of the heel cord and plantar fascia. A local corticosteroid injection, using a 25-gauge needle, often is beneficial.

Achilles Tendon Rupture

Spontaneous rupture of the Achilles tendon is well-known and occurs with a sudden onset of pain during forced dorsiflexion. An audible snap may be heard, followed by difficulty in walking and standing on toes. Swelling and edema usually develop over the area. Diagnosis can be made with the Thompson test, in which the patient kneels on a chair with the feet extending over the edge, and the examiner squeezes the calf and pushes toward the knee. Normally this produces plantar flexion, but in a ruptured tendon, no plantar flexion occurs. Achilles tendon rupture generally is due to athletic activity or trauma from jumps or falls. The tendon is more prone to tear in people having preexisting Achilles tendon disease or in those taking corticosteroids. Orthopaedic consultation should be obtained, and immobilization or surgery may be selected, depending on the situation.

Tarsal Tunnel Syndrome

In tarsal tunnel syndrome, the posterior tibial nerve is compressed at or near the flexor retinaculum. Just distally, the nerve divides into the medial plantar, lateral plantar, and posterior calcaneal branches. The flexor retinaculum is located posterior and inferior to the medial malleolus. Numbness, burning pain, and paresthesias of the toes and sole extend proximally to the area over the medial malleolus. Nocturnal exacerbation may be reported. The patient gets some relief by leg, foot, and ankle movements. A positive Tinel's sign may be elicited on percussion posterior to the medial malleolus, and loss of pinprick and two-point discrimination may be present. Women are affected more often than men are. Trauma to the foot, especially fracture, valgus foot deformity, hypermobility, and occupational factors may relate to development of this condition. An electrodiagnostic test may show prolonged motor and sensory latencies and slowing of the nerve conduction velocities. In addition, a positive tourniquet test and pressure over the flexor retinaculum can induce symptoms. Shoe corrections and corticosteroid injection into the tarsal tunnel may be beneficial, but surgical decompression often is required.

Posterior Tibial Tendinitis

Pain and tenderness posterior to the medial malleolus occur in posterior tibial tendinitis. This can be due to trauma, excessive pronation, RA, or spondyloarthropathy. Extension and flexion may be normal, but pain is present on resisted inversion or passive eversion. The discomfort usually is worse after athletic activity, and swelling and localized tenderness may be present. Treatment usually includes rest, NSAIDs, and possibly, a local injection of corticosteroid. Immobilization with a splint sometimes is needed.

Peroneal Tendon Dislocation and Peroneal Tendinitis

Dislocation of the peroneal tendon may be caused by a direct blow, repetitive trauma, or sudden dorsiflexion with eversion. Sometimes, a painless snapping noise is heard at the time of dislocation. Other patients report more severe pain and tenderness of the tendon area that lies over the lateral malleolus. The condition may be confused with an acute ankle sprain. Conservative treatment with immobilization often is satisfactory because the peroneal tendon usually reduces spontaneously. If the retinaculum supporting the tendon is ruptured, however, surgical correction may be needed. Peroneal tendinitis can occur and be manifested as localized tenderness over the lateral malleolus. Conservative treatment usually is indicated.

Hallux Valgus

In hallux valgus, deviation of the large toe lateral to the midline and deviation of the first metatarsal medially occurs. A bunion (adventitious bursa) on the head of the first metatarsophalangeal (MTP) joint may be present, often causing pain, tenderness, and swelling. Hallux valgus is more common in women. It may be caused by a genetic tendency or by wearing pointed shoes, or it can be secondary to RA or generalized OA. Stretching of shoes, use of bunion pads, or surgery may be indicated. Metatarsus primus varus, a developmental condition in which the first metatarsal is angulated medially, results in the hallux valgus.

Bunionette

A bunionette, or tailor's bunion, is a prominence of the fifth metatarsal head resulting from the overlying bursa and a localized callus. The fifth metatarsal has a lateral (valgus) deviation.

Hammertoe

In hammertoe, the PIP joint is flexed and the tip of the toe points downward. The second toe most commonly is involved. Calluses may form at the tip of the toe and over the dorsum of the IP joint, resulting from pressure against the shoe. Hammertoe may be congenital or acquired secondary to hallux valgus and may result from improper footwear. When the MTP joint is hyperextended, the deformity is known as cocked-up toes. This condition may be seen in RA.

Morton's Neuroma

Morton's neuroma, an entrapment neuropathy of the interdigital nerve occurring most often between the third and fourth toes, affects middle-aged women most frequently. Paresthesia and a burning, aching pain are experienced in the fourth toe. The symptoms are made worse by walking on hard surfaces or wearing tight shoes or high heels. Tenderness may be elicited by palpation between the third and fourth metatarsal heads. Occasionally, a neuroma is seen between the second and third toes. Compression of the interdigital nerve by the transverse metatarsal ligament and, possibly, by an intermetatarsophalangeal bursa or synovial cyst may be responsible for the entrapment. Treatment usually includes a metatarsal bar or a local steroid injection into the web space. Ultimately, surgical excision of the neuroma and a portion of the nerve may be needed.

Metatarsalgia

Pain arising from the metatarsal heads, known as metatarsalgia, is a symptom resulting from a variety of conditions. Pain on standing and tenderness on palpation of the metatarsal heads are present. Calluses over the metatarsal heads usually are seen. The causes of metatarsalgia are many, including foot strain, high-heeled shoes, everted foot, trauma, sesamoiditis, hallux valgus, arthritis, foot surgery, or a foot with a high longitudinal arch. Flattening of the transverse arch and weakness of the intrinsic muscles occur, resulting in a maldistribution of weight on the forefoot. Treatment is directed at elevating the middle portion of the transverse arch with an orthotic device, strengthening the intrinsic muscles, weight reduction, and use of metatarsal pads or a metatarsal bar.

Pes Planus

Pes planus, or flatfoot, often is asymptomatic, but may cause fatigue of the foot muscles and aching, with intolerance to prolonged walking or standing. There is loss of the longitudinal arch on the medial side and prominence of the navicular and head of the talus (Fig. 8D-3). The calcaneus is everted (valgus), and out-toeing can be seen on ambulation. The tendency for this condition largely is inherited and is seen with generalized hypermobility. A Thomas heel, firm shoes, and grasping exercises to strengthen the intrinsic muscles are helpful. A shoe orthosis may be needed. The asymptomatic flatfoot is left untreated.

Pes Cavus

Pes cavus, or claw foot, is characterized by an unusually high medial arch, and in severe cases, a high longitudinal arch, resulting in shortening of the foot. These abnormally high arches result in shortening of the extensor ligaments, causing dorsiflexion of the PIP joints and plantar flexion of the DIP joints, and giving a claw-like appearance to the toes. The plantar fascia also may be contracted. Generally, a tendency to pes cavus is inherited, and in a high percentage of cases, an underlying neurologic disorder is present. Although pes cavus can cause foot fatigue, pain, and tenderness over the metatarsal heads with callus formation, it can be asymptomatic. Calluses generally develop over the dorsum of the toes. Use of metatarsal pads or a bar is helpful, and stretching of the toe extensors usually is prescribed. In severe cases, surgical correction may be needed.

Posterior Tibialis Tendon Rupture

The rupture of the posterior tibialis tendon, not commonly recognized, is a cause of progressive flatfoot (24). Trauma, chronic tendon degeneration, or RA may cause it. An insidious onset of pain and tenderness may be noted along the course of the tendon just distal to the medial malleolus, along with swelling medial to the hindfoot. The unilateral deformity of hindfoot valgus and forefoot abduction is an important finding. The forefoot abduction can best be seen from behind; more toes are seen from this position than would be seen normally. The result of the single-heel rise test is positive when the patient is unable to rise onto the ball of the affected foot while the contralateral foot is off the floor. Orthopedic consultation should be obtained to determine whether the rupture should be treated with NSAIDs and casting or with a surgical repair.

Disorders of the Anterior Chest Wall

Chest wall pain of musculoskeletal origin is fairly common. It must be differentiated from chest pain of a cardiac nature, which usually is the main concern, or from pain due to pulmonary or gastrointestinal disease. Pain also can radiate to the chest as a result of cervical or thoracic spine disease. The musculoskeletal syndromes usually associated with chest wall pain are Tietze's syndrome and costochondritis. Both conditions are characterized by tenderness of one or more costal cartilages, and the terms sometimes are used interchangeably. However, the disorders generally are separated by the presence of local swelling in Tietze's syndrome, but not in costochondritis (25).

Tietze's syndrome is much less common than costochondritis and is of unknown etiology. Its onset may be gradual or abrupt, with swelling usually occurring in the second or third costal cartilage. Pain, which ranges

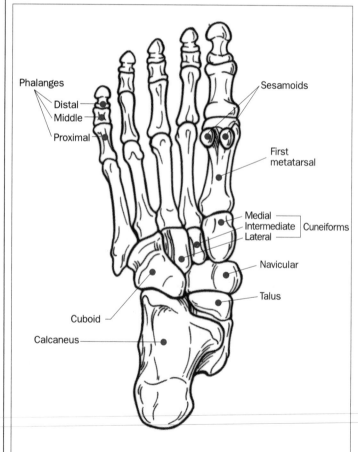

Fig. 8D-3. Bones of the feet.

from mild to severe, may radiate to the shoulder and be aggravated by coughing, sneezing, inspiration, or various movements affecting the chest wall. Tenderness is elicited on palpation, and approximately 80% of patients have a single site.

Costochondritis is more common and is associated with pain and tenderness of the chest wall, without swelling. Tenderness often is present over more than one costochondral junction, and palpation should duplicate the described pain. In a study of 100 patients with noncardiac chest pain, 69% were found to have local tenderness on palpation, and in 16%, palpation elicited the typical pain (26). Other names attached to costochondritis include anterior wall syndrome, costosternal syndrome, parasternal chondrodynia, and chest wall syndrome. Some individuals with chest wall pain are found to have fibromyalgia or localized myofascial pain. Chest wall pain can complicate heart or lung disease, so its presence does not exclude more serious problems.

Xiphoid cartilage syndrome or xiphoidalgia, also known as hypersensitive xiphoid or *xiphodynia*, is characterized by pain over the xiphoid area and tenderness on palpation. Pain may be intermittent and brought on by overeating and various twisting movements.

These three conditions often are self-limited. Treatment consists of reassurance, heat, stretching of chest wall muscles, and local injections of lidocaine, corticosteroid, or both.

A number of other disorders may produce chest wall pain. Sternocostoclavicular hyperostosis is manifested by a painful swelling of the clavicles, sternum, or ribs, and may be relapsing. It is associated with an elevated erythrocyte sedimentation rate, pustules on the palms and soles, and progression to ossification of the chest wall lesions. Condensing osteitis of clavicles is a rare, benign condition of unknown etiology, occurring primarily in women of child-bearing age. It is characterized by sclerosis of the medial ends of the clavicles, without involvement of the sternoclavicular joints. Pain and local tenderness are present.

Any condition involving the sternoclavicular joint, including spondyloarthropathy, OA, and infection, can cause chest wall pain. Stress fracture of the ribs, cough fracture, herpes zoster of the thorax, and intercostobrachial nerve entrapment are other causes of chest pain.

Thorough palpation of the chest wall, including the sternoclavicular joint, costochondral junctions, sternum, and chest wall muscles, must be performed. Such maneuvers as crossed-chest adduction of the arm and backward extension of the arm from 90° of abduction help in elucidating whether chest pain is of a musculoskeletal origin. Imaging studies may include plain radiography of the ribs, special radiography of the sternoclavicular joint, tomography, and bone scan. A computed tomography scan or MRI provides the most detail of the sternoclavicular joint.

JOSEPH J. BIUNDO, Jr., MD

References

1. Sheon RP, Moskowitz RW, Goldberg VM. Soft Tissue Rheumatic Pain: Recognition, Management, Prevention, 3rd edition. Philadelphia: Lippincott, Williams & Williams, 1996.
2. Neustadt DH. Local corticosteroid injection therapy in soft tissue rheumatic conditions of the hand and wrist. Arthritis Rheum 1991;34:923–925.
3. Kisner C, Colby LA. Therapeutic Exercise: Foundations and Techniques, 3rd edition. Philadelphia: FA Davis, 1996.
4. Biundo JJ, Hughes GM. Rheumatoid arthritis rehabilitation: practical guidelines, Part I. J Musculoskel Med 1991;8(8): 85–96.
5. Neer CR: Impingement lesions. Clin Orthop 1983;173:70–77.
6. Goupille P, Sibilia J. Local corticosteroid injections in the treatment of rotator cuff tendinitis (except frozen shoulder and calcific tendinitis). Clin Exp Rheumatol 1996;14: 561–566.
7. Frieman BG, Albert TJ, Fenlin JM Jr. Rotator cuff disease: a review of diagnosis, pathophysiology and current trends in treatment. Arch Phys Med Rehabil 1994;75:604–609.
8. Naredo AE, Aguado P, Padron M, et al. A comparative study of ultrasonography with magnetic resonance imaging in patients with painful shoulder. J Clin Rheumatol 1999;5: 184–192.
9. Dacre JE, Beeney N, Scott DL. Injections and physiotherapy for the painful stiff shoulder. Ann Rheum Dis 1989;48: 322–325.
10. Weinstein PS, Canoso JJ, Wohlgethan JR. Long-term follow up of corticosteroid injection for traumatic olecranon bursitis. Ann Rheum Dis 1984;43:44–46.
11. Cyriax J. Diagnosis of soft tissue lesions. In: Cyriax J (ed). Textbook of Orthopaedic Medicine, Vol. 1. London: Bailliere Tindall, 1982; pp 173.
12. Anderson BC, Manthey R, Brouns MC. Treatment of de Quervain's tenosynovitis with corticosteroids. Arthritis Rheumatol 1991;34:793–798.
13. Stern PJ. Tendinitis, overuse syndromes, and tendon injuries. Hand Clin 1990;6:467–475.
14. Kishner S, Biundo JJ. Posterior interosseous neuropathy in rheumatoid arthritis. J Clin Rheumatol 1996;2:1080–1084.
15. Burke DT, Burke MM, Stewart GW, Cambre A. Splinting for carpal tunnel syndrome: in search of the optimal angle. Arch Phys Med Rehabil 1994;75:1241–1244.
16. Wu JS, Morris JD, Hogan GR. Ulnar neuropathy at the wrist: case report and review of the literature. Arch Phys Med Rehabil 1985;66:785–788.
17. Anderson B, Kaye S. Treatment of flexor tenosynovitis of the hand ("trigger finger") with corticosteroids. Arch Intern Med 1991;151:153–156.
18. Williams CS, Riordan DC. Mycobacterium marinum infections of the hand. J Bone Joint Surg 1973;55A:1042–1050.
19. Shbeer MI, O'Duffy JD, Michet CJ Jr, O'Fallon WM, Matteson EL. Evaluation of glucocorticosteroid injection for the treatment of trochanteric bursitis. J Rheumatol 1996;23:2104–2106.

20. Wyant GM. Chronic pain syndromes and their treatment. III. The piriformis syndrome. Can Anaesth Soc J 1979;26:305–308.
21. Galloway MT, Jokl P. Patella plica syndrome. Ann Sports Med 1990;5:38–41.
22. Wang JC, Shapiro MS. Pellegrini-Stieda syndrome. Am J Orthop 1995;24:493–497.
23. Papagelopoulos PJ, Sim FH. Patellofemoral pain syndrome: diagnosis and management. Orthopedics 1997;20:148–157.
24. Churchhill RS, Sferra JJ. Posterior tibial tendon insufficiency. Its diagnosis, management, and treatment. Am J Orthop 1998;27:339–347.
25. Calabro JJ. Costochondritis. N Engl J Med 1977;296:946–947.
26. Wise CM, Semble L, Dalton CB. Musculoskeletal chest wall syndromes in patients with noncardiac chest pain: a study of 100 patients. Arch Phys Med Rehabil 1992;72:147–149.

MUSCULOSKELETAL SIGNS AND SYMPTOMS
E. Fibromyalgia and Diffuse Pain Syndromes

Diffuse pain is a defining symptom of fibromyalgia. The diagnostic evaluation of an individual with diffuse pain, which can be caused by a number of disorders, depends on the duration of symptoms and the findings in the history and physical examination. Diffuse pain that has been present for years is likely to be due to fibromyalgia, especially if accompanied by such subjective complaints as fatigue, memory difficulties, sleep disturbance, and irritable bowel symptoms. For people with these symptoms who have physical examination findings compatible with fibromyalgia (i.e., diffuse tender points) only a limited work-up is necessary.

In contrast, an individual who has had diffuse pain for a shorter period (weeks or months) needs a more extensive evaluation. Some disorders that may present with diffuse pain are listed in Table 8E-1. In performing the history, the clinician should focus on the onset and character of the pain, the accompanying symptoms, and any "exposures" that could cause the symptoms (particularly medications – prescription or over-the-counter – and dietary supplements). The examination should focus on identifying signs of inflammation (e.g., synovitis) or other findings (e.g., objective weakness) that are incompatible with fibromyalgia.

At a minimum, individuals who present with chronic, widespread pain should have a complete blood count; tests of liver, kidney, and thyroid function; and a sedimentation rate (or C-reactive protein) performed during the course of their illness. Because fibromyalgia occurs less frequently in males, it may be underdiagnosed. Some clinicians have suggested more aggressive diagnostic testing when a male presents with symptoms consistent with fibromyalgia, especially for conditions that are more common in males, such as sleep apnea and hepatitis C infection.

The overlap between fibromyalgia and autoimmune disorders deserves special mention. Early in the course of autoimmune disorders, many individuals present with symptoms suggesting fibromyalgia. Symptoms that may be seen in both fibromyalgia and autoimmune disorders include not only arthralgias, myalgias, and fatigue, but also morning stiffness and subjective swelling of the hands and feet. In addition, a Raynaud's-like syndrome (characterized by the entire hand turning pale or red, instead of just the digits), malar flushing (in contrast to a fixed malar rash), and livedo reticularis are common in fibromyalgia and can mislead the practitioner to suspect an autoimmune disorder.

Persons with established autoimmune disorders may experience symptoms of fibromyalgia. Studies have suggested that approximately 25% of people with systemic inflammatory disorders, such as systemic lupus erythematosus, rheumatoid arthritis, and ankylosing spondylitis, also meet American College of Rheumatology (ACR) criteria for fibromyalgia. Because both inflammatory and noninflammatory mechanisms may cause symptoms, fibromyalgia should be suspected when an individual with an autoimmune disorder has symptoms despite normal inflammatory indices, or when symptoms are unresponsive to anti-inflam-

TABLE 8E-1
Conditions that Simulate Fibromyalgia, or Occur Concurrently With Fibromyalgia

Common
Hypothyroidism
Medications (especially lipid-lowering drugs, antiviral agents)
Polymyalgia rheumatica
Hepatitis C
Sleep apnea
Parvovirus infection
Cervical stenosis/Chiari malformation

Less common
Autoimmune disorders (e.g., SLE, RA; especially early in course of disease)
Endocrine disorders (e.g., Addison's disease, Cushing's syndrome, hyperparathyroidism)
Lyme disease
Eosinophilia-myalgia syndrome
Tapering of corticosteroids
Malignancy

SLE, systemic lupus erythematosus; RA, rheumatoid arthritis.

matory regimens. Symptoms that mimic fibromyalgia also may occur when individuals are being tapered from high-dose corticosteroids (this phenomena previously had been called pseudo-rheumatism).

Etiology and Pathogenesis

Etiology

There is evidence of familial aggregation in fibromyalgia. First-degree relatives of people with fibromyalgia display a higher-than-expected frequency of fibromyalgia, as well as related conditions (1,2). One hypothesis holds that, like many rheumatic conditions, fibromyalgia may be expressed when a person who is genetically predisposed comes in contact with certain environmental exposures that can trigger the development of symptoms. Environmental exposures that generally are accepted to be triggers of fibromyalgia, all of which can be considered stressors, include physical trauma (especially to the axial skeleton), infections (e.g., parvovirus, hepatitis C), emotional distress (acute or chronic), endocrine disorders (e.g., hypothyroidism), and immune stimulation as may occur in a variety of autoimmune disorders (1,3). Although studies of groups of individuals suggest there are many stressors that can trigger the development of this illness, it usually is difficult to assess with certainty the role of a single exposure in a given patient.

Pathogenesis

Most investigators in this field believe that the primary abnormality leading to the expression of symptoms in fibromyalgia and related conditions is aberrant central nervous system function (4,5). Furthermore, there is a general belief that the central components of the stress response may play a major role in symptom expression. The principal components of the human stress response are corticotropin-releasing hormone and locus ceruleus-norepinephrine/autonomic nervous systems. These systems are capable of being activated by a variety of stressors; and disturbances in these systems can affect sensory processing as well as autonomic and neuroendocrine function. Finally, psychobehavioral factors may contibute to the pathogenesis of fibromyalgia.

Abnormalities in Sensory Processing

Several investigators have moved beyond determinations of tender point counts and dolorimeter values in fibromyalgia to examine more extensively the basis for widespread pain and tenderness in this condition. Such studies have demonstrated that people with fibromyalgia cannot *detect* electrical, pressure, or thermal stimuli at lower levels than normal, but these stimuli cause pain or unpleasantness at a lower threshold (6,7). Although nearly all of the research on sensory processing in fibromyalgia has focused on the processing of pain, some data suggest a more generalized sensory processing disturbance. For example, many patients experience sensitivity to loud noises, bright lights, odors, drugs, and chemicals. These

symptoms of generalized sensitivity to multiple stimuli account for the significant number of persons with fibromyalgia who also could be classified as having "multiple chemical sensitivity."

Other investigations have attempted to identify specific neurochemical abnormalities that may be associated with abnormal pain transmission. Several groups have demonstrated that people with fibromyalgia have approximately threefold higher concentrations of substance P (SP) in cerebrospinal fluid (CSF) than controls (8; Fig. 8E-1). There is remarkable consistency between the findings of these investigators, and in all cases, there is very little overlap in SP levels between the people with fibromyalgia and controls.

The meaning of these elevated CSF SP levels is not entirely clear. Substance P is a pro-nociceptive peptide stored in the secretory granules of sensory nerves and released upon axonal stimulation. The SP theoretically could be derived from overactive peripheral nociceptive fibers or from central neurons. An elevated CSF SP level is not specific for fibromyalgia, since this finding also has been noted in people with osteoarthritis of the hip and chronic low back pain. It is likely that these findings are related to the presence of pain, because people with chronic fatigue syndrome (CFS) do not display this finding. Russell et al (8) has demonstrated that SP levels in fibromyalgia are stable or rise over time, and do not change in response to acute pain. Also, the same magnitude of elevation of CSF SP is found in fibromyalgia patients with and without psychiatric comorbidities.

Hypothalamic-Pituitary and Autonomic Dysfunction

Substantial data indicate that the hypothalamic-pituitary axis functions abnormally in subsets of persons with fibromyalgia and related disorders (9). Each of these disorders differs somewhat with respect to the precise perturbations, and in all instances, hypothalamic function is abnormal only in a small subset of subjects. In fibromyalgia, most studies have revealed low 24-hour urinary free cortisol excretion, exaggerated adrenocorticotropic hormone release in response to corticotropin-releasing challenge, and abnormal diurnal rhythmicity in the secretion of cortisol and other hormones. Changes have also been noted in growth hormone (GH) reg-

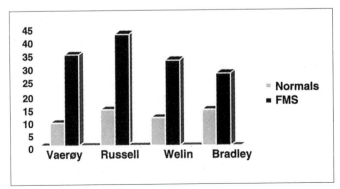

Fig. 8E-1. Mean cerebrospinal fluid levels of substance P in fibromyalgia are noted in four separate studies.

ulation, suggesting abnormal hypothalamic function. Insulin-like growth factor 1 (IGF-1) is very low in about one-quarter of people with fibromyalgia. Produced in the liver primarily in response to GH, IGF-1 is responsible for many of the biologic activities of GH. The defect in GH secretion that leads to low IGF-1 levels appears to be hypothalamic in origin, because these individuals fail to secrete GH in response to various types of stimulation. Although administration of recombinant GH to this subset of fibromyalgia patients has been demonstrated to be of clinical benefit, the expense of this treatment and the likelihood that other, less expensive treatments may be of similar efficacy has limited its use.

Autonomic Nervous System

Many people with diffuse-pain disorders have identifiable abnormalities in autonomic nervous system function. Just as with neuroendocrine function, however, only a subset of people with fibromyalgia have abnormal autonomic function, depending on how this is defined. A number of studies have demonstrated that subsets of people with fibromyalgia and such similar disorders as CFS display low baseline sympathetic tone and an inability to respond to stressors (10). Clinical manifestations related to autonomic dysfunction may include orthostatic intolerance (e.g., as in neurally mediated hypotension), vasomotor instability, and visceral dysfunction.

Psychiatric, Psychological, and Behavioral Factors

There has been a longstanding debate over the role of psychiatric, psychological, and behavioral factors in fibromyalgia. Some health professionals contend that all of the symptoms of fibromyalgia are supratentorial in origin or that fibromyalgia represents a state of distress or vulnerability, whereas others counter that the rate of psychiatric comorbidities in these conditions is similar to that found in any chronic disease.

Mood disorders clearly occur more commonly in individuals with fibromyalgia. Approximately 20%–40% of people with fibromyalgia seen in tertiary care centers have identifiable current mood disorders such as depression or anxiety (11). The lifetime incidence of psychiatric comorbidities in fibromyalgia patients from tertiary care centers ranges from 40% to 70%. Some of these differences in the current and lifetime history of mood disorders likely are due to health care seeking behaviors, because lower lifetime incidences of affective disorders typically are noted in individuals with fibromyalgia who are identified in the general population.

As with most chronic medical illnesses, other psychosocial factors play a significant role in some individuals with fibromyalgia. These factors include behavioral pathways, such as sick-role behavior and maladaptive coping mechanisms; cognitive pathways, such as victimization and loss of control; and social pathways, such as interference with role functioning and deterioration of social or other support networks. As pain progresses from acute to chronic, problems emerge, such as job loss, financial constraints, and the distancing of friends. If patients' responses to these problems are maladaptive (e.g., the avoidance of work, friends, financial responsibilities, and physical activity), the patient

may become distressed and overwhelmed by the pain and its negative impact. Increased stress, learned helplessness, depression, anxiety, anger, distrust, entitlement, and somatization can emerge and worsen symptoms. All of these factors are important in dictating how individuals report symptoms, how and when they seek health care, and how they respond to therapy. This also may explain why cognitive-behavioral therapy (CBT) generally has been effective in the treatment of fibromyalgia, as well as in nearly all other chronic medical conditions (12).

Clinical Features

To fulfill the criteria for fibromyalgia published by an ACR committee in 1990, an individual must have a history of chronic widespread pain involving all four quadrants of the body (and the axial skeleton) and the presence of 11 of 18 "tender points" on physical examination (13) (Fig. 8E-2). These classification criteria were never intended to be applied to individual patients for the purpose of diagnosis. At least half of the individuals who have the clinical diagnosis of fibromyalgia will not fulfill this definition.

There are problems with the ACR criteria, particularly the requirement for a certain number of tender points. Tender points are predefined anatomic points that are considered "positive" when an individual complains of pain upon the application of 4 kg (approximately 9 lbs) of pressure – the approximate amount of pressure required to blanch the examiner's nail. Although early studies suggested

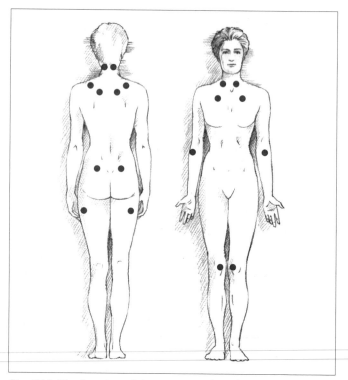

Fig. 8E-2. The location of the nine paired tender points that comprise the 1990 American College of Rheumatology criteria for fibromyalgia.

that people with fibromyalgia experienced tenderness only in these discrete regions, recent data show that individuals with fibromyalgia display increased sensitivity to pain throughout the body (4). Tender points (e.g., the midtrapezius region, epicondyles, etc.) appear to represent regions of the body where everyone is more tender, and individuals who are more diffusely tender generally will have greater numbers of tender points. Also, tender points measure not only how tender individuals are, but also how distressed they are. Finally, tenderness is influenced by many factors. Female gender, increasing age, poor aerobic fitness, and mood disorders all tend to increase cutaneous pressure sensitivity. Therefore, rigid adherence to the ACR criteria in clinical practice will skew the diagnosis of fibromyalgia toward older females with poor aerobic fitness and high levels of distress.

Although pain and tenderness are defining features of fibromyalgia, the latter rarely is a presenting complaint. The pain of fibromyalgia frequently waxes and wanes, may be quite migratory, and often is accompanied by dysesthesias or paresthesias following a nondermatomal distribution. In some instances, patients will present with "aching all over;" in other instances, patients experience several areas of chronic regional pain. Regional musculoskeletal pain typically involves the axial skeleton or areas of "tender points," and originally may be diagnosed as a local problem (e.g., low back pain, lateral epicondylitis). Regional pain involving nonmusculoskeletal regions also is common, including a higher-than-expected prevalence of tension and migraine headaches, temporomandibular joint syndrome, noncardiac chest pain, irritable bowel syndrome, several entities characterized by chronic pelvic pain, and plantar or heel pain.

In addition to pain and tenderness, most individuals experience a high prevalence of nondefining symptoms (15) (Fig. 8E-3). For example, most people with fibromyalgia experience fatigue, and at least half of individuals who meet ACR criteria for fibromyalgia also will meet criteria for CFS. The fatigue is worse after activities, and may be accompanied by memory difficulties. Mental difficulties, especially with attention span and short-term memory, may be the most debilitating aspect of the illness. Other constitutional complaints include fluctuations in weight, heat and cold intolerance, and the subjective sensation of weakness.

Patients with fibromyalgia and related illnesses also display a wide array of "allergic" symptoms, ranging from adverse reactions to drugs and environmental stimuli (as seen in multiple chemical sensitivity) to higher-than-expected incidences of rhinitis, nasal congestion, and lower respiratory symptoms. Although some of these individuals truly may be atopic, many of these symptoms are due to neural (e.g., hypersensitivities, vasomotor rhinitis) mechanisms. Hearing, ocular, and vestibular abnormalities have been noted, including a high incidence of sicca symptoms, a decreased painful-sound threshold, exaggerated nystagmus and ocular dysmotility, and asymptomatic, low-frequency, sensorineural hearing loss.

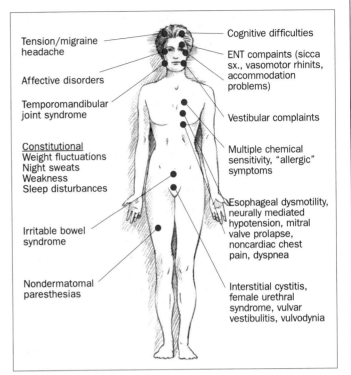

Fig. 8E-3. Nondefining features of fibromyalgia and related disorders. ENT, ear nose throat.

Individuals with fibromyalgia also experience many symptoms of functional disorders of visceral organs, including a high incidence of recurrent noncardiac chest pain, heartburn, palpitations, and irritable bowel symptoms. However, prospective studies of randomly selected individuals with fibromyalgia have detected a high frequency of *objective* evidence of dysfunction of several visceral organs, including echocardiographic evidence of mitral valve prolapse, esophageal dysmotility, and diminished static inspiratory and expiratory pressures on pulmonary function testing. Neurally mediated hypotension and syncope also occur more frequently in these individuals. Similar syndromes characterized by visceral pain and/or smooth-muscle dysmotility also are seen in the pelvis, including dysmenorrhea, urinary frequency urgency, interstitial cystitis, endometriosis, and vulvar vestibulitis or vulvodynia.

The physical examination generally is unremarkable in fibromyalgia, except for tender points. The tenderness may occur in virtually any part of the body, and is not confined to the regions identified in the ACR criteria. The concept of control points, previously described as areas of the body that should not be tender, has been abandoned.

Laboratory testing should be used judiciously. Even if the individual has acute or subacute onset of symptoms, ordering serologic assays such as antinuclear antibodies (ANA) and rheumatoid factor should be avoided unless there is strong evidence of an autoimmune disorder. Such tests have a low predictive value in the setting of nonspecific symptoms, and the rate of ANA positivity may be higher in people with these illnesses (16,17).

Treatment

General Approach

At present, the treatment of fibromyalgia is as much art as science. Once the diagnosis has been made, the practitioner must consider whether to "label" the individual. For the majority of patients, this label will help them understand their symptoms and the most appropriate treatment, but there may be some individuals for whom this label is harmful (18).

The practitioner should schedule a prolonged visit or series of visits when this diagnosis is considered. Although there are no data to support the hypothesis, it is likely that this "up-front" time is extremely useful for both patients and providers, as it helps the physician understand precisely what is bothering the patient, and assists the patient in understanding the goals and rationale of treatment. The physician should explore the symptoms that are most bothersome, the impact these symptoms are having on various aspects of life, perception about what is causing these symptoms, and the stressors that may be exacerbating the problem.

Education

Some people who present with symptoms of fibromyalgia want only to be told that this is a benign, nonprogressive condition. These patients generally have mild symptoms that have been present for some time, and they possess adequate strategies for improving symptoms and maintaining function. For all people with fibromyalgia, education about the nature of this disorder is critical. Physicians should describe the condition in terms with which they feel most comfortable, and then refer the patient to such reputable sources of information as the Arthritis Foundation, national patient support organizations (e.g., American Fibromyalgia Syndrome Association, National Fibromyalgia Research Association, and Fibromyalgia Alliance of America), and up-to-date Web sites (www.fms-cfs.org).

Pharmacologic Therapies

Tricyclic compounds, notably amitriptyline and cyclobenzaprine, have been the most extensively studied agents for the treatment of fibromyalgia. Low doses of tricyclic drugs have demonstrated short-term benefit in treating a number of other conditions and symptoms, including migraine and tension headaches, noncardiac chest pain, irritable bowel syndrome, rheumatoid arthritis, insomnia, and a variety of chronic pain conditions (19).

A problem with all controlled trials of tricyclic drugs in fibromyalgia is that there is tremendous variability in the optimal dosage across groups of patients, and blinded trials do not allow for the highly individualized dosing regimens that can be used in clinical practice. To increase the tolerance of cyclobenzaprine and amitriptyline, these compounds should be administered several hours before bedtime, begun at low doses (10 mg or less), and increased slowly (10 mg every one to two weeks) until the patient reaches the maximally beneficial dose (up to 40 mg of cyclobenzaprine, or 70–80 mg of amitriptyline).

Because of the side effects of tricyclic agents, recent studies have examined the efficacy of better-tolerated compounds in these conditions. Studies show conflicting results regarding the efficacy of fluoxetine in fibromyalgia. Trials have shown a beneficial effect (either alone or with amitriptyline), and the other studies have demonstrated no advantage over placebo. Single trials suggest that sertraline and venlafaxine may be of some benefit. Medications that augment central adrenergic tone may be more effective than drugs that work exclusively via serotonergic mechanisms. Anecdotally, other compounds with more prominent noradrenergic or dopaminergic mechanisms, such as buproprion, nefazodone, and pemoline, have shown some clinical utility, especially when given during the day to patients with prominent fatigue or cognitive complaints.

Other drugs may be useful for treating certain symptoms of fibromyalgia, without necessarily leading to a globally beneficial effect. For example, tramadol has been an effective analgesic in this disorder. Gabapentin may have some efficacy as a central analgesic when used at high doses (e.g., 1000–2000 mg/day), but it has not been tested in people with fibromyalgia. For treating insomnia in persons intolerant to tricyclic compounds, bedtime doses of trazadone and zolpidem may be of benefit. In people with symptoms suggestive of autonomic dysfunction, such as orthostatic intolerance, vasomotor instability, or palpitations, increased fluid and sodium/potassium intake or low doses of beta blockers may be useful.

Nonpharmacologic Therapies

Many clinicians believe that treatment programs combining symptom-based pharmacologic therapy with extensive use of nonpharmacologic therapies (e.g., CBT, aerobic exercise) are the most effective strategies in fibromyalgia.

Cognitive-Behavioral Therapy

Cognitive-behavioral therapy refers to a structured education program that focuses on teaching skills that individuals can use to cope with their illness. It has been shown to be effective in improving patient outcomes in nearly every chronic medical illness, including fibromyalgia, but it needs to be tailored to the specific condition being treated (19). The skills most commonly associated with CBT include relaxation training, activity pacing, pleasant activity scheduling, visual imagery techniques, distraction strategies, focal point and visual distraction, cognitive restructuring, problem solving, and goal setting. A goal of CBT is to give patients the tools to gain control over their illness.

Aerobic Exercise

Aerobic exercise improves outcomes for a wide range of conditions, including fibromyalgia (20). The reason for the benefit is likely multifactorial because aerobic exercise has analgesic and antidepressant effects, and it enhances the patient's sense of well-being and control. In designing an aerobic exercise program, careful planning is required to enhance tolerability and ensure long-term compliance. Patients may experience a worsening of symptoms immediately after exercise, especially in such illnesses as fibromyalgia, and thus fear that any form of exercise will exacerbate their condition. To reduce the pain associated with exercise, low-impact exercises such as aquatic exercise, walking, swimming, or stationary cycling are recommended. Just as with medication, a "start low, go slow" approach appears to be most effective, with emphasis on a gradual progression in exercise intensity and a focus on adherence to a lifelong program.

Complementary Therapies

Several types of complementary therapies are used by physicians and patients to treat fibromyalgia. These therapies include trigger-point injections, myofascial release therapy (or other "hands on" techniques), acupuncture, and chiropractic manipulation, each of which has some data supporting efficacy. Other techniques fall into a more dubious category.

Because there are very few controlled trials to guide the practitioner in choosing from such treatment modalities, a general approach is suggested. The practitioner should evaluate the safety of the proposed treatment, and point out to the patient any potentially harmful effects. The physician then should consider whether this treatment is reinforcing a maladaptive belief that will be harmful to the patient in the long run (e.g., a treatment program of prolonged bed rest or isolation). If the treatment is neither harmful nor maladaptive, the practitioner may suggest that the patient conduct the equivalent of an "n of 1" trial. In this setting, the patient begins a single treatment (keeping all other variables constant) and determines if the treatment is beneficial. If the patient judges the treatment to be helpful, the treatment should be discontinued to determine if the symptoms worsen. Even if the treatment withstands this test of efficacy, a placebo effect cannot be excluded. When managing a condition as enigmatic as fibromyalgia in clinical practice, however, it is difficult to argue with success.

DANIEL J. CLAUW, MD

References

1. Hudson JI, Goldenberg DL, Pope HG Jr, Keck PE Jr, Schlesinger L. Comorbidity of fibromyalgia with medical and psychiatric disorders. Am J Med 1992;92:363–367.
2. Buskila D, Neumann L. Fibromyalgia syndrome (FM) and nonarticular tenderness in relatives of patients with FM. J Rheumatol 1997;24:941–944.
3. Buskila D, Neumann L, Vaisberg G, Alkalay D, Wolfe F. Increased rates of fibromyalgia following cervical spine injury. A controlled study of 161 cases of traumatic injury. Arthritis Rheum 1997;40:446–452.
4. Yunus MB. Towards a model of pathophysiology of fibromyalgia: aberrant central pain mechanisms with peripheral modulation. J Rheumatol 1992;19:846–850.
5. Clauw DJ, Chrousos GP. Chronic pain and fatigue syndromes: overlapping clinical and neuroendocrine features and potential pathogenic mechanisms. Neuroimmunomodulation 1997;4:134–153.
6. Lautenbacher S, Rollman GB, McCain GA. Multi-method assessment of experimental and clinical pain in patients with fibromyalgia. Pain 1994;59:45–53.
7. Arroyo JF, Cohen ML. Abnormal responses to electrocutaneous stimulation in fibromyalgia. J Rheumatol 1993;20:1925–1931.
8. Russell IJ, Orr MD, Littman B, et al. Elevated cerebrospinal fluid levels of substance P in patients with the fibromyalgia syndrome. Arthritis Rheum 1994;37:1593–1601.
9. Crofford LJ. Neuroendocrine abnormalities in fibromyalgia and related disorders. Am J Med Sci 1998;315:359–366.
10. Petzke F, Clauw DJ. Sympathetic function in fibromyalgia. Curr Opin Rheumatol (in press).
11. Boissevain MD, McCain GA. Toward an integrated understanding of fibromyalgia syndrome. II. Psychological and phenomenological aspects. Pain 1991;45:239–248.
12. N.I.H. Technology Assessment Panel. Integration of behavioral and relaxation approaches into the treatment of chronic pain and insomnia. JAMA 1996;276:313–318.
13. Wolfe F, Smythe HA, Yunus MB, et al. The American College of Rheumatology 1990 Criteria for the Classification of Fibromyalgia. Report of the Multicenter Criteria Committee. Arthritis Rheum 1990;33:160–172.
14. Granges G, Littlejohn G. Pressure pain threshold in pain-free subjects, in patients with chronic regional pain syndromes, and in patients with fibromyalgia syndrome. Arthritis Rheum 1993;36:642–646.
15. Clauw DJ. Fibromyalgia: more than just a musculoskeletal disease. Am Fam Physician 1995;52:843–851.
16. Bates DW, Buchwald D, Lee J, et al. Clinical laboratory test findings in patients with chronic fatigue syndrome. Arch Intern Med 1995;155:97–103.
17. Pincus T. A pragmatic approach to cost-effective use of laboratory tests and imaging procedures in patients with musculoskeletal symptoms. Prim Care 1993;20:795–814.
18. Hadler NM. Fibromyalgia, chronic fatigue, and other iatrogenic diagnostic algorithms. Do some labels escalate illness in vulnerable patients? Postgrad Med 1997;102:161–172.
19. Godfrey RG. A guide to the understanding and use of tricyclic antidepressants in the overall management of fibromyalgia and other chronic pain syndromes. Arch Intern Med 1996;156:1047–1052.
20. Minor MA, Hewett JE, Webel RR, Anderson SK, Kay DR. Efficacy of physical conditioning exercise in patients with rheumatoid arthritis and osteoarthritis. Arthritis Rheum 1989;32:1396–1405.

MUSCULOSKELETAL SIGNS AND SYMPTOMS
F. Periodic Syndromes

Several forms of arthritis can present with episodes of exacerbation and remission that might be considered "periodic." This section focuses on four mendelian disorders that present with episodic fever and arthritis, and a group of disorders with unclear etiologies.

Hereditary Periodic Fever Syndromes

The hereditary periodic fever syndromes (Table 8F-1) are a group of four genetic diseases characterized by episodes of fever and serosal, synovial, and/or cutaneous inflammation. Two of these disorders, familial Mediterranean fever (FMF) and the hyperimmunoglobulinemia D with periodic fever syndrome (HIDS), are inherited in an autosomal recessive manner. The other two, the tumor necrosis factor (TNF) receptor-associated periodic syndrome (TRAPS) and the Muckle-Wells syndrome (MWS), are dominantly inherited. Each displays distinctive clinical features, and recent molecular genetic data corroborate the view that these are distinct entities. Because high-titer autoantibodies generally are not detected in these disorders, they sometimes are referred to as *autoinflammatory* diseases (1).

Familial Mediterranean Fever

FMF is a recessive autoinflammatory disease observed most frequently in Jewish, Armenian, Arab, Turkish, and Italian populations (2), with a male:female ratio of 1.5–2:1 (3,4). In 80%–90% of cases, the first episode occurs before the age of 20 years, sometimes as early as infancy. Attacks last one to three days and present as fever with or without abdominal pain, pleuritic chest pain, skin rash, and arthritis (3,4). The time between attacks ranges from days to years and can vary for an individual patient.

FMF (entry 249100 of Online Mendelian Inheritance in Man, OMIM, at http://www.ncbi.nlm.nih.gov/omim/) is caused by mutations in *MEFV*, a 10-exon gene encoded on the short arm of chromosome 16 (5). *MEFV* codes for a 781–amino-acid protein called pyrin, or alternatively, marenostrin. A total of 28 mutations have been identified, most of them clustered in exon 10. Haplotype studies indicate probable common founders for several of the mutations seen across populations (2,5,6). Carrier frequencies in high-risk populations can be as high as 1:3, suggesting a possible selective advantage (such as increased resistance to infection) for individuals bearing single mutant copies of the gene. Of the common mutations, M694V is thought to be associated with an increased risk of amyloidosis (7), and E148Q generally has been associated with a mild phenotype. *MEFV* is expressed predominantly in polymorphonuclear leukocytes and activated monocytes. Although pyrin

has been hypothesized to be a nuclear protein (5), the full-length pyrin protein has been shown to associate with the cytoskeleton, perhaps accounting for the effectiveness of colchicine therapy in FMF. Because mutations lead to an autoinflammatory state, pyrin is thought to be a negative regulator of inflammation, but its precise biochemical function remains unknown.

The availability of genetic testing provides a new tool for diagnosing FMF, but genetic testing is not necessary for people from high-risk ethnic groups who experience typical attacks and respond therapeutically to colchicine. Genetic testing can be a useful adjunct for atypical cases, or for physicians not familiar with FMF and related conditions. However, using current methods of mutational screening, as many as one-third of patients meeting clinical criteria for FMF may have only one demonstrable mutation (2), rather than the two that would be expected for a recessive condition. Furthermore, a small number of patients with clinical FMF may have no demonstrable mutations. These considerations raise the possibility that there is a second FMF gene, or that mutations exist in *MEFV* regions not accessible to current screening methods. The interpretation of genetic testing also is complicated by the existence of complex alleles (2), in which more than one mutation is found on a single carrier chromosome.

Clinical and Laboratory Features

The magnitude of fever in FMF varies, and fever may be overlooked if body temperature is not checked. Attacks resolve spontaneously after one to three days, and patients feel well during intercritical periods. During the attacks, laboratory abnormalities include leukocytosis and elevated acute-phase reactants, such as erythrocyte sedimentation rate, C-reactive protein, fibrinogen, and haptoglobin.

More than 90% of patients have abdominal symptoms that vary in severity from relatively mild to acute pain, sometimes prompting exploratory laparotomy. Peritoneal irritation and constipation are common. Pleural attacks, which are seen in 25%–50% of patients, usually are unilateral and sometimes lead to pleural effusions. The most common skin lesion of FMF is a demarcated, raised, erythematous, often painful rash on the lower leg, ankle, or dorsum of the foot, called *erysipeloid erythema*.

In some patients, arthritis is the presenting sign; arthralgia also is common, but nonspecific (3,4). The risk of arthritic attacks may be increased in patients who are homozygous for the M694V *MEFV* mutation (7). The arthritis of FMF most frequently is acute and monarticular or pauciarticular, with attacks lasting up to one week. The knee, ankle, and hip are the joints affected most often. Severe pain and effusions are common, but erythema and warmth may be disproportionately mild. Synovial fluid may contain large numbers of

TABLE 8F-1
The Hereditary Periodic Fever Syndromes

Feature	Familial Mediterranean fever	Hyper-IgD syndrome	TNF receptor-associated periodic syndrome	Muckle-Wells syndrome
Ethnic distribution	Jewish, Armenian, Arab, Turkish, Italian	Northern European	Multiple ethnic groups	Northern European
Mode of inheritance	Autosomal recessive	Autosomal recessive	Autosomal dominant	Autosomal dominant
Chromosome	16p13.3	12q24	12p13	1q44
Underlying gene	*MEFV*, encoding pyrin (alternatively, marenostrin)	*MVK*, encoding mevalonate kinase	*TNFRSF1A*, encoding p55 TNF receptor	Unknown
Duration of episodes	1–3 days	3–7 days	>1 week	1–2 days
Abdominal pain	Mild discomfort to peritonitis; constipation more common than diarrhea	Mild to severe pain, but peritonitis uncommon; diarrhea more common than constipation	Mild discomfort to peritonitis; diarrhea or constipation	Abdominal pain, vomiting, diarrhea
Pleurisy	Common	Rare	Common	Rare
Joints	Most often acute monarticular or pauciarticular arthritis; arthralgia; rarely, protracted arthritis	Symmetric polyarticular nondestructive arthritis; no protracted arthritis	Arthralgia; monarticular or pauciarticular nonerosive arthritis	Arthralgia; oligoarticular arthritis of large joints; persistent synovitis less common
Myalgia	Effort-associated myalgia; rarely, protracted febrile myalgia	Uncommon	Migratory myalgia common; due to fascial inflammation	Common
Cutaneous manifestation	Erysipeloid erythema most common	Erythematous macules and papules; urticaria less common	Migratory erythema	Urticaria
Lymphadenopathy	Uncommon	Prominent during attacks, particularly in cervical nodes	Sometimes present	Not prominent
Ocular	Rare	None reported	Periorbital edema, conjunctivitis	Conjunctivitis, episcleritis
Auditory	None reported	None reported	None reported	Sensorineural deafness
Amyloidosis	Risk associated with M694V/M694V genotype	None reported	~10% of cases	~25% of cases
Treatment	Daily colchicine prophylaxis	Statins investigational	Prednisone; etanercept investigational	Possibly prednisone, colchicine

polymorphonuclear leukocytes, but is sterile. Even after repeated acute episodes, radiographs usually are normal. Chronic arthritis of the sacroiliac joints, accompanied by radiographic changes, is seen with increased frequency in people with FMF, regardless of human leukocyte antigen B27 status. FMF patients may develop a protracted form of arthritis, usually involving the knee or hip, that sometimes necessitates joint replacement. However, this circumstance is unusual since the advent of colchicine prophylaxis.

Other, less common types of FMF attacks include unilateral acute scrotum, pericarditis, and febrile myalgia. These attacks may be brief or protracted, sometimes lasting four to six weeks. Henoch-Schönlein purpura is seen in up to 5% of children with FMF, and the frequency of polyarteritis nodosa is increased. Aseptic meningitis has been reported in FMF, but a firm causal relationship has not been established.

The most serious complication of FMF is systemic amyloidosis due to deposition of a product of the acute-phase reactant serum amyloid A (SAA). The organs affected most frequently are the kidneys, adrenal glands, intestine, spleen, lung, and testes, but not the peripheral nerves or joints. Before the use of colchicine, amyloid-induced renal failure was a major cause of death in FMF. Rarely, amyloidosis presents as the first manifestation of FMF (phenotype II). Factors that determine the risk of developing amyloidosis include a positive family history of amyloidosis, the M694V homozygous *MEFV* genotype (7), male gender, and the *SAA1a/a* genotype. Environmental factors also may be important. Urinalysis for protein is a rapid and inexpensive screen for amyloidosis. In patients with persistent proteinuria, amyloidosis can be evaluated directly by examination of a Congo-red–stained rectal or renal biopsy specimen under polarized light.

Treatment

The mainstay of treatment for FMF is daily colchicine. This agent has been demonstrated effective in preventing acute attacks and amyloidosis. In adults, the usual daily dose is 1.2–1.8 mg orally. In very young children, lower doses may be effective, but children over the age of 5 often require doses comparable to adults. Diarrhea is the most common side effect, but can be minimized by starting at a low dose and gradually increasing, and by splitting the daily dose. Myopathy and neuropathy have been reported, primarily in elderly patients with renal insufficiency. There may be a slightly increased risk of trisomy 21 in the offspring of parents taking colchicine at the time of conception. Intravenous colchicine generally is avoided in FMF, because the risk of serious toxicity (e.g., bone marrow suppression) is increased substantially in patients already taking oral colchicine.

Patients with breakthrough attacks sometimes benefit from interferon α administered subcutaneously at the earliest sign of an attack. FMF patients with Henoch-Schönlein purpura or protracted febrile myalgia may require corticosteroids, and those with polyarteritis nodosa may require cyclophosphamide and high-dose corticosteroids.

Hyperimmunoglobulinemia D with Periodic Fever Syndrome

HIDS is a recessively inherited autoinflammatory disorder described primarily in individuals of northern European ancestry (e.g., the Netherlands and northern France). Febrile episodes tend to be somewhat longer than in FMF, lasting three to seven days, on average (8). The median age of onset is 6 months, and early episodes sometimes are associated with childhood immunizations.

In 1999, HIDS (OMIM 260920) was shown to be caused by mutations in the mevalonate kinase (*MVK*) gene on the long arm of chromosome 12 (9,10). Mevalonate kinase is an enzyme that catalyzes the conversion of mevalonic acid to 5-phosphomevalonic acid in the synthesis of cholesterol and nonsterol isoprene compounds. Mutations leading to HIDS leave 1%–3% residual enzyme activity in fibroblasts, and patients exhibit elevated levels of mevalonic acid in their urine during acute attacks. *MVK* mutations leading to a complete loss of enzymatic activity cause mevalonic aciduria, a condition with markedly higher levels of mevalonic acid in the urine. Patients with this condition have not only the periodic fevers, lymphadenopathy, arthralgia, rash, and abdominal pain seen in HIDS, but also exhibit cataracts, mental retardation, hypotonia, and failure to thrive. The mechanism by which mutations in the MVK gene lead to inflammation is unknown. Current theories focus on downstream products of the mevalonate pathway, other than cholesterol.

Clinical and Laboratory Features

As in FMF, abdominal pain frequently accompanies febrile episodes, but peritoneal irritation is much less common, and diarrhea is observed more often than constipation. Pleuritic chest pain has not been reported in HIDS. A number of different skin rashes can be seen in HIDS, including urticaria, morbilliform lesions, and erythematous macules, papules, and nodules.

The joint manifestations of HIDS include arthralgia and a nondestructive arthritis. About 70% of patients develop articular complaints with their febrile episodes. As in FMF, arthritis tends to affect the large joints, and synovial fluid shows a predominance of polymorphonuclear leukocytes. HIDS arthritis, unlike that of FMF, is polyarticular and often occurs concomitantly with abdominal pain.

HIDS episodes usually are accompanied by a leukocytosis and elevated acute-phase reactants. Pericarditis, scrotal involvement, and amyloidosis appear to distinguish FMF from HIDS. Conversely, diffuse tender lymphadenopathy, which is most prominent in the neck during attacks, appears to be distinctive for HIDS. Before identification of the underlying genetic defect, the *sine qua non* for diagnosis of HIDS consisted of two observations of elevated serum IgD (>100 U/mL, or >14.1 mg/dL) at least one month apart. However, the absence of correlation between IgD levels and the frequency or intensity of attacks contradicts the view that IgD elevations are pathogenic. Moreover, about 80% of patients also have elevated serum IgA levels (8).

The diagnosis of HIDS can be established without the need for DNA testing in patients with a consistent clinical picture and an elevated IgD level. Rarely, however, patients may have typical HIDS attacks and HIDS-associated *MVK* mutations without an elevated serum IgD (9), raising the possibility of HIDS *sine* hyperimmunoglobulinemia D.

Because HIDS does not appear to be associated with systemic amyloidosis, this disorder does not have a major effect on longevity, and in some patients, the attacks ameliorate in adulthood.

Treatment

There is no satisfactory treatment for HIDS, although some patients have benefited from NSAIDs, colchicine, corticosteroids, cyclosporine, or intravenous immunoglobulin. Such HMG CoA reductase inhibitors as lovastatin and TNF inhibitors are under investigation in the treatment of this condition.

TNF Receptor-Associated Periodic Syndrome

TRAPS is a dominantly inherited autoinflammatory disease caused by mutations in *TNFRSF1A,* a gene on the short arm of chromosome 12 that encodes the 55-kDa receptor for TNF (1). People with TRAPS tend to have inflammatory episodes that are longer than those seen in FMF or HIDS, with self-limited attacks usually lasting at least one week and sometimes lasting as long as four to six weeks (4). Before identification of the *TNFRSF1A* mutations, case reports described this condition under a number of clinical names, including familial Hibernian fever (OMIM 142680) in a large kindred of Irish/Scottish ancestry (11), and benign autosomal dominant familial periodic fever in a family of Scottish descent (12). With the recognition that this disorder can be seen in people from a broad range of ancestries, nomenclature was adopted that emphasizes pathogenesis rather than ethnicity.

In 1999, the first six disease-associated mutations in *TNFRSF1A* were identified (1). Five of these mutations are single-nucleotide differences that cause amino-acid substitutions at highly conserved cysteine residues involved in disulfide bonding of the receptor's extracellular domain. The sixth mutation substitutes methionine for a threonine that participates in a conserved intrachain hydrogen bond. Nine additional mutations subsequently have been found, bringing the total to 15. Fourteen of these mutations cause single amino-acid substitutions in the protein's extracellular domain; eight of the substitutions involve cysteine residues. The remaining mutation adds four amino acids to the extracellular domain by creating an abnormal splice site.

TNF receptor mutations probably lead to a dominantly inherited condition because these receptors form homotrimers on the cell surface, and abnormalities in even one component of the trimer affect overall structure. In the initial report describing *TNFRSF1A* mutations, evidence indicated that the C52F mutation impaired the shedding of p55 TNF receptors that occurs upon cellular activation (1). This metalloprotease-mediated receptor cleavage may have a negative homeostatic effect on the inflammatory response by reducing the number of cell-surface receptors available for repeated stimulation and by creating a pool of soluble receptors that compete for TNF binding. By interfering with these normal regulatory processes, the C52F mutation could create a hyperinflammatory state. Subsequent studies indicate that this mechanism also is operative for several other mutations, but suggest that additional pathways are likely to be involved in the pathogenesis of TRAPS.

Clinical and Laboratory Features

Inflammatory episodes observed in TRAPS are characterized by fever with abdominal pain, pleurisy, arthralgia (or less commonly, arthritis), myalgia, and a characteristic skin rash (1,11,12). Local trauma, mild infections, physical exertion, and psychological stress may provoke episodes of TRAPS inflammation. In some female patients, pregnancy has resulted in reduced frequency or intensity of attacks. Clinical features that distinguish TRAPS from the recessively inherited periodic fever syndromes include the prolonged duration of attacks; the presence of conjunctival involvement or periorbital edema; a centrifugal, migratory, erythematous skin rash on the limbs or trunk (Fig. 8F-1); localized myalgia, sometimes associated with the rash (Fig. 8F-1); and a much more pronounced therapeutic response to corticosteroids than to colchicine.

As is the case for FMF and HIDS, the attacks of TRAPS are associated with a marked acute-phase response. Systemic AA amyloidosis, eventually leading to hepatic or renal failure, has been observed in approximately 10% of people with TRAPS (Fig. 8F-1). The risk of amyloidosis appears to be higher for patients with substitutions at cysteine residues in the p55 TNF receptor.

The diagnosis of TRAPS should be considered in people with unexplained inflammatory episodes as described, even when there is no positive family history. Although studies of the first seven reported families indicated that 95% of individuals with mutations have symptoms, suggesting that most patients would have a positive family history, more recent experience indicates a significant proportion of "sporadic" cases, including some in patients who have asymptomatic relatives with documented mutations. To make the diagnosis of TRAPS, a patient should have a documented *TNFRSF1A* mutation and a history of recurrent inflammatory episodes.

Although the attacks of TRAPS can be quite debilitating, they are self-limited. TRAPS is not life-threatening unless systemic amyloidosis develops.

Treatment

Daily colchicine sometimes ameliorates attacks, but is not nearly as effective as in FMF. Corticosteroids often are effective in treating the acute attacks, but many patients require escalating doses over the course of their illness. Preliminary experience with etanercept in preventing TRAPS episodes is encouraging, but the role of TNF inhibition in preventing TRAPS-induced amyloidosis remains to be established.

Muckle-Wells Syndrome

In 1962, Muckle and Wells (13) described a five-generation English family with a dominantly inherited syndrome of episodic inflammation, progressive sensorineural deafness beginning in childhood, and in some cases, amyloidosis (OMIM 191900). The attacks, termed "aguey bouts," typically lasted about 36 hours and consisted of fever, chills, malaise, urticarial rash, limb and joint pain, and sometimes, swelling of the hands and feet. In some cases, there were amyloid deposits in the kidneys, liver, adrenals, spleen, and testes. In two patients, post-mortem studies of the inner ear showed absence of the organ of Corti and vestibular sensory epithelium, but no amyloid deposits.

The MWS gene has been mapped to chromosome 1q44 by linkage analysis (14). In the three pedigrees studied, penetrance was complete, but there was variable expressivity, with some patients exhibiting only part of the syndrome. The pathophysiology of MWS episodes awaits identification of the underlying gene. Interleukin 6 levels are elevated during acute flares, but it is unknown if this is primary or secondary.

The susceptibility locus for familial cold urticaria (FCU; OMIM 120100), an inflammatory disorder characterized by cold-induced episodes of fever, rash, arthralgia, conjunctivitis, leukocytosis, and in some cases, amyloidosis, was mapped to the same region of chromosome 1 as the MWS gene (15). In contrast to MWS, episodes of FCU usually are cold-induced, and FCU is not associated with deafness. However, it is possible that allelic mutations at a single locus on chromosome 1 may account for both MWS and FCU.

Clinical and Laboratory Features

Since the original description of MWS, approximately 100 cases have been reported, predominantly from northern Europe. Most cases have been familial, with apparent dominant inheritance, although sporadic cases have been reported. Both heat and cold have been associated with attacks in individual patients. Conjunctivitis, episcleritis, and abdominal pain have been observed in some patients during acute episodes. Laboratory evaluation during the episodes reveals an accelerated erythrocyte sedimentation rate and leukocytosis. The arthropathy of MWS can range from intermittent arthralgia to an episodic (<48 hours) oligoarticular inflammatory arthritis, affecting predominantly the large joints. Persistent synovitis may be observed, but is less common. Amyloidosis of the AA type occurs in about one-quarter of people with MWS and, if present, usually develops in middle age. The prognosis in MWS depends largely on whether the patient develops systemic amyloidosis.

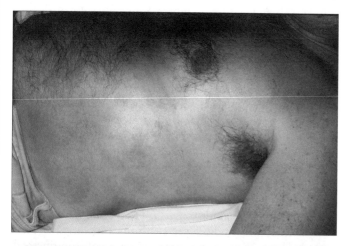

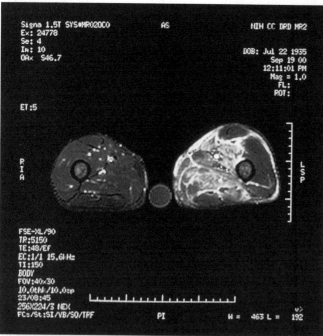

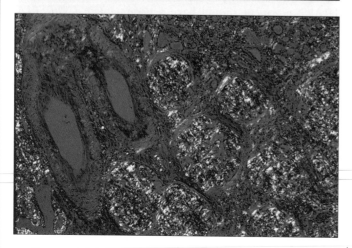

Fig. 8F-1. Clinical features of the tumor necrosis factor (TNF) receptor-associated periodic syndrome (TRAPS). **Top:** Typical migratory erythematous rash on the trunk of a patient with the T50M mutation. **Center:** Magnetic resonance image of a person with TRAPS (T50M), with skin rash and myalgia of the left thigh. Biopsy demonstrated fasciitis and panniculitis, but no myositis. **Bottom:** Photomicrograph demonstrating amyloidosis in the kidney of a TRAPS patient with the C52F mutation. The kidney section was stained with Congo red and viewed under polarized light.

The diagnosis of MWS is made on clinical grounds. In families that are sufficiently large, linkage analysis may corroborate the diagnosis, but a definitive molecular test awaits identification of the specific gene involved. Given the variable expressivity of MWS in known families, it is possible that MWS may be unrecognized in some individuals with unexplained joint complaints, skin rash, hearing loss, or amyloidosis.

Treatment

There is anecdotal evidence that colchicine and high dose corticosteroids may ameliorate MWS attacks, but it is unknown whether these agents prevent the development of amyloidosis in this disorder.

Periodic Disorders of Unknown Etiology

In contrast to the hereditary periodic fever syndromes, there are a group of periodic arthritides in which genetics plays a less important role (Table 8F-2).

Palindromic Rheumatism

Palindromic rheumatism (PR) is a term coined by Hench and Rosenberg (16) to describe intermittent, relatively brief episodes of arthritis and/or inflammation of the soft tissue around the joint (periarthritis). The prevalence of PR is roughly 20-fold less than that of rheumatoid arthritis (RA).

The mean age of onset is approximately 45 years, and the gender ratio is relatively even. A number of families have been reported with multiple cases of PR, or in which PR and RA occur together. The HLA-DR1 and -DR4 associations seen in RA have not been documented in PR (17).

Clinical and Laboratory Features

In PR, attacks occur suddenly and irregularly, unaccompanied by constitutional symptoms or identifiable inciting events. They usually last less than 48 hours. Typically, a single joint is affected in an attack, although multiple joints may be involved over time. Joint pain and tenderness can be substantial, with periarticular soft-tissue swelling and, sometimes, small, tender nodules on the tendons of the hands, fingers, and thumb pads. The joints most frequently affected are the interphalangeal joints of the hands and feet, wrists, shoulders, and ankles (17). Between attacks, patients feel well and have no residual disability. Radiographs are normal.

During the attacks, there is a mild to moderate acceleration in the erythrocyte sedimentation rate (16,17). Approximately one-half of patients with PR have a positive rheumatoid factor (17), but antinuclear antibodies usually are not present, and complement levels are normal. Synovial fluid taken during an attack may contain up to 10,000 white blood cells/mm^3, and synovial biopsies demonstrate an early influx of polymorphonuclear leukocytes (16). Subcutaneous nodules are inflammatory but, in contrast to rheumatoid nodules, lack areas of central fibrinoid necrosis and palisading mononuclear cells.

TABLE 8F-2
Idiopathic Periodic Syndromes

Feature	Palindromic rheumatism	Intermittent hydrarthrosis	Eosinophilic synovitis
Attacks	~2 days; monarticular arthritis or periarticular soft-tissue inflammation; usually irregular intervals	3–5 days; monarticular arthritis, large effusions	1–2 weeks; monarthritis triggered by trauma
Joints involved	MCPs, PIPs, wrists, shoulders, MTPs, ankles	Knee >> hip, ankle, elbow	Knee, MTP
Associated conditions	Familial aggregation with RA	Episodes sometimes coincide with menses	Personal or family history of allergy; dermatographism
Prognosis	~50% have persistent palindromic rheumatism; ~33% develop RA	Attacks often occur at predictable intervals; sometimes spontaneous remissions	Self-limited episodes; benign prognosis
Treatment	Injectable gold, antimalarials, D-penicillamine	NSAIDs, intra-articular steroids, synovectomy	Symptomatic

MCP, metacarpophalangeal; PIP, proximal interphalangeal; MTP, metatarsophalangeal; RA, rheumatoid arthritis; NSAIDs, nonsteroidal anti-inflammatory drugs

Approximately one-third of people with PR eventually develop RA, with conversion to seropositivity sometimes heralding the development of more aggressive disease. In one large series, 48% of patients had persistent PR, 33% developed RA, 4% went on to develop rheumatic diseases other than RA, and 15% experienced a prolonged remission (17). A recent retrospective study of 127 patients with PR identified rheumatoid factor seropositivity, involvement of the wrist and proximal interphalangeal joints, and female gender as the greatest risk factors for developing RA (18).

Treatment

There have been no large, controlled trials on the treatment of PR, although retrospective studies suggest that NSAIDs, injectable gold, antimalarials, and sulfasalazine may have a role.

Intermittent Hydrarthrosis

Intermittent hydrarthrosis is characterized by periodic episodes of monarticular or pauciarticular arthritis. The episodes typically last three to five days, often occur at very regular intervals, and are not accompanied by fever or constitutional symptoms. Spontaneous remission occurs in some cases (19).

It is a relatively rare condition, with no prevalence data available. The usual age of onset is between 20 and 50 years, and the gender ratio is relatively even. In some women, attacks coincide with menses, beginning at menarche and remitting during pregnancy or after menopause. Generally, intermittent hydrarthrosis does not cluster in families.

Clinical Features

Attacks involve joint pain, limitation of motion, and a massive effusion, but only minimal erythema or warmth over the involved joint. In individual patients, a limited number of joints are affected, with the knee most frequent, and the hip, ankle, and elbow involved less often. In some patients, the same joint is always involved, and in others, swelling may alternate in two or more joints.

Laboratory findings during attacks are minimal (19). The erythrocyte sedimentation rate and white count usually are normal. Synovial fluid is mildly inflammatory, usually with fewer than 5000 white blood cells/mm³. Edema, hyperemia, and inflammatory infiltrates may be present on synovial biopsies (19). Radiographs may show soft-tissue swelling during an attack, but there are no chronic radiographic changes, even after repeated attacks in the same joint.

Treatment

A number of therapeutic approaches have been used, including NSAIDs, intra-articular steroids, surgical synovectomy, and intra-articular radioactive gold.

Eosinophilic Synovitis

First described in seven individuals with a personal or family history of allergy (20), eosinophilic synovitis is an acute, recurring, painless monarthritis triggered by minor trauma.

The episodes are self-limited and require only symptomatic treatment. Like intermittent hydrarthrosis, eosinophilic synovitis is quite rare, and no useful prevalence data are available. The usual age of onset is between 20 and 50 years, with no gender bias.

Clinical and Laboratory Features

Large effusions develop over 12–24 hours with minimal associated erythema or warmth, and these effusions persist for one to two weeks. The knee and metatarsophalangeal joints are affected most frequently. The erythrocyte sedimentation rate, white blood cell count, and peripheral eosinophil counts are normal during attacks, although some patients have elevated serum IgE levels. Synovial fluid typically has 5000–20,000 white blood cells/mm³, with as many as 50% eosinophils. Wet preparations of synovial fluid incubated under a coverslip at 4°C overnight show Charcot-Leyden crystals, which are bipyramidal, hexagonal crystals formed by intracellular lipases in eosinophils (20). There are no long-term radiographic changes in eosinophilic synovitis.

The differential diagnosis of synovial eosinophilia is extensive and includes RA, psoriatic arthritis, rheumatic fever, parasitic arthritides, infectious arthritides (e.g., tuberculosis and Lyme disease), the hypereosinophilic syndrome, metastatic adenocarcinoma, and history of recent arthrography (20). Distinctive features of eosinophilic synovitis include a personal or family history of allergy and dermatographism. The authors of the original description of this syndrome speculated that eosinophilic effusions may be the synovial equivalent of dermatographism.

DANIEL L. KASTNER, MD, PhD

References

1. McDermott MF, Aksentijevich I, Galon J, et al. Germline mutations in the extracellular domains of the 55 kDa TNF receptor, TNFR1, define a family of dominantly inherited autoinflammatory syndromes. Cell 1999;97:133–144.
2. Aksentijevich I, Torosyan Y, Samuels J, et al. Mutation and haplotype studies of familial Mediterranean fever reveal new ancestral relationships and evidence for a high carrier frequency with reduced penetrance in the Ashkenazi Jewish population. Am J Hum Genet 1999;64:949–962.
3. Sohar E, Gafni J, Pras M, Heller H. Familial Mediterranean fever. A survey of 470 cases and review of the literature. Am J Med 1967;43:227–253.
4. Kastner DL. Intermittent and periodic arthritic syndromes. In: Koopman WJ (ed.) Arthritis and Allied Conditions, 14th edition. Philadelphia: Lippincott Williams & Wilkins, 2001; pp 1400–1441.
5. The International FMF Consortium. Ancient missense mutations in a new member of the RoRet gene family are likely to cause familial Mediterranean fever. Cell 1997;90:797–807.
6. The French FMF Consortium. A candidate gene for familial Mediterranean fever. Nat Genet 1997;17:25–31.

7. Cazeneuve C, Sarkisian T, Pêcheux C, et al. MEFV-gene analysis in Armenian patients with familial Mediterranean fever: diagnostic value and unfavorable renal prognosis of the M694V homozygous genotype – genetic and therapeutic implications. Am J Hum Genet 1999;65:88–97.

8. Drenth JP, Haagsma CJ, van der Meer JW. Hyperimmunoglobulinemia D and periodic fever syndrome. The clinical spectrum in a series of 50 patients. International Hyper-IgD Study Group. Medicine (Baltimore) 1994;73:133–144.

9. Houten SM, Kuis W, Duran M, et al. Mutations in MVK, encoding mevalonate kinase, cause hyperimmunoglobulinaemia D and periodic fever syndrome. Nat Genet 1999;22:175–177.

10. Drenth JP, Cuisset L, Grateau G, et al. Mutations in the gene encoding mevalonate kinase cause hyper-IgD and periodic fever syndrome. International Hyper-IgD Study Group. Nat Genet 1999;22:178–181.

11. McDermott EM, Smillie DM, Powell RJ. The clinical spectrum of familial Hibernian fever: a 14-year follow-up study of the index case and extended family. Mayo Clin Proc 1997;72:806–817.

12. Mulley J, Saar K, Hewitt G, et al. Gene localization for an autosomal dominant familial periodic fever to 12p13. Am J Hum Genet 1998;62:884–889.

13. Muckle TJ, Wells M. Urticaria, deafness, and amyloidosis: a new heredo-familial syndrome. Q J Med 1962;31:235–248.

14. Cuisset L, Drenth JP, Berthelot JM, et al. Genetic linkage of the Muckle-Wells syndrome to chromosome 1q44. Am J Hum Genet 1999;65:1054–1059.

15. Hoffman HM, Wright FA, Broide DH, Wanderer AA, Kolodner RD. Identification of a locus on chromosome 1q44 for familial cold urticaria. Am J Hum Genet 2000;66:1693–1698.

16. Hench PS, Rosenberg EF. Palindromic rheumatism. A "new," oft recurring disease of joints (arthritis, periarthritis, para-arthritis) apparently producing no articular residues. Report of thirty-four cases; its relation to "angioneural arthrosis," "allergic rheumatism" and rheumatoid arthritis. Arch Intern Med 1944;73:293–321.

17. Guerne P-A, Weisman MH. Palindromic rheumatism: part of or apart from the spectrum of rheumatoid arthritis. Am J Med 1992;93:451–460.

18. Gonzalez-Lopez L, Gamez-Nava JI, Jhangri GS, Ramos-Remus C, Russell AS, Suarez-Almazor ME. Prognostic factors for the development of rheumatoid arthritis and other connective tissue diseases in patients with palindromic rheumatism. J Rheumatol 1999;26:540–545.

19. Weiner AD. Periodic benign synovitis. Idiopathic intermittent hydrarthrosis. J Bone Joint Surg 1956;38A:1039–1055.

20. Brown JP, Rola-Pleszczynski M, Ménard HA. Eosinophilic synovitis: clinical observations on a newly recognized subset of patients with dermatographism. Arthritis Rheum 1986;29:1147–1151.

MUSCULOSKELETAL SIGNS AND SYMPTOMS
G. Sports and Occupational Injuries

Musculoskeletal injuries occurring at the workplace and in athletic pursuits are associated with significant socioeconomic, physical, and psychological ramifications. Computerized instruments have replaced some physically demanding occupations, but also have introduced a new spectrum of physical disabilities. Workplace demographics have changed to include an ever-increasing number of women, senior citizens, and disabled individuals. Productivity has increased while numbers of employees have decreased, creating an environment conducive to decreased morale and increased fatigue and physical injury.

Athletic activity has increased exponentially over the past two decades, largely because people are sensitized to the benefits of physical fitness. It is estimated that 30 million people participate in some form of organized sport annually in the United States (1). Countless millions more are involved in nonorganized sports and may have the same propensity to physical injury. Approximately 25% of high-school athletes will sustain an injury at some time. Direct costs of such injuries exceed $250 million per year (1).

Recognizing the impact on fiscal health-care dollars and on physical well-being, a federal initiative entitled Health 2000 has stimulated injury prevention research in sports with the goal of increasing overall health, fitness pleasure, and relaxation. To this end, conditioning and warm-up exercises have assumed greater priority, as have modifications to equipment and the physical environment in which sports are played. Similarly, the field of ergonomics has evolved to modify the workplace to the benefit of the employee.

Sports Injuries
Bone Injuries
Although considerably less common than injuries to soft tissue, bone injuries are becoming more common because more people are engaging in sports such as motorcross, hang-gliding, cycling, and snowmobiling. The spectrum of bone injuries encompasses contusion, stress fracture, avulsive injury, and fracture, including growth-plate injuries in the skeletally immature adolescent.

Contusions to bone generally occur upon direct impact with another player, surface, or object in the playing field. They also can occur indirectly when a ligament injury produces laxity of the contiguous joint, allowing excessive contact between joint surfaces. Such an indirect insult commonly is seen with an acute anterior cruciate ligament injury that allows the tibia to rotate and translate excessively on the femur, with subsequent impaction between the joint surfaces. Direct injuries tend to occur in subcutaneous locations, such as the distal and proximal fibula, femoral condyles at the knee, patella, condyles of the distal humerus, and styloid of the radius.

The player presents with an acute onset of pain in the vicinity of the contact, which may be obvious due to an abrasion, laceration, ecchymosis, or hematoma. Palpation directly over the area elicits discomfort but no evident underlying bone defect. Examination of the contiguous joint reveals no evidence of an effusion or ligament disruption, and although somewhat uncomfortable, full motion usually is possible.

If radiographs exclude associated ligament and osseous injuries, local treatment includes ice, elevation, a compressive dressing, and encouraging the patient to maintain and promote motion. The patient can gradually return to activities.

Stress fractures are incomplete fractures due to repetitive strains on normal bone from periarticular muscle contractions that exceed the bone's ability to withstand such forces. Three types of mechanical events may lead to stress fractures: an increased applied load; an increased number of applied stresses; and an increased surface area over which the load is applied. Stress fractures need to be distinguished from pathologic fractures due to osteoporosis, Paget's disease, hyperparathyroidism, or malignancy. Stress fractures can occur when an athlete suddenly changes activity, training, or equipment, including footwear (2). Some athletes are predisposed because of developmental or congenital abnormalities, such as genu varum, hindfoot varum, or forefoot varum, all of which place greater stresses on the compressive side of the bones of the lower extremity. The etiology of stress fracture likely is multifactorial, with contributing mechanical, hormonal, and nutritional factors (3). The most common sites of stress fractures include the metatarsals, calcaneus, tibia, fibula, and femoral neck. Spondylosis or stress fractures of the posterior vertebral elements are not uncommon causes of back pain, particularly in young female gymnasts, dancers, or figure skaters.

Patients present with localized pain, and often are unable to place full weight or hop on the involved limb. Examinations of the fibula, tibia, calcaneus, and metatarsals often demonstrate localized tenderness, swelling, and if callus already has developed, a local deformity of bone. Unlike other areas, the hip cannot be effectively palpated, and the clinician must rely on imaging to make the diagnosis. Plain radiographic evidence of injury is not present for at least two weeks and even as long as several months after symptom onset. Periosteal reaction, callus, and a linear sclerotic line will usually confirm the diagnosis. Bone scintigraphy often allows diagnosis in the early stages. Magnetic resonance imaging (MRI) for proximal femoral stress fracture can determine whether the injury was caused by tension or compression and whether the fracture pattern is complete or incomplete.

Treatment involves discontinuing the physical activity, adopting other means of aerobic exercise while protecting the limb, and modifying weight-bearing. A more global and comprehensive treatment approach addresses such intrinsic and extrinsic risk factors as skeletal malalignment, flexibility, muscular strength and endurance, and reviews hormonal and nutritional factors. When radiographic and clinical examination show that union is secure, the patient may return to the activity with a modified program that addresses any predisposing factors.

Proximal femoral neck stress fractures are unique (4). The inferior neck stress or compressive fracture generally heals with the previously described recommendations. However, the superior neck or vertically oriented fracture on the tensile side of the femoral neck has a propensity for completing the fracture and displacing. Most people with this complication require surgical stabilization to minimize the possibility of displacement, osteonecrosis, or malunion.

Avulsive injuries of the lower extremity are unique to adolescent athletes (5). This injury is a counterpart to the muscle tendon strain or disruption that occurs in the adult athlete. The avulsive injury involves secondary growth centers (apophyses) and causes the cartilaginous growth plate to separate from the underlying bone. These injuries may occur before ossification of the secondary growth center, and therefore may not be immediately evident on radiographs. The injury is a result of a sudden contracture of the muscle attached to the apophysis while the extremity is forced in the opposite direction, which suddenly and violently increases the length of the muscle-tendon unit. The most common sites of involvement are the ischial apophysis (hamstring origin), lesser trochanteric apophysis (iliopsoas insertion), anterior-superior iliac spine apophysis (sartorius origin), and anterior-inferior iliac spine apophysis (rectus femoris origin). Displacement of the avulsed segment is minimized due to the extensive periosteal and perichondral insertion.

The patient presents with severe sudden onset of pain at the site of the injury, inability to actively resist stretching of the involved muscle, ecchymosis and swelling at the avulsed site, and inability to place full weight on the involved extremity. The treatment of these conditions is directed toward minimizing any further displacement of the apophysis, and should be given in the following sequence: analgesics, ice, protected weight-bearing, and positioning the extremity to relax the involved muscle. After the acute pain has resolved, active excursion of the muscle is encouraged, progressing to recruiting muscles in close proximity. Resistive exercises can be initiated when active motion has returned fully. Patients can resume sports activities when full motion and muscle power is restored, which generally takes up to six weeks.

Definitive fractures of long bones, pelvis, and spine are rare among athletes. They usually are associated with high-speed motorized sporting activity or falls from heights (6). The patient presents with pain, inability to move the extremity, deformity, and crepitation at the fracture site. Local ecchymosis and swelling often are evident in such subcutaneous locations as the ankle and forearm, but these signs may be absent in fractures of the thigh, spine, and pelvis. Most of these injuries are treated at trauma centers and necessitate either closed reduction and immobilization or open reduction and internal fixation, depending on the nature of the injury.

Growth-plate injuries through epiphyses occur in skeletally immature adolescents (7). These injuries often are assumed to be ligament injuries because the physical findings are similar, including instability of the contiguous joint. Epiphyseal injuries usually are due to shearing and avulsive forces, although compressive stresses also play a significant role. Given that these injuries tend to occur in youngsters with remarkable healing potential, fractures that initially unite with some deformity can completely remodel with subsequent growth. Recognizing the skeletally immature status of the patient and the possibility of apophyseal injury should prompt stress views, which often can delineate the nature of the growth-plate injury. These injuries can be devastating because of the associated interruption of growth and maturation of the limb.

Muscle and Tendon Injuries

Because most sports require sudden, powerful, and repetitive muscle contractions, injuries to muscles and tendons are common in athletes. These injuries include muscle cramps, exercise-induced muscle soreness, contusions, strains, lacerations, and compartment syndromes.

Although the exact mechanism of *muscle cramps* is not well understood, the physical findings are uniformly similar (8). The patient experiences sudden onset of discomfort, muscle spasm with visible fasciculations, pain on palpation, and involuntary movement of contiguous joints. Muscle cramps more commonly involve the lower extremity than the upper limbs. Onset generally is due to sudden contracture of an already shortened muscle. It may occur in perfectly healthy young athletes and in those who have a significant electrolyte imbalance with alterations in serum sodium, calcium, or magnesium. The cramp can be aborted by forcefully stretching the muscle or by activating antagonistic muscles. Muscle excitability and fasciculations can last for several days, well after the process largely has been reversed.

Exercise-induced muscle soreness is experienced by most, if not all, athletes who start or resume a particularly demanding physical activity. Acute pain during exercise likely is the product of lactic acid accumulation within the muscle. Although unpleasant, it usually is not associated with any visible or palpable muscle spasm and resolves shortly after activity cessation. In contrast, delayed muscle soreness one or even two days after the activity likely is a product of microtears within the muscle. Local pain when contracting or stretching the muscle is typical. Applying ice and a compressive bandage may assist in resolving the discomfort. Graduated return to physical activity after the acute phase is recommended. Recurrence may be avoided by training less aggressively (8).

Direct muscle injury is common in contact sports (9). The anterior thigh is the site most frequently injured, usually due to contact with equipment or another player. The injury is marked by swelling, pain with any active or passive movement of the muscle, and sometimes, ecchymosis. Contusions are graded according to severity of the disability, which depends primarily on the degree of pain and swelling immediately after the injury. For example, a grade I quadriceps contusion is that in which knee flexion can be accomplished beyond 90°, grade II is flexion from 45° to 90°, and grade III is less than 45° of active flexion. Disability is minimized by applying ice immediately, elevating the limb, using a compressive dressing, and starting active movement early to promote gentle stretching of the involved muscle.

These preventive measures minimize the development of *myositis ossificans*, an ossification of the hematoma in muscle, which can be seen on radiograph two to three weeks after the injury. Myositis ossificans can prolong disability and discomfort. Myositis ossificans evolves through an inflammatory phase during which fibroblasts mature into chondrocytes, then ultimately into immature bone. With resolution of the acute inflammation, the newly developed bone matures histologically and radiographically. In spite of the presence of a sizable bulk of bone in the muscle, rarely does it cause symptoms sufficient to warrant surgical excision. Physical therapy with passive assisted motion or with constant passive motion machines has been associated with the development of myositis ossificans. Recent studies suggest that immobilizing the contused muscle in a maximum stretch position serves to reduce disability and return motion rapidly (10). Active motion promotes stretching of involved muscle as does keeping the immobilized muscle in its maximal stretched position.

In addition to these recommendations, stretch-induced muscle injuries or strains, muscle contusions, and delayed-onset muscle soreness often are treated with nonsteroidal anti-inflammatory drugs, which modestly inhibit the initial inflammatory response and associated symptoms. However, because these medications (and particularly corticosteroids) decrease or mitigate the inflammatory response of the healing phase, adverse or incomplete healing could occur (11).

Tendon disruption occurs from sudden, violent contracture of a muscle against sudden resistance. Common tendon injuries in the senior athlete involve the Achilles, quadriceps, patellar tendon, or the long head of the biceps at the shoulder or radial tuberosity. With the exception of the proximal biceps, rupture of these tendons is disabling and requires surgical repair. Achilles tendon rupture is most common in racquet sports and basketball, where sudden deceleration on the court produces such tension in the tendon as to rupture it several centimeters from the bony insertion. The athlete experiences immediate pain and is unable to put full weight on the lower limb. Findings on physical examination are ecchymosis and an obvious palpable deformity on the distal posterior aspect of the calf, positive

Thompson's sign, inability to plantar flex the foot with any power, and on rare occasions, decreased sensation of the sural nerve dermatome. Similarly, athletes who experience quadriceps or patellar tendon disruptions lose the extensor mechanism and are unable to walk. Disruption of the biceps tendon causes swelling and ecchymosis at the site. If proximal disruption occurs, the muscle portion of the biceps migrates distally, causing the muscle to bulge markedly. If a tear occurs at the radial styloid insertion, the muscle migrates proximally, which is more disabling than a proximal tear because it interferes more with elbow flexion and supination.

Compartment syndrome is characterized by a pathologic increase in the interstitial pressure within an anatomically confined muscle compartment, thereby interfering with neurovascular innervation, which can lead to myonecrosis. The sudden increase in intracompartmental pressure can be caused by hemorrhage or by intracellular or even extracellular edema. The clinical presentation includes an inordinate amount of pain (particularly on active and passive stretching of muscles within the compartment), paresthesias in the distribution of nerves coursing though the compartment, and a definitive and marked increase in resistance to palpation. The pulses may be intact distally and not diminished. Diagnosis is confirmed by measuring the intracompartmental pressure. Pressure in excess of 30–40 mm Hg or within 30 mm of the diastolic pressure is indicative of evolving or actual compartment syndrome and the need for emergent fasciotomy.

Chronic exertional compartment syndromes are more common and generally are seen in long-distance runners. Pain is isolated to the anterior or lateral compartment and begins early in the athlete's training program. It can be a difficult diagnosis to make and to differentiate from stress fractures, shin splints, popliteal entrapment syndrome, and other conditions remote from the calf, such as piriformis syndrome. The diagnosis is suggested by intracompartmental pressure elevations above normal during exercise and a slow return to resting levels at the conclusion of exercise. Once the diagnosis is confirmed, it may be necessary to perform fasciotomy.

Chronic overuse syndromes commonly are seen in senior athletes because repetitive demands on muscles and tendons eclipse the adaptive and healing capabilities of these structures (12). The pain associated with this phenomenon can occur during or after exercise, with or without alterations in performance level. The evolution of this process follows three stages: inflammation and edema, scarring, and thickening and fibrosis within the tendon. If medical intervention or activity modification is not initiated, continued injury to the tendon can result in partial or complete rupture. Several classic examples of repetitive overuse syndromes include impingement syndrome of the shoulder, deltoid tendinitis at its insertion on the mid to upper humerus, tendinitis of the common extensor muscle originating from the lateral epicondyle of the elbow, and tendinitis of the Achilles tendon at its insertion on the calcaneus.

People with overuse syndromes universally complain of pain when performing their activities, have localized discomfort, sometimes manifest crepitation, and may even have palpable thickness of the tendons as a result of edema and inflammation. Treatment consists of ice, modification of activities, nonsteroidal anti-inflammatory drugs, ultrasound treatment, and gentle eccentric stretching of the musculotendinous units. Modification of training or performance may minimize further insult (Table 8G-1). For those who have progressed to partial- or full-thickness tears, surgical reconstruction may be necessary to restore normal power and motion. Although stretching before exercise is recommended, basic science research suggests that it does not affect muscle compliance during eccentric activity, when most strains are believed to occur, and it can produce damage at the cytoskeleton level. There is, therefore, no convincing evidence that stretching before exercise reduces the risk of injury (13).

TABLE 8G-1
Chronic Overuse Syndromes

Grade	Symptoms	Treatment
I	Pain after activity only	Ice
II	Pain during and after activity, but no significant interference with performance	Ice and 10%–25% decrease in activity
III	Pain during and after activity, with interference with performance	Ice, 25%–75% decrease in activity, and NSAIDs
IV	Constant pain that interferes with activities of daily living	Ice, complete rest of involved area, and NSAIDs

NSAIDs, nonsteroidal anti-inflammatory drugs.

Injuries to Ligaments and Capsule

Joints are supported and stabilized by congruency of the articulating surfaces. The shoulder, hip, and knee are further reinforced by fibrocartilage extensions of the articulating segments in the form of a labrum or menisci. Additionally, there are well-defined ligaments that minimize excursion of the articulating segments in certain planes. One or all of these structures can be injured by force applied either to the joint directly or to the bone in such a way that it increases the distance between the articulating surfaces and overcomes the ability of ligaments to resist such forces. The degree of injury depends on the magnitude and direction of the force, the position of the joint at the time of injury, and the speed at which the force was applied.

Ligament injuries are classified according to the extent of tear and degree of laxity, which usually can be determined by a thorough clinical examination (Table 8G-2). Ligament injuries of the knee are common and likely to be disabling if tears are missed or misdiagnosed, because chronic instability precipitates further intra-articular damage in the form of meniscal tears, chondral contusions and disruptions, and possibly, premature degenerative arthritis. Knee ligament injuries should be diagnosed early and appropriate treatment initiated to minimize the sequelae. Varus or valgus force jeopardizes the lateral or medial collateral ligament, respectively. Likewise, anterior or posterior force may injure the anterior or posterior cruciate ligament. It is rare that force is applied in an isolated, unidirectional manner. Generally, the force includes a significant rotational element that contributes to a combination of ligament injuries or ligament and meniscal pathology.

Most athletes who sustain ligament injuries cannot continue to practice or play (14). They feel a tearing sensation or a "pop" that may be heard, even by people nearby, suggesting complete ligament disruption or significant bony injury. The patient has difficulty standing on the injured leg and often needs support. Acute swelling within the knee suggests intra-articular hemorrhage and the strong probability of cruciate ligament injury. Effusions that occur 24–36 hours after injury suggest meniscal tears without concomitant ligament injury.

Initial assessment should include a thorough neurovascular examination distal to the injury, an evaluation of the injured limb's orientation compared with the uninvolved limb, and a check of the extent of effusion. The orientation of the patella relative to the underlying femur may reveal a concomitant patellofemoral dislocation. Active and passive range of motion should be assessed. A knee that cannot be flexed passively or extended beyond the resting flexed position suggests the presence of a displaced, bucket-handle tear of the meniscus. Similarly, a knee that is "locked" in full extension and has what appears to be a soft mechanical block suggests displaced meniscal pathology, a loose fragment, or a torn anterior cruciate that has fallen between the articulating segments. Integrity of the collateral ligaments can be determined through varus/valgus stressing in extension and in 30° of flexion. Assessment of the anterior cruciate ligament should include the Lachman's test, anterior drawer test at 70°–90° flexion, and the pivot-shift test. Maximum flexion with rotation may elicit discomfort or a classic clicking sound, which are associated with a positive McMurray's sign for meniscal pathology. Pain elicited by palpation along either joint line suggests meniscal tears, and pain at the condylar insertion and origin of the collateral ligaments suggests injury to these structures.

Radiographs may show an avulsive injury of the collateral or cruciate ligaments, osteocartilaginous loose bodies within the knee joint, or previously undiagnosed osteochondritis dissecans. A flake of bone from the lateral tibial condyle (Segond's sign) is pathognomonic for an associated anterior cruciate injury. In the presence of acute hemarthrosis and pain, it may be impossible initially to ascertain the extent of ligament and associated injuries. By applying a knee immobilizer and initiating protective ambulation, the clinician can evaluate the knee after it becomes less irritable. An MRI may help to determine the full extent of injury and to develop a more effective treatment plan.

Most grade I and grade II isolated ligament injuries can be treated with ice, compressive bandage, protected ambulation, and functional bracing, as necessary, followed by early return of motion and resumption of routine activities.

TABLE 8G-2
Classification and Treatment of Ligament Tears

	1st Degree	2nd Degree	3rd Degree
Injury	Minimal tear	Partial tear	Complete tear
Laxity	None	Mild to moderate	Unstable
Treatment	Ice with rehabilitation and supportive care	Ice, muscle rehabilitation, functional bracing, and possible cast	Ice, splint, and possible surgery
Prognosis	Excellent	Good	Variable

Grade III isolated medial collateral ligament injuries generally can be treated conservatively in a similar manner. Ligaments will heal more rapidly if joint movement is initiated early, rather than keeping the knee immobilized.

It is estimated that 1 in 3000 individuals per year sustains an anterior cruciate ligament injury in the United States – corresponding to an overall injury rate of approximately 100,000 annually (15). This injury is almost epidemic among young female athletes, with anterior cruciate ligament injury rates reported to be two to eight times higher than in men participating in similar sports. Speculation on the possible etiology of anterior cruciate ligament injuries in women has identified joint laxity, hormonal alterations, training techniques, and anatomic differences (specifically the intercondylar distance, which is narrow in females, contributing to the extrinsic compression of the ligament with rotation). Women tend to maintain a more erect posture and extend their knees somewhat farther when they perform cutting and landing maneuvers, increasing the propensity for injuries to the anterior cruciate ligament.

Treatment of isolated anterior cruciate ligament injuries depends on the patient's age and anticipated future physical activities (14). It may be appropriate to initiate rehabilitation as described previously, incorporate closed kinetic chain exercises early to compensate for the cruciate deficiency, and have the patient wear a brace during athletic activities. Active individuals may elect to have anterior cruciate ligament reconstruction surgery. Multiligament injuries or anterior cruciate injuries associated with significant meniscal pathology are best treated by surgical reconstruction.

Another common site for ligament injury is the anterior lateral aspect of the ankle. An inversion plantar-flexed position of the foot, with sudden weight-bearing, principally injures the anterior talofibular ligament and, less often, the fibulocalcaneal and posterior talofibular ligaments. The subcutaneous position of these ligaments results in early significant swelling, ecchymosis, and discoloration. The pain is located on the anterolateral fibula, at the insertion site of the anterior talofibular ligament, and often on the distal tibiofibular ligament, just anterior to the ankle joint. Assessment should include other sites of discomfort, however, to exclude the possibility of associated osseous injuries. Ankle stability is assessed by placing the foot in 20°–30° of plantar flexion and pulling anteriorly on the posterior aspect of the hindfoot in an attempt to sublux the talar dome from the underlying tibia. Generally, disruption of the anterior talofibular ligament is marked by slight anterior translation of the talus from underneath the tibia in 30° of plantar flexion, but in neutral position, it stabilizes. Treatment is directed toward minimizing the edema and swelling; patients should be encouraged to resume ankle motion and to have confidence in weight-bearing. Extensive strengthening of the lateral structures of the ankle helps minimize future inversion injuries. The most common risk factor for ankle sprain in sports is a history of a previous sprain. As such, athletes with a sprained ankle should complete supervised rehabilitation before returning to practice or competition, and athletes suffering a moderate to severe sprain should wear an appropriate orthosis for at least six months.

When force applied to the joint surfaces exceeds the resistance of the ligaments and capsule, the joint may subluxate or dislocate. In subluxation, the joint partially separates but spontaneously reduces; in dislocation, the joint surfaces are dislodged. The patient complains of immediate pain, is unable to move the extremity in any effective direction, protects the extremity, and may or may not complain of dysthesias. The most common dislocations are those of the shoulder and patellofemoral joints; dislocations of the elbow, hip, and knee are distinctly uncommon.

Patients with a shoulder dislocation have a squared-off appearance, lack the usual deltoid contour, and have a prominence on the anterior aspect of the chest wall, a result of the dislocated humeral head lying anterior and inferior to the glenoid (16). Examination should include an extensive neurologic evaluation of the extremity, as well as assessment of the axillary nerve. Decreased sensation in a small patchy area over the lateral aspect of the upper arm suggests the possibility of concomitant injury. Relocation is accomplished with sedation and traction, but radiographic views should be made first to rule out the possibility of an associated fracture of the tuberosities or upper humeral shaft that could be displaced farther by aggressive traction. Neurologic examination should be repeated after reduction.

Considerably less common, but much more devastating, are dislocations of the hip and knee. In an effort to avoid osteonecrosis, a hip dislocation should be considered an emergency, and reduction accomplished within six to eight hours. Radiographic studies before and after reduction should be performed to identify associated fractures that could prevent a congruent reduction. If this condition is suspected, fine-cut computerized tomography scans of the pelvis should be performed to identify intra-articular loose fragments. In knee dislocations, the possibility of neurovascular injury always should be considered. All patients with knee dislocations should have an arteriogram to rule out concomitant vascular injury.

Given the interest and intensity of physical training among middle-aged and senior citizens, there is increasing concern that too much activity may lead to premature osteoarthritis. The continuous stress that physical activity places on the joints can result in microtrauma and degeneration of the articular cartilage. The onset of osteoarthritis appears to depend on the frequency, intensity, and duration of physical activity (17). There currently is no compelling evidence to suggest that moderate amounts of exercise without adverse consequence will accelerate the development of osteoarthritis. Excessive participation in high-impact sports, particularly over a prolonged period, could increase the risk of developing osteoarthritis and may need to be taken into consideration.

Occupational Injuries

In contrast to the prevalence of lower-extremity injuries among athletes, the upper extremity, back, and cervical spine are much more commonly affected by injuries sustained in the workforce. In addition, work-related injuries often are based on exposure to repetitive tasks over time. Such terms as cumulative trauma disorder and repetitive stress injury (RSI) are used to describe a wide spectrum of disorders, including many that are similar to chronic overuse syndromes in athletes.

Occupational injuries affect 15%–20% of all Americans, and RSIs account for 56% of all occupational injuries, with an incidence of 21 cases per 100,000 workers annually (18, 19). This incidence is an exponential increase from the 1980s, possibly a product of evolving workplace technology, generous changes in workers' compensation benefits, improved accuracy of reporting and diagnosis, increased awareness of employee rights, and with ever-increasing downsizing, pressure on employees to perform more tasks, more quickly, in a shorter period of time.

Muscles actively engaged in performing repetitive tasks and distant muscles that remain contracted for long periods of time to sustain an unsupported extremity are vulnerable to muscle fatigue and microtears, with associated inflammation, edema, and dysfunction. The following risk factors in the workplace are associated with RSI: repetition, high force, awkward joint position, direct pressure, vibration, and prolonged constrained posture. The incidence of musculoskeletal complaints and injury rise significantly if two or more risk factors are present (20). It is important to determine whether patients engage in avocational activities that also may predispose them to such injury. In addition, reviewing the nature of the work and possibly even visiting the job site allow the examiner to more accurately determine the association between work and physical injury (21).

RSIs cover a wide spectrum of disorders, many having a distinctive presentation, predisposing factors, findings on clinical examination, and well-defined and often successful treatment. These injuries include stenosing tenosynovitis of the fingers, deQuervain's tenosynovitis, intersection syndrome, lateral epicondylitis, and rotator cuff tendinitis. Less well-defined disorders include diffuse back and paraspinal complaints, numbness, tingling, perceived weakness, and fatigue. Many people with these complaints have several, if not all, risk factors. Persistent abnormal posture leads to muscle imbalance and increased tension within the peripheral nerves, which precipitates multilevel nerve compression and symptoms. A more extensive examination of these patients and their workplaces may have to be conducted, because the inciting factors are likely to be multiple. Evaluation of the patient's posture and position maintained at work often reveals poor support in the seating and arrangement of tools. Additionally, observing the patient at work may help identify both the muscle unit principally involved with the task and remote muscles that support the activity.

Generally, the treatment of RSI is to rest the affected part with such devices as night-time splints, neck braces, and lower-back supports. Acute management may include the application of ice, nonsteroidal anti-inflammatory drugs, judicious use of local corticosteroid injections, and referral to a physical therapist who can teach appropriate stretching and strengthening exercises and guide the patient through a progressive aerobic program to increase overall physical fitness.

Treatment of RSI is not limited to active medical intervention to reverse the disorder, but includes recommendations on alterations at the job site to minimize further injuries to the patient and his or her colleagues. Ergonomics, which is a discipline that devises ways to maximize comfort and productivity while minimizing injury in the workplace, has become a vital adjunct in the management of workplace injuries.

To prevent reinjury, assessment of risk factors in the workplace should suggest modifications, such as using different tools, reducing time on a high-risk task by job rotation, or using protective equipment, such as pads and splints (22,23). Reducing known risk factors and educating workers about intervention strategies including ergonomics will result in healthier, more informed employees and less financial burden on management. It also is imperative that workplace nurses be proactive in the development and implementation of injury prevention and educational programs related to RSIs (24).

Injuries to Muscle and Tendon

Sustained muscle contraction and repetitive use often precipitate muscle fatigue, which is associated with decreased strength, coordination, and ability to persist with the activity. This is particularly true in a working situation where arms are held at a distance from the body, without support. Such situations are common for automobile assembly workers, mechanics, and electricians who commonly work above their heads while holding heavy equipment. In a similar fashion, workers who are constantly in a static posture and must maintain an arm in abduction or extension for prolonged periods or must sustain a forward thrust of the neck can develop neck torsion syndrome. This syndrome is characterized by pain along the paravertebral segment of the cervical spine extending into the trapezius. On examination, these patients have bilateral trapezius spasm, pain on palpation in the area, decreased neck movement, and pain with extreme movement.

Repetitive use of an extremity often precipitates tenosynovitis. The most commonly involved sites are the first dorsal compartment (deQuervain's tenosynovitis), the area where the mobile wad (abductor pollicis, extensor pollicis longus, extensor pollicis brevis) crosses over the common extensors to the digits in the dorsal distal aspect of the forearm (intersection syndrome), lateral epicondylitis, deltoid tendinitis, and impingement syndrome. Typically, tendinitis is associated with localized discomfort that increases with passive stretching of the affected muscle-tendon unit. There often is pain-induced weakness and crepitation at the site of tendon excursion, and swelling may be apparent in subcutaneous areas.

Injuries of peripheral nerves caused by abnormal posture are common in many job situations and environments. Muscle hypertrophy and atrophy occur simultaneously in muscles challenged and not challenged, respectively. Common entrapments of the upper extremity include the median nerve at the wrist (carpal tunnel syndrome), ulnar nerve at the elbow (cubital tunnel syndrome), and Guyon's canal and radial nerve as it penetrates the supinator in the proximal aspect of the forearm. Direct injury of these nerves also can occur by repeated extrinsic compression.

One of the more common occupational injuries is carpal tunnel syndrome. Carpal tunnel syndrome is a clinical manifestation of compression of the median nerve as it passes through the carpal tunnel or canal. It is reported to be the most common entrapment neuropathy, and is commonly seen as a product of forceful use of the hands, repetitive use of the hands, and hand-arm vibration often seen in the workplace. Patients complain of a tingling sensation along the thumb, index, and middle finger, which may awaken them at night. They also experience weak pinch action and a sensation of spasm in the three digits. Physical examination reveals a positive Tinel's sign at the wrist, decreased muscle bulk in the thenar musculature, decreased sensation along the nerve distribution, and a positive Phalen's test in which wrist flexion reproduces the numbness and tingling. If the pain is not alleviated by splints worn at night, NSAIDs, and corticosteroid injections, and there appears to be evidence of electromyographic dysfunction, carpal tunnel release can be performed by either open surgery or endoscopy. However, one-quarter of patients experiencing carpal tunnel disease also have symptoms suggestive of other soft-tissue injuries, such as tendinitis at various sites or even peripheral nerve entrapment.

Although they consume literally billions of dollars a year due to loss of productivity and continued compensation, RSIs largely are preventable with appropriate assessment of the work environment by well-trained ergonomists.

MICHAEL G. ROCK, MD

References

1. Requa RK. The scope of the problem: the impact of sports-related injuries. In: Conference on Sports Injuries in Youth: Surveillance Strategies. National Inst. of Health, Bethesda MD, April 8-9, 1991.
2. Arendt EA, Clohisy DR. The stress injuries of bone. In: Nicholas JH, Hershman EB (eds). The Lower Extremity and Spine in Sports Medicine, 2nd ed. St Louis, MO: Mosby, 1995.
3. Bennell K, Matheson G, Meeuwisse W, Brukner P. Risk factors for stress fractures. Sports Med 1999;28:91–122.
4. Fullerton LR, Snowdy HA. Femoral neck stress fractures. Am J Sports Med 1988;16:365–377.
5. Sundar M, Carty H. Avulsion fractures of the pelvis in children: a report of 32 fractures and their outcome. Skeletal Radiol 1994;23:85–90.
6. Fink RA, Monge JJ. Snowmobiling injuries. Minn Med 1971;54:29-32.
7. Paletta GA, Andrish JT. Injuries about the hip and pelvis in the young athlete. Clin Sports Med 1995;14:591–628.
8. Abetakis PPM. Muscle soreness in rhabdomyolysis. In: Nicholas JA, Hershman EB (eds). The Lower Extremity and Spine in Sports Medicine, 2nd ed. St. Louis, MO: Mosby, 1995; pp 53–63.
9. Sim FH, Rock MG, Scott SG. Pelvis and hip injuries in athletes: anatomy and function. In: Nicholas JA, Hershman EB (eds). The Lower Extremity and Spine in Sports Medicine, 2nd ed. St. Louis, MO: Mosby, 1995; pp 1025–1065.
10. Ryan JB, Wheeler JH, Hopkinson WJ, Arciero RA, Kolakowski KR. Quadriceps contusions. West Point update. Am J Sports Med 1991;19:299-304.
11. Almekinders LC. Anti-inflammatory treatment of muscular injuries in sports. An update of recent studies. Sports Med 1999;28:383–388.
12. Mercier LR. Sports medicine. In: Mercier LR (ed). Practical Orthopedics, 4th ed. St. Louis MO: Mosby, 1995; pp 294–326.
13. Shrier I. Stretching before exercise does not reduce the risk of local muscle injury: a critical review of the clinical and basic science literature. Clin J Sport Med 1999;9:221–227.
14. Noyes FR, Basset RW, Grood ES, Butler DL. Arthroscopy in acute traumatic hemarthrosis of the knee. Incidence of anterior cruciate tears and other injuries. J Bone Joint Surg 1980;62:687–695, 797.
15. Huston LJ, Greenfield ML, Wojtys EM. Anterior cruciate ligament injuries in the female athlete. Potential risk factors. Clin Orthop 2000;2000:50–63.
16. Steinberg GG, Akins CM, Baran DT. Shoulder and upper arm. In: Steinberg GG, Akins CM, Baran DT (eds). Ramamurti's Orthopedics in Primary Care, 2nd ed. Baltimore: Williams and Wilkins, 1992; pp 26–61.
17. Saxon L, Finch C, Bass S. Sports participation, sports injuries and osteoarthritis: implications for prevention. Sports Med 1999;28:123–135.
18. Melhorn JM. Cumulative trauma disorders and repetitive strain injuries. The future. Clin Orthop 1998;1998:107–126.
19. Bureau of Labor Statistics reports on survey of occupational injuries and illnesses in 1977 through 1989, Washington DC, Bureau of Labor Statistics, U.S. Department of Labor, 1990.
20. Armstrong T, Fine LJ, Goldstein SA, Lifshitz YR, Silverstein BA. Ergonomics considerations in hand and wrist tendinitis. J Surg Hand [Am] 1987;12:830–837.
21. Rodgers SH. Job evaluation in worker fitness determination. Occupational Health: Occup Med 1988;3:219–239.
22. Rempel DM, Harrison RJ, Barnhart S. Work-related cumulative trauma disorders of the upper extremity. JAMA 1992;267: 838–842.
23. Higgs PE, Mackinnon SE. Repetitive motion injuries. Ann Rev Med 1995;46:1–16.
24. Fisher TF. Preventing upper extremity cumulative trauma disorders. An approach to employee wellness. AAOHN Journal 1998;46:296–301.

9

RHEUMATOID ARTHRITIS
A. Epidemiology, Pathology, and Pathogenesis

Rheumatoid arthritis (RA) is a systemic inflammatory disease that predominantly manifests in the synovial membrane of diarthrodial joints. The inflammation develops in a genetically predisposed host; exogenous events that precipitate disease development have not been identified. The chronic inflammatory process induces changes in the cellular composition and the gene expression profile of the synovial membrane, resulting in hyperplasia of synovial fibroblasts and structural damage of cartilage, bone, and ligaments. Extra-articular disease affecting a variety of organs occurs in the majority of patients and is a significant factor in morbidity and mortality of people with RA. The severity of RA encompasses a wide spectrum, ranging from self-limiting disease to chronic progressive disease, causing varying degrees of joint destruction and clinically evident extra-articular organ involvement. This clinical heterogeneity is determined by genetic and environmental factors that control the progression, degree, and pattern of inflammation.

Epidemiology

Rheumatoid arthritis has a worldwide distribution and affects all ethnic groups. The disease can occur at any age, but its prevalence increases with age; the peak incidence is between the fourth and sixth decades. In the absence of definitive tests to establish the diagnosis of RA, incidence and prevalence studies are based on a set of criteria developed for classification purposes. The most widely used criteria are the American College of Rheumatology 1987 revised criteria for the classification of RA (see Appendix I) (1). These criteria have a sensitivity and specificity of approximately 90%. Depending on the stringency of the criteria, the prevalence estimates have varied from 0.3%–1.5% in North America. The prevalence is about 2.5 times higher in women than in men. There are no reports of clustering in space or time that would support an infectious cause, and no environmental factors that precipitate disease onset have been identified. Support for a genetic predisposition for RA has come from studies reporting RA clusters in families. Formal genetic studies have confirmed this familial aggregation (2). Studies in monozygotic twins have shown a concordance rate of 15%–30% and a relative risk of 3.5 for RA developing in monozygotic versus dizygotic twins of affected cases. A high prevalence rate of 5%–6% has been described in some Native American populations, suggesting a higher genetic burden of RA risk genes. Differences in the prevalence rates in other ethnic groups are rather small and are partially explained by differences in disease ascertainment.

Pathology

The histologic changes in RA are not disease-specific and depend on the organ involved. In the joint, the primary inflammatory lesion involves the synovium. The normal synovial membrane consists of a synovial-lining layer formed by one or two layers of synoviocytes. Two cell types constitute the synovial lining: a bone marrow-derived type-A synoviocyte, which has macrophage features, and a mesenchymal type-B synoviocyte. The sublining layer, which is not separated from the synovial lining by a basement membrane, consists of loose connective tissue with numerous blood vessels (3).

The earliest changes in RA, as documented by electron microscopy, are injury to the synovial microvasculature with occlusion of the lumen, swelling of the endothelial cells, and the formation of gaps between endothelial cells. This inflammatory stage usually is associated with congestion, edema, fibrin exudation, and a mild hyperplasia of the superficial lining cell layer. Both type-A and type-B synoviocytes contribute to the synovial membrane hyperplasia, suggesting a paracrine interaction between them. Cellular infiltration occurs early in the disease, consists mainly of lymphocytes and macrophages, and is a consistent feature of patients with active RA irrespective of disease duration. In about one-third of people with RA, the cellular infiltrate acquires a topographical organization reminiscent of tertiary lymphoid tissues (4). In these tissues, T cells and B cells form focal aggregates with an interspersed diffuse infiltrate (Fig. 9A-1). The aggregates are enriched with CD4[+] T cells, and CD8[+] T cells dominate in the diffuse zones. In a substantial proportion of these patients, the aggregates display all characteristics of secondary lymphoid follicles, including germinal-center reactions with proliferating B cells grouped around a network of follicular dendritic cells; primary lymphoid follicles are absent (5). In another 10%–20% of cases, granuloma formation with histologic changes similar to rheumatoid nodules are seen. Plasma cells usually are found in the more advanced stages of inflammation, and multinucleated giant cells and mast cells are not uncommon. The sublining layer of the RA synovium is characterized by neoangiogenesis and tissue fibrosis. Synovial lining hyperplasia, lymphocytic infiltration, and neoangiogenesis are present in biopsies from people with early and late disease and correlate with disease activity rather than different stages of the disease.

The synovial membrane that extends to the cartilage and bone is known as pannus. It actively invades and destroys the periarticular bone and cartilage at the margin between synovium and bone. The major effector cells are synovial fibroblasts and macrophages. In the areas of focal bone erosion, resorption lacunae of multinucleated cells are found that have a gene expression profile identical to classical osteoclasts.

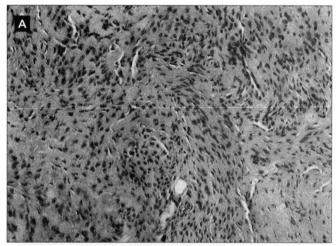
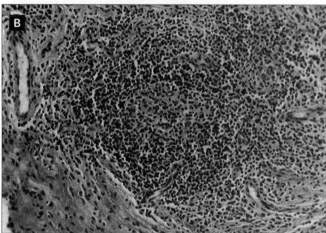
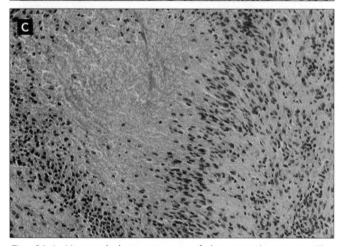

Fig. 9A-1. Histopathologic patterns of rheumatoid synovitis. The inflammatory infiltrate in the synovial membrane can acquire the topographical arrangement of a T-cell–B-cell aggregate, frequently with germinal center formation (**B**) or of a granulomatous lesion (**C**). In about 50% of all patients, the infiltrate is diffuse, lacking distinct structural organizations (**A**). Reprinted from Klimiuk et al (4), with permission of American Society for Investigative Pathology.

Extra-articular manifestations are common in people with RA; however, individuals differ in the pattern of tissues involved. The most characteristic lesions are rheumatoid nodules, which have the histologic appearance of a granulomatous reaction. Typically, multicentric fibrinoid necrosis is surrounded by palisading elongated cells arranged radially, followed by a layer of granulation tissue with inflammatory cells. The composition of the necrotic material can vary, and histology does not allow for any conclusions about the necrosis-inducing event. However, nodules frequently occur at pressure points, suggesting that minor trauma may precipitate the necrosis. The elongated cells in the second layer represent modified macrophages and are aligned parallel to collagen fibers.

Tenosynovitis is present in the majority of patients. Involvement of the tendons is frequent and usually represents a nonspecific inflammatory infiltrate and, less frequently, the formation of characteristic nodules with central necrosis. Similarly, pleurisy and pericarditis are characterized by a diffuse mononuclear infiltration and fibrinoid necrosis, with occasional nodule formation. Vascular involvement usually is confined to small segments of terminal arteries and lacks distinctive histologic characteristics. Infiltration of mid-sized and large arteries with mononuclear cells can occur; however, necrotizing arteritis is infrequent. The diffuse interstitial pulmonary fibrosis seen in RA cannot be distinguished from the fibrosis in other connective-tissue diseases or from primary idiopathic fibrosis. Sicca syndrome, frequently seen in RA patients, histologically resembles Sjögren's syndrome.

Pathogenesis

Rheumatoid arthritis is a disease of an aberrant immune response in a genetically predisposed host that leads to chronic progressive synovial inflammation and destruction of the joint architecture. Research efforts have shed light on the genetic factors, the immunoregulatory defects, and the effector mechanisms leading to tissue injury. Although the impact of genetic factors is obvious, the genetic basis is complex and not sufficient to explain the triggering of the immune insult. Precipitating factors have not been identified, and it remains a matter of debate whether the disease is triggered by an exogenous infectious agent, a breach in tolerance leading to classical autoimmunity, or merely stochastic events that have accumulated with age. Persistence and progression of the disease are regulated by immune mediators that continue to be defined and provide targets for immune intervention.

Genetic Basis of RA

Family studies and studies in monozygotic and dizygotic twins support the concept that genetic factors are important for the susceptibility of RA. However, RA does not frequently aggregate in families and does not show a segregation pattern found in disorders of single- and high-penetrance genes. Many different genes, each of which makes only a small contribution to disease susceptibility, appear to be involved. Interactive genetic effects are suspected to modulate the impact of individual disease-risk genes and likely contribute to the low penetrance. Genetic risk factors not only determine susceptibility for the disease but also correlate with disease severity and phenotype, providing the unique opportunity to use genetic markers as prognostic tools in the management of RA. A measure used to estimate the genetic component to disease is the coefficient of familial clustering, λs, defined as the ratio of the prevalence in affected siblings to the population prevalence. For RA, λs ranges from two to 12, depending on the published data set used. Although clearly supporting the influence of genetic factors, this λs is rather low compared with other autoimmune diseases or common genetic diseases, leaving considerable room for environmental or stochastic events in the pathogenesis of the disease. In part, λs may be rather low because RA is a heterogeneous syndrome that includes several genetically semi-homogenous subsets.

The genetic system studied most thoroughly is the major histocompatibility complex (MHC). In initial studies, RA was shown to be associated with human leukocyte antigen (HLA)-DR4 (6). Studies of the HLA-D region's genomic organization and of the molecular characterization of allelic polymorphisms are the basis for a model showing that the actual disease-conferring sequence is confined to a short sequence that encompasses amino acids 67–74 of the HLA-DRB1 gene (7). Comparing sequences of the disease-associated HLA-DRB1 allele demonstrates sharing of a sequence motif in the third hypervariable region. Association studies in different ethnic populations support the concept that HLA-DRB1 alleles expressing this sequence motif are over-represented among people with RA (2). The sequence polymorphism is characterized by a glutamine or arginine at position 70, a lysine or arginine at position 71, and an alanine at position 74. Alleles with a negatively charged amino acid at any one of these positions are not associated with the disease. The disease-associated alleles include HLA-DRB1*0401, *0404, and *0408. Additional disease-associated alleles include HLA-DRB1*0101/2 mainly in the Caucasian population, HLA-DRB1*0405 in the Asian population, HLA-DRB1*1402 in some Native American populations, and HLA-DRB1*10 in the Greek population.

Clinical-association studies have provided important information to place these genes in the pathophysiology of the disease. In essence, evidence has been provided that HLA-DRB1 alleles modify disease expression. Patients with a disease-associated HLA-DRB1 allele different from HLA-DR4 often develop mild and seronegative disease (8). Disease severity also appears to be influenced by the Lys/Arg dimorphism at position 71 of the disease-associated HLA-DRB1 sequence stretch. Patients with severe joint disease and/or extra-articular manifestations have the strongest HLA-DRB1 association. These patients frequently express two disease-associated HLA-DRB1*04 alleles (9). Family studies have emphasized the importance of the second haplotype. Concordance rates in siblings who share both disease-associated MHC haplotypes are higher than in siblings who share only one haplotype. These data suggest that the disease-associated HLA-DRB1 alleles are important not only in disease initiation, but also in disease progression. Sequence polymorphisms within these alleles and gene-dose effects are important variables influencing the expression of RA (Fig. 9A-2). The data further suggest that these alleles act in concert with other MHC genes as well as background genes.

Crystallographic studies of HLA-DR peptide complexes have mapped the conserved sequence stretch to an a helix that borders the antigen-binding cleft of the HLA-DR molecule (10). Side chains of the MHC molecules form pockets that interact with side chains of antigenic peptides, usually nine amino acids in length, thereby determining the peptide specificity of MHC binding. The polymorphic residues of the shared epitope form the pocket that interacts with the side chains of the fourth amino acid in the bound peptide. In particular, the positively charged amino acid at position 71 of the shared epitope favors the binding of peptides with a negatively charged amino acid. Amino acids of the shared epitope also can interact with the T-cell receptor (TCR) that recognizes the HLA-peptide complex. Depending on the peptide bound, the α-helical conformation is altered and the amino acid at position 70 points to the T-cell receptor.

Based on this structural knowledge, three models for the function of disease-associated polymorphisms have been proposed: 1) selective binding of autoantigenic peptides; 2) selective binding of TCR molecules; and 3) the HLA molecule functioning as a peptide donor. In the first model, antigenic peptides with a negatively charged amino acid in the middle would be prone to trigger a disease-inducing T-cell response. One possible scenario is that peptides derived from pathogenetic microorganisms cross-react with autoantigens. It is likely that different antigenic peptides would be involved in different patients because the peptide-binding profiles of the different disease-associated HLA-DRB1 alleles are quite different, except for their preference for a negatively charged amino acid at position 4. However, it is unclear what aspect could be unique for a particular set of peptides. In the second model, the disease-associated sequence stretch would be involved by directly interacting with contact residues of the TCR. TCR–HLA-DR contact residues contribute to the affinity of the complex formation. The shared epitope could be involved in the selection of a particular set of T cells, either during T-cell repertoire formation in the thymus or by influencing T-cell survival in the periphery (11). In the third model, the disease-associated sequence would not function as a part of the entire HLA-DR molecule but as a peptide. HLA-derived peptides are recognized in the thymus and influence the selection of T cells. Positive selection of such T cells could result in a repertoire that is biased toward the recognition of cross-reactive microbial peptides (12). Molecular mimicry between the disease-associated sequence and bacterial heat-shock proteins has been described. The RA-associated HLA-DRB1 amino acid sequence, QKRAA, also is present in the bacterial heat-shock protein *dnaJ,* which is able to trigger proliferative responses of synovial-fluid T cells from RA patients. Although elegant, all three models have limitations in explaining how MHC genes influence the induction or progression of RA. Understanding the role of the HLA-DRB1 polymorphisms remains one of the major challenges, but also one of the best prospects, to define the etiology of RA.

MHC genes are not the only germline-encoded genes influencing susceptibility to RA. Female sex clearly increases the risk, and female patients develop a different phenotype of the disease than do male patients. However, no sex-linked genes have been identified as disease-risk genes. Several consortiums have started genome-wide searches, using affected sibling pairs (13,14). In these studies, the role of the HLA region was evident and accounted for a λs of 1.7 (compared with a λs of two to 12 for the entire genetic load contributing to RA), suggesting that the λs of other susceptibility genes would be very small. Susceptibility regions have been proposed for chromosomes 1, 3, 8, and 18, which will require confirmation and further refinement by other investigators. Eventually, the candidate gene approach may be more sensitive for identifying risk genes, in particular when considering the heterogeneity of disease severity and phenotype. The recent definition of single nucleotide polymorphisms throughout the human genome has increased significantly the feasibility of this approach. Studies of TCR and immunoglobulin genes have not been revealing; several cytokine polymorphisms, including tumor necrosis factor (TNF)-α and interferon (IFN)-γ were described to influence disease severity, but studies are needed to confirm this hypothesis.

Nongenomic Risk Factors

Rheumatoid arthritis concordance rates in monozygotic twins are 15%–30%, clearly stressing the involvement of nongenetic factors in RA. Potential candidates include classic environmental factors, stochastic events accumulated during the aging process, and acquired genomic variability. The pos-

sibility of a bacterial or viral infection has been pursued vigorously. Infectious agents have been shown to induce chronic arthritis in animal models. This concept has received even more attention after several infectious agents were demonstrated to be able to induce a chronic arthropathy in humans that was histologically indistinguishable from RA. Lyme disease has been identified as a spirochete infection. Parvovirus infection in the adult frequently results in acute and, sometimes, protracted polyarthritis. Rubella virus has been recovered from people with seronegative chronic polyarthritis. The incorporation of the *tax* gene into synoviocytes has been postulated as a mechanism to explain the synovial proliferation in HTLV-1–associated arthropathy (15). Nevertheless, the search for a putative initiating agent of RA has been unrewarding. All efforts to associate an infectious agent with RA by isolation, electron microscopy, or molecular biology techniques have failed. Of lifestyle factors, only smoking has been associated with an increased risk of developing RA. Age is an important variable in RA; the risk of developing RA increases within the first six decades of life, and possibly throughout life. The contribution of the aging process to RA is emphasized in studies demonstrating an accelerated immunosenescence in RA patients. Finally, genetic variability not encoded in the germline is of particular relevance to the immune system, in which gene rearrangements generate the diverse antigen receptor repertoires of B cells and T cells. It is likely that such stochastic events contribute to disease susceptibility.

Antigen-Specific Immune Responses in the Synovium

Classic autoimmunity is defined as an antigen-specific immune response to an autoantigen that leads to disease. An autoantigen has not been unequivocally identified in RA, but the synovium clearly is the site of an antigen-specific T-cell response. Tissue-infiltrating T cells, in particular CD4 T cells, are a consistent feature of rheumatoid synovitis. This finding, together with the HLA-DRB1 association of RA, convincingly argues for a central role of the CD4+ T cell in the pathogenesis of RA. In approximately 30% of patients, tertiary lymphoid tissue, including classical germinal centers, is formed in the synovium (5). Germinal centers are the archetype

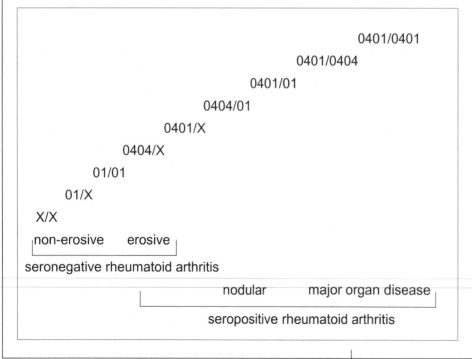

Fig. 9A-2. Hierarchy of HLA-DRB1 alleles in determining disease severity. HLA-DRB1 allelic polymorphisms correlate with aggressiveness of the rheumatoid synovitis and the risk of developing extra-articular manifestations. Gene-dosing of disease-associated alleles has an additional independent contribution to disease severity. Reprinted from Weyand et al (8), with permission.

of an antigen-specific response in which B cells recognize antigen on follicular dendritic cells and receive help from antigen-specific T cells. Furthermore, T cells are oligoclonally expanded in the rheumatoid synovium, and T cells expressing identical TCRs are found in distinct joints, consistent with the interpretation that they have proliferated in response to an antigen in the synovial lesion. Studies with human synovium-SCID mouse chimeras have confirmed that the synovial inflammation is maintained by an antigen-specific T-cell response (16). In these studies, rheumatoid synovium was engrafted into SCID mice. Subsequent treatment of these mice with T-cell–depleting antibodies reduced the production of T-cell–derived cytokines and of inflammatory mediators and metalloproteinases produced by synovial macrophages and fibroblasts. Conversely, the synovial inflammation was boosted by the adoptive transfer of HLA-DR–compatible T-cell clones derived from the synovium.

The concept of a synovial T-cell response as the critical step in RA pathophysiology has found clinical applications in studies using T-cell–depleting antibodies in patients. The results were disappointing, apparently for two reasons (17). First, the clonal expansion of T cells is such a widespread phenomenon that T-cell depletion was not sufficiently complete to achieve more than a transient suppression of the synovial T-cell response; and second, the restorative capacity of the lymphoid system in people with RA is exhausted (18). Patients were not able to generate new T-cell precursors after T-cell depletion. As a consequence, the synovial T-cell infiltrate was nearly unchanged in spite of profound peripheral lymphopenia.

The antigens recognized in the synovial tissue have remained elusive. Infectious agents that could act as exogenous antigen to drive a local immune response have not been found, and the role of different autoantigens remains a matter of debate (19). Circumstantial evidence indicates that in at least some synovial germinal centers, rheumatoid factors are produced. Cartilage-specific antigens, such as collagens and proteoglycans, have been implicated. GP39, a possible autoantigen that is expressed in a variety of tissues, is induced in cartilage after exposure to cytokines and may confer joint specificity. Although immunizations with self-antigens can break tolerance and induce erosive arthritis in animal models, they do not appear to be relevant for the majority of people with RA. Autoantibodies to these antigens are not consistently found. Studies with MHC class II antigenic peptide tetramers, used to estimate the frequencies of antigen-specific T cells, have failed to demonstrate a T-cell response to these antigens in the synovium (20). CD8 T cells have been found to respond to transcriptional transactivators encoded by the Epstein-Barr virus (EBV), but there is no evidence of increased transcription of EBV genes in the rheumatoid synovium, and such T-cell responses are found in a variety of inflammatory conditions (21). It is possible that the antigen maintaining the T-cell response is not preferentially expressed in the joint, but is ubiquitous. If so, mechanisms other than selective antigen expression would be responsible for tissue targeting in RA. In a recently described mouse model, an immune response to an enzyme of the glycolytic pathway, glucose-6-phosphate iso-

merase, induced a joint-specific inflammation that led to erosions and destruction of the joint architecture (22). This concept fits with the notion that RA is a systemic disease. Indeed, oligoclonal T-cell expansions, which can be used to indicate antigen-specific responses, are not restricted to the synovial lesion in people with RA.

The Cytokine Cascade in RA

Cytokines play a central role in the perpetuation of synovial inflammation. The cytokine system is a highly complex network with cytokines cross-regulating their expression and function. Many of these cytokines have redundant properties, with multiple cytokines apparently capable of exerting the same function. Numerous cytokines have been found in the rheumatoid synovium. The pathogenetic significance of each cytokine in RA is, therefore, difficult to assess. Data have been interpreted in the context of two concepts that are not mutually exclusive (23). The first model assumes a cascade of events in which some cytokines are higher in the hierarchy than others. The second model interprets the system as a balance between pro- and anti-inflammatory activities, with less emphasis on the action of single cytokines (Fig. 9A-3). These interpretations influence the decision of which cytokine may be a suitable target for clinical interventions, and clinical trials may provide insights into the validity of the models.

Based on the preferential cytokines produced, T-cell responses are categorized as T-helper 1 (IFN-γ) or Th2 (IL-4 and IL-13) responses, with Th1 responses being implicated in chronic inflammatory autoimmune diseases. T-cell–derived cytokines are not abundant in the rheumatoid synovium. Nevertheless, IFN-γ appears to be the key mediator controlling the production of monokines (TNF-α and IL-1β) and metalloproteinases by synovial macrophages and fibroblasts (16). However, the persistence of inflammation in RA cannot be interpreted as the consequence of a faulty commitment to the Th1 pathway. Lymphokine production is variable in RA and correlates with the type of tissue inflammation, rather than being specific for all forms of RA (4). Diffuse synovitis is characterized by very low production of IFN-γ and IL-4. In synovial tissues with lymphoid aggregates, IFN-γ and IL-10, but not IL-4, are produced; granuloma formation is associated with the highest production of IFN-γ and IL-4.

Cytokines produced by the innate immune system are involved in feedback loops that control the activity of cognitive immune responses and contribute to perpetuation of synovial inflammation (24). IL-15 and IL-18 have received the greatest attention. IL-15 can recruit, expand, and stimulate T cells that then interact with synovial macrophages in a contact-dependent, but possibly antigen-independent, manner to produce TNF-α and additional IL-15. Other cytokines, such as IL-18, act synergistically in this antigen-independent bystander T-cell activation.

TNF-α has been identified as a key player in synovial inflammation and is the direct target for several anti-cytokine agents approved for, or currently in clinical studies for, the treatment of RA. Initial studies gave rise to the hypothesis that TNF-α is at the top of a cascade of proinflammatory cytokines, and that TNF-α blockade would suppress the production of other inflammatory mediators, such as IL-1, IL-6, and IL-8 (25). Supportive evidence came from TNF-α transgenic mice, which developed erosive arthritis, and from treatment trials with anti–TNF-α agents in animal models and humans. Although anti–TNF-α is effective in controlling synovial inflammation, the disease relapses after treatment is discontinued. This observation demonstrates that the persistence of synovial inflammation in RA is not caused by an autocrine feedback loop of TNF-α production. Future studies must explore whether TNF-α has a unique position among the inflammatory cytokines or whether shifting the balance between pro- and anti-inflammatory cytokines (e.g., by blocking IL-1β or IL-6 activity or by providing IL-4, IL-10, IL-11, or IL-13) will be effective.

Rheumatoid Factors

Production of autoantibodies with specificity for the Fc fragment of immunoglobulin G (IgG) is a major immunologic abnormality in RA. Rheumatoid factors (RFs) are not specific for RA; they also can be detected in healthy individuals and in patients with a variety of conditions, including chronic bacterial infection, transplanted organs, and selected chronic inflammatory diseases. The prevalence in healthy individuals increases with age. RFs are not present in all people with RA and, therefore, are not a necessary requirement for the development of RA. In spite of these limitations, RFs are the major laboratory hallmark of RA. Rheumatoid factor production has been associated with a more severe disease course, and extra-articular manifestations are seen almost exclusively in RF-positive patients.

The mechanisms that initiate the production of RFs are unknown. No evidence has been provided for immunoglobulin gene polymorphisms as a genetic risk factor for the production of RF. In contrast to B-cell tumor-derived RFs that have a very restricted Vk gene segment usage, RFs in people with RA include a heterogeneous set of germline gene elements (26). Many RFs are of the IgM isotype and many of the Ig genes sequenced are in germline configuration. These data would suggest that a polyclonal B-cell activation is involved in early triggering of RF production. Polyclonal stimulators, including lectins and superantigens, have been shown to induce RF production. Rheumatoid factors undergo T-cell–driven isotype switch and affinity maturation in vivo. The antigen driving RF production may not be the Ig itself. It cannot be completely excluded that IgGs in people with RA have developed neoantigens, possibly secondary to a change in the glycosylation pattern. However, the recent crystal structure of an Ig with RF activity suggests that RFs interact with the Ig Fc molecule and not with their antigen-binding site, which may be occupied by a different antigen (27).

Rheumatoid factors may have several effector functions in the disease process. Deposition of immune complexes containing RFs have been shown in several tissues, and it is likely that activation of the complement cascade by immune complexes contributes to the inflammatory changes in the rheumatoid synovium and in rheumatoid vasculitis. However, the evidence for immune-complex–mediated tissue injury remains indirect and the clinical and pathologic features of RA are not suggestive for an immune-complex–mediated disease. The role of RFs in RA also may be closely related to their normal biologic function. Due to their ability to bind IgG, RF-expressing B cells capture antigens trapped in immune complexes. These B cells exist at high frequencies in healthy individuals and have a unique localization in the lymph node, where they are found in the mantle zone. Therefore, RF-producing B cells in RA may serve as antigen-presenting cells for IgG-complexed antigens, and increase the efficiency of immune responses to infrequent antigens.

The Response of the Synovial Membrane

In response to tissue inflammation, the synovial membrane undergoes dramatic changes that, by themselves, are important for the persistence and progression of the disease. Synovial lining hyperplasia develops, and extensive neoangiogenesis is seen in the sublin-

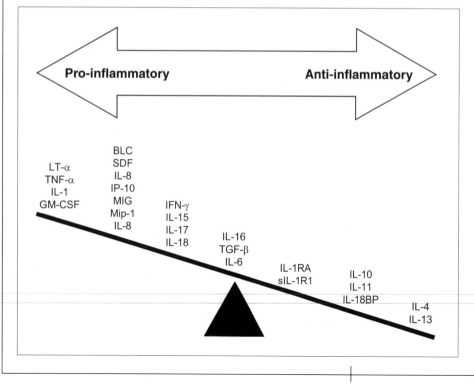

Fig. 9A-3. Dysequilibrium in the balance between pro- and anti-inflammatory cytokines in rheumatoid synovitis. Production of pro- and anti-inflammatory cytokines is increased in the RA synovium, but the balance is shifted toward pro-inflammatory cytokines.

ing. Endothelial cells are activated to express adhesion molecules and to produce chemokines that facilitate the influx of additional inflammatory cells. High endothelial venules are formed that usually are found in secondary lymphoid tissues and are specialized in lymphocyte recruitment. Proliferation of synovial fibroblasts and neoangiogenesis are controlled by growth factors produced during the inflammatory response. The invasive potential of the synovial membrane suggests the hypothesis that synovial fibroblasts have developed self-sufficiency in growth signals or mechanisms to evade regulation, reminiscent of a malignant transformation. Studies of transcription factors and oncogenes expressed in synovial fibroblasts are consistent with the interpretation that these cells are activated, but these studies have not provided any evidence of a deregulated proliferation program. Acquired evasiveness to apoptotic mechanisms has been suggested by the finding of p53 mutations in synovial fibroblasts. The mutations in the p53 tumor suppressor genes appear to result from oxidative damage, a consequence of the oxidative metabolism in the inflamed areas and the production of free oxygen radicals. Abnormalities in p53 function could contribute to synovial fibroblast proliferation, survival, and activation (28). In addition, immature mesenchymal cells are recruited that express embryonic growth factors of the *wingless* and *frizzled* families, and that have replaced normal synovial fibroblasts (29).

Mechanisms of Joint Destruction

The joint destruction in RA targets articular cartilage, ligaments, tendons, and bone. Several mechanisms contribute to this tissue-destruction process (Table 9A-1). Inflammatory mediators and enzymes in the synovial fluid have a direct effect on articular cartilage. Focal bone erosions develop at the margin between bone and cartilage that is invaded by the synovial membrane, also referred to as pannus. Subchondral osteolysis may come from the adjacent bone marrow, rather than the synovial inflammation. Cartilage and bone are not the only targets of the tissue-destruction process; chondrocytes and osteoclasts actively participate in the loss of extracellular matrix.

Neutrophils show a clear compartmentalization in RA (30). Very few neutrophils are present in the proliferating synovial tissue, but they constitute the major cellular component of the synovial fluid. The reasons for this compartmentalization are not entirely clear. However, it is known that neutrophils adhere to the endothelium of postcapillary venules, a process that is activation-dependent, and mediators with neutrophil-activating ability are abundant in the synovial fluid. Many of these chemoattractants are cytokines produced by the synovial tissue. The most important mediators for neutrophil adherence and transmigration are transforming growth factor (TGF)-β and IL-8. Classic chemoattractants present in the joint include the complement factor C5a, which is activated as a consequence of immune-complex formation, and the leukotriene B$_4$. The presence of cytokines and phagocytosis of soluble immune complexes by neutrophils result in prostaglandin and leukotriene production, neutrophil degranulation, and respiratory burst. Immune-complex deposition in the upper layers of the cartilage may target the neutrophils directly to the cartilage and may facilitate accumulation of a critical concentration of active proteinases and oxygen metabolites.

The tissue-destructive properties of the pannus are related closely to the production of metalloproteinases and

TABLE 9A-1
Mechanisms of Joint Destruction in Rheumatoid Arthritis

Mechanism	Effector molecule(s)	Cellular origin
Differentiation of synovial macrophages into osteoclasts	Osteoclast-differentiating factor	T cells, synovial fibroblasts
Osteoclast differentiation and activation	IL-1, TNF-α, IL-6, IL-11, IL-17	T cells, synovial macrophages
Decreased proteoglycan production by chondrocytes	IL-1, TNF-α	Synovial macrophages
Degradation of collagen, proteoglycans, laminin, fibronectin, elastin	Matrix metalloproteinases (MMPs)	Synovial macrophages and fibroblasts, chondrocytes
Degradation of collagen, proteoglycans, fibronectin, elastin	Cathepsins L and B	Synovial macrophages and fibroblasts
Degradation of type II collagen, osteocalcein	Cathepsin K, tartrate-resistant acid phosphatase	Osteoclasts

other proteinases that are able to degrade collagen and proteoglycans. The major metalloproteinase-producing cells are the synovial fibroblasts and monocytic phagocytes in the synovial-lining layer. The production of the proteinases is controlled by a number of different cytokines, including IL-1, TNF-α, and TGF-β. Most of these cytokines are secreted by tissue-residing macrophages. Chondrocytes respond to these cytokines with a decrease in collagen and proteoglycan synthesis, while simultaneously increasing synthesis of collagenase and stromolysin, which degrade type II collagen and proteoglycans of the cartilage. Extracellular matrix in the bone is protected from the assault of the enzymes as long as the extracellular matrix is mineralized. One of the first steps in focal bone erosions is the recruitment and differentiation of cells that express an osteoclast phenotype. The bony lesions include classical resorption lacunae of multinucleated giant cells that express the entire repertoire of genes of mature osteoclasts, including acid phosphatase, cathepsin K, and the calcitonin receptor. The origin of these cells is uncertain, but the adjacent pannus is rich in cells of the macrophage lineage that may differentiate into osteoclasts in response to such inflammatory mediators as IL-1, TNF-α, and the T-cell–derived cytokine IL-17. An additional potent regulator of osteoclast differentiation has recently been identified. Osteoclast differentiation factor is produced by T cells and fibroblast-like cells in the rheumatoid synovium (31). Studies in animal models have shown that treatment with the soluble receptor of osteoclast differentiation factor, osteoprotegerin, can prevent bone erosions.

The Systemic Component of Rheumatoid Arthritis

Although RA is characterized by synovial inflammation, people with RA generally have systemic manifestations, and a substantial fraction of patients develop tissue damage in organs other than the joints. These systemic manifestations appear to be mediated by immunologic processes. Studies of the immune system in people with RA have demonstrated signs of immune activation and, more importantly, have yielded evidence for profound and systemwide abnormalities (Fig. 9A-4). Specifically, patients with RA have an age-inappropriate reduction in thymic function (18). In RA, peripheral T cells have undergone extensive proliferation and show features of replicative senescence, such as shortened telomeres and limited ability to clonally expand. The diversity of the T-cell and B-cell compartments is contracted, and clonal T-cell and B-cell proliferation frequently is observed in the peripheral circulation (32). The senescence of the immune system is associated with a shift in the gene-expression profile of peripheral T cells. Although certain molecules, such as the important costimulatory molecule CD28, are lost, clonally expanded T cells gain natural killer cell functions, including cytotoxic activity and the expression of receptors usually expressed only on natural killer cells. It is not clear whether this immune exhaustion is a consequence of RA or actually is an important risk fac-

tor in the development of RA, raising the possibility that the primary immunopathogenic defect for RA lies in the failure of homeostatic control of the immune system. Irrespectively, effector functions acquired by presenescent T cells appear to have relevance for some of the extra-articular manifestations of RA, including Felty's syndrome and rheumatoid vasculitis. In addition, CD4 T cells phenotypically and functionally identical to those in people with RA have been identified in patients with acute coronary syndromes, in which they infiltrate the "culprit" atherosclerotic lesion causing acute coronary thrombosis (33). Sharing of disease mechanism in RA and coronary artery disease may provide an explanation for the recent recognition that excess mortality in RA can be attributed to cardiovascular complications.

JÖRG J. GORONZY, MD
CORNELIA M. WEYAND, MD

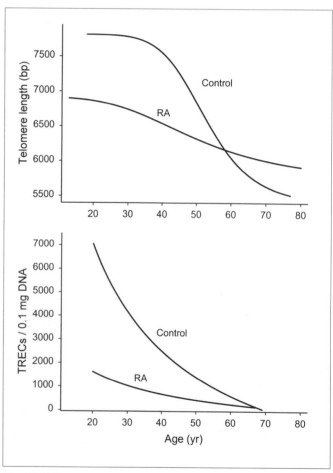

Fig. 9A-4. Premature immunosenescence in rheumatoid arthritis. In people with RA, the global T-cell system has characteristics of immunosenescence. Compared to age-matched controls, peripheral T cells of RA patients have shortened telomeres, indicative of an increased replicative history (upper panel). Also, thymic function declines earlier in life, resulting in a reduced production of new T cells that express T-cell receptor excision circles. Reprinted from Goronzy and Weyand (34), with permission.

References

1. Arnett FC, Edworthy SM, Bloch DA, et al. The American Rheumatism Association 1987 revised criteria for the classification of rheumatoid arthritis. Arthritis Rheum 1988;31: 315–324.

2. Ollier W, Winchester R. The germline and somatic genetic basis for rheumatoid arthritis. In: Theofilopoulos AN (ed). Genes and Genetics of Autoimmunity. Basel, Switzerland: Karger, 1999; pp 166–193.

3. Harris ED. Rheumatoid Arthritis. Philadelphia: W.B. Saunders Company, 1997.

4. Klimiuk PA, Goronzy JJ, Bjornsson J, Beckenbaugh RD, Weyand CM. Tissue cytokine patterns distinguish variants of rheumatoid synovitis. Am J Pathol 1997;151:1311–1319.

5. Schroder AE, Greiner A, Seyfert C, Berek C. Differentiation of B cells in the nonlymphoid tissue of the synovial membrane of patients with rheumatoid arthritis. Proc Natl Acad Sci USA 1996;93:221–225.

6. Stastny P. Association of the B-cell alloantigen DRw4 with rheumatoid arthritis. N Engl J Med 1978;298:869–871.

7. Gregersen PK, Silver J, Winchester RJ. The shared epitope hypothesis. An approach to understanding the molecular genetics of susceptibility to rheumatoid arthritis. Arthritis Rheum 1987;30:1205–1213.

8. Weyand CM, McCarthy TG, Goronzy JJ. Correlation between disease phenotype and genetic heterogeneity in rheumatoid arthritis. J Clin Invest 1995;95:2120–2126.

9. Weyand CM, Hicok KC, Conn DL, Goronzy JJ. The influence of HLA-DRB1 genes on disease severity in rheumatoid arthritis. Ann Intern Med 1992;117:801–806.

10. Sinigaglia F, Nagy ZA. Structural basis for the HLA-DR association of rheumatoid arthritis. In: Goronzy JJ, Weyand CM (eds). Rheumatoid Arthritis. Basel, Switzerland: Karger, 2000; pp 36–50.

11. Walser-Kuntz DR, Weyand CM, Weaver AJ, O'Fallon WM, Goronzy JJ. Mechanisms underlying the formation of the T cell receptor repertoire in rheumatoid arthritis. Immunity 1995;2:597–605.

12. Albani S, Carson DA. A multistep molecular mimicry hypothesis for the pathogenesis of rheumatoid arthritis. Immunol Today 1996;17:466–470.

13. Seldin MF, Amos CI, Ward R, Gregersen PK. The genetics revolution and the assault on rheumatoid arthritis. Arthritis Rheum 1999;42:1071–1079.

14. Cornelis F. Susceptibility genes in rheumatoid arthritis. In: Goronzy JJ, Weyand CM (eds). Rheumatoid Arthritis. Basel, Switzerland: Karger, 2000; pp 1–16.

15. Nakajima T, Aono H, Hasunuma T, et al. Overgrowth of human synovial cells driven by the human T cell leukemia virus type I tax gene. J Clin Invest 1993;92:186–193.

16. Klimiuk PA, Yang H, Goronzy JJ, Weyand CM. Production of cytokines and metalloproteinases in rheumatoid synovitis is T cell dependent. Clin Immunol 1999;90:65–78.

17. Matteson EL. Recent clinical trials in the rheumatic diseases. Curr Opin Rheumatol 1997;9:95–101.

18. Koetz K, Bryl E, Spickschen K, O'Fallon WM, Goronzy JJ, Weyand CM. T cell homeostasis in patients with rheumatoid arthritis. Proc Natl Acad Sci USA 2000;97:9203–9208.

19. Cope AP, Sonderstrup G. Evaluating candidate autoantigens in rheumatoid arthritis. Springer Semin Immunopathol 1998;20:23–39.

20. Kotzin BL, Falta MT, Crawford F, et al. Use of soluble peptide-DR4 tetramers to detect synovial T cells specific for cartilage antigens in patients with rheumatoid arthritis. Proc Natl Acad Sci USA 2000;97:291–296.

21. Scotet E, David-Ameline J, Peyrat MA, et al. T cell response to Epstein-Barr virus transactivators in chronic rheumatoid arthritis. J Exp Med 1996;184:1791–1800.

22. Matsumoto I, Staub A, Benoist C, Mathis D. Arthritis provoked by linked T and B cell recognition of a glycolytic enzyme. Science 1999;286:1732–1735.

23. Feldmann M, Brennan FM, Maini RN. Rheumatoid arthritis. Cell 1996;85:307–310.

24. McInnes IB, Leung BP. Innate response cytokines in inflammatory synovitis: a role for interleukin-15. In: Goronzy JJ, Weyand CM (eds). Rheumatoid Arthritis. Basel, Switzerland: Karger, 2000; pp 200–215.

25. Brennan FM, Maini RN, Feldmann M. Role of pro-inflammatory cytokines in rheumatoid arthritis. Springer Semin Immunol 1998;20:133–147.

26. Randen I, Thompson KM, Pascual V, et al. Rheumatoid factor V genes from patients with rheumatoid arthritis are diverse and show evidence of an antigen-driven response. Immunol Rev 1992;128:49–71.

27. Sutton B, Corper A, Bonagura V, Taussig M. The structure and origin of rheumatoid factors. Immunol Today 2000;21:177–183.

28. Firestein GS, Echeverri F, Yeo M, Zvaifler NJ, Green DR. Somatic mutations in the p53 tumor suppressor gene in rheumatoid arthritis synovium. Proc Natl Acad Sci USA 1997;94:10895–10900.

29. Sen M, Lauterbach K, El-Gabalawy H, Firestein GS, Corr M, Carson DA. Expression and function of wingless and frizzled homologs in rheumatoid arthritis. Proc Natl Acad Sci USA 2000;97:2791–2796.

30. Pillinger MH, Abramson SB. The neutrophil in rheumatoid arthritis. Rheum Dis Clin North Am 1995;21:691–714.

31. Goldring SR, Gravallese EM. Pathogenesis of bone erosions in rheumatoid arthritis. Curr Opin Rheumatol 2000;12:195–199.

32. Wagner UG, Koetz K, Weyand CM, Goronzy JJ. Perturbation of the T cell repertoire in rheumatoid arthritis. Proc Natl Acad Sci USA 1998;95:14447–14452.

33. Liuzzo G, Goronzy JJ, Yang H, et al. Monoclonal T-cell proliferation and plaque instability in acute coronary syndromes. Circulation 2000;101:2883–2888.

34. Goronzy JJ, Weyand CM. Thymic function and peripheral T-cell homeostasis in rheumatoid arthritis. Trends in Immunol 2001;22:251-255

RHEUMATOID ARTHRITIS
B. Clinical and Laboratory Features

Clinical features of rheumatoid arthritis (RA) vary not only from one patient to another, but also in an individual patient over the disease course. The most common mode of onset is the insidious development of symptoms over a period of several weeks (1,2). Explosive, acute polyarticular onset that evolves over several days also occurs, but acute monarticular arthritis as the initial manifestation is decidedly rare. The initial presentation often lacks the characteristic symmetry seen as the disease progresses to a more chronic state.

Diagnosis

Diagnosis during the early weeks of the disease essentially is one of exclusion, although characteristic features, such as symmetric sterile synovitis with typical serologic findings, strongly suggest RA. Radiographic evidence of erosions becomes apparent only after the disease has been present for several months or more than a year.

The American College of Rheumatology has established criteria for the diagnosis of RA, the classification of severity by radiography, functional classes, and the definition of remission (see Appendix I). Although not designed for managing individual patients, the criteria are useful as a frame of reference and in describing clinical phenomena.

By definition, the diagnosis of RA cannot be made until the disease has been present for at least several weeks. Many extra-articular features of RA, the characteristic symmetry of inflammation, and the typical serologic findings may not be evident in the first month or two of the disease. Therefore, the diagnosis of RA usually is presumptive early in its course.

Although extra-articular manifestations may dominate in some patients, documentation of an inflammatory synovitis is essential for a diagnosis. Inflammatory synovitis can be documented by demonstrating synovial-fluid leukocytosis, defined as white blood cell (WBC) counts greater than 2000/mm^3, histologic evidence of synovitis, or radiographic evidence of characteristic erosions.

Other causes of synovitis must be excluded. Although this determination often is possible upon initial evaluation, such conditions as systemic lupus erythematosus (SLE), psoriatic arthritis, arthritis associated with parvovirus or hepatitis B virus, and the seronegative spondyloarthropathies initially may be indistinguishable from RA. Usually, it is the development of extra-articular features of these disorders, rather than characteristics of the synovitis, that allows a differential diagnosis.

Synovial biopsies seldom are performed or required for diagnosis, and radiographic changes are not apparent in early disease, when the diagnosis is in doubt. If a palpable effusion is detected, the joint should be aspirated to document synovial-fluid leukocytosis and to exclude the presence of crystals.

Effusions and synovial thickening are difficult to detect in joint spaces deep below the surface, such as in the hip; often, the shoulder; and occasionally, the metatarsophalangeal (MTP) joints. For this reason, the examiner must depend on demonstrations of the joint's limited motion. The presence of a joint deformity is not specific evidence of inflammatory synovitis because deformities can occur in other inflammatory conditions, such as SLE, and in noninflammatory disorders, such as osteoarthritis. However, if the disorder involves a non–weight-bearing joint, such as the elbow or wrist, the examiner usually can assume that, unless a patient has a history of unique joint trauma, the deformity results from synovitis.

Laboratory Features

No laboratory test, histologic finding, or radiographic feature confirms a diagnosis of RA. Rather, the diagnosis is established by a constellation of findings observed over a period of time.

Rheumatoid factor (RF) is found in the serum of about 85% of people with RA. Studies indicate that RF titers tend to correlate with severe and unremitting disease, nodules, and extra-articular lesions. In the individual patient, however, the RF titer is of little prognostic value, and serial titers are of no value in following the disease process. When a patient is known to be RF-positive, repeating the test at a later date serves no purpose. However, a small percentage of patients who initially are RF-negative become RF-positive as the disease progresses, and the clinical features and prognosis parallel those of patients who were RF-positive in early disease. Rheumatoid factor can be found in other diseases, including several other inflammatory disorders associated with synovitis (Table 9B-1).

The erythrocyte sedimentation rate (ESR) is a measurement of the rate at which red blood cells settle and is related to several factors in the serum (see Chapter 7C). Typically, the ESR correlates with the degree of synovial inflammation, but this correlation varies greatly from patient to patient, and rarely, a patient with active inflammatory RA may have a normal ESR. However, the ESR generally is a useful objective measure for following the course of inflammatory activity in an individual patient. C-reactive protein, an acute-phase reactant, also may be used to monitor the level of inflammation.

Other laboratory abnormalities observed in people with RA include hypergammaglobulinemia, hypocomplementemia, thrombocytosis, and eosinophilia. These states occur more often in patients with severe disease, high RF titer, rheumatoid nodules, and extra-articular manifestations.

TABLE 9B-1
Selected Diseases Associated With Elevated Serum Rheumatoid Factors

Chronic bacterial infections
  Subacute bacterial endocarditis
  Leprosy
  Tuberculosis
  Syphilis
  Lyme disease

Viral diseases
  Rubella
  Cytomegalovirus
  Infectious mononucleosis
  Influenza

Parasitic diseases

Chronic inflammatory disease of uncertain etiology
  Sarcoidosis
  Periodontal disease
  Pulmonary interstitial disease
  Liver disease

Mixed cryoglobulinemia

Hypergammaglobulinemic purpura

Modified from Koopman WJ, Schrohenber RE: Rheumatoid factor. In: Utsinger PD, Zvaifler NJ, Ehrlich GE (eds). Rheumatoid Arthritis: Etiology, Diagnosis and Therapy. Philadelphia: JB Lippincott, 1985; pp 217–241.

Articular Manifestations

The articular manifestations of RA can be placed in two categories: reversible signs and symptoms related to inflammatory synovitis and irreversible structural damage caused by synovitis. This concept is useful for staging disease, determining prognosis, and selecting medical or surgical treatment. Structural damage in the typical patient begins sometime between the first and second year of the disease (3). Although synovitis tends to follow a fluctuating pattern, structural damage progresses as a linear function of the amount of prior synovitis (Fig. 9B-1).

Morning Stiffness

Morning stiffness is an almost universal feature of synovial inflammation, in RA and in other systemic rheumatic disorders. In contrast to the brief (five to 10 minutes) period of gelling seen in osteoarthritis, morning stiffness in RA is prolonged, usually lasting more than two hours. This phenomenon relates to the immobilization that occurs during sleep and is not a function of the hour of the day or periods of sunlight. The duration tends to correlate with the degree of synovial inflammation and disappears when a remission occurs. For this reason, the presence and length of morning stiffness is useful in following the disease course and should be documented in the patient's database. Patients can be asked, "After you have gotten up, how long does it take until you're feeling as good as you'll feel for the day?"

Synovial Inflammation

Clinical signs of synovitis may be subtle and often are subjective. Warm, swollen, obviously inflamed joints usually are seen only in the most active phases of inflammatory synovitis. These observations usually are restricted to superficial joints with an easily distensible capsule, such as the knee and, occasionally, the wrist and proximal interphalangeal (PIP) joints. Deeply buried joints, such as the hip, rarely present with a tense effusion that is apparent on physical examination. Ankle effusions also are difficult to detect because numerous tendons and retinacula restrict the joint capsule. Even when swelling is present, it often is difficult to distinguish an ankle effusion from edema or cellulitis.

The pathologic and clinical picture of chronic rheumatoid synovitis differs considerably from synovitis in early disease. As the inflammation continues, granulation tissue and fibrosis develop, and vascularity of the synovium decreases. The joint immobility brought on by the disease process further reduces synovial vascularity, and the degree of obvious inflammation apparent on examination is reduced significantly. This phenomenon has been called "burned-out" RA, a faulty concept describing patients with long-standing RA whose joints are not warm or noticeably swollen. Further observation of these patients reveals that they continue to experience prolonged morning stiffness, general malaise, and chronic fatigue; have anemia and elevated ESR; and, most importantly, demonstrate progressive joint destruction on serial radiographs. Therefore, clinical assessments based on decreased joint swelling and tenderness in the later stages of RA may be overly optimistic (4). In fact, RA rarely remits spontaneously after the first year (5).

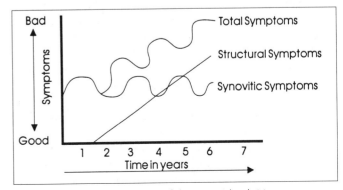

Fig. 9B-1. Symptomatic course of rheumatoid arthritis.

Structural Damage

Cartilage loss and erosion of periarticular bone are the characteristic features of structural damage. The clinical features related to structural damage are marked by progressive deterioration, functionally and anatomically. Structural damage to the joint is irreversible and additive. Objective evidence of cartilage destruction can be obtained by radiographs showing total loss of joint space or by demonstrating bone-on-bone crepitus, a high-pitched screech detectable on palpation or auscultation. Nothing else makes this sound.

Symptoms that fail to respond to aggressive anti-inflammatory therapy indicate that irreversible structural damage exists. When such damage is suspected, corticosteroids may be injected into the joint. Failure to benefit from this treatment provides good evidence that other anti-inflammatory therapies are unlikely to be beneficial.

Manifestations in Specific Joints

Principles of the role of synovitis in joint destruction are applicable to all joints. However, certain aspects are pertinent to specific joints.

Cervical Spine

Although RA of the thoracic and lumbar spine is exceptionally rare, cervical spine involvement is common. The inflammatory process involves diarthrodial joints and is neither palpable nor visible to the examiner. Clinical manifestations of early disease consist primarily of neck stiffness that is perceived through the entire arc of motion, and general loss of motion also may develop. Tenosynovitis of the transverse ligament of C1, which stabilizes the odontoid process of C2, may produce significant C1–C2 instability. Cervical myelopathy may develop as a result of erosion of the odontoid process, ligament laxity, or ligament rupture. Disease of the apophyseal joints also contributes to cervical instability. Clinical evaluation of people with RA should include a careful neurologic examination. Neck pain without neurologic features tends to be self-limited and usually improves, even when radiographic evidence of joint destruction is present. This may be related to the fact that the neck is a non–weight-bearing structure. Conversely, pain does not always accompany cervical instability, even when myelopathy is significant. Frequently, the course of neck pain and neurologic symptoms are not synchronous.

Shoulders

Because the shoulder capsule lies beneath the muscular rotator cuff, an effusion is difficult to detect on physical examination. Typically, the only objective finding is loss of motion. The patient responds to shoulder pain by unconsciously restricting shoulder motion. Because basic activities of daily living do not require extremes of shoulder movement, frozen shoulder syndrome can develop rapidly. An aggressive program of range of motion exercises may prevent this. Symptoms related to frozen shoulder usually are much more severe at night, when movements during

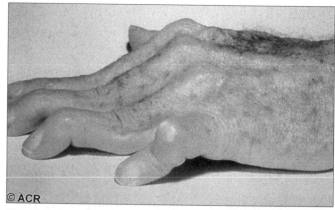
© ACR

Fig. 9B-2. Swan-neck deformities are seen in the second, third, and fourth digits of a patient with chronic rheumatoid arthritis. A boutonniere deformity of the fifth digit is present. Reprinted from the Revised Clinical Slide Collection on the Rheumatic Diseases, with permission of the American College of Rheumatology.

sleep stretch the tightened joint capsule. If irreversible joint damage occurs, the shoulder symptoms do not necessarily parallel cartilage destruction, possibly because the shoulder is a relatively unconstrained and non–weight-bearing joint that is not as dependent as other joints on the cartilage surface for useful function (6).

Elbow

The elbow is one of the easiest of all joints in which to detect inflammation. Because this joint is superficial, synovitis is evident by palpating fullness and thickening in the radiohumeral joint. Flexion deformities of the elbow may develop in early RA. The ulnar nerve passes posteromedially to the elbow, and compressive neuropathies related to the synovitis may develop at this site. Symptoms include paresthesia over the fourth and fifth fingers and weakness in the flexor muscle of the little finger. If structural symptoms begin to develop, and surgical intervention is considered, the physician should distinguish symptoms of radiohumeral disease (which is accentuated by pronation-supination) from those related to ulnohumeral disease (which is brought on by flexion-extension).

Hand

The wrists are affected in virtually all people with RA. The metacarpophalangeal (MCP) and PIP joints often are involved, but the distal interphalangeal (DIP) joints usually (although not always) are spared. Ulnar deviation at the MCP joints often is associated with radial deviation at the wrists. Swan-neck deformities (Fig. 9B-2) can develop, as can the boutonniere deformity, in which flexion at the PIP and hyperextension at the DIP joints occur.

Pain or dysfunction may be caused by compression of a peripheral nerve entrapped in a confined area by synovitis. The most common site is the carpal tunnel of the wrist. Patients with early wrist disease may develop carpal tunnel syndrome from compression of the median nerve. As the

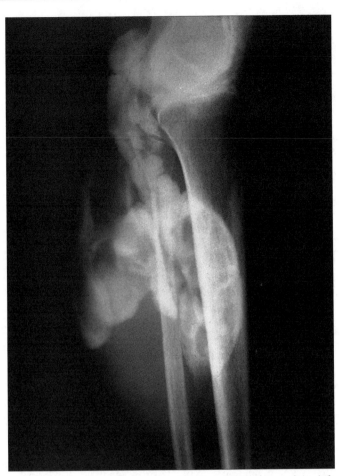

Fig. 9B-3. This is the lateral projection of the arthrogram of the left knee of a patient with a popliteal cyst. Good filling is noted of the suprapatellar bursa and knee joint proper. The contrast medium extends posteriorly into the distended gastrocnemio-semimembranosus bursa with extension and/or rupture distally into the calf.

disease progresses, the retinaculum distends and symptoms may improve. A similar neuropathy involves the ulnar nerve, which passes through Guyon's canal within the wrist. Guyon's canal syndrome may be distinguished from entrapment neuropathy at the elbow by the absence of weakness of the fifth finger when flexed against resistance.

Tenosynovitis and the formation of rheumatoid nodules within tendon sheaths can interfere with finger flexion. Nodular thickening, which may be palpated along the flexor tendons of the palm, may cause symptoms that patients describe as "locking and catching," as the nodule slides along its sheath. Tendon rupture may occur if inflammatory tenosynovitis erodes through the tendon, an event that is most common in the extensor muscle of the DIP joint of the thumb. Another cause of tendon rupture at the wrist is the so-called attrition rupture of extensor tendons in the third, fourth, and fifth fingers. This rupture occurs because these tendons, which cross the dorsal surface of the ulnar styloid process, are subjected to abrasion if the ulnar styloid erodes to jagged bone. Tendon ruptures present with a history of an abrupt, usually painless loss of a highly specific function

(e.g., inability to flex or extend) on active motion, although passive range of motion is unaffected.

Hip

Although hip involvement is common in RA, early manifestations of hip disease often are not apparent by history or physical exam. Because the joint is located deep within the pelvis, evidence of palpable distention or synovial thickening is absent. Early hip disease often is asymptomatic, although a subtle reduction in range of motion may be observed. Typically, the dysfunction is first noticed when the patient has difficulty putting on shoes or socks on the affected side. When pain develops, it usually appears in the groin or thigh, but may also be felt in the buttock, low back, or medial aspect of the knee. If cartilage destruction occurs, the symptoms may accelerate more rapidly than in other joints.

Knee

Effusions and synovial thickening of the knee usually are detected easily on examination. Posterior herniation of the capsule creating a popliteal (Baker's) cyst may be associated with dissection or rupture into the calf, producing symptoms suggestive of thrombophlebitis. However, the characteristic history, absence of engorged collateral veins, and a distinct border of edema below the knee distinguish this syndrome from thrombophlebitis. Ultrasonography can readily define a Baker's cyst, but may show little after rupture or dissection has occurred. Arthrography with a film of the calf musculature taken after a brief period of exercise may be required to demonstrate a herniation of the calf musculature (Fig. 9B-3).

Foot and Ankle

Because lower-extremity joints are weight-bearing structures, involvement of the foot and ankle causes greater dysfunction and pain than occur in upper-extremity joints. In descending order of frequency, RA characteristically affects the MTP, talonavicular, and ankle joints. MTP arthritis causes cock-up deformities of the toes and subluxations of the MTP heads on the sole. As a result, the normally smooth, flowing transmission of forces across the metatarsal heads is interrupted, causing gait problems. Inflammation of the talonavicular joint causes pronation and eversion of the foot. Flexion and extension of the ankle usually are preserved in early RA. The tarsal tunnel, which is posteroinferior to the medial malleolus and contains the posterior tibial nerve, often is compressed by synovitis. Entrapment of this nerve causes burning paresthesia on the sole of the foot, which is made worse by standing or walking (7).

Joint Deformities

Joint deformities in RA occur from several different mechanisms, all related to synovitis and the patient's attempt to avoid pain by keeping the joint in the least painful position. These mechanisms are joint immobilization, destruction of cartilage and bone, and alterations in muscles, tendons, and ligaments.

Any joint, healthy or impaired, that is subjected to prolonged immobilization will lose motion because of tendon shortening and contraction of the articular capsule. By maintaining motion, the development of deformities may be avoided. The value of continued movement is illustrated by the fact that such joints as the knee and ankle seldom lose motion in early RA because walking, sitting, and climbing stairs put these joints through their full range of motion. In contrast, joints whose full range of motion is less critical to basic function, such as the shoulder, wrist, and elbow, often develop deformities in early disease because patients are able to function with reduced range of motion. By holding these joints in a position that maximizes the volume within the joint cavity, patients reduce pain by decreasing intra-articular pressure.

Muscles and tendons around an inflamed joint may undergo spasm and shorten in response to inflammation. This phenomenon is easiest to observe in abnormalities of intrinsic muscles of the hand and anterior peroneal muscle tendons over the arch of the foot. Spasms and shortening in these areas contribute to deformities of MCP flexion and tarsal pronation.

Ligaments that stabilize the joint may be weakened or severed by the erosive properties of inflamed synovium or pannus and the inflammatory mediators they release. Damaged ligaments lead to instability, altering the lines of force and the axis of rotation of the joint involved. MCP subluxations and ulnar deviation are related to this mechanism.

The tenosynovium lining the tendon sheath commonly is inflamed in RA, leading to joint deformities related to thickening of the tendon sheath, the formation of obstructing tendon nodules, or tendon ruptures. Characteristically, tendon ruptures are abrupt and painless. On physical examination, tendon dysfunction is detected by a discrepancy between active and passive motion.

Persistent synovitis and pannus may denude the surface of cartilage and erode juxta-articular bone, creating incongruous articular surfaces. Once cartilage is completely gone, the opposing bone surfaces may fuse if immobilized, much as a bone fracture fuses when splinted.

Extra-Articular Manifestations

Rheumatoid arthritis is a systemic disease, and most patients experience general malaise or fatigue. Significant inflammation of organ systems occurs, predominantly in RF-positive patients. Other risk factors that generally correlate with the development of extra-articular manifestations include rheumatoid nodules, severe articular disease, and probably, the major histocompatibility complex (MHC) class II HLA-DRB1*0401 allele (8).

Skin Manifestations

Rheumatoid nodules develop in up to 50% of people with RA. Virtually all patients with nodules are RF-positive. The nodules tend to develop in crops during active phases of the disease, and form subcutaneously, in bursae, and along tendon sheaths. Although they have been described in almost every region and may occur in the viscera, nod-

ules typically are located over pressure points, such as the extensor surface of the forearm (Fig. 9B-4), Achilles tendon, ischial area, the MTP joint, and the flexor surfaces of the fingers. These lesions may develop gradually or abruptly, and generally are associated with some sign of inflammation. Nodules and gouty tophi both have a predilection for the olecranon, but tophi tend to develop insidiously and grow slowly, often without apparent inflammation. Biopsy of the nodule may be necessary if the diagnosis is uncertain. In gout, crystals are found in the aspirate. Over time, rheumatoid nodules often disappear or involute. Methotrexate may enhance or accelerate the development of rheumatoid nodules (9).

Vasculitic lesions, particularly various forms of dermal vasculitis, often are seen in RA. The most common is leukocytoclastic vasculitis, with resulting palpable purpura on physical exam. Although dermal vasculitis generally does not indicate a coexistent systemic vasculitis, patients should be examined for evidence of involvement of other organ systems, especially renal and neurologic dysfunction. Ischemic ulcers often occur with systemic involvement.

Drugs used to treat RA can create skin abnormalities. Ecchymoses may occur as a consequence of either platelet dysfunction related to nonsteroidal anti-inflammatory drugs (NSAIDs) or capillary fragility from corticosteroids. Petechiae may be a sign of thrombocytopenia from disease-modifying drugs, such as gold, penicillamine, or sulfasalazine. Chrysiasis, a cyanotic hue most apparent on the forehead, is a manifestation of long-term gold therapy. A similar grayish hue, most prominent on the face, can result from chronic use of minocycline.

Ocular Manifestations

Keratoconjunctivitis sicca as a manifestation of associated Sjögren's syndrome is common in RA. Because patients are not always aware of the symptoms, clinicians should ask questions about eye dryness and institute prophylactic meas-

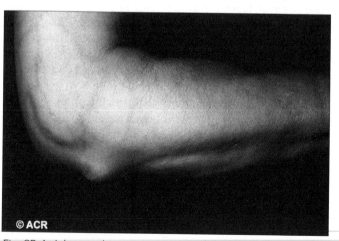

Fig. 9B-4. A large subcutaneous nodule is located on the extensor surface of the forearm near the elbow. Reprinted from the Revised Clinical Slide Collection on the Rheumatic Diseases, with permission of the American College of Rheumatology.

ures. Episodes of episcleritis are common and usually run a benign, self-limited course. Scleritis has a more morbid prognosis, however. This inflammation, which histologically resembles that of rheumatoid nodules, may erode through the sclera into the choroid, causing scleromalacia perforans.

Respiratory Manifestations

Inflammation of the cricoarytenoid joint is a common finding in RA. The symptoms usually are episodic and consist of laryngeal pain, dysphonia, and occasionally, pain on swallowing, all of which may be accentuated in the morning (10). Laryngeal obstruction is rare, but may occur after extubation for endotracheal anesthesia.

Autopsy studies show some degree of interstitial lung disease in the majority of people with RA (11). Clinical symptoms of pulmonary insufficiency occur less frequently than the histologic changes. Because RA imposes limitations that make physical exertion difficult (11), respiratory involvement may be asymptomatic. However, the mortality from pulmonary disease in RA is twice that of the general population (12). Radiographic features of respiratory involvement include interstitial fibrosis, which has a predilection for basal involvement, and solitary or multiple nodules in the lung parenchyma. Cavitation of these nodules can be identified on computed tomography. On rare occasions, a subpleural nodule may rupture, creating a bronchopleural fistula, which may progress to a pneumothorax or empyema.

Pulmonary involvement identical to that seen in RA alone has been described in association with penicillamine and with gold therapy, but the significance of this observation is uncertain. A similar process has been reported with methotrexate therapy; respiratory symptoms tend to improve when the drug is stopped. Bronchiolitis obliterans may be associated with RA or a complication of drug therapy.

Inflammation of the pleura may occur, causing typical symptoms and findings of pleurisy. This event usually is self-limited and episodic. Inflammatory pleural disease also may be asymptomatic, and the small pleural effusions are discovered incidentally on chest radiographs. Laboratory evaluation of the pleural fluid demonstrates markedly low glucose levels, compared with serum levels, and a WBC count usually less than 5000/mm^3.

Cardiac Manifestations

Echocardiographic evidence of a pericardial effusion or other pericardial abnormality is seen in almost 50% of people with RA who have no clinical symptoms of heart involvement (13). Symptomatic pericarditis, manifested by pain or altered cardiovascular physiology, is rare. Although pericarditis may occur at any time, these episodes usually develop during a disease flare. Occasionally, a patient's disease may progress to chronic constrictive pericarditis, manifested by peripheral edema and signs of right-sided heart failure. Inflammatory lesions similar to rheumatoid nodules may develop on the myocardium and valve leaflets. Clinical manifestations include valvular dysfunction, embolic phenomena, conduction defects, and possibly, myocardiopathy. Aortitis involving

segments of or the entire aorta has been described and is associated with aortic insufficiency related to dilation of the aortic root and with aneurysmal rupture (14).

Gastrointestinal Manifestations

No gastrointestinal abnormalities are related specifically to RA, with the exception of xerostomia seen in patients with associated Sjögren's syndrome and ischemic bowel complications of rheumatoid vasculitis. However, gastritis and peptic ulcer disease are major complications of NSAID therapy and a significant cause of morbidity and mortality in RA.

Renal Manifestations

In contrast to SLE, glomerular disease is exceedingly rare in RA. Proteinuria, if it develops, usually is related to drug toxicity (gold or penicillamine) or is secondary to amyloidosis. Interstitial renal disease may occur in Sjögren's syndrome, but in RA patients, it is related more often to the use of NSAIDs, acetaminophen, or other analgesics. Papillary necrosis may occur as a result of chronic exposure to these agents.

Neurologic Complications

Nervous system involvement is common in RA, but usually is subtle in presentation, which can make it difficult to distinguish between articular and neuropathic lesions (15). The pathogenesis of neurologic disorders is related fundamentally to one of three mechanisms: cervical spine instability, peripheral nerve entrapment, and vasculitis resulting in mononeuritis multiplex.

Cervical spine instability, most commonly occurring at C1–C2, is related to destruction of the transverse ligament of C1 or the odontoid process itself. A "step-off" subluxation related to apophyseal joint destruction may occur, most commonly at C4–C5 or C5–C6. Lateral radiographs taken in flexion and extension are required to demonstrate the instability. Magnetic resonance imaging or computed tomography then is performed to further evaluate the precise anatomy and to document spinal cord compression.

Symptoms of cervical myelopathy typically are gradual in onset and often are unrelated to the development of or accentuation in neck pain. When neck pain does occur, it frequently radiates over the occiput in the distribution of the C1–C3 nerve roots. L'hermitte's sign, the sudden development of tingling paresthesia that descends the thoracolumbar spine as the cervical spine is flexed, may occur. In patients with long-standing destructive RA, the most common symptom of cervical myelopathy is the development over weeks to months of bilateral sensory paresthesia of the hands and motor weakness. Physical examination may demonstrate pathologic reflexes, such as Babinski's sign, Hoffmann's sign, and hyperactive deep-tendon reflexes.

When a peripheral nerve passes through a compartment that also is occupied by synovium or tendon sheaths, the potential exists for nerve compression by synovitis or tenosynovitis. Symptoms often vary with fluctuations in synovial inflammation and the joint posture. The diagnosis of a compressive neuropathy related to local synovial inflammation may be confirmed clinically by demonstrating a response to either temporary splinting or the use of intra-articular corticosteroids. In addition to causing compression of the median nerve in the carpal tunnel or the ulnar nerve in Guyon's canal, neuropathies may involve the posterior interosseous nerve in the antecubital fossa, the femoral nerve anterior to the hip joint, the peroneal nerve adjacent to the fibular head, and the interdigital nerve at the MTP joint. Compression syndromes of these nerves may be confirmed by neurophysiologic studies.

The syndrome of mononeuritis multiplex is marked by abrupt onset of a persistent peripheral neuropathy that is unaltered by change in the joint position or reduction in synovial inflammation, distinguishing it from a compression neuropathy. Concurrent evidence of rheumatoid vasculitis often is seen. Neurophysiologic studies reveal an axonal lesion and frequently demonstrate several clinically inapparent mononeuropathies. A sural nerve biopsy may confirm the diagnosis.

Hematologic Manifestations

A hypochromic-microcytic anemia with low serum ferritin and low or normal iron-binding capacity is an almost universal finding in people with active RA. Because most patients are taking ulcerogenic NSAIDs, and therefore, often test positive for occult blood on stool tests, distinguishing this anemia from an iron-deficiency anemia is difficult. To compound the problem, patients with iron deficiency may fail to respond vigorously to iron therapy with a brisk reticulocytosis. Serum ferritin levels also fail to distinguish the two. Only an examination of the bone marrow for iron stores provides a definitive answer. More aggressive evaluation generally should be restricted to patients whose pattern of gastrointestinal symptoms, degree of anemia, or documented loss of blood via the gastrointestinal tract seems to require gastrointestinal or hematologic studies.

Felty's syndrome originally was described as the combination of RA, splenomegaly, leukopenia, and leg ulcers. Subsequent observations have shown an association with lymphadenopathy, thrombocytopenia, and the HLA-DR4 haplotype (16). Felty's syndrome is most common in people with severe, nodule-forming RA. The precise pathogenesis of the leukopenia, which selectively involves neutrophils, is poorly understood. The large granular lymphocyte (LGL) syndrome shares many of the same features of Felty's syndrome (17), but it is not exclusive to RA. LGL syndrome may represent a process that permits RA to develop, rather than being a result of the disease. An increased incidence of non-Hodgkin's lymphoma has been reported in people with Felty's syndrome (18).

Thrombocytopenia may occur in RA as a result of marrow suppression due to immunosuppressive or cytotoxic therapy, or it may be related to an autoimmune process in gold, penicillamine, or sulfasalazine therapy.

Course and Prognosis

Studies of prognosis in people with RA are difficult because of the chronic nature of the disease, its inherent variability,

and the difficulty of identifying milder or subclinical forms. Many patients never seek medical care, and the diagnosis of RA often is not included on the death certificate.

Criteria for remission have been established (see Appendix I), but the prevalence of remission is unknown. A population study on the prevalence of RA was unable to substantiate the diagnosis in more than one-half of patients who had been diagnosed with the disease several years earlier (19). Although some of these patients may have experienced spontaneous remission, interpreting such studies is difficult because therapy and patient selection can influence epidemiologic findings. In a classic monograph on the clinical picture of RA patients treated with only salicylates and simple orthopedic measures, Short and Bauer found that only 10% of patients experienced clinical remission during more than a decade of follow-up (20). This observation is similar to that of Ragan, who found a low rate of spontaneous remission and noted that when remissions did occur, they did so in the first two years of disease onset (5). Both studies, which focused on patients seeking medical care from rheumatologists, seem to closely parallel current clinical observations. Factors that predict a more severe, persistent disease course are the presence of rheumatoid factor, nodules, and the HLA-DR4 haplotype (21). In patients who do not undergo spontaneous remission, the prognosis in regard to joint destruction seems to depend on the severity of synovial inflammation (22).

Almost 90% of the joints ultimately affected in a given patient are involved during the first year of disease (6). Therefore, a patient who has had RA for several years may be assured, given the worst-case scenario, which joints will or will not be involved in the future.

Several studies over the past decade have demonstrated increased mortality rates in people with RA and have shown that patients with severe forms of the disease die 10–15 years earlier than expected. The causes of death that were disproportionately high, compared with the total US population, were infections, pulmonary and renal disease, lymphoproliferative disorders, gastrointestinal bleeding, and possibly, cardiovascular disease (12,23).

RONALD J. ANDERSON, MD

References

1. Fleming A, Benn RT, Corbett M, Wood PH. Early rheumatoid disease. Patterns of joint involvement. Ann Rheum Dis 1976;35:361–364.
2. Schumacher HR. Palindromic onset of rheumatoid arthritis. Arthritis Rheum 1982;25:361–365.
3. van der Heijde DM, van Riel PL, van Leeuwen MA, van't Hof MA, van Rijswijk MH, van de Putte LB. Prognostic factors for radiographic damage and physical disability in early rheumatoid arthritis. A prospective study of 147 patients. Br J Rheumatol 1992;31:519–525.
4. Pincus T, Brooks RH, Callahan LF. Measurements of inflammatory activity in rheumatoid arthritis may indicate no change or improvement over 5 years while measures of dam-

age indicate disease progression: implications for assessment of long-term outcomes. *Arthritis Rheum* 1995;38:S630.

5. Ragan C, Farrington E. The clinical features of rheumatoid arthritis. Prognostic indices. *JAMA* 1959;2:16.

6. Roberts WN, Daltroy LH, Anderson RJ. Stability of normal joint findings in persistent classical rheumatoid arthritis. *Arthritis Rheum* 1988;31:267–271.

7. McGuigan L, Burke D, Fleming A. Tarsal tunnel syndrome and peripheral neuropathy in rheumatoid disease. *Ann Rheum Dis* 1983;42:128–131.

8. Weyand CM, Hicok KC, Conn DL, Goronzy JJ. The influence of HLA-DR B1 genes on disease severity in rheumatoid arthritis. *Ann Intern Med* 1992;117:801–806.

9. Kerstens PJ, Boerbooms AM, Jeurissen ME, Fast JH, Assman KJ, van de Putte LB. Accelerated nodulosis during long term methotrexate therapy for rheumatoid arthritis: an analysis of 10 cases. *J Rheumatol* 1992;19:867–871.

10. Bienenstock H, Ehrlich GE, Freyberg RH. Rheumatoid arthritis of the cricoarytenoid joint: a clinicopathological study. *Arthritis Rheum* 1963;6:48–63.

11. Walker WC, Wright V. Pulmonary lesions and rheumatoid arthritis. *Medicine (Baltimore)* 1968;47:501–520.

12. Pincus T, Callahan LF. Early mortality in RA predicted by poor clinical status. *Bull Rheum Dis* 1992;41(4):1–4.

13. John JT Jr, Hough A, Sergent JS. Pericardial disease in rheumatoid arthritis. *Am J Med* 1979;66:385–390.

14. Gravallese EM, Corson JM, Coblyn JS, Pinkusas, Weinblatt ME. Rheumatoid aortitis: a rarely recognized but clinically significant entity. *Medicine (Baltimore)* 1989;68:95–106.

15. Nakano KK, Schoene WC, Baker RA, Dawson DM. The cervical myelopathy associated with rheumatoid arthritis. *Ann Neurol* 1978;3:144-151.

16. Dinant HJ, Hissink Muller W, van den Berg-Loonen EM, Nijenhuis LE, Engelfriet CP. HLA DRW4 in Felty's syndrome. *Arthritis Rheum* 1980;23:1336.

17. Barton JC, Prasthofer EF, Egan ML, Heck LW, Koopman WJ, Grossi CE. Rheumatoid arthritis associated with expanded populations of granular lymphocytes. *Ann Intern Med* 1986;104:314–323.

18. Gridley G, Klippel JH, Hoover RN, Fraumeni JF. Incidence of cancer among men with Felty syndrome. *Ann Intern Med* 1994;120:35–39.

19. O'Sullivan JB, Cathcart ES. The prevalence of rheumatoid arthritis. Follow-up evaluation of the effect of criteria on rates in Sudbury, Mass. *Ann Intern Med* 1972;76:573–577.

20. Short CL, Bauer W, Reynolds WE. Rheumatoid Arthritis. Boston: Harvard University Press, 1957.

21. van Zeben D, Hazes JM, Zwinderman AH, et al. Association of HLA-DR4 with a more progressive disease course in patients with rheumatoid arthritis. Results of a follow-up study. *Arthritis Rheum* 1991;34:822–830.

22. Drossaers-Bakker KK, de Buck M, van Zeben D, et al. Long-term prognosis and outcome of functional capacity in rheumatoid arthritis. *Arthritis Rheum* 1999;42:1854–1860.

23. Wolfe F, Mitchell DM, Sibley JT, et al. The mortality of rheumatoid arthritis. *Arthritis Rheum* 1994;37:481–494.

RHEUMATOID ARTHRITIS
C. Treatment

There have been major advances in the treatment of rheumatoid arthritis (RA) over the past several years, due to three trends: 1) recognition that drug therapies, especially when used early in the disease, can alter the outcome and reduce severity, disability, and mortality; 2) improved understanding of the pathogenetic mechanisms involved in immunologic and inflammatory processes; and 3) development of therapies that target more specifically the pathophysiologic processes and mediators involved in the pathogenesis of RA. As a consequence, rheumatologists and other practitioners are more willing to prescribe medications that may ameliorate symptoms, slow or even halt disease progression, and modify the disease course, preventing damage to the joints and resultant functional limitations. An accurate diagnosis is the foundation for proper management of RA. Appropriate and timely therapeutic intervention can not only alleviate the symptoms, but also improve the prognosis (1).

The most effective treatment regimens for RA focus on the (incomplete) understanding of the pathogenetic mechanisms of the disease and, most importantly, on the individual patient. Clinicians who understand determinants of disease outcome can devise a treatment strategy that will be useful and acceptable to the individual patient. These determinants include presence of rheumatoid factor, early onset of severe synovitis with functional limitation, joint erosions, persistent elevation of erythrocyte sedimentation rate or C-reactive protein, presence of extra-articular manifestations, and a family history of severe RA.

Rheumatoid arthritis is a pleomorphic disease with variable expression. Gradual onset occurs in more than 50% of patients, and as many as 20% of patients have a monocyclic course that will abate within two years. The remainder will have a polycyclic or progressive course (2). The long-term prognosis of people with abrupt onset of disease is similar to that for people with gradual disease onset. Management strategies appropriate to the disease course must account for this variability to avoid overtreating or undertreating patients with RA.

In the future, knowledge of genetic factors may provide useful information on the likely disease course and help guide treatment. Poor socioeconomic status and educational achievement are important predictors of poor disease outcome. The health-related beliefs, goals, and desires of patients are important predictors of compliance with treatment and outcome. A willingness on the part of health care providers to understand and work with these beliefs, and to educate patients about the disease, is as fundamental to the successful treatment of RA as any medication that can be prescribed. Access to rheumatologists and other health care professionals skilled in the treatment of RA is fundamental to lessening the burden of disease (3). This is important for correct diagnosis and initiation of patient-specific treatment early in the disease course; both are critical factors in the successful management of RA. Although joint destruction progresses at variable rates and with variable intensity, many patients experience joint damage evident by radiography early in the disease, emphasizing the need for timely and aggressive use of disease-modifying agents to prevent long-term disability (1). Still, the median time between the onset of symptoms of RA and its diagnosis is 36 weeks (4).

People with RA see health care providers because of pain, functional limitation, and concern and fear about their diagnosis and prognosis. Initial therapeutic efforts must address these concerns and patients' beliefs about their disease. Failure to place these concerns at the center of the relationship will adversely affect the patient's ability to cope with the disease. Communication and constant reassessment of the patient's progress through open dialogue and quantitative measures are vital for monitoring the disease course and patient distress. Communication helps patients understand the need for proposed therapies, including disease-modifying agents.

Clinical tools for monitoring a patient's well-being and the efficacy of therapy include patient assessments of the duration of morning stiffness and severity of fatigue, as well as functional, social, emotional, and pain status, as measured by a health assessment questionnaire. A patient-derived global assessment using a visual analog scale is a simple and effective means of recording patient well-being. The number of tender and swollen joints is a useful measure of disease activity, as are the presence of anemia, thrombocytosis, and elevated sedimentation rate or C-reactive protein. Serial radiographs of target joints, including the hands, are useful in assessing disease progression.

Management Principles

The major goals of therapy are to relieve pain, swelling, and fatigue; improve joint function; stop joint damage, and prevent disability and disease-related morbidity. These goals are constant throughout the disease course, although the emphasis may shift to address specific patient needs. For example, some patients with advanced joint damage experience minimal swelling or constitutional symptoms, and benefit most from physical therapy, joint reconstruction, and pain control. Most patients, however, require continued efforts to control the inflammatory process through disease-modifying therapy.

Patient education is essential early in the disease course and on an ongoing basis. Educational topics include the nature of the disease and its prognosis, vocational and avocational counseling, lifestyle and family counseling, enhancement of self-esteem, home modifications, and disease treatment. This process includes family members, who often are overlooked. Patients are best served by a multidisciplinary approach with early referral to a rheumatologist and other specially trained medical personnel, including nurses, counselors, and occupational and physical therapists who are skilled and knowledgeable about RA. Appropriate medical care of people with RA encompasses attention to smoking cessation, immunizations, prompt treatment of infections, and management of comorbid conditions, including diabetes, hypertension, and osteoporosis.

Modalities pursued by occupational and physical therapists focus on improving function and reducing disability. These modalities include joint protection; functional enhancement; use of splints, orthotics, and adaptive and adequate footwear, and other adaptive devices; and exercises, including range-of-motion, stretching, strengthening, and conditioning. All people with RA must be taught the most fundamental treatment of joint inflammation, which is, quite simply, adequate rest. An afternoon nap and nighttime rest are integral components of an effective treatment program to reduce the fatigue that patients with active RA experience. Immobilization of individual joints will lessen the symptoms of inflammation. Range-of-motion exercises to preserve function, increase muscle strength, and improve overall endurance should be maintained through a therapy program appropriate to the patient's level of function and extent of joint inflammation.

Drug Therapy

Drugs for the management of RA have been traditionally, but imperfectly, divided into two groups: those used primarily for the control of joint pain and swelling, and those intended to limit joint damage and improve long-term outcome. Symptoms of pain and swelling in RA are mediated, at least in part, by intense cytokine activity. Nonsteroidal anti-inflammatory drugs (NSAIDs) inhibit proinflammatory prostaglandins and are effective treatments for pain, swelling, and stiffness, but have no effect on the disease course or risk of joint damage. On the other hand, anti-inflammatory properties have been noted for several disease-modifying antirheumatic drugs (DMARDs), which are used principally to control disease and to limit joint damage. These include methotrexate and biologic response modifiers with actions targeted against specific cytokines, such as tumor necrosis factor α (TNF-α). Corticosteroids are powerful, nonspecific inhibitors of cytokines and, in some studies that compared them with placebos, are reported to delay joint erosions effectively (5).

As treatment of RA becomes more effective and more complex, more attention will be given to drug costs and side effects with respect to disease control and remission. Drugs that improve the long-term outcome of the disease will be prescribed more frequently, and efforts will be made to limit the use of NSAIDs to people coping with joint pain and swelling.

Nonsteroidal Anti-Inflammatory Drugs

NSAIDs, including salicylates, act quickly to reduce inflammation and pain, but they do not prevent tissue injury or progressive joint damage, nor do they completely eliminate signs and symptoms of active arthritis. NSAIDs inhibit one or both types of cyclooxygenase (COX) enzymes. COX-1 is expressed constitutively in the gastrointestinal (GI) mucosa, kidneys, platelets, and vascular endothelium. COX-2 is expressed functionally and promotes the elaboration of prostaglandins in inflamed tissues.

NSAIDs are used primarily for symptom control, and may be discontinued in the asymptomatic patient. Patients are more likely to adhere to therapy when the agents used are affordable, demonstrate relatively low toxicity, and follow a simple dosing schedule. Although some NSAIDs are more efficacious and/or better tolerated than others, NSAID therapy ultimately must be tailored to the individual, and the appropriate NSAID for a particular patient may not be the least toxic or most efficacious choice. A guide to currently available salicylates and NSAIDs is provided in Appendix III.

When considering NSAID therapy, the patient's age, sex, and medical history (including a history of upper GI bleeding and renal function) must be taken into account. Older patients, especially those who are female or have a history of GI bleeding, are at a higher risk for GI complications from NSAIDs. Use of nonselective NSAIDs generally is contraindicated in these patients. If NSAIDs are prescribed, these patients should receive gastric protective agents, such as proton pump blockers, misoprostol, or a more selective COX-2 inhibitory agent.

NSAID gastropathy is common, and people with RA have about a 30% chance of hospitalization or death from GI toxicity during the course of their disease. Selective inhibition of COX-2 may lead to an improved safety profile for these agents by reducing major GI toxicity, especially bleeding. Celecoxib, rofecoxib and valdecoxib are the first agents available in the United States that selectively block COX-2, other agents are likely to follow. Although less gastrotoxic, the efficacy of COX-2 inhibitors does not differ substantially from that of conventional NSAIDs. Despite their advantages, COX-2 inhibitors may be associated with significant adverse reactions, including allergy, fluid retention, and renal failure. Like other NSAIDs, they should be used cautiously or avoided in patients with renal insufficiency. Use of NSAIDs in rheumatic disease is discussed in Chapter 45.

Corticosteroids

Corticosteroids are potent suppressors of inflammation, and they are effective in managing the pain and functional limitations of people with active inflammatory joint disease (see Chapter 46). However, most studies, and 50 years of experience with their use, attest to the inadequacy of corticosteroids as the sole therapy for RA.

It is desirable, but often not possible, to avoid continuous corticosteroid therapy in people with RA. Because of the well-appreciated side affects of these drugs, long-term use generally should be avoided. Brief courses of corticosteroids (15–20 mg of prednisone a day, tapering over one to three weeks) may be effective for controlling disease flares or as a "bridge" of disease control until DMARD therapy becomes effective.

For severe polyarticular disease, corticosteroids may be needed in doses typically ranging from 2 mg to 15 mg per day of prednisone, often given in divided doses (for example, 2 mg three times a day). The split dosing regimen often is necessary because of the short half-life of the anti-inflammatory effect of oral corticosteroids. In systemic disease, such as rheumatoid vasculitis, prednisone doses of 40–60 mg/day may be necessary, tapering according to response (6). Intra-articular injection of corticosteroid is an effective means for reducing pain and inflammation in individual recalcitrant joints.

Disease-Modifying Antirheumatic Drugs

DMARDs differ greatly in their mechanisms of action. These actions are well-understood for some agents, including such biologic response modifiers as the TNF-α antagonists, but less understood for others, such as gold or hydroxychloroquine. DMARDs also vary greatly in their chemical structure, toxicity, and indications for use. An effective DMARD should prevent joint erosions and damage, and control the active synovitis and constitutional features of the disease. There is increasing evidence that some DMARDs can achieve these goals in short-term clinical trials, and some, in longer-term observational follow-up. However, there is no evidence that any available DMARD can heal erosions, reverse joint deformities, or "cure" the disease.

Estimating DMARD utility is difficult because, with the notable exception of methotrexate (7), there are few studies of these agents that extended more than one year. An additional problem in translating results of clinical trials to clinical practice is that long-term use of a given DMARD by an individual patient is uncommon, due to primary and secondary treatment failure, and more commonly, because of drug toxicity. After five to 12 years of treatment with methotrexate, about 50% of patients still are on therapy (8), whereas fewer than 20% of patients remain on other DMARDs for five years or longer.

Ideally, DMARDs should be used when the diagnosis of RA is established and before erosive changes appear on radiographs. Patients requiring DMARDs have experienced functional compromise, chronic pain, and persistent synovitis. DMARDs may be used with NSAIDs and/or corticosteroids, if needed. A complete discussion of the mechanisms of action and toxicity profiles of individual DMARDs is described in Chapter 47 and Appendix III.

TABLE 9C-1
Practical Application of Therapeutic Strategies for Rheumatoid Arthritis

1. Newly diagnosed RA in a young woman with positive rheumatoid factor and mild disease (few joints involved and sedimentation rate less than 30 mm/h).	1. Hydroxychloroquine, 400 mg/day with or without an NSAID, and prednisone, 3–5 mg/day over a 1–3 month period. Sulfasalazine, up to 3 g per day in two divided doses, would be an acceptable alternative.
2. Patient with new-onset RA and marked symptoms including fatigue and low-grade fever, weight loss, and polyarticular disease.[a]	2. Methotrexate, with an NSAID, and prednisone, 5–15 mg/day; tapering prednisone over a 3–4 month period if possible. If unable to achieve control over the initial 6–8 weeks of therapy, consider adding hydroxychloroquine and/or sulfasalazine to this regimen.
3. Patient with established mild disease.	3. Same as scenario #1.
4. Patient with established rheumatoid arthritis in whom methotrexate is partially effective.[a]	4. Add NSAIDs or prednisone 5–15 mg/day.
a. Initiate combination therapy.	a. Add hydroxychloroquine, sulfasalazine, or both, or add a TNF-α antagonist or leflunomide.
b. Combination therapy with hydroxychloroquine, sulfasalazine, or both is ineffective.	b. Discontinue hydroxychloroquine and sulfasalazine; add leflunomide, azathioprine, cyclosporine, or a TNF-α antagonist.
c. Combination therapy with methotrexate and cyclosporine, leflunomide, or azathioprine is poorly tolerated or ineffective.	c. Continue methotrexate but discontinue the combination drug and add a TNF-α antagonist.
5. Patient with established RA in whom methotrexate is ineffective, not tolerated, or contraindicated[a]	5. Mild disease: leflunomide, sulfasalazine, azathioprine. Severe disease: cyclosporine and combinations of DMARDs such as sulfasalazine, hydroxychloroquine, and others; or add a TNF-α antagonist. Gold is also occasionally used. Oral prednisone, 5–15 mg/day may be needed.

[a] The role of TNF-α antagonists is evolving; some rheumatologists may institute therapy with these agents at different points in these scenarios. These agents are being increasingly used in early disease.

There are two basic approaches to the use of DMARDs in early disease. A "step-up" approach of monotherapy consists of selecting a DMARD appropriate to the disease severity, as estimated by the presence of prognostic markers. These markers include a poor health assessment questionnaire score, presence of rheumatoid factor, female sex, and perhaps, in future clinical practice, genotypic profiles (such as HLA-DR shared disease epitopes in relevant populations) If disease control fails to improve with monotherapy, the DMARD is switched or one or two other DMARDs are added. The second approach is to give a combination of DMARDs and corticosteroids at the outset of disease to people with an expected poor prognosis, with a "step down" elimination of corticosteroids and DMARDs as disease control improves. In people with established disease, estimates of disease activity and severity can guide treatment decisions.

The choice of a DMARD is complex, and depends on the patient and disease-related factors, including immediate and long-term costs. Unfortunately, people with RA of longer disease duration do not respond as well to treatment as do patients with early disease, so that results of studies of early disease cannot easily be applied to all patients. Examples of drug treatment regimens for patients at different stages of disease are given in Table 9C-1. Advances in joint surgery can help these patients to partially overcome critical functional limitations caused by the disease.

The costs of DMARD therapy consist of the cost of the drug, the expense of monitoring for and treating toxicities, and years of life lost due to the disease and treatment complications. A simulation analysis compared people with RA to healthy controls during the first 25 years after diagnosis. Adjustments were made for differential survival among people with RA, and it was determined that the median lifetime incremental costs of RA in 1995 US dollars range approximately from $61,000 to $122,000 (higher for younger individuals) (9). Interventions (such as autologous bone marrow transplantation) costing up to $60,000 may be cost-saving if they eliminate the downstream incremental costs of RA, especially if they can be shown to be effective at the outset of disease (9).

Hydroxychloroquine

For people with early, mild, and/or seronegative disease, the antimalarial hydroxychloroquine often is the first drug of choice because of its favorable toxicity profile and ease of use. The onset of activity occurs within three to four months in about 50% of patients, although it may take up to one year for the full benefit of drug treatment to be realized. Retinopathy due to hydroxychloroquine rarely develops when appropriate dosages are used.

Sulfasalazine

Like hydroxychloroquine, this DMARD has an acceptable toxicity profile and often is used as initial treatment for early, mild, and/or seronegative disease. The initial dose is 500–1000 mg/day, escalating to a maximum of 1500 mg twice a day. Toxicities include GI upset, which may be lessened by using an enteric-coated preparation, and myelosuppression. It frequently is used in combination with other agents, including hydroxychloroquine and methotrexate.

Methotrexate

For people with established disease or severe, newly diagnosed disease, methotrexate is a preferred choice. As a single therapy, it has been shown to be superior or equivalent to other standard DMARDs, providing about 60%–70% objective improvement. It often is used in combination with other standard DMARDs, as well as with newer agents, including leflunomide and such biologic response modifiers as the TNF-α antagonists. It has a well-recognized, long-term efficacy and toxicity profile, and the lowest long-term drug discontinuation rate of any DMARD currently available (8). The initial dosage usually is 7.5–10.0 mg/week, titrated upward to an average dosage of 12.5–17.5 mg/week. A therapeutic effect usually is evident after four to 10 weeks. Dosages of 20–25 mg/week may be necessary to realize this drug's therapeutic potential before response is deemed "inadequate."

Methotrexate may be given orally, in tablet or liquid form; the liquid preparation is substantially less expensive than tablets. In some patients, however, injection may be associated with less stomatitis and GI upset. Although methotrexate generally is well-tolerated, side effects may occur in as many as 70% of patients (10). Methotrexate can cause GI upset and, rarely, hepatotoxicity, including liver fibrosis and cirrhosis. People taking this drug should not use alcohol. Other side effects include the possibility of opportunistic infections and, rarely, development of a B-cell non-Hodgkin's lymphoma. Accelerated nodulosis may occur, for which there are no clearly effective treatments. Methotrexate should not be used in pregnant patients because of its teratogenicity, or in patients with hepatic or renal insufficiency; it should be used cautiously, if at all, in those with severe lung disease. Supplemental folate (usually 1 mg/day) seems to reduce the occurrence of other adverse effects, including stomatitis, hair thinning, and to some extent, bone marrow suppression. The use of such antifolate drugs as sulfamethoxazole, which may precipitate pancytopenia, should be avoided in people taking methotrexate.

Despite the success of methotrexate, alone and in combination with other DMARDs, methotrexate use may slow, but does not halt, the progression of disease (11). Methotrexate is likely to remain a major therapy for RA for the foreseeable future. Newer drugs will be compared with it, and added to it, because the safety and efficacy of long-term treatment is well-known for methotrexate. Methotrexate also is much less expensive than newer agents. Patients with established disease who respond to methotrexate have significantly increased life expectancy, compared with patients who do not respond (12). Newer agents will challenge methotrexate's use in early aggressive disease only if their use can establish remission, limit joint damage, and demonstrate a favorable long-term safety and cost profile.

Azathioprine

Azathioprine traditionally has been prescribed for people with moderate or severe RA. It has an adequate toxicity and safety profile, but generally has been displaced by methotrexate and newer DMARDs. There is no convincing evidence that it has true disease-modifying capability. Its greatest utility in patients may be with refractory disease or severe extra-articular disease manifestations, such as vasculitis.

Cyclosporine

Cyclosporine is effective in low dosages (2.5–5.0 mg/kg/day), as solo therapy or in combination with methotrexate, and can slow the progression of joint damage even in patients with severe, refractory RA (13,14). Its high cost, potential for causing hypertension and renal toxicity, and need for close monitoring have limited the acceptance of cyclosporine as a treatment for RA.

Cyclophosphamide

This alkylating agent is of limited benefit for the treatment of synovitis and has a poor toxicity profile, including bone marrow toxicity, infertility, bladder toxicity, and oncogenicity. Its use in RA generally is restricted to treatment of corticosteroid-refractory systemic vasculitis.

Leflunomide

Leflunomide is a pyrimidine synthesis inhibitor, with clinical efficacy generally equivalent to that of methotrexate. In a 12-month study, leflunomide was shown to slow the rate of radiographic progression of erosive disease (15). Additional benefit may be achieved when it is used in combination with methotrexate. Side effects reported with leflunomide include rash, alopecia, allergy, weight loss, thrombocytopenia, and diarrhea. The diarrhea often occurs early in the treatment course and may abate, but if dosage reduction or concomitant use of antidiarrheal agents cannot ameliorate it, leflunomide use may need to be discontinued.

Anti-TNF-α Antibody Agents

Etanercept and infliximab are TNF-α antagonists that have powerful anti-inflammatory effects in people with both early and established RA (16,17,18). Tumor necrosis factor is a potent inflammatory cytokine expressed in increased amounts in the serum and synovial fluid of people with RA. It promotes the release of other proinflammatory cytokines, particularly interleukin (IL)-1, IL-6, and IL-8, and stimulates protease production.

Etanercept is a fusion protein composed of two identical chains of recombinant human TNF-α receptor fused with the Fc portion of human IgG1. In vitro, it binds to soluble TNF-α. Approximately 70% of patients receiving subcutaneous etanercept at dosages of 25 mg twice a week have substantial decreases of joint inflammation, often within one to two weeks after initiation of therapy. This improvement can be enhanced by combining etanercept with methotrexate (16). Adverse effects of etanercept are influenza-like symptoms and reactions at the injection site, which usually abate after the first few injections.

Infliximab is a chimeric monoclonal antibody to TNF-α that is administered intravenously (17). The usual maintenance dose after initiation of therapy is 3 mg/kg every eight weeks. It is used in combination with methotrexate, and has efficacy roughly equivalent to etanercept. Infliximab is now indicated for "inhibiting the progression of joint damage and improving physical function" in patients with RA. Infliximab may be associated with development of autoantibodies such as antinuclear antibodies.

Potential long-term risks of these TNF-α antagonists have not been established. To date, neither drug has been associated with an increased risk of malignancy or autoimmune disease. Case reports suggest an increased risk of active tuberculosis and demyelinating syndromes in patients treated with these agents. These issues are the subject of ongoing post-marketing surveillance (see Chapter 48). The cost of these drugs, more than $12,000 per year, is a significant barrier to use for many patients. Although TNF-α antagonists appear to significantly benefit patients with early RA and may have longer-term ameliorative effects for such patients, they should be considered only for people with recalcitrant disease that is not controlled by one or more DMARDs, usually including methotrexate. Indications for the use of TNF-α antagonists are in flux; initial reports of disease-modifying activity, with slowed radiographic progression, eventually may prompt their use earlier in the disease course (17). These agents should lead to significant improvement in symptoms in eight to 12 weeks. They should not be used in patients with active serious infections, such as septic arthritis, sepsis, osteomyelitis, or systemic fungal infections, and they should be avoided in patients with a history of tuberculosis or myeloproliferative disease, including lymphoma.

Other Therapies

Because of its slow onset of action, high frequency of side effects, and lack of DMARD properties, *penicillamine* is used infrequently to treat RA. *Gold* preparations are useful for long-term symptom control in a very small percentage of patients, but there are a few studies documenting their ability to prevent joint damage. Only one parenteral and one oral formulation are available in the United States.

TABLE 9C-2
Treatment of Rheumatoid Vasculitis

1. General measures	Stop smoking, and treat such comorbid conditions as hypertension and diabetes mellitus.
2. In all cases, manage rheumatoid arthritis and constitutional features.	NSAIDs, low-dose prednisone, disease-modifying drugs.
3. Localized vasculitis manifestations a. Nail fold infarcts b. Distal sensory neuropathy c. Leg ulcers d. Digital tip gangrene without other manifestations and no clinical evidence of inflammation	a. Manage the rheumatoid arthritis as in 2. b. Manage the rheumatoid arthritis as in 2. c. Local care for leg ulcers, possibly skin graft. d. Antiplatelet drugs, vasodilating agents.
4. Systemic vasculitis a. Progressive manifestations with clinical evidence of inflammation, mononeuritis multiplex, digital tip infarcts, CNS, and/or visceral involvement b. Resistant progressive inflammatory multisystem disease	a. High-divided-dose prednisone, azathioprine, chlorambucil, mycophenolate mofetil or cyclophosphamide, or antiplatelet drugs. b. Addition of IV immunoglobulin. Trial of a TNF-α antagonist.

NSAIDs, nonsteroidal anti-inflammatory drugs; CNS, central nervous system; TNF-α, tumor necrosis factor α.

Minocycline, the only antibiotic to be carefully studied for use in RA (19), can improve mild-to-moderate symptoms, but has no documented DMARD properties. Clinical experience suggests a high rate of drug discontinuation due to lack of long-term efficacy and the presence of such side effects as skin discoloration, dizziness, GI upset, and autoimmune phenomena, including hepatitis.

Chlorambucil has a poor toxicity/efficacy profile, although it sometimes is useful in treating severe extra-articular disease manifestations, such as systemic vasculitis and severe scleritis.

An *immunosorbent column* (Prosorba) has been approved for treatment of RA (20). Weekly exchanges for an initial period of 12 weeks may be useful for a minority of patients with established disease. Side effects include the risk of thrombophlebitis, syncope, and thromboembolism.

Complementary therapies are overwhelmingly endorsed by the lay public. However, rigorous scientific studies of the safety and efficacy of these treatments are lacking (see Chapter 50).

Combination Therapies

In people with moderate to severe disease activity, methotrexate often is used in combination with other agents. In patients who have acute and severe disease, initial therapy often consists of a combination of DMARDs, corticosteroids, and NSAIDs. Combinations of DMARDs also are used to improve disease control; approximately 50% of people with RA treated by rheumatologists are prescribed combination therapies with two or three DMARDs. The combination of methotrexate, hydroxychloroquine, and sulfasalazine is among the most popular regimens, although study results are not readily duplicated among prescribing physicians. Other successful combination therapies include methotrexate used with such agents as cyclosporine, TNF-α antagonists, leflunomide, and azathioprine.

Treating Extra-Articular Disease Manifestations of RA

Serious extra-articular disease manifestations, including vasculitis, scleritis, and recalcitrant serositis, generally require systemic corticosteroids and may necessitate the use of such immunosuppressive agents as cyclophosphamide or cyclosporine (7). When the disease is controlled, methotrexate (15–25 mg/week) may be substituted for the immunosuppressive agent. Table 9C-2 contains suggestions for managing vasculitis in RA.

Subcutaneous rheumatoid nodules may, rarely, require excision because of severe pain, inconvenient location, or infection. Nodules occurring in parenchymal organs are treated by managing the underlying disease. Sicca symptoms are treated with preparations to moisturize the eyes and mouth, and with attention to dental hygiene (See Chapter 20 on Sjögren's syndrome). Serositis (pleuritis and pericarditis) is treated with NSAIDs or oral corticosteroids. Pericardiocentesis, local steroid injection, or a pericardial window may be needed for treatment of pericardial tamponade, and pericardiectomy may be needed for management of constrictive pericarditis. Felty's syndrome may be treated with DMARDs, such as gold or methotrexate, and supportive therapy, including granulocyte colony-stimulating factor. Splenectomy may be required for people with recurrent infections and pancytopenia, but is effective in only about 50% of patients.

Surgery

Advances in orthopedic surgery have substantially improved the function, mobility, pain control, and quality of life for people with RA. Surgeries include tendon repair and transfer, carpal tunnel release, total joint replacement, and stabilization of unstable cervical vertebrae. Many rheumatologists and orthopedic surgeons recommend discontinuing such therapies as methotrexate, immunosuppressives, and TNF-α antagonists in the perioperative period, but no data support this practice.

Conclusion

Significant challenges face patients with RA and the physicians who treat them. On the one hand, DMARDs are becoming more accepted by physicians and their patients. Yet, due to side effects or failure to effect long-term disease control, it is unusual for a patient with RA to take any given DMARD for more than three to five years. Understanding the relationship between genetic factors of disease susceptibility and severity may provide an avenue for individualized treatment in the future.

ERIC L. MATTESON, MD

References

1. Fries JF, Williams CA, Morfeld D, Singh G, Sibley J. *Reduction in long-term disability in patients with rheumatoid arthritis by disease-modifying antirheumatic drug-based treatment strategies. Arthritis Rheum 1996;39:616–622.*

2. Masi AT. *Articular patterns in the early course of rheumatoid arthritis. Am J Med 1983;75:16–26.*

3. Ward MM, Leigh JP, Fries JF. *Progression of functional disability in patients with rheumatoid arthritis. Associations with rheumatology subspecialty care. Arch Int Med 1993;153:2229–2237.*

4. Chan KW, Felson DT, Yood RA, Walker AM. *The lag time between onset of symptoms and diagnosis of rheumatoid arthritis. Arthritis Rheum 1994;37:814–820.*

5. Kirwan JR. *The effect of glucocorticoids on joint destruction in rheumatoid arthritis. The Arthritis and Rheumatism Council Low-dose Glucocorticoid Study Group. N Engl J Med 1995;333:142–146.*

6. Matteson EL, Conn DL. Extra-articular manifestations of rheumatoid arthritis. In: Weisman MH, Weinblatt ME, Louie JS (eds). Treatment of the Rheumatic Diseases. Philadelphia: WB Saunders, 1995; pp 236-248.

7. Weinblatt ME, Maier AL, Fraser PA, Coblyn JS. Longterm prospective study of methotrexate in rheumatoid arthritis: conclusion after 132 months of therapy. J Rheumatol 1998;25:238–242.

8. Wluka A, Buchbinder R, Mylvaganam A, et al. Longterm methotrexate use in rheumatoid arthritis: 12 year followup of 460 patients treated in community practice.J Rheumatol 2000;27:1864-1871.

9. Gabriel SE, Crowson CS, Luthra HS, Wagner JL, O'Fallon WM. Modeling the lifetime costs of rheumatoid arthritis. J Rheumatol 1999;26:1269–1274.

10. Weinblatt ME, Kaplan H, Germain BF, et al. Low-dose methotrexate compared with auranofin in adult rheumatoid arthritis: a thirty-six week, double-blind trial. Arthritis Rheum 1990;33:330–338.

11. Rich E, Moreland LW, Alarcon GS. Paucity of radiographic progression in rheumatoid arthritis treated with methotrexate as the first disease modifying antirheumatic drug. J Rheumatol 1999;26:259–261.

12. Krause D, Schleusser B, Herborn G, Rau R. Response to methotrexate treatment is associated with reduced mortality in patients with severe rheumatoid arthritis. Arthritis Rheum 2000;43:14–21.

13. Pasero G, Priolo F, Marubini E, et al. Slow progression of joint damage in early rheumatoid arthritis treated with cyclosporin A. Arthritis Rheum 1996;39:1006–1015.

14. Tugwell P, Pincus T, Yocum D, et al. Combination therapy with cyclosporine and methotrexate in severe rheumatoid arthritis: The Methotrexate-Cyclosporine Combination Study Group. N Engl J Med 1995;333:137–141.

15. Sharp JT, Strand V, Leung H, Hurley F, Loew-Friedrich I. Treatment with leflunomide slows radiographic progression of rheumatoid arthritis. Arthritis Rheum 2000;43:495–505.

16. Weinblatt ME, Kremer JM, Bankhurst AD, et al. A trial of etanercept, a recombinant tumor necrosis factor receptor:Fc fusion protein, in patients with rheumatoid arthritis receiving methotrexate. N Engl J Med 1999;340:253–259.

17. Lipsky PE, van der Heijde DM, St. Clair EW, et al. Infliximab and methotrexate in the treatment of rheumatoid arthritis. N Engl J Med 2000;343:1594-1602.

18. Bathon JM, Martin RW, Fleischmann AM, et al. A comparison of etanercept and methotrexate in patients with early rheumatoid arthritis. N engl J Med 2000;343:1586-1593.

19. O'Dell JR, Haire CE, Palmer W, et al. Treatment of early rheumatoid arthritis with minocycline or placebo: results of a randomized, double-blind, placebo-controlled trial. Arthritis Rheum 1997;40:842–848.

20. Felson DT, LaValley MP, Baldassare AR, et al. The Prosorba column for treatment of refractory rheumatoid arthritis: a randomized, double-blind, sham-controlled trial. Arthritis Rheum 1999;42:2153–2159.

10 PSORIATIC ARTHRITIS

Psoriatic arthritis is a heterogeneous disease with features typical of the spondyloarthropathies in some patients, features of rheumatoid arthritis (RA) in others, and features of both diseases coexisting in yet others. The disease presents with a variety of forms, including monarthritis, asymmetric oligoarthritis, or symmetric polyarthritis. Clinical, epidemiologic, genetic, and radiographic studies suggest that psoriatic arthritis is a separate disease entity, distinct from other inflammatory arthritides.

Epidemiology

The overall prevalence of psoriatic arthritis is approximately 0.1% in the United States. Arthritis occurs in approximately 5%–7% of people with psoriasis, but it may affect up to 40% of hospitalized patients with extensive skin involvement (1). Psoriasis is common in Caucasians (overall prevalence is approximately 2%), but it is relatively uncommon in Asians. Psoriatic arthritis has been described in African blacks, but adequate prevalence data are not available for this population. The male-to-female ratio is equal, but this ratio varies in different subsets of the disease. In contrast to psoriasis, where the peak age of onset is between 5 and 15 years, the peak age of onset for psoriatic arthritis is between 30 and 55 years.

Pathogenesis

The etiology of psoriasis and psoriatic arthritis is not known. Genetic, environmental, and immunologic factors appear to influence susceptibility and disease expression. In view of the similarities of the disease to RA and the spondyloarthropathies, etiopathogenetic mechanisms involved in these diseases are likely to be involved in the distinct subgroups of patients.

Genetic Factors
Convincing evidence of a genetic basis for psoriasis comes from population surveys, twin studies, and analysis of individual pedigrees (2). Inheritance does not follow single-gene Mendelian patterns, but is suggestive of a polygenic influence with ubiquitous genetic or environmental factors contributing to phenotype diversity. Although the concordance between monozygotic twins with psoriasis is high (about 70%, compared with about 30% in RA), the lack of complete concordance suggests a role for environmental factors. Formal twin studies have not been undertaken in people with psoriatic arthritis, and thus the relative importance of

genetic and environmental factors is not known. Family studies suggest an approximate 50-fold increased risk of psoriatic arthritis in first-degree relatives of people with the disease. Within a family, there may be some members who develop only psoriasis or arthritis and some who develop both conditions. Affected fathers are twice as likely to transmit the disease as are affected mothers (3).

An important role for class I human leukocyte antigens (HLA) in the pathogenesis of psoriatic arthritis is supported by data derived from the HLA-B27 transgenic rat model where psoriasiform skin and nail lesions have been observed (4). HLA class I antigens B13, B16 (B38/B39), B17, and Cw6 have been related to psoriasis with or without arthritis (2). The primary association is with HLA-Cw*0602; the association of the remaining HLA class I antigens is due to linkage disequilibrium between these antigens and Cw6 (5). Recently a MICA [class I major histocompatibility chain (MHC)-related gene A] polymorphism, which associates with the MICA-002 allele, has been found to confer susceptibility to polyarticular psoriatic arthritis independent of Cw*0602 (6). HLA-B27 also is associated with the peripheral arthropathy and the spinal disease. HLA class II antigens also have been reported to be associated with psoriasis and psoriatic arthritis. Relationships have been described between HLA-DR7 and psoriasis, and between HLA-DR4 and psoriatic arthritis, although these results have not been confirmed in all populations studied. A gene associated with psoriasis has been mapped to the distal end of the long arm of chromosome 17 (7).

Environmental Factors
Environmental factors including infectious agents and physical trauma are likely to be important in the pathogenesis of psoriatic arthritis. The clinical similarities of reactive arthritis and psoriatic arthritis, and the precipitation of guttate psoriasis by streptococcal infections in children support a role for infectious agents in the pathogenesis of the disease. The notion that psoriatic arthritis may be a reactive arthritis due to psoriatic plaque flora (*Streptococci* and *Staphylococci*) has been discussed extensively, with little evidence to support it. Moreover, the hypothesis that, similar to guttate psoriasis, microbial antigens act as superantigens leading to widespread polyclonal T-cell activation and expansion (8) has not been supported by T-cell receptor (TCR) repertoire analysis (9). The possibility that trauma may precipitate psoriatic arthritis (the deep Koebner effect) has been suggested by several case series. Trauma could

result in the release of putative autoantigens or the expression of heat-shock proteins resembling bacterial antigens.

Immunologic Factors

The histopathologic changes in the skin and synovium are remarkably similar, with activation and expansion of tissue-specific cell subsets (keratinocytes and synoviocytes), accumulation of inflammatory cells (T cells, B cells, macrophages, and neutrophils), and angiogenesis (10). Recent studies using magnetic resonance imaging have highlighted the importance of entheseal inflammation in psoriatic arthritis (11).

T cells play an important pathogenic role in the skin and joint manifestations of psoriatic arthritis. There is T-cell activation with skewing of TCR repertoire consistent with an ongoing Th1 phenotype. In addition to CD4 T cells, an important role for CD8 T cells is suggested by the association of the disease with class I MHC antigens and the observed association of human immunodeficiency virus (HIV)-1 infection with an explosive onset of psoriasis and psoriatic arthritis (12). Psoriasis improves following T-cell–directed therapies (10), such as cyclosporine, interleukin (IL)-2 fusion toxins (which preferentially eliminate IL-2 receptor-bearing cells), and the inhibitor of T-cell costimulation CTLA4Ig (which inhibits costimulatory signals for T-cell activation) (13,14).

The cytokine network in the psoriatic skin and synovium is dominated by the monocyte-derived cytokines tumor necrosis factor (TNF)-α, IL-1α, IL-1β, IL-6, IL-15, and IL-10. Compared with rheumatoid synovium, the TNF-α:IL-10 ratio in psoriatic arthritis patients is elevated, suggesting that a relative deficiency in IL-10 may play a significant role in psoriatic arthritis (15). Cytokines such as IL-15 may play an important role in the pathogenesis of psoriatic skin lesions by inhibiting keratinocyte apoptosis and promoting keratinocyte accumulation (16).

Clinical Features

From a diagnostic and therapeutic point of view, patients may be classified into the following three groups: 1) mono- or oligoarthritis with enthesitis resembling reactive arthritis (observed in about 30%–50% of patients); 2) symmetric polyarthritis resembling RA (about 30%–50%); and 3) predominantly axial disease (spondylitis, sacroiliitis, and/or arthritis of hip and shoulder joints resembling ankylosing spondylitis) with or without peripheral joint disease (about 5%).

Distal interphalangeal (DIP) joint involvement (overall prevalence about 25%), arthritis mutilans (about 5%), sacroiliitis (about 35%), and spondylitis (about 30%) may occur with any of these subgroups (Fig. 10-1). Transition of one pattern into another is not uncommon and may result in heterogenous combinations of joint disease.

Clinical Presentation

In about 70% of patients, psoriasis is present many years before the onset of arthritis; in about 15%, it appears con-

comitantly. Although the arthritis usually is insidious in onset, approximately one-third of patients have an acute onset. Constitutional symptoms are uncommon. In about 15% of adults, and more often in children, the arthritis appears before the skin or nail changes (arthritis *sine* psoriasis). Most patients have a family history of psoriasis, as well as certain clinical features that may provide important clues for its diagnosis.

Joint Disease

Monarticular or oligoarticular arthritis

The most common initial manifestation, observed in up to two-thirds of patients, is a mono- or oligoarticular arthritis similar to the peripheral arthritis seen in the spondyloarthropathies. In approximately one-third to one-half of these patients, this arthritis will evolve into a more symmetric polyarthritis indistinguishable from RA. A classic presentation includes oligoarticular arthritis involving a large joint, such as a knee, with one or two interphalangeal joints and a dactylitic digit or toe. Dactylitis occurs as a result of a combination of tenosynovitis and arthritis of the DIP or proximal interphalangeal (PIP) joints. In some cases, the arthritis may follow an episode of trauma, leading to the erroneous diagnosis of "post-traumatic" or "mechanical" arthritis. If a careful history reveals either a family his-

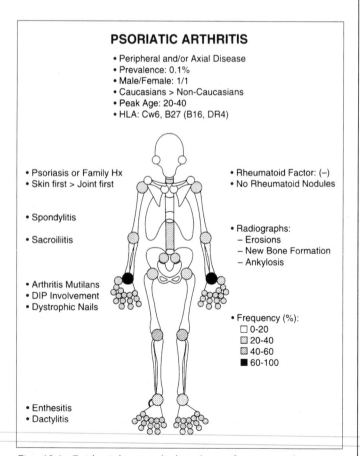

PSORIATIC ARTHRITIS
- Peripheral and/or Axial Disease
- Prevalence: 0.1%
- Male/Female: 1/1
- Caucasians > Non-Caucasians
- Peak Age: 20-40
- HLA: Cw6, B27 (B16, DR4)

- Psoriasis or Family Hx
- Skin first > Joint first

- Spondylitis

- Sacroiliitis

- Arthritis Mutilans
- DIP Involvement
- Dystrophic Nails

- Enthesitis
- Dactylitis

- Rheumatoid Factor: (–)
- No Rheumatoid Nodules

- Radiographs:
  – Erosions
  – New Bone Formation
  – Ankylosis

- Frequency (%):
  - ☐ 0-20
  - ▦ 20-40
  - ▨ 40-60
  - ■ 60-100

Fig. 10-1. Epidemiology and clinical manifestations of psoriatic arthritis. The disease combines features of rheumatoid arthritis and the spondyloarthropathies. DIP, distal interphalangeal.

tory of psoriasis or guttate psoriasis in childhood, a search for hidden areas of psoriasis (scalp, umbilicus, and perianal area) and characteristic radiographic findings (discussed later in this section) will provide important clues to the correct diagnosis. Psoriatic lesions may be limited to one or two small psoriatic patches, with or without nail involvement. Involvement of the DIP joints is characteristic of the disease; DIP joint involvement is almost always associated with psoriatic changes in the nails.

Polyarthritis
Symmetric polyarthritis involving the small joints of the hands and feet, wrists, ankles, knees, and elbows is the most common pattern of psoriatic arthritis. The arthritis may be indistinguishable from RA, but there is a higher frequency of DIP joint involvement and a tendency for bony ankylosis of the DIP and PIP joints, which may lead to "claw" or "paddle" deformities of the hands.

Arthritis Mutilans
Arthritis mutilans is a rare, but highly characteristic feature of the psoriatic arthritis, in which osteolysis of the phalanges and metacarpals of the hand (or in rare cases of the phalanges and metatarsals of the feet) results in "telescoping" of the involved finger (or toe). It occurs in about 5% of patients with psoriatic arthritis.

Axial Disease
Axial disease may occur in people with rheumatoid factor-negative peripheral arthritis. It often is asymptomatic, and both genders are affected equally. Although axial disease may occur independent of peripheral arthritis, usually it manifests itself after several years of peripheral arthritis. Spine symptoms rarely are a presenting feature. Symptoms of inflammatory low-back pain or chest-wall pain may be absent or minimal, despite advanced radiographic changes. Sacroiliitis, observed in up to one-third of patients, frequently is asymptomatic and asymmetric, and may occur independent of spondylitis. Spondylitis also may occur without sacroiliitis, may affect any portion of the spine in a random fashion, and may result in fusion of the spine. In rare cases, involvement of the cervical spine results in atlantoaxial and subaxial subluxations.

Other Manifestations
Inflammation at the site of attachment of tendons and ligaments to bones (enthesitis), a characteristic feature of the spondyloarthropathies, is common, especially at the insertions of the Achilles tendon and plantar fascia into the calcaneus. Enthesopathies tend to occur more frequently in the oligoarthritis form of disease. Ocular involvement, predominantly conjunctivitis, has been observed in up to one-third of patients. As with ankylosing spondylitis, complications such as aortic insufficiency, uveitis, pulmonary fibrosis involving the upper lobes, and amyloidosis may occur, but are rare.

Dermatologic Features
The typical psoriatic skin lesion is a sharply demarcated erythematous plaque with a well-marked, silvery scale. The lesions typically appear on the extensor surfaces of the elbows and knees, in the scalp, and on the ears and presacral areas, but they may be found anywhere on the body, including palms and soles, flexor sites, low back, hair line, perineum, and genitalia. Their size is variable, ranging from 1 mm or less in early acute psoriasis to several centimeters in well-established disease. Gentle scraping usually produces pinpoint bleeding (Auspitz's sign).

Nail involvement is the only clinical feature that identifies patients with psoriasis who are likely to develop arthritis. Clinical signs of psoriatic involvement of the nails include pitting, onycholysis (separation of the nail from the underlying nail bed), transverse depression (ridging) and cracking, subungual keratosis, brown-yellow discoloration (oil-drop sign), and leukonychia. None of these dystrophic nail abnormalities are specific for psoriatic arthritis. Although nail pitting is not uncommon in healthy individuals, multiple pits (usually more than 20) in a single nail of a digit affected by dactylitis or an inflamed DIP joint is characteristic of psoriatic arthritis.

Radiographic Features
Several radiographic features are characteristic for the disease (Fig. 10-2). The bone changes in psoriatic arthritis are a unique combination of erosion, which helps in differentiating it from ankylosing spondylitis, and bone production in a specific distribution, which distinguishes it from RA. The distinguishing features are fusiform soft-tissue swelling in a bilateral asymmetric distribution, with maintenance of normal mineralization; dramatic joint-space loss, with or without ankylosis of the IP joints of the hands and feet; destruction of IP joints, with widening of the joint spaces; bone proliferation of the base of the distal phalanx and resorption of the tufts of the involved distal phalanges; joint erosion, with tapering of the proximal phalanx and bone proliferation of the distal phalanx (pencil-in-cup deformity); and "fluffy" periostitis. In decreasing order of frequency, the radiographic abnormalities are distributed in the hands, feet, sacroiliac joints, and spine. Sacroiliitis may be unilateral or symmetric in early stages, but may progress to bilateral fusion. Spondylitis may occur with or without involvement of the sacroiliac joints. Isolated, sometimes unusually bulky and irregular marginal or nonmarginal syndesmophytes may appear at any portion of the spine.

Differential Diagnosis
Helpful features in distinguishing psoriatic arthritis from rheumatoid arthritis include the presence of dactylitis and enthesitis, signs of psoriatic skin or nail disease, involvement of the DIP joints, and the presence of spinal or sacroiliitis disease. Much more problematic is the distinction between psoriatic arthritis and other seronegative spondyloarthropathies. Spine disease is less severe than in ankylosing spondylitis and appears at a later age (30 years

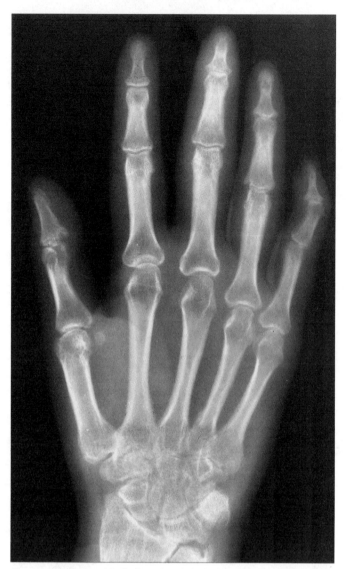

Fig. 10-2. Radiographic findings in psoriatic arthritis. Marginal erosions are seen at the distal and proximal interphalangeal joints, with new bone formation. Involvement of the carpus, with joint-space narrowing and new bone formation around the ulnar styloid are also present. (Courtesy of Dr. Mark D. Murphy, Armed Forces Institute of Pathology.)

or older). Other differences that help distinguish between psoriatic arthritis and ankylosing spondylitis are psoriatic skin or nail disease, a family history of psoriasis, and less-symmetric radiographic features. Reactive arthritis and psoriatic arthritis share many common features, but the lack of a preceding infectious episode, the predilection for joints of the upper extremities, and the absence of balanitis and urethritis suggest psoriatic arthritis Keratoderma blennorrhagica and palmoplantar pustural psoriasis are clinically and histologically identical, but hyperkeratotic changes that occur in reactive arthritis typically involve only the soles and palms, not the nails. Because both psoriasis and psoriatic arthritis may be presenting features of undiagnosed HIV infection, this diagnosis should be ruled out, especially in patients with unusually severe disease.

Treatment

Skin Disease

The initial treatment for stable plaque psoriasis is topical. However, topical therapy may be impractical for patients with extensive psoriasis (more than 20% involvement) and systemic therapy may be indicated at the onset (17). Topical treatment includes emollients and keratolytic agents alone or in combination with anthralin, corticosteroids, vitamin D derivatives such as calcipotriene, and topical retinoids. Emollients (aqueous creams or petrolatum) are the cornerstone of topical therapy and are best used twice daily. Emollients hydrate skin, soften scales, and reduce itching.

Patients with extensive skin disease may benefit from photochemotherapy (PUVA therapy) under the care of a dermatologist. In PUVA therapy, a psoralen, such as methoxsalen 0.6 mg/kg, is applied to the skin and followed two hours later with ultraviolet A radiation. PUVA therapy is initiated three times weekly and, after significant improvement occurs (approximately within eight to 12 weeks), is maintained with sessions every two to four weeks for an additional two to three months (18).

Joint Disease

The general principles of managing RA and the spondyloarthropathies also apply to psoriatic arthritis. The treatment depends on the type of the joint disease (axial versus peripheral) and the severity of joint and skin involvement. Physical or occupational therapy should be considered early in the disease. Regular therapeutic exercise, splinting for persistent synovitis or enthesitis, and assistive devices alleviate pain and preserve function. Nonsteroidal anti-inflammatory agents (NSAIDs) are effective in most patients and should be the initial therapy for people with mild disease, with instructions to return for an evaluation a few weeks later. Regular evaluation, especially at the beginning of the disease, is essential to assess disease severity and response to treatment. Disease activity that involves only one or two joints can be treated effectively with local corticosteroid injections. Intra-articular injections into psoriatic lesions should be avoided because the skin may be colonized with *Staphylococci* and *Streptococci*. If such injections are unavoidable, careful preparation of the skin is essential.

Disease-modifying antirheumatic drugs (DMARDs) should be initiated as early as possible (preferably within a few weeks) for patients whose conditions don't respond adequately to NSAIDs, and those who have progressive, erosive, polyarticular disease or oligoarticular disease involving large joints that does not respond to local corticosteroid injections. Methotrexate is effective for both the skin disease and peripheral arthritis in patients with oligo- or polyarticular disease. In general, dosage and monitoring are the same as for patients with RA.

Sulfasalazine (2–3 g/day) is helpful for peripheral arthritis (19) but not for axial disease (20), and it has no significant effect on the skin disease. PUVA therapy may be especially helpful for patients with extensive skin involvement and is effective for both skin and joint disease, but only in nonspondylitic disease (18). Results from small, open-label, uncontrolled trials suggest that antimalarials, gold, azathioprine, cyclosporine, mycophenolate mofetil, leflunomide, retinoids, and vitamin D may be effective. Etretinate probably should be avoided in patients with axial disease because spinal ligamentous calcification is associated with long-term use. Corticosteroids can be used safely in low doses, either in combination with DMARDs or as bridge therapy while waiting for onset of action of DMARDs. Rare reports of generalized pustular psoriasis upon tapering of high-dose corticosteroids used to treat psoriasis dictate caution, especially in patients with extensive skin disease.

In patients with aggressive, destructive disease whose response to single-agent therapy is inadequate, combination therapy (i.e., methotrexate with sulfasalazine, cyclosporine, or leflunomide) may be considered. Etanercept, a genetically engineered soluble TNF receptor (sTNFR) that inhibits TNF action, administered twice weekly by subcutaneous injections (25 mg/dose) resulted in a significantly higher response rate, compared with placebo, in patients with oligo- or polyarticular psoriatic arthritis (response rate 87% in the treatment group versus 23% in the placebo group). Both joint and skin disease improved at the end of this 12-week study (21). Additional data are required to better define the exact role of TNF inhibitors in the treatment of psoriatic arthritis and their long-term efficacy, tolerability, and safety. Etanercept was approved for the treatment of psoriatic arthritis by the FDA in January 2002.

For patients with intractable pain or loss of joint function, surgery is indicated. Although several reports have raised concerns about a higher risk of infection, recurrent contracture or stiffness, or excessive bone formation after surgery, most of these fears are ill-founded, and surgery should not be withheld.

Prognosis

In general, people with psoriatic arthritis have a more benign course of disease than do people with RA, and earlier studies may have overestimated the actual disease morbidity because of referral biases (22). However, morbidity from disease is substantial and comparable to RA in people with polyarticular or oligoarticular psoriatic arthritis involving large joints (23). Clearly defined prognostic factors are not available, but a family history of psoriatic arthritis, disease onset before age 20, the presence of HLA-DR3 or HLA-DR4, erosive or polyarticular disease, and extensive skin involvement have been associated with a worse prognosis, and patients who exhibit these factors may require more aggressive treatment.

DIMITRIOS T. BOUMPAS, MD
GABOR G. ILLEI, MD
IOANNIS O. TASSIULAS, MD

References

1. Cuellar ML, Silveira LH, Espinoza LR. Recent developments in psoriatic arthritis. Curr Opin Rheumatol 1994;6:378–384.
2. Eastmont CJ. Genetics and HLA antigens. Bailliere's Clin Rheumatol 1994;8:263–276.
3. Rahman P, Gladman DD, Schentag CT, Petronis A. Excessive paternal transmission in psoriatic arthritis. Arthritis Rheum 1999;42:1228–1231.
4. Hammer RE, Maika SD, Richardson JA, Tang JP, Taurog JD. Spontaneous inflammatory disease in transgenic rats expressing HLA-B27 and human β2m: an animal model of HLA-B27-associated human disorders. Cell 1990;63:1099–1112.
5. Ozawa A, Ohkido M, Inoko H, Ando A, Tsuji K. Specific restriction fragment length polymorphism on the HLA-C region and susceptibillity to psoriasis vulgaris. J Invest Dermatol 1988;90:402–405.
6. Gonzalez S, Martinez-Borra J, Torre-Alonso JC, et al. The MICA-A9 triplet repeat polymorphism in the transmembrane region confers additional susceptibility to the development of psoriatic arthritis and is independent of the association of Cw* 0602 in psoriasis. Arthritis Rheum 1999;42:1010–1016.
7. Tomfohrde J, Silverman A, Barnes R, et al. Gene for familial psoriasis susceptibility mapped to the distal end of human chromosome 17q. Science 1994;264:1141–1145.
8. Leung DYM, Travers JB, Giorno R, et al. Evidence for a streptococcal superantigen-driven process in acute guttate psoriasis. J Clin Invest 1995;96:2106–2112.
9. Tassiulas I, Duncan SR, Centola M, Theofilopoulos AN, Boumpas DT. Clonal characteristics of T cell infiltrates in skin and synovium of patients with psoriatic arthritis. Hum Immunol 1999;60:479–491.
10. Panayi GS. Immunology of psoriasis and psoriatic arthritis. Baillieres Clin Rheumatol 1994;8:419–427.
11. McGonagle D, Conaghan PG, Emery P. Psoriatic arthritis: a unified concept twenty years on. Arthritis Rheum 1999;42:1080–1086.
12. Calabrese LH. Human immunodeficiency virus (HIV) infection and arthritis. Rheum Dis Clin North Am 1993;19:477–488.
13. Schon MP, Detmar M, Parker CM. Murine psoriasis-like disorder induced by naïve CD4+ T cells. Nat Med 1997;3:183–188.
14. Abrams JR, Lebwohl MG, Guzzo CA, et al. CTLA4Ig-mediated blockade of T-cell costimulation in patients with psoriasis vulgaris. J Clin Invest 1999;103:1243–1252.
15. Danning CL, Illei GG, Hitchon C, Greer MR, Boumpas DT, and McInnes IB. Macrophage-derived cytokine and nuclear factor kB p65 expression in synovial membrane and skin of patients with psoriatic arthritis. Arthritis Rheum 2000;43:1244–1256.
16. Ruckert R, Asadullah K, Seifert M, et al. Inhibition of keratinocyte apoptosis by IL-15: a new parameter in the pathogenesis of psoriasis? J Immunol 2000;165:2240–2250.
17. Greaves MW, Weinstein GD. Treatment of psoriasis. N Engl J Med 1995;332:581–588.
18. Perlman SG, Gerber LH, Roberts RM, Nigra TP, Barth WF. Photochemotherapy and psoriatic arthritis. A prospective study. Ann Intern Med 1979;91:717–722.

19. Clegg DO, Reda DJ, Mejias E, et al: Comparison of sulfasalazine and placebo in the treatment of psoriatic arthritis. A Department of Veterans Affairs Cooperative Study. Arthritis Rheum 1996;39:2013–2020.

20. Clegg DO, Reda DJ, Abdellatif M. Comparison of sulfasalazine and placebo for the treatment of axial and peripheral articular manifestations of the seronegative spondylarthropathies. A Department of Veterans Affairs cooperative study. Arthritis Rheum 1999;42:2325–2329.

21. Mease PJ, Goffe BS, Metz J, VanderStoep A, Finck B, Burge DJ. Etanercept in the treatment of psoriatic arthritis and psoriasis: a randomised trial. Lancet 2000;356:385–390.

22. Shbeeb M, Uramoto KM, Gibson LE, O'Fallon WM, Gabriel SE. The epidemiology of psoriatic arthritis in Olmsted County, Minnesota, USA, 1982-1991. J Rheumatol 2000;27:1247–1250.

23. Gladman DD, Stafford-Brady F, Chang CH, Lewandowski K, Russell ML. Longitudinal study of clinical and radiological progression in psoriatic arthritis. J Rheumatol 1990;17:809–812.

11 SERONEGATIVE SPONDYLOARTHROPATHIES A. Epidemiology, Pathology, and Pathogenesis

The seronegative spondyloarthropathies include a heterogeneous group of diseases characterized by inflammatory axial spine involvement (e.g., sacroiliitis and spondylitis), asymmetric peripheral arthritis, enthesopathy, inflammatory eye disease, and overlapping mucocutaneous features occurring in the absence of serum rheumatoid factor. There is a tendency toward familial aggregation and associations with certain human leukocyte antigen (HLA) class I genes, particularly HLA-B27. This group of diseases includes ankylosing spondylitis (AS), reactive arthritis (ReA), psoriatic arthritis/spondylitis, the arthritis/spondylitis of inflammatory bowel disease, juvenile spondyloarthropathy, and a heterogeneous group of disorders known as the undifferentiated spondyloarthropathies (uSpA). It has been proposed that other isolated HLA-B27–associated syndromes, such as acute anterior uveitis and isolated atrioventricular block, be included in the category of spondyloarthropathy.

Criteria

The criteria currently used for most clinical studies of ankylosing spondylitis are the modified New York criteria (Table 11A-1) (1). These criteria demand the presence of radiographic sacroiliitis in combination with at least one of three clinical criteria. Recently, it has been suggested

that the diagnosis of ReA be based on a documented urogenital infection with *Chlamydia trachomatis* or a gastrointestinal infection with a relevant enteric pathogen (2). Patients in whom this documentation is not available are classified as having uSpA.

Validated criteria for psoriatic arthritis have not been established. However, it has been proposed that psoriatic arthritis be classified as an enthesopathy-associated disease, rather than a disease, such as rheumatoid arthritis, that is associated with primary synovial involvement (3).

In people with spondyloarthropathy, radiographic changes occur later in the disease course and axial involvement may not always occur. The European Spondyloarthropathy Study Group (ESSG) criteria, established in the early 1990s, are based on clinical findings and do not depend specifically on radiographic confirmation (Table 11A-2) (4).

Epidemiology

Manifestations of spondyloarthropathy have been described in every ethnic group. In general, frequency parallels that of the presence of HLA-B27. Among North American Caucasians, where the frequency of HLA-B27 is 7%, AS occurs at a prevalence of 0.2% (5). In Europe, where the frequency of HLA-B27 ranges between 7% and 20%, the

TABLE 11A-1
The Modified New York Criteria for Ankylosing Spondylitis (1984)

A. Diagnosis
   1. Clinical criteria
      a. Low back pain and stiffness for more than 3 months, which improves with exercise, but is not relieved by rest.
      b. Limitation of motion of the lumbar spine in both the sagittal and frontal planes.
      c. Limitation of chest expansion relative to normal values corrected for age and sex.
   2. Radiologic criterion
      Sacroiliitis: Grade >2 bilaterally or Grade 3–4 unilaterally

B. Grading
   1. Definite ankylosing spondylitis if the radiologic criterion is associated with at least one clinical criterion.
   2. Probable ankylosing spondylitis if:
      a. The three clinical criteria are present.
      b. The radiologic criterion is present without any sign or symptoms satisfying the clinical criteria. (Other sources of sacroiliitis should be considered.)

Modified from van der Linden et al (1), with permission.

TABLE 11A-2
European Spondyloarthropathy Study Group Criteria for Spondyloarthropathy

Inflammatory spinal pain
            or
Synovitis (asymmetrical or predominantly in the lower limbs)
                plus

Any one or more of the following:
Positive family history
Psoriasis
Inflammatory bowel disease
Alternate buttock pain
Enthesopathy
Sacroiliitis[a]

a Without sacroiliitis: sensitivity 77%, specificity 89%. With sacroiliitis: sensitivity 86%, specificity 87%. Data from Dougados et al (4).

prevalence is higher (6). The highest prevalence of AS has been described in certain native American groups, such as the Haidas and Bella Coolas in British Columbia, where the frequency of HLA-B27 is as high as 50%. The spondyloarthropathies occur uncommonly in African Americans, in whom the frequency of HLA-B27 is likewise much lower (1%–2%). Among Asians, HLA-B27 occurs at approximately the same frequency as North American Caucasians (7%) and the prevalence of AS is similar (0.26%) (7). Using ESSG criteria, spondyloarthropathy has been reported to occur in as many as 13.6% of HLA-B27–positive individuals or, in one recent study, at an overall prevalence of 1.9% in Caucasians (6).

HLA-B27 Structure and Function

Nearly 30 years have passed since HLA-B27 was first associated with AS and other spondyloarthropathies, and this relationship still is one of the best examples of the association between an inflammatory arthritis and a hereditary marker. The molecular structure of the HLA-B27 molecule has been determined, and the function of it and other HLA class I molecules in antigen presentation has been explored. HLA class I molecules present protein antigens that have been synthesized within the cell (viral, tumor, or self-derived) to $\alpha\beta$ T-cell receptors on cytotoxic (CD8[+]) T lymphocytes. The newly synthesized HLA class I heavy chain is taken up in the endoplasmic reticulum of the cell, where its folding is mediated by "chaperone" molecules, such as calnexin and calreticulin. The TAP gene complex mediates loading of the nonameric peptide (nine amino acids in length) into the peptide-binding groove, and transport of the trimolecular complex of peptide, HLA class I heavy chain, and β_2-microglobulin to the cell surface. The HLA-class I molecule is folded into five domains: two outermost domains (α1 and α2) that form the peptide-binding groove (Fig. 11A-1); the membrane-proximal domain (α3), which works with β_2-microglobulin to stabilize the molecule on the cell surface; and the smaller transmembrane and intracytoplasmic domains, which function in anchoring the molecule to the cell surface and also in signal transduction to the cytoplasm. The peptide-binding groove itself is comprised of six "pockets" that serve to anchor the peptide in the groove and to configure it for optimal presentation to and contact with the T-cell receptor. The "B" pocket is unique in the HLA-B27 molecule. Critical in peptide anchoring, it has an absolute requirement for an *arginine* residue in the second position (P2) of the nonameric peptide. This pocket is formed by a lysine residue at position 70, cysteine at position 67, isoleucine at position 66, aspartic acid at position 45, threonine at position 24, and a histidine at position 9 of the outermost (α1) domain of the HLA-B27 molecule. The cysteine residue at position 67 is unique to HLA-B27 alleles, and gives HLA-B27 the capacity to form homodimers through disulfide bonds at cysteine 67, both in vitro and in vivo, in the absence of β_2-microglobulin. Although this process has been described in B27 transgenic mice (8) and in vitro, its biologic significance is unclear.

It is thought that HLA molecules in general, and class I molecules in particular, evolved in response to specific environmental stresses, and polymorphisms of HLA class I molecules deal with infectious stresses, such as viruses, with varying efficiencies. HLA-B27–positive individuals are more effective in dealing with influenza viruses and the human immunodeficiency virus (HIV-1) than are HLA-B27–negative individuals. However, HLA-B27–positive individuals are associated with less efficient intracellular elimination of *Chlamydia* and certain enteric bacteria than are B27–negative individuals. This finding is thought to be important in the pathogenesis of ReA, and also suggests a secondary role for the HLA-B27 molecule, in addition to antigen presentation.

The role of HLA-B27 in the pathogenesis of the spondyl-oarthropathies has not been defined. It had been speculated that the association of AS and other spondyloarthropathies with B27 might better be explained by another gene linked to HLA-B27. This theory was largely laid to rest by the development of the HLA-B27 transgenic rat model by Hammer et al (9). This model is a Lewis rat line that has been made transgenic for the HLA-B27 gene. When HLA-B27 is expressed in high copy number on the surface of antigen-presenting cells, these rats develop peripheral arthritis, mucocutaneous lesions, and inflammatory bowel disease characteristic of the spondyloarthropathies. They do not, however, develop spondylitis. The spondyloarthropathies in these transgenic rats is T-cell mediated, specifically by CD4[+] cells. The presence of gut flora appears to be necessary for the development of disease, as transgenic rats raised in a germ-free environment fail to develop gut and joint inflammation.

Whether the HLA-B27 molecule contributes to disease susceptibility by its failure to eliminate intracellular organisms or by presentation of an "arthritogenic peptide" has not been determined. HLA class I molecules can present a variety of antigens, including self-peptides, to the cytotoxic T cells. As noted above, there are certain requirements about the nature of the peptides that can fit in the peptide-binding groove, and computer modeling has identified peptides derived from causative microorganisms that could be presented by HLA-B27–positive antigen-presenting cells. However, none of these peptides actually has been found in the antigenic cleft of the HLA-B27, and none has been proved to constitute an "arthritogenic peptide." It also has been suggested that intracellular misfolding of HLA-B27 could cause disease (8).

HLA-B27 Subtypes

To date, 23 different subtypes of HLA-B27 have been described (10) (Table 11A-3). Most of these are quite rare. One, *HLA-B*2705*, is not only the most common B27 subtype and is present is all populations, but is believed to represent the "ancestral" or "parent" B27 genotype. Other subtypes tend to be more ethnic-specific. *HLA-B*2702* accounts for approximately 10% of B27 subtypes in Caucasians. *HLA-B*2703* is uniquely West African in origin. *HLA-B*2704* occurs in eastern Asians, *HLA-B*2706* in southeast Asians (particularly in Indonesia, where it is the most common B27 subtype), *HLA-B*2707* in southern Asia and the Middle East, *HLA-B*2708* in western Europeans, and *HLA-B*2709* in Sardinians. The other B27 subtypes (*B*2701, B*2710-*2723*) are too rare to comment on differential ethnic frequencies. *HLA-B*2713* does not differ from other HLA-B27 subtypes in exons 2 and 3, but shows a glutamic acid substitution for an alanine in the signal peptide (exon 1). Although most of the HLA-B27 subtypes do not affect the "B" pocket, *HLA-B*2718* is distinct from other B27 subtypes in having a serine instead of a cysteine at position 67 of the first domain, which would have a major effect on the peptide-binding properties of the B pocket.

It has been demonstrated that two of these subtypes, *HLA-B*2706* and *B*2709*, are not associated with the spondyloarthropathies (although rare cases are described of patients with both of these subtypes). These two subtypes differ from other B27 subtypes in the lack of binding of peptides with a tyrosine in the C-terminal position. *HLA-B*2703* also may be less disease-associated, although confirmatory epidemiologic data is sparse. The presence of spondyloarthropathy in general is accounted for by either *HLA-B*2705, B*2704, B*2702*, or *B*2707* worldwide. The other subtypes are too rare to comment on vis-a-vis disease susceptibility. The idea that one of these subtypes may be more disease-associated (i.e., a hierarchical ranking may exist in disease susceptibility) is controversial.

Genetics of the Seronegative Spondyloarthropathies

Fewer than 5% of HLA-B27–positive individuals ever develop a seronegative spondyloarthropathy. If an individual is HLA-B27–positive and has a family member with AS, that person's risk of developing spondylitis is significantly higher than that of other HLA-B27–positive people. This increased risk suggests that other genes, in addition to HLA-B27, are involved in the pathogenesis of the spondyloarthropathies. Family studies have suggested that HLA-B27 contributes only 16%–50% of the total genetic risk for AS. Other MHC genes have been implicated. For example, HLA-B60 has been shown to increase the risk for AS threefold, regardless of HLA-B27 status (11). Certain HLA class II genes also have been implicated. In some studies, HLA-DR1 has been suggested to independently increase the risk for AS, although other studies have suggested that this finding is better explained by linkage disequilibrium with HLA-B27 (12). The presence of HLA-DR8 in some studies has been found to increase the risk for uveitis, as does the presence of certain alleles of low molecular-weight proteasome (LMP) genes (13), also found in the class II region. Studies of tumor necrosis factor (TNF) genes, located in the MHC class III region not far from HLA-B27, have shown associations of varying strength with AS, which may or may not be due to linkage with HLA-B27 (14).

Family studies have shown that MHC genes account for only part of the risk for AS (15). The only non-MHC gene found associated with AS in more than one group is the "*pm*" (poor metabolizer) genotype of the cytochrome P450 2D6 gene, located on chromosome 22q, found in German and British AS patients (16). This gene is involved in the metabolism of certain drugs, although how this polymorphism contributes to AS is not clear. Results are pending for three genome-wide screens in Britain, mainland Europe, and North America to identify other non-MHC genes (17).

The genetics of psoriatic spondylitis are less clear. The associations of HLA-B13, -B17, and -Cw6 with psoriasis and HLA-B16 (now split into -B38 and -B39) and -B27 with psoriatic arthritis have been known for nearly three decades. HLA-B27 is found in 60%–70% of people with psoriatic spondylitis, and approximately 25% of those with peripheral psoriatic arthritis. More recently, the HLA-Cw6 association with psoriasis (most specifically, the *Cw*0602* allele) was thought to be explained better by a novel psoriasis locus, near Cw6 in the HLA-class I region, whose gene has not been identified (tentatively called *PSOR1*). One possible candidate for this psoriasis-susceptibility allele is *MICA* (class I major histocompatibility complex chain-related gene A), an allele of which (*MICA-002*) has been associated with the development of psoriatic arthritis even independent of HLA-*Cw*0602* (18). Genome-wide screens also have implicated regions on other chromosomes, such as on 17q, although the identity of these non-MHC genes remains to be established.

Up to 70% of people with spondylitis occurring in the setting of inflammatory bowel disease express HLA-B27.

TABLE 11A-3
Amino Acid Sequences of HLA-B27

	10	20	30	40	50	60
B*2705	GSHSMRYFHT	SVSRPGRGEP	RFITVGYVDD	TLFVRFDSDA	ASPREEPRAP	WIEQEGPEYW
B*2701	—————	—————	—————	—————	—————	—————
B*2702	—————	—————	—————	—————	—————	—————
B*2703	—————	—————	—————	—————	—————	—————H—
B*2704	—————	—————	—————	—————	—————	—————
B*2706	—————	—————	—————	—————	—————	—————
B*2707	—————	—————	—————	—————	—————	—————
B*2708	—————	—————	—————	—————	—————	—————
B*2709	—————	—————	—————	—————	—————	—————
B*2710	—————	—————	—————	—————	—————	—————
B*2711	—————	—————	—————	—————	—————	—————
B*2712	—————	—————	—————	—————	—————	—————
B*2713	—————	—————	—————	—————	—————	—————
B*2714	—————	—————	—————	—————	—————	—————
B*2715	—————	—————	—————	—————	—————	—————
B*2716	—————	—————	—————	—————	—————	—————
B*2717	—————	—————	—————	—————	—————	—————
B*2718	—————	—————	—————	—————	—————	—————
B*2719	—————	—————	—————	—————	—————	—————
B*2720	—————	—————	—————	—————	—————	—————
B*2721	—————	—————	—————	—————	—————	—————
B*2722	—————	—————	—————	—————	—————	—————
B*2723	—————	—————	—————	—————	—————	—————

Second domain (α2)

	100	110	120	130	140	150
B*2705	GSHTLQNMYG	CDVGPDGRLL	RGYHQDAYDG	KDYIALNEDL	SSWTAADTAA	QITQRKWEAA
B*2701	—————	—————	—————	—————	—————	—————
B*2702	—————	—————	—————	—————	—————	—————
B*2703	—————	—————	—————	—————	—————	—————
B*2704	—————	—————	—————	—————	—————	—————
B*2706	—————	—————	—D-Y—	—————	—————	—————
B*2707	——S—	—————	—HN-Y——	R—	—————	—————
B*2708	—————	—————	—————	—————	—————	—————
B*2709	—————	—————	——H—	—————	—————	—————
B*2710	—————	—————	—————	—————	—————	—————
B*2711	——S—	—————	—HN-Y—	—————	—————	—————
B*2712	—————	—————	—————	—————	—————	—————
B*2713	—————	—————	—————	—————	—————	—————
B*2714	——T—	—L—	—————	—————	—————	—————
B*2715	—————	—————	—————	—————	—————	—————
B*2716	—————	—————	—————	—————	—————	—————
B*2717	—————	—————	—————	—————	—————	—————
B*2718	—————	—————	—————	—————	—————	—————
B*2719	——R—	—————	—————	—————	—————	—————
B*2720	—————	—————	—HN-Y—	—————	—————	—————
B*2721	——R—	—————	—D-Y—	—————	—————	—————
B*2722	—————	—————	—D-Y—	—————	—————	—————
B*2723	—————	—————	—————	—————	—————	—————

Amino acid sequences of the two outermost domains of the currently known subtypes of HLA-B27.

70 DRETQICKAK	80 AQTDREDLRT	90 LLRYYNQSEA
	Y---N	A
	---N-I	A
	---S-	
	---S-	
	---S--N	-RG-
-----TN	T---S--N	-RG-
	-----S-	
-----TN	T-	
-----S-TN	T---Y--S--N	-RG-
	-----S-	
	-----S-	
	-----S-	
-N-----TN-	T---Y--S-	

160 RVAEQLRAYL	170 EGECVEWLRR	180 YLENGKETLQ
-E-		
-E-		
-E-		
-E-	-T-	
-E-		
-E-		
-E-		

There is no HLA class I association with either asymptomatic sacroiliitis or with peripheral arthritis. One group reported an increased frequency of HLA-DR1 in those with peripheral arthritis.

Infection's Role in Triggering Spondyloarthropathy

Probably the best example of infectious triggers in the rheumatic diseases is reactive arthritis (Reiter's syndrome). In general, ReA falls into two etiologic categories: that triggered by enteric infections and that by urogenital infections.

Since the original descriptions by Brodie in the 19th century and Reiter during World War I, it has been known that attacks of dysentery could trigger ReA. Probably the best example was the large number of cases of "epidemic" ReA occurring in Finland during World War II that were caused by a widespread outbreak of *Shigella flexneri* dysentery. Since then, ReA has also been attributed to various species of *Salmonella* (*typhimurium* and *enteritidis*), *Campylobacter* (*jejuni* and *fetus*), and in Europe, *Yersinia* (*enterocolitica*) and possibly *Clostridium*.

Most frequently, ReA follows urogenital infections with *Chlamydia trachomatis* (so-called endemic reactive arthritis). Less commonly encountered is *Chlamydia pneumonia* (at about one-tenth the frequency of *Chlamydia trachomatis*). There are no differences clinically between the two types of infection, and the finding of a primary respiratory pathogen in the joints of people with ReA raises the possibility of a route of infection in addition to the gut and urogenital systems.

An important clue to the cause of ReA came with the identification of bacterial antigens in synovial tissue in the early and middle 1990s, despite negative synovial-fluid cultures. Urogenital bacterial triggers (i.e., *Chlamydia*) differ from enteric triggers; viable bacterial DNA from the bacterial triggers has been identified by polymerase chain reaction (PCR) in synovial cells (predominantly in monocytes and macrophages), which is not the case for the enteric triggers. These *Chlamydia* microorganisms are not only viable but also metabolically active, with demonstrated up-regulation of the bacterial hsp60 and down-regulation of the *omp1* genes. HLA-B27 also is thought to be involved in pathogenesis by prolonging the intracellular survival (and hence escape from immune surveillance) of these causative microorganisms (19).

Recent findings have raised doubts whether it is the persistence of the Chlamydial infection, per se, that causes ReA. Positive PCR results for Chlamydial DNA also have been found in other joint diseases, including rheumatoid arthritis and even osteoarthritis (20). Of particular concern is the report by Wilkinson et al that there was no correlation between the presence of Chlamydial DNA in synovial tissue and the specific cellular and humoral response to the infection (21). This raises the issue whether it is the infection itself or the host response to the infection that is etiologic in ReA.

No specific infectious trigger has been established for psoriatic arthritis, although old studies have suggested a role for group A streptococci. One recent report found ribosomal RNA of group A streptococci in the peripheral blood and synovial fluid of people with psoriatic arthritis (22).

Despite early findings of increased fecal carriage of *Klebsiella* in patients with AS, recent studies have failed to demonstrate any strains of *Klebsiella* that are specific for this disorder, and it has not been established that this bacteria plays a role in the causation of spondyloarthropathy.

The Role of Gut Inflammation in Spondyloarthropathy

AS and the spondylitis of inflammatory bowel disease affect the axial skeleton in a similar manner. Ileocolonoscopy has revealed asymptomatic gut inflammation in up to half of people with primary AS, particularly in the terminal ileum (23). Studies of people with spondyloarthropathy have shown features of Crohn's disease in up to 26% (24), and antibodies to enteric organism-derived proteins, particularly from *Klebsiella pneumonia*, frequently are found in people with AS. This leads to speculation that chronic inflammation may increase the permeability of the intestinal mucosa to enteric organisms. This hypothesis has been fueled by the recent finding of increased small intestinal (but not gastric) permeability that is not explained by NSAID use in AS patients and their first-degree relatives (25). The precise mechanism of this increased permeability has not been determined, although its elucidation potentially would offer a route for disease prevention.

JOHN D. REVEILLE, MD

References

1. van der Linden S, Valkenburg HA, Cats A. Evaluation of diagnostic criteria for ankylosing spondylitis. A proposal for modification of the New York criteria. Arthritis Rheum 1984;27: 361–368.

2. Inman RD. Classification criteria for reactive arthritis. J Rheumatol 1999;26:1219–1221.

3. McGonagle D, Conaghan PG, Emery P. Psoriatic arthritis: a unified concept twenty years on. Arthritis Rheum 1999;42: 1080–1086.

4. Dougados M, van der Linden S, Juhlin R et al. The European Spondyloarthropathy Study Group preliminary criteria for the classification of spondyloarthropathy. Arthritis Rheum 1991; 34:1218–1227.

5. Lawrence RC, Helmick CG, Arnett FC, et al. Estimates of the prevalence of arthritis and selected musculoskeletal disorders in the United States. Arthritis Rheum 1998;41:778–799.

6. Braun J, Bollow M, Remlinger G, et al. Prevalence of spondyloarthropathies in HLA-B27 positive and negative blood donors. Arthritis Rheum 1998;41:58–67.

7. Wigley RD, Zhang NZ, Zeng QY, et al. Rheumatic diseases in China: ILAR-China study comparing the prevalence of rheumatic symptoms in northern and southern rural populations. J Rheumatol 1994;21:1484–1490.

8. Mear JP, Schreiber KL, Munz C, et al. Misfolding of HLA-B27 as a result of its B pocket suggests a novel mechanism for its role in susceptibility to spondyloarthropathies. J Immunol 1999;163:6665–6670.

9. Hammer RE Maika SD, Richardson JA, et al. Spontaneous inflammatory disease in transgenic rats expressing HLA-B27 and human beta 2m: an animal model of HLA-B27-associated human disorders. Cell 1990;63:1099–1112.

10. Ball EJ, Khan MA. HLA-B27 polymorphism. Submitted, 2001.

11. Robinson WP, van der Linden SM, Khan MA, et al. HLA-Bw60 increases susceptibility to ankylosing spondylitis in HLA-B27+ patients. Arthritis Rheum 1989;32:1135–1141.

12. Brown MA, Kennedy LG, Darke C, et al. The effect of HLA-DR genes on susceptibility to and severity of ankylosing spondylitis. Arthritis Rheum 1998;41:460–465.

13. Maksymowych WP, Wessler A, Schmitt-Egenolf M, et al. Polymorphism in an HLA linked proteasome gene influences phenotypic expression of disease in HLA-B27 positive individuals. J Rheumatol 1994;21:665–669.

14. Hohler T, Schaper T, Schneider PM, et al. Association of different tumor necrosis factor alpha promoter allele frequencies with ankylosing spondylitis in HLA-B27 positive individuals. Arthritis Rheum 1998;41:1489–1492.

15. Brown MA, Kennedy LG, MacGregor AJ, et al. Susceptibility to ankylosing spondylitis in twins: the role of genes, HLA, and the environment. Arthritis Rheum 1997;40:1823–1828.

16. Beyeler C, Armstrong M, Bird HA, et al. Relationship between genotype for cytochrome P450 CYP2D6 and susceptibility to ankylosing spondylitis and rheumatoid arthritis. Ann Rheum Dis 1996;55:66–68.

17. Brown MA, Pile KD, Kennedy LG, et al. A genome-wide screen for susceptibility loci in ankylosing spondylitis. Arthritis Rheum 1998;41:588–595.

18. Gonzalez S, Martinez-Borra J, Torre-Alonso JC, et al: The MICA-A9 triplet repeat polymorphism in the transmembrane region confers additional susceptibility to the development of psoriatic arthritis and is independent of the association of Cw*0602 in psoriasis. Arthritis Rheum 1999;42:1010–1016.

19. Laitio P, Virtala M, Salmi M, Pelliniemi LJ, Yu DT, Granfors K. HLA-B27 modulates intracellular survival of Salmonella enteritidis in human monocytic cells. Eur J Immunol 1997;27:1331–1338.

20. Schumacher HR Jr, Arayssi T, Crane M, et al. Chlamydia trachomatis nucleic acids can be found in the synovium of some asymptomatic subjects. Arthritis Rheum 1999;42:1281–1284.

21. Wilkinson NZ, Kingsley GH, Sieper J, et al: Lack of correlation between the detection of Chlamydia trachomatis DNA in synovial fluid from patients with a range of rheumatic diseases and the presence of an antichlamydial immune response. Arthritis Rheum 1998;41:845–854.

22. Wang Q, Vasey FB, Mahfood JP, et al. V2 regions of 16S ribosomal RNA used as a molecular marker for the species identification of streptococci in peripheral blood and synovial fluid from patients with psoriatic arthritis. Arthritis Rheum 1999;42:2055–2059.

23. Mielants H, Veys EM, Cuvelier C, De Vos M, Botelberghe L. HLA-B27 related arthritis and bowel inflammation. Part 2. Ileocolonoscopy and bowel histology in patients with HLA-B27-related arthritis. J Rheumatol 1985;12:294–298.

24. Leirisalo-Repo M, Turunen U, Stenman S, Helenius P, Seppala K. High frequency of silent inflammatory bowel disease in spondyloarthropathy. Arthritis Rheum 1994;37:23–31.

25. Vaile JH, Meddings JB, Yacyshyn BR, Russell AS, Maksymowych WP. Bowel permeability and CD45RO expression on circulating CD20+ B cells in patients with ankylosing spondylitis and their relatives. J Rheumatol 1999;26: 128–135.

SERONEGATIVE SPONDYLOARTHROPATHIES
B. Reactive Arthritis and Enteropathic Arthritis

Reactive Arthritis

Reactive arthritis (ReA) refers to a form of peripheral arthritis, often accompanied by one or more extra-articular manifestations, that appears shortly after certain infections of the genitourinary or gastrointestinal tracts (1). The majority of affected individuals, usually young men, have inherited the human leukocyte antigen (HLA) B27. The original description of reactive arthritis was in a young German officer who, following a bout of bloody dairrhea, developed the clinical triad of nongonococcal urethritis, conjunctivitis, and arthritis (2). Cases have been observed following epidemics or sporadic outbreaks of diarrheal illnesses caused by *Shigella*, *Salmonella*, and *Campylobacter* microorganisms, as well as by venereally acquired genitourinary infections, usually *Chlamydia trachomatis*.

A high frequency of HLA-B27 was discovered in people with ReA in 1973–1974 (1). HLA-B27 typing was used to confirm that ReA syndrome occurred frequently in the absence of clinically apparent urethritis or conjunctivitis (3). Because of many overlapping clinical, epidemiologic, and genetic features, ReA is classified as a seronegative spondyloarthropathy that is distinct from rheumatoid arthritis (Table 11B-1) (4).

Clinical Presentation

Reactive arthritis typically begins acutely two to four weeks after venereal infections or bouts of gastroenteritis (1). Reports of either infection in the month preceding onset of ReA are useful diagnostically, but venereal infection frequently is asymptomatic. Most endemic cases of ReA occur in young men, and the ratio of male to female patients is 9:1. These cases are believed to result from venereally acquired infections (1,5); cases following food-borne enteric infections affect both genders equally. Whites are affected more commonly than African Americans or other racial groups that have a lower frequency of HLA-B27. Recent evidence suggests that respiratory infections with *Chlamydia pneumoniae* also may trigger the disease (6).

Nongonococcal urethritis, when present, usually is the first manifestation and occurs in both postvenereal and postenteric forms of the disease. Mild dysuria and a mucopurulent urethral discharge are the most typical symptoms in men, but

occasionally, prostatitis and/or epididymitis are present. Women may have dysuria, vaginal discharge, and purulent cervicitis and/or vaginitis. Patients who are asymptomatic for genital inflammation often have sterile pyuria, especially when a first-voided morning urine sample is examined. *C. trachomatis* frequently is the cause of the urethritis or cervicitis and is the triggering agent of the ReA. *Neisseria gonorrhoeae* also may be found in the genital tract, as it frequently coexists with *Chlamydia* infections, but does not cause ReA. *Ureaplasma urealyticum* may be a cause of ReA, but a definite etiologic role has not been established. Sterile genital inflammation may occur in postenteric ReA as an inherent disease feature and is unrelated to any sexually acquired infection.

Conjunctivitis, when present, usually accompanies urethritis or develops within several days. Because symptoms and signs often are mild and transient, patients should be questioned about recent crusting of the eyelids, especially in the morning, which suggests subtle ocular inflammation. Some patients develop obvious conjunctival redness, usually bilateral, with a burning sensation and exudation. Acute anterior uveitis (iritis), typically affecting one eye, may occur simultaneously with, later than, or instead of conjunctivitis and is characterized by severe ocular erythema, pain, and photophobia.

Articular manifestations typically appear last, often after symptoms of urethral and ocular inflammation have subsided. In cases following gastroenteritis, the bowel symptoms usually have resolved one to three weeks earlier, and the inciting enteric pathogen cannot be cultured from the stool.

Articular Manifestations

Reactive arthritis characteristically is additive, asymmetric, and oligoarticular, affecting an average number of four joints (Table 11B-1). Lower limb joints – especially knees, ankles, and small joints of the feet – are affected more commonly than are joints of the upper extremities (wrists, elbows, and hand joints). At least one-third of patients have an exclusively lower-limb arthritis; rarely does a patient have only upper-extremity involvement (3). Hip disease is uncommon, but sternoclavicular, shoulder, and temporomandibular joints occasionally are affected.

Joints affected with ReA typically are swollen, warm, tender, and painful on active and passive movement. They

TABLE 11B-1
Demographic, Clinical, Laboratory, and Radiographic Features of Reactive Arthritis[a]

Demographic Features	
Age at onset	
Range	13–60 years
Mean	26 years
Median	24 years
Male	87%
Race	
White	80%
African American	20%
Preceding diarrhea	6%
Clinical features	
Nongonococcal urethritis	46%
Conjunctivitis	31%
Peripheral arthritis	
Upper limbs only	0
Lower limbs only	39%
Both upper and lower limbs	61%
Knees	68%
Ankles	49%
Small joints of feet	64%
Small joints of hands	42%
Wrists	25%
Elbows	22%
Shoulders	19%
Temporomandibular joints	6%
Sternoclavicular joints	6%
Hips	<1%
Mean number of affected joints	4.5
Sausage digits	52%
Heel pain	61%
x-ray changes of calcaneus	16%
Spinal arthritis	
Low back pain	61%
Sacroiliitis (on x-ray)	17%
Spondylitis (on x-ray)	7%
Mucocutaneous lesions (any)	43%
Keratoderma blenorrhagicum	23%
Circinate balanitis	26%
Oral ulcers	14%
Nail changes	13%
Other clinical features	
Fever ≥101°F	32%
Weight loss (≥4.5 kg)	19%
Uveitis	12%
Amyloidosis	<1%
Laboratory findings	
Anemia	39%
Leukocytosis (>10,000/mm³)	34%
Thrombocytosis (>400,000/mm³)	27%
Elevated erythrocyte sedimentation rate	72%
Rheumatoid factor	0
HLA-B27 positive	81%

[a] Frequencies in 69 consecutive patients with reactive arthritis evaluated at a referral medical center. Adaped from Arnett (3), with permission.

often display a dusky blue discoloration or frank erythema accompanied by exquisite tenderness suggestive of a septic joint. When toes or fingers are affected, the entire digit usually is diffusely swollen, a phenomenon referred to as "sausage" digits or dactylitis.

Typically, inflammation also occurs at bony sites where tendons, ligaments, or fascia have their attachments or insertions (entheses). Enthesitis (or enthesopathy) most commonly occurs at the insertions of the plantar aponeurosis and Achilles tendon on the calcaneus, leading to one of the most frequent, distinctive, and disabling manifestations of the disease: heel pain. Other common sites for enthesitis include ischial tuberosities, iliac crests, tibial tuberosities, and ribs, thus causing musculoskeletal pain at sites other than joints.

Low back and buttock pain are common in ReA, occurring in approximately 50% of cases. Low back symptoms probably are caused primarily by sacroiliac or other spinal-joint involvement; however, radiographically demonstrable sacroiliitis eventually develops in only 20% of patients. Other potential causes of back pain are enthesitis or prostatitis. With time, approximately 10%–12% of patients progress to clinically evident ankylosing spondylitis, but it is unclear whether this represents the continuation of ReA or the independent development of ankylosing spondylitis, which also is genetically linked to HLA-B27 (3,7).

Extra-Articular Manifestations

Several other mucocutaneous and visceral manifestations are highly associated with ReA (Table 11B-1). *Keratoderma blennorrhagicum* is a papulosquamous skin rash that appears most commonly on the soles or palms but may affect any cutaneous area (Fig. 11B-1). Raised, waxy, papular lesions that resemble mollusk shells or pustules usually are the earliest findings. Later, these lesions become hyperkeratotic and scaly, often coalescing into large patches indistinguishable from psoriasis. In fact, keratoderma blennorrhagicum is a form of pustular psoriasis that may occur in the absence of ReA, but which also is associated with HLA-B27. In a few people with ReA, the rash affects large areas of the skin and/or evolves into a generalized exfoliative dermatitis.

Toenails and fingernails may become thickened and opaque, and may crumble, resembling nail changes that resemble mycotic infection or psoriatic onychodystrophy. However, "Reiter's nails" do not demonstrate the pitting seen in psoriasis.

Circinate balanitis is the characteristic lesion involving the glans or shaft of the penis. In uncircumcised men, the lesions appear as moist, shallow ulcers that often are serpiginous and surround the meatus. In circumcised men, the rash is dry, plaque-like, hyperkeratotic, and resembles keratoderma or psoriasis (Fig. 11B-2). Oral ulcers, which are shallow and usually painless, may appear on the tongue or hard palate. The patient may be unaware of their presence. All of these mucocutaneous manifestations are similar histopathologically, showing spongiosiform changes similar to the changes seen in psoriasis and differing only in the degree of hyperkeratosis. Profound weight loss and even cachexia occur in some patients, and the cause is unknown.

Acute anterior uveitis occurs episodically in 20% of patients at any time during the course of ReA. A few patients develop chronic uveitis that ultimately results in visual impairment or loss.

Aortitis occurs in 1%–2% of patients, typically after longstanding active arthritis, but occasionally earlier, during the acute phase. Aortic valve regurgitation and heart block are the clinical consequences when the proximal aortic root and valves sustain inflammatory thickening, which may extend to the atrioventricular node or adjacent conducting system (8). Less commonly, the interventricular septum also is involved, leading to mitral valve regurgitation. The majority of patients with aortic regurgitation have relentless progression of valvular incompetence, leading to left-sided heart failure and ultimately, to aortic valve replacement. Those who develop complete heart block need immediate cardiac pacemaker placement.

Amyloidosis of the *serum amyloid A* (SAA) variety has been reported in a few cases and usually presents as proteinuria or the nephrotic syndrome. An immunoglobulin A (IgA) nephropathy occurs occasionally.

Some people with ReA have been reported to have neurologic complications, including peripheral neuropathies, encephalopathy, and transverse myelitis. However, it is unclear whether these nervous-system syndromes truly were related to the ReA process.

Clinical Course and Prognosis

Reactive arthritis runs a self-limited course of three to 12 months in the majority of patients; however, some studies suggest that many people continue to have minor residual musculoskeletal symptoms beyond 12 months (7,9). Relapses may occur in up to 15% of cases, but it is unclear whether this is the result of reinfection. Approximately 15% of patients continue to have chronic, often destructive and disabling arthritis or enthesitis. Long-term disability

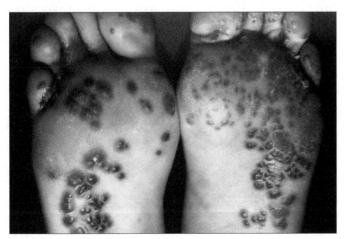

Fig. 11B-1. Typical cutaneous lesions of keratoderma blennorrhagicum on the feet of a person with reactive arthritis.

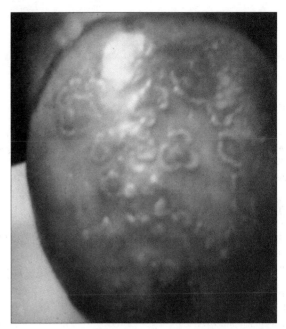

Fig. 11B-2. Circinate balanitis in a person with reactive arthritis.

usually is related to chronic foot pain or deformities from arthritis, heel pain (enthesitis), or vision loss. Ankylosing spondylitis develops in approximately 10% of cases. Mortality from ReA is infrequent and results most often from the cardiac complications or amyloidosis (1,3).

Relation to HIV Infection

Reactive arthritis has been reported frequently in people with human immunodeficiency virus (HIV) infection (10). Recent epidemiologic surveys suggest that HIV itself does not cause the disease, but rather, the association is an indirect one due to sexually acquired diseases caused by microorganisms (such as *C. trachomatis* or enteric pathogens) that are common to both HIV and ReA (11).

Observations that ReA is likely to be more severe in HIV-positive individuals, especially those with AIDS, probably are correct. Severe polyarticular arthritis and disabling enthesitis, as well as extensive cutaneous manifestations, have been described in such patients. HLA-B27 occurs in the same frequency (approximately 75%) in HIV-positive patients with ReA as in HIV-negative cases (10).

Laboratory Features

A mild normocytic, normochromic anemia due to chronic inflammation is not uncommon. Leukocytosis with total white blood cell counts of 10,000–15,000/mm^3 is typical during the acute phase, and thrombocytosis with platelet counts of 400,000–600,000/mm^3 is not unusual. Acute-phase reactants, including C-reactive protein and erythrocyte sedimentation rate, typically are abnormal. Serum globulins, especially IgA, frequently are elevated. In fact, IgA antibodies against the specific bacterium triggering the disease can be detected (12). Tests for rheumatoid factor and antinuclear antibodies are negative.

Typing for HLA-B27 is positive in approximately 65%–75% of white patients with ReA, but is less common (30%–50%) in African Americans. HLA-B27 is more likely to be found in patients with a chronic or relapsing course, as well as those with complicating sacroiliitis, spondylitis, iritis, or aortitis (7).

Synovial fluid typically shows highly inflammatory changes, including turbidity, poor viscosity or poor mucin clot tests; white blood cell counts ranging from 5000 to 50,000/mm³, with a polymorphonuclear cell predominance; and high total protein and complement levels. Compared with serum levels, the synovial fluid glucose level is not reduced significantly, as it is in true septic arthritis. Gram stains show no microorganisms, and bacterial cultures are sterile. Occasionally, synovial fluid contains "Reiter's cells," which are large mononuclear cells that contain several ingested polymorphonuclear leukocytes, which in turn contain inclusion bodies. Recent data have shown that the intracellular inclusions represent bacterial antigens. In fact, even after years of disease, bacterial antigens and viable microorganisms have been detected in synovial fluid, but more often in synovial tissue, of people with ReA (13–15). Research techniques such as polymerase chain reaction to detect bacterial RNA or DNA in joint fluid and tissue can identify the specific bacteria causing ReA. These technologies are likely to be adapted for clinical testing.

Radiographic Manifestations

Abnormalities on joint X-ray should not be expected early in disease, but only after symptoms have been present for at least several months (16). The most distinctive radiographic findings are a fluffy periosteal reaction and, at times, bony erosions of the calcaneus at the insertions of the plantar and/or Achilles tendons in people who have symptoms of heel pain (Fig. 11B-3). Similar radiographic findings occasionally may be found in people with ankylosing spondylitis or psoriatic arthritis. Periostitis and new bone formation also may be seen at other symptomatic sites of enthesitis or around affected joints or adjacent bony shafts. Such changes are seen most commonly in the feet, involving metatarsophalangeal bones and joints where there may be destruction with or without bony fusion. "Pencil-in-cup" deformities of small joints in feet or hands occasionally are found resembling deformities more typically seen in psoriatic arthritis.

Spinal radiographic abnormalities include sacroiliitis, which often is unilateral, and atypical ossified ligaments (syndesmophytes), which tend to be more asymmetrical and spotty than those seen in ankylosing spondylitis.

Diagnosis

The diagnosis of ReA is made on clinical grounds, based on the disease manifestations and laboratory findings (1). The presence of a seronegative, asymmetrical oligoarthritis, especially in a young person, should alert the physician to the possibility of ReA. The presence of an antecedent diarrheal illness or venereal exposure adds additional weight to the diagnosis, but such conditions often are absent. The

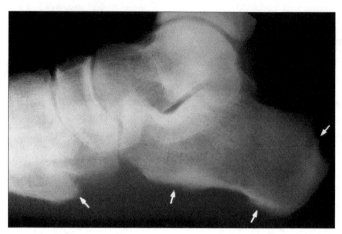

Fig. 11B-3. Radiograph of the lateral foot in a person with reactive arthritis and heel pain, indicating enthesitis with periosteal reaction (arrows) at sites of tendon insertions.

presence of heel pain or other symptoms of enthesitis, sausaging of digits, or any of the mucocutaneous lesions increases the likelihood of ReA. Testing for HLA-B27 may be a useful adjunct in diagnosis and shows a reasonable predictive value only if the clinical data support a strong likelihood of the disease. However, only two-thirds of white patients with ReA are HLA-B27-positive.

Care must be taken to exclude gonococcal and other forms of septic arthritis. All people with symptoms or signs of genital tract inflammation should have urethral or cervical smears tested for *N. gonorrhoeae* and *C. trachomatis* using Gram stain, culture, or molecular probes. When possible, synovial fluid should be cultured for *N. gonorrhoeae* and other pathogens, because gonococcal or other septic arthritides may mimic ReA. Psoriatic arthritis may be difficult or impossible to discriminate from ReA, although it usually is a more indolent process. The presence of distal interphalangeal joint involvement, pitting of the nails, and plaque-like psoriatic lesions over elbows or knees are strongly supportive of psoriatic arthritis. Atypical presentations of ankylosing spondylitis that begin with peripheral joint symptoms or so-called undifferentiated spondyloarthropathies, which have overlapping clinical features of several of these diseases, may be impossible to distinguish from ReA unless a specific bacterium can be identified.

Idiopathic Inflammatory Bowel Disease
Clinical Features

Peripheral arthritis occurs in approximately 10%–20% of people with Crohn's disease or ulcerative colitis (17,18). Not infrequently, arthritis with or without other extraintestinal manifestations is the first clinical symptom of inflammatory bowel disease (IBD), especially Crohn's disease. However, in retrospect, the patient may recall subtle symptoms of abdominal cramping, occasional diarrhea, and weight loss. IBD most often affects young adults and children, both males and females.

The typical pattern of joint inflammation is migratory arthralgias or arthritis. Less often, the arthritis is additive, oligoarticular, usually asymmetric, and affects predominantly the lower-extremity joints. Knees, ankles, and feet are affected most commonly, but any peripheral joint may be involved, including the hip. Large-joint effusions, especially of the knee, are common. Deformities are rare. Peripheral arthritis can reflect active IBD and can subside with treatment of the bowel inflammation. In fact, surgical colectomy in ulcerative colitis may result in permanent remission of the arthritis; however, this is not the case in Crohn's disease, in which other bowel areas may be affected. Rare instances of a chronic granulomatous synovitis, which may be destructive, have been described in Crohn's disease. HLA-B27 is not associated with Crohn's disease, ulcerative colitis, or the peripheral arthritis of IBD.

Spinal arthritis, including sacroiliitis or frank spondylitis, occurs in approximately 10% of people with IBD and frequently is asymptomatic (17,18). Males develop this complication more often than females (3:1). Unlike peripheral arthritis, spondylitis does not necessarily reflect active bowel inflammation, and it tends to run an independent course. Even colectomy does not halt its progression. The clinical symptoms, signs, and radiographic features of IBD-associated spondylitis are indistinguishable from those of idiopathic ankylosing spondylitis, except that HLA-B27 is found less frequently in the former (approximately 50%).

Extra-articular manifestations of IBD also typically reflect active bowel disease and tend to occur at the same time as the peripheral arthritis. The most common cutaneous complication of Crohn's disease is erythema nodosum, while that of ulcerative colitis is pyoderma gangrenosa. Painful, deep oral ulcers may occur in both disorders, as may attacks of acute anterior uveitis. Fever and weight loss also are common during active disease periods.

Laboratory Features
Anemia is common in IBD and reflects chronic inflammation and chronic gastrointestinal blood loss. Leukocytosis also is common, and an extreme thrombocytosis (platelet counts of 700,000/mm³ to more than 1 million/mm³) sometimes occurs. Acute-phase reactants, such as C-reactive protein and erythrocyte sedimentation rate, typically are elevated. Serum rheumatoid factor and antinuclear antibodies are not found; however, positive tests for antineutrophil cytoplasmic antibodies (ANCA), usually perinuclear (p)-ANCA, have been reported in approximately 60% of people with ulcerative colitis and, less commonly, in people with Crohn's disease (19). P-ANCA, rather than proteinase-3 (cytoplasmic ANCA) or myeloperoxidase (the usual p-ANCA), is directed against lactoferrin autoantigens. The frequency of HLA-B27 is no greater in people with IBD or with IBD-associated arthritis than in the general population. However, approximately half of the patients with complicating spondylitis are B27-positive. Synovial fluid findings have been reported infrequently, but show nonspecific inflammatory changes and are sterile on culture.

Whipple's Disease
Whipple's disease is a rare multisystem disease, usually affecting men, characterized by fever, diarrhea, steatorrhea, and profound weight loss. A variety of extra-intestinal manifestations may occur, especially joint disease, which can appear as migratory arthralgias or transient episodes of an additive, symmetrical polyarthritis. Rarely, the arthritis is chronic, but typically, it is nondeforming. There are some reports of sacroiliitis and HLA-B27 positivity, but it is unclear whether these are true associations. Other features may include serositis (pleural effusions), lymphadenopathy, cutaneous hyperpigmentation, anterior and/or posterior uveitis, nervous system disease (ocular palsies or encephalopathy), leukocytosis, and thrombocytosis.

Diagnosis traditionally has been based on finding characteristic, periodic acid-Schiff staining deposits in macrophages of the small intestine and, less commonly, in biopsies of lymph nodes or joint synovia. On electron microscopy, rod-shaped bacillary organisms have been seen in the same cells. A unique bacterial RNA sequence has been found, which has been classified as a Gram-positive actinomycete and named *Tropheryma whippelii*. Thus, Whipple's disease appears to be a systemic infection. Diagnosis is possible using polymerase chain reaction of affected tissues or blood samples (20), and remission can be achieved using long-term antibiotic treatment with tetracyclines.

FRANK C. ARNETT, MD

References
1. Amor B. Reiter's syndrome. Diagnosis and clinical features. *Rheum Dis Clin North Am* 1998;24:677–695.
2. Reiter H. Ueber eine bisher unbekannte Spirochaeten Infektion (spirochaetosis arthritica). *Dtsche Med Wschr* 1916;42: 1535–1536.
3. Arnett FC. Incomplete Reiter's syndrome: clinical comparisons with classical triad. *Ann Rheum Dis* 1979; 38(Suppl 1): 73–78.
4. Moll JM, Haslock I, MacRae IF, Wright V. Associations between ankylosing spondylitis, psoriatic arthritis, Reiter's disease, the intestinal arthropathies, and Behcet's syndrome. *Medicine* 1974;53:343–364.
5. Iliopoulos A, Karras D, Ioakimidis D, et al. Change in the epidemiology of Reiter's syndrome (reactive arthritis) in the post-AIDS era? An analysis of cases appearing in the Greek army. *J Rheumatol* 1995;22:252–254.
6. Hannu T, Puolakkainen M, Leirisalo-Repo M. Chlamydia pneumoniae as a triggering infection in reactive arthritis. *Rheumatology* 1999;38:411–414.
7. Leirisalo M, Skylv G, Kousa M, et al. Followup study on patients with Reiter's disease and reactive arthritis, with special reference to HLA-B27. *Arthritis Rheum* 1982;25: 249–259.

8. Bergfeldt L. HLA-B27-associated cardiac disease. Ann Intern Med 1997;127:621–629.
9. Thomson GTD, DeRubeis DA, Hodge MA, Rajanayagam C, Inman RD. Post-salmonella reactive arthritis: late clinical sequelae in a point source cohort. Am J Med 1995;98: 13–21.
10. Winchester R, Bernstein DH, Fischer HD, Enlow R, Solomon G. The co-occurrence of Reiter's syndrome and acquired immunodeficiency. Ann Intern Med 1987;106: 19–26.
11. Clark MR, Solinger AM, Hochberg MC. Human immunodeficiency virus infection is not associated with Reiter's syndrome. Data from three large cohort studies. Rheum Dis Clin North Am 1992;18:267–276.
12. Kingsley G, Panayi G. Antigenic responses in reactive arthritis. Rheum Dis Clin North Am 1992;18:49–66.
13. Nikkari S, Rantakokko K, Ekman P, et al. Salmonella-triggered reactive arthritis. Arthritis Rheum 1999;42:84–89.
14. Gaston JS, Cox C, Granfors K. Clinical and experimental evidence for persistent Yersinia infection in reactive arthritis. Arthritis Rheum 1999;42:2239–2242.
15. Schumacher HR Jr, Gerard HC, Arayssi TK, et al. Lower prevalence of Chlamydia pneumoniae DNA compared with Chlamydia trachomatis DNA in synovial tissue of arthritis patients. Arthritis Rheum 1999;42:1889–1893.
16. Brower AC, Flemming DJ. Reiter's disease. In: Brower AC, Flemming DJ (eds). Arthritis in Black and White, 2nd Edition. Philadelphia: W.B. Saunders Company, 1997; pp 245–255.
17. DeKeyser F, Elewaut D, DeVos M, et al. Bowel inflammation and the spondyloarthropathies. Rheum Dis Clin North Am 1998;24:785–813.
18. Suh CH, Lee CH, Lee J, et al. Arthritis manifestations of inflammatory bowel disease. J Korean Med Sci 1998;13: 39–43.
19. Duerr RH, Targan SR, Landers CJ, et al. Neutrophil cytoplasmic antibodies: a link between primary sclerosing cholangitis and ulcerative colitis. Gastroenterol 1991;100:1385–1391.
20. O'Duffy JD, Griffing WL, Li CY, Abdelmalek MF, Persing DH. Whipple's arthritis: direct detection of Tropheryma whippelii in synovial fluid and tissue. Arthritis Rheum 1999; 42:812–817.

SERONEGATIVE SPONDYLOARTHROPATHIES
C. Ankylosing Spondylitis

Ankylosing spondylitis (AS) is a chronic inflammatory disease of the sacroiliac joints and spine that may be associated with characteristic extraspinal lesions. It is, essentially, a disease of young adults. Progressive stiffening of the spine is usual, with ankylosis (fusion of some or all spinal joints) occurring after some years of disease in many, but not all, patients. Patients with long-standing severe disease are at increased risk of premature death, but overall, the life span of individuals with ankylosing spondylitis appears to be normal. AS shares many features with the arthritides associated with psoriasis, inflammatory bowel disease, and reactive arthritis, and these conditions comprise the spondyloarthritis family (1). Typical spondylitis may be present in each of the other spondyloarthropathies.

Epidemiology

The prevalence of AS in different populations varies from 0.1% in some African and Eskimo populations, through 0.5%–1.0% among white populations in the UK and USA, to around 6% in the Haida Native Americans in Northern Canada. The prevalence generally, but not exclusively, reflects the prevalence of human leukocyte antigen (HLA)-B27 in the different populations. Because few population surveys have been undertaken, much of the available data has been drawn from selective hospital-based surveys and from information on other related spondyloarthropathies.

Ankylosing spondylitis is more common in men, with a male:female ratio of approximately 5:1. Expression of disease may vary slightly between men and women, but earlier reports exaggerated this variance to the detriment of women with AS, many of whom experienced unnecessary delays in reaching a diagnosis (2). Some investigators have suggested that the true sex ratio is closer to unity.

Etiology

In spite of dramatic advances in recent years, the etiology of AS remains unclear. A strong multigenic inherited component is evident, although HLA-B27 remains the strongest association in almost all populations (3). Animal and laboratory studies suggest that the HLA-B27 molecule itself plays a key role, and that involvement of class 1 major histocompatibility complex (MHC) antigens in the presentation of microbial peptides is central to the pathogenic mechanism (4).

Infective mechanisms also have been proposed. However, aside from the undoubted development of AS in a minority of people with reactive arthritis, no clear evidence implicates specific infection. Klebsiella aeruginosa has been implicated on the basis of molecular mimicry with HLA-B27 and clinical studies, although its real significance remains unclear. Subclinical mucosal inflammation in the large and small bowel undoubtedly is present in many individuals with AS; this finding could provide the basis for an immune or infective mechanism for the spinal disease.

Although prostatitis and salpingitis have been described in many patients, identification of these lesions is more problematic, and their relevance, if any, remains uncertain.

Clinical Features

The principal musculoskeletal lesions associated with AS are enthesitis and synovitis, with sacroiliitis also involving adjacent bone. Inflammatory eye lesions, myocardial changes, gut mucosal lesions, and genitourinary inflammation are inconsistent, but characteristic, features of AS.

Presenting Features

Spinal features of AS seldom appear before the age of 16–18 years. Before this age, children and teenagers may develop oligoarthritis – typically a swollen knee or metatarsophalangeal joint – sometimes associated with iritis and/or enthesitis (5). Juvenile AS is remarkable because it does not involve the spine.

For many, symptoms begin early in the third decade of life, and the average age at onset is 26 years. It is rare for AS to begin after the age of 40 years, but not uncommon for evidence of the disease to be discovered later in life, since earlier symptoms often are mild or ignored.

The usual presenting symptom is inflammatory back pain that is insidious in onset, persistent for more than three months, worsened by such inactivity as overnight rest, and improved by exercise. Sacroiliitis, the most common initial feature, causes pain in the buttocks that sometimes radiates down the thighs, but never below the knee. Although clinical examination is unreliable as a means of diagnosing sacroiliitis, pain in the buttocks may be elicited in some patients by pushing firmly with both hands on the sacrum when the patient is prone. A minority of patients present with oligoarthritis or enthesitis that particularly affects the heel, or hip pain due to aggressive synovitis. Fatigue is a common and troublesome symptom, and impaired sleep, due to pain and stiffness, is a major contributor to this fatigue. Other constitutional features may include fever and weight loss. Overt or subclinical depression, with loss of libido and reduced capacity for work, also may contribute to lack of well-being.

Typically, spinal discomfort and stiffness gradually ascend the spine over a period of years to produce progressive spinal pain and restriction. This progression affects the costovertebral joints, reducing respiratory excursion, and the cervical spine, limiting neck movement. Thoracic spine involvement may be associated with anterior chest pain and sternal/costal cartilage tenderness, which can be particularly distressing for patients. During the early phase of disease, osteoporosis develops in many patients and, without adequate treatment or prophylaxis, leads to vertebral and other fractures later in life (6). Spinal fractures are more common in patients who have severe involvement with rigidity.

Enthesitis

The central feature of AS is inflammation at entheses, the sites where tendons and ligaments attach to bone. These inflammatory lesions initially lead to radiographic appearances of osteopenia or "lytic lesions," but subsequently, reactive bone forms a new, more superficial enthesis, which develops into a radiologically detectable bony overgrowth or spur (7). In the spine, enthesitis occurs at capsular and ligamentous attachments and discovertebral, costovertebral, and costotransverse joints, with involvement also at bony attachments of interspinous and paravertebral ligaments.

Enthesitis accounts for much of the pain, stiffness, and restriction at sacroiliac and other spinal joints. It also occurs at extraspinal sites, producing troublesome symptoms. Most commonly, such lesions affect the plantar fascia and Achilles tendon insertions to the calcaneus, producing disabling heel pain. Plantar fasciitis typically leads to the formation of fluffy calcaneal spurs, visible on heel radiographs after six to 12 months. Similar lesions may occur around the pelvis, costochondral junctions, tibial tubercles, and elsewhere, causing marked local tenderness. More widespread diffuse lesions lead to insidious stiffness and generalized discomfort. Sternal and costochondral pain also reflect a combination of local enthesitis and referred pain from the thoracic spine. This development frequently produces worrying chest pain, which should be distinguished carefully from myocardial ischemia.

Sacroiliitis

Inflammation of the sacroiliac joints develops most frequently in the late teens or in the third decade of life, producing bilateral or occasionally unilateral buttock pain, usually worse after inactivity and sometimes aggravated by weight-bearing. Changes principally affect the lower anterior (synovial) portion of the sacroiliac joints and are associated with juxta-articular osteopenia and osteitis. This condition leads to radiographic appearances of widening of the sacroiliac joint. Enchondral ossification as a consequence of the osteitis gives the radiographic appearance of "erosion" along the lower part of the sacroiliac joints. Osteitis appears as increased water content of adjacent bone, as seen on magnetic resonance imaging (MRI). Capsular enthesopathy also occurs over the anterior and posterior aspect of the joint throughout its length, leading to sheets of ossification that ultimately obscure the joint completely on standard radiographs.

Synovitis

Peripheral synovitis is characterized by the distribution of joints affected rather than by histologic changes. Synovitis is indistinguishable histologically and immunohistochemically from typical rheumatoid disease.

Peripheral joint synovitis may precede, accompany, or follow the onset of spinal symptoms. Hips, knees, ankles and metatarsophalangeal joints may be affected, but upper-limb joints are almost never involved, except when psoriasis also is present. In further contrast to rheumatoid arthritis, peripheral joint synovitis usually is oligoarticular, often asymmetrical, and may be episodic rather than persistent. Joint erosion may occur, especially at the metatarsophalangeal joints, leading to subluxation and deformity. Peripheral joint involvement is indistinguishable from that seen in the other spondyloarthropathies. Temporomandibular joints may be affected, leading to reduced mouth opening and discomfort on chewing. Dactylitis may lead to pain at one or more toes lasting many months, but usually resolves spontaneously.

Eye Lesions

Eye discomfort, a common problem in people with AS, typically occurs as nonspecific dryness; conjunctivitis also may occur. Acute anterior uveitis (iritis) develops at some time in approximately one-third of patients with AS, and may be recurrent. Acute anterior uveitis usually is unilateral, asynchronous with arthritis flares, and associated with pain, redness, lacrimation, photophobia, and blurred vision. Untreated or inadequately treated iritis may lead rapidly to considerable scarring, irregularity of the pupil, and visual impairment. Red, sore, gritty eyes or blurring of vision require urgent ophthalmologic examination.

Enteritis and Colitis

Sacroiliitis, with or without typical AS, occurs in 6%–25% of people with Crohn's disease or ulcerative colitis. Similarly, inflammatory bowel disease may be present or develop in people with preexisting AS. Indeed, approximately 60% of people with AS have subclinical changes in the small or large bowel (8). There is speculation that these changes may relate to the pathogenesis of AS, but their true significance is unknown.

Altered bowel habits with diarrhea and abdominal discomfort, with or without passage of blood or mucus, requires investigation. Ulcerative colitis and Crohn's disease are associated closely with AS. Even though some AS lesions closely resemble those of Crohn's disease, it would appear that for the vast majority, such lesions never become symptomatic. The link between AS and inflammatory bowel disease appears to be indirect, as variations in inflammatory activity of each disease appear to occur independently.

In a minority of people with colitis and peripheral arthritis, peripheral joint disease may settle after total colectomy. Conversely, however, many patients complain of a fibromyalgia-like disorder that produces mild but widespread discomfort, even after colectomy. Active inflammatory bowel disease increases the risk and severity of osteoporosis. Crohn's disease with extensive small-bowel involvement also may lead to impaired vitamin D absorption and osteomalacia, producing ill-defined musculoskeletal pain and difficulty walking.

Prostatitis and Salpingitis

Both prostatitis and salpingitis have been described in people with AS and isolated sacroiliitis. Sexually transmitted infection of the lower genital tract is well-recognized in the initiation of reactive arthritis. No clear infectious explanation for these lesions has emerged, and the link between them and spondylitis itself is unclear. Unfortunately, diagnostic criteria for both of these conditions have been some-

what imprecise, and the true prevalence and significance of these lesions are unknown. Chronic prostatitis may produce recurrent perineal pain and dysuria, and is extremely difficult to treat successfully.

Cardiovascular Involvement

Cardiac conduction abnormalities and myocardial dysfunction have been recorded in a significant minority of people with AS (9). Aortitis with dilatation of the aortic valve ring and aortic regurgitation has been demonstrated in approximately 1% of patients.

Pulmonary Involvement

Approximately 1% of patients develop progressive upper-lobe fibrosis of the lungs (10). Breathlessness on exertion is not uncommon, especially in those with extensive, severe disease. Rigidity of the chest wall, with or without apical lung fibrosis, is the most common factor, but cardiac dysrhythmias and aortic valve disease should be considered. Cavitation may be followed by secondary fungal or bacterial infection.

Neurologic Lesions

Neurologic deficit is associated most often with cord or root lesions following spinal fracture. Nerve root pain may arise from the cervical spine, especially when there is marked flexion deformity. Long-tract signs, including quadriplegia, may follow spinal fracture dislocation after relatively minor trauma and complicate spontaneous atlantoaxial subluxation. Subluxation also may lead to severe occipital headache.

Weakness of the legs occasionally occurs in association with a cauda equina syndrome. This syndrome is particularly associated with the development of dural ectasia demonstrable on MRI.

Other Clinical Features

Kidney function seldom is affected in AS, but immunoglobulin A nephropathy and amyloidosis are well-described.

Diagnosis and Differential Diagnosis

Strict diagnosis depends on conformity with the New York criteria (11). In clinical practice, however, diagnosis at either the "definite" or "probable" level often is required at an early stage of disease, before classical radiographic changes have occurred. Probable AS can be diagnosed based on inflammatory back or buttock pain that is relieved by exercise or nonsteroidal anti-inflammatory drugs (NSAIDs), with restricted spinal movements. A history of iritis, psoriasis, or inflammatory bowel disease, or a family history of a spondyloarthropathy increases the confidence of the diagnosis. Early evidence of bilateral sacroiliitis is best achieved by MRI or computed tomography scanning; the classic radiographic appearances of juxta-articular osteoporosis, followed by irregular bone erosion and sclerosis, often take several months or years to become apparent

(12). The presence of definite bilateral sacroiliitis effectively confirms the diagnosis. Isotope bone scanning is less readily interpretable and should not be used in diagnosing AS, except to exclude other conditions. Early radiographic changes in the spine include squaring of lumbar vertebrae, with sclerosis at the corners of the vertebrae (shiny corners) and subsequent development of vertical syndesmophytes and loss of definition of apophyseal joints (13).

When the clinical suspicion of AS is high, the presence of the HLA-B27 antigen enhances the likelihood of this diagnosis. In patients with ill-defined back pain, testing for HLA-B27 antigen may be misleading and should be avoided.

Virtually the whole gamut of causes of spinal pain need to be considered in the differential diagnosis of AS (see Table 11C-1). Although usually diagnosed in young adults in their third decade, symptoms may arise or first be noticed in older people. True spondylitis and sacroiliitis generally do not occur before the age of 16; the term "juvenile AS" refers to a peripheral spondyloarthropathy that may progress to include spinal involvement.

The greatest diagnostic difficulty may be differentiating AS from idiopathic pain syndromes; indeed, the two conditions occasionally coexist. Tenderness over the ribs and costal cartilage is common in both conditions, but tenderness over many or all of the vertebra, with relatively less pain on direct sacral pressure, is atypical of AS and strongly characteristic of a fibromyalgia-like illness.

Course and Outcome

Ankylosing spondylitis tends to produce progressive stiffness and spinal restriction, with intermittent exacerbations and remissions (14). Some patients, especially those with early aggressive disease, hip involvement, and poor adherence to treatment, develop profound spinal rigidity, with flexion deformity of the spine. The majority of patients, however, have mild or moderate disease and maintain some mobility and independence throughout life (14).

Most individuals remain at work, although many experience difficulties with pain and fatigue. In consequence, many patients must carefully select their type of work and adjust working hours to cope with fatigue.

Overall survival of individuals with AS probably is comparable to that of the general population (15,16). Individuals with long-standing, severe disease, however, have reduced life expectancy as a result of amyloidosis, malignancies following multiple courses of radiotherapy, aortic valve disease, traumatic spinal fractures, and the risks of drug and surgical treatments. Similarly, complications of associated conditions, such as ulcerative colitis and Crohn's disease, may contribute to premature death in some patients.

Pregnancy may pose particular problems for young women with AS (17). Unlike rheumatoid arthritis, there is no tendency for AS to remit during pregnancy. Sacroiliitis may produce severe pain during delivery and fused sacroiliac joints may hinder the process. Nonsteroidal anti-inflammatory drugs should be avoided, if possible, because of the

TABLE 11C-1
Differential Diagnosis of Ankylosing Spondylitis

Prolapsed intervertebral disc
Fibromyalgia/idiopathic musculoskeletal pain syndrome
Spinal tumors: chordoma, ependymoma
Bone tumors: osteoid osteoma, plasmacytoma,
  secondary carcinoma, leukemic infiltration
Infection in spinal or sacroiliac joint: tuberculosis,
  brucellosis
Pelvic inflammatory disease
Metabolic bone disease: osteomalacia, hypophos
  phatemic rickets
Diffuse interstitial spinal hyperostosis (Forrestier's
  disease)

theoretical possibility of fetal abnormalities and the real possibility of oligohydramnios and premature closure of the *ductus arteriosus*. Steroids may be acceptable for symptom control during this period. Every effort should be made to maintain spinal mobility, which will aid symptom control and help prevent a step-wise reduction in spinal mobility.

Assessment of Disease Activity and Severity

Clinical assessment of disease activity and severity, as well as response to treatment, is complex and difficult in AS. It is essential to separate activity of spinal, peripheral joint, and other extraspinal lesions. Traditional measures of acute-phase response, such as the erythrocyte sedimentation rate and C-reactive protein levels, may be valuable for extraspinal lesions but correlate poorly with activity of spinal disease. Judgement of inflammatory activity of spondylitis per se is largely subjective. Functional state can be assessed by modifications of the Health Assessment Questionnaire devised for rheumatoid arthritis (18). Several instruments have been introduced to measure activity of AS using composite scores of patient symptoms and physical findings, and a degree of consensus has been achieved over the establishment of a core data set (19).

Treatment

The fundamental prerequisite of effective management is establishing and communicating the diagnosis and its implications to the patient. Although no cure or treatment shows proven efficacy in preventing disease progression, an assiduous approach to management usually can maintain acceptable comfort and lifestyle.

Treatment is aimed at maintaining normal upright posture and spinal mobility, minimizing the impact of hip and peripheral manifestations, and reducing pain and stiffness.

Of all therapeutic modalities, only regular exercise has been shown to curtail progression of spinal stiffness and restriction. It is essential that patients understand the role of stretching and spinal exercise in minimizing the long-term impact of their condition. Ideally, patients should undertake a daily period of spinal exercise. This exercise may take the form of prescribed stretching, gym exercises, or participation in a favored sport, such as swimming or badminton. Contact sports should be considered with caution, although suboptimal regular exercise is better than no regular exercise. Regular treatment by a physical therapist may be helpful, but patient-driven treatment is more likely to be maintained. Physical therapists, however, may be crucial in establishing a sustainable pattern of beneficial exercise and in imparting confidence that no harm will come from gradually increased activity. Participating in regular group exercises, such as those provided by self-help groups, is beneficial. Attention to posture is crucial, especially for those with sedentary occupations or tendencies. After a prolonged period of sitting, as at a desk or computer, spinal extension may be encouraged by a period of lying flat on the floor. The principal role of the physician is to sustain the patient's resolve to keep up regular exercise and stretching and to provide sufficient medication to make this possible.

Pain and spinal stiffness may be reduced by NSAID use, and the choice of drug depends largely on individual preference and tolerance. Long-acting NSAIDs taken at night may be valuable in promoting sound sleep and reducing morning stiffness. Local corticosteroid injections may relieve enthesitis at peripheral sites, such as the Achilles' tendon or plantar fascia attachments at the heel. Brief courses of oral or parenteral steroid treatment may be extremely helpful in overcoming severe spinal or peripheral inflammatory disease and may help maximize progress at the beginning of an exercise program. Second-line drugs have been disappointing in AS. Sulfasalazine and methotrexate may be beneficial in peripheral joint disease, but have little, if any effect on spinal disease (20).

Hip and knee arthroplasty have revolutionized life for many with AS, because disease at these sites is a major cause of disability. Excess new bone formation postoperatively, however, may gradually impair joint function and necessitate revision. Corrective spinal surgery has become a safer prospect since the advent of preoperative MRI scanning and may be extremely helpful in carefully selected patients with spinal deformity or pseudoarthrosis.

Any patient with a spondyloarthropathy developing a painful red eye requires urgent specialist ophthalmologic examination to diagnose or exclude acute anterior uveitis (iritis).

Constitutional problems of fatigue, poor sleep, depression, and low self-esteem, as well as practical difficulties at work, travelling, at home, and in bed, may plague patients and merit the attention of physicians and therapists. Readiness to explore these issues and to use appropriate antidepressant drugs, including tricyclics in low dosages, frequently yields substantial dividends.

ANDREW KEAT, MD

References

1. Khan MA. An overview of clinical spectrum and heterogeneity of spondyloarthropathies. Rheum Dis Clin N Am 1992;18:1–10.

2. Kidd B, Mullee M, Frank A, Cawley M. Disease expression of ankylosing spondylitis in males and females. J Rheumatol 1988;15:1407–1409.

3. Wordsworth P. Genes in the spondyloarthropathies. Rheum Dis Clin North Am 1998;24:845–863.

4. Gonzalez S, Martinez-Borra J, Lopez-Larrea C. Immunogenetics, HLA-B27 and spondyloarthropathies. Curr Opin Rheumatol 1999;11:257–264.

5. Burgos-Vargos R, Vazquez-Mellado J. The early recognition of juvenile onset ankylosing spondylitis and its differentiation from juvenile rheumatoid arthritis. Arthritis Rheum 1995;38:835–844.

6. Will R, Palmer R, Bhalla A, Ring F, Calin A. Osteoporosis in early ankylosing spondylitis: a primary pathological event? Lancet 1989;2:1483–1485.

7. Vernon-Roberts B. Ankylosing spondylitis; pathology. In: Klippel JH, Dieppe PA (eds). Rheumatology. 2nd edition. London: Mosby, 1998; pp 6.18.1–6.18.6.

8. Leirisalo-Repo M, Repo H. Gut and spondyloarthropathies. Rheum Dis Clin North Am 1992;18:23–35.

9. O'Neill TW, Bresnihan B. The heart in ankylosing spondylitis. Ann Rheum Dis 1992;51:705–706.

10. Rosenow E, Strimlan CV, Muhm JR, Ferguson RH. Pleuropulmonary manifestations of ankylosing spondylitis. Mayo Clin Proc 1977;52:641–649.

11. Khan MA. Ankylosing spondylitis: clinical features. In: Klippel JH, Dieppe PA (eds). Rheumatology, 2nd edition. London: Mosby, 1998; pp 6.16.1–6.16.10.

12. Blum U, Buitrago-Tellez C, Mundinger A, et al. Magnetic resonance imaging for detection of active sacroiliitis. A prospective study comparing conventional radiography, scintigraphy and contrast enhanced MRI. J Rheumatol 1996;23:2107–2115.

13. Resnick D, Niwayama G. Ankylosing spondylitis. In: Resnick D (ed). Diagnosis of Bone and Joint Disorders, 3rd edition. Philadelphia: WB Saunders, 1995; pp 1008–1074.

14. Carette S, Graham D, Little H, Rubinstein J, Rosen P. The natural disease course of ankylosing spondylitis. Arthritis Rheum 1983;26:186–190.

15. Khan MA, Khan MK, Kushner I. Survival among patients with ankylosing spondylitis: a life-table analysis. J Rheumatol 1981;8:86–90.

16. Callahan LF, Pincus T. Mortality in the rheumatic diseases. Arthritis Care Res; 1995;8:229–241.

17. Ostensen M, Ostensen H. Ankylosing spondylitis – the female aspect. J Rheumatol 1998;25:120–124.

18. Daltroy LH, Larson MG, Roberts NW, Liang MH. A modification of the health assessment questionnaire for the spondyloarthropathies. J Rheumatol 1990;17:946–950.

19. Van der Heijde D, Calin A, Dougados M, Khan MA, van der Linden S, Bellamy N. Selection of instruments in the core set for DC-ART, SMARD, physical therapy and clinical record keeping in ankylosing spondylitis. Progress report of the ASAS Working Group. J Rheumatol 1999;26:951–954.

20. Creemers MC, Franssen MJ, Van de Putte LB, Gribnau FW, van Riel PL. Methotrexate in severe ankylosing spondylitis: an open study. J Rheumatol 1995;22:1104–1107.

SERONEGATIVE SPONDYLOARTHROPATHIES
D. Treatment

The seronegative spondyloarthropathies include ankylosing spondylitis (AS), reactive arthritis (ReA), psoriatic arthritis (PsA), and colitic arthropathy associated with inflammatory bowel disease (IBD). These conditions necessitate a global approach to management in which patient education is the cornerstone. With the typical onset during young adulthood and with a male predominance, people with these diagnoses frequently display frustration and depression when it becomes apparent that they have a chronic rheumatic disease that can significantly impair their functional capabilities and quality of life. Validated measures of disease activity – the Bath Ankylosing Spondylitis Functional Index (BASFI), Dougados Functional Index (DFI), and an AS-specific version of the Health Assessment Questionnaire (HAQ-S) – have proved useful in determining functional status and response to therapy (1). An AS-specific Arthritis Impact Measurement Scale 2 (AS-AIMS2), which includes measurements of spine pain and mobility, has correlated with a marked deterioration in these patients' quality of life (2). Stiffness, pain, fatigue, poor sleep, concerns about appearance, and worry about the future are extremely common in people with the spondyloarthropathies. Clinicians treating people with these diseases should be aware that these psychosocial aspects of the disease are part of the burden of illness.

Exercise is an important part of treatment for people with AS. Generally, high-impact sports should be avoided. Swimming is an ideal exercise, and biking often is well-tolerated, unless restricted neck extension limits the field of view, which often is the case in more advanced AS. Stretching to maintain mobility and posture should be emphasized, and an experienced physiotherapist can instruct the patient in daily exercises. Long car trips and air travel should include periodic stretching. Sleeping with a straight back position is better than sleeping curled on the side. Deep breathing exercises and avoidance of cigarettes should be stressed.

Education is a key element in the comprehensive care of a person with ReA. If the ReA has been preceded by a sexually transmitted disease (STD), there may be an important emotional element for the patient that needs to be addressed. Genitourinary manifestations, such as balanitis (which is as likely to occur after a gastrointestinal infection as after an STD), can be of particular concern for patients and their sexual partners, and current concepts of triggering infections should be discussed. Another area of concern is prognosis, because ReA and other spondyloarthropathies often occur in individuals for whom athletic activity is a priority. There is general recognition that ReA has a greater propensity for chronicity than was appreciated previously, and this knowledge should temper an overly optimistic projection. In a review of 63 patients with post-*Salmonella* ReA, with a mean of 11 years disease duration, 10 had mild joint symptoms, 11 had recurrent acute arthritis, five had acute iritis, and eight had developed a chronic spondyloarthropathy (3).

Particularly perplexing for clinician and patient alike is the variability in prognosis for the many patients who fall into the diagnostic category of undifferentiated spondyloarthropathy. This heterogeneous cluster of articular and extra-articular features lack reliable predictors of progression, and this uncertainty influences the clinician's discussions with patients, and the interpretation of therapeutic outcomes.

Steroidal and Nonsteroidal Therapy

In general, people with a spondyloarthropathy experience significant improvement in joint inflammation after administration of NSAIDs, and newer NSAIDs often are more effective than salicylates. Indomethacin or diclofenac (up to 200 mg daily, in divided doses) generally is well-tolerated in this patient population. No trials have specifically addressed the use of selective COX-2 inhibitors, such as rofecoxib and celecoxib, in the spondyloarthropathies, but these medicines may form an important part of the therapeutic regimen in patients who do not tolerate conventional NSAID therapy. In the case of AS, the goal of anti-inflammatory treatment is to achieve sufficient control of pain and stiffness to allow an active, sustained program of exercise and physical activity, and to improve quality of life.

Corticosteroid therapy for spondyloarthropathy usually consists of intra-articular injections into actively inflamed joints. The response to local steroid injection often is neither as dramatic nor as sustained as it is in people with rheumatoid arthritis. Corticosteroid injection into the sacroiliac joints usually is performed under imaging guidance (fluoroscopy or computed tomography). This procedure can, on occasion, obviate the need for initiating second-line agents. Systemic corticosteroids (administered orally or as an intravenous bolus protocol) have been used with some success for severe symptomatic flares, but lack any controlled trials to validate effectiveness. The goal should be prompt taper of the dose when symptomatic control is achieved. Topical steroids usually are effective for treating the mucous membrane and skin manifestations of ReA. For uveitis, topical corticosteroid eye drops are an integral component of management, and treatment should be monitored jointly with an ophthalmologist.

Antibiotic Therapy

The current concept of the pathogenesis of ReA postulates that a bacterial infection, usually gastrointestinal or genitourinary, is the triggering event in an immunogenetically susceptible host. For the other spondyloarthropathies, there is less compelling evidence to implicate infection in a causal role. It is sound clinical practice to treat any culture-proven *Chlamydia* urethritis. The patients' sexual partners also should be treated. In this regard, azithromycin, 1 g as a single dose, is as effective as doxycycline, 100 mg twice per day for seven days (4).

The role of antibiotics in the management of the spondyloarthropathies has been controversial. In an uncontrolled experience, a retrospective review of 109 patients with urethritis concluded that 37% of episodes of urethritis not treated with anti-*Chlamydia* agents were associated with subsequent ReA, whereas only 10% of such episodes when treated with tetracycline progressed to ReA (5). Lymecycline (a form of tetracycline) was evaluated in a three-month, double-blind, placebo-controlled study of 40 people with chronic ReA (6). The antibiotic therapy significantly decreased the duration of illness in patients with *Chlamydia*-induced ReA, but not in patients with ReA triggered by enteric pathogens. These observations provide indirect support for the notion that *Chlamydia* may persist in the joints for prolonged periods of time in an altered metabolic state that is, however, still viable.

Wakefield et al reported results of a randomized, placebo-controlled trial of 12 months of treatment with ciprofloxacin (750 mg twice per day) in 56 people with ReA and 42 people with anterior uveitis (7). There was no difference between treatment and placebo arms with respect to disease relapse, joint inflammation, or ocular inflammation. A three-month, randomized, placebo-controlled trial examined the effect of ciprofloxacin (500 mg twice per day) in patients with ReA or undifferentiated oligoarthritis (8). There were 49 people with undifferentiated oligoarthritis and 52 people with ReA whose antecedent infection could be identified: 14 had post-*Yersinia* ReA, 13 had post-*Chlamydia* ReA, and 25 had post-*Salmonella* ReA. No difference was seen in patients with disease duration fewer than three months. No overall difference in outcome was found between ciprofloxacin treatment and placebo. Ciprofloxacin was not effective in *Yersinia*- or *Salmonella*-induced arthritis, but seemed to be better than placebo in *Chlamydia*-induced arthritis. This difference was not significant, however, possibly due to the small sample size. Definitive conclusions on the role of antibiotic treatment in *Chlamydia*-induced ReA await a controlled trial.

Second-Line Agents
Sulfasalazine

A six-month, randomized, placebo-controlled, double-blind, multicenter study examined sulfasalazine (SSZ), at a dosage of 3 g/day, in spondyloarthropathy patients who had not achieved disease control with NSAID treatment alone (9). A majority (75% of participants) completed the trial, and the dropout rate was comparable between placebo and treatment arms. Of the four primary outcome variables, only patient global assessment reached statistical significance; 60% of patients receiving SSZ, versus 44% receiving placebo noted an improvement of one point on a five-point scale. In subgroup analysis, the most impressive effects were seen in people with PsA.

Subsequently, three 36-week, randomized, double-blind, multicenter studies of people with AS, PsA, and ReA were undertaken, comparing SSZ (2 g/day) to placebo. Patients had active disease, defined by morning stiffness, inflammatory back pain, and patient and physician global assessments reflecting at least moderate disease activity. In the AS cohort, there was a trend favoring SSZ in the middle of treatment, but no difference at the end of treatment (10); final response rates were 38% for SSZ and 36% for placebo. Participants with AS with associated peripheral arthritis showed improvement that favored SSZ. In the ReA cohort, longitudinal analysis revealed improvement with SSZ over placebo, a trend that appeared at four weeks and continued throughout the trial (11). At the end of treatment, the response rates were 62% for SSZ and 48% for placebo. In the PsA cohort, longitudinal analysis revealed a trend favoring SSZ, and response rates at the end of treatment were 58% for SSZ and 47% for placebo (12). The response rates in the placebo arms of these trials highlight the variability in clinical course in the spondyloarthropathies, and complicate study design for definitive trials in the future.

A recent re-analysis of this experience with SSZ stratified the patients into those having axial or peripheral disease (13). Of 187 patients with only axial disease, response criteria were met in 40% of the SSZ group and 43% of the placebo group. Of the 432 patients with peripheral arthritis, responses were seen in 59% of the SSZ group and 43% of the placebo group ($P < 0.0005$). Besides guiding patient selection for SSZ treatment options, these studies suggest that the axial:peripheral stratification of people with the spondyloarthropathies may be more biologically based than the traditional division into AS:ReA:PsA:IBD subcategories.

Methotrexate

Concurrent with the widespread use of methotrexate (MTX) in people with rheumatoid arthritis, there has been increasing use of MTX in people with the spondyloarthropathies. Generally, responses have been good, particularly for peripheral joint disease, but there have been few trials to substantiate these clinical impressions. In people with ReA, where there is a predominance of young male patients, the hazards of alcohol intake while on MTX must be discussed.

In a 24-week, open study of 11 people with AS, clinical improvement over baseline was observed at the end of treatment (14). Of the five patients who discontinued treatment, three had disease flares and restarted MTX. More recently, a three-year, open study of MTX in AS was reported (15). Sixteen patients completed the three-year trial. A good response was seen, as defined by clinimetrics and laboratory markers of inflammation, except for patients with peripheral disease and uveitis. There was no radiographic progression of disease in the spine or the sacroiliac joints. The axial:peripheral aspect of this trial is the reciprocal of the SSZ trials discussed previously, and suggests that combination treatment protocols may have value, as has proved to be the case for rheumatoid arthritis. The caveat in this study, however, is the increased response rate in placebo-treated patients, as compared to the controlled trials above.

Experience with long-term MTX therapy for 38 people with PsA has been reported (16). In 45% of these patients there was greater than a 40% improvement in active joint count at six and 24 months. Radiographic analysis at 24 months showed an increase in damage score in 63% of the MTX-treated patients, which was comparable to radiographic progression in a control group of PsA patients not receiving MTX. Longer-term follow-up may resolve whether MTX has a joint-sparing effect in PsA.

Other Disease-Modifying Agents

Several therapeutic approaches for controlling PsA have been studied. Of 24 patients treated with chloroquine for six months, 75% had greater than a 30% reduction in active joint count, which was superior to results from a control group (17). Clinical efficacy by joint count measures was observed with intramuscular gold treatment in 18 people with PsA (18). However, the gold therapy did not alter progression of radiographic damage, compared with clinic control patients.

Cyclosporine has been studied extensively in people with psoriasis, with some assessments of drug effects on joint disease. One study randomized 210 people with psoriasis to either cyclosporine or etretinate therapy (19). After 10 weeks of therapy, greater control of skin disease was achieved with cyclosporine than with etretinate. There was significant improvement of joint disease in both groups. Recent trials using intermittent short courses of cyclosporine (20) or combination therapy with MTX and cyclosporine (21) have shown encouraging results for severe, recalcitrant psoriasis, and these results may warrant formal trials in refractory PsA.

The response of the spondyloarthropathies to SSZ may be attributable to the antibiotic moiety of this compound (sulfapyridine) or to the anti-inflammatory moiety [5-aminosalicylic acid (5-ASA)]. A recent study reported on 20 spondyloarthropathy patients who had been taking SSZ and then were switched to 5-ASA (22). Of these patients, 85% responded, as measured by physician global assessment, compared with the previous SSZ-treatment period. These results support the notion that 5-ASA may be the active moiety in SSZ and suggest that 5-ASA warrants a formal prospective trial in the spondyloarthropathies.

An open study of intravenous pamidronate in 22 people with refractory AS has been reported (23). After three monthly infusions of pamidronate, there was a significant improvement in disease activity scores, and after six monthly infusions, there were improvements in metrology measurements and erythrocyte sedimentation rates. A controlled trial is in progress to follow up the encouraging results from this open study.

Anti-TNF Therapy

The role of immunomodulatory cytokines in the pathogenesis of the spondyloarthropathies has not been resolved. Some studies have implicated tumor necrosis factor (TNF)-α as an AS-susceptibility-marker genetic polymorphism associated with a relative impairment of TNF-α production, but not all studies have supported this notion. Despite uncertainties about the role of pro-inflammatory cytokines in AS, some of the newer biologic agents, such as the chimeric monoclonal antibody to TNF-α (infliximab) or the soluble TNF receptor (etenercept), seem to promise more effective treatment for spondyloarthropathies. An open pilot study that examined the effect of three infusions (weeks 0, 2, and 6) of infliximab (5 mg/kg) in 21 people with active spondyloarthropathy (24) showed prompt response in clinical outcome measures and laboratory indicators of inflammation. The response was sustained to day 84, when the final assessment was made. In the eight patients with PsA, there was a significant improvement in skin involvement. The treatment was well-tolerated and no adverse events were seen. A similar treatment regimen was reported in 11 people with active AS of relatively short duration (median, five years; range, 0.5–13 years) (25). Of 10 patients completing the three infusions, nine were observed to have ≥50% improvement in activity, function, and pain scores. There was significant decrease in serum C-reactive protein and interleukin 6 levels. In eight of the 10 patients, the clear-cut benefit lasted for six weeks after the third infusion. A more recent study described a significant improvement in 21 AS patients treated with infliximab (26). Whether these encouraging results will be borne out in the long-term management of AS, and whether anti-TNF treatment can alter the progressive ankylosis of this disease over time, awaits further study.

ROBERT D. INMAN, MD

References

1. Ruof J, Sangha O, Stucki G. Comparative responsiveness of 3 functional indices in ankylosing spondylitis. J Rheumatol 1999;26:1959–1963.
2. Guillemin F, Challier B, Urlacher F, Vancon G, Pourel J. Quality of life in ankylosing spondylitis: validation of the AS-AIMS2, a modified arthritis impact measurement scales questionnaire. Arthritis Care Res 1999;12:157–162.

3. Leirisalo-Repo M, Helenius P, Hannu T, et al. Long term prognosis of reactive salmonella arthritis. Ann Rheum Dis 1997;56:516–520.

4. Martin DH, Mroczkowski TF, Dalu ZA, et al. A controlled trial of a single dose of azithromycin for the treatment of chlamydial urethritis and cervicitis. N Engl J Med 1992;327:921–925.

5. Bardin T, Enel C, Cornelis F, et al. Antibiotic treatment of venereal disease and Reiter's syndrome in a Greenland population. Arthritis Rheum 1992;35:190–194.

6. Lauhio A, Leirisalo-Repo M, Lahdevirta J, Saikku P, Repo H. Double-blind, placebo-controlled study of three-month treatment with lymecycline in reactive arthritis, with special reference to Chlamydia trachomatis. Arthritis Rheum 1991;34:6–14.

7. Wakefield D, McCluskey P, Verma M, Aziz K, Gatus B, Carr G. Ciprofloxacin treatment does not influence course or relapse rate of reactive arthritis and anterior uveitis. Arthritis Rheum 1999;42:1894–1897.

8. Sieper J, Fendler C, Laitko S, et al. No benefit of long-term ciprofloxacin treatment in patients with reactive arthritis and undifferentiated oligoarthritis. Arthritis Rheum 1999;42:1386–1396.

9. Dougados M, van der Linden S, Leirisalo-Repo M, et al. Sulfasalazine in the treatment of spondyloarthropathy. Arthritis Rheum 1995;38:618–627.

10. Clegg DO, Reda DJ, Weisman MH, et al. Comparison of sulfasalazine and placebo in the treatment of ankylosing sponylitis. Arthritis Rheum 1996;39:2004–2012.

11. Clegg DO, Reda DJ, Mejias E, et al. Comparison of sulfasalazine and placebo in the treatment of psoriatic arthritis. Arthritis Rheum 1996;39:2013–2020.

12. Clegg DO, Reda DJ, Weisman MH, et al. Comparison of sulfasalazine and placebo in the treatment of reactive arthritis. Arthritis Rheum 1996;39:2021–2027.

13. Clegg DO, Reda DJ, Abdellatif M. Comparison of sulfasalazine and placebo for the treatment of axial and peripheral articular manifestations of the seronegative spondyloarthopathies. Arthritis Rheum 1999;42:2325–2329.

14. Creemers MC, Franssen MJ, van de Putte LB, Gribnau FW, van Riel PL. Methotrexate in severe anklyosing spondylitis: an open study. J Rheumatol 1995;22:1104–1107.

15. Biasi D, Carletto A, Caramaschi P, Pacor ML, Maleknia T, Bambara LM. Efficacy of methotrexate in the treatment of anklyosing spondylitis: a three-year open study. Clin Rheumatol 2000;19:114–117.

16. Abu-Shakra M, Gladman DD, Thorne JC, Long J, Gough J, Farewell VT. Longterm methotrexate in psoriatic arthritis: clinical and radiological outcome. J Rheumatol 1995;22:241–245.

17. Gladman DD, Blake R, Brubacher B, Farewell VT. Chloroquine therapy in psoriatic arthritis. J Rheumatol 1992;19:1724–1726.

18. Mader R, Gladman DD, Long J, Gough J, Farewell VT. Does injectable gold retard radiologic evidence of joint damage in psoriatic arthritis? Clin Invest Med 1995;18:129–143.

19. Mahrle G, Schulze HJ, Farber L, Weidinger G, Steigleder GK. Low-dose, short-term cyclosporine versus etretinate in psoriasis: improvement of skin, nail, and joint involvement. J Am Acad Derm 1995;32:78–88.

20. Ho VC, Griffiths CE, Albrecht G, et al. Intermittent short courses of cyclosporin (Neoral) for psoriasis unresponsive to topical therapy: a 1-year multicentre, randomized study. Br J Dermatol 1999;141:283–291.

21. Clark CM, Kirby B, Morris AD, et al. Combination treatment of methotrexate and cyclosporin for severe recalcitrant psoriasis. Br J Dermatol 1999;141:279–282.

22. Dekker-Saeys BJ, Dijkmans BA, Tytgat GN. Treatment of spondyloarthropathy with 5-aminosalicylic acid (mesalazine): an open trial. J Rheumatol 2000;27:723–726.

23. Maksymowych WP, Jhangri GS, Leclerq S, Skeith K, Yan A, Russell AS. An open study of pamidronate in the treatment of refractory ankylosing spondylitis. J Rheumatol 1998;25:714–717.

24. Van den Bosch F, Kruithof E, Baeten D, De Keyser F, Mielants H, Veys EM. Effects of loading dose regimen of three infusions of chimeric monoclonal antibody to tumor necrosis factor alpha (infliximab) in spondyloarthropathy: an open pilot study. Ann Rheum Dis 2000;59:428–433.

25. Brandt J, Haibel H, Cornely D, et al. Successful treatment of active ankylosing spondylitis with the anti-tumor necrosis factor-α monoclonal antibody infliximab. Arthritis Rheum 2000;43:1346–1352.

26. Stone M, Salonen D, Lax M, Payne U, Lapp V, Inman D. Clinical and imaging correlates of response to treatment with infliximab in patients with Ankylosing spondylitis. J Rheumatol, in press.

12 INFECTIOUS DISORDERS
A. Septic Arthritis

Normal joints, diseased joints, and prosthetic joints are all vulnerable to bacterial infection, albeit to different degrees. Mortality rates among adults who contract nongonococcal joint infections range from 10% to greater than 50%. Among those who are accurately diagnosed and promptly treated, full recovery is possible, but poor outcome is common among those with preexisting arthritis, especially rheumatoid arthritis (RA). This chapter discusses the risk factors, pathogenesis, microbiology, clinical features, diagnosis, treatment, prognosis, outcome, and preventive measures of acute bacterial arthritis. Septic arthritis in children, gonococcal joint infection, and septic bursitis are discussed at the end of the chapter.

Risk Factors

A number of host factors predispose to septic arthritis. Compared with diseased or prosthetic joints, a normal joint is very resistant to infection. Independent risk factors identified in a prospective study of people attending an arthritis clinic include age older than 80 years, comorbid conditions (especially diabetes mellitus), rheumatoid arthritis, the presence of a prosthetic joint in the knee or hip, recent joint surgery, and skin infection (1).

Another important host factor that predisposes to septic arthritis is the immunosuppressed state, either as the result of illness or due to therapies that impair the immune system. Additional comorbid conditions that predispose to septic arthritis include liver cirrhosis, chronic renal failure, malignancies such as multiple myeloma and lymphoproliferative disorders, acquired immunodeficiency syndrome (AIDS), hemophilia, and transplanted organs. The association of mycoplasmal joint infection with hypogammaglobulinemia is intriguing (2). Adults with common variable immunodeficiency are susceptible to such infections.

People undergoing hemodialysis and intravenous drug abusers appear to be predisposed to bacterial joint infection at sites in the axial skeleton such as the sternoclavicular and sacroiliac joints.

Pathogenesis

In the primary care setting, septic arthritis occurs most commonly as a result of bacteremic seeding of the affected joint from an extra-articular site of infection. For example, *Staphylococcus aureus* in a knee joint may be the result of an infected skin lesion, or *Escherichia coli* septic arthritis may result from pyelonephritis caused by the *E. coli* microorganism. Less commonly, direct inoculation of the pathogen into a joint leads to septic arthritis. Examples include *Pasteurella multocida* infection of a finger joint or wrist as the result of a cat bite; *Pseudomonas aeruginosa* infection of a foot as the result of a nail puncturing the sole; or in rare instances, infection of a joint resulting from arthrocentesis or joint injection that introduces bacteria residing on the skin. The latter situation is estimated to occur at a rate 0.0002% (3). Other uncommon scenarios include injection of a drug or solution contaminated by microorganisms and the spread of infection into a joint from neighboring soft-tissue infection or periarticular osteomyelitis.

Orthopedic surgeons are more likely to encounter patients with joint infections as a result of trauma or surgical procedures. Examples of these include a penetrating injury or foreign body accidentally introduced into a joint, arthroscopic surgery (4), open reduction of fractures that involve the joint, and arthroplasties, including total joint replacement. Contamination of the wound at the time of elective surgery is rare because of the meticulous attention to aseptic techniques, the ultra-clean environment of operating rooms, and the common practice of perioperative antibiotic prophylaxis.

Late infections of prosthetic joints, usually defined as occurring one year or later after successful joint replacement, can result from contamination at the time of the implant surgery or as the result of bacterial seeding by transient or sustained bacteremia. Fortunately, this complication is uncommon. Patients with this late complication may present to their primary care physicians complaining of pain in a previously painless total joint replacement. Aseptic loosening of a prosthetic joint must be distinguished from infection causing prosthesis failure because the management of each requires different strategies.

Microbiology

The microbiology of agents infecting native joints differs in several ways from that of microorganisms causing prosthetic joint infections. Among nongonococcal causes of acute bacterial arthritis, the Gram-positive cocci are the major pathogens. The relative frequencies of the causative microorganisms for nongonococcal septic arthritis in adults are 75%–80% Gram-positive cocci and 15%–20% Gram-negative bacilli. *S. aureus* is the most common infective agent in both native and prosthetic joints. *S. epidermidis* is common in prosthetic infections but almost unheard of in native joint infections. Other than *S. aureus*, the streptococci including the pneumococcus are the most common Gram-positive aerobes. Anaerobic infections and coagulase-negative staphylococci are more common in prosthetic joint infections.

In the elderly, the Gram-negative bacilli may be a relatively more common cause of septic arthritis because people in this population are more likely to have comorbidities that predispose them to systemic Gram-negative bacillary infections. The elderly with chronic arthritis also have a high incidence of joint damage, making their joints more susceptible to infection. As a result, microorganisms usually regarded as nonpathogenic have been reported to cause septic arthritis. Invariably, in these cases, the hosts are severely immunocompromised and have many comorbidities.

Clinical Features

Septic arthritis is monarticular in 80%–90% of cases and polyarticular in 10%–20%. Large peripheral joints are infected more commonly than small ones. The tendency is for involvement of a single large joint, typically the knee. Thus, in the evaluation of a person presenting with an acute monoarthritis, septic arthritis always is a consideration, especially if the patient is febrile, appears toxic, or has an extra-articular site of bacterial infection (5). In the patient with an underlying inflammatory arthritis, such as rheumatoid arthritis, an acute exacerbation of joint inflammation, whether monarticular or polyarticular, must raise the suspicion of superimposed infection.

If septic arthritis is suspected, arthrocentesis is mandatory, and the synovial fluid should be examined carefully for evidence of bacterial infection. If the synovial-fluid cell count is extremely high – e.g., 100,000 white blood cells (WBC) per mm³ or greater – treatment for presumed septic arthritis should be initiated, pending result of the fluid culture. Pseudoseptic arthritis, an extremely inflammatory arthritis not due to bacterial infection, can be diagnosed only when one is confident that infectious causes have been excluded (6). The causes of pseudoseptic arthritis are listed in Table 12A-1. To confirm this diagnosis, a negative Gram-stained smear or a negative culture of the synovial fluid should be corroborated by negative blood cultures and perhaps, in the future, by a negative polymerase chain reaction (PCR) test for bacterial DNA in the synovial fluid (7).

Bacterial infection involving more than one joint is less common. In literature reviews, polyarticular infection may be more common in people with preexisting arthritis and may portend a less favorable outcome (8). *S. aureus* is again the major pathogen. People with rheumatoid arthritis and polyarticular septic arthritis have a mortality rate of >50% (9). More than one joint should be aspirated when infection is suspected to be present in multiple joints of a person with acute polyarthritis.

Laboratory Findings

The synovial fluid of a septic joint usually is purulent, with extremely high WBC counts where polymorphonuclear cells predominate (90% or greater). The WBC range can vary widely from a few thousand cells to more than 100,000 cells/mm³. The Gram-stained smear of the infected synovial fluid is positive 60%–80% of the time. Gram-positive microorganisms are identified more easily than Gram-negative ones. Although low glucose levels in synovial fluid suggest infection, these levels are neither very sensitive nor specific for a bacterial infection. Protein and glucose levels in synovial fluids often do not provide specific, useful data in the differential diagnosis of acute synovitis, and these measurements generally are no longer recommended (10). In addition to culturing for microorganisms, other tests that must be performed immediately on the synovial fluid include a cell count and its differential, a Gram-stained smear, and a wet preparation examined under polarizing microscopy. Using blood culture bottles to culture synovial fluid specimens may increase the yield of the offending microorganism (11). The main reasons for "false negative" culture results are prior use of antibiotics that can suppress microorganism growth and some microorganisms' fastidious growth requirements that may not be met in the laboratory. Blood cultures are positive in about one-half of the patients with nongonococcal septic arthritis (3).

The coexistence of crystal-induced inflammation and bacterial infection must not be overlooked. Fever can be due to acute crystal-induced synovitis or acute flare of rheumatoid arthritis without infection (12), but fever must not be attributed to underlying rheumatic disease without a diligent search for complicating bacterial infection in the inflamed joint.

The PCR test is an extremely sensitive technique and a powerful tool in molecular biology. Its utility in the diagnosis and management of many infectious diseases, includ-

TABLE 12A-1
Conditions that May Present as Pseudoseptic Arthritis

Rheumatoid arthritis
Juvenile rheumatoid arthritis
Gout
Pseudogout
Apatite-related arthropathy
Reactive arthritis
Psoriatic arthritis
Systemic lupus erythematosus
Sickle cell disease
Dialysis-related amyloidosis
Transient synovitis of the hip
Plant thorn synovitis
Metastatic carcinoma
Pigmented villonodular synovitis
Hemarthrosis
Neuropathic arthropathy

ing septic arthritis, still is being defined (13). To date, it appears useful in detecting bacterial DNA in joint infections where the pathogens are fastidious, slow-growing, or not able to be cultured. *Neisseria gonorrhoeae* and *Mycoplasma* are examples of microorganisms with fastidious growth requirements, and cultures may be negative in the presence of infection. The PCR test may be useful for detecting unculturable bacteria in a prosthetic joint, where the distinction between septic and aseptic loosening must be made before any revision can be undertaken (14). Determination by PCR test of bacterial DNA in serial samples of synovial fluid from an infected joint can confirm the eradication of infection (PCR becomes negative) or the persistence of infection (PCR remains positive, with high-intensity signal).

Treatment

Prompt treatment will cure infection, speed recovery, and decrease morbidity. If a presumptive diagnosis of septic arthritis has been made, and the appropriate samples for microbiologic studies have been collected, antibiotic treatment should begin immediately, even before the identity of the microorganism is known. The choice of antibiotic agent depends on results of the Gram-stained smear of the synovial fluid and the most likely causative microorganism, based on the entire clinical picture.

Narrow antibiotic coverage is provided if one suspects staphylococci and Gram-positive cocci are found on the synovial fluid smear. On the other hand, if the Gram-stained smear is nonrevealing and no clue is found after searching for an extra-articular source of infection in an elderly debilitated patient, broad antibiotic coverage against Gram-positive cocci and Gram-negative bacilli should be given. If an otherwise healthy, young, sexually active person presents with tenosynovitis and swelling of a wrist following two days of migratory joint pain, and if the Gram-stained smear reveals no visible bacteria, monotherapy against gonococcal infection is appropriate after culturing all portals of possible infection.

Knowing the antibiotic susceptibility profiles of bacteria and the prevalence of antibiotic resistance in one's geographic region facilitates selection of the best antimicrobial agent, pending culture and sensitivity data. After the microorganism is identified and any sensitivities to antimicrobial agents are known, therapy should continue with the most effective, safest, and least expensive agent. Whether to use home intravenous antibiotic services or change from intravenous to oral administration are decisions that should be made on a case-by-case basis, with the help of an infectious diseases consultant, if necessary.

During the initial few days, immobilization of the affected joint and effective analgesic medication will ensure patient comfort. Physical therapy should be instituted as soon as the patient can tolerate and undergo therapy to mobilize the inflamed joint. Involving the orthopedic surgeon and the physical therapist early in the course of treatment will facili-

tate the best choice of drainage procedure and result in the best functional outcome.

The infected joint space must be drained adequately to eradicate the infection, hasten recovery of lost function, and reduce pain. If sterilization of the joint space can be achieved rapidly, repeated needle aspirations may prove sufficient in some patients. However, surgical drainage may be necessary if needle aspiration is technically difficult or does not provide thorough drainage of the joint, sterilization of the joint fluid is delayed, the infected joint has been damaged by preexisting arthritis, or infected synovial tissue or bone needs debridement (15). Tidal lavage and arthroscopic procedures are intermediate steps that may benefit some patients and avoid the morbidity of arthrotomy. Clinical judgement and experience, accurate assessment of the patient's course, and willingness to explore other available and effective means of treatment will provide the best care.

The duration of antibiotic treatment has not been prospectively studied. For native joint infections, antibiotic treatment can be as brief as two weeks for uncomplicated infection by susceptible microorganisms. Treatment duration typically is more prolonged, between four and six weeks, for more serious infection in a compromised host. For prosthetic joint infections, the antibiotic course usually is quite protracted. Most cases will require that the infected prosthesis be removed. Antibiotic treatment is continued until the site is sterile before reimplantation is considered. Antibiotic-impregnated cement or beads sometimes are used in the reimplantation, during multistaged procedures or an exchange arthroplasty. In rare cases, antibiotic treatment is continued indefinitely when the risk of removing the infected prosthesis is too great and the microorganism responsible for the infection can be reasonably suppressed with an oral antibiotic.

Outcome

Common wisdom from retrospective observations suggests that certain factors portend poor outcome. Some of these factors are old age, virulent microorganism, delay in diagnosis or treatment, underlying joint disease, and site of infection (e.g., shoulder, hip). However, a prospective study identified only old age, preexisting joint disease, and the presence of a prosthetic device as negative prognostic factors (16).

Avoiding delays in diagnosis, ensuring adequate decompression to prevent osteonecrosis (e.g., infected hips in children), willingness to consider alternative drainage methods when progress is not being made, and being proactive with rehabilitation are within our control. Although evidence-based data are lacking, intuition suggests that these are important variables that may improve the outcome of patients with unfavorable prognostic factors.

Prevention

Opportunities to prevent septic arthritis are limited but should be kept in mind when treating patients with underlying arthritis, especially RA, or patients with total joint replacements. The American Dental Association (ADA) and American Academy of Orthopedic Surgeons (AAOS) in 1997 issued an advisory statement regarding the use of antibiotic prophylaxis for patients with total joint replacement when they undergo invasive dental procedures (17). The advisory states that antibiotic prophylaxis is not routinely indicated for most dental patients with total joint replacements. However, all people who have had a total joint replacement within two years and some immunocompromised patients with total joint replacements (who may be at higher risk for hematogenous infections) should be considered for antibiotic prophylaxis before undergoing dental procedures with a high bacteremic risk. The recommended antibiotic agents are based on an empiric regimen directed against the microorganisms most commonly responsible for late prosthetic joint infections.

The issue of the cost-effectiveness of antibiotic prophylaxis to prevent late infections in prosthetic joints remains extremely controversial. Clinical decision-making is difficult, if not impossible, due to the lack of accurate data about the incidence of this complication, the choice of antimicrobial agent, the effectiveness of prophylaxis when antibiotics are used, and the cost of the morbidity and mortality associated with an infected joint prosthesis. Arguments cited by the various medical societies and organizations are based on opinions of respected authorities, descriptive studies, and reports of expert committees. However, no long-term observational studies or prospective trials have been done, and the attitudes and practices of physicians and dentists regarding antibiotic prophylaxis vary widely. The incidence of late infection of a prosthetic joint as a result of procedure-related bacteremia appears to be extremely low, perhaps 10–100 cases per 100,000 patients with total joint replacement per year. The cost of providing antibiotic prophylaxis to all patients with total joint replacement before all procedures that are associated with transient bacteremia (any degree of bleeding at a site that normally is not sterile) is substantial. Until future studies provide definitive data on cost-effectiveness, the decision regarding the use of antibiotic prophylaxis must be based on the physician's estimation of the potential risks and benefits involved for a particular patient and the patient's understanding and decision after communicating with the physician (18).

A possible approach to antibiotic prophylaxis for people with prosthetic joints is outlined in Table 12A-2. Patients with total joint replacements should be aware that there is a small but real risk of the prosthesis becoming infected. Any local or systemic bacterial infections must be treated promptly to minimize the possible spread of the infection to the artificial joint. Common infections are skin lesions (e.g., abrasions and abscesses), urinary tract infections, and respiratory tract infections. When confronted with an elective procedure that is likely to lead to transient bacteremia, the opportunity to take an antibiotic agent beforehand is offered and discussed.

Septic Arthritis in Children

Septic arthritis in children is monarticular >90% of the time. The knee and the hip account for about two-thirds of all cases (19). A bacterial etiology is identified in 70% of the cases. Bacterial infections affecting the joints of neonates, infants, young children, and older children differ in clinical features and microbiology. Children younger than two years appear to be more susceptible to septic arthritis than are older children. Signs of joint disease in the neonate and infant may be minimal or absent. Failure to thrive or irritability may be the only clues to this serious infection. Fever may be absent or low-grade. Besides S. aureus, which is the most common cause of septic arthritis in all children, group B streptococci and Gram-negative microorganisms are important pathogens in the neonate and young infant. Candida and Gram-negative bacilli should be considered if the infection is nosocomially acquired.

In children aged 6 months to 5 years, Haemophilus influenzae had been a significant microorganism until the widespread use of the HIB vaccine. The conjugated vaccine was licensed in 1987, and has been approved since 1990 for use in infants younger than two months. Consequently, the incidence of H. influenzae septic arthritis in children has been declining since 1988. This is a gratifying success story for preventive medicine.

With the decline in H. influenzae septic arthritis, other microorganisms, such as Kingella kingae, may be seen more commonly. Gonococcal infection always must be considered in the sexually active adolescent with migratory arthritis and hemorrhagic or pustular skin lesions. As in adults, this disease is polyarticular in children in up to 50% of cases.

Osteomyelitis that complicates septic arthritis or results in septic arthritis is seen more frequently in the very young because the metaphyseal and epiphyseal blood vessels communicate, and the metaphyses of some long bones are within the joint capsule. Osteonecrosis can complicate septic arthritis of the hip in children. This can be prevented by early and effective decompression of the infected hip to reduce high intra-articular pressure that compromises the blood flow to the femoral head. The treatment outcome for septic arthritis in children is more favorable than in the adult. Late sequelae, such as leg-length discrepancy, limitation of joint mobility, and secondary degenerative joint disease, may be seen in 25% of cases.

Gonococcal Joint Disease

Whether joint infection caused by gonococcus (GC) is more common than nongonococcal septic arthritis depends on the population treated. Certainly, migratory arthritis and/or tenosynovitis with or without skin lesions in a sexually active adult should raise the suspicion of disseminated gonococcal infection (DGI). Besides the clinical presentation, infections caused by N. gonorrhoeae differ from nongonococcal disease in several ways. The person with GC

TABLE 12A-2
Counseling About Antibiotic Prophylaxis

1. You have these conditions (this condition or no condition) that may make you more susceptible to infections.

2. The procedure that you are about to undergo may cause bacteria to enter your bloodstream briefly. This normally results in no problems. Brushing your teeth or moving your bowel may result in a small number of bacteria entering your bloodstream briefly in a similar manner.

3. Taking this antibiotic drug beforehand may reduce the likelihood of the bacteria causing problems in the replaced joint, but there is no proof or guarantee that this preventive step is 100% effective.

4. The antibiotic medication is not very expensive, but taking it is associated with a slight risk of unpredictable side effects, similar to what you may encounter when taking other medications.

5. The risk of total joint replacement infection as the result of the procedure is very small (estimated to be between 1 in 10,000 and 1 in 1,000), and taking an antibiotic beforehand will reduce the risk.

6. If the artificial joint becomes infected, it usually means that it has to be removed, the infection has to be treated until it is cured, and then another total joint replacement undertaking can be considered.

7. In my opinion (recommend one of the three choices):
   You most likely do not need an antibiotic before this procedure.

   I don't have a strong feeling one way or the other. In other words, your choices of taking or not taking the antibiotic are equally reasonable.

   I believe that taking the antibiotic beforehand is worthwhile in your case.

arthritis often is a young, healthy adult, whereas the patient with nongonococcal arthritis usually has an underlying serious illness or is elderly. Women appear to be more susceptible to DGI than men.

In a recent series of 41 representative cases, only 13% of blood cultures were positive for GC (20). Synovial-fluid Gram stains often were negative and the culture yield from the synovial fluid also was relatively low (44%). Culture for GC at extra-articular sites may help confirm the diagnosis; genitourinary tract cultures were positive for GC in 86%, rectal culture in 39%, and throat culture in 7% of the 41 patients (20). Using PCR to detect Neisserial DNA in the joint fluid may be a rapid and sensitive means of diagnosing GC arthritis in the future (7).

Prompt response to antibiotic therapy is the rule, and residual problems in the affected joint are uncommon. Because resistance to penicillin is on the rise, it is wise to use a third-generation cephalosporin as the initial treatment of DGI.

Septic Bursitis

The bursae throughout the body facilitate joint mobility, and many are located in close proximity to the synovial joints. The superficial bursae are more susceptible than the deep bursae to bacterial infection (21). However, septic bur-

sitis does not place the adjacent joint at risk of damage by the infection unless the infection also affects the joint through an anatomic connection between the bursa and the joint. An example of this uncommon occurrence is the communication between an infected subacromial bursa and a septic shoulder. Other, rarer instances include communication of septic olecranon bursitis with a septic elbow in severe rheumatoid arthritis, and septic prepatellar bursitis with the knee joint through a traumatic fracture of the patella.

The most common sites of septic bursitis are the olecranon and the prepatellar bursa. The pathogenesis of septic bursitis is the direct extension of a superficial skin infection into the adjacent bursa. The activities that cause trauma or chronic pressure against the superficial bursae are many and varied. A partial list includes carpet laying, mining, plumbing, roofing, gardening, wrestling, and gymnastics. Trauma results in a bursal effusion that subsequently becomes infected. The same traumatic event frequently abrades the skin, which becomes colonized or infected by bacteria commonly found on the skin. *S. aureus* is therefore the most common bacteria responsible for >80% of all cases.

An accurate diagnosis begins with the history, followed by a physical examination that pinpoints the bursal swelling and sparing of the adjacent joint. A careful search for skin lesions at the portal of bacterial invasion often is informative. Extensive cellulitis surrounding the bursa and distal edema on the affected limb may be misleading. A bursal effusion or fluctuance should lead to aspiration of the content, which in septic bursitis, usually is inflammatory. If *S. aureus* is the culprit, the WBC counts vary widely, and the Gram-stained smear is positive for Gram-positive cocci. A bactericidal antistaphylococcal agent generally is the initial drug of choice. In mild infections, an oral agent may suffice, with outpatient follow-up to monitor the response and the need for repeat drainage. If the infection is severe and the patient appears toxic, admission to the hospital is advisable. Parenteral antibiotic treatment may be changed to the oral route once clinical response is achieved; the course of antibiotic treatment is then completed at home. A large-bore needle is necessary to drain the bursa when the content is thick or contains particulate matter. Rarely will surgical drainage or bursectomy be necessary. Treatment outcome for septic bursitis of the superficial bursae usually is satisfactory.

GEORGE HO, Jr., MD

References

1. Kaandorp CJ, Van Schaardenburg D, Krijnen P, Habbema JD, van de Laar MA. Risk factors for septic arthritis in patients with joint disease. A prospective study. Arthritis Rheum 1995; 38:1819–1825.

2. Franz A, Webster AD, Furr PM, Taylor-Robinson D. Mycoplasmal arthritis in patients with primary immunoglobulin deficiency: clinical features and outcome in 18 patients. Br J Rheumatol 1997;36:661–668.

3. Esterhai JL Jr, Gelb I. Adult septic arthritis. Orthop Clin North Am 1991;22:503–514.

4. Armstrong RW, Bolding F, Joseph R. Septic arthritis following arthroscopy: clinical syndromes and analysis of risk factors. Arthroscopy 1992;8:213–223.

5. Baker DG, Schumacher HR. Acute monoarthritis. N Engl J Med 1993;329:1013–1020.

6. Ho G Jr. Pseudoseptic arthritis. R I Med 1994;77:7–9.

7. Louie JS, Liebling MR. The polymerase chain reaction in infectious and post-infectious arthritis: a review. Rheum Dis Clin North Am 1998;24:227–236.

8. Dubost JJ, Fis I, Denis P, Lopitaux R, Soubrier M, Ristori JM, Bussiere JL, Sirot J, Sauvezie B. Polyarticular septic arthritis. Medicine 1993;72:296–310.

9. Epstein JH, Zimmermann B, Ho G Jr. Polyarticular septic arthritis. J Rheumatol 1986;13:1105–1107.

10. Shmerling RH, Delbanco TL, Tosteson ANA, Trentham DE. Synovial fluid tests. What should be ordered? JAMA 1990;264:1009–1014.

11. Von Essen R. Culture of joint specimens in bacterial arthritis. Impact of blood culture bottle utilization. Scand J Rheumatol 1997;26:293–300.

12. Pinals RS. Polyarthritis and fever. N Engl J Med 1994;330: 769–774.

13. Post JC, Ehrlich GD. The impact of the polymerase chain reaction in clinical medicine. JAMA 2000;283:1544–1546.

14. Mariani BD, Martin DS, Levine MJ, Booth RE Jr, Tuan RS. The Coventry Award. Polymerase chain reaction detection of bacterial infection in total knee arthroplasty. Clin Orthop 1996;331:11–22.

15. Ho G Jr. How best to drain an infected joint. Will we ever know for certain? J Rheumatol 1993;20:2001–2003.

16. Kaandorp CJ, Krijnen P, Moens HJ, Habbema JD, van Schaardenburg D. The outcome of bacterial arthritis: a prospective community-based study. Arthritis Rheum 1997; 40:884–892.

17. American Dental Association/American Academy of Orthopaedic Surgeons. Advisory statement: antibiotic prophylaxis for dental patients with total joint replacements. J Am Dent Assoc 1997;128:1004–1008.

18. Deacon JM, Pagliaro AJ, Zelicof SB, Horowitz HW. Prophylactic use of antibiotics for procedures after total joint replacement. J Bone Joint Surg Am 1996;78:1755–1770.

19. Fink CW, Nelson JD. Septic arthritis and osteomyelitis in children. Clin Rheum Dis 1986;12:423–435.

20. Wise CM, Morris CR, Wasilauskas BL, Salzer WL. Gonococcal arthritis in an era of increasing penicillin resistance: presentations and outcomes in 41 recent cases (1985–1991). Arch Intern Med 1994;154:2690–2695.

21. Zimmermann B III, Mikolich DJ, Ho G Jr. Septic bursitis. Semin Arthritis Rheum 1995;24:391–410.

INFECTIOUS DISORDERS
B. Viral Arthritis

Acute arthritis has long been recognized as a feature of some viral infections. Development of chronic arthralgia or arthritis following acute infection has spurred investigators to search for virus-induced immune-system alterations or persistent viral infections to explain chronic sequelae. The number of people in the rheumatic disease population with post-viral arthralgia/arthritis may be significant, but diagnosis of the acute infection rarely is confirmed by acute-phase serology or viral isolation because patients often present late in the disease course. As improvements in biotechnology provide simpler, more sensitive tests for viral diagnosis, and new antiviral treatments become available, specific viruses must be considered in the differential diagnosis of arthritis.

Parvovirus B19

Infection with human parvovirus, designated B19, may be responsible for as many as 12% of people presenting with recent-onset polyarthralgia or polyarthritis (1). B19 causes the common childhood exanthem erythema infectiosum, or fifth disease, which is characterized by "slapped cheeks" and a lacy or blotchy rash of the torso and extremities (Fig. 12B-1). The virus is widespread, and up to 60% of adults have serologic evidence of past infection. Outbreaks of erythema infectiosum typically occur in late winter and in spring, but summer and fall outbreaks also have been observed. Sporadic cases may occur throughout the year (2).

The B19 infection usually is asymptomatic or mild in children, but adults tend to have a more severe, flu-like illness. Adults usually lack the "slapped cheeks," and the reticular rash on the torso or extremities may be subtle or absent. Approximately 10% of children with fifth disease have arthralgias, and 5% have arthritis, usually short-lived. However, as many as 78% of infected, symptomatic adults develop joint symptoms. Arthralgia is more prominent than frank arthritis, but the distribution of involved joints is rheumatoid-like. Symmetric involvement of metacarpophalangeal, proximal interphalangeal, knee, wrist, and ankle joints is prominent. Patients usually experience sudden-onset polyarthralgia/arthritis, followed by improvement in two weeks. Joint symptoms in infected adults usually are self-limited, but up to 10% of symptomatic adults may have prolonged symptoms. Chronic arthropathy may last up to nine years, the longest follow-up that has been reported. Patients with chronic symptoms have intermittent flares, and only one-third are symptom-free between flares (1). Morning stiffness is prominent. About one-half of patients with chronic symptoms meet American College of Rheumatology diagnostic criteria for rheumatoid arthritis (see Appendix I).

Rheumatoid factor usually is absent in parvovirus B19 arthropathy, but transient, low-to-moderate titer rheuma-

toid factor, anti-DNA, antilymphocyte, or anticardiolipin antibodies may be found in some patients. Joint erosions and rheumatoid nodules have not been reported. Specific serologic diagnosis is possible only during a brief window of opportunity because anti-B19 IgM antibodies may be elevated for only two months following an acute infection. Joint symptoms occur one to three weeks following initial infection; anti-B19 IgM antibodies usually are present at the time of onset of rash or joint symptoms. The high prevalence of anti-B19 IgG antibodies in the adult population limits the diagnostic usefulness of IgG detection.

B19 has also been shown to cause most cases of transient aplastic crisis in patients with chronic hemolytic anemias, some cases of hydrops fetalis with fetal loss, and in immunocompromised patients, chronic bone-marrow suppression (3). B19 infection also has been associated with cases of Henoch-Schönlein purpura; thrombotic thrombocytopenic purpura; vasculitis; hepatitis; acute non-A, non-B, and non-C fulminant liver failure; and hemophagocytic syndrome. Treatment is limited to nonsteroidal anti-inflammatory agents.

Hepatitis Viruses

Hepatitis B virus (HBV) infection may cause an immune-complex–mediated arthritis. Significant viremia occurs early in infection; soluble immune complexes with circulating antihepatitis B surface antigen are formed as antihepatitis B surface-antigen antibodies are produced. Arthritis

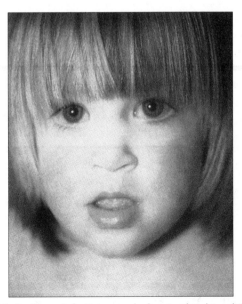

Fig. 12B-1. Erythema infectiosum rash showing bright red "slapped cheeks." Note that the rash spares the nasolabial folds. There may be circumoral pallor. Reprinted from Feder HM Jr. Fifth disease. N Engl J Med 1994;331:1062, with permission.

onset usually is sudden and often is severe. Joint involvement usually is symmetric and migratory, but it may start with simultaneous involvement of several joints and be additive. The joints of the hand and knee are affected most often, but wrists, ankles, elbows, shoulders, and other large joints may be involved. Arthritis and urticaria may precede jaundice by days or weeks and may persist several weeks after jaundice. Although arthritis usually is limited to the preicteric prodrome, patients who develop chronic active hepatitis or chronic HBV viremia may have recurrent arthralgias or arthritis. Polyarteritis nodosa frequently is associated with chronic HBV viremia (4). In rare cases, arthralgia and rash are associated with acute hepatitis A infection, and cryoglobulinemia is associated with chronic hepatitis A infection (5).

Hepatitis C virus (HCV) infection is the leading cause of chronic hepatitis, cirrhosis, and liver transplantation in the United States. Between 2.7 and 4 million Americans are estimated to be infected. HCV is acquired parenterally. Sexually transmitted infection is unusual. HCV became epidemic in the 1960s, rising from 18 cases per 100,000 population before 1965, to 130 cases per 100,000 in 1989. The introduction in 1989 of serologic tests for blood donors helped decrease the incidence of new infections. However, because the latent period from infection to symptomatic liver disease or extrahepatic manifestations may be as long as 15 to 20 years, only now are late sequelae beginning to present in significant numbers.

The pathologic hallmark of chronic HCV infection is inflammatory destruction of hepatocytes and progressive fibrosis. Serum transaminases may be normal despite active liver disease, especially early in the course of disease. Mixed cryoglobulinemia, types II and III, is a common extrahepatic sequela of HCV infection. Rheumatoid factor often is present and titers may be high. The classic triad of essential mixed cryoglobulinemia consisting of arthritis, palpable purpura, and cryoglobulins is caused in most cases by HCV infection. Cutaneous vasculitis often occurs, and larger vessels also may be affected. Membranoproliferative glomerulonephritis occurs in people with HCV infection and type II cryoglobulinemia. Interferon-α (3–5 million units subcutaneously twice weekly) has been used to some effect in controlling viral titers and cryoglobulinemia. Interferon-α and ribavirin combination therapy is being evaluated for therapy of HCV infection, but its efficacy in cryoglobulinemia remains to be determined. There is concern that interferon-α may exacerbate underlying autoimmune processes, such as autoimmune thyroiditis or rheumatoid arthritis. Corticosteroids and cyclophosphamide often are required for control of vasculitis, despite reservations about using these agents in the setting of chronic viral infection (6).

Rubella Virus

Rubella virus is the sole member of the genus rubivirus in the Togaviridae family of RNA viruses. Rubella infection leads to a high incidence of joint complaints in adults, espe-

cially in women. Joint symptoms may occur one week before or after onset of the characteristic rash. Joint involvement usually is symmetric and may be migratory, resolving over a few days to two weeks. Arthralgias are more common than frank arthritis, and stiffness is prominent. The proximal interphalangeal and metacarpophalangeal joints of the hands, knees, wrists, ankles, and elbows are involved most frequently. Periarthritis, tenosynovitis, and carpal tunnel syndrome are known complications. In some patients, symptoms may persist for several months or years (7,8).

Live attenuated vaccines have been used in rubella vaccination. A high frequency of postvaccination arthralgia, myalgia, arthritis, and paresthesia has been associated with all vaccine preparations. The HPV77/DK12 strain was the most arthritogenic of the vaccine strains available in the United States. The currently used vaccine, RA 27/3, may cause postvaccination joint symptoms in as many as 15% or more of recipients (8). The pattern of joint involvement is similar to that of natural infection. Arthritis usually occurs two weeks postinoculation and lasts less than a week. However, symptoms may persist in some patients for more than a year. In children, two syndromes of rheumatologic interest may occur. In "arm syndrome," a brachial radiculoneuritis causes arm and hand pain and dysesthesias that are worse at night. "Catcher's crouch" syndrome is a lumbar radiculoneuropathy characterized by popliteal fossa pain on arising in the morning. Those affected assume a catcher's crouch position with flexed knees. The pain gradually decreases through the day. Both syndromes occur one to two months postvaccination. The initial episode may last up to two months, but recurrences usually are shorter in duration. Episodes of catcher's crouch syndrome may recur for up to one year, but there is no permanent damage (8,9).

Retroviruses

Several musculoskeletal syndromes have been described in people infected with human immunodeficiency virus (HIV) (10). The incidence and prevalence of these rheumatic diseases, such as Reiter's syndrome and psoriatic arthritis, may vary between populations studied and may depend on geography, mode of HIV transmission, exposure to different infectious agents, other risk factors, and patient ascertainment (11). Reiter's syndrome may have a prevalence as high as 11% in some HIV-infected populations. These cases differ from idiopathic Reiter's syndrome in that sacroiliitis and anterior uveitis are not present, and patients do not present with the classic triad of arthritis, urethritis, and uveitis. The prevalence of HLA-B27 positivity appears to be lower in the HIV-infected patients, compared with non-HIV–associated Reiter's patients (12,13).

In Africa, where the route of HIV transmission is predominantly heterosexual, approximately 40% of HIV patients with joint symptoms have Reiter's syndrome, and another 40% have a pauciarticular presentation without extra-articular features characteristic of Reiter's syndrome

(14,15). In the United States, psoriatic arthritis limited to a pattern of asymmetric oligoarthritis may be seen in as many as one-third of HIV infected patients with psoriasis, but the overall incidence of psoriasis does not appear to be increased significantly. Whether the different patterns of rheumatic disease expression are attributable to HIV infection itself or coinfection with other agents remains controversial. The caprine arthritis-encephalitis virus, a goat retrovirus, causes an inflammatory destructive arthritis and lends support to the notion that HIV infection alone may have musculoskeletal manifestations.

Initial HIV infection may be associated with a transient flu-like illness with arthralgias. Later, four pain syndromes not associated with synovitis may be seen. An acute symmetric polyarthritis involving the small joints of the hands and the wrists, with periosteal new bone formation around the involved joints, has been described in a very small number of patients. Periosteal new bone formation is a feature not seen in rheumatoid arthritis. A subacute oligoarticular arthritis, primarily of the knees and ankles, may cause severe arthralgia and disability, but it is transient, peaks in intensity within one to six weeks, and responds to nonsteroidal anti-inflammatory agents. The synovial fluid is noninflammatory, although mononuclear cell infiltrates may be seen in the synovium of the involved joints. As many as 10% of people infected with HIV may experience a "painful articular syndrome," which is characterized by intermittent severe joint pain predominantly of the shoulders, elbows, and knees. The pain may be incapacitating and require short-term narcotic analgesics, but episodes typically last less than a day. Fibromyalgia also has been reported in HIV-infected people, with prevalence cited at 29% in one series. The role of HIV and other agents in these pain syndromes remains to be clarified (11).

Human T-cell leukemia virus (HTLV) is endemic in Japan, where it has been associated with oligoarthritis and a nodular rash. Patients have positive serologies for anti-HTLV antibodies, and type-C viral particles may be seen in skin lesions. The presence of atypical synovial cells with lobulated nuclei and T-cell synovial infiltrates suggests direct involvement of the synovial tissue by the leukemic process (16). People infected with HTLV may have sialadenitis, but typically lack the autoantibodies, such as anti-SSA or anti-SSB, seen in Sjögren's syndrome.

Alphaviruses

The alphavirus genus of the Togaviridae family includes a number of arthritogenic viruses responsible for major epidemics of febrile polyarthritis in Africa, Australia, Europe, and Latin America. All are mosquito-borne, the specific species depending on the virus and the locale. The known major viral pathogens in this genus include Sindbis virus, Chikungunya fever virus, O'nyong-nyong virus, Ross River virus, Barmah Forest virus, and Mayaro virus (17,18). Although these viruses are not endemic to the United States, the recent emergence of the West Nile virus in the north-

eastern United States underscores the need to be cognizant of these infections.

Sindbis virus, discovered in a *Culex univittatus* mosquito in Egypt in 1952, was associated with five cases of vesicular rash in Uganda in 1961 and, subsequently, with epidemic arthralgia and rash in South Africa and Australia. There is a high seroprevalence of anti-Sindbis virus antibody in Africa and Asia, where sporadic cases and small outbreaks occur. In Europe, disease occurs in northern European forests; it is known as Okelbo disease in Sweden, Pogosta disease in Finland, and Karelian fever in the Karelian Isthmus of Russia. Sindbis virus infection is characterized by low-grade fever, malaise, joint and tendon pain, myalgia, and rash. The rash is maculopapular, and it involves the torso and extremities but spares the face. The rash can evolve to include vesicles and pustules that may be hemorrhagic, especially on the hands and feet. Diagnosis is confirmed by specific serology. Recovery is full, but may be prolonged. The rash may recur during convalescence.

Chikungunya (Swahili for "that which bends up") fever virus causes sporadic cases and large-scale outbreaks of febrile arthritis. It is transmitted from its reservoir hosts (baboons, monkeys, and, in Senegal, *Scotophilus* bats) to man by *Aedes* mosquitoes in south Africa, west-central Africa, Thailand, Vietnam, and India. Following a three- to 12-day incubation period, Chikungunya fever virus causes abrupt onset of fever (as high as 104° F) that lasts two to four days, a flushed appearance for one to two days, headache, myalgia, nausea, vomiting, coryza, lymphadenopathy, conjunctivitis, photophobia, retrobulbar pain, and sudden severe pain in one or more joints. The wrists and ankles are affected most commonly, followed by metacarpophalangeal and proximal interphalangeal joints, knee, distal interphalangeal joints, shoulders, elbows, and neck. Synovial fluid shows decreased viscosity with poor mucin clot and 2000–5000 white cells/mm³. Joint erosions do not occur. A maculopapular skin eruption occurs two to four days after onset. Petechiae may occur, and tourniquet sign may be positive. Diagnosis is confirmed by serology showing high-titer Chikungunya antibody. Acute disease resolves within 10 days, but joint pain and swelling may last weeks to months. Approximately 10% of patients have chronic or recurrent joint symptoms.

O'nyong-nyong virus first appeared in an outbreak in northwest Uganda in 1959 and quickly spread by *Anopheles* mosquitoes to Kenya, Tanzania, Sudan, Nyasaland, Zaire, and the Central African Republic at a rate of spread of 1.7 km/day, ultimately affecting 2 million people before the outbreak ended in 1962. The infection rate was 90%, with a greater than 70% clinical attack rate. Following an incubation period of up to 28 days, infected individuals developed sudden onset headache, retro-orbital pain, chills, and symmetric, severe polyarthralgia. The polyarthralgia was disabling, hence the term O'nyong-nyong ("joint breaker" in the Ugandan Acholi dialect). A majority of patients developed a morbilliform rash, often pruritic, by day four of the illness. Facial involvement, including conjunctivitis, was seen in 60%–70% of patients. Postcervical lymphadenitis often was prominent. Mild fever lasted as long as five days; one-third had fever greater than 101° F. Residual joint pain often persisted. After the resolution of the 1959–1962 epidemic, O'nyong-nyong fever was not detected again until a new outbreak in northwestern Uganda in 1997.

Ross river virus is responsible for epidemics of acute febrile polyarthritis in the islands of the South Pacific, including Australia and New Zealand, where it is endemic. The *Aedes vigilex* mosquito transmits the virus. Outbreaks occur most frequently in the late summer and fall. Patients experience sudden-onset chills, arthralgias, myalgias, mild fever, and joint pain. Wrist, ankle, metacarpophalangeal, interphalangeal, knee, and elbow joints are affected most commonly. The majority of patients develop a macular, papular, or maculopapular rash, and vesicular or petechial lesions also may be seen. Most patients improve within two to three days, but for as long as one year, some may have numerous recurrences of arthralgias, joint swelling, and weakness that steadily decrease in severity. Barmah Forest virus is another alphavirus originally isolated from mosquitoes in Australia and recently shown to cause febrile polyarthritis (17).

Haemogogus mosquitoes transmit Mayaro virus from its monkey reservoir to humans in the South American tropical rain forest. Mayaro virus was first recognized in Trinidad in 1954. It causes epidemics and sporadic cases in the Bolivia, Brazil, and Peru nexus. An outbreak in Belterra, Brazil, in 1988 affected 800 of 4,000 exposed latex gatherers with a clinical attack rate of 80%. Patients had sudden onset of fever, headache, dizziness, chills, and arthralgias in the wrists, fingers, ankles, and toes. About 20% had joint swelling. Unilateral inguinal lymphadenopathy was seen in some patients. Leukopenia was common. During the first one to two days of illness, viremia was present. After two to five days, fever resolution was associated with onset of a maculopapular rash on the trunk and extremities. The rash lasted about three days. Recovery was complete, although some patients had persistent arthralgias at two months. Mayaro virus has been isolated from a bird in Louisiana, and the diagnosis has been made in Americans who return from travel in the endemic area.

Other Viruses

Apart from specific viral infections in which arthralgia and/or arthritis typically is a prominent feature, joint involvement occasionally is seen in a host of commonly encountered viral syndromes. Children with varicella have been reported, rarely, to develop brief monarticular or pauciarticular arthritis that is thought to be viral in origin. This condition is different from the occasional septic arthritis that is due to contiguous bacterial spread from an infected vesicle. Adults who develop mumps occasionally develop small-joint and large-joint synovitis that may last for several weeks. Arthritis may precede or follow parotitis by up to four weeks.

Infection with adenovirus and coxsackieviruses A9, B2, B3, B4, and B6 have been associated with recurrent episodes of polyarthritis, pleuritis, myalgia, rash, pharyngitis, myocarditis, and leukocytosis. Epstein-Barr virus-associated mononucleosis frequently is accompanied by polyarthralgia, but frank arthritis is rare. Polyarthritis, fever, and myalgias due to echovirus infection have been reported in only a few cases. Arthritis associated with herpes simplex virus or cytomegalovirus infection also is rare. A severe inflammatory arthritis with cytomegalovirus in synovial fluid may occur after bone-marrow transplantation. Vaccinia virus has been associated with postvaccination knee arthritis in only two reported cases.

STANLEY J. NAIDES, MD

References

1. White DG, Woolf AD, Mortimer PP, Cohen BJ, Blake DR, Bacon PA. Human parvovirus arthropathy. Lancet 1985;1: 419–421.
2. Naides SJ. Parvoviruses. In: Spector S, Hodinka RL, Young SA (eds). Manual of Clinical Virology, 3rd edition. New York: Elsevier, 2000.
3. Naides SJ, Scharosch LL, Foto F, Howard EJ. Rheumatologic manifestations of human parvovirus B19 infection in adults. Initial two-year clinical experience. Arthritis Rheum 1990;33: 1297–1309.
4. Sergent JS. Extrahepatic manifestations of hepatitis B infection. Bull Rheum Dis 1983;33:1–6.
5. Inman RD, Hodge M, Johnston ME, Wright J, Heathcote J. Arthritis, vasculitis, and cryoglobulinemia associated with relapsing hepatitis A virus infection. Ann Intern Med 1986; 105:700–703.
6. Liang TJ, Hoofnagle JH (eds). Hepatitis C. San Diego: Academic Press, 2000.
7. Weibel RE, Benor DE. Chronic arthropathy and musculoskeletal symptoms associated with rubella vaccines. A review of 124 claims submitted to the National Vaccine Injury Compensation Program. Arthritis Rheum 1996;39:1529–1534.
8. Howson CP, Howe CJ, Fineberg HV, eds. Adverse Effects of Pertussis and Rubella Vaccines. A Report of the Committee to Review the Adverse Consequences of Pertussis and Rubella Vaccines. Washington, DC: National Academy Press, 1991.
9. Schaffner W, Fleet WF, Kilroy AW, et al. Polyneuropathy following rubella immunization: a follow-up study and review of the problem. Am J Dis Child 1974;127:684–688.
10. Cuellar ML. HIV infection-associated inflammatory musculoskeletal disorders. Rheum Dis Clin North Am 1998;24: 403–421.
11. Calabrese LH. Human immunodeficiency virus (HIV) infection and arthritis. Rheum Dis Clin North Am 1993;19:477–488.
12. Itescu S. Adult immunodeficiency and rheumatic disease. Rheum Dis Clin North Am 1996;22:53–73.
13. Berman A, Reboredo G, Spindler A, Lasala ME, Lopez H, Espinoza LR. Rheumatic manifestations in populations at risk for HIV infection: the added effect of HIV. J Rheumatol 1991;18:1564–1567.

14. *Adebajo A, Davis P. Rheumatic diseases in African blacks. Semin Arthritis Rheum 1994;24:139–153.*
15. *Davis P, Stein M. Human immunodeficiency virus related connective tissue diseases: a Zimbabwean perspective. Rheum Dis Clin North Am 1991;17:89–97.*
16. *Nishioka K, Nakajima T, Hasunuma T, et al. Rheumatic manifestation of human leukemic virus infection. Rheum Dis Clin North Am 1993;19:489–503.*
17. *Johnston RE, Peters CJ. Alphaviruses. In: Fields BN, Knipe DM, Howley PM, et al. (eds). Virology, 3rd edition. New York: Raven Press, 1996; pp 843-898.*
18. *Nash P, Harrington T. Acute Barmah Forest polyarthritis. Aust N Z J Med 1991;21:737–738.*

INFECTIOUS ARTHRITIS
C. Lyme Disease

Lyme disease is a multisystem inflammatory disease caused by the tick-borne spirochete *Borrelia burgdorferi* (1). It first was called Lyme arthritis in a report describing a cluster of cases of "juvenile rheumatoid arthritis" in three towns – including Lyme, Connecticut – on the east bank of the Connecticut River (2). It was noted that the arthritis often was preceded by a distinctive skin rash, subsequently recognized as erythema migrans (EM). In time, the term Lyme disease was adopted to describe the multisystem nature of the illness.

Epidemiology

Currently, more than 90% of all Lyme disease in the United States is reported from eight states: New York, New Jersey, Connecticut, Rhode Island, Massachusetts, Pennsylvania, Wisconsin, and Minnesota. Within these states, the distribution is not uniform; there are endemic areas and areas where the risk of Lyme disease is negligible. Visitors to an endemic area can acquire infection and return to their homes in nonendemic areas for clinical presentation and diagnosis.

In 1982, a spirochete was isolated from ticks captured on eastern Long Island (an area endemic for Lyme disease), and the same type of spirochete was grown from plasma and clinical samples of infected humans (3,4). The spirochete was named *Borrelia burgdorferi*. Three etiologic agents for Lyme disease are included within the category *B. burgdorferi sensu lato*: *B. burgdorferi sensu stricto*, *B. afzelii* (formerly known as VS461), and *B. garinii*. All are present in Europe and Asia, but only *sensu stricto* has been identified in North America. Differences between the organisms and the immunogenetics of the affected human populations have been implicated as causes for the differences between European and North American Lyme disease.

Recent polymerase chain reaction (PCR) studies have identified the DNA of *B. burgdorferi* in museum specimen rodents obtained on Cape Cod at the turn of the century. There is reason to believe that Lyme disease has been present from at least the 1960s in the Northeast, e.g., "Montauk knee" and reports of EM-like lesions. The recent increase in Lyme disease likely is related to a number of factors, including growth of deer and tick populations, expansion of endemic areas due to changes in land use, and movement of people into endemic areas. As the endemic areas grow and the number of cases and concern about the disease increase, there has been an alarming trend toward over-diagnosis.

When Lyme disease first was described, the vector in the Northeast was identified as *I. dammini*, which was thought to be different from *I. scapularis* in the Southeast and Midwest. Subsequent studies suggest that there is only a single species, with the morphologic variation *I. scapularis*. The vector in the Pacific states is *I. pacificus* (the black-legged tick). *I. ricinus* and *I. persulcatus* are the vectors in Europe and Asia, respectively. Only Ixodid ticks are known to spread *B. burgdorferi*.

Pathogenesis

How *B. burgdorferi* causes Lyme disease is unclear. The organism does not make toxins or cause local tissue damage. It may bind to and activate host proteolytic enzymes, allowing it to escape the inoculation site and disseminate (5), possibly within days of the local infection. *B. burgdorferi* has been identified in EM lesions, myocardium, and spinal and synovial fluids, by culture, PCR, and histologic examination. It is likely that poorly degraded antigens on dead or effete organisms perpetuate inflammation. Local cytokine production may cause persistence of the local immune reaction and may modify local cells' immune and other functions. There is an immunogenetic linkage of chronic Lyme arthritis with HLA-DR4 and secondarily with HLA-DR2 (6), although how this link is involved in the pathogenesis of the synovitis and its persistence is not clear.

Vasculitis has been implicated in some cases of peripheral neuropathy, and a vascular lesion resembling *endarteritis obliterans* has been identified in meninges and synovium. Early in Lyme disease there is polyclonal B-cell activation, with immune complex and cryoglobulin production. However, because no illness resembling serum sickness occurs, the immune complexes do not appear to be pathogenic. In neurologic Lyme disease, in vitro evidence implicates molecular mimicry as a mechanism; the organism's flagellin contains an epitope that cross-reacts with a human axonal protein, and a monoclonal antibody to this epitope modifies neural cell lines in vitro (7).

Clinical Features

The clinical manifestations of Lyme disease can be divided into three phases: early localized, early disseminated, and late disease. This division is somewhat arbitrary because a patient can have features of different phases at the same time. There are many examples of patients presenting with late-disease features as the first manifestations of Lyme disease.

Early Localized Disease

Early localized disease includes EM and associated findings (8). Erythema migrans occurs in up to 90% of patients, essentially always within one month of the tick bite. Only about 30% of patients recall the tick bite at the site of the EM lesion, which generally is found in or near the axilla, inguina, or belt line. Erythema migrans usually is asymptomatic, although it may burn, itch, or hurt. Typically, the rash expands over the course of a few days, and there may be central clearing, or the EM may be uniformly red. Only a minority of patients have the so-called "classic" bull's-eye lesion. Mimics of EM include fixed drug eruption, ringworm, tick- or arthropod-bite reaction, granuloma annulare, and cellulitis. Approximately one-half of patients with EM have multiple skin lesions due to spirochetemia.

Patients with early localized disease may describe nonspecific complaints resembling a viral syndrome, including fever, fatigue, malaise, headache, myalgias, and arthralgias. Physical examination occasionally reveals regional or generalized lymphadenopathy or hepatosplenomegaly. Musculoskeletal complaints were reported by approximately 80% of people with EM (including 20% with arthralgias) who had not received prior antibiotic therapy (9). Intermittent, migratory episodes of polyarthritis in a pattern that mimicked juvenile rheumatoid arthritis occurred in 50% of the original cluster of cases of "Lyme arthritis."

Early Disseminated Disease

Early disseminated disease occurs days to months after the tick bite, and may occur without preceding EM. The two most common manifestations are cardiac and neurologic involvement. In the absence of treatment, approximately 8% of people with EM will develop cardiac manifestations, including heart block of any degree (or combination of degrees) and mild myopericarditis. In the vast majority of cases, cardiac disease begins to resolve during or even before antibiotic therapy, although there is evidence suggesting that B. burgdorferi, in rare cases, can cause persisting heart block. In Europe, B. burgdorferi is said to cause chronic cardiomyopathy, although that has not been the experience in the United States.

Neurologic damage occurs in about 10% of people with untreated EM and includes lymphocytic meningitis, cranial nerve palsies (especially the facial nerve, occasionally bilateral), and radiculoneuritis. Meningitis typically resolves spontaneously. Treatment of early disseminated neurologic disease can speed resolution and prevent progression to later features of Lyme disease. In addition to the more common neurologic findings, mononeuritis multiplex, plexitis, and myelitis have been described.

Late Disease

Late disease occurs months to years after onset of infection and is not necessarily preceded by other features of Lyme disease. The chronic arthritis of Lyme disease usually is monarticular, affecting the knee. It occurs in approximately 10% of patients and can cause erosion of cartilage and bone. Chronic arthritis due to B. burgdorferi typically lasts for five to eight years, although brief episodes of arthralgia may persist thereafter. By the time patients develop Lyme arthritis, they typically are strongly seropositive. The incidence of arthritis in patients appropriately treated with antibiotics for earlier features of Lyme disease is not known, but is certainly quite low.

Late neurologic features of B. burgdorferi infection, called tertiary neuroborreliosis (drawing on possible analogies with tertiary neurosyphilis), include encephalopathy, neurocognitive dysfunction, and peripheral neuropathy (10). The encephalopathy may be subtle, causing cognitive, mood, and sleep disturbances. Neuropsychological testing can demonstrate changes suggestive (but not diagnostic) of Lyme disease, and such testing also can provide the basis for cognitive rehabilitation, should it prove necessary. Patients may complain of distal paresthesias or radicular pain; for the former, somatosensory evoked potentials may be useful in identifying changes, whereas nerve conduction velocity/electromyography studies help with the latter. Spinal fluid changes include elevated levels of protein and specific antibodies; lymphocytic pleocytosis usually is not present. People with neuroborreliosis due to B. Burgdorferi typically are strongly seropositive.

Lymphocytoma and acrodermatitis chronica atrophicans, more common in Europe than in the United States, are established cutaneous features of B. burgdorferi infection (11,12). Other clinical problems linked to Lyme disease include panniculitis resembling erythema nodosa, myositis, bursitis and tendinitis, liver disease (mild hepatitis in early Lyme disease), inflammation of various structures of the eye, and splenitis (13). Nonspecific complaints, such as headache, fatigue, and arthralgia, may persist after treatment of Lyme disease, often lingering for months with slow, unaided resolution.

Lyme Disease and Pregnancy

Pregnancy complicated by Lyme disease remains a major concern. Initial case reports suggest that maternal–fetal transmission might cause congenital anomalies or fetal demise (14). However, where Borrelial forms have been found in fetal tissues, there was no inflammation, in marked contrast to the histologic findings of inflammation in congenital lues. Large-scale prospective studies have suggested that there is little, if any, risk to the fetus, and have concluded that there is no definable "congenital Lyme disease syndrome" (15,16).

Laboratory Findings

The diagnosis of Lyme disease should be based on a history and objective physical findings explicitly suggesting the diagnosis, which then can be confirmed by serologic testing. An enzyme-linked immunosorbent assay (ELISA) is used to screen for antibodies to *Borrelia*. The current practice is to confirm all positive or equivocal ELISA results with Western blot analysis. Individuals with positive ELISA not corroborated by Western blot are considered to have false-positive ELISA results. False-positive ELISA results occur in up to 5% of the population, and they have been reported in patients with other spirochetal infections (e.g., relapsing fever, syphilis, pinta, yaws, bejel, leptospirosis), Epstein-Barr virus infection, nonspirochetal endocarditis, rheumatoid arthritis, and systemic lupus erythematosus. Even if a positive ELISA is corroborated by a positive Western blot, the significance of true seropositivity in a healthy person has not been established. Criteria for interpreting a Western blot analysis were proposed by the Centers for Disease Control and Prevention (Table 12C-1).

There are numerous considerations for laboratory testing for Lyme disease. Antibody responses may be undetectable early in infection for a number of reasons. If disease duration is less than six weeks, the person may be seronegative simply because the immune system has not had sufficient time to mount a humoral response to the organism. Early, even incomplete, antibiotic therapy may abrogate the humoral response, rendering the patient permanently seronegative, despite infection. Because serologic reactivity may persist long after the infection has been eradicated, follow-up testing may give clinically irrelevant information; most people with later manifestations are strongly seropositive, even if they have received antibiotics. Thus, seronegativity in patients with features indicative of late Lyme disease should raise doubts about that diagnosis. Finally, it is possible to be seropositive and have clinical problems that are explained by another disease. That is, seropositivity does not prove causality, and current problems may not be due to *B. burgdorferi*.

Neuropsychologic testing, electrophysiologic testing (cardiac and neurologic), and brain magnetic resonance imaging can be helpful in documenting objective abnormalities, but none is a specific marker of damage due to *B. burgdorferi*. Testing of inflammatory fluids (e.g., synovial or spinal fluid) for the presence of specific antibodies is the only way to be assured that inflammation is due to *B. burgdorferi*. Typical joint fluid findings include a white cell count of 25,000 cells/mm^3, most of which are polymorphonuclear cells. In spinal fluid, the predominant cell type is mononuclear.

Treatment

Antibiotic treatment of *B. burgdorferi* infection in early disease usually prevents progression and is curative (1). Suggested drug regimens for each feature of Lyme disease are given in Table 12C-2. There is no evidence to suggest the need for oral therapy in follow-up to intravenous therapy, nor for more prolonged, higher dose, or combination therapies. Of note, 5%–10% of patients with early disease experience a mild Jarisch-Herxheimer reaction within the first days of treatment, lasting for less than a day. There are unsubstantiated reports of patients with "recurrent Herxheimer reactions" every four weeks, due to a hypothesized in vivo cyclicity of the organism, but there is no proof that such a phenomenon really exists. Therapy during pregnancy should be as is appropriate for the features of Lyme disease, although some clinicians treat such women parenterally. Current studies suggest that the risk of contracting Lyme disease from a known tick bite is very small,

TABLE 12C-1
Criteria For Positive Western Blot (Immunoblot) Analysis in the Serologic Confirmation of *Borrelia burgdorferi* Infection (Lyme Disease)[a]

	Isotype tested	Bands to be considered
First few weeks of infection	IgM	Two of the following eight: 18, 21, 28, 37, 41, 58, 93 kDa OR Two of the following three: ospC (23), 39, 41[b] kDa
After first weeks of infection	IgG	Five of the following 10: 18, 21, 28, 30, 39, 41, 45, 58, 66, 93 kDa

[a] Criteria derived from Dressler F, Whalen JA, Reinhardt BN, Steere AC. Western blotting in the serodiagnosis of Lyme disease. J Infect Dis 1993;167:392–400.

[b] Alternative criteria for immunoglobulin M reactivity, proposed by a Centers for Disease Control and Prevention conference. Other points noted at that conference were the need for standardization of antigen preparation and techniques.

TABLE 12C-2
Current Recommendations for Therapy in Lyme Disease

Oral therapy of early localized Lyme disease

Adults Drug	Dosage	Duration
Doxycycline[a]	100 mg p.o., b.i.d.	3–4 weeks[d]
Tetracycline[a,b]	250–500 mg p.o., q.i.d.	3–4 weeks[d]
Amoxicillin[b,c]	250 to 500 mg p.o., q.i.d.	3–4 weeks[d]
Children		
Amoxicillin	40 mg/kg/day, divided dose	3–4 weeks[d]
Erythromycin	30 mg/kg/day, divided dose	3–4 weeks[d]
Penicillin G	25–50 mg/kg/day, divided dose	3–4 weeks[d]

Intravenous therapy of early disseminated and late Lyme disease[e]

Adults Drug	Dosage	Duration
Third generation cephalosporins		
Ceftriaxone	2 g q.d. or 1 g b.i.d.	2–4 weeks
Cefotaxime	3 g b.i.d.	2–4 weeks
Penicillin		
Penicillin G	20 million U in 6 divided doses	2–4 weeks
Chloramphenicol	50 mg/kg/day in 4 divided doses	2–4 weeks
Children		
Third generation cephalosporins		
Ceftriaxone	75–100 mg/kg/day	2–4 weeks
Cefotaxime	90–180 mg/kg/day, in 2 or 3 divided doses	2–4 weeks
Penicillin		
Penicillin G	300,000 U/kg/day in 6 divided doses	2–4 weeks

[a] No studies comparing doxycycline with tetracycline have been done.

[b] Dosage determined by size of patient.

[c] No studies comparing amoxicillin with amoxicillin plus probenecid have been done; cefuroxime axetil and azithromycin have also been studied in Lyme disease.

[d] There is no proof that this the optimal duration of therapy or that more than 10–14 days of treatment is necessary.

[e] There is no proof that isolated facial nerve palsy or carditis must be treated with intravenous therapy. Oral doxycycline for early Lyme neuroborreliosis has been shown to be effective in European studies. Especially in children, oral treatment for Lyme arthritis may suffice.

Adapted with permission from: Sigal LH. Current drug therapy recommendations for the treatment of Lyme disease. Drugs 1992;43:683–699.

so prophylactic therapy is not recommended (17). Lyme arthritis refractory to antibiotic therapy may benefit from intra-articular corticosteroid injections, hydroxychloroquine, or synovectomy.

In evaluating response to therapy, it is important to recognize that there may be persistent nonspecific complaints for many months following adequate treatment. Recovery from neurologic damage, in particular, may be very slow because peripheral neurons regenerate at a rate of 1–2 mm/day. There are no examples of antibiotic-resistant *B. burgdorferi*, nor is there evidence that the organism

can hide in vivo or become dormant, thereby avoiding antibiotics. Lack of response to appropriate antibiotic therapy should prompt a re-examination of the initial and current diagnoses.

It is important, therefore, that clinicians differentiate between four commonly confused entities: true infection (Lyme disease); post-Lyme disease syndromes; Lyme anxiety; and concurrent, unrelated medical occurrences. Post-Lyme disease syndromes occur in patients with prior, cured infection, but who have ongoing complaints unrelated to active infection. These syndromes do not respond to further antibiotic therapy (18). Examples include fibromyalgia, sleep disorder, patellofemoral joint dysfunction, and poorly defined autoimmune phenomena. Lyme anxiety is concern about having Lyme disease, despite the absence of objective clinical or serologic findings of infection or response to antibiotic therapy. Coexisting, unrelated medical problems in patients with Lyme disease are common.

Prevention

The best technique for avoiding Lyme disease is to take precautions when in an endemic area. Perform careful and frequent tick checks; remove ticks before they can bite; shower with a washcloth at the end of the day to dislodge ticks; wear long pants, long-sleeved shirts, and light-colored clothes so that ticks will be visible; and tuck pants legs into socks so that ticks cannot gain access to the skin. Proper use of repellants, e.g., DEET (*N,N*-diethyl-*m*-toluamide) is suggested. Most cases of Lyme disease are acquired peridomestically. By eliminating or limiting the tick's preferred habitat (moist, shaded areas), one can decrease the number of ticks on one's property. Methods include clearing brush, especially at the edge of an adjoining forest, spreading wood chips at the forest edge, and applying acaricide (especially particulate preparations) at these sites.

Lyme Vaccine

The rationale for vaccine development included clinical observations that patients who had late features of Lyme disease rarely, if ever, experienced subsequent EM. In addition, a recent retrospective study suggested that patients with a history of Lyme disease had milder, not more severe, manifestations with their second *B. burgdorferi* infection (19).

In animal studies, inoculation with the *B. burgdorferi* outer-surface protein OspA has been shown to prevent subsequent infection (20). Large field trials of an OspA vaccine have demonstrated a high level of efficacy, and a very mild and uncommon side-effect profile (21,22), despite concerns that the heterogeneity of OspA might mean that a single OspA vaccine may not be effective in different geographic areas. There recently has been concern raised about the possibility that OspA inoculation might cause autoimmune reactivity directed at articular structures, based on a molecular mimicry between OspA and the human integrin lymphocyte function-associated antigen-1 (23). However, there is no evidence to date that such reactivity has caused immune-mediated damage to vaccine recipients or that the molecular mimicry is of clinical significance.

Other molecules, including Borrelial proteins (e.g., the decorin binding protein), chimeric constructs of various Borrelial proteins, and specific peptides (rather than whole proteins) are candidates for a next-generation vaccine.

LEONARD H. SIGAL, MD

References

1. Steere AC. Lyme disease. New Engl J Med 1989;321:586–596.
2. Steere AC, Malawista SE, Snydman DR, et al. Lyme arthritis: an epidemic of oligoarticular arthritis in children and adults in three Connecticut communities. Arthritis Rheum 1977; 20:7–17.
3. Steere AC, Grodzicki RL, Kornblatt AN, et al. The spirochetal etiology of Lyme disease. N Engl J Med 1983;308:733–740.
4. Benach JL, Bosler EM, Hanrahan JP, et al. Spirochetes isolated from the blood of two patients with Lyme disease. N Engl J Med 1983;308:740–742.
5. Coleman JL, Sellati TJ, Testa JE, Kew RR, Furie MB, Benach JL. Borrelia burgdorferi binds plasminogen, resulting in enhanced penetration of endothelial monolayers. Infect Immun 1995;63:2478–2484.
6. Steere AC, Dwyer E, Winchester R. Association of chronic Lyme arthritis with HLA-DR4 and HLA-DR2 alleles. N Engl J Med 1990;323:219–223.
7. Sigal LH. Immunopathogenesis of Lyme Borreliosis. Clin Dermatol 1993;11:415–422.
8. Steere AC, Bartenhagen NH, Craft JE, et al. The early clinical manifestations of Lyme disease. Ann Intern Med 1983;99:76–82.
9. Steere AC, Schoen RT, Taylor E. The clinical evolution of Lyme arthritis. Ann Intern Med 1987;107:725–731.
10. Logigian EL, Kaplan RF, Steere AC. Chronic neurological manifestations of Lyme disease. N Engl J Med 1990;323:1438–1444.
11. de Koning J. Histopathologic patterns of erythema migrans and Borrelial lymphocytoma. Clin Dermatol 1993;11:377–383.
12. Asbrink E. Acodermatitis chronica atrophicans. Clin Dermatol 1993;11:369–375.
13. Ilowite NT. Musculoskeletal, reticuloendothelial and late skin manifestations of Lyme disease. Am J Med 1995;98(suppl 4A):63S–68S.
14. Markowitz LE, Steere AC, Benach JL, Slade JD, Broome CV. Lyme disease during pregnancy. JAMA 1986;255:3394–3396.
15. Strobino BA, Williams CL, Abid S, Chalson S, Spierling P. Lyme disease and pregnancy outcome: a prospective study of two thousand prenatal patients. Am J Obstet Gynecol 1993;169:367–374.
16. Williams CL, Strobino B, Weinstein A, Spierling P, Medici F. Maternal Lyme disease and congenital malformations: a cord blood serosurvey in endemic and control areas. Pediatr Perinat Epidemiol 1995;9:320–330.
17. Shapiro ED, Gerber MA, Holabird NB, et al. A controlled trial of antimicrobial prophylaxis for Lyme disease after deer-tick bite. N Engl J Med 1992;327:1769–1773.
18. Shadick NA, Phillips CB, Logigian EL, et al. The long-term clinical outcomes of Lyme disease. A population-based retrospective cohort study. Ann Intern Med 1994;121:560–567.
19. Asch ES, Bujak DI, Weiss M, Peterson MG, Weinstein A. Lyme disease: an infectious and postinfectious syndrome. J Rheumatol 1994;21:454–461.
20. Fikrig E, Barthold SW, Kantor FS, Flavell RA. Long-term protection of mice from Lyme disease by vaccination with OspA. Infect Immun 1992;60:773–777.

21. Sigal LH, Zahradnik JM, Lavin P, et al. A vaccine consisting of recombinant Borrelia burgdorferi outer-surface protein A to prevent Lyme disease. N Engl J Med 1998;339:216–222.

22. Steere AC, Sikand VK, Meurice F, et al. Vaccination against Lyme disease with recombinant Borrelia burgdorferi outer-surface lipoprotein A with adjuvant. N Engl J Med 1998;339:209–215.

23. Gross DM, Forsthuber T, Tary-Lehmann M, et al. Identification of LFA-1 as a candidate autoantigen in treatment-resistant Lyme arthritis. Science 1998;281:703–706.

INFECTIOUS DISORDERS
D. Mycobacterial, Fungal, and Parasitic Arthritis

Mycobacteria, fungi, and parasites infrequently cause musculoskeletal infections. However, they are becoming more prevalent because more people are immunosuppressed due to human immunodeficiency virus infection, aging, or debilitating diseases, and immigration from developing countries endemic for these infections is increasing. These agents should be considered in people with chronic monarticular arthritis, but they also may present with other disorders, including spondylitis, osteomyelitis, tendinitis, and erythema nodosum (Table 12D-1). Definitive diagnosis usually depends on identification of the responsible organism in pus, synovial fluid, or tissue.

Mycobacteria
Mycobacterium tuberculosis

Infection with *M. tuberculosis* usually is acquired by inhalation and begins as nonspecific pneumonitis, followed by lymphatic and hematogenous spread to upper lobes and other organs. In immunocompetent hosts, infection is limited by cellular immunity. Reactivation may occur during a period of diminished host immunity, with multiplication of bacilli in dormant foci, and may spread via lymphatics or blood. Osteoarticular involvement occurs in 1%–5% of people with tuberculosis (1). Of these, up to 30% have infection in other organs. Bone infection typically occurs via hematogenous seeding, during primary pulmonary infection (in children), or from a quiescent pulmonary focus or an extrapulmonary site (in adults). Tuberculin skin tests are positive in most patients with osteoarticular tuberculosis, but chest radiographs often are normal. The definitive diagnosis is made by the demonstration of *M. tuberculosis* in tissue or synovial fluid. Polymerase chain reaction identification has been introduced as a more rapid means of detection and, in the future, may facilitate diagnosis of tuberculosis and other infections (2).

The classic presentation of osteoarticular infection is spinal tuberculosis, or Pott's disease. Infection of peripheral joints, especially weight-bearing joints, tendons, bursae, or bones, may occur, and reactive arthritis (Poncet's disease) has been reported. Tuberculosis also must be considered in cases of chronic arthritis in people with underlying connective-tissue disease.

Spinal Tuberculosis

Tuberculous spondylitis, or Pott's disease, is the most common form of osteoarticular infection with *M. tuberculosis* (3). Thoracic vertebrae are involved most frequently, followed by lumbar, and less commonly, cervical and sacral vertebrae. In endemic areas, spinal tuberculosis primarily is a disease of children and young adults. In the United States and Europe, most cases occur in adults, due to reactivation of dormant foci (4).

Infection characteristically begins in the anterior portion of the vertebral

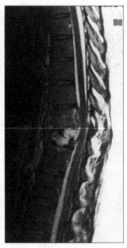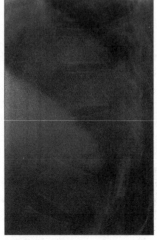

Fig. 12D-1. Tuberculous spondylitis (Pott's disease). **Right:** A lateral radiograph of the thoracic spine shows destruction of adjacent vertebral endplates of the T10 and T11 vertebrae with disc-space narrowing and vertebral collapse, resulting in a gibbus deformity. **Center:** A lateral T2-weighted MRI image of the thoracic spine in the same patient demonstrates inflammation in the area of collapse and extension anteriorly. **Left:** An AP T2-weighted MRI image of the thoracic spine of the same patient demonstrates a multilocular soft-tissue mass extending above and below the area of vertebral collapse. Figure provided by Dr. Timothy Maus, Mayo Clinic, Rochester, MN.

TABLE 12D-1
Typical Presentations of Osteoarticular Infections Caused by Mycobacteria and Fungi

Mycobacteria	
Tuberculosis	Spondylitis (Pott's disease)
	Monarticular arthritis of large weight-bearing joints
	Osteomyelitis and dactylitis
	Bursitis and tenosynovitis
	Reactive arthritis (Poncet's disease)
BCG treatment	Migratory arthritis or arthralgias
Atypical mycobacteria	Arthritis or tendinitis of hand or wrist
	Multifocal bone, joint or tendon infection
Leprosy	Polyarticular arthritis with erythema nodosum leprosum
	Destructive arthritis of small bones and joints of hands and feet
	Neuropathic arthritis of wrists or ankles
Fungi	
Candidiasis	Polyarticular arthritis with osteomyelitis in seriously ill infants
	Monarticular arthritis of knee in seriously ill patients past infancy
Coccidioidomycosis	Polyarticular arthritis with erythema nodosum
	Monarticular arthritis of knee
	Osteomyelitis
Sporotrichosis	Monarticular arthritis of knee, wrist, or hand
	Polyarticular arthritis with disseminated cutaneous lesions
Blastomycosis	Osteomyelitis
	Spondylitis
	Monarticular arthritis of weight-bearing joints with lung and cutaneous lesions
Cryptococcosis	Osseous infection
	Spondylitis
	Rare monarticular arthritis
Histoplasmosis	Polyarticular arthritis with erythema nodosum

BCG, Bacillus Calmette-Guerin.

bodies, with subsequent disc involvement, disc-space narrowing, vertebral end-plate destruction, and collapse of the anterior portion of the vertebral body, causing the characteristic gibbus deformity (Fig. 12D-1) (5). Infection often extends to adjoining discs or vertebrae, or to distant sites. Localized soft-tissue inflammation or abscesses, such as paravertebral or psoas abscesses, may occur; sinus tracts may be formed; and neurologic injury may ensue.

Most patients experience back pain and tenderness, but signs of inflammation usually are absent. Neurologic manifestations from spinal cord or root compression occur in 12%–50% (5). Active pulmonary tuberculosis may be absent, but there often is evidence of past disease.

Radiographs typically show disc-space narrowing with vertebral collapse and paraspinous abscess (6,7). Computerized tomography (CT) can define the bony anatomy and paraspinal masses, and magnetic resonance imaging can show impingement on neural structures. The differential diagnosis is broad, including other infections, neoplasm, and sarcoidosis; bacteriologic confirmation is recommended. Diagnosis is best made by examination of biopsy specimens obtained by CT-guided or open biopsy.

Therapy is complicated by the increase in drug-resistant tuberculosis. Combination chemotherapy lasting nine to 12 months is recommended (8). Indications for surgery include motor deficits, spinal deformity, a nondiagnostic needle biopsy, and nonadherence or lack of response to medical therapy (4).

Tuberculous Arthritis
Tuberculous arthritis occurs mainly in the hips and knees, but may involve other joints (9). Most patients are middle-aged or older, often with underlying medical disorders or previous intra-articular corticosteroid injections. Arthritis

typically is monarticular and insidious. Joint pain and swelling usually are present, but signs of inflammation may be limited. A delay in diagnosis of three to four years is not unknown. Articular tuberculosis usually is due to reactivation of a hematogenously seeded focus and need not be associated with active disease elsewhere; it can spread from adjacent osteomyelitis. Tuberculous osteomyelitis can occur without joint involvement. In adults, a single lesion is most common, usually involving the metaphysis of a long bone. In children, the hands and feet may be involved, causing tuberculous dactylitis.

Characteristic radiographic findings of tuberculous arthritis are juxta-articular osteoporosis, marginal erosions, and gradual joint-space narrowing (Phemister's triad). Similar changes can occur in other forms of infection or rheumatoid arthritis. Additional radiographic findings include soft-tissue swelling, subchondral cysts, bony sclerosis, periostitis, and calcifications.

Synovial-fluid white blood cell count generally is elevated, with a predominance of polymorphonuclear cells and low glucose levels. Synovial-fluid acid-fast smears are positive in approximately 20% of cases, and culture is positive in up to 80% (1). The diagnosis of tuberculous arthritis is best made by histologic and microbiologic examination of synovium. Histology may demonstrate caseating or noncaseating granulomas.

Tuberculous arthritis usually responds to combination chemotherapy (9). Surgery may be needed for synovectomy, debridement, joint stabilization, or to remove infected prostheses.

Poncet's Disease

Poncet's disease is a form of reactive arthritis occurring during active tuberculosis (10). Polyarticular arthritis typically involves the hands and feet. Joint fluid and tissue samples are sterile. Symptoms abate with antituberculous treatment.

Mycobacterium bovis and Bacillus Calmette-Guerin

M. bovis infection is now rare, but musculoskeletal symptoms have been related to attenuated M. bovis as a component of Bacillus Calmette-Guerin (BCG) (11). Intravesicular BCG instillation for bladder cancer has been associated with fever, malaise, and migratory polyarticular arthralgias or arthritis in up to 6% of patients. Symptoms worsen with repeated treatments, but can be prevented by isoniazid. Other syndromes include systemic BCG infection, including monarticular arthritis with M. bovis isolated from joints, and reactive arthritis. M. bovis infection of a prosthetic joint also has been described.

Atypical Mycobacteria

Musculoskeletal involvement with atypical (nontuberculous) mycobacteria can mimic tuberculosis and include bone, joint, tendon, and bursal infection. Infections are indolent with insidious onset. The peak age incidence is 40–69 years, with a male-to-female ratio of 3:1 (12). M. marinum, M. kansasii,

and M. avium complex cause the majority of infections. Various other mycobacterial species are identified in the remaining cases. A history of prior trauma, operation, or intra-articular injection is usual, but occasionally hematogenous seeding occurs. Corticosteroid use and underlying arthritis are additional risk factors. M. marinum infection often is associated with aquatic exposure.

Any joint, bursa, or tendon sheath may be infected, but the hands are involved most frequently, followed by the wrists and knees. Polyarticular involvement occurs in less than one-fourth of patients. The most common presenting complaint is joint swelling, followed by joint pain and limited motion. Carpal tunnel syndrome may arise from synovitis involving the flexor tendons of the wrist. A slow-healing wound may be present. Constitutional symptoms, such as fever, chills, weight loss, and malaise, are infrequent.

Radiographs of affected joints often are normal. If abnormalities are identified, they usually are soft-tissue swelling, joint destruction, effusion, bony erosion, or bone destruction. A pattern of preservation of the central joint space, marginal erosion, and sclerotic borders of adjacent bone has been described.

Synovial fluid may be noninflammatory or markedly inflammatory. Pathology typically demonstrates noncaseating granulomatous inflammation, but the absence of granulomas does not exclude the diagnosis. Diagnosis is made by demonstration of the responsible mycobacterium in synovial fluid or tissue. Negative cultures do not rule out infection, as these organisms can be difficult to cultivate.

Treatment of atypical mycobacterial joint infections involves a combination of chemotherapy and surgery. Most strains of nontuberculous mycobacteria are resistant to antituberculous drugs to some degree; combination chemotherapy usually is required (1).

Mycobacterium leprae

Leprosy can cause several forms of arthritis (13). Erythema nodosum leprosum occurs in people with lepromatous leprosy. Manifestations include crops of subcutaneous nodules, fever, and polyarticular arthralgias or arthritis; joint symptoms are immunologically mediated. Septic arthritis, with M. leprae in synovial fluid, occurs infrequently. Chronic erosive arthritis of large and small joints resembles rheumatoid arthritis and improves with treatment of the leprosy. A classic finding in late stages of leprosy is the development of Charcot joints due to sensory neuropathy and repeated trauma.

Fungi

Most fungal musculoskeletal infections have an insidious onset, indolent course, and generally mild inflammation. Other than positive cultures, most laboratory findings are nonspecific.

Candidae

Candida species rarely cause septic arthritis, but arthritis can arise from direct inoculation or hematogenous dissemination of organisms (14,15). Intra-articular inoculation may occur during arthrocentesis or joint surgery. When related to injection, arthritis typically is chronic, monarticular, and caused by species other than *C. albicans*. Fungi cause only 1% of infected prosthetic joints; *C. albicans* is the most frequent organism (15). Infection usually is indolent, monarticular, and chronic. Symptoms may not develop until two years after surgery. Radiographs demonstrate loosening of prosthetic components.

Hematogenous spread of *C. albicans* to joints can occur with disseminated candidiasis. Disseminated candidiasis is associated with drug abuse; among non-drug abusers, it is seen in seriously ill patients receiving intensive medical care, notably hospitalized infants (15). In infants, *Candida* arthritis usually is polyarticular and associated with local osteomyelitis. Beyond infancy, people with disseminated candidiasis typically have a serious illness treated with antibiotics, chemotherapy, and/or immunosuppressive agents. The clinical course may be acute, with marked synovitis, or more indolent and milder. Arthritis is monarticular in about 75% of cases, most often involving a knee. Bursitis also has been associated with disseminated candidiasis.

The diagnosis is made by culture of synovial fluid or tissue. Treatment with systemic or intra-articular amphotericin B has been successful. 5-Fluorocytosine may be helpful as an adjunct to amphotericin B, but should not be used alone because of resistance. Ketoconazole and fluconazole have been successful in treating candidal infection, but the *Candida* species causing infection must be identified, as some species other than *C. albicans* are resistant (16). Treatment of infected prosthetic joints usually requires removal of the prosthesis and debridement.

Coccidioidomycosis
Coccidioidomycosis is caused by *Coccidioides immitis*, a soil fungus found in semi-arid areas of the southwestern United States, Central America, and South America. Osteoarticular involvement can occur during primary or disseminated infection.

Primary infection often is asymptomatic; about 40% of infected patients develop self-limited symptoms ranging from flu-like complaints to pneumonia. "Valley fever" or "desert rheumatism" are terms used for erythema nodosum, erythema multiforme, and arthralgias or arthritis caused by coccidioidomycosis. Arthritis usually is polyarticular and migratory, lasting less than four weeks (17).

Chronic pulmonary infection occurs in about 2% of patients, and disseminated disease is seen in about 0.2%. Arthritis and osteomyelitis can occur during disseminated infection. Chronic arthritis of one knee is the most frequent articular manifestation. Pathologic features include villous hypertrophy, pannus formation, and bony erosions. Delay in diagnosis averages more than four years. Osteomyelitis, most often involving ends of long bones, the skull, vertebrae, and ribs, occurs in 10% to 20% of patients with disseminated disease.

Synovial-fluid samples rarely yield *C. immitis*. The diagnosis is best made by demonstration of organisms in tissue. Amphotericin B followed by ketoconazole, or long-term ketoconazole can treat osteoarticular coccidioidomycosis, but infection may recur after therapy ends (1). Intra-articular amphotericin B has been reported to be useful. Surgical drainage of pus, debridement, or synovectomy may be necessary.

Sporotrichosis
Sporotrichosis, caused by *Sporothrix schenckii*, usually is limited to cutaneous disease, presenting as a painful erythematous nodule at the site of a thorn scratch or puncture. Infection is spread by lymphatic drainage or local extension.

Extracutaneous disease primarily affects musculoskeletal structures, causing arthritis, tenosynovitis, osteitis, or granulomatous myositis (17). Cutaneous findings are present in most patients with musculoskeletal involvement. Arthritis usually is chronic, and it may be mono- or polyarticular, involving knees, wrists, small joints of the hands, ankles, and elbows (18). Disseminated sporotrichosis is rare, usually occurring in immunosuppressed or systemically ill people. Most people with disseminated sporotrichosis have bone or joint involvement, or both. Radiographs show single or multiple lytic lesions with minimal periostitis.

Synovium demonstrates chronic noncaseating granulomatous inflammation. Diagnosis is based on culture of organisms from joint fluid or tissue. Amphotericin B, with or without surgical debridement, often is curative, but prolonged treatment may be necessary. Intra-articular amphotericin B, itraconazole, and ketoconazole have been reported effective.

Blastomycosis
Blastomyces dermatitidis is endemic in the Ohio and Mississippi River valleys, and mid-Atlantic states of the United States. Primary pulmonary infection occurs after inhalation of infectious spores; other sites are seeded by hematogenous or lymphatic spread. Skeletal infection occurs in most patients (17). Osteomyelitis is most common, involving vertebrae, ribs, tibia, and skull. Vertebral infection mimics tuberculosis. Arthritis typically is monarticular, but can be polyarticular, and usually is associated with pulmonary disease and cutaneous abscesses. In contrast to other fungal causes of arthritis, blastomycosis usually causes constitutional symptoms, and arthritis more often is acute, leading to quick diagnosis. A knee is involved most frequently, followed by an ankle or elbow. In most cases, articular disease arises from hematogenous spread, but about one-third of cases are due to nearby osteomyelitis.

Synovial-fluid smears and stains may reveal organisms, but definitive diagnosis requires culture. Blastomycosis can be treated with amphotericin B, ketoconazole, or itraconazole. Surgery may be required if treatment with these drugs fails.

Cryptococcosis
Inhalation of *Cryptococcus neoformans* can cause clinically silent or overt pulmonary infection. Hematogenous spread

may seed other organs, notably the central nervous system. Most clinically apparent disseminated cases occur in immunosuppressed patients. Osseous infection occurs in 5%–10% of disseminated cases, and involves the long bones, vertebrae, ribs, tarsals, and carpals, with a subacute or chronic course (17). Vertebral infection may mimic tuberculosis. Radiographs show lytic lesions with little periosteal reaction. Cryptococcal arthritis is infrequent and usually is due to direct extension of adjacent osteomyelitis (17). The diagnosis is made by demonstration of organisms in synovial fluid or tissue. Treatment usually is with amphotericin B, with or without 5-fluorocytosine. Fluconazole may be sufficient for immunocompetent hosts.

Histoplasmosis

Histoplasmosis, caused by *Histoplasma capsulatum,* is endemic in the Mississippi and Ohio River valleys. Most infections are subclinical and self-limited. Dissemination occurs in less than 0.1% of cases, usually in the elderly or immunosuppressed (17). During primary infection, acute, self-limited, migratory, polyarticular arthralgia or arthritis may occur, with or without erythema nodosum or erythema multiforme. Arthritis in these cases is mediated immunologically. Arthritis, osteomyelitis, tenosynovitis, and carpal tunnel syndrome occur infrequently in disseminated histoplasmosis. Diagnosis is based on the culture of *H. capsulatum* from tissue or histologic demonstration of organisms. Successful treatment has been accomplished with amphotericin B, itraconazole, and fluconazole, but surgical debridement may be required.

Other Fungal and Related Organisms

Maduromycosis, or mycetoma, is a chronic infection of skin, subcutaneous tissue, and bone, most often involving the foot. Maduromycosis is caused by a variety of organisms, including *Actinomyces* or true fungi. Infection begins with subcutaneous inoculation of organisms and local extension, with eventual development of granule-draining sinus tracts.

Invasive *Aspergillus* infection can involve a variety of organs, most often the lungs and sinuses. Direct extension of infection can result in osteomyelitis of vertebrae, ribs, or skull. Vertebral involvement can mimic Pott's disease. Articular involvement is rare.

A variety of other fungi have been reported as rare causes of infectious arthritis, including *Pseudallescheria boydii, Fusarium solani, Saccharomyces cerevisiae, Torulopsis glabrata* (17).

The actinomycetes are strictly anaerobic bacilli, but have properties similar to fungi. Actinomycosis, caused most often by *Actinomyces israelii,* is manifest as abscess formation in the abdomen, lung, or soft tissues of the neck. Skeletal infection occurs by local extension, involving the mandible or spine. Usually, several vertebrae are involved, with sparing of discs. Diagnosis is made by demonstration of characteristic sulfur granules on Gram stain and culture of organisms. The actinomycetes are sensitive to penicillin and tetracycline.

Parasites

Parasites are organisms that live on or in another organism and derive their nourishment from the host. They can be grouped as protozoa, helminths, and arthropods (19). Some parasites may persist in the host for extended periods. Immune responses induced by parasitic infections can cause tissue injury and musculoskeletal manifestations, including hypersensitivity reactions and immune-complex deposition. Such manifestations usually are benign and often resolve with treatment of the underlying infection. Arthralgia is more common than arthritis, but the frequency of joint involvement is not clearly known.

Among protozoa, *Giardia lamblia* has been reported as a cause of acute-onset, mild, recurrent seronegative arthritis, similar to reactive arthritis (20). Other protozoa associated with arthralgias and arthritis include *Entamoeba histolytica, Trichomona vaginalis,* and *Toxoplasma gondii.*

Several helminths have been associated with joint symptoms. *Strongyloides stercoralis* can cause reactive arthritis. *Taenia saginata* (beef tapeworm) has been associated with oligo- and polyarticular findings, with an immune-mediated mechanism and response to antiparasitic therapy. Cysticercosis has been associated with localized myalgias and arthralgias. *Echinococcus granulosus,* which causes hydatid cysts, can involve the spine or long bones. Schistosomiasis has been associated with arthritis and sacroiliitis. Articular involvement occurs in about 10% of patients with filariasis, usually monarticular arthritis of the knee or ankle (19). Nonsteroidal anti-inflammatory drugs are not helpful, but symptoms improve with anti-infective agents. Dracunculosis can produce a variety of musculoskeletal symptoms, including myalgias, arthralgia, and acute or chronic monarticular arthritis.

STEVEN R. YTTERBERG, MD

References

1. Meier JL, Hoffman GS. *Mycobacterial and fungal infections. In: Sledge CB, Ruddy S, Harris ED Jr, Kelley WN (eds). Arthritis Surgery. Philadelphia: WB Saunders, 1994; pp 513–529.*
2. Louie JS, Liebling MR. *The polymerase chain reaction in infectious and post-infectious arthritis. A review. Rheum Dis Clin North Am 1998;24:227–236.*
3. Martini M, Ouahes M. *Bone and joint tuberculosis: a review of 652 cases. Orthopedics 1988;11:861–866.*
4. Rezai AR, Lee M, Cooper PR, Errico TJ, Koslow M. *Modern management of spinal tuberculosis. Neurosurgery 1995;36: 87–97.*
5. Mahowald ML, Messner RP. *Arthritis due to mycobacteria, fungi and parasites. In: Koopman WJ (ed). Arthritis and Allied Conditions, 13th edition. Baltimore: Williams & Wilkins, 1997; pp 2305–2320.*

6. Perronne C, Saba J, Behloul Z, et al. Pyogenic and tuberculous spondylodiskitis (vertebral osteomyelitis) in 80 adult patients. Clin Infect Dis 1994;19:746–750.

7. Ridley N, Shaikh MI, Remedios D, Mitchell R. Radiology of skeletal tuberculosis. Orthopedics 1998;21:1213–1220.

8. Bass JB Jr, Farer LS, Hopewell PC, et al. Treatment of tuberculosis and tuberculosis infection in adults and children. American Thoracic Society and The Centers for Disease Control and Prevention. Am J Respir Crit Care Med 1994;149:1359–1374.

9. Garrido G, Gomez-Reino JJ, Fernandez-Dapica P, Palenque E, Prieto S. A review of peripheral tuberculous arthritis. Semin Arthritis Rheum 1988;18:142–149.

10. Dall L, Long L, Stanford J. Poncet's disease: tuberculous rheumatism. Rev Infect Dis 1989;11:105–107.

11. Clavel G, Grados F, Cayrolle G, et al. Polyarthritis following intravesical BCG immunotherapy. Report of a case and review of 26 cases in the literature. Rev Rheum Engl Ed 1999;66:115–118.

12. Yangco BC, Espinoza CG, Germain BF. Nontuberculous mycobacterial joint infections. In: Espinosa L (ed). Infections in the Rheumatic Diseases. Orlando, FL: Grune & Stratton, 1988; pp 139–157.

13. Gibson T, Ahsan Q, Hussein K. Arthritis of leprosy. Br J Rheumatol 1994;33:963–966.

14. Cuende E, Barbadillo C, E-Mazzucchelli R, Isasi C, Trujillo A, Andreu JL. Candida arthritis in adult patients who are not intravenous drug addicts: report of three cases and review of the literature. Semin Arthritis Rheum 1993;22:224–241.

15. Silveira LH, Cuellar ML, Citera G, Cabrera GE, Scopelitis E, Espinoza LR. Candida arthritis. Rheum Dis Clin North Am 1993;19:427–437.

16. Perez-Gomez A, Prieto A, Torresano M, et al. Role of the new azoles in the treatment of fungal osteoarticular infections. Semin Arthritis Rheum 1998;27:226–244.

17. Cuellar ML, Silveira LH, Citera G, Cabrera GE, Valle R. Other fungal arthritides. Rheum Dis Clin North Am 1993;19:439–455.

18. Howell SJ, Toohey JS. Sporotrichal arthritis in south central Kansas. Clin Orthop 1998;346:207–214.

19. Bocanegra TS. Rheumatic manifestations of parasitic diseases. In: Espinoza L (ed). Infections in the Rheumatic Diseases. Orlando: Grune & Stratton, 1988; pp 243–261.

20. Tupchong M, Simor A, Dewar C. Beaver fever - a rare cause of reactive arthritis. J Rheumatol 1999;26:2701–2702.

INFECTIOUS DISORDERS
E. Rheumatic Fever

Acute rheumatic fever is a delayed, nonsuppurative sequela of a pharyngeal infection with the group A streptococci. Onset usually is characterized by an acute febrile illness that may manifest itself in migratory arthritis predominantly involving the large joints, clinical and laboratory signs of carditis and valvulitis, central nervous system involvement (e.g., Sydenham's chorea), or a combination of these manifestations. The clinical episodes are self-limiting, but damage to the valves may be chronic and progressive, resulting in cardiac dysfunction.

The severity and mortality of acute rheumatic fever declined dramatically during the 20th century, but reports of its resurgence in the United States (1) are a reminder that the disease remains a public health problem, even in developed countries. The disease continues essentially unabated in many developing countries, and estimates suggest there will be 10–20 million new cases per year in those countries, where two-thirds of the world population lives.

Epidemiology

The incidence of rheumatic fever began to decline before the introduction of antibiotics into clinical practice, decreasing from 250 per 100,000 to 100 per 100,000 from 1862–1962 in Denmark (2). The introduction of antibiotics in 1950 rapidly accelerated this decline; in 1980, the incidence ranged from 0.23 to 1.88 patients per 100,000, and occurred primarily in children and teenagers. A notable exception to this decline has been seen in the Hawaiian, New Zealand, and Maori populations, which are predominantly of Polynesian ancestry, where the rate continues to be 13.4 per 100,000 hospitalized children per year (3).

Pathogenesis

Although affected tissues of patients with acute rheumatic fever show little evidence of direct involvement of group A streptococci, there is significant epidemiologic evidence indirectly implicating the bacteria in the initiation of disease. It is well-known that outbreaks of acute rheumatic fever closely follow epidemics of streptococcal sore throat and scarlet fever. In patients with documented streptococcal pharyngitis, adequate antibiotic treatment markedly reduces the incidence of subsequent rheumatic fever, and appropriate antimicrobial prophylaxis prevents disease recurrence (4). When tested for three antistreptococcal antibodies (i.e., streptolysin O, hyaluronidase, and streptokinase), the sera of most people with acute rheumatic fever shows elevated antibody titers to these antigens, whether or not the patient recalls an antecedent streptococcal sore throat.

Caution is necessary when documenting, either clinically or microbiologically, an antecedent streptococcal infection. The rate of isolation of group A streptococci from the oropharynx is extremely low, even in populations who generally do not have access to microbial antibiotics. There also appears to be an age-related discrepancy in the clinical documentation of an antecedent pharyngitis. In older children and young adults, the rate approaches only 20% (5), but it reaches 70% in younger children. Rheumatic fever should be suspected in children or young adults presenting with signs of arthritis and/or carditis, even in the absence of a documented pharyngitis.

Another intriguing and unexplained observation is the association of rheumatic fever with only one type of streptococcus, streptococcal pharyngitis. Group A streptococci are divided into two main classes based on differences in the C-repeat regions of the M protein (6). One class clearly is associated with streptococcal pharyngeal infection, but the other class, with some exceptions, belongs to strains commonly associated with impetigo. Because rheumatic fever rarely occurs following infection with impetigo-associated streptococcal strains, the particular strain of streptococcus may be crucial in initiating the disease process.

The pharyngeal site of infection, with its large repository of lymphoid tissue, may be important in initiating the host's abnormal humoral response to antigens that cross-react with target organs. Although impetigo strains do colonize the pharynx, they do not appear to elicit as strong an immunologic response to the M-protein moiety as do the pharyngeal strains (7). Streptococcal strains capable of causing pharyngitis almost always are capable of causing rheumatic fever. Whether certain strains are more "rheumatogenic" than others remains unresolved.

Only a few M serotypes (types 5, 14, 18, and 24) have been implicated in outbreaks of rheumatic fever. During an outbreak in Utah, several different M types isolated from patients were both mucoid and nonmucoid in character (8). In Trinidad, types 41 and 11 have been the strains most commonly associated with rheumatic fever.

Increased frequencies of the major histocompatibility complex (MHC) class II alleles HLA-DR4 and -DR2 have been noted in Caucasian and black patients with rheumatic heart disease (9). Other studies have implicated HLA-DR1 and -DRw6 as susceptibility factors in South African black patients with rheumatic heart disease (10). Most recently, associations of HLA-DR7 and -Dw53 have been noted in rheumatic fever patients in Brazil (11). These varying results concerning HLA antigens and rheumatic fever susceptibility prompt speculation that the reported associations might be for genes close to, but not identical to, the rheumatic fever susceptibility gene.

Monoclonal antibodies have been prepared by immunizing mice with B cells from people with rheumatic fever. One of these antibodies, D8/17, was found to identify a marker expressed on increased numbers (>20%) of B cells in all rheumatic fever patients of diverse ethnic origins (12). Approximately 90%–95% of unaffected individuals had a range of 4%–6% D8/17$^+$ B cells. However, a distinct population of unaffected individuals (4%–7%) had D8/17 B cells that were one standard deviation above normal (i.e., 10%–12% positive cells); these individuals could be considered susceptible to rheumatic fever. The antigen defined by this monoclonal antibody showed no association with or linkage to any known MHC allele, nor did it appear to be related to B-cell activation antigens.

Clinical Features

Arthritis

In the classic, untreated case, the arthritis of rheumatic fever affects several joints in quick succession, each for a short time. The legs usually are affected first, and later, the arms. The terms migrating and migratory often are used to describe the polyarthritis of rheumatic fever because the various localizations usually overlap, and pain during the onset, in contrast to pain experienced during the full course of the arthritis, migrates from joint to joint.

Joint involvement is more common and more severe in adolescents and young adults than in children. This involvement occurs early in the rheumatic illness and usually is the earliest symptomatic manifestation of the disease, although asymptomatic carditis may precede it. Rheumatic polyarthritis may be painful but almost always is transient. The pain usually is more prominent than are the objective signs of inflammation. Each joint is inflamed for a week at the most, and inflammation may be present in multiple joints. The inflammation decreases and then disappears. Radiographs taken at this point may show a slight effusion, but most likely will be unremarkable.

In routine practice, many patients with arthritis and/or arthralgias are treated empirically with salicylates or other nonsteroidal anti-inflammatory drugs. Accordingly, arthritis subsides quickly in the joints already affected and does not migrate to new joints, depriving the diagnostician of a useful sign.

Carditis

Cardiac valvular and muscle damage can be manifested in a variety of signs and symptoms. These manifestations include heart murmurs, cardiomegaly, congestive heart failure, and pericarditis. Mild to moderate chest discomfort, pleuritic chest pain, and pericardial friction rub are indications of pericarditis. On clinical examination, the patient may have new or changing murmurs. Severe valve damage that occurs concurrently with cardiac dysfunction may lead to congestive heart failure, the most life-threatening clinical syndrome of acute rheumatic fever. Electrocardiographic abnormalities encompass all degrees of heart block, including atrioventricular dissociation. The most common radiologic manifestation of carditis is cardiomegaly. Studies using echocardiographic techniques suggest that when these more sensitive measurements of cardiac dysfunction are used, nearly all patients with acute rheumatic fever have signs of acute carditis.

Rheumatic Heart Disease

Rheumatic heart disease is the most severe sequela of acute rheumatic fever. Occurring 10 to 20 years after the original attack, it is the major cause of acquired valvular disease worldwide (13). The mitral valve is involved most commonly, with aortic valve involvement occurring less often. Mitral stenosis due to severe calcification of the mitral valve is a classic finding and needs to be treated surgically, especially when symptoms of left atrial enlargement are seen. However, younger patients who have mitral stenosis without valvular calcification may be spared valve replacement for some time by the use of percutaneous (balloon) mitral valvuloplasty. This therapy may have great potential in countries where cardiac surgery is not readily available.

The incidence of rheumatic heart disease in patients with a history of acute rheumatic fever has varied. Valve damage manifesting as organic murmur later in life is likely to occur in almost one-half of patients who show evidence of carditis at initial diagnosis.

Chorea

Sydenham's chorea, chorea minor, or St. Vitus dance is a neurologic disorder consisting of abrupt, purposeless, non-rhythmic involuntary movements, muscle weakness, and emotional disturbances. The movements commonly are more marked on one side and occasionally are completely unilateral (hemichorea).

The muscle weakness is best revealed by asking the patient to squeeze the examiner's hands; the pressure of the patient's grip increases and decreases continuously and capriciously, a phenomenon known as relapsing grip, or "milking sign." Emotional changes manifest themselves in outbursts of inappropriate behavior, including crying and restlessness. In rare cases, the psychological manifestations may be severe and may result in transient psychosis.

The neurologic examination fails to reveal sensory losses or involvement of the pyramidal tract. Diffuse hypotonia may be present. Chorea may follow streptococcal infections after a latent period that is longer, on average, than the latent period of other rheumatic manifestations. Some patients with chorea have no other symptoms, but careful examination of the heart may reveal murmurs.

Subcutaneous Nodules

The subcutaneous nodules of rheumatic fever are firm and painless. They range from a few millimeters to 1 cm or even 2 cm in diameter. The overlying skin is not inflamed and usually can be moved over the nodules. The nodules are located most commonly over bony surfaces or prominences, or near tendons, and their number varies from a single nodule to a few dozen. When numerous, they usually are symmetric. These nodules are present for one or more weeks, but rarely for more than a month. They are smaller and more short-lived than the nodules of rheumatoid arthritis. Although the elbows are the joints most frequently involved in both diseases, rheumatic fever nodules occur more commonly on the olecranon, and nodules of rheumatoid arthritis usually are found 3 cm or 4 cm distal to it. Rheumatic subcutaneous nodules generally appear only after the first weeks of illness, usually in patients with carditis.

Erythema Marginatum

Erythema marginatum is an evanescent, nonpruritic skin rash, pink or faintly red, that usually affects the trunk, and sometimes involves the proximal parts or the limbs, but does not occur on the face (Fig. 12E-1). This lesion extends centrifugally, while the skin in the center returns to normal, resulting in a sharp lesion with a diffuse inner edge. Because the margin of the lesion usually is continuous and forms a ring, the lesion also is known as *erythema annulare*. Individual lesions may appear and disappear in a matter of hours, usually to return. A hot bath or shower may make them more evident or reveal them for the first time.

Erythema marginatum usually occurs early in the disease. It often persists or recurs, even after all other manifestations of disease have disappeared. Occasionally, the lesions appear for the first time or, more likely, are noticed for the first time, late in the course of the illness or during convalescence. This disorder usually occurs only in patients with carditis.

Laboratory Findings

The diagnosis of rheumatic fever cannot be established readily by laboratory tests. However, serial chest radiographs may be helpful in following the course of carditis, and electrocardiograms may reflect the effects of the inflammatory process on the conduction system.

Throat cultures usually are negative by the time rheumatic fever appears, but an attempt should be made to isolate the organism. The antibody usually tested for is the antistreptolysin O titer. If results are negative, the patient should be tested for anti-DNAse B, anti-DNAse, and anti-

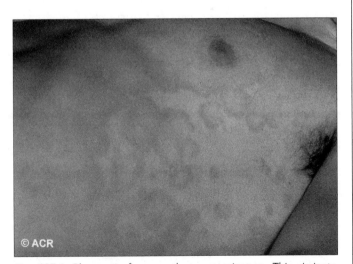

Fig. 12E-1. Rheumatic fever: erythema marginatum. This circinate eruption extends centrifugally, sometimes leaving residual hyperpigmentation. Individual lesions appear principally as open or closed rings with sharp outer edges, but macular rings with pale centers also occur. Fusion of adjacent rings produces a polycyclic configuration. Although it is a major criterion for the diagnosis of acute rheumatic fever, erythema marginatum is not often seen. Reprinted from the Clinical Slide Collection on the Rheumatic Diseases, with permission from the American College of Rheumatology.

hyaluronidase antibodies. Streptococcal antibodies are more useful because they reach a peak titer around the time of rheumatic fever onset, indicate true infection rather than transient carriage, and allow detection of recent streptococcal infection by several tests of different antibodies. It is useful to compare an initial serum specimen with a second specimen, taken two weeks later.

Titers of antistreptolysin vary with age, season, and geography. Titers of 200 to 300 Todd units/mL are common in healthy children of elementary school age. After onset of streptococcal pharyngitis, Antibody response peaks at about four to five weeks, which usually is during the second or third week of rheumatic fever. Antibody titers decline rapidly during the next several months, and after six months, they decline more slowly. Because 80% of patients with rheumatic fever show a rise in the titer of antistreptolysin, it is recommended that other antistreptococcal antibody tests be made in the absence of a positive titer for antistreptolysin. Increased streptococcal antibodies support, but do not prove, the diagnosis of acute rheumatic fever.

Acute-Phase Reactants

Acute-phase reactants are increased during acute rheumatic fever, just as they are during other inflammatory conditions. The C-reactive protein and erythrocyte sedimentation rate (ESR) invariably are abnormal during the active rheumatic process, if not suppressed by antirheumatic drugs. When treatment has been discontinued or is being tapered, the C-reactive protein or ESR can help monitor inflammation. If the C-reactive protein or ESR remain normal for a few weeks after discontinuing antirheumatic therapy, the attack may be considered ended, unless chorea appears.

Anemia

A mild, normochromic, normocytic anemia of chronic inflammation may be seen during acute rheumatic fever. Suppressing the inflammation usually improves the anemia, and iron therapy usually is not indicated.

Treatment

The mainstay of treatment for acute rheumatic fever has been anti-inflammatory agents, most commonly aspirin. Dramatic improvement in symptoms usually is seen after the start of therapy. Usually 80 to 100 mg/day in children and 4 to 8 g/day in adults are required to achieve a serum salicylate concentration of 20–30 mg/dL. Anti-inflammatory therapy should be maintained until all symptoms are absent and ESR or C-reactive protein is normal. If severe carditis is present, as indicated by significant cardiomegaly, congestive heart failure, or third-degree heart block, corticosteroid therapy can be instituted. The usual dosage is 2 mg/kg/day of oral prednisone during the first one to two weeks. Depending on clinical and laboratory improvement, the dosage of prednisone is tapered over the next several weeks. As the dose of prednisone is tapered, aspirin may be added in the dosage recommended previously.

Whether or not signs of pharyngitis are present at the time of diagnosis, antibiotic therapy with penicillin should be started and maintained for at least 10 days, in doses recommended for eradication of streptococcal pharyngitis. In addition, all family contacts should be cultured, and individuals positive for beta-hemolytic streptococci also should be treated. If compliance is an issue, depot penicillins, e.g., benzathine penicillin G (600,000 units in children, 1.2 million units in adults) should be given. Recurrence of acute rheumatic fever is most common within two years of the original attack but can happen at any time. The risk of recurrence decreases with age. Recurrence rates have been decreasing, from 20% to between 2% and 4% in recent outbreaks. This decrease may be due to better surveillance and treatment.

Prophylaxis

Antibiotic prophylaxis with penicillin should start immediately after resolution of the acute episode. The optimal regimen consists of oral penicillin VK (250,000 units twice daily) or intramuscular injection of depot penicillin G (1.2 million units every four weeks). If the patient is allergic to penicillin, erythromycin (250 mg/day) can be substituted.

Although guidelines for long-term prophylaxis are unclear, most clinicians believe it should continue at least until the patient is a young adult (18–20 years), which usually is 10 years after an acute attack with no recurrence.

TABLE 12E-1
Revised Jones Criteria for Diagnosis of Acute Rheumatic Fever[a]

Major manifestations	Minor manifestations
Carditis	Clinical findings
Polyarthritis	Arthralgia
Chorea	Fever
Erythema marginatum	Laboratory findings
Subcutaneous nodules	Elevated acute-phase reactants
	Erythrocyte sedimentation rate
	C-reactive protein
	Prolonged PR interval on EKG

Plus:

Supporting evidence of antecedent group A streptococcal infection.

Positive throat culture or rapid streptococcal antigen test.

Elevated or rising streptococcal antibody titer.

[a] If supported by evidence of preceding group A streptococcal infection, the presence of two major manifestations or of one major and two minor manifestations indicates a high probability of acute rheumatic fever.

However, it has been suggested that individuals with documented evidence of rheumatic heart disease should be continued on prophylaxis indefinitely, as rheumatic fever can recur as late as the fifth or sixth decade of life. An attractive alternative to long-term prophylaxis in an individual with rheumatic fever would be a streptococcal vaccine designed to prevent recurrent infections in rheumatic-susceptible individuals and to prevent streptococcal disease.

Post-Streptococcal Reactive Arthritis

Several arguments favor regarding post-streptococcal reactive arthritis as a distinct clinical entity from acute rheumatic fever. For example, the one- to two-week latent period between the antecedent streptococcal infection and the onset of migratory arthritis is shorter than the two to three weeks usually seen in classic acute rheumatic fever. The response of the arthritis to aspirin and other nonsteroidal drugs is poor, compared with the dramatic response seen in acute rheumatic fever. Evidence of carditis usually is not seen in patients with post-streptococcal reactive arthritis, and the severity of the arthritis is quite marked. Extra-articular manifestations, such as tenosynovitis and renal abnormalities, often are seen in these patients.

Recently, however, several investigators have speculated that post-streptococcal reactive arthritis, in adults and children, actually may be acute rheumatic fever (14,15). Varying responses to aspirin, especially in children, often are not documented with serum salicylate levels, and an unusual clinical course is not sufficient to exclude the diagnosis of acute rheumatic fever. Migratory arthritis without evidence of other major Jones Criteria (Table 12E-1), supported by two minor manifestations, must be considered acute rheumatic fever, and appropriate antibiotic prophylaxis should be prescribed (16).

ALLAN GIBOFSKY, MD
JOHN B. ZABRISKIE, MD

References

1. Veasy LG, Tani LY, Hill HR. Persistence of acute rheumatic fever in the intermountain area of the United States. J Pediatr 1994;124:9–16.
2. Gordis L. The virtual disappearance of rheumatic fever in the United States: lessons in the rise and fall of disease. Circulation 1985;72:1155–1162.
3. Pope RM. Rheumatic fever in the 1980s. Bull Rheum Dis 1989;38:1–8.
4. Shulman ST, Gerber MA, Tanz RR, Markowitz M. Streptococcal pharyngitis: the case for penicillin therapy. Pediatr Infect Dis J 1994;13:1–7.
5. Veasy LG, Wiedmeier SE, Orsmond GS, et al. Resurgence of acute rheumatic fever in the intermountain of the United States. N Engl J Med 1987;316:421–427.
6. Bessen D, Jones KF, Fischetti VA. Evidence for the distinct classes of streptococcal M protein and their relationship to rheumatic fever. J Exp Med 1989;169:269–283.
7. Kaplan EL, Anthony BF, Chapman SS, Ayoub EM, Wannamaker LW. The influence of the site of infection on the immune response to group A streptococci. J Clin Invest 1970;49:1405–1414.
8. Kaplan EL, Johnson DR, Cleary PP. Group A streptococcal serotypes isolated from patients and sibling contacts during the resurgence of rheumatic fever in the United States in the mid-1980s. J Infect Dis 1989;159:101–103.
9. Ayoub EM, Barrett DJ, Maclaren NK, Krischer JP. Association of class II human histocompatibility leucocyte antigens with rheumatic fever. J Clin Invest 1986;77:2019–2026.
10. Maharaj B, Hammond MG, Appadoo B, Leary WP, Pudifin DJ. HLA-A, B, DR and DQ antigens in black patients with severe chronic rheumatic heart disease. Circulation 1987;765:259–261.
11. Guilherme L, Weidenbach W, Kiss MH, Snitcowsky R, Kalil J. Association of human leucocyte class II antigens with rheumatic fever or rheumatic heart disease in a Brazilian population. Circulation 1991;83:1995–1998.
12. Khanna AK, Buskirk DR, Williams RC Jr, Gibofsky A, Crow MK, Mennon A. Presence of a non-HLA B cell antigen in rheumatic fever patients and their families as defined by a monoclonal antibody. J Clin Invest 1989;83:1710–1716.
13. United Kingdom and United States joint report on rheumatic heart disease. The natural history of rheumatic fever and rheumatic heart disease. Circulation 1965;32:457–476.
14. Schaffer FM, Agarwal R, Helm J, Gingell RL, Roland JM, O'Neil KM. Poststreptococcal reactive arthritis and silent carditis: a case report and review of the literature. Pediatrics 1994;93:837–839.
15. Arnold MH, Tyndall A. Poststreptococcal reactive arthritis. Ann Rheum Dis 1989;48:686–688.
16. Gibofsky A, Zabriskie JB. Rheumatic fever: new insights into an old disease. Bull Rheum Dis 1993;42:5–7.

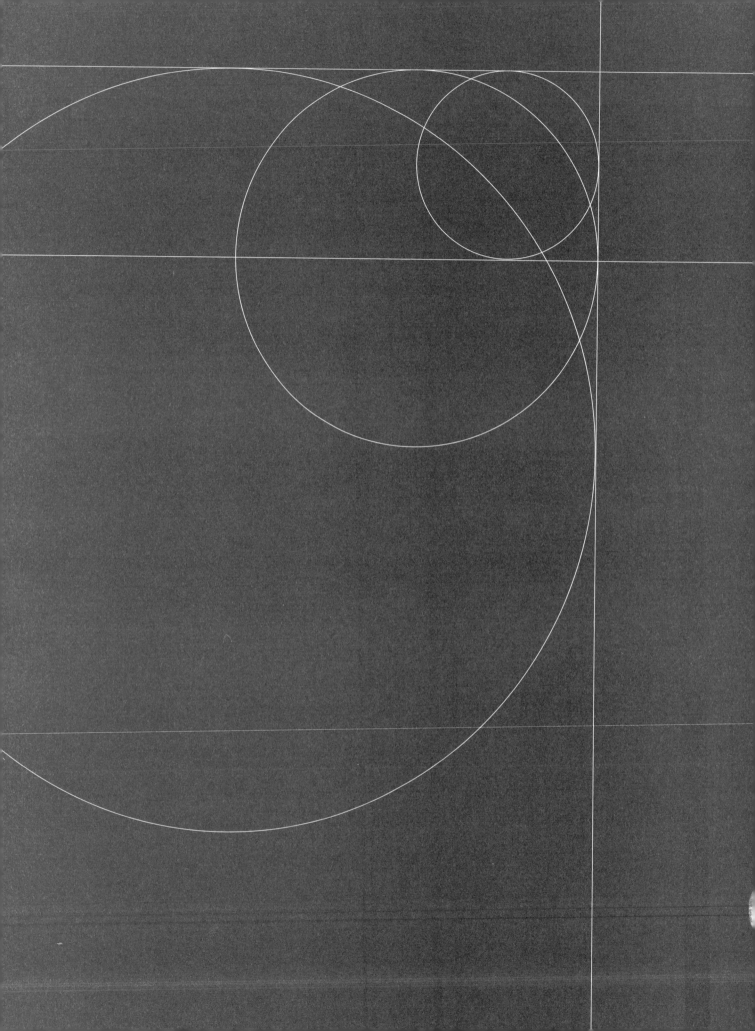

13 OSTEOARTHRITIS
A. Epidemiology, Pathology, and Pathogenesis

Epidemiology

Osteoarthritis (OA) is by far the most common joint disorder in the United States and throughout the world, and is one of the leading causes of disability and pain in the elderly (1). People with OA account for one of every eight days of restricted activity among the elderly in the United States. Although the disease commonly affects the cervical and lumbar spine, most epidemiologic studies report that it has a predilection for weight-bearing joints in the leg and certain joints in the hand. The prevalence of OA in all joints correlates strikingly with age. One-third of people aged 65 years and older have knee OA that is evident by radiograph. Before the age of 50, men are more likely to have OA than women, but after age 50, it is women who are more likely to be affected.

Not all people with radiographic OA develop symptomatic OA. The discrepancy between radiographic and symptomatic OA accounts for differing results of epidemiologic studies designed to define risk factors; most studies have surveyed only asymptomatic radiographic disease. These investigations have implicated systemic factors (age, sex, race, heredity, and obesity) and local factors (certain physical activities, injury, and developmental deformity) as risks for developing radiographic OA (2).

Local Factors
Excess Weight
Population-based studies of OA consistently have shown that overweight people are at greater risk of developing knee OA than average-weight controls. Obese women are four to five times more likely to have knee OA than persons of average weight. Longitudinal studies suggest that obese people with knee OA are at greater risk than thinner people for disease progression. Weight reduction is likely to lessen the symptoms of knee OA.

Although the association with body weight is not as strong for hip OA as it is for knee OA, overweight people appear to be at increased risk of OA in all weight-bearing joints, including hip OA. Surprisingly, there also is a positive association between obesity and OA in the hand, suggesting that obesity is a systemic risk factor for OA.

Injury and Occupation
Major acute knee injuries, including cruciate ligament and meniscal tears, are common causes of knee OA. Osteoarthritic changes have been reported in up to 89% of people after meniscectomy (3). Most people who have experienced complete anterior cruciate ligament rupture will develop knee OA. OA is associated with a variety of sport activities, including marathon running (hip OA), soccer playing (knee and hip OA), and American football playing (knee OA). However, there are conflicting data, because information on joint injury in this population often is unavailable. Standing, bending, walking long distances over rough ground, lifting, and moving heavy objects appear to increase the high risk of hip OA. Occupations associated with high rates of OA include farmer (hip OA), jackhammer operator (elbow), miner (knee and spine OA), and cotton mill worker (hand OA).

TABLE 13A-1
Factors Leading to Secondary Osteoarthritis

Local secondary forms	Generalized secondary forms
Joint injury	Hemochromatosis
Developmental deformities	Ochronosis
Osteonecrosis	Hyperparathyroidism
Rheumatoid arthritis (following cartilage damage)	Wilson's disease
Gout (following cartilage damage)	Gout
Chondrocalcinosis (following cartilage damage)	Chondrocalcinosis
Septic arthritis (following cartilage damage)	Acromegaly
Hemophilia-induced arthropathy	Amyloidosis
Neuropathic arthropathy	Hyperlaxity syndromes
Osteochondritis	Ehlers-Danlos disease
Paget's disease	

Developmental Deformities

Anatomic abnormalities of the knee and the hip that are present at birth or that develop during childhood may result in accelerated or premature OA. These abnormalities include genu varum, genu valgum, congenital hip subluxation, slipped capital femoral epiphysis, Legg-Calvé-Perthes disease, and acetabular dysplasia.

Other Local Factors

Strength of the lesser quadriceps, after adjustment for body weight, age, and sex, is predictive of both radiographic and symptomatic OA of the knee. Knee laxity, defined as abnormal displacement or rotation of the tibia with respect to the femur, may increase the risk of OA and contribute to progression. Damage to other local cartilage also can lead to OA (Table 13A-1).

Systemic Factors

Sex Hormones

Osteoarthritis occurs more frequently in women over the age of 50 than in age-matched men. Epidemiologic studies of women who take estrogen replacement therapy report that these women are less likely to have OA than women not taking estrogen (4).

Genetic Susceptibility

Many studies have demonstrated that genetic factors influence the incidence of OA. Heritability of primary OA of the hands has been reported to be as high as 65% (5). The existence of familial forms of certain OA, such as hand OA, implies the involvement of one or more genetic factors. Early studies focused on the alterations in type II and IX collagen, but no significant abnormalities were detected, except for mutations in COL2A1 in some families that had a phenotype distant from the common primary OA. More recent studies on other matrix components, such as aggrecan or the vitamin D receptor, have revealed no significant genetic abnormality in people with primary OA. In fact, twin and familial studies have shown OA to be a multigenic trait, with several genes involved (6).

Racial Differences

There is conflicting evidence as to whether African Americans have different rates of OA than Caucasians. The incidence of knee OA could be higher in African-American women (7).

Other Systemic Factors

Low vitamin D and vitamin C intakes are associated with increased risk of knee OA progression. Metabolic and endocrine disorders are associated with secondary forms of OA (Table 13A-1).

Pathology

Osteoarthritis can be defined as a gradual loss of articular cartilage, combined with thickening of the subchondral bone; bony outgrowths (osteophytes) at joint margins; and mild, chronic nonspecific synovial inflammation. The difference between "physiologic" aging of the cartilage and OA cartilage is not sharp. However, three cartilage stages can be identified: stage I, normal cartilage; stage II, aging cartilage; and stage III, OA cartilage.

Normal Cartilage

Normal cartilage has two main components. One is the extracellular matrix, which is rich in collagens (mainly types II, IX, and XI) and proteoglycans (mainly aggrecan). Aggrecan is a central core protein bearing numerous glycosaminoglycan chains of chondroitin sulfate and keratan sulfate, all capable of retaining molecules of water. The second component consists of isolated chondrocytes, which lie in the matrix. The matrix components are responsible for the tensile strength and resistance to mechanical loading of the articular cartilage. For a more detailed description of articular cartilage, see Chapter 2B.

Passage of Normal Cartilage to Aging Cartilage

Several structural and biochemical changes involving the noncollagenous component of the matrix occur during aging. These changes alter biomechanical properties of the cartilage that are essential for the distribution of forces in the weight-bearing zone. Glycosaminoglycans are modified qualitatively; they become shorter as the cartilage ages. The concentration of type 6 keratan sulfate (KS) increases during aging, to the detriment of type 4 KS. These quantitative and qualitative changes in proteoglycan reduce the capacity of the molecules to retain water. Thus, aging cartilage contains less water, which alters the biomechanical properties of the cartilage. Fissures that develop in cartilage during aging are due mainly to stress fractures of the collagen network.

Ostoearthritic Joints

Osteoarthritic joints have abnormal cartilage and bone, with synovial and capsular lesions (8). Macroscopically, the most characteristic elements are reduced joint space; formation of osteophytes (protrusions of bone and cartilage) mostly at the margins of joints; and sclerosis of the subchondral bone. These changes are the result of several histologic phases.

Phase 1: edema and microcracks. The first recognizable change in OA is edema of the extracellular matrix, principally in the intermediate layer. The cartilage loses its smooth aspect, and microcracks appear. There is a focal loss of chondrocytes, alternating with areas of chondrocyte proliferation.

Phase 2: fissuring and pitting. The microcracks deepen perpendicularly in the direction of the forces of tangential cutting and along fibrils of collagen. Vertical clefts form in the subchondral bone cartilage. Clusters of chondrocytes appear around these clefts and at the surface.

17. Schumacher HR Jr. Secondary osteoarthritis. In: Moskowitz RW, Howell DS, Goldberg VM, Mankin HJ (eds). Osteoarthritis: Diagnosis and Surgical Management. Philadelphia: WB Saunders, 1993; pp 367–398.
18. Kellgren JH, Moore R. Generalized osteoarthritis and Heberden's nodes. Br Med J 1952;1:181–187.
19. Altman RD, Asch E, Bloch D, et al. Development of criteria for the classification and reporting of osteoarthritis: classification of osteoarthritis of the knee. Arthritis Rheum 1986;29: 1039–1049.
20. Altman R, Alarcon G, Appelrough D, et al. The American College of Rheumatology criteria for the classification and reporting of osteoarthritis of the hand. Arthritis Rheum 1990; 33:1601–1610.
21. Altman R, Alarcon G, Appelrough D, et al. The American College of Rheumatology criteria for the classification and reporting of osteoarthritis of the hip. Arthritis Rheum 1991; 34:505–514.

OSTEOARTHRITIS
C. Treatment

Osteoarthritis (OA) is a serious and often disabling condition. The severity and impairment of OA may range from mild to severe. In addition, the number and distribution of involved joints varies significantly. Because of the heterogeneous nature of this disease, the treatment of OA must be individualized. Selecting the best treatment for each patient requires a mutual effort by the patient and the physician. As with all interventions, the potential benefits of treatment must be balanced against the possible risks. When both patient and physician understand the possible benefits and risks of therapy, an individualized treatment plan can be developed to achieve predefined goals and provide a framework for monitoring potential adverse events. The underlying principles of managing OA are relieving symptoms, maintaining and/or improving function, limiting physical disability, and avoiding drug toxicity (Table 13C-1). The American College of Rheumatology (ACR) originally published guidelines for the medical management of OA of the hip (1) and knee (2) in 1995. An update to these guidelines was published in 2000 (3). These guidelines provide practical recommendations on implementing the principles underlying medical management of OA.

Nonpharmacologic Therapy

The ACR guidelines recommend initial treatment with nonpharmacologic modalities in the management of OA. The 2000 update of the ACR guidelines again emphasizes the need for nonpharmacologic therapy and cites the increasing evidence that people with OA benefit from weight loss, physical therapy, muscle strengthening, and aerobic exercise.

TABLE 13C-1
General Principles of Osteoarthritis Treatment

Relieving symptoms
Maintaining and/or improving function
Limiting physical disability
Avoiding drug toxicity

This initial emphasis is to encourage interventions that can provide significant benefit with little associated risk to people with OA. Although these interventions frequently will not give sufficient relief as the only therapy, they often provide a beneficial foundation to which additional treatment can be added (Table 13C-2).

Patient Education and Support

A foundation of education must be established before patients can participate effectively in their care. Patient education materials, including pamphlets and online resources by the Arthritis Foundation, provide basic information to help people understand and cope with OA (4). Patients should be encouraged to participate in self-management programs, such as the Arthritis Self-Help Course, which is administered by local chapters of the Arthritis Foundation.

TABLE 13C-2
Nonpharmacologic Therapy of Osteoarthritis

Patient education
  Self-management programs
  Social support

Physical therapy
  Exercises
    Range of motion
    Muscle strengthening
    Aerobic conditioning
  Modalities
  Assistive Devices

Occupational therapy
  Assessment of activities of daily living
  Assistive devices for ambulation and activities of daily living

Weight loss

Studies have shown that people who participate in this program have better outcomes and lower health care costs than people who receive only traditional care (5).

Physical Therapy

Physical therapy can help patients build strength, improve range of motion, and use therapeutic modalities (6). Exercise programs stress range of motion and muscle strengthening (e.g., quadriceps-strengthening exercises to improve stability for people with knee OA). Although weight-bearing exercise generally is well-tolerated in people with healthy joints, high-impact activities that involve a joint with OA may accelerate the disease in this joint. Physical therapy can assist with the development of a non-impact aerobic exercise program for people with OA. An effective aerobic exercise program helps manage OA, provides significant general health benefits, and may assist in weight reduction, if needed. Local chapters of the Arthritis Foundation often sponsor aquatic exercise programs in heated pools under the direction of a trained therapist. Pre- and postoperative physical therapy for people undergoing reconstructive orthopedic surgery also plays a crucial role.

Occupational therapy

People with physical disabilities and difficulties in performing activities of daily living may benefit from consultation with an occupational therapist. The occupational therapist evaluates the patient's ability to perform activities of daily living, provides assistive devices as needed, and teaches joint protection techniques and energy conservation skills. Splints can be designed to stabilize and reduce pain and inflammation in finger joints, especially the thumb base. Braces, canes, walkers, other ambulation aids (including wedged shoe insoles), patella taping, and other assistive devices can be provided.

Weight reduction

Obesity clearly is associated with an increased incidence of OA. Although the data supporting weight loss as a means of reducing OA symptoms is not without limitations, and no prospective studies have unequivocally demonstrated that weight loss can arrest disease progression, overweight patients should be encouraged to lose weight. General health benefits are associated with achieving ideal weight. Epidemiologic data demonstrating the relationship between OA and obesity supports this recommendation. In patients being considered for total joint replacements, weight reduction is particularly important to reduce associated operative morbidity and mortality. Referral for dietary instruction and enrollment in an aerobic exercise program, such as fitness walking or swimming, may be helpful.

Systemic Pharmacologic Therapy

The main indication for drug therapy in OA is pain relief. Although inflammation may have a role in OA, analgesia is the primary benefit of most medications in OA, including traditional nonsteroidal anti-inflammatory drugs (NSAIDs)

and specific cyclooxygenase-2 (COX-2) inhibitors. The principal goal of systemic therapy has been to provide the most effective pain relief with the least associated toxicity (Table 13C-3).

Analgesic Medication
Nonnarcotic Analgesia
Acetaminophen is the initial systemic pharmacologic therapy recommended by ACR guidelines for the treatment of OA of the hip and knee. The 2000 update of these guidelines emphasizes the important role for acetaminophen in the treatment of OA and continues the recommendation that this agent be considered for initial therapy. However, the 2000 update recognizes that acetaminophen may not be as effective as NSAIDs in some patients. Two studies demonstrated that the short-term (7) and long-term (8) efficacy of acetaminophen is comparable with that of ibuprofen and naproxen in people with knee OA. Because these studies reported similar clinical benefit in people receiving acetaminophen, compared with people receiving NSAIDs, the ACR guidelines recommend the use of acetaminophen initially because of the lower toxicity associated with this agent. The comparable efficacy of these two classes of medication has been the subject of significant debate. Recent surveys of patient preference and practice patterns have suggested that NSAIDs may have a greater clinical benefit in OA patients (9). This controversy highlights the need for individualized therapy and the observation that clinical response to these agents will vary among patients. The data demonstrate that some patients will have a significant clinical benefit with acetaminophen that is comparable, in these patients, to the benefit with NSAIDs.

Narcotic Analgesia
Oral narcotic analgesia has been used in people with advanced and severe OA that has failed to respond to other

Table 13C-3
Pharmacologic Therapy of Osteoarthritis

Systemic
  Analgesia agents
    Non-narcotic analgesic (e.g., acetaminophen)
    Narcotic analgesics
  Anti-inflammatory agents
    Nonsteroidal anti-inflammatory drugs
    Specific cyclooxygenase-2 inhibitors

Local
  Intra-articular
    Corticosteroid injections
    Viscosupplementation
    Closed tidal lavage
  Topical therapy

measures. Although not technically a narcotic, tramadol has narcotic-like action and pain-relieving properties. The use of tramadol has been reported to reduce NSAID use and successfully treat breakthrough pain for people with OA. Recent advances in the management of acute and chronic malignant pain have lead to guidelines for treatments that have provided great benefit to patients with these conditions. The management of chronic nonmalignant pain has been a much more challenging issue. Although some guidelines are published to assist in the management of these conditions (10), the use of narcotic medication generally should be considered as a last resort and avoided if other effective therapy is available.

Anti-Inflammatory Agents

Mechanical abnormalities clearly play a significant role in OA pain. The significance of inflammation in the pathophysiology and clinical manifestation of OA is less clear. Powerful anti-inflammatory agents, such as corticosteroids, do not significantly improve OA symptoms, except in the case of localized injection, and thus are not indicated in OA. In contrast, NSAIDs, which have both analgesic and anti-inflammatory properties, are effective in OA. If symptoms do not respond to acetaminophen, NSAID use should be considered, unless contraindicated. The 2000 ACR guidelines highlight the increased understanding of NSAID-induced toxicity and the need to avoid this serious medication complication. These revised guidelines emphasize the risk stratification of patients for NSAID-induced complications, particularly gastrointestinal (GI) toxicity, and the use of specific COX-2 inhibitors or the addition of gastroprotective agents with traditional NSAIDs in patients at risk for GI complications.

Nonsteroidal Anti-Inflammatory Drugs

Several studies have demonstrated that NSAIDs are effective in OA. Because the different NSAIDs are about equally effective in relieving pain, the choice of a specific NSAID largely is influenced by differences in toxicity profiles, frequency of drug dosing, patient risk factors, and cost (11). The major concern about the routine use of NSAIDs in OA patients is the increased risk of upper GI toxicity, such as gastric and duodenal ulcers; GI bleeding; and renal toxicity, such as reversible renal insufficiency, fluid retention, and hyperkalemia. NSAIDs also can disrupt platelet function. For a more detailed review of NSAID toxicity, see Chapter 45.

The concern for NSAID-induced drug toxicity has been a major factor in the recommendation that other forms of analgesia be used first in the treatment of OA. Despite these concerns, NSAIDs provide important symptomatic relief. The 2000 ACR guidelines recommend the inclusion of either misoprostol or a proton-pump inhibitor if a nonselective NSAID is used in a patient at increased risk for an adverse GI event. If patients at low risk for GI events are to receive a nonselective NSAID, ACR guidelines recommend using the lowest effective dose, but do not recommend the addition of gastroprotective therapy. When considering the use of NSAID agents in the treatment of OA, the patient and physi-

cian must discuss the associated risks and benefits to determine if these agents should be used. This discussion should include a review of the GI and renal toxicity of NSAIDs.

Specific COX-2 Inhibitors

Specific COX-2 inhibitors have been evaluated in people with OA. These investigations have demonstrated that specific COX-2 inhibitors have clinical benefit similar to that of traditional NSAIDs and are more effective than placebo (12,13). In addition, studies of OA patients and healthy controls have demonstrated that the incidence of endoscopically proven GI toxicity with specific COX-2 inhibitors is much less than the incidence of endoscopically proven GI toxicity seen with traditional NSAIDs, and is similar to the incidence of GI toxicity seen with placebo (13). For a more detailed review of COX-2 inhibitors, see Chapters 4E and 45.

The place for specific COX-2 inhibitors in the treatment of OA is being established. The recent ACR guidelines recommend the use of specific COX-2 inhibitors or traditional NSAIDs with a gastroprotective agent in OA patients with an increased risk for GI toxicity. All available data suggest that these agents will provide clinical efficacy similar to that of traditional NSAIDs, but with less toxicity, particularly GI adverse events. Specific COX-2 inhibitors clearly represent an important option in the treatment of OA. Their appropriate role will be determined with more experience regarding their clinical efficacy, a greater understanding of their ability to avoid serious adverse drug events seen with traditional NSAIDs, and evaluations of the comparative efficacy of specific COX-2 inhibitors to acetaminophen. The costs associated with these new medications are important in determining their role. Currently, each practitioner will need to assess the risk and benefits, including cost, when determining which agent is most appropriate for each patient.

Localized Therapy

Intra-Articular Pharmacologic Therapy

Corticosteroid Injections

Intra-articular corticosteroid injections may be helpful for some OA patients with joint effusion or local inflammation. Local injections are beneficial as an adjunct to systemic therapy and may be used for those who are unable to take NSAIDs or specific COX-2 inhibitors. Injections must be performed using aseptic technique, and aspirated fluid should be cultured appropriately, if infection is suspected. Repeated intra-articular injections at a frequency of more than two or three times per year into the same joint have been discouraged because of concern about the potential for progressive cartilage damage and pseudo-Charcot arthropathy. In reality, very few such complications have been reported.

Viscosupplementation

Hyaluronan is a large glycosaminoglycan composed of repeating disaccharides of glucuronic acid and *N*-acetylglucosamine. In OA, the concentration and size of hyaluronan is reduced. Viscosupplementation therapy is the intra-articular injection of hyaluronan or its derivatives. Clinical trials comparing multiple joint injections of viscosupplementation therapy to placebo injections and/or NSAIDs have been conducted. Although some studies have failed to demonstrate clinically and statistically significant differences between the active and sham therapies, other studies have demonstrated a greater reduction in joint symptoms with viscosupplementation therapy than with placebo injections and a response similar to that seen with systemic NSAID treatment. The therapy has been reported effective for knee OA for periods of up to one year. A recent review of viscosupplementation therapy concluded that even if the improvement with viscosupplementation therapy is significantly better statistically than placebo injections, it is not clear that viscosupplementation therapy is significantly better clinically than placebo injections (14). The most common adverse events are injection-site reactions. Because of the nature of this therapy, viscosupplementation is regulated and approved in the United States as a medical device. The mechanism of action through which these compounds might reduce OA pain and their effect on joint cartilage is unknown.

Closed Tidal Lavage

Some patients with knee OA that has not responded to other therapies have been reported to benefit from closed tidal joint lavage. Tidal lavage of the knee involves the insertion of two large cannulae with the inflow and removal of a large fluid volume, usually one liter of normal saline. Tidal lavage has been reported to provide clinical benefit similar to intra-articular corticosteroid injection and arthroscopic debridement of the knee, although the duration of response with these different interventions is variable.

Topical Therapy

Topical therapies have been advocated as an adjuvant to systemic therapy or a replacement for systemic therapies. Topical NSAIDs and salicylates, and capsaicin creams have been reported effective for some people with OA.

Surgery

Patients whose symptoms are not controlled adequately with medical therapy and who have moderate to severe pain and functional impairment should be considered for orthopedic surgery. The majority of people with OA who will benefit from orthopedic surgery will have significant radiographic abnormalities.

Total joint arthroplasty has markedly improved the quality of life of patients with knee and hip OA and is one of the major advances in the management of OA over the past 30 years (15). These operations almost always provide significant, if not excellent, pain relief, but function is not always restored. Therefore, the most satisfying results are obtained when the operation is performed for the primary purpose of pain relief. Perioperative mortality generally is below 1%, and short-term complications, including thromboembolic disease and infection, occur in fewer than 5% of patients. A major concern with total joint arthroplasty is the long-term complication of loosening due to deterioration of the bone-cement interface. The developments of cementless prostheses and newer techniques for cementing prostheses eventually may reduce the frequency and severity of this complication. Despite these advances, total joint arthroplasties can fail and will require revision. Revision arthroplasty is a more complicated procedure than an initial joint arthroplasty.

Because one of the major factors leading to failure of a total joint replacement is the duration for which the artificial joint is in place, these procedures should be avoided in young patients who have other acceptable options. Other procedures often delay the need for a total joint replacement until an older age. OA of the knee complicated by internal derangement may be treated with arthroscopic debridement and, if indicated, lavage with meniscectomy. High tibial osteotomy is indicated for young patients in whom it is desirable to delay a total-joint replacement. For similar reasons, femoral osteotomy may be indicated for some younger patients with unilateral OA of the hip.

Alternative and Experimental Therapies

An estimated 23% of people with OA regularly use alternative and complementary therapies (16). Most patients using unconventional remedies are willing to discuss these therapies with their physician when asked (16). A description of the vast array of alternative therapies used by OA patients is beyond the scope of this review, but is the subject of Chapter 50 and Appendix IV in this book and other Arthritis Foundation publications (17). Understanding these alternative therapies can allow the physician to educate the patient with the information available about their use in OA and possible risks of treatment. These discussions can help patients use judgement when considering alternative treatments and avoid potentially harmful interventions.

Glucosamine and Chondroitin

Glucosamine and chrondroitin preparations are used commonly by people with OA and are widely advocated in lay publications. Multiple sources distribute these compounds. Because they are not classified as medications, but rather regulated as nutritional supplements, the quality and constitution of the different preparations varies. Fortunately, only minimal adverse events with glucosamine and chondroitin sulfate have been described.

Although several studies of these therapies in OA have been published, the quality of these investigations is not optimal. Limitations in these investigations include methodologic weaknesses, proprietary sponsorship, and possible publication bias (18). Despite these limitations, there is the possibility that these compounds may improve OA symptoms and even reduce the radiographic progression of OA. Large-scale, ongoing investigations of these agents may answer important questions.

Cartilage Repair and Transplantation

Extensive work has attempted to promote cartilage repair and restore normal cartilage tissue (19). Experimental procedures used to promote cartilage repair include penetration of subchondral bone, osteotomy, joint distraction, soft-tissue grafts of periosteum or perichondrium, cell transplantation, and use of growth factors. Unfortunately, these procedures generally are not successful in promoting cartilage repair. Results of early clinical experience with cartilage transplantation of autografts and allografts suggest that these procedures may benefit selected patient populations with focal cartilage defects. Currently, these procedures are not sufficiently successful for general application in people with OA.

Summary

Osteoarthritis is a serious and disabling condition. Many patients benefit significantly from a well-designed management program. A partnership between the patient and health care provider is the key to developing an individualized and effective treatment plan. Patient education, physical therapy, and occupational therapy form an important foundation in a comprehensive program. These activities can lead to an effective exercise program, use of assistive devices as necessary, and weight reduction if needed. Systemic and local therapies also are an effective component of treatment. Pharmacologic interventions include analgesic medications, NSAIDs, specific COX-2 inhibitors, intra-articular injections, and topical therapies. An assessment of the risks of GI complications should be considered in the selection of medical therapy. The major goal of these medical treatments is to provide optimal pain relief with minimal toxicity. Some people with OA, particularly those with more advanced disease, benefit from surgery. The development of an individualized treatment plan can help patients achieve the goals of relieving symptoms, maintaining and/or improving function, limiting physical disability, and avoiding drug toxicity.

GRANT W. CANNON, MD

References

1. Hochberg MC, Altman RD, Brandt KD, et al. Guidelines for the medical management of osteoarthritis: Part I. Osteoarthritis of the hip. Arthritis Rheum 1995;38:1535–1540.
2. Hochberg MC, Altman RD, Brandt KD, et al. Guidelines for the medical management of osteoarthritis: Part II. Osteoarthritis of the knee. Arthritis Rheum 1995;38:1541–1546.
3. American College of Rheumatology Subcommittee on Osteoarthritis Guidelines. Recommendations for the medical management of osteoarthritis of the hip and knee: 2000 Update. Arthritis Rheum 2000;43:1905–1915.
4. Fries JF, Carey C, McShane DJ. Patient education in arthritis: randomized controlled trial of a mail-delivered program. J Rheumatol 1997;24:1378–1383.
5. Kruger JM, Helmick CG, Callahan LF, Haddix AC. Cost-effectiveness of the arthritis self-help course. Arch Intern Med 1998;158:1245–1249.
6. Deyle GD, Henderson NE, Matekel RL, Ryder MG, Garber MB, Allison SC. Effectiveness of manual physical therapy and exercise in osteoarthritis of the knee. A randomized, controlled trial. Ann Intern Med 2000;132:173–181.
7. Bradley JD, Brandt KD, Katz BP, Kalasinski LA, Ryan SL. Comparison of an inflammatory dose of ibuprofen, an analgesic dose of ibuprofen and acetaminophen in the treatment of patients with osteoarthritis of the knee. N Engl J Med 1991; 325:87–91.
8. Williams HJ, Ward JR, Egger MJ, et al. Comparison of naproxen and acetaminophen in a two-year study of treatment of osteoarthritis of the knee. Arthritis Rheum 1993;36:1196–1206.
9. Wolfe F, Zhao S, Lane N. Preference for nonsteroidal anti-inflammatory drugs over acetaminophen by rheumatic disease patients: a survey of 1,799 patients with osteoarthritis, rheumatoid arthritis, and fibromyalgia. Arthritis Rheum 2000;43:378–385.
10. AGS Panel on Chronic Pain in Older Persons. Clinical practice guidelines: the management of chronic pain in older persons. JAGS 1998;46:635–651.
11. Furst DE. Are there differences among nonsteroidal anti-inflammatory drugs? Comparing acetylated salicylates, nonacetylated salicylates, and nonacetylated nonsteroidal anti-inflammatory drugs. Arthritis Rheum 1994;37:1–9.
12. Crofford LJ, Lipsky PE, Brooks P, Abramson SB, Simon LS, Van De Putte LBA. Basic biology and clinical application of specific cyclooxygenase-2 inhibitors. Arthritis Rheum 2000; 43:4–13.
13. Feldman M, McMahon AT. Do cyclooxygenase-2 inhibitors provide benefits similar to those of traditional nonsteroidal anti-inflammatory drugs, with less gastrointestinal toxicity? Ann Intern Med 2000;132:134–143.
14. Brandt KD, Smith GN Jr, Simon LS. Intraarticular injection of hyaluronan as treatment for knee osteoarthritis: what is the evidence? Arthritis Rheum 2000;43:1192–1203.
15. Crawford RW, Murray DW. Total hip replacement: indications for surgery and risk factors for failure. Ann Rheum Dis 1997;56:455–457.
16. Rao JK, Mihaliak K, Kroenke K, Bradley J, Tierney WM, Weinberger M. Use of complementary therapies for arthritis among patients of rheumatologists. Ann Intern Med 1999; 131:409–416.
17. Horstman J. The Arthritis Foundation's Guide to Alternative Therapies. Atlanta: Arthritis Foundation, 1999.
18. McAlindon TE, LaValley MP, Gulin JP, Felson DT. Glucosamine and chondroitin for treatment of osteoarthritis: a systematic quality assessment and meta-analysis. JAMA 2000;283:1469–1475.
19. Buckwalter JA, Mankin HJ. Articular cartilage repair and transplantation. Arthritis Rheum 1998;41:1331–1342.

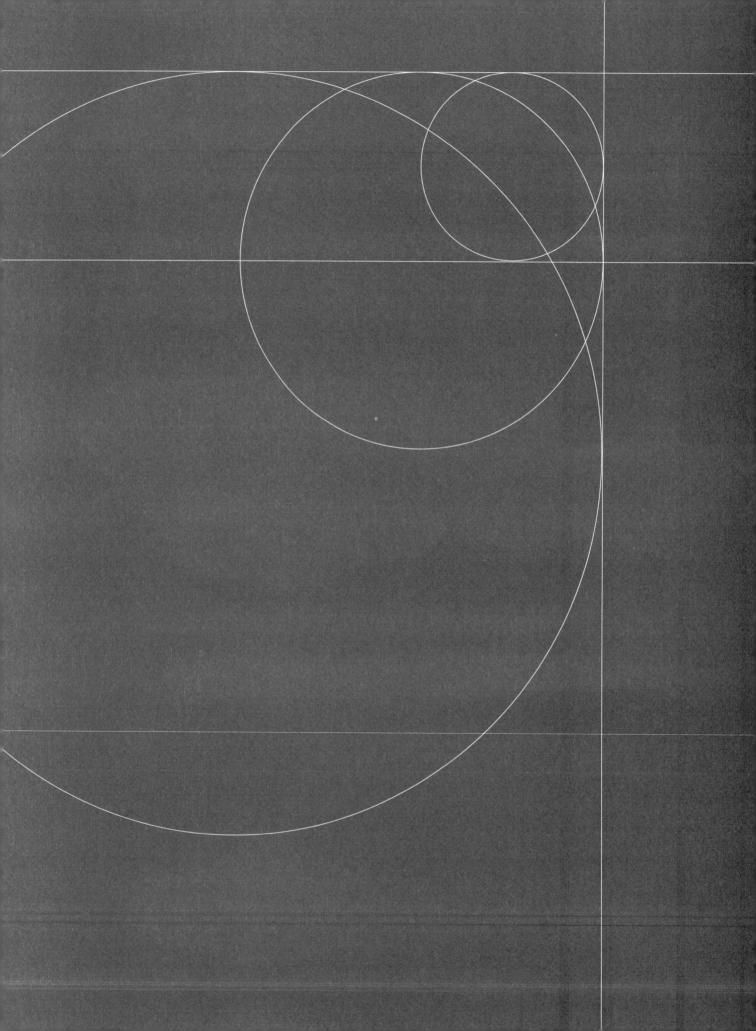

14 ARTHRITIS ASSOCIATED WITH CALCIUM-CONTAINING CRYSTALS

Calcium Pyrophosphate Dihydrate Crystal Deposition Disease

Specific identification of calcium pyrophosphate dihydrate (CPPD) crystals ($Ca_2P_2O_7 \bullet H_2O$) in synovial fluid or articular tissue allows the clinician to differentiate between CPPD crystal deposition disease and other inflammatory and degenerative arthritides (1). The term *chondrocalcinosis* refers to the presence of calcium-containing crystals detected as radiodensities in articular cartilage. Calcium-containing crystals other than CPPD may also deposit in articular cartilages, producing radiographically detectable densities in cartilage, and joint inflammation or degeneration. Deposition of CPPD crystals is not limited to articular cartilage; less frequently, CPPD crystals are deposited in synovial lining, ligaments, tendons, and on rare occasions, periarticular soft tissue (much like gouty tophi).

CPPD crystal deposition disease may be asymptomatic or may manifest in a variety of ways. The term *pseudogout* refers to the acute, gout-like attacks of inflammation that occur in some people with CPPD crystal deposition disease. CPPD deposition also may cause symptoms similar to septic arthritis, polyarticular inflammatory arthritis, or osteoarthritis (OA).

Pathologic surveys indicate that about 4% of the adult population have articular CPPD deposits at the time of death (1). Radiologic surveys show a steadily increasing prevalence with age, and by their ninth decade, nearly 50% of individuals have chondrocalcinosis.

Classification

Arthritis associated with CPPD crystal deposition can be classified as hereditary, sporadic (idiopathic), or associated with various metabolic diseases or trauma. Most patients with familial disease show an autosomal dominant pattern of inheritance. Susceptibility to familial CPPD crystal deposition disease has been most commonly localized to the short arm of chromosome 5 (2). A thorough study of patients with sporadic disease likely would result in reclassifying many people as having heritable or disease-associated deposition. Because of the high prevalence of CPPD crystal deposition, the condition often has been reported as associated with other conditions. The most likely "true" associations include hyperparathyroidism, hemochromatosis, hypothyroidism, amyloidosis, hypomagnesemia, and hypophosphatasia. However, none of these associations has been proved in rigorously controlled studies. An association with aging is well-documented.

The routine study of a patient newly diagnosed with CPPD crystal deposition should include evaluation of serum calcium, ferritin, magnesium, phosphorous, alkaline phosphatase, and thyroid-stimulating hormone. Further studies should be obtained if abnormal values are found. Hypomagnesemia and hypophosphatasia are uncommon associations in people over age 60 years at the time of first clinical symptoms.

Pathogenesis of Inflammation and Cartilage Degeneration

Acute pseudogout is thought to represent a dose-related inflammatory host response to CPPD crystals shed from cartilaginous tissues contiguous to the synovial cavity (3). Phagocytosis of crystals by neutrophils results in release of lysosomal enzymes and cell-derived chemotactic factors. Phagocytosis by synovial-lining cells leads to cell proliferation and release of prostaglandins, cytokines, and proteases able to degrade cartilage matrix, such as collagenase and stromelysin.

Colchicine in therapeutic concentrations is remarkably effective in blocking the release of chemotactic factors for neutrophils and mononuclear cells, and it inhibits neutrophil–endothelial cell binding, a step in the ingress of neutrophils into the synovial space.

The frequency of association of CPPD crystal deposits and degenerative joint disease may result from the biologic properties of cell interaction with calcium-containing crystals (4,5). Ingestion of such crystals by fibroblasts or mononuclear synovial-lining cells is followed by intracellular dissolution, raising intracellular free-calcium levels. This sequence predictably engenders a mitogenic response, resulting in tissue hypertrophy. Stimulated lining cells secrete proteolytic enzymes (matrix metalloproteinases), which may damage cartilage and other articular structures. Cytokine release can lead to further protease release by lining cells or chondrocytes. Such effects have been demonstrated for CPPD crystals in vitro. That these events occur in vivo is suggested by synovial-fluid studies indicating that fluids containing CPPD crystals have, on average, the highest concentration of proteoglycan breakdown products, and the highest ratio of protease-to-protease inhibitor of all forms of arthritis tested.

Pathogenesis of Crystal Deposition

Plasma levels and urinary excretion of inorganic pyrophosphate (PPi) are not elevated in patients with CPPD crystal deposition disease. Synovial fluid PPi concentration, however, is elevated in most joints afflicted with CPPD crystal deposition. Articular chondrocytes likely contribute to PPi, which accumulates in joint fluids, because cartilage slices and chondrocyte cell cultures liberate PPi into the ambient media, while nonarticular tissues do not. The liberation of PPi is stimulated by ascorbate (6), transforming growth factor beta (7), retinoic acid (8), and thyroid hormones (9); it is inhibited by probenecid (10), insulin-like growth factor-1 (11), inhibitors of protein synthesis (6), isoforms of parathyroid hormone-related peptide (12), and interleukin 1 (13). Signaling pathways involved in PPi generation include protein kinase C (up-regulates) and adenylyl cyclase (down-regulates) (14). Kinetic studies indicate that much of the extracellular PPi may be generated by an ectoenzyme, NTPPase. This enzyme is found in elevated amounts in cartilage extracts (15), synovial fluids (16), and cell cultures (17) from people with CPPD crystal deposits. It generates PPi from nucleoside triphosphate substrates, such as adenosine triphosphate (ATP), which also is present in elevated concentrations in joint fluids containing CPPD crystals (18). Vesicles derived from chondrocytes are particularly enriched in NTPPase activity and are able to nucleate and grow monoclinic CPPD crystals in vitro in the presence of ATP (19). ATP added to cartilage explants likewise induces formation of perichondral CPPD-like crystals, many of which appear to form within membranous structures (20). The vesicle-associated form of NTPPase is distinct from two other forms found on many cells, including chondrocytes (21,22) The vesicle-associated form of NTPPase is identical to intermediate-layer cartilage protein (23). Recent studies of murine ankylosis suggest that the ANK protein is important in increasing extracellular PPi formation. Mutation of this protein underlies murine ankylosis, suggesting that extracellular PPi has a physiologic role in preventing excess articular structure apatite mineralization (24).

Unlike gout, a disease generally associated with a systemic abnormality of excess anion (hyperuricemia), CPPD crystal deposition is driven by a local abnormality of excess articular anion production. In either condition, local factors determine the foci of crystal deposition. Local factors favoring CPPD crystal deposition could include bursts of increased PPi generation by selected chondrocytes, leading to a pericellular increase in anion; synthesis of molecules or particulates capable of heterologous CPPD crystal nucleation; or absence of physiologic crystal inhibitors.

Clinical Features

Acute pseudogout is marked by inflammation in one or more joints that lasts for several days to two weeks. These self-limited attacks can be as abrupt in onset and as severe as acute gout. Almost one-half of all attacks involve the knees, although attacks have been documented in nearly all joints, including the first metatarsophalangeal (the most common site for gout). As with gout, pseudogout attacks can occur spontaneously or can be provoked by trauma, surgery, or severe illness, such as stroke or myocardial infarction. Patients usually are asymptomatic between episodes. Differentiation from gout or joint infection may be difficult and requires

arthrocentesis, examination of the synovial fluid for crystals, and culture. About 25% of people with CPPD crystal deposition disease exhibit the pseudogout pattern of disease.

About 5% of people with CPPD deposition manifest a "pseudorheumatoid" presentation, including multiple joint involvement with symmetric distribution and low-grade inflammation. Accompanying morning stiffness, fatigue, synovial thickening, flexion contractures, and elevated erythrocyte sedimentation rate often lead to a misdiagnosis of rheumatoid arthritis. In addition, 10% of people with CPPD crystal deposits have low titers of rheumatoid factor, which provide further diagnostic confusion. The presence of high-titer rheumatoid factor and radiographic evidence of typical rheumatoid bony erosions favor the diagnosis of "true" rheumatoid arthritis.

Nearly one-half of people with CPPD crystal deposits have progressive degeneration of numerous joints. The knees are affected most commonly, followed by the wrists, metacarpophalangeal joints, hips, shoulders, elbows, and ankles. Although there is some overlap with the pattern of joint involvement in primary OA (e.g., hip and knee), the distribution of joint degeneration with CPPD crystal deposition is distinctive. Involvement of distal interphalangeal and proximal interphalangeal joints (manifested by Heberden's and Bouchard's nodes) and the first carpometacarpal joint – all characteristic of primary OA – are no more common in patients with CPPD deposition disease than would be expected by chance alone in an elderly population. Symmetric involvement is the rule, although degeneration may be more advanced on one side. Flexion contractures of the affected joints and deformities of the knees are common. Valgus knee deformities are especially suggestive of underlying CPPD crystal deposits. Patients with chronic symptoms of this pseudo-OA pattern may have superimposed episodes of joint inflammation.

Neurologic manifestations of CPPD crystal deposition in the axial skeleton can occur. A syndrome of acute neck pain ascribed to CPPD (or to basic calcium phosphate) crystal deposits, associated with a tomographic appearance of calcification surrounding the odontoid process, has been called the *crowned dens* syndrome (25). At times, neck pain may be accompanied by stiffness and fever that mimic meningitis. This may occur in the postoperative period after parathyroidectomy. Other patients have developed long tract signs and symptoms related to deposits of CPPD crystals and adjacent tissue hypertrophy in the cervical or lumbar spine. The ligamentum flavum has been the cervical site most regularly reported for CPPD crystal deposition (26). Crystal deposits, ligament hypertrophy, chondroid metaplastic growths, facet joint osteophytes, and bulging discs contribute to encroachment on the cord.

Systemic findings during an acute attack of pseudogout are frequent but not invariable. These include a fever of 99°–103°F, leukocytosis of 12,000–15,000 cells/mm^3, and elevated erythrocyte sedimentation rate and serum acute-phase reactants. Interleukin 6 may mediate some of these systemic effects (27).

Many people with CPPD crystal deposits have no joint symptoms. Even patients who have symptoms in some joints have other joints with CPPD crystal deposits that are completely asymptomatic and clinically normal.

Radiologic Features

The typical appearance of punctate and linear densities in articular hyaline or fibrocartilaginous tissues is helpful diagnostically. The most characteristic sites of crystal deposition are illustrated in Fig. 14-1. When the deposits are typical and unequivocal (Fig. 14-2), the radiologic appearance is nearly specific, but interpretation of atypical or faint deposits often is difficult. Calcific deposits also may appear in the articular capsule, ligaments, and tendons. Although the earliest calcific deposits occur in radiographically normal cartilage, degenerative changes often supervene. A person can be screened for CPPD crystal deposits with four radiographs: an anteroposterior (AP) view of both knees (preferably not standing), an AP view of the pelvis for visualization of the symphysis pubis and hips, and a posteroanterior (PA) view of each hand to include the wrists. If these views show no evidence of crystal deposits, it is most unlikely that further study will prove fruitful.

Changes in the metacarpophalangeal joints, such as squaring of the bone ends, subchondral cysts, and

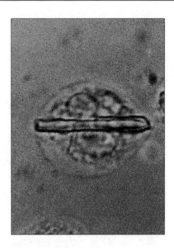

Fig. 14-2. Neutrophilic leukocyte in fresh preparation of synovial fluid from an 84-year-old woman with acute inflammation of the knee (pseudogout). Note rod-shaped crystal of calcium pyrophosphate dihydrate.

hook-like osteophytes, are characteristic features of the arthritis associated with hemochromatosis, but also are found in patients with CPPD crystal deposition alone. These changes occur more frequently in people with CPPD crystal deposits and hemochromatosis than in those with only crystal deposits. In addition to the difference in the pattern of affected joints, the finding of isolated patellofemoral joint space narrowing or isolated wrist degeneration differentiates CPPD from OA. Such differences may provide helpful clinical clues and are incorporated into the diagnostic criteria given in Table 14-1.

Treatment

In contrast to monosodium urate crystals in gout, there is no practical way to remove CPPD crystals from joints. Treatment of putative associated diseases, such as hyperparathyroidism, hemochromatosis, or myxedema, does not result in resorption of CPPD crystal deposits. Acute attacks in large joints can be treated through aspiration alone or aspiration combined with injection of microcrystalline corticosteroid esters. Intravenous colchicine is effective in the treatment of pseudogout, but nonsteroidal anti-inflammatory drugs (NSAIDs) are recommended for most patients. The effectiveness of oral colchicine is less predictable in pseudogout than in gout, but the number and duration of acute attacks are reduced significantly by colchicine taken on a daily basis for prophylaxis. Corticotropin or corticosteroid treatment has been used successfully in patients with gout and pseudogout (28). Although in development, phosphocitrate is a promising agent that inhibits CPPD crystal formation and cellular responses (mitogenesis and protease secretion) to CPPD crystals (29). Whether crystal removal prevents or slows the degenerative cartilaginous and bony changes is an important but unanswered question.

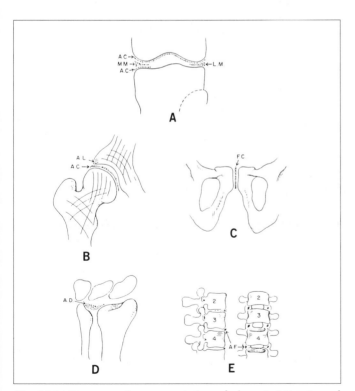

Fig. 14-1. Diagrammatic representation of characteristic sites of CPPD crystal deposition. A: AC, articular cartilage; LM and MM, lateral and medial meniscus in knee joint shown in anteroposterior (AP) projection. B: AL, acetabular labrum in AP projection of hip joint. C: FC, fibrocartilaginous symphysis pubis in AP projection of pelvis. D: AD, articular disc of the wrist in AP projection. E: AF, anulus fibrosus of intervertebral discs in AP and lateral views. Reprinted from Bulletin on the Rheumatic Diseases, with permission.

Basic Calcium Phosphates

A wide variety of crystals may deposit in joints and periarticular tissues (Table 14-2). Basic calcium phosphate crystals (BCP), consisting of carbonate-substituted hydroxyapatite, octacalcium phosphate, and rarely, tricalcium phosphate,

TABLE 14-1
Revised Diagnostic Criteria for CPPD Crystal Deposition Disease

Criteria

I. Demonstration of CPPD crystals in tissue or synovial fluid by definitive means (e.g., characteristic X-ray diffraction or chemical analysis)

II. (a) Identification of monoclinic or triclinic crystals showing weakly positive or no birefringence by compensated polarized light microscopy

   (b) Presence of typical radiographic calcification

III. (a) Acute arthritis, especially of knees or other large joints

   (b) Chronic arthritis, especially of knee, hip, wrist, carpus, elbow, shoulder, or metacarpophalangeal joint, especially if accompanied by acute exacerbations. The following features help differentiate chronic arthritis from osteoarthritis:

   1. Uncommon site – wrist, metacarpophalangeal, elbow, shoulder
   2. Radiographic appearance – radiocarpal or patellofemoral joint space narrowing, especially if isolated (patella "wrapped around" the femur)
   3. Subchondral cyst formation
   4. Severity of degeneration – progressive, with subchondral bony collapse and fragmentation with formation of intra-articular radiodense bodies
   5. Osteophyte formation – variable and inconstant
   6. Tendon calcifications, especially triceps, Achilles, obturators

Categories

A. Definite disease: Criteria I or II(a) plus II(b) must be fulfilled.

B. Probable disease: Criteria II(a) or II(b) must be fulfilled.

C. Possible disease: Criteria III(a) or III(b) should alert the clinician to the possibility of underlying CPPD crystal deposition

frequently deposit in articular tissues, but also may be found in skin, arteries, and other tissues (30). In the musculoskeletal system, crystals may be found in tendons, intervertebral discs, joint capsule, synovium, and cartilage. Usually, calcifications are single, but multiple deposits may occur. Rarely, a familial relationship is identified.

The role of BCP crystals in the pathogenesis of such joint diseases as OA remains uncertain. Several hypotheses have been formulated that account for possible roles of BCP crystals, as follows: 1) BCP crystals may directly cause arthritis; 2) BCP crystals may accelerate or exacerbate preexisting arthritis; 3) BCP crystals may exist as an epiphenomenon without a significant role in arthritis. Despite a lack of defin-

itive knowledge about BCP crystals, several associations have been made in which a pathogenic role is possible.

Etiology and Pathogenesis of BCP-Related Conditions

Although physiologic concentrations of calcium and phosphate are close to saturation, tissue calcification is unusual because of endogenous inhibitors of calcification. Metastatic calcification occurs with a high calcium × phosphate product (e.g., renal failure with elevated levels of phosphate). Dystrophic calcification occurs in tissues that have been altered in some way to promote calcification, but with normal levels of calcium and phosphate. Pathophysiologic changes that promote calcification may include tissue damage, hypovascularity and tissue hypoxia, age-related tissue changes, and genetically determined predispositions favoring calcification. Calcification could occur with the loss of inhibitors or the appearance of calcification promoters (e.g., crystal nucleators). Actual mechanisms of calcification remain poorly understood, and in individual patients, the exact cause of calcification is unlikely to be determined. In calcific tendinitis/periarthritis, chondrocytes or metaplastic synoviocytes may produce calcifying matrix vesicles, partially reproducing the mechanism of enchondral ossification in growing bones (31).

If a sufficient number of BCP crystals are released into a joint space or surrounding tissues, it is presumed that polymorphonuclear leukocytes are attracted, crystals are phagocytosed, and an inflammatory response results. This mechanism, which is similar to that seen in gout and pseudogout, is unusual with BCP crystals. More commonly, BCP crystals are found in osteoarthritic synovial fluids that are not inflammatory. The synovial-fluid leukocyte count is low, and the cells are predominantly mononuclear. Low-grade inflammation may be present, with manifestations that include the formation of an effusion within an affected joint and synovial-lining cell hypertrophy (32). Chronic damage may occur when BCP crystals are phagocytosed by synovial-lining cells with subsequent induction of cell proliferation and the synthesis and release of prostaglandins, collagenase, stromelysin, and other proteases and biologically active substances that directly or indirectly damage cartilage (33,34).

BCP Crystal Identification

Although BCP crystals are common, particularly in OA, their presence is recognized infrequently because of the lack of a simple, reliable test for detection. Polarized light microscopy, which effectively identifies monosodium urate and CPPD crystals, is unable to detect BCP crystals, which are too small to be resolved by light microscopy (length, 50–500 nm). Despite the small size of individual crystals, they tend to aggregate into larger masses that occasionally may be observed by light microscopy as refractile "shiny coins" up to 5 mm in diameter. The larger BCP aggregates have been detected by Alizarin red S staining, but this method lacks sensitivity and specificity (35). Techniques

TABLE 14-2
Some Crystals and Other Particles Identified in Joint Tissues and Synovial Fluids[a]

Monosodium urate monohydrate crystals
Spherulites of urates
Calcium pyrophosphate dihydrate crystals
Basic calcium phosphates
    Apatites
    Tricalcium phosphate
    Octacalcium phosphate
Dicalcium phosphate dihydrate (brushite)
Calcium magnesium phosphate (whitlokite)
Calcium carbonates (calcite and aragonite)
Calcium oxalates (monohydrate and dihydrate)
Lipids
    Cholesterol crystals
    "Liquid lipid crystals"
    Lipid spherulites
Protein crystals, such as cryoglobulins, hematoidin
    crystals, and Charcot-Leyden crystals
Steroid crystals
Plant thorns, sea urchin spines, and other extrinsic particles
Metal, plastic, and cement fragments from implants
Cartilage fragments

[a] Combinations or mixtures of two or more types of particle in the same joint are seen more commonly than would be expected by chance.

that are more specific for BCP-crystal identification include x-ray diffraction, scanning or transmission electron microscopy with energy dispersive analysis, electron microprobe, Fourier transform infrared spectroscopy, Raman spectroscopy, atomic force microscopy, and a binding assay utilizing [^{14}C]ethane-1-hyroxy-1,1-diphosphonate (36). Unfortunately, these methods typically are unavailable or too costly for the handling of routine clinical specimens.

Clinical Features
Large-Joint Destructive Arthritis
Shoulder disease is common in the elderly, usually taking the form of rotator cuff tendinitis, a rotator cuff tear, bursitis, or glenohumeral OA. Occasionally, cases of extreme shoulder joint damage are encountered. Typically, these patients are elderly women and manifest large, cool synovial effusions, severe radiographic damage, and large rotator cuff tears. Patients have variable pain, frequent night pain, limited range of motion, and in some cases, subluxation of the glenohumeral joint. Synovial-fluid leukocyte counts are low, and most fluids contain BCP crystals. Some have CPPD crystals in addition to BCP crystals in the synovial fluid. Radiographs show periarticular calcifications, upward subluxation of the humeral head, and deformity of the humeral head (Fig. 14-3). Various terms have been used to describe this shoulder

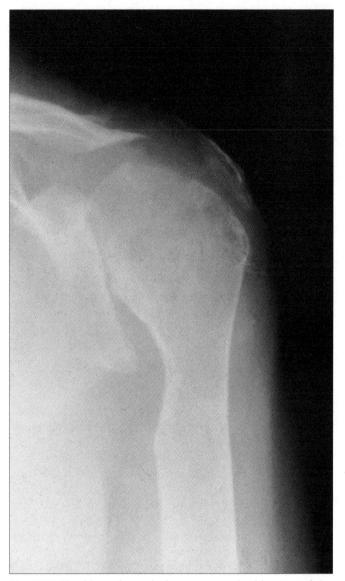

Fig. 14-3. Shoulder radiograph showing upward subluxation of the humerus and extensive bony destruction of the acromium and of both sides of the glenohumeral joint, with soft-tissue evidence of an effusion and calcific deposits. These are the characteristic features of advanced apatite-associated destructive arthritis or Milwaukee shoulder.

disorder, including l'arthropathie destructice rapide de l'epaule, idiopathic destructive arthritis, Milwaukee shoulder syndrome, and cuff tear arthropathy (37–40).

Calcific Periarthritis
Periarticular calcifications occasionally are observed on shoulder or other radiographs (Fig. 14-4). The most common site of calcification is in the rotator cuff. Most calcifications remain asymptomatic. If a patient has chronic shoulder pain, the radiographic finding of a calcification in the supraspinatus tendon or another tendon in the rotator cuff supports a diagnosis of chronic calcific tendinitis. In a few cases, particularly in those with large calcific deposits, a severe attack of joint pain is precipitated by dispersal of

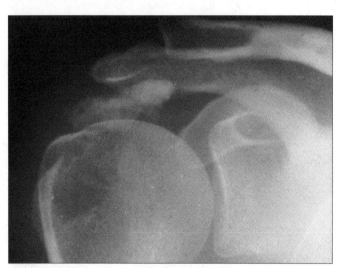

Fig. 14-4. Shoulder radiograph showing a large periarticular deposit of calcific material in the area of the supraspinatus tendon and subacromial bursa. Note that the deposit has no trabeculae (indicating that it is not bony) and that it has clear edges. When an acute attack of calcific periarthritis occurs, the edges become blurred and the deposit smaller, as crystals are shed into the surrounding soft tissues.

crystals into surrounding tissues, the subdeltoid bursa, or the shoulder joint. These crystals elicit a major local inflammatory response. Patients present with severe pain and joint swelling, with warmth and erythema. The diagnosis is suspected upon radiographic observation of a rotator cuff calcification. Other diagnoses are likely to be considered, including sepsis, trauma, fracture, gout, or pseudogout. The radiographic features may evolve over time, with the calcific deposit becoming smaller, fragmenting, or disappearing. In some cases, particularly involving areas other than the shoulder, computed tomography or magnetic resonance imaging may suggest the diagnosis. Needle aspiration of a calcific deposit may yield chalky material, and in the case of the shoulder, may shorten the course of the attack. Improvement also occurs following administration of NSAIDs or a local steroid injection. Ultrasound has been suggested as a method of breaking up calcific deposits (41). Untreated, the involved area may remain symptomatic for a few days or several weeks. Smaller joints, such as the first metatarsal of the foot (hydroxyapatite pseudopodagra) and small joints of the hand, may undergo similar inflammatory attacks, particularly in younger women (42,43).

Osteoarthritis

BCP crystals are present in 30%–60% of osteoarthritic joints but, for the most part, remain undetected by routine synovial-fluid analysis (44). The severity of the osteoarthritic lesion correlates with the presence and amount of BCP crystals. With a more sensitive technique for detection of BCP crystals, BCP was found in nearly all osteoarthritic fluids (45). BCP crystals most likely arise from exposed bone or from metaplastic synovial tissue. BCP crystals also have been observed in hyaline articular cartilage, but not in the

large deposits that occur with CPPD crystals. Whether or not BCP crystals associated with OA actually contribute to the pathogenesis of the arthritis remains undetermined. (In a similar way, monosodium urate crystals and CPPD crystals also may be found in joint fluids from joints without significant inflammation, and the same question applies to these crystals.) There is no known therapy for prevention or removal of calcium-containing crystals from joints.

Acute Arthritis

In rare situations, BCP crystals may cause acute inflammation in joints. BCP crystals have been found in finger joints that exhibit inflammation and erosive changes (46). BCP crystals may have a role in "inflammatory OA," a subgroup of OA associated with erythema, synovial thickening, and severe radiographic damage in proximal and distal interphalangeal joints of the hands.

Calcinosis

Calcinosis is the soft-tissue deposition of BCP crystals. A wide variety of diseases has been associated with dystrophic calcification. Some of these conditions include the connective-tissue diseases (limited scleroderma, myositis, systemic lupus erythematosus), calcification following severe neurologic injury, and calcification following triamcinolone hexacetonide injection of joints.

PAUL B. HALVERSON, MD
LAWRENCE M. RYAN, MD

References

1. Ryan LM, McCarty DJ. Calcium pyrophosphate dihydrate crystal deposition disease; pseudogout; articular chondrocalcinosis. In: Koopman WJ (ed). Arthritis and Allied Conditions. Baltimore: Williams & Wilkins, 1997; pp 2103.

2. Andrew LJ, Brancolini V, de la Pena LS, et al. Refinement of the chromosome 5p locus for familial calcium pyrophosphate dihydrate deposition disease. Am J Hum Genet 1999;64:136–145.

3. Terkeltaub RA. Pathogenesis and treatment of crystal-induced inflammation. In: Koopman WJ (ed). Arthritis and Allied Conditions. Baltimore: Williams & Wilkins, 1997; pp 2085.

4. Cheung HS, Ryan LM. Role of crystal deposition in matrix degradation. In: Woessner FJ, Howell DS (eds). Joint Cartilage Degradation: Basic and Clinical Aspects. New York: Marcel Dekker, 1995; pp 209.

5. Ryan LM, Cheung HS. The role of crystals in osteoarthritis. Rheum Dis Clin North Am 1999;25:257–267.

6. Ryan LM, Kurup I, Cheung HS. Stimulation of cartilage inorganic pyrophosphate elaboration by ascorbate. Matrix 1991;11:276–281.

7. Rosenthal AK, Cheung HS, Ryan LM. Transforming growth factor β1 stimulates inorganic pyrophosphate elaboration by porcine cartilage. Arthritis Rheum 1991;34:904–911.

8. Rosenthal AK, Henry LA. Retinoic acid stimulates pyrophosphate elaboration by cartilage and chondrocytes. Calcif Tissue Int 1996;59:128–133.

9. Rosenthal AK, Henry LA. Thyroid hormones induce features of the hypertrophic phenotype and stimulate correlates of CPPD crystal formation in articular chondrocytes. J Rheumatol 1999;26:395–401.

10. Rosenthal AK, Ryan LM. Probenecid inhibits transforming growth factor beta1 induced pyrophosphate elaboration by chondrocytes. J Rheumatol 1994;21:896–900.

11. Olmez U, Ryan LM, Kurup IV, Rosenthal AK. Insulin-like growth factor-1 suppresses pyrophosphate elaboration by transforming growth factor beta1-stimulated chondrocytes and cartilage. Osteoarthritis Cartilage 1994;2:149–154.

12. Terkeltaub R, Lotz M, Johnson K, et al. Parathyroid hormone-related protein is abundant in osteoarthritic cartilage, and the parathyroid hormone-related protein 1-173 isoform is selectively induced by transforming growth factor β in articular chondrocytes and suppresses generation of extracellular inorganic pyrophosphate. Arthritis Rheum 1998;41:2152–2164.

13. Lotz M, Rosen F, McCabe G, et al. Interleukin 1 beta suppresses transforming growth factor-induced inorganic pyrophosphate (PPi) production and expression of the PPi-generating enzyme PC-1 in human chondrocytes. Proc Natl Acad Sci USA 1995;92:10364–10368.

14. Ryan LM, Kurup IV, Cheung HS. Transduction mechanisms of porcine chondrocyte inorganic pyrophosphate elaboration. Arhtritis Rheum 1999;42:555–560.

15. Tenenbaum J, Muniz O, Schumacher HR, Good AE, Howell DS. Comparison of pyrophosphohydrolase activities from articular cartilage in calcium pyrophosphate deposition disease and primary osteoarthritis. Arthritis Rheum 1981;24:492–500.

16. Rachow JW, Ryan LM, McCarty DJ, Halverson PB. Synovial fluid inorganic pyrophosphate concentration and nucleotide pyrophosphohydrolase activity in basic calcium phosphate deposition arthropathy and Milwaukee shoulder syndrome. Arthritis Rheum 1988;31:408–413.

17. Ryan LM, Wortmann RL, Karas B, Lynch MP, McCarty DJ. Pyrophosphohydrolase activity and inorganic pyrophosphate content of cultured human skin fibroblasts. Elevated levels in some patients with calcium pyrophosphate dihydrate deposition disease. J Clin Invest 1986;77:1689–1693.

18. Ryan LM, Rachow JW, McCarty DJ. Synovial fluid ATP: a potential substrate for the production of inorganic pyrophosphate. J Rheumatol 1991;18:716–720.

19. Derfus BA, Rachow JW, Mandel NS, et al. Articular cartilage vesicles generate calcium pyrophosphate dihydrate-like crystals in vitro. Arthritis Rheum 1992;35:231–240.

20. Ryan LM, Kurup IV, Derfus BA, Kushnaryov VM. ATP-induced chondrocalcinosis. Arthritis Rheum 1992;35:1520–1525.

21. Masuda I, Hamada J, Haas AL, Ryan LM, McCarty DJ. A unique ectonucleotide pyrophosphohydrolase associated with porcine chondrocyte-derived vesicles. J Clin Invest 1995;95:699–704.

22. Huang R, Rosenbach M, Vaughn R, et al. Expression of the murine plasma cell nucleotide pyrophosphohydrolase PC-1 is shared by human liver, bone and cartilage cells. J Clin Invest 1994;94:560–567.

23. Lorenzo P, Bayliss MT, Heinegard D. A novel cartilage protein (CILP) present in the mid-zone of human articular cartilage increases with age. J Biol Chem 1998;273:23463–23468.

24. Ho AM, Johnson MD, Kingsley DM. Role of the mouse ank gene in control of tissue calcification and arthritis. Science 2000;289:265–270.

25. Bouvet JP, le Parc JM, Michalski B, Benlahrache C, Auquier L. Acute neck pain due to calcifications surrounding the odontoid process: the crowned dens syndrome. Arthritis Rheum 1985;28:1417–1420.

26. Baba H, Maezawa Y, Kawahara N, Tomita K, Furusawa N, Imura S. Calcium crystal deposition in the ligamentum flavum of the cervical spine. Spine 1993;18:2174–2181.

27. Guerne PA, Terkeltaub R, Zuraw B, Lotz M. Inflammatory microcrystals stimulate interleukin-6 production and secretion by human monocytes and synoviocytes. Arthritis Rheum 1989;32:1443–1452.

28. Ritter J, Kerr LD, Valeriano-Marcet J, Spiera H. ACTH revisited: effective treatment for acute crystal induced synovitis in patients with multiple medical problems. J Rheumatol 1994;21:696–699.

29. Cheung HS, Sallis JD, Struve JA. Specific inhibition of calcium phosphate and calcium pyrophosphate dihydrate crystal-induced collagenase and stromelysin synthesis by phosphocitrate. Biochim Biophys Acta 1996;1315:105–111.

30. McCarty DJ, Lehr JR, Halverson PB. Crystal populations in human synovial fluid. Identification of apatite, octacalcium phosphate, tricalcium phosphate. Arthritis Rheum 1983;26:1220–1224.

31. Sarkar K, Uthoff HK. Rotator cuff tendinopathies with calcification. In: Rubin RP, Weiss G, Putney JW (eds). Calcium in Biological Systems. New York: Plenum Press, 1984; pp 725.

32. Doyle DV. Tissue calcification and inflammation in osteoarthritis. J Pathol 1982;136:199–216.

33. Cheung HS, Story MT, McCarty DJ. Mitogenic effects of hydroxyapatite and calcium pyrophosphate dihydrate crystals on cultured mammalian cells. Arthritis Rheum 1984;27:668–674.

34. McCarthy GM, Mitchell PG, Struve JA, Cheung HS. Basic calcium phosphate crystals cause co-ordinated induction and secretion of collagenase and stromelysin. J Cell Physiol 1992;153:140–146.

35. Paul H, Reginato AJ, Schumacher HR. Alizarin red S staining as a screening test to detect calcium containing compounds in synovial fluid. Arthritis Rheum 1983;26:191–200.

36. Halverson PB, McCarty DJ. Basic calcium phosphate (apatite, octacalcium phosphate, tricalcium phosphate) crystal deposition disease; calcinosis. In: Koopman WJ (ed). Arthritis and Allied Conditions. Baltimore, MD: Williams & Wilkins, 1997; pp 2127.

37. Lequesne M, Fallut M, Coulomb R, Magnet JL, Strauss J. L'arthropathie destructrice rapide de l'epaule. Rev Rheum Mal Osteoartic 1982;49:427–437.

38. Campion GV, McCrae F, Alwan W, Watt I, Bradfield J, Dieppe PA. Idiopathic destructive arthritis of the shoulder. Semin Arthritis Rheum 1988;17:232–245.

39. Halverson PB, Carrera GF, McCarty DJ. Milwaukee shoulder syndrome: fifteen additional cases and a description of contributing factors. Arch Intern Med 1990;150:677–682.

40. Neer CS, Craig EV, Fukuda H. Cuff tear arthropathy. J Bone Joint Surg 1983;65:1232–1244.

41. Ebenbichler JR, Erdogmus CB, Resch KL, et al. Ultrasound treatment for calcific tendinitis of the shoulder. N Engl J Med 1999;340:1533–1538.

42. Fam AG, Rubenstein J. Hydroxyapatite pseudopodagra. a syndrome of young women. Arthritis Rheum 1989;32:741–747.

43. McCarthy GM, Carrera GF, Ryan LM. Acute calcific periarthritis of the finger joints: a syndrome of women. J Rheumatol 1993;20:1077–1080.

44. Halverson PB, McCarty DJ. Patterns of radiographic abnormalities associated with basic calcium phosphate and calcium pyrophosphate dihydrate crystal deposition in the knee. Ann Rheum Dis 1986;45:603–605.

45. Swan A, Chapman B, Heap P, Seward H, Dieppe P. Submicroscopic crystals in osteoarthritic synovial fluids. Ann Rheum Dis 1994;53:467–470.

46. Schumacher HR, Miller JL, Ludivico C, Jessar RA. Erosive arthritis associated with apatite crystal deposition. Arthritis Rheum 1981;24:31–37.

15 GOUT
A. Epidemiology, Pathology, and Pathogenesis

Gout is a heterogeneous group of diseases resulting from monosodium urate (MSU) crystal deposition in tissues or from supersaturation of uric acid in extracellular fluids. Clinical manifestations include 1) recurrent attacks of articular and periarticular inflammation, also called gouty arthritis; 2) accumulation of articular, osseous, soft tissue, and cartilaginous crystalline deposits, called tophi; 3) uric acid calculi in the urinary tract; and 4) interstitial nephropathy with renal function impairment, called gouty nephropathy (1). The metabolic disorder underlying gout is hyperuricemia, which is defined as serum urate concentration more than two standard deviations (SD) above the mean, as established by individual laboratories according to gender (generally, more than 7.0 mg/dL for men and 6.0 mg/dL for women). By itself, hyperuricemia is not sufficient for the expression of gout, and asymptomatic hyperuricemia in the absence of gout is not a disease.

Epidemiology

Gout predominantly is a disease of adult men, with a peak incidence in the fifth decade. As cited by Hippocrates, the disease rarely occurs in men before adolescence or in women before menopause. It is a common disorder that frequently results in significant short-term disability, occupational limitations, and utilization of medical services. In 1986, the prevalence of self-reported gout in the United States was estimated to be 13.6 per 1000 men and 6.4 per 1000 women. The prevalence has increased over the past few decades in the United States, as well as in other countries that have a high standard of living. Prevalence among African-American men may be higher than among Caucasian men, possibly reflecting the relative prevalence of hypertension (2).

Beginning in puberty, serum urate concentrations in males rise from childhood mean values of 3.5 mg/dL and reach adult levels of 4.0 mg/dL. In contrast, serum urate levels remain rather constant in females until menopause, at which time concentrations begin to rise. This discrepancy during the reproductive years appears to stem from the action of estrogen, which promotes renal excretion of uric acid (1). Because of increased longevity and frequent long-term use of thiazide diuretics, the prevalence of gout is rising among elderly women in Western countries, particularly in association with chronic renal insufficiency.

Hyperuricemia is present in at least 5% of asymptomatic Americans on at least one occasion during adulthood. However, it appears that fewer than one in four hyperuricemic individuals will, at any point, develop clinically apparent urate crystal deposition. The most likely reasons, at least in part, are that increases in urate levels are relatively mild in most individuals (serum urate less than 9.0 mg/dL) and often are transient, due to dietary alterations or to ingestion of certain drugs.

The duration and magnitude of hyperuricemia directly correlate with the likelihood of developing gouty arthritis and uric acid urolithiasis, and with age at onset of initial clinical gouty manifestations (1). Nevertheless, in the absence of uric acid overproduction, severe hyperuricemia (at least 13 mg/dL in men and 10 mg/dL in women) is tolerated with little apparent jeopardy to renal function.

Pathogenesis of Hyperuricemia

Uric acid is the normal end product of the degradation of purine compounds (1). The limit of solubility of MSU in plasma is approximately 6.7 mg/dL at 37°C. Normal adult mean (±SD) serum urate concentrations (5.1 ± 1.0 mg/dL in men and 4.0 ± 1.0 mg/dL in women) provide a narrow margin of safety for urate deposition. In humans, gout is a consequence of the specieswide lack of the enzyme uric acid oxidase, or uricase. Uricase oxidizes uric acid, which is only sparingly soluble in body fluids, to the highly soluble compound allantoin.

Knockout mice that are homozygous for absence of the uricase gene exhibit a marked increase in serum urate – from approximately 1.0 mg/dL to about 11.0 mg/dL – and develop severe uric acid nephrolithiasis and renal dysfunction during the first month of life (3). Multiple genetic and environmental influences prompt the chain of events that governs uric acid formation, transport, and disposal. Single or combined derangements in these delicately balanced processes can lead to hyperuricemia and gout. Environmental factors that modify serum urate concentration include body weight, diet, lifestyle, social class, and hemoglobin level. The interplay of genetic and environmental factors in determining hyperuricemia is demonstrated by the higher mean serum urate levels encountered among Filipinos living in the United States versus individuals of identical racial background living in the Philippines. The limited ability of members of this ethnic population to excrete uric acid supports the hypothesis that a tendency toward hyperuricemia is inherited and is manifested when a diet with a relatively high purine content, such as the typical American diet, is ingested. The familial occurrence of gout, known for nearly 2000 years, is reported by about 20% of affected patients, and hyperuricemia has been demonstrated in one-fourth of first-degree relatives of people with gout (1).

Purine Metabolism and Biochemistry

In humans, uric acid is derived both from the ingestion of foods containing purines and from the endogenous synthesis of purine nucleotides, which are building blocks in the synthesis of nucleic acids. The synthesis of purine nucleotides involves closely regulated biochemical pathways (Fig. 15A-1). In the pathway of purine synthesis de novo, a purine ring is synthesized from small-molecule precursors. These precursors are added sequentially to a ribose–phosphate backbone donated by 5-phosphoribosyl-1-pyrophosphate (PRPP), a substrate usually present in limited concentrations in the cell. The first reaction of the pathway is catalyzed by amidophosphoribosyltransferase (Fig. 15A-1). This reaction is the main site of pathway regulation by means of an antagonistic interaction involving inhibition by purine nucleotide products and activation by PRPP. Other sites for control of purine nucleotide production have been identified at the level of PRPP synthesis and at the distal branch point governing distribution of newly formed nucleotides into adenylate and guanylate derivatives (1).

Purine nucleotide synthesis also can occur through the activities of adenine phosphoribosyltransferase and hypoxanthine–guanine phosphoribosyltransferase (HGPRT)

(Fig. 15A-1). Each enzyme catalyzes the reaction between PRPP and the respective purine base substrate in the single-step synthesis of purine nucleotides. Factors that govern the relationship between rates of purine-base salvage and purine synthesis include the availability of PRPP and concentrations of the nucleotide products common to both pathways (1).

The catabolic steps that generate uric acid from nucleic acids and free purine nucleotides involve degradation to hypoxanthine and xanthine through purine nucleoside intermediates. These intermediates ultimately are oxidized to uric acid in sequential reactions catalyzed by the enzyme xanthine oxidase.

Urate circulates in the plasma mainly in unbound form. The total miscible urate pool averages about 1200 mg (range 800–1600 mg) in healthy men and about one-half this value in healthy women. Since uric acid synthesis averages about 750 mg/day in men, an estimated two-thirds of the urate pool is turned over daily (1). Chronic hyperuricemia in gout invariably is characterized by substantial expansion of the total body urate, uric-acid pool, and urate supersaturation of the extracellular space.

The major route of uric acid disposal is renal excretion, which accounts for about two-thirds of urate loss. Adult men who eat a purine-free diet excrete about 425 ± 80 mg/day in the urine. Substantial increases in urinary uric

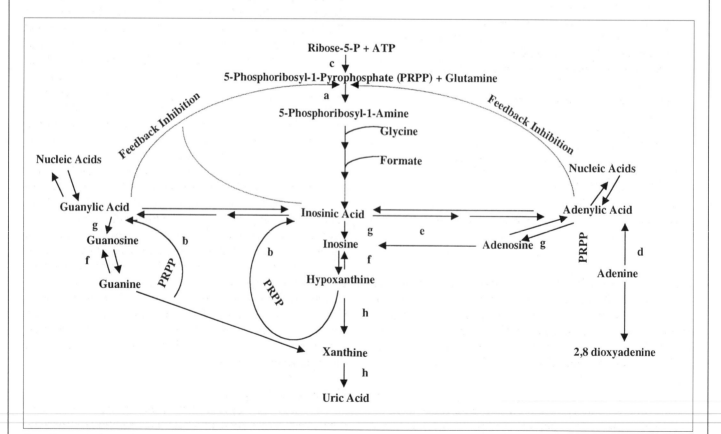

Fig. 15A-1. Mechanisms regulating uric acid production in purine metabolism. a, amidophosphoribosyltransferase; b, hypoxanthine–guanine phosphoribosyltransferase; c, 5-phosphoribosyl-1-pyrophosphate (PRPP) synthetase; d, adenine phosphoribosyltransferase; 3, adenosine deaminase; f, purine nucleoside phosphorylase; g, 5'-nucleotidase; h, xanthine oxidase.

TABLE 15A-1
Classification of Hyperuricemia

Uric acid overproduction
  Primary hyperuricemia
    Idiopathic
    HGPRT deficiency (partial and complete)
    PRPP synthetase superactivity
  Secondary hyperuricemia
    Excessive dietary purine intake
    Increased nucleotide turnover (e.g., myeloproliferative
      and lymphoproliferative disorders, hemolytic
      diseases, psoriasis)
    Accelerated ATP degradation
      Glycogen storage diseases (types I, III, V, and VII)
      Fructose ingestion and hereditary fructose
        intolerance
      Hypoxemia and tissue underperfusion
      Severe muscle exertion
      Ethanol abuse

Uric acid underexcretion
  Primary hyperuricemia
    Idiopathic
  Secondary hyperuricemia
    Diminished renal function
    Inhibition of tubular urate secretion
      Competitive anions (e.g., keto- and lactic acidosis)
    Enhanced tubular urate reabsorption
      Dehydration, diuretics, and insulin resistance
        (syndrome X)
    Mechanism incompletely defined
      Hypertension
      Hyperparathyroidism
      Certain drugs (e.g., cyclosporine, pyrazinamide,
        ethambutol, and low-dose salicylates)
      Lead nephropathy

HGPRT, hypoxanthine–guanine phosphoribosyltransferase; PRPP, 5-phosphoribosyl-1-pyrophosphate.

acid excretion normally are possible in response to increased filtered urate load. Bacterial oxidation of urate secreted into the gut is the principal mechanism of extrarenal urate disposal. This pathway has a relatively limited ability to compensate for changes in urate-pool size until serum urate values rise above 14.0 mg/dL.

Causes and Classification of Hyperuricemia

Increased uric acid production and diminished uric acid excretion by the kidney, operating alone or in combination, contribute substantially to the hyperuricemia of people with gout. Thus, people with hyperuricemia and gout can be subclassified according to the mechanism responsible for

hyperuricemia – that is, overproduction or underexcretion of uric acid, or both (Table 15A-1). In this scheme, primary hyperuricemia refers to inherently disordered uric acid metabolism not associated with another acquired disorder. Such classification is particularly useful in diagnosis and may be used to guide therapy.

Urate Overproduction

In 24-hour urine collections, approximately 10% of people with hyperuricemia or gout excrete excessive quantities of uric acid, commonly defined as more than 800 mg of uric acid excreted while on a typical Western diet. Isotopic labeling studies generally demonstrate increased rates of uric acid synthesis (overproduction) in such individuals. Overproduction of urate occurs with some frequency in a variety of acquired and genetic disorders characterized by excessive rates of cell and, therefore, nucleic-acid turnover. These disorders, which include myeloproliferative and lymphoproliferative diseases, hemolytic anemias, anemias associated with ineffective erythropoiesis, Paget's disease of bone, and psoriasis, constitute examples of secondary hyperuricemia and gout with uric acid overproduction.

People with inherited derangements in mechanisms that regulate purine nucleotide synthesis account for a very small fraction of people with urate overproduction. Early adult-onset gout and a high incidence of uric acid urinary tract stones constitute the usual clinical phenotype in partial deficiency of HGPRT and in milder forms of superactivity of PRPP synthetase (1,4). Severe HGPRT deficiency is associated with spasticity, choreoathetosis, mental retardation, and compulsive self-mutilation (Lesch-Nyhan syndrome) (1,4). In some individuals, regulatory defects in PRPP synthetase are accompanied by sensorineural deafness and neurodevelopmental defects (1).

Intracellular accumulation of PRPP is a result of diminished utilization of this regulatory substrate in purine-base salvage. This circumstance drives purine synthesis at an increased rate in HGPRT deficiency (Fig. 15A-1). In the case of variant forms of PRPP synthetase with excessive activity, increased PRPP availability for purine synthesis results from increased rates of PRPP generation (1). Thus, aberrations of each of these enzymes can result in increased uric acid synthesis by increasing PRPP availability and altering the balance of control of purine synthesis toward increased production. Because both of these enzymes are produced from X-linked genes, homozygous males are affected. In addition, postmenopausal gout and urinary tract stones can occur in carrier females. Hyperuricemia in prepubertal boys always suggests one of these enzymatic defects.

Uric Acid Underexcretion

More than 90% of people with primary hyperuricemia or gout have a relative deficit in the renal excretion of uric acid. Excretion of normal amounts of uric acid is accomplished in these individuals only when serum urate concentrations are inappropriately high (1).

Virtually all plasma urate is filtered at the glomerulus, with more than 95% of the filtered load undergoing proximal tubular (presecretory) reabsorption (1). Subsequent proximal tubular secretion (about 50% of the filtered urate load) contributes the major share of excreted uric acid. Postsecretory tubular reabsorption (about 40% of the filtered urate load) is another primary mechanism of renal uric acid handling.

Renal urate excretion can be influenced by heredity, and a number of kindreds with relatively early-onset gout and a reduced fractional excretion of urate have been described (5). A renal urate transporter gene has been identified and partly characterized functionally (6). However, there is no evidence to suggest that most primary uric acid underexcreters with gout constitute a population with a single genetic or acquired renal defect. A diminished tubular secretory rate may contribute to hyperuricemia in some patients, and increased tubular reabsorption or diminished uric acid filtration may contribute to renal urate retention in other patients.

Pharmacologic agents that alter renal tubular function can contribute to the occurrence of gout with uric acid underexcretion. Among the offending agents (Table 15A-1) are diuretics, cyclosporine (7), and low-dose salicylates (1). Cryptic forms of acquired renal impairment can also be manifested initially by gouty arthritis, as exemplified by the high incidence of this disorder in people with chronic lead intoxication. Decreased excretion of uric acid also occurs in diabetic ketoacidosis, starvation, ketosis, ethanol intoxication, and lactic acidosis. The organic acids that accumulate in these conditions compete with urate tubular secretion.

People with gout tend to have a relatively high incidence of other diseases that predispose to renal insufficiency, such as hypertension, which by itself can increase tubular urate reabsorption, and diabetes mellitus (1). With respect to diabetes mellitus, insulin stimulates the renal tubular sodium-hydrogen exchanger, which promotes urate reabsorption. Insulin resistance as a component of "syndrome X" can be associated with elevated circulating insulin levels, glucose intolerance or non–insulin-dependent diabetes, abdominal (visceral) obesity, hypertension, low levels of high-density lipoprotein cholesterol, hypertriglyceridemia (which can promote uric acid generation via the increased provision of acetate), and an increased risk of atherosclerosis. A substantial fraction of people with primary gout may have syndrome X (8).

Combined Overproduction and Underexcretion

Alcohol consumption promotes hyperuricemia by increasing urate production and decreasing uric acid excretion. The higher purine content in some alcoholic beverages is a factor. Excessive alcohol consumption causes accelerated hepatic breakdown of adenosine triphosphate (ATP) and increased urate production (9). High alcohol intake also may lead to hyperlactic acidemia, which blocks uric acid secretion.

Two inborn errors of metabolism can produce hyperuricemia by a combined mechanism. Glucose-6-phosphatase deficiency accelerates purine biosynthesis, and fructose-1-phosphate aldolase deficiency accelerates purine nucleotide degradation. Lactic acidemia is a consequence of each defect.

Pathogenesis of Tissue Manifestations

In most instances, urate crystallizes as a monosodium salt in oversaturated joint tissues (1). As mentioned, however, only a minority of individuals with sustained hyperuricemia develop tophi and gouty arthropathy. Furthermore, gout has been observed in a few individuals who have not shown previous evidence of hyperuricemia (10). The reasons for these exceptions are poorly understood. The decreased solubility of sodium urate at the lower temperatures of peripheral structures, such as toes and ears, may help explain why urate crystals deposit in these areas (1,11). However, the predilection for marked urate crystal deposition in the first metatarsophalangeal (MTP) joint may also relate to repetitive minor trauma.

Hemiplegia appears to have a sparing effect on the development of tophi and acute gout on the paretic side, and tophi and acute gout occur in interphalangeal joints at the location of Heberden's nodes. These observations suggest the potential importance of connective-tissue structure and turnover in urate crystal deposition. Provocative findings have raised the possibility that immunoglobulin plays a role in urate crystal deposition in vivo (11).

Urate tophi usually can be found in the synovial membrane at the time of the first gouty attack, and also may be found in cartilage (11). Urate crystals in joint fluid at the time of the acute attack may derive from rupture of preformed synovial deposits, or they may have precipitated de novo. Declines in serum urate levels, as effected by antihyperuricemic drugs, may promote the release of urate crystals from tophi by decreasing the size of crystals; packed crystals consequently may loosen, forming gaps at the periphery of deposits.

In some individuals with gout, urate crystals can be found in MTP and knee joints that have never been involved in an acute attack (11). Furthermore, asymptomatic patients with hyperuricemia may have urate crystals in MTP joint fluid. These findings confirm that gout can exist in an asymptomatic state.

Pathology of Gout

The histopathology of the tophi (Fig. 15A-2) shows a foreign-body granuloma surrounding a core of MSU crystals. The inflammatory reaction around the crystals consists mostly of mononuclear cells and giant cells. Erosion of cartilage and cortical bone may occur at the sites of tophi. A fibrous capsule usually is prominent around tophi. Crystals within the tophi are needle-shaped and often are arranged radially in small clusters. Because formalin-based fixatives can dissolve these crystals, specimens must be handled carefully. The De Galantha stain can be used to stain urates black; crystals also can be identified by compensated polarized light microscopy in frozen or alcohol-fixed specimens. Other potentially important components in tophi include lipids, glycosaminoglycans, and plasma proteins.

In the parenchymal renal disease of gout, the kidneys usually are small and equally affected. The cortical area is reduced in width, and scars can be seen throughout the capsule. Many of these changes can be related to associated hypertension and infection (1). The renal pelvis may contain uric acid stones.

Histologic examination of kidneys from people with gouty nephropathy reveals urate crystals located primarily in the medullary interstitium, papillae, and pyramids. Like other tophi, they may be surrounded by a chronic inflammatory reaction with foreign-body giant cells. Nephrosclerosis and other evidence of hypertensive disease also are common.

Gouty renal parenchymal disease is uncommon. Even before the availability of effective urate-depleting drugs, renal parenchymal urate deposits were present only occasionally.

Pathogenesis of Gouty Inflammation

Gout was the first disease in which crystals were identified in joint effusions and subsequently incriminated in the pathogenesis of the arthritis. Intra-articular injection of urate crystals was shown to induce gout-like attacks, even in healthy subjects. However, the finding of crystals in synovial fluids of asymptomatic joints illustrates that factors other than the presence of crystals may be important in modulating the inflammatory reaction (11).

Urate crystals are able to initiate and maintain intense attacks of acute inflammation because of their capacity to stimulate the release of numerous inflammatory mediators (12). The crystals induce phagocytes and synovial cells to generate and release such mediators as cyclooxygenase and lipoxygenase metabolites of arachidonic acid, phospholipase A_2-activating protein, lysosomal proteases, tumor necrosis factor (TNF)-α, interleukin (IL)-1, IL-6, and IL-8. In addition, urate crystals generate soluble mediators, including C5a, bradykinin, and kallikrein, via proteolysis of serum proteins (11).

The ability of urate crystals to activate cells appears to be due to nonspecific activation of certain signal transduction pathways (including membrane G protein activation; cytosolic calcium mobilization; and the signaling of various protein kinases, including Src-family tyrosine kinases and the mitogen-activated protein kinases ERK1/ERK2, JNK, and p38). These pathways are used in a more specific manner by receptor-mediated signals, such as growth factors, adhesion proteins, and immune complexes (11–14).

In acute gout, neutrophil influx is believed to be promoted both by endothelial–neutrophil adhesion triggered by IL-1 and TNF-α and by inducting expression of chemotactic factors (12, 15–17). The major mediators promoting neutrophil ingress into the joint in acute gout appear to be IL-8 and closely related chemokines that bind the IL-8 receptor CXCR2 (such as GROβ and GROγ) (15,16). The ingress of neutrophils appears to be the most important

event for developing acute urate crystal-induced synovitis, and effects at the level of neutrophil–endothelial interaction likely represent a major locus for the prophylactic and therapeutic effects of colchicine (18).

Intra-articular neutrophils can be activated by direct contact with crystals and by exposure to the rich soup of soluble mediators, including not only chemokines, but also platelet-activating factor, C5a, and leukotriene B_4 (11). Such activation supports continuing ingress of neutrophils, which probably is vital for perpetuating acute gouty inflammation, because of the limited functional life span (days) of normal neutrophils. In this regard, the rate at which neutrophils undergo apoptosis in the acute gouty joint is believed to be accelerated by some of the mediators, such as TNF-α, in the inflamed gouty joint.

The systemic release from the gouty joint into the venous circulation of IL-1, TNF-α, IL-6, and IL-8 appears to be responsible for systemic manifestations (e.g., fever, leukocytosis, hepatic acute-phase protein response), and it may help explain the capacity of the acute gouty attack to affect joints in more than one region.

The acute gouty attack may be self-limited not only by neutrophil apoptosis and a cessation of neutrophil influx within the joint, but also by certain changes in the physical properties and proteins coating intra-articular urate crystals (11). A change in the balance between pro- and anti-inflammatory factors (e.g., generation of lipoxins, and release of IL-1 receptor antagonist and transforming growth factor β) is likely to be the cornerstone of resolution of the acute phase of gouty inflammation (11,19,20). However, low-level synovitis may persist in affected joints, with evidence of ongoing intra-articular phagocytosis of crystals by leukocytes (21). Full-blown gouty synovitis may erupt subsequently in response to local tissue trauma and other factors. The precise mechanisms that spontaneously initiate and limit acute gouty inflammation have not been defined. Chronic gouty

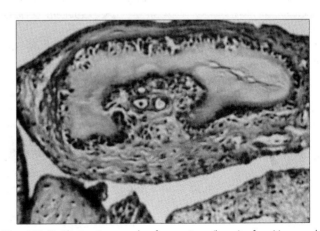

Fig. 15A-2. Photomicrograph of synovium (knee) of a 46-year-old man who sustained repeated attacks of gouty arthritis for 15 years. Note large tophaceous deposits in the synovial villus with surrounding histiocytic reaction. Crystals are dissolved from tophi unless tissue is processed with absolute alcohol.

inflammation can be associated with cytokine-driven synovial proliferation, cartilage loss, and bone erosion, and can thereby carry some clinical resemblance to synovitis seen in rheumatoid arthritis.

ROBERT A. TERKELTAUB, MD

References

1. Becker MA, Levinson D. Clinical gout and pathogenesis of hyperuricemia. In Koopman, WJ (ed). Arthritis and Allied Conditions, 13th ed. Baltimore: Williams & Wilkins, 1996; pp 2041–2072.

2. Hochberg MC, Thomas J, Thomas DJ, Mead L, Levine DM, Klag MJ. Racial differences in the incidence of gout: the role of hypertension. Arthritis Rheum 1995;38:628–632.

3. Wu X, Wakamiya M, Vaishnav S, et al. Hyperuricemia and urate nephropathy in urate oxidase-deficient mice. Proc Natl Acad Sci USA 1994;91:742–746.

4. Nyhan WL. The recognition of Lesch-Nyhan syndrome as an inborn error of purine metabolism. J Inherit Metab Dis 1997;20:171–178.

5. Emmerson BT, Nagel SL, Duffy DL, Martin NG. Genetic control of the renal clearance of urate: a study of twins. Ann Rheum Dis 1992;51:375–377.

6. Leal-Pinto E, Cohen BE, Abramson RG. Functional analysis and molecular modeling of a cloned urate transporter/channel. J Membr Biol 1999;169:13–27.

7. Laine J, Holmberg C. Mechanisms of hyperuricemia in cyclosporine-treated renal transplant children. Nephron 1996;74:318–323.

8. Dessein PH, Shipton EA, Stanwix AE, Joffe BI, Ramokgadi J. Beneficial effects of weight loss associated with moderate calorie/carbohydrate restriction, and increased proportional intake of protein and unsaturated fat on serum urate and lipoprotein levels in gout: a pilot study. Ann Rheum Dis 2000;59:539–543.

9. Eastmond CJ, Garton M, Robins S, Riddoch S. The effects of alcoholic beverages on urate metabolism in gout sufferers. Br J Rheumatol 1995;34:756–759.

10. McCarty DJ. Gout without hyperuricemia. JAMA 1994;271:302–303.

11. Terkeltaub R. Pathogenesis and treatment of crystal-induced inflammation. In: Koopman WJ (ed). Arthritis and Allied Conditions, 13th edition. Baltimore: Williams & Wilkins, 1996; pp 2085–2102.

12. Liu R, O'Connell M, Johnson K, Pritzker K, Mackman N, Terkeltaub R. Extracellular signal-regulated kinase 1/extracellular signal-regulated kinase 2 mitogen-activated protein kinase signaling and activation of activator protein 1 and nuclear factor kappaB transcription factors play central roles in interleukin-8 expression stimulated by monosodium urate monohydrate and calcium pyrophosphate crystals in monocytic cells. Arthritis Rheum 2000;43:1145–1155.

13. Roberge C, Gaudry M, Medicis R, Lussier A, Poubelle P, Naccache P. Crystal-induced neutrophil activation. IV. Specific inhibition of tyrosine phosphorylation by colchicine. J Clin Invest 1993; 92:1722-1729.

14. Barabe F, Gilbert C, Liao N, Bourgoin SG, Naccache PH. Crystal-induced neutrophil activation VI. Involvement of FcgammaRIIIB (CD16) and CD11b in response to inflammatory microcrystals. FASEB J 1998;12:209–220.

15. Terkeltaub R, Baird S, Sears P, Santiago R, Boisvert W. The murine homolog of the interleukin-8 receptor CXCR-2 is essential for the occurrence of neutrophilic inflammation in the air pouch model of acute urate crystal-induced gouty synovitis. Arthritis Rheum 1998;41:900–909.

16. Nishimura A, Akahoshi T, Takahashi M, et al. Attenuation of monosodium urate crystal-induced arthritis in rabbits by a neutralizing antibody against interleukin-8. J Leukoc Biol 1997;62:444–449.

17. Matsukawa A, Yoshimura T, Maeda T, Takahashi T, Ohkawara S, Yoshinaga M. Analysis of the cytokine network among tumor necrosis factor alpha, interleukin-1beta, interleukin-8, and interleukin-1 receptor antagonist in monosodium urate crystal-induced rabbit arthritis. Lab Invest 1998;78:559–569.

18. Cronstein BN, Molad Y, Reibman J, Balakhane E, Levin RI, Weissmann G. Colchicine alters the quantitative and qualitative display of selectins on endothelial cells and neutrophils. J Clin Invest 1995;96:994–1002.

19. Liote F, Prudhommeaux F, Schiltz C, et al. Inhibition and prevention of monosodium urate monohydrate crystal-induced acute inflammation in vivo by transforming growth factor beta-1. Arthritis Rheum 1996;39:1192–1198.

20. Clish CB, O'Brien JA, Gronert K, Stahl GL, Petasis NA, Serhan CN. Local and systemic delivery of a stable aspirin-triggered lipoxin prevents neutrophil recruitment in vivo. Proc Natl Acad Sci USA 1999;96:8247–8252.

21. Pascual E, Batlle-Gualda E, Martinez A, Rosas J, Vela P. Synovial fluid analysis for diagnosis of intercritical gout. Ann Int Med 1999;131:756–759.

GOUT
B. Clinical and Laboratory Features

Gout is a disease caused by the deposition of monosodium urate (MSU) crystals around and in the tissues of joints.

Stages of Classic Gout

The course of classic gout passes through three distinct stages: asymptomatic hyperuricemia, acute intermittent gout, and chronic tophaceous gout (Fig. 15B-1). The rate of progression from asymptomatic hyperuricemia to chronic tophaceous gout varies considerably from one person to another and is dependent on numerous endogenous and exogenous factors.

Asymptomatic Hyperuricemia

Hyperuricemia is a very common biochemical abnormality that can be defined in either physiologic or epidemiologic terms. In extracellular fluids, 98% of uric acid is in the form of MSU at pH 7.4. Clinical laboratories define hyperuricemia in epidemiologic terms as a serum urate level that is greater than two standard deviations above the mean value in a gender- and age-matched healthy population. Using this standard, the upper limit for normal serum urate frequently is listed as 8.0–8.5 mg/dL. In physiologic terms, any level above 6.8 mg/dL is hyperuricemia, since it exceeds the soluble concentration of MSU in body fluid. In males, adult levels of serum uric acid are reached during puberty. Serum urate levels for women are approximately 1 mg/dL lower than levels for men, but rise to a similar level after menopause.

The incidence of gout increases with age as well as with the degree of hyperuricemia. In the Normative Aging Study,

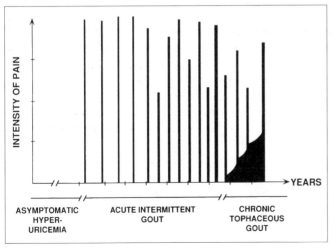

Fig. 15B-1. The three stages of disease progression in classic gout. The period of asymptomatic hyperuricemia lasts decades, followed by acute intermittent gout with painless intercritical segments, leading to chronic tophaceous gout with progressive background pain and joint destruction.

3% of subjects with urate levels between 7.0 and 8.0 mg/dL had a cumulative incidence of gouty arthritis, and subjects with urate levels of 9.0 mg/dL or more had a five-year cumulative incidence of 22% (1). However, the vast majority of people with hyperuricemia never develop symptoms associated with uric acid excess, such as gouty arthritis, tophi, or kidney stones.

Acute Intermittent Gout

The initial episode of acute gout usually follows decades of asymptomatic hyperuricemia (Fig. 15B-1). Thomas Sydenham, the famous 17th-century physician who wrote of his personal experiences with gout (2), eloquently described the initial hours of an acute attack:

> He goes to bed and sleeps well, but about Two a Clock in the Morning, is waked by the Pain, seizing either his great Toe, the Heel, the Calf of the Leg, or the Ankle; this Pain is like that of dislocated Bones, with the Sense as it were of Water almost cold, poured upon the Membranes of the part affected; presently shivering and shaking follow with a feverish Disposition; the Pain is first gentle, but increased by degrees-till dash towards Night it comes to its height, accompanying itself neatly according to the Variety of the bones of the Tarsus and Metatarsus, whose Ligaments it seizes, sometimes resembling a violent stretching or tearing of those ligaments, sometimes gnawing of a dog, and sometimes a weight; more over, the Part affected has such a quick and exquisite Pain, that it is not able to bear the weight of the cloths upon it, nor hard walking in the Chamber (2).

This classic description captures the intense pain frequently associated with acute gouty arthritis, and it is this clinical picture most commonly evoked by the term *gout*.

The onset of a gouty attack usually is heralded by the rapid development of warmth, swelling, erythema, and pain in the affected joint. Pain escalates from the faintest twinges to its most intense level over an eight- to 12-hour period. The initial attack usually is monarticular and, in one-half of patients, involves the first metatarsophalangeal joint. This joint eventually is affected in 90% of individuals with gout. Other joints that frequently are involved in this early stage are the midfoot, ankles, heels, and knees, and less commonly, the wrists, fingers, and elbows. The intensity of pain characteristically is very severe, but may vary among subjects. Classically, patients find walking difficult or impossible when lower-extremity joints are involved.

Systemic symptoms, such as fever, chills, and malaise, may accompany acute gout. The cutaneous erythema associated with the gouty attack may extend beyond the

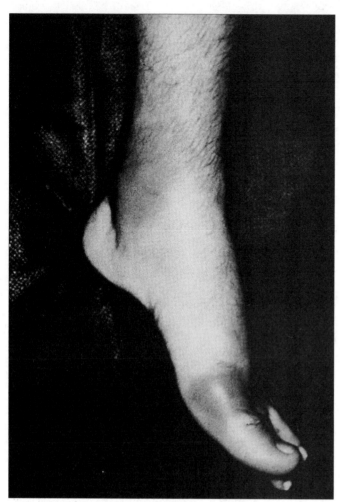

Fig. 15B-2. Acute gouty arthritis involving the first metatarsopha-langeal joint and ankle joint.

involved joint and resemble bacterial cellulitis (Fig. 15B-2). The natural course of untreated acute gout varies from episodes of mild pain that resolve in several hours ("petit attacks") to severe attacks that last one to two weeks. Early in the acute intermittent stage, episodes of acute arthritis are infrequent, and intervals between attacks sometimes last for years. Over time, the attacks typically become more frequent, longer in duration, and involve more joints.

Intercritical periods of acute intermittent gout are just as characteristic of this stage as are the acute attacks. Previously involved joints are virtually free of symptoms. Despite this, MSU crystals often can be identified in the synovial fluid. In one study, these crystals were found in the synovial fluids of 36 of 37 knees that previously had been inflamed. Synovial fluids containing crystals also had a higher mean cell count than those with no crystals, 449 cells/mm^3 versus 64 cells/mm^3 (3). These subtle differences may reflect ongoing subclinical inflammation.

Chronic Tophaceous Gout

Chronic tophaceous gout usually develops after 10 or more years of acute intermittent gout, although patients have been

reported with tophi as their initial clinical manifestation (4). The transition from acute intermittent gout to chronic tophaceous gout occurs when the intercritical periods no longer are free of pain. The involved joints become persistently uncomfortable and swollen, although the intensity of these symptoms is much less than during acute flares. Gouty attacks continue to occur against this painful background, and without therapy, they may recur as often as every few weeks. The amount of background pain also steadily increases with time if appropriate intervention is not started (Fig 15B-3). Clinically evident tophi may or may not be detected on physical examination during the first few years of this stage of gout. However, periarticular tophi detected by magnetic resonance imaging (5) and synovial "micro-tophi" discovered through the arthroscope certainly are present early in this stage of gout. Polyarticular involvement becomes much more frequent during this time. With diffuse and symmetric involvement of small joints in the hands and feet, chronic tophaceous gout can occasionally be confused with the symmetric polyarthritis of rheumatoid arthritis.

The development of tophaceous deposits of MSU is a function of the duration and severity of hyperuricemia (6). Hench found that untreated patients developed tophi 11.7 years after the onset of acute gout, on average, (7). In a study of 1165 people with primary gout, those without tophi had serum uric acid levels of 10.3 ± 1.3 mg/dL and those with extensive deposits had levels of 11.0 ± 2.0 mg/dL. Other factors associated with the development of tophi include early age of gout onset, long periods of active but untreated gout, an average of four attacks per year, and a greater tendency toward upper-extremity and polyarticular episodes (8).

Subcutaneous gouty tophi may be found anywhere over the body, but occur most commonly in the fingers, wrists, ears, knees, olecranon bursa, and such pressure points as the ulnar aspect of the forearm and the Achilles tendon. In people with nodal osteoarthritis, tophi have a propensity for forming in Heberden's nodes. Tophi also may occur in connective tissues at other sites, such as renal pyramids, heart valves, and sclerae. Before antihyperuricemic agents were available, as many as 50% of patients with gout eventually developed clinical or radiographic evidence of tophi. Since the introduction of allopurinol and the uricosuric agents, the incidence of tophaceous gout has declined.

Much of the knowledge about sequential development of the mature, multilobulated gouty tophus comes from the classic histopathologic descriptions of Sokoloff (9) and Schumacher (10), and the more recent immunohistochemical studies of Palmer et al. (11). Figure 15B-4 represents a theoretical sequence of how a noncrystalline, cellular locus (macrophage acinus) progresses through stages of crystal precipitation, coronal hypertrophy, and finally, crystal coalescence and cellular atrophy, to eventually form the clinically observable subcutaneous tophus (6). The macrophage acinus (Fig. 15B-4A) is the earliest structure observed by light microscopy in tophus development. The acinus has a core of noncrystalline, amorphous material surrounded by a rosette of mononuclear phagocytes. The central amorphous material is believed to be detritus from a collection of monocytes that conjugated at the locus in response to some inciting event.

Some time after the acinus is formed, a small, eccentric collection of radially arranged MSU crystals form in the amorphous core of monocyte-derived material (Fig. 15B-4B). The macrophages do not phagocytize the MSU crystal, but as the crystalline mass expands and contacts the surrounding cells, this shell that is one- to two-cells thick proliferates to form a tightly packed, eight- to 10-cell–thick corona (Fig. 15B-4C). As the tophus matures, this corona is lost and replaced by fibrous septae (Fig. 15B-4D) that contain some fibroblastic cells and occasional multinucleated giant cells. Adjacent crystalline deposits coalesce to form multilobulated tophi (Fig. 15B-4E) measuring 1–10 cm in diameter, interlaced with fibrous strands containing few cells and encapsulated by a sometimes-tenuous and sometimes-thick fibrous tissue. The cellular and crystalline components of a gouty tophus are easily demonstrated by magnetic resonance imaging (Fig. 15B-5).

Unusual Presentations

Early-Onset Gout

Between 3% and 6% of patients with gout have symptom onset before age 25. Early-onset gout represents a special subset of cases that generally have a genetic component, show a more accelerated clinical course, and require more aggressive antihyperuricemic therapy. In large epidemiologic studies of classic gout, a family history of gout and/or nephrolithiasis is present in 25%–30% of cases. In early-onset gout, the incidence of family history is approximately 80%. In this younger group, detailed questioning about the kindred over several generations may yield enough information to suggest a mode of inheritance (X-linked or autosomal dominant or recessive).

Like classic gout, early-onset gout may be caused by overproduction of urate or reduced renal clearance of uric acid. Diseases associated with overproduction of urate in children and young adults include enzymatic defects in the purine pathway, glycogen storage diseases, and hematologic disorders, such as hemoglobinopathies and leukemias. The complete deficiency of hypoxanthine-guanine phosphoribosyltransferase (HGPRT) is an X-linked inherited inborn error of purine metabolism with a characteristic clinical presentation known as the Lesch–Nyhan syndrome. These boys have severe neurologic abnormalities, and if not treated early with allopurinol, develop gout and kidney stones in the first decade of life. The partial deficiency of HGPRT (the Kelley–Seegmiller syndrome) results in early-onset gout or uric acid nephrolithiasis and also is X-linked in its inheritance. People with this syndrome have minor or no neurologic problems.

Glycogen storage disease types I, III, V, and VII are associated with early-onset gout and are inherited as autosomal recessive diseases. Sickle cell disease, β-thalassemia, and nonlymphocytic leukemias may be complicated by gouty arthritis in the young adult years.

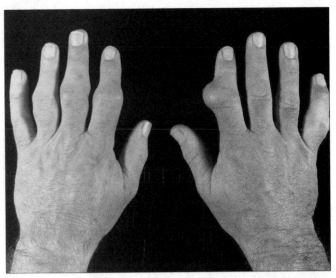

Fig. 15B-3. The hands of a patient with chronic tophaceous gout reveal large tophi over the right second and fifth proximal interphalangeal (PIP) joints and the left second through fourth PIPs.

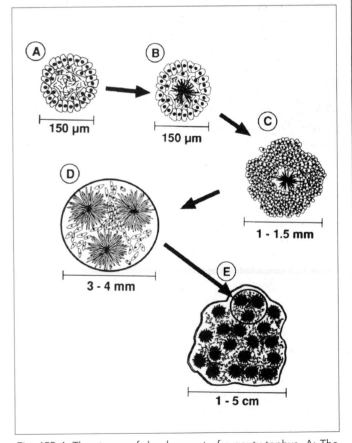

Fig. 15B-4. The stages of development of a gouty tophus. A: The crystal-free macrophage acinus probably is the earliest organized phase of a gouty tophus. B: The amorphous center of the acinus fosters urate crystal formation. C: As the crystalline mass expands, the surrounding corona of macrophages likewise undergoes hypertrophy. D: Further crystallization results in a thinning of the corona, until only fibrous septae separate one nidus of crystal formation from another. E: A fully mature tophus.

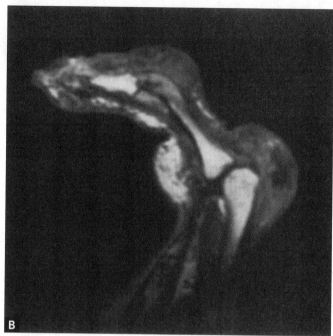

Fig. 15B-5. **A:** Midline sagittal section magnetic resonance image of a finger with advanced tophaceous deformities. **B:** T1-weighted, spin-echo technique with gadolinium contrast reveals the deep soft-tissue anatomy. The heterogenous composition of the tophus dorsal to the proximal interphalangeal joint and distal phalanx is revealed clearly. The central crystalline deposit remains low-intensity, but surrounding inflammatory tissue enhances.

Conditions associated with uric acid underexcretion in young patients include a specific renal tubular disorder known as familial urate nephropathy (12). This autosomal dominant disorder causes hyperuricemia from a very young age, before any evidence of renal insufficiency. The condition may lead to progressive renal failure and end-stage kidney disease by age 40. Other nephropathies associated with early-onset gout include polycystic kidney disease, chronic lead intoxication, medullary cystic disease, and focal tubulointerstitial disease.

Transplantation Gout

Hyperuricemia reportedly develops in 75%–80% of heart transplant recipients who routinely take cyclosporine to prevent allograft rejection (13). A slightly lower frequency (approximately 50%) of kidney and liver transplant recipients develop hyperuricemia, presumably because lower doses of cyclosporine are used in these individuals. In the general population, asymptomatic hyperuricemia progresses to clinical gout in one of 30 subjects, and cyclosporine-induced hyperuricemia leads to gout in one of six patients (14). Other differences between primary and cyclosporine-induced gout include the marked shortening of the asymptomatic hyperuricemia and acute intermittent gout stages, with the rapid appearance of tophi. The stage of asymptomatic hyperuricemia lasts for 20–30 years in classic gout, but is present for only six months to four years in cyclosporine-induced disease. Similarly, the duration of the acute intermittent stage is only one to four years in transplant recipients, but it may last eight to 15 years in classic gout. Because organ transplant

recipients use other medications, such as systemic corticosteroids and azathioprine, their gouty symptoms frequently are less dramatic than those of patients with classic gout.

Gout in Women

Unlike most other rheumatic conditions, gout is less common in women than in men. In most large reviews, women account for no more than 5% of all people with gout (15). Ninety percent of women are postmenopausal at the time of their initial attack. Postmenopausal gout is similar clinically in presentation and course to classic gout, except that the age of onset is later in women than in men. Conditions that are much more commonly associated with gout in postmenopausal women than with gout in men include diuretic use (95%), hypertension (73%), renal insufficiency (50%), and preexisting joint disease, such as osteoarthritis (16).

Premenopausal gout has a strong hereditary component, as does early-onset gout in men. Most women who develop gout before menopause have hypertension and renal insufficiency but are not using diuretic therapy. The rare woman with premenopausal gout and normal renal function should be evaluated for the autosomally inherited familial hyperuricemia nephropathy (9) or the even more rare non–X-linked inborn errors of purine metabolism (16).

"Normouricemic" Gout

The most frequent explanations for apparent gout with normal levels of uric acid are that the patient doesn't have gout, or that the serum urate is normal at the time measured, but the patient actually is chronically hyperuricemic.

Several articular conditions can mimic gout closely, including crystalline arthropathies of calcium pyrophosphate dihydrate, basic calcium (apatite), and liquid lipid (17). Other causes of acute monarthropathies, such as infection, sarcoidosis, and trauma, also should be considered (18). The clinical suspicions of gout should be confirmed by crystal analysis of synovial fluid. Without this confirmation, the diagnosis remains in question.

Misunderstanding the definition of hyperuricemia also can contribute to misdiagnosis of normouricemic gout. A sustained serum urate level above 7.0 mg/dL provides a permissive environment for MSU crystal formation, but people with acute and chronic gout may have urate values below this biochemical definition of hyperuricemia. It is, in fact, rather common for a person presenting with acute gout to have a normal serum urate during the episode of severe pain. This condition probably results from uricosuric effects of ACTH release and adrenal stimulation, which are caused by the stress of the painful process. Normalization of serum urate values during acute gouty flares may be more common in alcoholics than in nondrinkers. Aside from standard urate-lowering agents, such as allopurinol, probenecid, and sulfinpyrazone, such drugs as high-dose salicylates, corticosteroids, dicumarol, glycerol guaiacolate, and x-ray contrast agents also may lower serum urate values in people with gout and lead to the false impression of normouricemic gout.

Yü reported that 1.6% of 2145 gout patients had sustained normouricemia months after discontinuing use of allopurinol or uricosuric agents (19). In most of these cases, hyperuricemia eventually returned, although several patients with very mild gouty symptoms remained normouricemic over a prolonged period.

Provocative Factors of Acute Attacks

Why crystals form in some hyperuricemic fluids and not in others is unclear. When synovial fluids are balanced for urate concentrations, the fluids from gouty patients have a far greater propensity for promoting crystal formation than similar fluids from people with osteoarthritis or rheumatoid arthritis. A number of synovial-fluid proteins have been reported to function as promoters or inhibitors of crystal nucleation. The current list of physiologically important "nucleators" is short, with the leading contenders being type I collagen and a gamma globulin subfraction (20).

The degree of hyperuricemia correlates positively with the overall risk of acquiring gout. However, rapid increases or decreases in the concentration of synovial-fluid urate are related more closely to actual precipitation of the acute gouty attack. A rapid flux in urate level is a triggering mechanism in gout induced by trauma, alcohol ingestion, and drugs.

Trauma frequently is reported to be an inciting event for acute gouty episodes. The trauma may be as minor as a long walk and may not have caused pain during the activity, but it caused intra-articular swelling. When the joint is allowed to rest, there is a relatively rapid efflux of free water from the joint fluid. This results in a sudden increase in synovial fluid-urate concentration, which may allow precipitation of urate crystals and a gout attack. This mechanism may explain why gouty attacks commonly occur at night.

Alcohol ingestion may predispose to gout through several mechanisms. The consumption of lead-tainted moonshine results in chronic renal tubular damage that leads to secondary hyperuricemia and "saturnine" gout. The ingestion of any form of ethanol can raise uric acid production acutely by accelerating the breakdown of intracellular adenosine triphosphate (21). Beer consumption has an added impact on gout because it contains large quantities of guanosine, which is catabolized to uric acid.

Drugs may precipitate gout by rapidly raising or lowering urate levels. Thiazide diuretics are frequent offenders by selectively interfering with urate excretion at the proximal convoluted tubule. Low-dose aspirin (less than 2 g/day) also can raise serum urate levels, but higher doses have a uricosuric effect and may lower the serum urate concentration. A rapid increase or reduction in the serum urate level can provoke gouty attacks; allopurinol is the drug most often responsible for this effect. The mechanism for this paradoxic response appears to be the destabilizing of microtophi in the gouty synovium when the urate concentration of the synovial fluid is changed rapidly. As the microtophi break apart, crystals are shed into the synovial fluid and the gouty episode is initiated (22).

Clinical Associations

Renal Disease

The only consistent visceral damage caused by hyperuricemia is its effect on the kidneys. Several distinct forms of hyperuricemia-induced renal disease are recognized, including chronic urate nephropathy, acute uric acid nephropathy, and uric acid nephrolithiasis.

Progressive renal failure is common in people with gout and accounts for up to 10% of deaths in gouty subjects. Hypertension, diabetes, obesity, and ischemic heart disease are the most important comorbid factors contributing to this complication; the role of hyperuricemia as a single factor in chronic parenchymal disease of the kidney remains controversial. Chronic urate nephropathy is a distinct entity caused by deposition of MSU crystals in the renal medulla and pyramids and is associated with mild albuminuria. Although chronic hyperuricemia is thought to be the cause of urate nephropathy, this form of kidney involvement is essentially never seen in the absence of gouty arthritis.

Acute renal failure can be caused by hyperuricemia in the acute tumor lysis syndrome, which occurs in patients given chemotherapy for rapidly proliferating lymphomas and leukemias. With massive liberation of purines during cell lysis, uric acid precipitates in the distal tubules and collecting ducts of the kidney. Acute uric acid nephropathy can result in oliguria or anuria. This form of acute renal failure can be distinguished from other forms by a ratio of uric acid to creatinine greater than 1.0 in a random or 24-hour urine collection.

Uric acid renal stones occur in 10%–25% of all people with gout. The incidence correlates strongly with the serum urate level, and the likelihood of developing stones reaches 50% when the serum urate is above 13 mg/dL. Symptoms of renal stones precede the development of gout in 40% of patients. Calcium-containing renal stones occur 10 times more frequently in gouty subjects than in the general population.

Hypertension

Hypertension is present in 25%–50% of people with gout, and 2%–14% of people with hypertension have gout. Because serum urate concentration correlates directly with peripheral and renal vascular resistance, reduced renal blood flow may account for the association between hypertension and hyperuricemia. Factors such as obesity and male gender also link hypertension and hyperuricemia.

Obesity

Hyperuricemia and gout correlate highly with body weight for both men and women, and individuals with gout commonly are overweight, compared with the general population. Obesity may be a factor linking hyperuricemia, hypertension, hyperlipidemia, and atherosclerosis.

Hyperlipidemia

Serum triglycerides are elevated in 80% of people with gout. The association between hyperuricemia and serum cholesterol is controversial, although serum levels of high-density lipoprotein generally are decreased in patients with gout. These abnormalities of serum lipids likely reflect overindulgence rather than a genetic link.

Radiographic Features

The radiographic findings of gout often are unremarkable early in the disease course. In acute gouty arthritis, the only finding may be soft-tissue swelling around the affected joint. In most instances, bone and joint abnormalities develop only after many years of disease and are indicative of the deposition of urate crystals. Most frequently, the abnormalities are asymmetric and seen in the feet, hands, wrists, elbows, and knees.

The bony erosions of gout are radiographically distinct from the erosive changes of other inflammatory arthritides. Gouty erosions usually are slightly removed from the joint, but rheumatoid erosions typically are in the immediate proximity of the articular surface (Fig. 15B-6). The characteristic gouty erosion has features that are both atrophic and hypertrophic, leading to erosions with an "overhanging edge." The joint space is preserved in gout until very late in the disease process. Juxta-articular osteopenia, a common and early finding in rheumatoid arthritis, is absent or minimal in gout.

Laboratory Features and Diagnosis

An elevated serum urate level has long been considered a cornerstone in the diagnosis of gout. In reality, this laboratory finding is of limited value in establishing the diagnosis. The vast majority of hyperuricemic subjects will not develop gout, and serum urate levels may be normal during gouty attacks (23). Far too many patients are diagnosed with gout based on the clinical triad of an acute monarthritis, hyperuricemia, and a dramatic improvement of articular symptoms in response to colchicine. A diagnosis by these parameters is presumptive only, and the physician should remain alert to other possibilities. A clinical response to colchicine, once considered strong evidence of gout, frequently is observed with other types of arthritis, including calcium pyrophosphate pseudogout and basic calcium phosphate (hydroxyapatite) tendinitis. Serum urate determinations are helpful and necessary in following the effects of antihyperuricemic therapy.

The definitive diagnosis of gout is possible only by aspirating and inspecting synovial fluid or tophaceous material and demonstrating characteristic MSU crystals (Fig. 15B-7). The crystals usually are needle- or rod-shaped. On compensated polarized microscopy, they appear as bright, birefringent crystals that are yellow when parallel to the axis of slow vibration marked on the first-order compensator. The crystals usually are intracellular during acute attacks, but small, truncated, extracellular crystals commonly appear as the attack

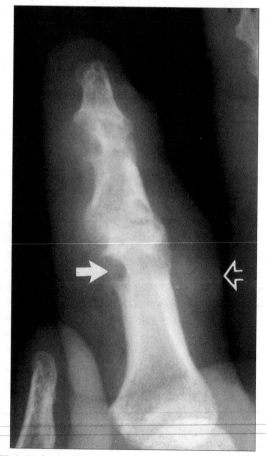

Fig. 15B-6. Radiographic changes of chronic gout include a typical gouty erosion with overhanging edge (solid arrow) and a soft-tissue tophus (open arrow).

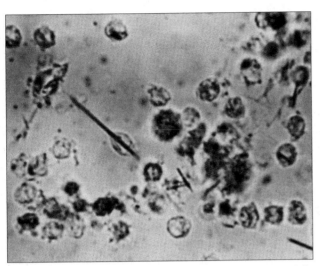

Fig. 15B-7. Photomicrograph of fresh preparation of synovial fluid obtained from the inflamed knee of a 45-year-old man with acute gouty arthritis. Note numerous small and large needle-shaped crystals of monosodium urate monohydrate that have been engulfed by neutrophilic leukocytes.

subsides and during the intercritical periods. See Chapter 7D for more information on visualizing crystals in synovial fluid.

The synovial-fluid findings are consistent with moderate to severe inflammation. The leukocyte count usually falls between 5000 and 80,000 cells/mm³, with the average count between 15,000 and 20,000 cells/mm³. The cells are predominantly neutrophils. Synovial aspirates should be sent for culture if there is any hint of a septic process. Bacterial infection can coexist with gouty crystals.

A 24-hour urine uric acid measurement is not required of all people presenting with gout. This measurement is useful for patients being considered for uricosuric therapy (probenecid or sulfinpyrazone) or when the cause of marked hyperuricemia (>11 mg/dL) is being investigated. On a regular diet, urinary uric acid excretion of more than 800 mg in 24 hours suggests a problem of urate overproduction. In children and young adults, this overproduction may be caused by enzymatic defects. In older patients, this level of urinary uric acid suggests one of the diseases associated with rapid cellular turnover, such as the myelo- or lymphoproliferative disorders. Certain drugs, contrast dyes, and alcohol interfere with urinary uric acid measurements and should be avoided for several days before the study.

N. LAWRENCE EDWARDS, MD

References

1. Campion EW, Glynn RJ, DeLabry LO. Asymptomatic hyperuricemia: risks and consequences in the Normative Aging Study. Am J Med 1987;82:421–426.
2. Sydenham T. The whole works of that excellent practical physician, Dr. Thomas Sydenham. 7th edition translated by John Pechey. London: Feales, 1717.
3. Pascual E. Persistence of monosodium urate crystals and low-grade inflammation in the synovial fluid of patients with untreated gout. Arthritis Rheum 1991;34:141–145.
4. Wernick R, Winkler C, Campbell S. Tophi as the initial manifestation of gout: report of six cases and review of the literature. Arch Intern Med 1992;152:873–876.
5. Popp JD, Bidgood WD, Edwards NL. Magnetic resonance imaging of tophaceous gout in the hands and wrists. Semin Arthritis Rheum 1996;25:282–289.
6. Popp JD, Bidgood WD, Edwards NL. The gouty tophus. Rheumatology Rev 1993;2:163–168.
7. Hench PS. The diagnosis of gout and gout arthritis. J Lab Clin Med 1936;22:48–55.
8. Nakayama DA, Barthelemy C, Carrera G, Lightfoot RW Jr, Wortmann RL. Tophaceous gout: a clinical and radiographic assessment. Arthritis Rheum 1984;27:468–471.
9. Sokoloff L. The pathology of gout. Metabolism 1957;6: 230–243.
10. Schumacher HR. Pathology of the synovial membrane in gout. Arthritis Rheum 1975;18 (Suppl):771–782.
11. Palmer DG, Highton J, Hessian PA. Development of the gout tophus. An hypothesis. Am J Clin Pathol 1989;91:190–195.
12. Moro F, Ogg CS, Simmonds HA, et al. Familial juvenile gouty nephropathy with renal urate hypoexcretion preceding renal disease. Clin Nephrol 1991;35:263–269.
13. Burack DA, Griffith BP, Thompson ME, Kahl, LE. Hyperuricemia and gout among heart transplant recipients receiving cyclosporine. Am J Med 1992;92:141–146.
14. Howe S, Edwards NL. Controlling hyperuricemia and gout in cardiac transplant recipients. J Musculoskel Med 1995;12: 15–24.
15. Lally EV, Ho G, Kaplan SR. The clinical spectrum of gouty arthritis in women. Arch Intern Med 1986;146:2221–2225.
16. Puig JG, Michán AD, Jiménez ML, et al. Female gout: clinical spectrum and uric acid metabolism. Arch Intern Med 1991; 151:726–732.
17. Reginato AJ, Schumacher HR, Allan DA, Rabinowitz JL. Acute monarthritis associated with lipid liquid crystals. Ann Rheum Dis 1985;44:537–543.
18. Baker DG, Schumacher HR Jr. Acute monarthritis. N Engl J Med 1993;329:1013–1020.
19. Yü TF. Diversity of clinical features in gouty arthritis. Semin Arthritis Rheum 1984;13:360–368.
20. McGill NW, Dieppe PA. The role of serum and synovial fluid components in the promotion of urate crystal formation. J Rheumatol 1991;18:1042–1045.
21. Puig JG, Fox IH. Ethanol-induced activations of adenine nucleotide turnover. Evidence for a role of acetate. J Clin Invest 1984;74:936–941.
22. Popp JD, Edwards NL. New insights into gouty arthritis. Contemp Intern Med 1995;7:55–64.
23. Schlesinger N, Baker DG, Schumacher HR Jr. How well have diagnostic tests and therapies for gout been evaluated? Curr Opin Rheumatol 1999;11:441–445.

GOUT
C. Treatment

Gout almost always can be treated successfully and without complications. Therapeutic goals include terminating acute attacks; providing rapid, safe relief of pain and inflammation; averting future attacks; and preventing such complications as formation of tophi, kidney stones, and destructive arthropathy (1). Management of gout can be challenging, given that the disease frequently presents in association with other disorders; patient compliance can be difficult to achieve, particularly if lifestyle changes are indicated; and the effectiveness and safety of therapies can vary widely from patient to patient, and over the course of the disease in an individual patient. However, with early intervention, careful monitoring, and patient education, the prognosis is excellent.

Acute Gout

An acute gout attack is marked by intense inflammation. Many agents, including nonsteroidal anti-inflammatory drugs (NSAIDs), colchicine, and systemic and intra-articular corticosteroids, can be used to eliminate the pain and associated symptoms. Timely administration of these agents is essential. Colchicine, for example, works best when instituted within minutes or hours of an attack. The number and location of joints affected and the existence of comorbid conditions influence the choice of agents. Urate-lowering drugs should not be instituted during an acute attack. However, patients presenting with an acute attack who have been taking allopurinol or a uricosuric drug should continue taking the medication to avoid a recurrent cycle of withholding and reinstitution.

Nonsteroidal Anti-Inflammatory Drugs
For many physicians, NSAIDs are the first choice to treat acute gout. Indomethacin usually is preferred, but other NSAIDs may be as effective. In general, NSAIDs are initiated at the maximum dosage at the first sign of an attack, and the dosage is lowered as symptoms abate. However, medication should be continued until pain and inflammation have been absent for at least 48 hours.

NSAIDs may cause significant side effects, most commonly gastrointestinal (GI) complications. Compared with NSAID use to treat other conditions, however, side effects appear to be less common in treatment of acute gout. The use of selective cyclooxygenase (COX)-2 inhibitors could provide the advantage of less GI toxicity in high-risk patients, but their use has not been reported in acute gout. Parenteral NSAIDs, such as ketorolac, offer no advantage in terms of lessening the likelihood of GI bleeding. For more information on NSAID use and toxicity, see Chapter 45.

Colchicine
Colchicine effectively treats acute gout, providing pain relief within 48 hours for most patients (1). Colchicine inhibits microtubule polymerization by binding microtubule protein subunits and preventing their aggregation, setting the stage for disruption of such membrane-dependent functions as chemotaxis and phagocytosis. Colchicine also hinders crystal-induced production of chemotactic factors and interleukin (IL)-6. Plasma levels decay rapidly after an intravenous dose, as colchicine is concentrated intracellularly. Only 10% of colchicine is excreted during the first 24 hours after administration, and sensitive assays can detect it in granulocytes and urine for up to 10 days afterward. Thus, toxicity mainly is a function of the cumulative dose, relative to renal function, during the seven to 10 days of administration (2). Colchicine also enters enterohepatic circulation, and its toxic effects may be amplified in people with liver disease or extrahepatic biliary obstruction.

Colchicine can be administered orally in hourly doses of 0.5-mg or 0.6-mg until pain and inflammation are alleviated. This regimen of small, repeated doses is intended to minimize GI toxicity, which occurs in up to 80% of patients. Symptoms of GI toxicity include severe nausea, vomiting, diarrhea, cramping, and abdominal pain, potentially leading to hypovolemia, electrolyte disturbances, and metabolic alkalosis. Dosage should be discontinued if such symptoms occur. In patients with normal renal and hepatic function, the maximum cumulative dose for oral colchicine is 6.0 mg.

Intravenous colchicine offers rapid onset of action, avoids GI toxicity, and is a useful method of delivery for postoperative patients whose oral intake is restricted, but it requires careful administration (3). The drug should be diluted in 20 mL of 0.9% sodium chloride solution which does not contain a bacteriostatic agent (not 5% dextrose in water) and administered over 10–20 minutes through a secured intravenous line. If intravenous colchicine is not diluted properly, thrombophlebitis can develop, and dislodgement of the intravenous line can cause extravasation, with potential skin sloughing at the site of leakage.

A single intravenous dose of colchicine should not exceed 3 mg, and the cumulative dose should not exceed 4 mg in a 24-hour period. Patients who receive a full intravenous dose should not receive additional colchicine by any route for at least seven days afterward, and a reduced dosage is indicated for patients with renal or hepatic disease and older patients with apparently normal renal function. Absolute contraindications to intravenous colchicine include combined renal and hepatic disease, a glomerular filtration rate of <10 mL/min, and extrahepatic biliary obstruction. Relative contraindications include significant intercurrent infection, preexisting bone marrow suppression, and immediate prior use of oral colchicine. Dosage should be halved for patients with estimated glomerular filtration rates of <50–60 mL/min (4). Concurrent use of oral and intravenous colchicine during an attack or for seven to 10 days after is advised against.

Excessive colchicine dosage may result in bone marrow suppression, renal failure, disseminated intravascular coagulation, hypocalcemia, cardiopulmonary failure, seizures, and death (2–5). Overdose can be treated successfully with colchicine-specific Fab antibody fragments (6). In patients with toxicity, colchicine-induced granulocytopenia is a major contributor to a fatal outcome. All reported cases of death, severe toxicity, or neuromuscular disease have involved unusually high doses of colchicine, renal insufficiency, advanced age, or the use of both oral and intravenous preparations during a short period of time.

Corticosteroids and Adrenocorticotropic Hormone

For patients in whom colchicine or NSAIDs are contraindicated or ineffective, corticosteroids or adrenocorticotropic hormone (ACTH) can be used. Although relapse or early recurrence has been reported, one study of corticosteroids in acute gout noted infrequent relapse (7). A single unblinded trial that compared ACTH with indomethacin for patients with monarticular gout reported similar efficacy (8).

Patients with acute gout typically receive daily doses of prednisone (20–40 mg) or its equivalent for three to four days. Dosage then is tapered gradually over one to two weeks. ACTH is given as an intramuscular injection of 40–80 IU, and some clinicians recommend following the initial dose with 40 IU every six to 12 hours for several days, if necessary.

A person with gout in one or two large joints may benefit from joint drainage, followed by intra-articular injection with 10–40 mg of triamcinolone or 2–10 mg dexamethasone, in combination with lidocaine. This regimen is appropriate for recalcitrant gout and also provides a nontoxic therapeutic option for the elderly patient with renal insufficiency, peptic ulcer disease, or other intercurrent illness. To maximize the concentration of medication in the joint, as much fluid as possible should be aspirated before instilling corticosteroids and lidocaine. If septic arthritis is suspected, injection should be deferred until synovial fluid has been cultured. Arthrocentesis can be performed safely on individuals taking anticoagulants if a small-bore needle (22-gauge or smaller) is used, needle manipulation is minimized, and direct pressure is held on the injection site for five minutes after the procedure is completed.

Gout usually will respond to colchicine, NSAIDs, or corticosteroids alone. However, if therapy is delayed or the attack is severe, one agent may not be sufficient. In such situations, these agents may be used in combination, and pain medications (including narcotics) may be added.

Prophylaxis

Diet and lifestyle modification may reduce the frequency of acute attacks and decrease or negate the need for medication. Weight loss may reduce serum urate, and dietary purine restriction also may be helpful, although resultant urate reduction usually is modest. Alcohol should be avoided because it increases production of urate and impairs its excretion. Dehydration and repetitive trauma that may occur in certain exercises or occupations should be avoided, and medications known to contribute to hyperuricemia, including thiazide and loop diuretics, low-dose salicylates, cyclosporine, niacin, ethambutol, pyrazinamide, and didanosine, should be eliminated, if possible.

Prophylactic Colchicine

Prophylactic colchicine may be appropriate for some patients, but such issues as potential toxicity, cost, difficulty of adherence, and patient tolerance of attacks must be considered. Prophylactic therapy reduces the frequency of attacks by 75%–85% and mitigates the severity of attacks that do occur. However, a single acute attack of gout does not justify lifelong use of prophylactic colchicine.

Some rheumatologists believe that prophylactic therapy should be initiated only after an antihyperuricemic agent has been added to the regimen. It is believed that prophylactic use of colchicine without control of hyperuricemia may allow tophi to develop without the usual warning signs of acute gouty attacks. If, however, a patient does not meet the criteria for prescribing a uricosuric agent or allopurinol, or has contraindications to these drugs, the use of colchicine alone can be considered. Furthermore, because initiation of urate-lowering drugs may precipitate attacks in people with hyperuricemia and intercritical gout, it may be appropriate to use colchicine (0.6 mg once or twice daily) until the dosage of urate-lowering drug is optimized. Once serum urate levels are in the desired range, prophylactic colchicine should be discontinued.

The efficacy of prophylactic colchicine is based on a double-blind, placebo-controlled study in which one 0.5-mg colchicine tablet was administered twice daily (9). Clinical experience, however, has shown that 0.6 mg once a day may work as well as the twice-daily regimen. To minimize the risk of toxicity, patients should use the smallest daily dose that will provide acceptable control of attacks.

Long-term use of small daily doses of colchicine appears to be relatively safe. However, a neuromuscular syndrome that occurs exclusively in patients with chronic renal insufficiency (serum creatinine ≥ 1.6 mg/dL) has been associated with prophylactic therapy (10). Colchicine-induced myopathy resembles polymyositis, exhibiting proximal muscle weakness, elevated creatine kinase levels, and abnormalities on electromyogram. Muscle biopsy characteristically reveals vacuolated myopathy. The myopathy may resolve spontaneously within several weeks, but the more subtle polyneuropathy caused by colchicine takes longer to resolve (5).

Urate-Lowering Agents

Treating hyperuricemia in people with recurrent or chronic gout requires long-term commitment to daily therapy and lifestyle change. However, antihyperuricemic agents are sufficiently potent that it usually is not necessary to restrict dietary purines or avoid medications that have hyperuricemic properties.

The goal of therapy with urate-lowering drugs is to maintain serum urate at <6.0 mg/dL. However, one study that examined radiographic changes over 10 years of urate-lowering therapy (11) found that achieving normal serum urate levels did not translate into radiographic improvement of intraosseous tophi as often as expected. The findings suggest that greater reductions of serum urate may be necessary, even when symptoms are controlled. Urate-lowering therapy should not be initiated during an acute attack because any change in serum urate may exacerbate or prolong the attack (12).

Appropriate antihyperuricemic agents, including uricosuric drugs and xanthine oxidase inhibitors, should be used at the lowest dosage necessary to maintain acceptable serum urate levels. Although uricosuric therapy is rarely inappropriate, given that fewer than 10% of patients are overproducers of urate, allopurinol is recommended more often because it offers the convenience of a single daily dose and is effective in both overproducers and underexcreters. Both allopurinol and uricosuric drugs are available in generic form, with roughly comparable prices for average effective doses. For these reasons, a 24-hour urine collection to determine overproducer versus underexcreter status is seldom performed in clinical practice.

Studies have been conducted to determine the advisability of lifelong urate-lowering therapy. In one study of 10 patients, five experienced no recurrence 33 months after discontinuation of urate-lowering therapy (13). The other five patients had their first recurring attacks at 15.8 months on average. Such data suggest that discontinuation of urate-lowering therapy may be well-tolerated after years of normouricemia and presumed depletion of total body urate. However, another study of 21 patients found that nine (43%) had tophi recur a mean of 39.6 months after discontinuation of antihyperuricemic drugs (14). Seventeen patients (81%) had subsequent attacks of acute arthritis. These data suggest that it is prudent to continue urate-lowering drugs indefinitely in individuals with chronic tophaceous gout who tolerate the medication, even if they have not had symptoms for years.

Allopurinol

For people with urate overproduction, tophus formation, nephrolithiasis, or other contraindications to uricosuric therapy, allopurinol is the agent of choice. It is the preferred drug in cases of renal insufficiency, but its toxicity occurs most frequently when the glomerular filtration rate is reduced. Toxicity usually can be avoided if dosages are adjusted appropriately. Therapy typically is initiated at a dosage of 300 mg/day; however, dosages of 100 mg or less are appropriate in the elderly, in those with frequent attacks, or in patients with glomerular filtration rates of <50 ml/min (1). A weekly check of serum urate levels, with a dosage increase of 100 mg/day where indicated, can help achieve optimum serum urate levels. Although the maximum recommended dosage is 800 mg/day, some patients may require and tolerate higher doses (15).

Prolonged treatment with sufficient doses of allopurinol often leads to resolution of even large, draining tophi. For this reason, and the likelihood of poor wound healing, surgical removal of tophi seldom is indicated. The degree of resolution and its pace are determined in part by the characteristics of the tophus. Soft tophi, in which urate crystals can be aspirated easily, may resolve quickly. Other tophi may be hard and resistant to dissolution, presumably because they have been present for a longer time and they include fibrous tissue (15). A combination of uricosuric agent and allopurinol may be indicated in patients with extensive tophi and adequate renal function. The urate diuretic enhances excretion of large quantities of solubilized urate, and allopurinol reduces the formation of new urate (15).

Dyspepsia, headache, and diarrhea are allopurinol's most common side effects. A pruritic papular rash occurs in 3%–10% of patients. If the rash is mild and nonpurpuric, the patient may tolerate a dose of allopurinol sufficient to maintain normalization of the serum urate level. In some patients with a minor rash, allopurinol can be discontinued and restarted later at low doses without complication (15). Additional toxicities include fever, urticaria, eosinophilia, interstitial nephritis, acute renal failure, bone marrow suppression, granulomatous hepatitis, vasculitis, and toxic epidermal necrolysis.

Allopurinol hypersensitivity syndrome is a rare but serious toxicity with a mortality rate of 20%–30% (1). If the need to reduce hyperuricemia is great, allopurinol hypersensitivity may be overcome through cautious desensitization. In an oral regimen, daily escalations of dose from 8 μg to 300 mg within 30 days may be successful (16). A rapid regimen for intravenous desensitization may be considered for patients in whom oral desensitization has failed (17). In one such patient, a 0.1-μg intradermal skin test was followed by allopurinol infusion at 15-minute intervals in five increments from 0.1 μg to 500 μg. In five further increments, dosage was advanced at 30-minute intervals from 1.0 mg to 50 mg. One hour later, 100 mg was given intravenously; the following morning, 300 mg was given orally. Thereafter, daily 300-mg doses of allopurinol were tolerated without incident. Symptoms of hypersensitivity can recur after desensitization and resumption of the drug at full dosage (18). Some patients sensitive to allopurinol may tolerate oxypurinol, the active metabolite of allopurinol. The U.S. Food and Drug Administration (FDA) lists an orphan indication for oxypurinol as the treatment of hyperuricemia in patients intolerant of allopurinol (19). However, if serious toxicities are encountered with allopurinol, oxypurinol also should be avoided.

Uricosuric Agents

Uricosuric agents are effective for patients who have a glomerular filtration rate exceeding 50–60 mL/min; are willing to drink at least two liters of fluids daily and maintain good urine flow, even at night; have no history of nephrolithiasis or excessive urine acidity; and can avoid ingestion of all salicylates, which can inhibit the uricosuric agent's effect. With advancing age, glomerular filtration rates fall, and few patients older than 65 years respond adequately to most uricosuric drugs.

Probenecid is the most commonly used uricosuric agent. Initial dosage is 0.5 g/day; dosages are increased slowly to not more than 1 g twice daily, or until target urate levels are reached. Common side effects include rash and GI upset, as well as urate nephrolithiasis, the adverse effect of greatest concern. Formation of stones despite efforts to maintain high urine volume indicates that uricosuric therapy may be inappropriate, and allopurinol is preferred in such patients. If a uricosuric is absolutely necessary, urinary alkalinization to pH 6.0–6.5 may increase urate solubility. Potassium citrate (30–80 mEq/day) may help prevent nephrolithiasis.

Similar precautions should be used with sulfinpyrazone, a potent uricosuric agent that promotes urate nephrolithiasis and also causes gastrointestinal side effects in approximately 5% of patients (1). As a congener of phenylbutazone, sulfinpyrazone may be ulcerogenic; in rare cases, bone marrow suppression may occur. Dosage is increased slowly from 100 mg to approximately 800 mg daily in divided doses until the desired level of serum urate is reached. Benzbromarone, available in Europe, is an even more potent uricosuric agent that may be effective in instances of moderate renal insufficiency or salicylate use. Losartan, an angiotensin II receptor antagonist, may be particularly useful for treating elderly people with both gout and hypertension. Losartan promotes urate diuresis and may even normalize serum urate levels (15).

Drug Interactions

Several drug interactions involving urate-lowering agents should be noted. The concomitant administration of allopurinol and ampicillin is associated with increased frequency of rash. Probenecid inhibits the excretion of the penicillins, indomethacin, dapsone, and acetazolamide. Probenecid also may affect metabolism of rifampin and heparin. Because allopurinol may increase the half-life of probenecid, and probenecid accelerates the excretion of allopurinol, careful dosage adjustment is necessary when the drugs are to be used in combination. For example, a patient with tophaceous gout who is taking allopurinol and is prescribed probenecid to enhance urate excretion may need higher doses of allopurinol, while probenecid may be effective in relatively low doses. Because the uricosuric effect of probenecid is antagonized by salicylates and pyrazinamide, these compounds should be avoided.

In the future, there may be a treatment option for patients with tophaceous gout who cannot take uricosuric agents or allopurinol. The gene encoding the enzyme uricase, or urate oxidase, is present in many animals, but not in humans. Uricase oxidizes urate to allantoin, which is highly soluble and excreted in the urine. Urate oxidase has been used successfully in the prevention and treatment of tumor lysis syndrome in people with cancer who undergo chemotherapy (20).

Asymptomatic Hyperuricemia

Hyperuricemia alone rarely requires treatment. However, moderate hyperuricemia over a period of years may lead to gouty arthritis, tophus formation, and less commonly, nephrolithiasis. Although there is little long-term risk of tophus formation in a person with a plasma urate level of 7–8 mg/dL, there is increasing risk with higher levels. Up to 50% of gout patients may develop tophi if not treated. Because individuals almost always experience attacks of acute gout before tophi develop, the finding of asymptomatic hyperuricemia is not an indication for treatment with urate-lowering drugs. The cause for hyperuricemia should be determined, and associated problems, such as hypertension, alcoholism, hyperlipidemia, or obesity, should be addressed.

Gout in the Transplant Recipient

The prevalence of gout in organ recipients has increased with the use of cyclosporine, which inhibits urate excretion. Hyperuricemia develops in more than 50% of kidney, liver, and heart transplant hosts (15). Treatment of an acute gout attack may be difficult because renal function often is impaired in any organ transplant patient. NSAIDs and cyclosporine may interfere with renal prostaglandin formation, decreasing renal blood flow, and when used together, they may have an additive effect on renal function (21). Colchicine use may be hazardous in patients on azathioprine whose granulocyte count is decreased. ACTH or corticosteroids at dosages of 20–30 mg/day may be effective in patients not already taking corticosteroids, but most transplant recipients are taking corticosteroids at the time of their attack. Thus, an initial dosage of 40–60 mg/day may be necessary in transplant recipients already receiving prednisone (15). In patients with marginal renal function or white blood cell count, intra-articular injection may be the safest alternative to colchicine and NSAIDs. Synovial fluid culture should be performed routinely in such patients.

Managing hyperuricemia in the transplant host is similarly complex. When the glomerular filtration rate is <50 mL/min, patients do not respond to uricosuric agents. Tophi may be present, mandating the use of allopurinol, even in patients with adequate glomerular filtration rates. However, allopurinol causes potentiation of azathioprine, which, as a purine analog, is metabolized by xanthine oxidase. The use of allopurinol requires a 50%–75% reduction of azathioprine dose (21), and even with frequent monitoring of white blood cell count, the therapeutic margin between leukopenia and inadequate immunosuppression is dangerously narrow. Mycophenolate mofetil has supplanted azathioprine in many antirejection regimens, which makes the treatment of hyperuricemia in these individuals less problematic because this drug is not metabolized by xanthine oxidase.

S. LOUIS BRIDGES, Jr., MD, PhD

References

1. Emmerson BT. The management of gout. N Engl J Med 1996;334:445-451.

2. Moreland LW, Ball GV. Colchicine and gout. Arthritis Rheum 1991;34:782-786.

3. Wallace SL, Singer JZ. Review: systemic toxicity associated with the intravenous administration of colchicine – guidelines for use. J Rheumatol 1988;15:495-499.

4. Roberts WN, Liang MH, Stern SH. Colchicine in acute gout: reassessment of risks and benefits. JAMA 1987;257:1920-1922.

5. Putterman C, Ben-Chetrit E, Caraco Y, Levy M. Colchicine intoxication: clinical pharmacology, risk factors, features, and management. Semin Arthritis Rheum 1991;21:143-55.

6. Baud FJ, Sabouraud A, Vicaut E, et al. Brief report: treatment of severe colchicine overdose with colchicine-specific Fab fragments. N Engl J Med 1995;332:642-645.

7. Groff GD, Franck WA, Raddatz DA. Systemic steroid therapy for acute gout: a clinical trial and review of the literature. Semin Arthritis Rheum 1990;19:329-336.

8. Axelrod D, Preston S. Comparison of parenteral adrenocorticotropic hormone with oral indomethacin in the treatment of acute gout. Arthritis Rheum 1988;31:803-5.

9. Paulus HE, Schlosstein LH, Godfrey RG, Klinenberg JR, Bluestone R. Prophylactic colchicine therapy of intercritical gout. A placebo-controlled study of probenecid-treated patients. Arthritis Rheum 1974;17:609-614.

10. Kuncl RW, Duncan G, Watson D, Alderson K, Rogawski MA, Peper M. Colchicine myopathy and neuropathy. N Engl J Med 1987;316:1562-1568.

11. McCarthy GM, Barthelemy CR, Veum JA, Wortmann, RL. Influence of antihyperuricemic therapy on the clinical and radiographic progression of gout. Arthritis Rheum 1991;34:1489-1494.

12. Yu TF, Gutman AB. Effect of allopurinol (4-hydroxypyrazolo(3,4-d)pyrimidine) on serum and urinary uric acid in primary and secondary gout. Am J Med 1964;37:885-98.

13. Gast LF. Withdrawal of longterm antihyperuricemic therapy in tophaceous gout. Clin Rheumatol 1987;6:70-73.

14. Lieshout-Zuidema MF, Breedveld FC. Withdrawal of longterm antihyperuricemic therapy in tophaceous gout. J Rheumatol 1993;20:1383-1385.

15. Jones RE, Ball EV. Gout: beyond the stereotype. Hosp Pract (Off Ed) 1999;34:95-102.

16. Fam AG, Dunne SM, Iazzetta J, Paton TW. Efficacy and safety of desensitization to allopurinol following cutaneous reactions. Arthritis Rheum 2001, 44:231-238.

17. Walz-LeBlanc BA, Reynolds WJ, MacFadden DK. Allopurinol hypersensitivity in a patient with chronic tophaceous gout: Success of intravenous desensitization after failure of oral desensitization. Arthritis Rheum 1991;34:1329-1331.

18. Unsworth J, Blake DR, d'Assis Fonseca AE, Beswick DT. Desensitisation to allopurinol: a cautionary tale. Ann Rheum Dis 1987;46:646.

19. U.S. Food and Drug Administration. List of Orphan Designations and Approvals. Available at: www.fda.gov/orphan/designat/list.htm. Accessed June 4, 2001.

20. Pui CH, Relling MV, Lascombes F, et al. Urate oxidase in prevention and treatment of hyperuricemia associated with lymphoid malignancies. Leukemia 1997;11:1813-1816.

21. West C, Carpenter BJ, Hakala TR. The incidence of gout in renal transplant recipients. Am J Kidney Dis 1987;10:369-372.

16 CONNECTIVE-TISSUE DISEASES

As pathologists grappled with an understanding of disseminated lupus erythematosus in the first half of the 1900s, they became aware of limitations of Morgagni's idea that diseases reside in certain organs in the body. Rather, they began to appreciate the interdependence of organs and tissue systems. From this perspective, diseases such as rheumatic fever, periarteritis nodosa, disseminated lupus erythematosus, and diffuse scleroderma presented a challenge. The work of Klemperer and colleagues during this time was seminal in developing the conceptual framework that still strongly influences the approach to these conditions (1):

> "The apparent heterogeneous involvement of various organs in this disease [disseminated lupus erythematosus] had no logic until it became apparent that the widespread lesions were identical in that they were mere local expressions of a morbid process affecting the entire collagenous tissue system. The most prominent of these alterations is fibrinoid degeneration...

> "It is evident, then, that fibrinoid degeneration and collagen sclerosis are the morphologic expression of different phases of a disturbed colloidal collagen system ... [which is] the result of a fundamental alteration of the collagenous tissues.

> It is reasonable to consider these maladies as systemic diseases of the connective tissues."

But even as Klemperer, in the terms of his day, conceptualized the connective tissues of the body as "a well defined, widely dispersed colloidal system" and invoked a "colloidal imbalance within the collagenous tissues," he cautioned that "to identify this system as the seat of certain diseases is *by no means to identify these diseases with one another or even to relate them*" (1).

Klemperer's descriptive and theoretical work focused on fibrinoid degeneration as a fundamental underpinning of this process (2). Fibrinoid degeneration was a term used to describe "deeply eosinophilic substance disposed among the fibers . . . associated with a striking and unequivocal change in the fibers themselves [which] become straight and irregularly thickened ... highly refractive. Their massiveness is augmented by the accretion of adherent clumps of ground substance. The alteration of fibers and ground substance is accompanied by a conspicuous proliferation of fibroblasts . . . infiltration of histiocytes and leukocytes"

(2). Fibrinoid degeneration was recognized as a common characteristic frequently associated with inflammation. In addition, what attracted Klemperer's attention in the context of disseminated lupus erythematosus was the systemic occurrence of the connective-tissue changes and the absence of an identifiable "palpable injurious" agent.

With these observations, the essential character of disseminated lupus was defined as an idiopathic, inflammatory, systemic disease affecting multiple organs. Furthermore, "a similar widespread alteration of collagen also [was] noted in certain cases of diffuse scleroderma. Here, however, the collagen disturbance is manifest not only as fibrinoid degeneration but also as an increase in the bulk and density of the connective tissue. . . . [T]his sclerosing type of lesion has also been observed in disseminated lupus erythematosus. It is evident, then, that fibrinoid degeneration and collagen sclerosis are the morphologic expression of different phases of a disturbed colloidal collagen system" (1). Thus, "an ill-defined group, referred to as collagen diseases, in which fibrinoid alteration of the connective tissue is the determining diagnostic feature" was created (3).

Reflecting on this nomenclature nearly 20 years later, one of Klemperer's colleagues, Abou Pollack, commented that the term connective-tissue disease was not intended to "evoke the idea of a single nosological entity having several different manifestations [e.g.,] SLE, rheumatoid arthritis, scleroderma, etc." (4). In Pollack's view, the term was intended to focus attention on the common pathologic findings, although he and Klemperer had championed the idea of a fundamental connective-tissue injury. Their perspective led to the interpretation of vascular thrombi as accretions of subendothelial fibrinoid and of vascular lesions as a "mere local expression of the fundamental connective-tissue injury" (2). A possible primary endothelial nature of the vascular injury was dismissed as untenable (2). With the benefit of hindsight, however, it seems that the enthusiasm for the newly defined connective-tissue system and for the rubric of fundamental connective-tissue injury leading to fibrinoid degeneration or sclerosis may have overstepped the bounds of descriptive pathology as it tried to superimpose mechanism.

Current texts of the rheumatic diseases approach the connective-tissue diseases in varied fashion (Table 16-1). In some texts, systemic lupus erythematosus (SLE), progressive systemic sclerosis, inflammatory muscle disease, Sjögren's syndrome, and the systemic vasculitides are grouped together loosely. In other texts, these diseases stand in separate sections. What then, does the term "connective-tissue diseases" mean?

TABLE 16-1
Idiopathic Connective-Tissue Diseases

Systemic lupus erythematosus
Inflammatory muscle disease (polymyositis, dermatomyositis)
Progressive systemic sclerosis
Overlap syndromes
Sjögren's syndrome
Systemic vasculitides
Relapsing polychondritis
Eosinophilic fasciitis

Inflammation and Immunity

Sustained inflammation is the hallmark of this group of diseases. Inflammatory effector mechanisms can engage mast cells, platelets, neutrophils, endothelial cells, mononuclear phagocytes, and lymphocytes, and can trigger the complement, kinin, and coagulation cascades. From an immunologic perspective, the traditional boundary between natural (innate) and cognate (acquired) immune mechanisms has been blurred as the roles have expanded for immune-system cells in pathogenesis of disease. For example, mast cells, typically associated with antigen-specific immunoglobulin E (IgE)-mediated allergic reactions, contribute to IgG immune-complex–initiated disease, independent of antigen specificity (5), and to nonimmune host defense against bacteria (6,7). Neutrophils and mononuclear phagocytes, the quintessential effector cells of the innate immune system and acute inflammation, influence acquired immunity through their action on T cells. Furthermore, studies in atherosclerosis point to an important role for CD4[+] T cells, B cells, and macrophages in the proliferation of fibroblasts in connective tissue, leading to concentric neointimal expansion and luminal narrowing (8). Diversity in the potential mechanisms activated during inflammation and the potential for substantial interplay among elements of the immune system in the inflammatory response provide the basis for a broad spectrum of clinical manifestations.

Environmental Factors

The particular mechanisms activated depend, at least in part, on the properties of the initiating stimulus (Table 16-2). The ability of different stimuli to lead to inflammation with some common features, however, is not the same as the imperative that all stimuli lead to identical programs of inflammation and tissue injury. The erosive synovitis of rheumatoid arthritis, the glomerulonephritis of systemic lupus, the myositis of polymyositis, and the vasculitis of classical polyarteritis nodosa reflect some fundamental differences in the targeting of the inflammatory process.

Presumably, many of these differences reflect the biology of the initiating event. For some diseases, this event may be infection with a biologic agent – a bacterium (*Streptococcus* and rheumatic fever), a spirochete (*Borrelia burgdorferi* and Lyme disease), or a virus (parvovirus and rheumatoid arthritis-like disease). For other diseases, this event may be a biologically active compound (L-tryptophan and eosinophilia myalgia syndrome; rapeseed oil and progressive systemic sclerosis) or other environmental exposure (ultraviolet radiation and flares of SLE).

Genetic Factors

The models of rheumatic fever and Lyme arthritis point directly to specific etiologic agents, and they have sharpened the focus of theory and research in the hunt for specific inciting antigens. However, both of these diseases and many other animal and human models incorporate the equally important lesson of differential host susceptibility. Not all individuals with streptococcal infection get rheumatic fever (9), and even in the context of more highly controlled animal models, different inbred strains of rodents show marked differences in their susceptibility to a range of model diseases, including Lyme arthritis, collagen-induced arthritis, and adjuvant arthritis.

Genetic differences in the ability of major histocompatibility class (MHC) I and II molecules to present disease-related antigens to the immune system clearly play an important role in determining susceptibility in many models (10,11); however, non-MHC genes are emerging from their "background" role into the forefront of investigative efforts (12,13). Recognition of genetically defined differences in opsonins, such as complement components and mannose binding lectin, and in immunoglobulin receptors, cytokine promoters, and many intracellular signaling molecules, expand the perspective of antigen "nonspecific" genes and their potential to influence the reactivity of the immune system (14–18) (Table 16-3).

TABLE 16-2
Environmental Factors Associated With Connective-Tissue Diseases

Biologic agents
  Group A β-hemolytic streptococci (rheumatic fever)
  Borrelia burgdorferi (Lyme arthritis)

Drugs
  Hydralazine, procainamide, others (drug-induced lupus)
  Penicillamine (myasthenia and lupus-like syndromes)
  Bleomycin, pentazocine (fibrosing syndromes)

Uncommon exposures and ingestions
  Vinyl chloride (progressive systemic sclerosis)
  L-tryptophan (eosinophilia myalgia syndrome)
  Rapeseed oil (toxic oil syndrome)

Clinical Phenotype

Within the interplay between the immune system, genetically determined variation in its function, and various environmental stimuli, certain themes emerge among the diseases often grouped as connective-tissue diseases. The sustained inflammation typically is systemic, rather than limited to a single organ. The engagement of the immune system involves natural and acquired effector functions, and often is characterized by autoreactive cells and autoantibodies reacting with self-determinants. From a clinical perspective, disease manifestations often overlap with fever, weight loss, synovitis, pleuropericarditis, myositis, and skin rashes. Laboratory evaluation often shows signs of inflammation, with elevated erythrocyte sedimentation rate and C-reactive protein, as well as certain markers of autoreactivity, including the presence of antinuclear antibodies. This overlap, now conceptualized as undifferentiated connective-tissue or autoimmune disease, typically is more pronounced early in the course of disease (19). Over time, it may evolve into one of the recognized connective-tissue diseases, although such evolution is not obligatory. Alternatively, the disease process may dissipate.

If the clinical syndrome evolves, one can anticipate circumstances in which more distinct manifestations of two or more diseases may be present. The concept of mixed connective-tissue disease, marked by clinical elements of SLE, inflammatory myositis, and scleroderma, and by the frequent presence of autoantibodies to the nuclear ribonucleoprotein or U_1 RNP antigens, has generated substantial controversy in the literature. However, the variable occurrence of clinical manifestations and certain autoantibodies might not have surprised Klemperer and his contemporaries.

Clinical experience teaches us that there are connective-tissue diseases that are characterized by distinctive features. The synovitis of rheumatoid arthritis is more proliferative than that of SLE, inflammatory muscle disease, or progressive systemic sclerosis. With rheumatoid arthritis, synovial pannus formation leads to invasion of cartilage and bone with erosions and joint destruction. Such events are uncommon in SLE, polymyositis, and progressive systemic sclerosis.

Renal involvement is common in SLE and typically is an immune-complex–related glomerulonephritis, with features that may be seen much less commonly in Sjögren's syndrome. However, renal disease is not a feature of myositis, and renal involvement in progressive systemic sclerosis reflects primary vascular involvement without significant antibody deposition. Similarly, the skin is affected by many of the connective-tissue diseases, but each may have quite distinctive findings that are sufficiently characteristic to play an important role in differential diagnosis. The butterfly rash of lupus, the violaceous heliotrope discoloration of the eyelids in dermatomyositis, and the tightening of the skin in progressive systemic sclerosis clearly reflect different processes.

Different profiles of autoantibody reactivities also underscore distinctive features of the connective-tissue diseases. Antibodies to double-stranded DNA, Sm, and

TABLE 16-3
Proposed Genetic Factors in Connective-Tissue Diseases

Opsonins and opsonin receptors
Complement component deficiencies
Mannose binding lectin
Complement receptors (CR1)
Fcγ receptors (FcγRIIA, FcγRIIIA)

Antigen processing/presentation
Opsonin pathway components
MHC class I and II
Transporters associated with antigen processing
T-cell receptors for antigen

Cytokine-related genes
TNF-α promoter polymorphisms
IL-1, IL-1Ra, IL-6, IL-10 polymorphisms
Cytokine receptor γc chain deficiency
(immunodeficiency)

Apoptosis-related genes
Fas, Fas ligand, caspase 10
TNF receptor

MHC, major histocompatibility complex; TNF, tumor necrosis factor; IL, interleukin.

ribosomal P proteins are seen almost exclusively in SLE, whereas antibodies to certain nucleolar antigens, such as topoisomerase I (anti-Scl70) and centromere antigens, occur in systemic sclerosis. In patients with polymyositis, especially with interstitial lung disease, antibodies to histidyl, threonyl, and alanyl transfer RNA synthetases (Jo-1, PL-7, and PL-12, respectively) and to the translation component KJ are found. In contrast, antibodies to the signal recognition particle occur in SLE patients without interstitial lung disease. Antibodies to Mi2, a nuclear protein complex, appear to occur specifically in patients with dermatomyositis.

ROBERT P. KIMBERLY, MD

References

1. Klemperer P, Pollack AD, Baehr G. Diffuse collagen disease. Acute disseminated lupus erythematosus and diffuse scleroderma. JAM 1942;119:331–332.
2. Klemperer P, Pollack AD, Baehr G. Pathology of disseminated lupus erythematosus. Arch Pathol 1941;32:569–609.
3. Klemperer P. The significance of the intermediate substances of the connective tissue in human disease. Harvey Lectures 1953;XLIX:100–121.

4. Pollack AD. Some observations on the pathology of systemic lupus erythematosus. In: Baehr G, Klemperer P (eds). Systemic Lupus Erythematosus. New York: Grune and Stratton, 1959; pp 1–16.

5. Sylvestre DL, Ravetch JV. Fc receptors initiate the Arthus reaction: redefining the inflammatory cascade. Science 1994; 265:1095–1098.

6. Echtenacher B, Mannel DN, Hultner L. Critical protective role of mast cells in a model of acute septic peritonitis. Nature 1996;381:75–77.

7. Malaviya R, Ikeda T, Ross E, Abraham SN. Mast cell modulation of neutrophil influx and bacterial clearance at sites of infection through TNF-α. Nature 1996;381:77–80.

8. Shi C, Lee WS, He Q, et al. The immunologic basis of transplant-associated arteriosclerosis. Proc Natl Acad Sci USA 1996;93:4051–4056.

9. Khanna AK, Buskirk DR, Williams RC Jr, et al. Presence of a non-HLA B cell antigen in rheumatic fever patients and their families as defined by a monoclonal antibody. J Clin Invest 1989;83:710–716.

10. Hammer J, Gallazzi F, Bono E, et al. Peptide binding specificity of HLA-DR4 molecules: correlation with rheumatoid arthritis association. J Exp Med 1995;181:1847–1855.

11. Nagaraju K, Raben N, Loeffler L, et al. Conditional up-regulation of MHC class I in skeletal muscle leads to self-sustaining autoimmune myositis and myositis-specific autoantibodies. Proc Natl Acad Sci USA 2000;97:9209–9214.

12. Kimberly RP. Genetics of human lupus. In: Theofilopoulos AN (ed). Genes and Genetics of Autoimmunity. Basel, Switzerland: Karger, 1999; pp 99–120.

13. Wakeland EK, Wandstrat AE, Liu K, Morel L. Genetic dissection of systemic lupus erythematosus. Current Opin Immunol 1999;11:701–707.

14. Gibson AW, Wu J, Edberg JC, Kimberly RP. Fcγ receptor polymorphisms, insight into pathogenesis. In: Kammer GM, Tsokos GC (Eds). Lupus: Cellular and Molecular Pathogenesis. Totowa, NJ: Humana Press, 1999; pp 557–573.

15. Moulds JM, Krych M, Holers VM, Liszewski MK, Atkinson JP. Genetics of the complement system and rheumatic diseases. Rheum Dis Clin North Am 1992;18:893–914.

16. Feldmann M, Brennan FM, Maini RN. Role of cytokines in rheumatoid arthritis. Annu Rev Immunol 1996;14:397–440.

17. Murphy KM, Ouyang W, Farrar JD, et al. Signaling and transcription in T helper development. Annu Rev Immunol 2000; 18:451–494.

18. Shirakawa I, Deichmann KA, Izuhara I, Mao I, Adra CN, Hopkin JM. Atopy and asthma: genetic variants of IL-4 and IL-13 signaling. Immunol Today 2000;21:60–64.

19. LeRoy EC, Maricq HR, Kahaleh MB. Undifferentiated connective tissue syndromes. Arthritis Rheum 1980;23:341–343.

17 SYSTEMIC LUPUS ERYTHEMATOSUS
A. Epidemiology, Pathology, and Pathogenesis

Epidemiology

Systemic lupus erythematosus (SLE) is a prototypic autoimmune disease with a diverse array of clinical manifestations, which is characterized by the production of antibodies to components of the cell nucleus. SLE primarily is a disease of young women. Peak incidence occurs between the ages of 15 and 40, with a female:male ratio of 6–10:1. However, age at onset can range from infancy to advanced age; in both pediatric and older-onset patients, the female:male ratio is approximately 2:1. In a general outpatient population, SLE affects approximately one in 2000 individuals, although the prevalence varies with race, ethnicity, and socioeconomic status (1).

Systemic lupus erythematasus shows a strong familial aggregation, with a much higher frequency among first-degree relatives of patients. The disease occurs concordantly in approximately 25%–50% of monozygotic twins and 5% of dizygotic twins. Moreover, in extended families, SLE may occur with other autoimmune conditions, such as hemolytic anemia, thyroiditis, and idiopathic thrombocytopenia purpura. Despite the influence of heredity, most cases of SLE appear sporadic.

Immunopathology

The pathologic findings of SLE occur throughout the body and are manifested by inflammation, blood vessel abnormalities that encompass bland vasculopathy and vasculitis, and immune-complex deposition. The best-characterized

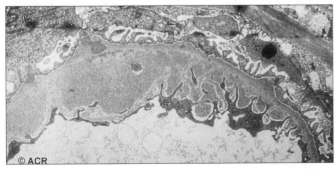

Fig. 17A-1. Immune deposits in lupus nephritis. This electron micrograph illustrates large granular subendothelial immune deposits, as well as smaller subepithelial and intramembranous deposits. Broadening and fusion of the foot processes also are present. Reprinted from the Revised Clinical Slide Collection on the Rheumatic Diseases, with permission of American College of Rheumatology.

organ pathology involves the kidney, which displays increases in mesangial cells and mesangial matrix, inflammation, cellular proliferation, basement membrane abnormalities and immune-complex deposition. These deposits are comprised of immunoglobulins M, G, and A (IgM, IgG and IgA), as well as complement components. On electron microscopy, the deposits can be seen in the mesangium and the subendothelial and subepithelial sides of the glomerular basement membrane (Fig. 17A-1).

Renal pathology is classified according to two grading schemes, which provide information for clinical staging. The World Health Organization (WHO) system is based on the extent and location of proliferative changes within glomeruli as well as alterations in the basement membrane. These patterns are not static, and transitions between categories can be observed. A second classification system is based on signs of activity and chronicity (2). This system is useful in predicting outcome because it distinguishes signs of active inflammation, which can be reversible, from those of scarring, which generally are irreversible (Table 17A-1). With either scheme, lupus nephritis exhibits marked variability, differing in severity and pattern among patients, as illustrated in Fig 17A-2.

Skin lesions in SLE demonstrate inflammation and degeneration at the dermal–epidermal junction, and the basal or germinal layer is the primary site of injury. In these lesions, granular deposits of IgG and complement components in a band-like pattern can be seen by immunofluorescence microscopy. Necrotizing vasculitis also may cause skin lesions.

Other organ systems affected by SLE usually display nonspecific inflammation or vessel abnormalities, although pathologic findings sometimes are minimal. For example, despite the severity of central nervous system involvement, the

TABLE 17A-1
Histologic Classification of Lupus Nephritis

Activity index	Chronicity index
Proliferative change	Sclerotic glomeruli
Necrosis/karyorrhexis	Fibrous crescents
Cellular crescents	Tubular atrophy
Leukocyte infiltration	Interstitial fibrosis
Hyaline thrombi	
Interstitial inflammation	

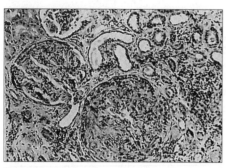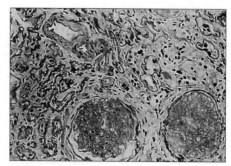

Fig. 17A-2. Left, Signs of "active" lupus nephritis showing glomerular proliferation, crescents, abundant inflammatory cell infiltration, and interstitial cell infiltrates (hematoxylin-eosin). Right, Signs of "chronic" lupus nephritis showing glomerular sclerosis, vascular thickening, tubular atrophy, and interstitial febrosis (periodic acid–Schiff).

typical findings are cortical microinfarcts and a bland vasculopathy with degenerative or proliferative changes; inflammation and necrosis indicative of vasculitis are found only rarely.

The heart may also show nonspecific foci of inflammation in the pericardium, myocardium, and endocardium, even in the absence of clinically significant manifestations. Verrucous endocarditis, known as Libman-Sacks endocarditis, is a classic pathologic finding of SLE and is manifested by vegetations, most frequently at the mitral valve. These vegetations consist of accumulations of immune complexes, inflammatory cells, fibrin, and necrotic debris.

Occlusive vasculopathy causes venous and arterial thrombosis in SLE and is a common pathologic finding. Although coagulation can result from inflammation, autoantibodies also may trigger thrombotic events. These autoantibodies represent a spectrum of specificities designated as antiphospholipid antibodies, anticardiolipin antibodies, and lupus anticoagulants. Although some of these antibodies bind lipid antigens, others are directed to the serum protein β_2-glycoprotein 1, a protein that can form complexes with lipids (3). Vessel abnormalities in SLE may also result from increases in endothelial cell adhesiveness by a mechanism analogous to the Schwartzman reaction (4).

Other pathologic findings prominent in SLE have an uncertain relationship to inflammation. Patients with longstanding disease, including women without the usual risk factors for cardiovascular disease, frequently develop atherosclerosis. It is unclear whether these lesions result from corticosteroid-induced metabolic abnormalities, hypertension, or vascular changes caused by a chronic burden of immune complexes and other pro-inflammatory mediators. Similarly, osteonecrosis, as well as neurodegeneration in people with chronic severe disease, may arise from vasculopathy, drug side effects, or persistent immunologic insults.

Immunopathogenesis of Antinuclear Antibodies

The central immunologic disturbance in SLE is autoantibody production. These antibodies are directed to a host of self molecules in the nucleus and cytoplasm of cells, as well

as on the cell surface. In addition, SLE sera contain antibodies to such soluble molecules as IgG and coagulation factors. Because of the wide range of its antigenic targets, SLE is classified as a disease of generalized autoimmunity.

Among autoantibodies expressed in patient sera, those directed against components of the cell nucleus (antinuclear antibodies, or ANA) are the most characteristic of SLE and are found in more than 95% of patients (5). These antibodies bind DNA, RNA, nuclear proteins, and protein–nucleic-acid complexes (Table 17A-2). As a group, the molecules targeted by ANA are highly conserved among species, serve important cellular functions, and exist inside cells as part of large complexes comprised of various protein and nucleic-acid components (e.g., nucleosomes). Antibodies to certain nuclear antigens (e.g., DNA and histones) frequently occur together, a phenomenon known as linkage. Linkage suggests that the complex, rather than the individual components, serves as the target of autoreactivity, as well as its driving antigen.

Among ANA specificities in SLE, two appear unique to this disease. Antibodies to double-stranded (ds) DNA and a nuclear antigen called Sm essentially are found only in people with SLE, and are included as serologic criteria in the classification of SLE (see Appendix I). Although both anti-DNA and anti-Sm are serologic markers, they differ in their pattern of expression and clinical associations. These antibodies are produced independently by patients, and although anti-DNA levels frequently fluctuate over time and may disappear with disease quiescence, anti-Sm levels remain more constant. The anti-Sm and anti-DNA responses also differ in the nature of their target antigens. The Sm antigen, which is designated an snRNP (small nuclear ribonucleoprotein), is composed of a set of uridine-rich RNA molecules complexed with a common group of core proteins as well as unique proteins that are specifically associated with the RNA molecules. In contrast to anti-DNA antibodies, which react to a conserved nucleic-acid determinant widely present on DNA, anti-Sm antibodies specifically target snRNP proteins and not RNA.

Perhaps the most remarkable feature of the anti-DNA response is its association with immunopathologic events in SLE, especially glomerulonephritis. This role has been established by correlating anti-DNA serum levels with periods of disease activity, isolating anti-DNA in enriched form from glomerular eluates of patients with active nephritis, and inducing nephritis by administering anti-DNA antibodies to normal animals. The relationship between levels of anti-DNA and active renal disease is not invariable; some patients with active nephritis may lack serum anti-DNA, and others with high levels of anti-DNA are clinically discordant and escape nephritis (6).

The occurrence of nephritis without anti-DNA may be explained by the pathogenicity of other autoantibody specificities (e.g., anti-Ro or anti-Sm). The converse situation of clinical quiescence despite serologic activity suggests that only some anti-DNA provoke glomerulonephritis. Antibodies with this property are denoted as pathogenic or nephritogenic. Studies to delineate the basis of renal pathogenicity initially focused on the role of antibodies to single-stranded (ss) DNA and dsDNA. Although anti-dsDNA antibodies essentially are exclusive to SLE, anti-ssDNA antibodies have wider expression among inflammatory and infectious diseases. Both specificities frequently coexist in SLE, however, because many anti-DNA antibodies bind a common antigenic determinant present on both ssDNA and dsDNA. Since renal eluates show antibody activity to both DNA forms, it appears likely that both anti-dsDNA and antibodies to ssDNA have similar pathogenic roles.

Studies correlating the properties of anti-DNA antibodies with nephritis suggest that several features promote pathogenicity. These features include isotype, charge, ability to fix complement, and capacity to bind glomerular preparations (7). In this regard, anti-DNA antibodies appear to be a subset of pathogenic antibodies that bind to nucleosomes, the likely form of DNA in the circulation as well as in immune deposits. These antibodies can bind to such components as DNA or histones, or to higher-order structures requiring an intact nucleosome or various components together. Unless the full range of anti-nucleosomal antibodies is assessed, the presence of nephritogenic antibodies may be missed (8). In contrast to their role in nephritis, anti-DNA antibodies have not been clearly associated with other clinical events.

Although many ANAs never have been adequately evaluated for pathogenicity, there is evidence that certain autoantibodies other than anti-DNA have a clinical impact. Associations of other autoantibodies with disease events include antibodies to ribosomal P proteins (anti-P) with neuropsychiatric disease and hepatitis; antibodies to Ro with neonatal lupus and subacute cutaneous lupus; antibodies to phospholipids with vascular thrombosis, thrombocytopenia, and recurrent abortion; and antibodies to blood cells with cytopenias.

The contribution of ANAs to clinical events in SLE has been difficult to understand because the intracellular location of the target antigens should protect them from antibody interactions. The location of these antigens may not be fixed, however, and some antigens may translocate to the membrane and become accessible to antibody attack. Damage to cells by ultraviolet radiation, for example, may lead to such movement. There also is evidence to suggest that ANAs may enter cells, bind nuclear antigens, and perturb cell function (9). Furthermore, ANAs may mediate injury by cross-reactive binding to a molecule with tissue-specific expression.

Because of the impact of kidney disease on morbidity and mortality, nephritis has been the clinical event in SLE

TABLE 17A-2
Principle Antinuclear Antibodies in Systemic Lupus Erythematosus

Specificity	Target antigen	Function	Frequency in SLE (%)
Native DNA	dsDNA	Genetic information	40
Denatured DNA	ssDNA	Genetic information	70
Histones	H1, H2A, H2B, H3, H4	Nucleosome structure	70
Sm	snRNP proteins B, B', D, E	Splicesome component, RNA processing	30
U1RNP	snRNP proteins, A, C, 70K	Splicesome component, RNA processing	32
SSA/Ro	60- and 52-kDa proteins, complexed with Y1–Y5 RNAs	Unknown	35
SSB/La	48-kDa protein complexed with various small RNAs	Regulation of RNA polymerase-3 transcription	15
Ku	86- and 66-kDa proteins	DNA binding	3
PCNA/cyclin	36-kDa protein	Auxillary protein of	10
Ribosomal RNP	38-, 16-, and 15-kDa phospho-proteins, associated with ribosomes	DNA polymerase d Protein synthesis	10

ds, double-stranded; ss, single-stranded; snRNP, small nuclear ribonucleoprotein.
Modified from Tan (5), with permission.

most intensively studied mechanistically. Clinical observations strongly suggest that SLE renal disease results from the deposition of immune complexes containing anti-DNA, since active nephritis is marked by elevated anti-DNA levels with a depression of total hemolytic complement. Because anti-DNA shows preferential renal deposition, these findings suggest that DNA–anti-DNA immune complexes are a major pathogenic species. DNA in these complexes likely is in the form of nucleosomes, suggesting that antibodies to other components of this structure may participate in immune-complex formation. Because of their charged structure, nucleosomes themselves may have affinity for glomerular macromolecules, leading to renal localization (8).

Although immune complexes may provoke renal injury in SLE, the amounts of such complexes in the serum appear limited. This finding has suggested that complexes may form in situ, rather than within the circulation, accounting for the paucity of complexes in the serum. According to this mechanism, immune complexes would be assembled in the kidney on DNA or other nucleosomal components adherent to the glomerular basement membrane.

Another mechanism for nephritis in SLE is the direct interaction of autoantibodies with glomerular antigens. Many anti-DNA antibodies are polyspecific and interact with molecules other than DNA. The binding of anti-DNA to these molecules could activate complement, inciting inflammation; this binding also could anchor immune complexes to kidney sites, whether the complexes are formed in the circulation or in situ.

The pathogenesis of other SLE manifestations is less well-understood, although immune-complex deposition at relevant tissue sites generally has been considered a likely mechanism. Indeed, the frequent association of depressed complement levels and signs of vasculitis with active SLE suggests that immune complexes are important agents for initiating or exacerbating organ damage. These considerations do not exclude the possibility that tissue injury results from either cell-mediated cytotoxicity or direct antibody attack on target tissues.

Determinants of Disease Susceptibility

Studies of patients suggest that SLE is caused by genetically determined immune abnormalities that can be triggered by exogenous and endogenous factors. Although the predisposition to disease is hereditary, it is likely to be multigenic and to involve different sets of genes in different individuals. Analysis of genetic susceptibility has been based primarily on the search for gene polymorphisms occurring with greater frequency in people with SLE than in control populations. Most of the markers tested have involved genes for known immune-response phenomena. The study of genetic factors predisposing to SLE also has involved genome-wide scans of siblings with SLE or multiplex families. Although this approach has led to identification of chromosomal regions associated with disease, the actual genes leading to susceptibility are not known (10).

Of genetic elements that could predispose to autoimmunity, the major histocompatibility complex (MHC) has been most intensively scrutinized for its contribution to human SLE. Using a variety of MHC gene markers, population-based studies indicate that the susceptibility to SLE, like many other autoimmune diseases in humans, involves class II gene polymorphisms. An association of human leukocyte antigen (HLA)-DR2 and HLA-DR3 (and recently defined subspecificities) with SLE has been commonly observed, with these alleles producing a relative risk of disease that ranges approximately from 2 to 5.

This analysis of MHC gene associations is complicated by the existence of extended HLA haplotypes in which class II genes are in linkage disequilibrium with other potential susceptibility genes. Because the MHC is rich in genes for immune-system elements, the association of disease with a class II marker does not denote a specific functional abnormality promoting pathogenesis. Indeed, the contribution of class II genes to SLE susceptibility has been difficult to conceptualize because these genes regulate responses in an antigen-specific manner, whereas SLE is characterized by responses to a host of self antigens of unrelated sequence and structure. In contrast to their uncertain role in disease susceptibility, class II genes appear to exert a more decisive influence on the production of particular ANAs.

Among other MHC gene systems, inherited complement deficiencies also influence disease susceptibility. Like class I and II molecules, complement components, in particular C4a and C4b, show striking genetic polymorphism, with a deficiency of C4a molecules (null alleles) a common occurrence in the population. As many as 80% of people with SLE have null alleles irrespective of ethnic background, with homozygous C4a deficiency conferring a high risk for SLE. Since C4a null alleles are part of an extended HLA haplotype with the markers HLA-B8 and HLA-DR3, the influence of these class I and class II alleles of disease susceptibility may reflect linkage disequilibrium with complement deficiency. SLE also is associated with inherited deficiency of C1q, C1r/s, and C2 (11).

An association of SLE with inherited complement deficiency may seem surprising because of the prominence of immune-complex deposition and complement consumption during disease. However, a decrease in complement activity could promote disease susceptibility by impairing the neutralization and clearance of foreign antigen, thus leading to prolonged immune stimulation. Furthermore, the complement system plays a role in the clearance of apoptotic cells. Apoptosis, or programmed cell death, is associated with the breakdown of DNA and the rearrangement of intracellular constituents. Although this process likely occurs commonly at sites of inflammation, the finding of apoptotic cells is rare, suggesting that clearance is rapid and efficient.

Clearance of apoptotic cells involves a number of pathways, including the complement system. C1q, for example, binds to apoptotic cells, initiating complement's role in clearance. In the absence of complement, apoptotic cells may persist and stimulate autoantibody responses. The importance of complement deficiency to autoimmunity is illustrated by the features of mice in which C1q has been eliminated by genetic knockout techniques. C1q-deficient mice have elevated anti-DNA levels, glomerulonephritis, and increased apoptotic cells in the tissue (12). Although complement deficiency could lead to generalized immune-system changes, its effects may be confined to certain responses. Thus, C4a and C4b differ in their interaction with antigens based on chemical composition; the absence of either molecule would create only a selective deficiency state, without jeopardizing overall host defenses.

Genetics of Murine SLE

Several strains of inbred mice with inherited lupus-like disease have been studied as models to elucidate the human disease. These mice mimic human SLE in ANA production, immune complex glomerulonephritis, lymphadenopathy, and abnormal B-cell and T-cell function. These strains differ in the expression of certain serologic and clinical findings (e.g., anti-Sm, hemolytic anemia, and arthritis), as well as in the occurrence of disease among males and females. Among various lupus strains described (NZB, NZB/NZW, MRL-*lpr/lpr*, BXSB, and C3H-*gld/gld*), the development of a full-blown lupus syndrome requires multiple unlinked genes (13).

In mice, single mutant genes (*lpr, gld,* and *Yaa*) can promote anti-DNA production and abnormalities in the number and function of B and T cells. In *lpr* and *gld* mice, these abnormalities result from mutations in proteins involved in apoptosis. Apoptosis plays a critical role in the development of the immune system, as well as in the establishment and maintenance of tolerance. The *lpr* mutation leads to the absence of Fas, a cell-surface molecule that triggers apoptosis in lymphocytes, and *gld* affects a molecule that interacts with Fas, the Fas ligand. These gene defects appear to operate in peripheral, in contrast to central, tolerance and allow the persistence of autoreactive cells (14).

Although defects in Fas may predispose to abnormal immune-cell function in mice, the occurrence of clinical disease manifestations (e.g., nephritis) requires other genes in the strain background. Only MRL-*lpr/lpr* mice of *lpr* congenic strains show immune-mediated glomerulonephritis in association with high-level production of pathogenic anti-DNA. A similar situation exists in humans, in whom mutations in Fas are associated with defects in apoptosis and with lymphoproliferation of an unusual population of CD4[-], CD8[-], Thy.1[+], and B220[+] cells. Although patients with this autoimmune lymphoproliferative syndrome display some autoantibodies, clinical and serologic findings of SLE are uncommon, suggesting that in humans, as in the mouse, SLE requires more than one gene (15).

The interaction of genes in SLE also is observed in New Zealand mice. NZB/NZW F1 mice develop an SLE-like illness that results from genes contributed by both NZB and NZW parents. Although the nature of these genes is not known, studies on congenic mice developed from the NZM2410 strain have shown a series of genes that can promote as well as suppress autoimmunity. Individually, genes that promote autoimmunity (denoted *sle2, sle2, sle3*) lead to distinct immune disturbances, including expression of ANA. When these genes are coexpressed because of genetic crosses, the clinical and serologic features of SLE occur. Importantly, other genes can suppress the development of SLE in mice, indicating complexity in the genetic predisposition for disease (16).

In contrast to human SLE, the lupus strains lack a common MHC class I or II marker that can be identified as a susceptibility factor. MHC molecules may, nevertheless, contribute to pathogenesis, as shown by genetics of disease in New Zealand mice (NZB, NZB/NZW), as well as the pattern of disease expression in congenic NZB mice with mutations in their class II genes. Such mice have nephritis and enhanced anti-DNA production, suggesting that self-antigen presentation may be influenced by the structure of the class II molecules. Among lupus mice, New Zealand strains have an MHC-linked deficiency in the expression of the pro-inflammatory cytokine tumor necrosis factor α (TNF-α). This deficiency, which has a counterpart in humans, may be pathogenic because administration of TNF-α to mice with low endogenous production ameliorates disease (17).

A variety of new SLE models have been created using molecular genetic techniques. These models reflect aberrant patterns of gene expression that occur in mice in which specific genes are eliminated by knockout techniques or enhanced by transgene expression. Studies of these mice suggest that a variety of genetic abnormalities may predispose to autoimmunity, and genes regulating immune-cell life span or signaling threshold may lead to autoantibody production. These genetic defects may affect the establishment of tolerance or the persistence of autoreactive cells.

Immune-Cell Disturbances

Autoantibody production in SLE occurs in the setting of generalized immune-cell abnormalities that involve the B-cell, T-cell, and monocyte lineages. These immune-cell disturbances appear to promote B-cell hyperactivity, leading to hyperglobulinemia, increased numbers of antibody-producing cells, and heightened responses to many antigens, both self and foreign. Another consequence of B-cell and T-cell disturbance in SLE may be abnormal tolerance. In healthy individuals, anti-DNA precursors are tolerized by anergy or deletion; however, people with SLE or animals with SLE models may retain such precursors, which can be stimulated to generate high-affinity autoantibody responses.

Although nonspecific immune activation can provoke certain ANA responses, it does not appear to be the major mechanism for inducing pathogenic autoantibodies, especially anti-DNA. Levels of these antibodies far exceed the extent of hyperglobulinemia. In addition, anti-DNA antibodies have features indicative of in vivo antigen selection by a receptor-driven mechanism. These features include variable-region somatic mutations that increase DNA binding activity and specificity for dsDNA (18). The generation of such responses also may be affected by the composition of the preimmune repertoire and the content of precursors that can be mutated under influence of self antigen drive.

The ability of DNA to drive autoantibody production in SLE contrasts with the poor immunogenicity of mammalian DNA when administered to normal animals. This discrepancy suggests that SLE patients either have a unique capacity to respond to DNA or are exposed to DNA in a form with enhanced immunogenicity (e.g., surface blebs on apoptotic cells or nucleosomes). Although serologic profiles of people with SLE and mice with murine models of SLE point to nucleosomes as the driving antigen, bacterial or viral DNA may stimulate this response. Bacterial DNA, because of characteristic sequence motifs lacking in mammalian DNA, has potent adjuvant properties. As a result, bacterial DNA is immunogenic and may be able to elicit anti-DNA autoantibodies in a genetically susceptible host (19).

The specificity of ANA directed to nuclear proteins supports the hypothesis that these responses are antigen-driven, since these antibodies bind multiple independent determinants found in different regions of these proteins. The pattern of ANA binding minimizes the possibility that molecular mimicry is the exclusive etiology for autoimmunity in SLE. According to this theory, autoantibody production might be stimulated by a foreign antigen bearing an amino acid sequence or antigenic structure resembling a self molecule. This type of cross-reactivity has been hypothesized for many different autoimmune diseases, and it has been suggested for SLE because of the sequence similarity between certain nuclear antigens and viral and bacterial proteins. However, if SLE autoantibodies resulted from molecular mimicry, they would be expected to bind self antigen only at sites of homology with foreign antigen, rather than throughout the entire molecule.

These arguments suggest that self antigen, rather than a mimic, sustains autoantibody production, but they do not eliminate the possibility that a cross-reactive response to a foreign antigen initiates an ANA response. Thus, a foreign antigen may induce a population of B cells with Ig receptors that bind both foreign and self antigen. These B cells could process self antigen and present determinants that are not subject to tolerance and can stimulate autoreactive T-cell responses. The possibility that infection triggers SLE is illustrated by the finding that people with SLE are infected more commonly with Epstein-Barr virus than are control populations (20).

Studies analyzing the genetics of SLE and the pattern of ANA production both strongly suggest that T cells are critical to disease pathogenesis. In murine models of lupus, the depletion of helper T cells by monoclonal antibody treatment abrogates autoantibody production and clinical disease manifestations. However, the nature of the T cells helping ANA responses, the mechanisms by which they escape tolerance, and the process of self-antigen presentation have not been elucidated. It is unclear whether self antigen is presented from endogenous sources or whether it is first released from damaged or dying cells, and then processed and presented by conventional antigen-presenting cells.

The basis of T-cell help in autoantibody responses may differ from conventional responses because of the nature of the antigens. Most SLE antigens exist as complexes or particles, such as nucleosomes, containing multiple protein and nucleic-acid species. Because these antigens may effectively trigger B-cell activation by multivalent binding, T-cell help for autoimmune responses could be delivered by nonspecifically activated T cells. Alternatively, T-cell reactivity to these antigens could be elicited to only one protein on a complex, allowing a single helper T cell to collaborate with B cells for multiple protein and nucleic-acid determinants.

Triggering Events

Although inheritance and the hormonal milieu may create a predisposition toward SLE, the initiation of disease and its temporal variation in intensity likely result from environmental and other exogenous factors. Among these potential influences are infectious agents, which could induce specific responses by molecular mimicry and perturb overall immunoregulation; stress, which can provoke neuroendocrine changes affecting immune-cell function; diet, which can affect production of inflammatory mediators; toxins, including drugs, which could modify cellular responsiveness and the immunogenicity of self antigens; and physical agents, such as sunlight, which can cause inflammation and tissue damage. The impingement of these factors on the predisposed individual is likely to be highly variable, which could provide a further explanation for the disease's heterogeneity and its alternating periods of flare and remission.

DAVID S. PISETSKY, MD, PhD

References

1. Ward MM, Pyun E, Studenski S. Long-term survival in systemic lupus erythematosus. Patient characteristics associated with poorer outcomes. Arthritis Rheum 1995;38:274–283.
2. Austin HA III, Boumpas DT, Vaughan EM, Balow JE. Predicting renal outcomes in severe lupus nephritis: contributions of clinical and histologic data. Kidney Int 1994;45:544–550.
3. Roubey RA. Immunology of the antiphospholipid antibody syndrome. Arthritis Rheum 1996;39:1444–1454.
4. Belmont HMN, Buyon J, Giorno R, Abramson S. Up-regulation of endothelial cell adhesion molecules characterizes disease activity in systemic lupus erythematosus. The Schwartzman phenomenon revisited. Arthritis Rheum 1994;37:376–383.
5. Tan EM. Antinuclear antibodies: diagnostic markers for autoimmune diseases and probes for cell biology. Adv Immunol 1989;44:93–151.

6. Pisetsky DS. Antibody responses to DNA in normal immunity and aberrant immunity. Clin Diagn Lab Immunol 1998;5:1–6.

7. Lefkowith JB, Gilkeson GS. Nephritogenic autoantibodies in lupus. Arthritis Rheum 1996;39:894–903.

8. Amoura Z, Piette JC, Bach JF, Koutouzov S. The key role of nucleosomoes in lupus. Arthritis Rheum 1999;42:833–843.

9. Reichlin M. Cell injury mediated by autoantibodies to intracellular antigens. Clin Immunol Immunopath 1995;76:215–219.

10. Gaffney PM, Kearns GM, Shark KB, et al. A genome-wide search for susceptibility genes in human systemic lupus erythematosus sib-pair families. Proc Natl Acad Sci 1998;95: 14875–14879.

11. Walport MJ, Davies KA, Morley BJ, Botto M. Complement deficiency and autoimmunity. Ann NY Acad Sci 1997;815: 267–281.

12. Botto M, Dell'Agnola C, Bygrave AE, et al. Homozygous C1q deficiency causes glomerulonephritis associated with multiple apoptotic bodies. Nature Gen 1998;19:56–59.

13. Theofilopoulos AN, Kofler R, Singer PA, Dixon FJ. Molecular genetics of murine lupus models. Adv Immunol 1989;46: 61–109.

14. Nagata S, Suda T. Fas and Fas ligand: lpr and gld mutations. Immunol Today 1995;16:39–43.

15. Vaishnaw AK, McNally JD, Elkon KB. Apoptosis in the rheumatic diseases. Arthritis Rheum 1997;40:1917–1927.

16. Morel L, Mohan C, Yu Y, et al. Functional dissection of systemic lupus erythematosus using congenic mouse strains. J Immunol 1997;158:6019–6028.

17. Jacob CO. Tumor necrosis factor and interferon gamma: relevance for immune regulation and genetic predisposition to autoimmune disease. Sem Immunol 1992;4:147–154.

18. Radic MZ, Weigert M. Genetic and structural evidence for antigen selection of anti-DNA antibodies. Annu Rev Immunol 1994;12:487–520.

19. Gilkeson GS, Pippen AMM, Pisetsky DS. Induction of cross-reactive anti-dsDNA antibodies in preautoimmune NZB/NZW mice by immunization with bacterial DNA. J Clin Invest 1995; 95:1398–1402.

20. James JA, Kaufman KM, Farris AD, Taylor-Albert E, Lehman TJA, Harley JB. An increased prevalence of Epstein-Barr virus infection in young patients suggests a possible etiology for systemic lupus erythematosus. J Clin Invest 1997;100:3019–3026.

SYSTEMIC LUPUS ERYTHEMATOSUS
B. Clinical and Laboratory Features

In sharp distinction to organ-specific autoimmune diseases such as thyroiditis, diabetes, or myasthenia gravis, systemic lupus erythematosus (SLE) is a constellation of signs and symptoms classified as one nosologic entity. It is the diversity of presentation, accumulation of manifestations over time, and undulating disease course that challenge clinicians. With rare exception, the unifying laboratory abnormality is the presence of circulating antinuclear antibodies (ANAs). Acknowledging the complexity of this disease, its broad differential diagnosis, and the need to develop better and more specific therapies, the American College of Rheumatology (ACR) has designated 11 diagnostic criteria (see Appendix I) (1) that reflect the major clinical features of the disease (mucocutaneous, articular, serosal, renal, neurologic) and incorporate the associated laboratory findings (hematologic and immunologic). The presence of four or more criteria is required for diagnosis. They need not necessarily present simultaneously: a single criterion such as arthritis or thrombocytopenia may recur over months or years before the diagnosis can be confirmed by the appearance of additional features. Although rheumatologists do not completely agree as to whether these criteria need to be strictly applied in a practice setting, or reserved only for formal academic studies, the criteria do facilitate a methodologic approach for evaluating patients.

Not only is just about every bodily part potentially affected by SLE, but in each organ different structural components can be involved with varying frequencies, as exemplified in evaluating a large Canadian cohort (Fig. 17B-1) (2).

In addition, nonspecific constitutional features of SLE, some of which dominate the clinical picture, are fatigue, fever, and weight loss. Demographic characteristics, such as female predominance (female:male ratio of 9:1), typical onset during the reproductive years, and over-representation of some minority groups (e.g., African-Americans) are helpful clues to diagnosis. Factors to consider that might precipitate the onset or exacerbation of systemic disease or isolated organ involvement include recent sun exposure, emotional stress, infection, and certain drugs such as sulfonamides.

More than 90% of people with SLE survive at least two years after diagnosis, compared to only about 50% three decades ago (3). Recent data support an 80%–90% survival at 10 years (4). A bimodal mortality curve is prevalent in SLE (5). Patients who die within five years of diagnosis usually have active disease requiring high doses of corticosteroids and intense immunosuppression, and commonly develop concomitant infections. In contrast, late deaths are often the result of cardiovascular disease. Although SLE is not considered curable, patients can enjoy periods of extended remission with virtually no clinical activity, and even the disappearance of ANAs.

Commonly Involved Organ Systems
Mucocutaneous

The cutaneous system is one of the most commonly affected, approaching 80%–90%. In parallel with the myriad of

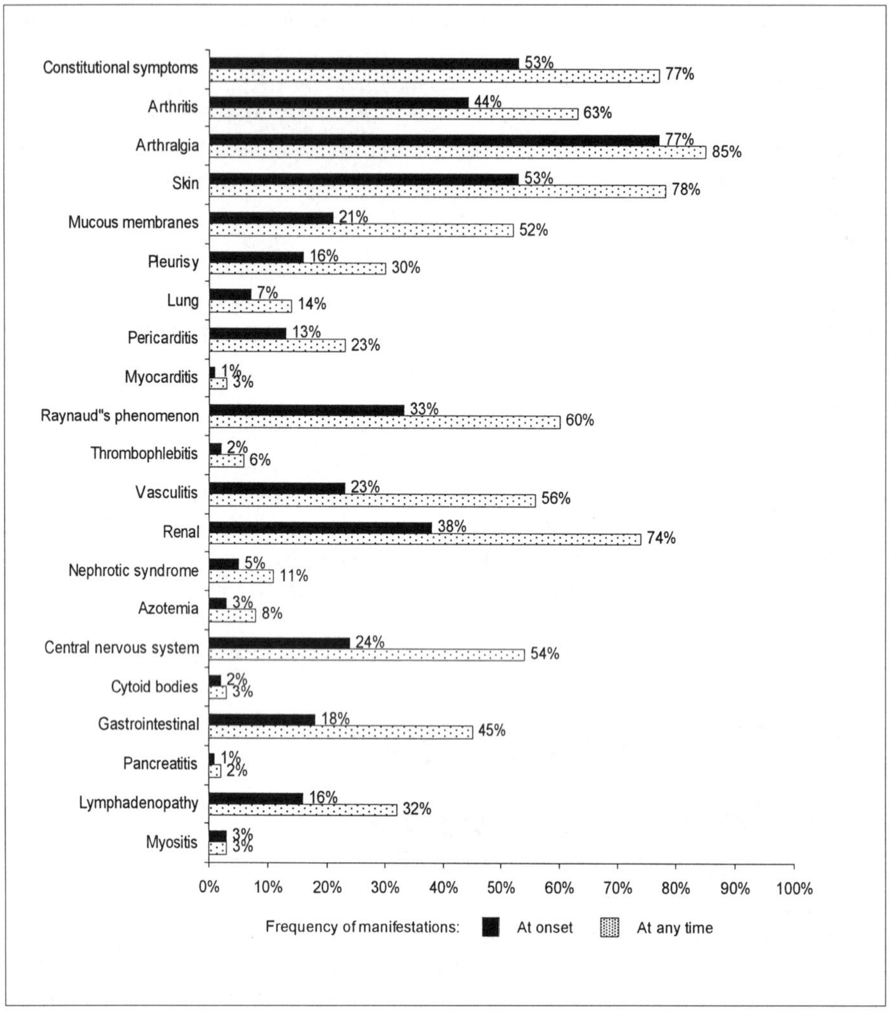

Fig. 17B-1. Frequency of manifestations at onset and at any time during the course of SLE, in a large Canadian cohort (2). The frequency at onset is based on 376 patients diagnosed at Lupus Clinic (University of Toronto), and frequency at anytime is for 750 patients registered prior to July 1995.

signs and symptoms of SLE itself, the skin and mucous membranes can be involved in a variety of ways (6). Notably, four of the 11 formal criteria can be fulfilled in this system alone. SLE-specific skin lesions are classified into three types – chronic, subacute, and acute – based strictly on clinical appearance and duration, without considering the extracutaneous manifestations or laboratory features of the overall disease.

The most common form of chronic disease is discoid lupus (DLE), which occurs in 15%–30% of people with SLE (Fig. 17B-2, Panel A). It can occur as part of the systemic disease or it can exist in isolation in the absence of any autoantibodies (2%–10% will develop SLE). DLE lesions are discrete plaques, often erythematous, covered by scale that extend into dilated hair follicles. These lesions most typically occur on the face, scalp, in the pinnae, behind the ears, and on the neck. They can be seen in areas not exposed to the sun. The lesions can progress, with active indurated erythema at the periphery. Central atrophic

scarring is characteristic. Irreversible alopecia can result from follicular destruction. Albeit rare, prominent dermal mucin accumulation in the early course of DLE can result in the succulent, edematous lesions of tumid lupus.

Lupus panniculitis-lupus profundus is a less-common form of chronic disease. These lesions spare the epidermis and represent involvement of the deep dermis and subcutaneous fat. The lesions of lupus panniculitis are firm nodules generally without surface changes. In time, the overlying skin becomes attached to the subcutaneous nodular lesions and is drawn inward, resulting in deep depressions.

Subacute cutaneous lupus erythematosus (SCLE) lesions are seen in 7%–27% of patients (Fig. 17B-2, Panels B and C). SCLE primarily affects Caucasian women. The lesions are typically symmetric, widespread, superficial, and nonscarring, and are most often present in sun-exposed areas, e.g., the shoulders, extensor surfaces of the arms, upper chest, upper back, and neck. The lesions begin as small, erythematous, scaly papules or plaques that can evolve into papulosquamous (psoriasiform) or annular polycyclic forms. The latter often coalesce to produce large confluent areas with central hypopigmentation. Generally, both forms are nonscarring. Antibodies to SSA/Ro ribonucleoproteins are commonly found in people with SCLE.

Perhaps the most classic of all the rashes in SLE is the malar, or butterfly, rash, which is categorized among the acute rashes (Fig. 17B-2, Panel D). It occurs in 30%–60% of all patients. This erythematous and edematous eruption simulates the shape of a butterfly with its body bridging over the base of the nose and wings spreading out over the malar eminences. At times the same rash can be seen on the forehead and chin, but it classically spares the nasolabial folds. The absence of discrete papules and pustules distinguishes it from acne rosacea. The rash is abrupt in onset and can last for days. Postinflammatory changes are common, particularly in patients with pigmented skin. The butterfly rash is often initiated and/or exacerbated by exposure to sunlight. However, patients can have a photosensitive erythematous rash elsewhere on the body in the absence of a butterfly rash. The criteria for photosensitivity and butterfly rash are thus independent of each other. A more widespread, morbilliform or exanthemous eruption is another acute cutaneous manifestation of SLE.

Alopecia is a feature of SLE. It may be diffuse or patchy, reversible or permanently scarring as a result of discoid lesions in the scalp. The breakage of hairs at the temples – so-called "lupus frizz" – can be observed.

Mucosal lesions are also part of the clinical spectrum of SLE and can affect the mouth (most commonly), nose, and anogenital area. Although oral lesions can be seen on the buccal mucosa and tongue, sores on the upper palate are particularly characteristic (Fig. 17B-2, Panel E). They typically are described as painless, but need not be. Central depression often occurs and painful ulcerations develop.

Vasculitis is another component of skin disease in SLE. It may be manifest as urticaria, palpable purpura, nailfold or digital ulcerations, erythematous papules of the pulps of the fingers and palms, or splinter hemorrhages (Fig. 17B-2, Panel F).

Because the skin can be an important marker of disease activity in SLE, the physical examination should always include inspection of often overlooked areas: the scalp, pinnae, behind the ears, palate, fingertips, and palms.

Musculoskeletal System

Painful joints are the most common presenting symptom of SLE, with frequencies reported between 76% and 100%. In some cases, the pain is more characteristic of arthralgia because it is unaccompanied by traditional signs of inflammation. In others, the classic signs of true arthritis are present: swelling, erythema, heat, and decreased range of motion. Notably, the patient's complaint of pain may be out of proportion to the degree of synovitis present on physical examination. Although arthritis can affect any joint, it is most often symmetric with involvement of the small joints of the hands (proximal interphalangeal and metacarpal phalangeal), wrists, and knees, but sparing the spine. The arthritis can be evanescent, resolving within 24 hours, or more persistent.

Many of these features account for the initial diagnostic consideration of early rheumatoid arthritis (RA) in some patients. In contrast to RA, the arthritis in SLE is nonerosive and generally nondeforming. In those patients who do appear to have deforming features such as ulnar deviation, hyperflexion, and hyperextension, the deformities generally are reducible (Fig. 17B-3). These hypermobile digits with reducible deformities are secondary to involvement of para-articular tissues such as the joint capsule, ligaments, and tendons, and are referred to as Jaccoud-like arthropathy. Exceptions are certainly possible and, when present, erosions may be clinically difficult to distinguish from RA; however, they are usually nonprogressive and likely result from capsular pressure and an altered mechanical situation caused by subluxation.

Effusions tend to be modest. The synovial fluid is clear to slightly cloudy with good viscosity and mucin clot, reflecting the absence of major inflammation. ANAs can be present. White blood cell (WBC) counts are usually <2,000/mm³ with a predominance of mononuclear cells. The fluid can be transudative or exudative. The serum/synovial fluid ratios of complement, total protein, and immunoglobulin (Ig) G can all be 1, indicating a proportional escape of proteins into the joint space, or >1 for complement levels only, indicating local consumption, not simply reflecting decreased serum complement. Larger effusions with warmth should prompt the consideration of septic arthritis.

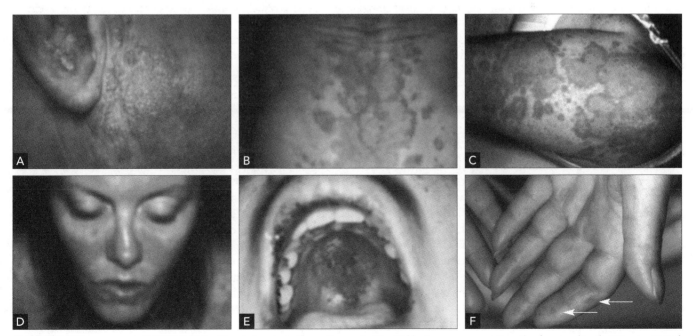

Fig. 17B-2. Cutaneous manifestations of systemic lupus erythematosus. **A:** Discoid lesions are present on the face and in the pinnae. **B and C:** Examples of the lesions of subacute cutaneous lupus erythematosus on the back and arm. **D:** Classic malar rash. **E:** Extensive acute perforating ulcer on the upper palate. **F:** Erythematous lesions consistent with cutaneous vasculitis on the digits. (Photographs provided by Dr. Andrew G. Franks, Jr. Associate Professor of Clinical Dermatology, New York University School of Medicine.)

Rheumatoid nodules can occur in SLE accompanied by the presence of rheumatoid factor, but this is not common.

Rheumatic complaints localized to the hips should raise serious consideration of osteonecrosis, the frequency of which has been reported at 5%–10%. Although the femoral head is the most common site of involvement, other sites include the femoral condyles, talus, humeral head, and occasionally the metatarsal heads, radial head, carpal bones, and metacarpal bones. Bilaterality is frequent but not necessarily simultaneous. Most cases are associated with the use of corticosteroids, but causality has also been attributed to Raynaud's phenomenon, small vessel vasculitis, fat emboli, or the presence of anti-phospholipid antibodies. Typically, people with osteonecrosis complain of persistent painful motion localized to a single joint, often relieved by rest.

Generalized myalgia and muscle weakness, frequently involving the deltoids and quadriceps, can be accompanying features of disease flares. Overt myositis with elevations of creatine phosphokinase occurs in <15% of patients. Electromyogram and muscle biopsy findings range from normal to those seen in dermatomyositis/polymyositis. Exceptionally high levels of creatine phosphokinase are rare. Patients with SLE can develop myopathy as a consequence of corticosteroid or antimalarial use.

Renal

The kidney is considered by many the signature organ affected by SLE. Essentially all studies of prognosis have identified lupus nephritis as an important predictor of poor outcome. Renal disease is present in one-half to two-thirds of patients, and with rare exception is based on the presence of proteinuria (dipstick 2+, >500 mg/24 hour). There is a spectrum of renal injury that can be assessed, in part on clinical grounds, and more definitively by biopsy (Table 17-1). Classification by the World Health Organization is based on histology and location of immune complexes. Renal biopsy results are abnormal in most patients, especially when tissue is evaluated by electron microscopy and immunofluorescence. Both diffuse proliferative nephritis and progressive forms of focal proliferative nephritis are associated with a poorer prognosis than membranous or mesangial disease.

Clinical evaluation initially includes urine dipstick and microscopic analysis. A baseline 24-hour urine analysis for measurement of protein and creatinine, even in the presence of 1+ dipstick, is common practice, especially in a patient with antibodies to double-stranded (ds) DNA and low complement levels. The sediment can be bland (consistent with mesangial or membranous disease) or active containing red blood cell (RBC) casts (consistent with proliferative lesions). Persistent hematuria with more than five RBCs per high-power field (in the absence of other causes such as menstruation) and/or pyuria with more than five WBCs per high-power field (excluding infection) would each be an unusual reflection of lupus nephritis in the absence of proteinuria (unless pathology is limited to the mesangium in the case of RBC and interstitium in case of WBC). An elevated creatinine without

TABLE 17B-1
World Health Organization Classification of Lupus Nephritis

Class	Pattern	Site of immune complex deposition
I	Normal	None
II	Mesangial	Mesangial only
III	Focal and segmental proliferative	Mesangial, subendothelial,
IV	Diffuse proliferative	Mesangial, subendothelial
V	Membranous	Subepithelial intramembranous

concomitant proteinuria is unexpected unless advanced renal insufficiency is present. Although renal disease is frequently insidious, symptoms that occur with progressive activity include swollen ankles, puffy eyes upon waking in the morning, and frequent urination. A low serum albumin level is an indicator of persistent proteinuria. Isolated hypertension outside of the norms for age, race, and gender should raise suspicion of underlying renal disease.

Biopsies are not required to diagnose lupus nephritis, but are extremely helpful in certain settings because clinical parameters are not absolute. Given the importance of identifying pathologic features suggestive of more aggressive disease, such as crescents, some clinicians believe kidney biopsy to be the fulcrum for therapeutic decisions. Thus, treatment with alkylating agents, which can result in premature ovarian failure, becomes readily justified in circumstances where the clinical picture may have suggested a more favorable histology. For example, there are patients who have rapidly rising titers of anti-dsDNA and falling complement levels, but only modest proteinuria (400 mg to 1 g), bland sediment, normal creatinine, and no other systemic manifestations to warrant intense immunosuppression. Other patients may have nephrotic-range proteinuria and an active sediment, yet serologic parameters are normal. Renal biopsies in these somewhat ambiguous situations can be quite informative. In contrast, the decision to withhold aggressive therapy is also important and may be appropriate for irreversible late-stage sclerotic disease. The "take-home" point is that renal biopsies should be performed when the result will make a clear difference in the approach and/or is required as part of a research study. Renal ultrasound is another helpful guide to therapy because the chances of reversible disease become smaller with decreased size and increased echogenicity of the kidneys.

Clinical Clues[a]

Sediment	Proteinuria (24-hr)	Serum creatinine	BP	Anti-dsDNA	C3/C4
Bland	<200 mg	Normal	Normal	Absent	Normal
RBC or bland	200–500 mg	Normal	Normal	Absent	Normal
RBC, WBC	500–3500 mg	Normal to mild elevation	Normal to elevated	Positive	Decreased
RBC, WBC, RBC casts	1000–>3500 mg	Normal to dialysis-dependent	High	Positive to high titer	Decreased
Bland	>3000 mg	Normal to mild elevation	Normal	Absent to modest titer	Normal

[a] These are only guidelines, and parameters may vary, substantiating the need for biopsy when precise diagnosis is required.
Table prepared in consultation with Dr. James A. Tumlin, Associate Professor of Medicine, Renal Division, Emory University School of Medicine.
BP, blood pressure; dsDNA, double-stranded DNA; RBC, red blood cells; WBC, white blood cells.

Urine protein is a critical measurement of ongoing renal lupus activity. Although new proteinuria of 500 mg is significant, patients with membranous nephropathy can have continued proteinuria between 500 mg and 2 g and still be considered stable. In such cases, an exacerbation is best defined as at least a doubling of baseline proteinuria. It is essential to monitor blood pressure because hypertension can be a reflection of renal disease activity and, as such, accelerates functional impairment.

Renal transplantation in lupus has been successful. However, lupus nephritis can recur (~10%), even in the absence of clinical or serologic evidence of active SLE (7), but is not always associated with allograft loss. Clinical and serologic activity in SLE may improve in patients who have end-stage renal disease (8), although this paradigm has been challenged recently (9).

Nervous System

Approximately two-thirds of people with SLE have neuropsychiatric manifestations. The pathophysiology of this broad clinical category is not well understood, which probably reflects the inaccessibility of the tissue involved. Proposed mechanisms include vascular occlusion due to vasculopathy; vasculitis, although rare; leukoaggregation or thrombosis; and antibody-mediated neuronal cell injury or dysfunction (10). Neuropsychiatric systemic lupus includes neurologic syndromes of the central, peripheral, and autonomic nervous systems, and psychiatric disorders in which other causes have been excluded. These manifestations may occur as single or multiple events in the same

person. Symptoms can be present concomitantly with activity in other systems, or exist in isolation. Although the formal ACR criteria for neuropsychiatric lupus include only seizures and psychosis, it has become increasingly clear that

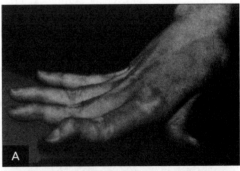
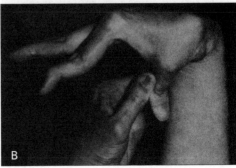

Fig. 17B-3. **A:** Swan neck deformity of the second and third digits. **B:** Hyperextension of the first interphalangeal joint. (Courtesy of Dr. Harry Fischer, Beth Israel Medical Center, New York, NY)

additional descriptors might be important in diagnosis. In an effort to expand the criteria, reporting standards, recommendations for laboratory and imaging evaluation, and case definitions for 19 neuropsychiatric syndromes observed in SLE have been developed (11).

A variety of psychiatric disorders are reported and include mood disorders, anxiety, and psychosis. Unequivocal attribution to lupus is difficult because such disorders may be related to the stress of having a major chronic illness, or may be due to drugs, infections, or metabolic disorders. Patients can demonstrate significant cognitive defects such as attention deficit, poor concentration, impaired memory, and difficulty in word finding. These abnormalities are best documented by neuropsychological testing and a decline from a higher former level of functioning. Another syndrome of diffuse neurologic dysfunction is acute confusional state, defined as disturbance of consciousness or level of arousal with reduced ability to focus, maintain, or shift attention, accompanied by cognitive disturbance and/or changes in mood, behavior, or affect. The syndrome often develops over a brief timeframe, fluctuates over the day, and covers a wide spectrum, ranging from mild alterations of consciousness to coma.

Inclusive in the neurologic manifestations of the central nervous system are seizures, which may be focal or generalized. Headache is a common complaint in patients, but there is still debate as to whether this is a feature attributable to SLE. The "lupus headache" has been operationally defined as severe, disabling, persistent, and not responsive to narcotic analgesics. However, severe migraine in the absence of lupus may have these same characteristics. Benign intracranial hypertension is also included in the case definition of headache. The term "lupoid sclerosis" has been used to describe a rare condition in which patients exhibit complex neurologic deficits similar to those observed in multiple sclerosis. Myelopathy and aseptic meningitis are rare. Chorea, albeit infrequent, is the most common movement disorder observed in SLE. This and cerebrovascular accidents have been related to the presence of antiphospholipid antibodies.

Disturbances of the cranial nerves can result in visual defects, blindness, papilledema, nystagmus or ptosis, tinnitus and vertigo, and facial palsy. Peripheral neuropathy may be motor, sensory, mixed motor-sensory, or mononeuritis multiplex. Transverse myelitis presenting with lower-extremity paralysis, sensory deficits, and loss of sphincter control has been observed in a limited number of people with SLE. An acute inflammatory demyelinating polyradiculoneuropathy (Guillain-Barre syndrome) has been described.

Examination of the cerebrospinal fluid is useful for ruling out infection. However, with regard to neuropsychiatric lupus, the findings often are nonspecific: Elevated cell counts, protein levels, or both, are found in only about one-third of patients. The fluid may be completely normal in the face of acute disease. Computerized tomography is sufficient for the initial diagnosis of most mass lesions and intracranial hemorrhages. The findings of magnetic reso-

nance imaging (MRI) reflect the histopathologic findings of vascular injury and may involve the white or gray matter. Abnormalities on MRI are more likely with focal findings (12). Unfortunately, the correlation between MRI findings and clinical presentation is low.

Cardiovascular System

A variety of cardiac complications are seen in SLE, but the most common is pericarditis, reported in various series as occurring in 6%–45% (most series approximately 25%). The clinical picture is typical, with the patient complaining of substernal or pericardial pain, aggravated by motion such as inspiration, coughing, swallowing, twisting, and bending forward. Symptoms may either be mild or severe. A pericardial rub may or may not be present and can be heard in an asymptomatic patient. Although the electrocardiogram may show the typical T-wave abnormalities, echocardiography is the best diagnostic test. Most effusions are small to moderate. The pericardial fluid is straw-colored to serosanguinous, exudative, and can have a high WBC count (up to 30,000 cells/mm^3) with a predominance of neutrophils. LE cells can be seen in the centrifuged cell sediment. Cardiac tamponade is rare, as is constrictive pericarditis.

Primary myocardial involvement in SLE is uncommon (<10%). The patient may have fever, dyspnea, palpitations, heart murmurs, sinus tachycardia, ventricular arrhythmias, conduction abnormalities, or congestive heart failure. Percutaneous endomyocardial biopsy may be helpful. It is now well recognized that hemodynamically and clinically significant valvular disease occurs and may require prosthetic valve replacement. Aortic insufficiency represents the most commonly reported lesion and may be the result of multiple factors, including fibrinoid degeneration, distortion of the valve by fibrosis, valvulitis, bacterial endocarditis, aortitis, and Libman-Sacks endocarditis. Libman-Sacks "atypical verrucous endocarditis," the classic cardiac lesion of SLE, is comprised of verrucous vegetations ranging from 1 mm to 4 mm in diameter, initially reported to be present on the tricuspid and mitral valves. Interestingly, it has been noted that neither the usual clinical and immunologic markers of lupus activity, nor its treatment, are temporally related to the presence of or changes in valvular disease (13). Prophylactic antibiotics for surgical and dental procedures are recommended for all people with SLE.

Accelerated atherosclerosis has received considerable attention and is an important cause of morbidity and mortality in SLE. It has been established that the proportionate mortality from myocardial infarction is approximately 10 times greater in people with SLE than in the general age- and sex-matched population (5,14). Autopsy studies support the clinical data, showing severe coronary artery atherosclerosis in up to 40% of people with SLE, compared with 2% of control subjects, matched for age at the time of death (15). Studies have identified hypercholesterolemia, hypertension, and lupus itself as risk factors in these patients (16). Corticosteroid therapy contributes to the elevation of plasma lipids, while antimalarials may result in a reduction of plasma cholesterol, low-density lipoprotein, and very low-density lipoprotein. Coronary arteritis is rare and may coexist with atherosclerotic heart disease. Studies of clinical outcomes for atherosclerotic disease, including angina and myocardial infarction, have shown a prevalence of 6%–12% in a number of SLE cohorts (5,16). More sensitive investigations, including carotid plaque and intima-media wall thickness (IMT) measured by B-mode ultrasound, revealed that 40% of 175 women with SLE had focal plaque (17).

The Pleura and Lungs

The lungs and contiguous structures involved in normal respiration are commonly affected by SLE. More than 30% of patients have some form of pleural disease in their lifetime, either as pleuritis with chest pain or frank effusion. Pleurisy is a more common feature of serositis than pericarditis. The pain of pleuritis can be quite severe and must be distinguished from pulmonary embolus or infection. Pleural rubs are less common than either clinical pleurisy or radiographic abnormalities. Pleural effusions are most often small and bilateral. The fluid is usually clear and exudative, has increased protein, and normal glucose. The WBC count is elevated but <10,000 with a predominance of neutrophils or lymphocytes, and decreased levels of complement.

Pulmonary involvement includes pneumonitis, pulmonary hemorrhage, pulmonary embolism, pulmonary hypertension, and shrinking-lung syndrome. The term acute lupus pneumonitis has been applied to an abrupt febrile pneumonitic process when infection has been ruled out. Prominent features are pleuritic chest pain, cough with hemoptysis, and dyspnea. Diffuse alveolar hemorrhage is considered a manifestation of acute lupus pneumonitis and is associated with a 50% mortality rate. It can occur in the absence of hemoptysis and is suggested by a falling hematocrit and pulmonary infiltrates. Rarely (<10%), patients develop a more chronic syndrome characterized by progressive dyspnea, nonproductive cough, basilar rales, and diffuse interstitial lung infiltrates.

Pulmonary hypertension should be suspected in patients complaining of progressive shortness of breath and in whom the chest radiograph is negative and profound hypoxemia is absent. Pulmonary function studies show a restrictive pattern with a reduction in the diffusing capacity for carbon monoxide. Doppler ultrasound studies and cardiac catheterization confirm the diagnosis. Frequently, these patients also have Raynaud's phenomenon. Intrapulmonary clotting and/or multiple pulmonary emboli must be addressed, especially in the setting of anti-phospholipid antibodies. Recent studies suggest that pulmonary hypertension is gradually progressive over time and is related to an increase in pulmonary resistance (18).

Less-Commonly Involved Organ Systems

Gastrointestinal Tract and Liver

Involvement of the gastrointestinal tract can, as in other organ systems, be varied, but for most patients is not the source of any diagnostic criteria. The peritoneum is the least likely of the serosal linings to be affected in SLE. Symptoms include rebound tenderness, fever, nausea, vomiting, and diarrhea. Confusion with serious abdominal pathology or infection can unfortunately prompt surgical intervention. Abdominal pain in SLE can also be caused by pancreatitis and bowel vasculitis. Rectal bleeding can be present in mesenteric vasculitis. Protein-losing enteropathy is quite uncommon, but should be considered in the face of low serum albumin, pedal edema, and the absence of proteinuria.

Parenchymal liver disease as a result of SLE is rare. However, elevated transaminases can be encountered during periods of active disease and/or following the use of many medications used to treat lupus, such as NSAIDs, azathioprine, and methotrexate. In the absence of known offending drugs, persistent signs of hepatitis may require a liver biopsy. The term "lupoid hepatitis" was coined by Bearn in 1956 and initially believed to be a manifestation of SLE. However, an individual need not have lupus; it is defined serologically and histologically and is a subset of chronic, active hepatitis. It is seen in fewer than 10% of patients who fulfill the ACR criteria for SLE.

Ocular

With regard to the eye itself, cotton-wool spots in the retina are generally cited as being the most common lesion, followed in frequency by corneal and conjunctival involvement, with patients only rarely exhibiting uveitis or scleritis. Although also quite uncommon, retinal damage from antimalarials used in treating SLE is probably a greater cause of vision loss than is retinal involvement occurring in the natural course of the disease. Cotton-wool spots (an ophthalmologic term) result from focal ischemia and are not pathognomonic for lupus. They occur preferentially in the posterior part of the retina and often involve the optic nerve head. Each spot appears as a grayish-white soft, fluffy exudate, averaging about one-third of a disc diameter in width. Cytoid bodies refer to the histologic features of the cotton-wool spot.

Laboratory Features

Hematologic Abnormalities

Each cellular element in the blood can be affected by SLE. Accordingly, the complete blood count is a critical part of the initial and continued evaluation of all people with SLE. In the absence of offending medications, the "penias" are generally secondary to peripheral destruction, and not marrow suppression.

Autoimmune hemolytic anemia is present in <10% of patients. A Coombs test can be positive (both direct and indirect) without active hemolysis. A nonspecific anemia reflecting chronic disease is present in up to 80% of patients. Leukopenia is seen in more than 50% of patients. Absolute lymphopenia is more common than neutropenia. Unfortunately, the criterion for lymphopenia (<1500 cells/mm^3) is not very stringent and, in most laboratories, is not highlighted as abnormal. Although leukopenia does represent some degree of disease activity, and has been described as a signal of more systemic activity, there are patients whose low WBC counts do not associate with disease flares in other organs and do not predispose them to infection. Thrombocytopenia can be modest (platelet counts of 50,000–100,000 cells/mm^3), chronic and totally asymptomatic, or profound (<20,000 cells/mm^3) and acute, with gum bleeding and petechiae. In some cases, thrombocytopenia is the sole manifestation of disease activity at a given point in time. Fortunately, there rarely are qualitative defects in the platelets and, therefore, life-threatening bleeding is unusual. Analogous to the other cell lines, antiplatelet antibodies may be present without thrombocytopenia.

The erythrocyte sedimentation rate frequently is elevated in SLE and is generally not considered a reliable marker of clinical activity. A rise in the C-reactive protein may be an indicator of infection, but this has not proven to be absolute.

The Hallmark Autoantibodies and Complement

Measuring the so-called "serologic parameters" is an integral part of the baseline evaluation and follow-up of people with SLE. The term refers to those tests performed using the serum component of whole blood, although testing for antibodies and functional assays of complement can be done using plasma. The presence of a positive ANA is one of the most important abnormalities to identify at presentation because it establishes that the differential diagnosis includes autoimmunity. However, a positive ANA, particularly in young women, can be detected in about 2% of healthy individuals. This test should be considered a valuable guide, but by no means diagnostic. Once documented, continued measurement of ANA is not useful as a gauge of disease activity. In contrast, the presence of antibodies to dsDNA (not single-stranded DNA) is not only of major diagnostic significance but in select patients, particularly those with renal involvement (see below), a valuable means of predicting and assessing disease activity. Anti-Sm antibodies, which recognize determinants on proteins associated with small ribonucleoproteins involved in processing of messenger RNA, are of diagnostic importance but do not track disease. Antibodies reactive with SSA/Ro and SSB/La ribonucleoproteins also do not correlate with activity, but are often seen in patients who may have one or more of the following: photosensitivity, dry eyes and dry mouth (secondary Sjögren's syndrome), subacute cutaneous lesions, and risk of having child with neonatal lupus. Anti-SSA/Ro antibodies, depending on the methodology used for screening, can stain the cytoplasmic component of the cell and therefore account for some ANA-negative lupus. While ANA-negative lupus is considered, it is difficult to conceptualize a situation in which an individual is said to have SLE, a prototypic autoimmune disease, yet has no detectable autoantibodies. It has recently been suggested that antinucleosome antibodies constitute a selective biologic marker of active SLE, specifically for lupus nephritis (19). The frequency of various autoantibodies and their clinical relevance are summarized in Table 17B-2.

Complement proteins, the "bullets" of the antibodies and intrinsic components of immune complexes, can be measured both functionally (CH50) and antigenically (C3, C4). Most laboratories measure the C3 and C4 because they are stable and do not require special handling. None of these traditional measures of the complement system discriminate between accelerated consumption of complement or decreased synthesis. Such distinction requires measurement of the complement split products (e.g., C3a), which is still considered a research tool and is not readily available in most commercial laboratories.

TABLE 17B-2
Autoantibodies and Clinical Features

Antibodies (%)	Frequency	Clinical associations	Relationship to disease activity
ANA	>90	Nonspecific	For diagnostic purposes only
Anti-dsDNA	40–60	Nephritis	May predict disease flare and associates with flare
Anti-RNP	30–40	Raynaud's, musculoskeletal	Does not track disease
Anti-ribosomal P	10–20	Diffuse CNS, psychosis, major depression	Does not track disease
Anti-SSA/Ro	30–45	Dry eyes and mouth, SCLE, neonatal lupus, photosensitivity	Does not track disease
Anti-SSB/La	10–15	Dry eyes and mouth, SCLE, neonatal lupus, photosensitivity	Does not track disease
Antiphospholipid	30	Clotting diathesis	Varied

ANA, antinuclear antibodies; dsDNA, double-stranded DNA; RNP, ribonucleoprotein; SCLE, subacute cutaneous lupus erythematosus

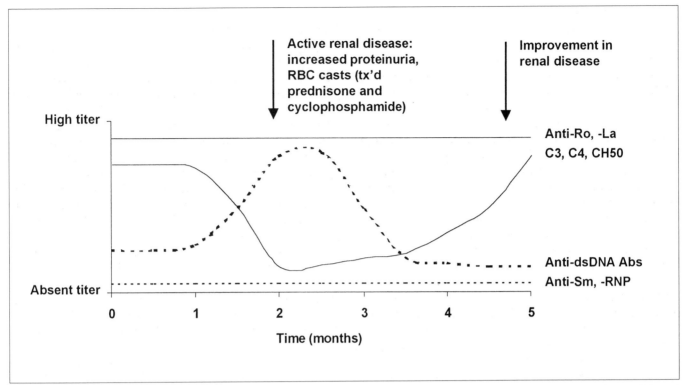

Fig. 17B-4. Longitudinal clinical and autoantibody profile in a patient with a lupus flare. This patient demonstrates concordance of clinical and serologic activity with regard to anti-double-stranded DNA and complements. Note that despite changes in disease activity, titers of anti-Ro/La (elevated throughout) and anti-Sm/RNP (absent throughout) remain stable.

A challenge in the management of SLE is identifying parameters that will stratify those at risk for disease flares, particularly flares that might lead to permanent damage in major organs. The presumption is that earlier treatment in the high-risk patient might have an impact on subsequent morbidity and mortality. Interest in measuring the complement system and anti-DNA antibodies originates from the long-standing observation that decreased complement levels and rising titers of anti-DNA are often associated with severe disease (20). These findings are linked to the notion that immune complexes result in complement activation products that are present locally or in the circulation, and are capable of stimulating inflammatory cells with resultant vascular injury.

Measurements of anti-DNA antibodies and complement are an essential part of baseline evaluation, but treatment is dictated by the clinical picture, not necessarily the serologic one. Over time it should become obvious in an individual patient whether these parameters predict and accompany disease flares. It is well-appreciated that in certain patients low complements and elevated anti-DNA antibodies persist, despite relative clinical quiescence. In contrast, there are patients who repeatedly demonstrate concordance of clinical and serologic activity (an illustrative case is provided in Fig. 17B-4). In these individuals, treatment may be considered solely on the basis of change in serologic parameters in advance of overt clinical disease, thus preventing relapse (21). These issues are currently being addressed in an ongoing trial to evaluate serologically active clinically stable (SACS) patients

and determine whether anti-DNA, C3, C4, or the complement split product C3a are predictive of flare, and whether a short trial of corticosteroids can avert major disease.

Special Considerations
SLE and Pregnancy
Sterility and fertility rates for women with SLE are comparable to control groups without disease. However, increased disease activity can be associated with secondary amenorrhea. Moreover, menstrual irregularities have been noted in women taking high doses of corticosteroids, and age-dependent premature ovarian failure occurs in those receiving cyclophosphamide. Women with SLE have a higher rate of spontaneous abortion, intrauterine fetal death, and premature birth compared to otherwise healthy women.

In contrast to the rule of remission during pregnancies in women with RA, the influence of pregnancy on SLE disease activity is variable. There are two principal areas of concern. The first is that the clinical and serologic expression of SLE may be adversely altered by pregnancy. The second is that the placenta and fetus may become targets of specific attack by maternal autoantibodies, resulting in a generalized failure of the pregnancy or specific syndromes of passively acquired autoimmunity such as neonatal lupus (see below).

Pregnancy outcome is optimal when disease is in complete clinical remission for six to 12 months (22,23). Whether flare rates increase during or after pregnancy is still unsettled, because individual patient series vary in the characteristics of patients accepted for study and in the definitions of flare. Current definitions of flare are imprecise, and accepted instruments used to measure disease activity, such as the Systemic Lupus Erythematosus Disease Activity Index (SLEDAI) or Systemic Lupus Activity Measurement (SLAM), do not account for the physiologic adaptations of pregnancy and have not been validated for pregnant lupus patients (24). Suggestions for valid criteria attributable to a flare during pregnancy are characteristic dermatologic involvement, arthritis, fever not secondary to infection, lymphadenopathy, leukopenia, alternative-pathway hypocomplementemia, and rising titers of antibodies to DNA. In contrast, invalid markers of disease activity include alopecia, facial or palmar blush, arthralgia, musculoskeletal aching, mild anemia, and fatigue, each of which may be present as part of the normal physiologic changes of pregnancy. Additionally, thrombocytopenia and proteinuria emerge in the setting of preeclampsia and cannot be unambiguously attributed to active lupus. In one major study comparing pregnant and nonpregnant SLE patients, the flare rates in both groups were similar (25). Despite a high overall flare rate in one series approaching 60% (22), recorded flares usually were not severe. In general, if all possible abnormalities are presumed due to SLE, disease exacerbation occurs in approximately 25%, and if only SLE-specific abnormalities are considered, disease exacerbation occurs in <13% (26).

In counseling a patient about the maternal risks of a prospective pregnancy, a major issue is the presence of active nephritis and/or deterioration of renal function. Newly diagnosed lupus nephritis in the first trimester is associated with a poor fetal outcome. In a patient with established membranous nephritis, the normal increase in glomerular filtrate rate may result in protein excretion greater than 300 mg in 24 hours, the upper limit accepted for an otherwise normal pregnancy. In some cases there will be coexistent hypertension, which then must be differentiated (if possible) from preeclampsia, especially if first evident in the third trimester. In other patients, proteinuria will more clearly represent an exacerbation of lupus nephritis, as suggested by cellular casts in the urinary sediment. Activation of the alternative complement pathway with a concomitant decrease in CH50 accompanies disease flares in SLE, a laboratory finding that may be useful in distinguishing active lupus nephritis from preeclampsia or pregnancy-induced hypertension (27). The presence of active lupus nephritis and/or preeclampsia increases the risk for preterm delivery and fetal death. Encouragingly, women in whom renal disease is stable (serum creatinine <1.5 and 24-hour protein <2 g) prior to pregnancy can experience an uncomplicated course during pregnancy, despite a history of severe histopathologic changes and heavier proteinuria.

Neonatal Lupus

This illness of the fetus and neonate is considered a model of passively acquired autoimmunity, in which immune abnormalities in the mother lead to the production of anti-SSA/Ro

and anti-SSB/La antibodies that cross the placenta and presumably injure fetal tissue (28). The most serious manifestation is damage to the cardiac conducting system resulting in congenital heart block (CHB), which is most often third-degree, although less-advanced blocks have been observed. CHB is generally identified between 16 and 24 weeks of gestation. The mortality rate is ~20% and the majority of children require pacing. Cutaneous involvement (erythematous and often annular lesions with a predilection for the periorbital region, face, and scalp; photosensitivity) and, to a lesser extent, hepatic and hematologic involvement are also associated with maternal anti-SSA/Ro and anti-SSB/La antibodies and are grouped under the heading of neonatal lupus syndromes. Neonatal lupus – so termed because the dermatologic lesions of the neonate resembled those seen in SLE – is a misnomer in that less than one-third of mothers of affected children actually have SLE (many are asymptomatic) and the neonatal disease is frequently only manifest as heart block, a problem rarely reported in adults with lupus. To date, complete heart block is irreversible. In contrast, the noncardiac manifestations are transient, resolving at about six months of life, coincident with the disappearance of maternal autoantibodies from the neonatal circulation.

The incidence of neonatal lupus in an offspring of a mother with anti-SSA/Ro antibodies is estimated at 1%–2%. No serologic profile is unique to mothers of affected children, but compared with mothers of healthy children, anti-SSA/Ro antibodies are usually of high titer (frequently anti-52-kDa SSA/Ro positive by immunoblot) and associated with anti-SSB/La antibodies (29). Reports of discordant dizygotic and monozygotic twins and low recurrence rates of CHB (in our series, 12 of 78 next pregnancies following the birth of a child with CHB) indicate that factors (likely fetal) in addition to anti-SSA/Ro and anti-SSB/La antibodies contribute to the development of neonatal lupus. The Research Registry for Neonatal Lupus was established in 1994. With the current enrollment of 269 mothers and their 318 affected children, this database (along with available serum and DNA) provides a valuable resource for basic researchers and clinicians.

Antiphospholipid Antibody Syndrome

Anti-phospholipid antibodies (aPL), ascertained by a variety of different assays, are associated with the risk of clotting. The clinical consequences include venous and arterial thromboses and placental insufficiency resulting in recurrent fetal loss. Except for manifestations of active SLE, lupus patients with aPLs do not appear to have different pregnancy courses from women with the primary aPL syndrome. Paradoxically, thrombocytopenia can also be part of the clinical spectrum because the surface of activated platelets display the anionic phospholipid target antigens. Patients can have aPLs and one of the above clinical features in the absence of any other manifestations of SLE (primary aPL syndrome). Alternatively, a patient can have these antibodies in the context of SLE (secondary aPL syndrome).

Currently assessment of aPL is done by ELISA to measure

reactivity with cardiolipin, or prolonged clotting in an in vitro system that is not corrected by mixing studies. The latter is a paradox because the readout is the inability to form a clot due to interference with proper assembly of the clotting factors, but in vivo these antibodies are thrombogenic. Experimental data suggest that "anti-phospholipid" antibodies are not directed against anionic phospholipids, as initially hypothesized, but are part of a larger group of autoantibodies that recognize phospholipid-binding proteins. At present, the best-characterized antigenic target is β_2-glycoprotein I (B2GPI) (30), which has been shown to possess multiple inhibitory functions in coagulation pathways. Although the measurement of aPLs by ELISA is now well-standardized, these new observations on B2GPI will require large-scale testing, the outcome of which may substantially alter current recommendations.

Drug-Related Lupus

The term drug-related lupus (DRL) refers to the development of a lupus-like syndrome that follows exposure to chlorpromazine, hydralazine, isoniazid, methyldopa, minocycline, procainamide, or quinidine. In addition to these definitively associated drugs, there is a long list of other potential offending agents such as diphenylhydantoin, penicillamine, and gold salts (31). There are no specified ACR criteria for DRL, but, in general, these patients present with fewer than four SLE criteria. A temporal association (generally a matter of weeks or months) between ingestion of an agent and development of symptoms is required. Following removal of the offending agent, there should be rapid resolution of the clinical features, although autoantibodies may persist for six months to one year. Drugs capable of causing DRL do not seem to aggravate idiopathic SLE. The demographic features of DRL tend to reflect those of the diseases for which the offending drug has been prescribed. Accordingly, DRL occurs more frequently in the elderly, occurs only slightly more frequently in females than males, and is more common in Caucasians than African Americans.

People with DRL frequently present with constitutional symptoms such as malaise, low-grade fever, and myalgia, which may occur acutely or insidiously. Articular complaints are present in more than 80%, with arthralgia being more common than arthritis. Pleuropulmonary disease and pericarditis are present most often in procainamide-related lupus. Other clinical manifestations of idiopathic SLE such as dermatologic, renal, and neurologic symptoms are rare in DRL. ANAs should be present to diagnose DRL. However, the development of an ANA without accompanying clinical features is insufficient for the diagnosis and not reason by itself to discontinue medication. Typically, the ANA is a diffuse-homogenous pattern that represents binding of autoantibodies to chromatin, which consists of DNA and histones. Anti-dsDNA and anti-Sm are not characteristic of DRL.

Conclusions

SLE is a composite of clinically unrelated manifestations often accumulated over time that are unified, with rare exception, by presence of antibodies directed against one or more self components of the nucleus. Greater awareness of the clinical features and advances in the laboratory evaluation of autoantibodies have facilitated diagnosis and eliminated much of the frustration previously experienced both by the patient and physician. In many patients, flares are mimetic. The accurate prediction of flares in clinically quiescent patients is likely to result in longer periods of remission. Attention to predictors of future morbidity and mortality offers unparalleled promise.

JILL P. BUYON, MD

References

1. Tan EM, Cohen AS, Fries JFet al. The 1982 revised criteria for the classification of systemic lupus erythematosus. Arthritis Rheum 1982;25:1271–1277.

2. Gladman DD. Systemic lupus erythematosus: Clinical features. In: Klippel JH, Weyand CM, Wortmann RL (eds). Primer on the Rheumatic Diseases, 11th edition. Atlanta: Arthritis Foundation, 1997; pp 267–272.

3. Ginzler EM, Schorn K. Outcome and prognosis in systemic lupus erythematosus. Rheum Dis Clin North Am 1988;14:67-78.

4. Boumpas DT, Fessler BJ, Austin HA III, Balow JE, Klippel JH, Lockshin MD. Systemic lupus erythematosus: emerging concepts. Part 2: Dermatologic and joint disease, the antiphospholipid antibody syndrome, pregnancy and hormonal therapy, morbidity and mortality, and pathogenesis. Ann Intern Med 1995;123:42-53.

5. Urowitz MB, Gladman DD. Accelerated atheroma in lupus – background. Lupus 2000;9:161-165.

6. Sontheimer RD. Systemic lupus erythematosus and the skin. In: Lahita R (ed). Systemic Lupus Erythematosus, 3rd edition. San Diego: Academic Press, 1998; pp. 631-656.

7. Stone JH, Millward CL, Olson JL, Amend WJ, Criswell LA. Frequency of recurrent lupus nephritis among ninety-seven renal transplant patients during the cyclosporine era. Arthritis Rheum 1998;41:678-686.

8. Nossent HC, Swaak TJ, Berden JH. Systemic lupus erythematosus: analysis of disease activity in 55 patients with end-stage renal failure treated with hemodialysis or continuous ambulatory peritoneal dialysis. Am J Med 1990;89:169-174.

9. Krane NK, Burjak K, Archie M, O'Donovan R. Persistent lupus activity in end-stage renal disease. Am J Kidney Dis 1999;33:872-879.

10. Boumpas DT, Austin HA, Fessler BJ, Balow JE, Klippel JH, Lockshin MD. Systemic lupus erythematosus: emerging concepts. Part 1: Renal, neuropsychiatric, cardiovascular, pulmonary and hematologic disease. Ann Int Med 1995; 122:940-950.

11. ACR Ad Hoc Committee on Neuropsychiatric Lupus Nomenclature. The American College of Rheumatology nomenclature and case definitions for neuropsychiatric lupus syndromes. Arthritis Rheum 1999;42:599-608.

12. West SG, Emlen W, Wener M, Kotzin BL. Neuropsychiatric lupus erythematosus: A 10-year prospective study on the value of diagnostic tests. Am J Med 1995;99:153-163.

13. Roldan CA, Shively BK, Crawford MH. An echocardiographic study of valvular heart disease associated with systemic lupus erythematosus. New Engl J Med 1996;335:1424-1430.

14. Rosner S, Ginzler EM, Diamond HS, et al. A multicenter study of outcome in systemic lupus erythematosus. II. Causes of death. Arthritis Rheum 1982;25:612-617.

15. Haider YS, Roberts WC. Coronary arterial disease in systemic lupus erythematosus; quantification of degrees of narrowing in 22 necropsy patients (21 women) aged 16 to 37 years. Am J Med 1981;70:775-781.

16. Petri M. Detection of coronary artery disease and the role of traditional risk factors in the Hopkins Lupus Cohort. Lupus 2000;9:170-175.

17. Manzi S, Selzer F, Sutton-Tyrrell K, et al. Prevalence and risk factors of carotid plaque in women with systemic lupus erythematosus. Arthritis Rheum 1999;42:51-60.

18. Winslow TM, Ossipov MA, Fazio GP, Simonson JS, Redberg RF, Schiller NB. Five-year follow-up study of the prevalence and progression of pulmonary hypertension in systemic lupus erythematosus. Am Heart J 1995;129:510-515.

19. Amoura Z, Koutouzov S, Chabre H, et al. Presence of antinucleosome autoantibodies in a restricted set of connective tissue diseases. Antinucleosome antibodies of the IgG3 subclass are marker of renal pathogenicity in systemic lupus erythematosus. Arthritis Rheum 2000;43:76-84.

20. Schur PH, Sandson J. Immunologic factors and clinical activity in systemic lupus erythematosus. New Engl J Med 1968;278:533-538.

21. Bootsma H, Spronk P, Derksen R, et al. Prevention of relapses in systemic lupus erythematosus. Lancet 1995;345:1595-1599.

22. Petri M, Howard D, Repke J. Frequency of lupus flares in pregnancy. The Hopkins Lupus Pregnancy Center experience. Arthritis Rheum 1991;34:1538-1545.

23. Urowitz MB, Gladman DD, Farewell VT, Stewart J, McDonald J. Lupus and pregnancy studies. Arthritis Rheum 1993;36:1392-1397.

24. Buyon J, Kalunian K, Ramsey-Goldman R, et al. Assessing disease activity in SLE patients during pregnancy. Lupus 1999;8:677-684.

25. Lockshin MD, Reinitz E, Druzin ML, Murrman M, Estes D. Lupus pregnancy. Case-control prospective study demonstrating absence of lupus exacerbation during or after pregnancy. Am J Med 1984;77:893-898.

26. Lockshin MD. Pregnancy does not cause systemic lupus erythematosus to worsen. Arthritis Rheum 1989;32:665-670.

27. Buyon JP, Tamerius J, Ordorica S, Abramson SB. Activation of the alternative complement pathway accompanies disease flares in systemic lupus erythematosus during pregnancy. Arthritis Rheum 1992;35:55-61.

28. Buyon JP, Hiebert R, Copel J, et al. Autoimmune-associated congenital heart block: demographics, mortality, morbidity, and recurrence rates obtained from a national neonatal lupus registry. J Am Coll Cardiol 1998;31:1658-1666.

29. Buyon JP, Winchester RJ, Slade SG, et al. Identification of mothers at risk for congenital heart block and other neonatal lupus syndromes in their children. Comparison of enzyme-linked immunosorbent assay and immunoblot for measurement of anti-SS-A/Ro and anti-SS-B/La antibodies. Arthritis Rheum 1993;36:1263-1273.

30. McNeil HP, Simpson RJ, Chesterman CN, Krilis SA. Antiphospholipid antibodies are directed against a complex antigen that includes a lipid-binding inhibitor of coagulation: beta 2-glycoprotein I (apolipoprotein H). Proc Natl Acad Sci USA 1990;87:4120-4124.

31. Mongey AB, Hess EV. Drug and environmental lupus: Clinical manifestations and differences. In: Lahita R (ed). Systemic Lupus Erythematosus, 3rd edition. San Diego: Academic Press, 1998; pp. 929-943.

32. Lahita R. Systemic Lupus Erythematosus, 3rd edition. San Diego: Academic Press, 1998.

33. Wallace DJ, Hahn BH (eds). Dubois' Lupus Erythematosus, 4th edition. Baltimore: Williams & Wilkins, 1996.

SYSTEMIC LUPUS ERYTHEMATOSUS
C. Treatment

In 1908, London dermatologist J.M. MacLeod was one of the first clinicians to write about treatment for the visceral manifestations of systemic lupus erythematosus (SLE): "As the exact nature of the toxins responsible where the disease is associated with such general toxins as result from nephritis, disease of the liver, rheumatism, etc., is uncertain, the appropriate antitoxin is not available..." (1). Major advances over the past century in the management of SLE have resulted in significant improvement in survival and quality of life. These advances have included nonpharmacologic strategies and drug therapies. Milestones in the treatment of lupus have included the discovery and use of corticosteroids in the 1950s and renal dialysis and cyclophosphamide in the 1960s and 1970s. A critical component of therapeutic advances in SLE has been the recognition that lupus comprises a spectrum of diseases and that individual manifestation rather than the primary diagnosis should guide treatment.

General Management

The value of patient education should not be underestimated in any chronic illness. Health professional-guided education is critical. Physicians should be prepared to help patients navigate the sea of information available through such modern technology as the Internet. Conveying the message that the manifestations and severity of disease vary may help alleviate fear and confusion caused by learning about worst-case scenarios from concerned friends, family members, and textbooks. For some patients, support groups are comforting and educational.

Fatigue is a prominent feature for many people with SLE. It is important to identify and treat conditions that could contribute to fatigue, particularly hypothyroidism, fibromyalgia, and depression. Adequate rest and energy conservation should be emphasized. Skin rashes or systemic disease flares following exposure to ultraviolet light are common. Patients who are photosensitive should be instructed to avoid excessive exposure to sunlight and routinely use sunscreen and wear photoprotective clothing. Ultraviolet radiation through windows and exposure to fluorescent lighting also may induce lupus activity. Protective window films and fluorescent lighting shields can minimize this risk. Prescription drugs, including certain antibiotics, can exacerbate photosensitive reactions and other manifestations of systemic disease. Patients must recognize this possibility and may need to avoid these agents.

Infections are common in lupus, and patients should be advised to seek medical attention for unexplained fevers. The risk of infections can be minimized with judicious use of immunosuppressive agents, corticosteroids, and appropriate immunizations, including influenza and pneumococcal vaccine, particularly following splenectomy. In general, pregnancies in women with SLE should be considered high-risk, due to potential disease flares in the mother and risk to the fetus. Effective birth control, planning pregnancy during times of minimal disease activity, and careful monitoring of the mother and baby during pregnancy can minimize poor outcomes.

People with SLE are at increased risk of premature cardiovascular disease, and it is critical to minimize risk factors, such as tobacco use, obesity, sedentary lifestyle, hyperlipidemia, and hypertension. Similarly, SLE is associated with an increased risk for osteoporosis, and it is essential to institute primary and secondary prevention measures. Although it is unclear whether people with SLE have an increased malignancy risk, routine, age-appropriate health maintenance, including gynecological evaluations and breast examinations, is recommended.

Nonsteroidal Anti-Inflammatory Drugs

Nonsteroidal anti-inflammatory drugs (NSAIDs) are used widely for the treatment of musculoskeletal complaints, pleuritis, pericarditis, and headache. The effectiveness of these agents varies for individual patients, and the choice of agent is dictated by cost, availability, tolerance, and effectiveness. Adverse effects of NSAIDs on the kidneys, liver, and central nervous system (CNS) may be confused with worsening lupus activity (2). For example, prostaglandins

and prostacyclins are important for maintenance of renal blood flow and tubular transport, but may be inhibited by NSAIDs. Therefore, new proteinuria or worsening renal function may be due to either SLE activity or NSAIDs. NSAIDs also can cause aseptic meningitis, headache, psychosis, and cognitive dysfunction, effects that may be confused with CNS symptoms caused by lupus. Mild, reversible elevations of serum transaminases are the most common hepatic side effect of NSAIDs.

Gastrointestinal toxicities are the most common side effects of the nonselective cyclooxygenase (COX) inhibitors at doses that effectively control inflammation. Although there are no published studies specifically examining the safety and efficacy of the selective COX-2 inhibitors in SLE, these agents are expected to reduce gastrointestinal side effects, as they have in other populations. Because there is measurable COX-2 activity in the brain and kidney, selective COX-2 inhibitors are not expected to provide protection from the adverse renal and CNS effects of these agents in people with SLE. The role of the selective COX-2 inhibitors in lupus, beyond gastrointestinal protection, is unknown. Recognition of common side effects and appropriate monitoring are recommended.

Table 17C-1 gives recommendations for monitoring the effects of NSAIDs and other agents commonly used in the management of SLE. Because of the unique and variable clinical manifestations of lupus, these general guidelines for drug monitoring may need to be modified for individual patients.

Corticosteroids

Corticosteroids are effective in the management of many different manifestations of SLE (3). Topical or intralesional preparations often are used for cutaneous lesions; intra-articular corticosteroids, for arthritis; and oral or parenteral therapy, for systemic disease. Most of the efficacy data for corticosteroids in lupus have been gathered from case reports and open trials; few controlled trials have been conducted. Oral administration ranging from 5 mg to 30 mg prednisone daily, in single or divided doses, is effective in treating constitutional symptoms, cutaneous disease, arthritis, and serositis. Often, corticosteroids are used to obtain immediate relief, and then tapered after institution of slower-acting agents, such as antimalarials or immune-modulatory therapies. More serious organ involvement, particularly nephritis, cerebritis, hematologic abnormalities, or systemic vasculitis, generally requires high-dose prednisone in the range of 1–2 mg/kg/day. Parenteral corticosteroid preparations in equivalent doses sometimes are used. In severe, life-threatening situations, bolus methylprednisolone (1000 mg) can be used for three consecutive days.

Numerous potential side effects of corticosteroid therapy suggest caution for long-term use. Some of the more problematic toxicities include weight gain, emotional lability, myopathy, osteonecrosis, hypertension, striae, hyperlipidemia, diabetes mellitus, glaucoma, peptic ulcer disease, osteoporosis,

TABLE 17C-1
Recommended Monitoring Strategy for Drugs Commonly Used in Systemic Lupus Erythematosus[a]

Drug	Toxicities requiring monitoring	Baseline evaluation
Salicylates, NSAIDs	Gastrointestinal bleeding, hepatic toxicity, renal toxicity, hypertension	CBC, creatinine, urinalysis, AST, ALT
Corticosteroids	Hypertension, hyperglycemia, hyperlipidemia, hypokalemia, osteoporosis, osteonecrosis, cataract, weight gain, infections, fluid retention	BP, bone densitometry, glucose, potassium, cholesterol, triglycerides (HDL, LDL)
Hydroxychloroquine	Macular damage	None unless patient is over 40 years of age or has previous eye disease
Azathioprine	Myelosuppression, hepatotoxicity, lymphoproliferative disorders	CBC, platelet count, creatinine, AST or ALT
Cyclophosphamide	Myelosuppression, myeloproliferative disorders, malignancy, immunosuppression, hemorrhagic cystitis, secondary infertility	CBC and differential and platelet count, urinalysis
Methotrexate	Myelosuppression, hepatic fibrosis, cirrhosis, pulmonary infiltrates, fibrosis	CBC, chest radiograph within past year, hepatitis B and C serology in high-risk patients, AST, albumin, bilirubin, creatinine

[a] Reproduced with permission from Guidelines for referral and management of systemic lupus erythematosus in adults. Arthritis Rheum 1999;42:1785–1796.

and increased risk of infections. Once disease activity is controlled, corticosteroids typically are tapered to discontinuation or a minimal daily or alternate-day dosing regimen.

Corticosteroids generally are well-tolerated during pregnancy, although they may exacerbate diabetes and hypertension. There is no evidence that corticosteroids cause congenital defects, but decreased birth weight and premature rupture of membranes have been associated with use of these agents in pregnancy.

Antimalarials

Antimalarial agents are some of the most commonly prescribed medications for SLE and include hydroxychloroquine, chloroquine, and quinacrine. They frequently are used in the management of constitutional symptoms, cutaneous and musculoskeletal manifestations, and in some cases, serositis. Combinations of antimalarials are thought to be synergistic and are commonly used when one agent alone is not effective. Particular benefit, including steroid-sparing effect, has been reported with hydroxychloroquine (200–400 mg/day) and quinacrine (100 mg/day); the only adverse effect is a reversible, yellowish skin discoloration often seen with quinacrine (4).

The landmark trial in lupus demonstrating clinical efficacy of hydroxychloroquine, the antimalarial agent used most commonly in the United States, was a 24-week, randomized, double-blind, placebo-controlled withdrawal trial (5). Patients who discontinued hydroxychloroquine were 2.5 times more likely to have a mild clinical flare than were patients who continued treatment. Flares included skin rashes, oral ulcers, arthritis, and constitutional signs and symptoms. Long-term follow-up of the participants in the original study suggested a trend toward reduction in flares for those who remained on hydroxychloroquine, although the results were not statistically significant (6).

The role of antimalarials in preventing major organ disease in SLE is unclear. Beneficial roles of hydroxychloroquine include lipid-lowering and possible anti-thrombotic effects.

Because antimalarials generally are well-tolerated, extended use of these agents is common practice. It is estimated that only 10% of patients have difficulties tolerating hydroxychloroquine; mild side effects include gastric upset, headache, myalgia, or rash. Much of the concern over use of antimalarial agents centers around the risk of ophthal-

Monitoring	
System review	Laboratory
Dark/black stool, dyspepsia, nausea/vomiting, abdominal pain, shortness of breath, edema	CBC yearly, creatinine yearly
Polyuria, polydipsia, edema, shortness of breath, BP at each visit, visual changes, bone pain	Urinary dipstick for glucose every 3–6 months, total cholesterol yearly, bone densitometry yearly to assess osteoporosis
Visual changes	Fundoscopic and visual fields every 6–12 months
Symptoms of myelosuppression	CBC and platelet count every 1–2 weeks with changes in dose (every 1–3 months thereafter), AST yearly, Pap test at regular intervals
Symptoms of myelosuppression, hematuria, infertility	CBC and urinalysis monthly, urine cytology and Pap test yearly for life
Symptoms of myelosuppression, shortness of breath, nausea/vomiting, oral ulcer	CBC and platelet count, AST or ALT, and albumin every 4–8 weeks, serum creatinine, urinalysis

CBC, complete blood cell count; AST, aspartate transaminase; ALT, alanine transaminase; BP, blood pressure; HDL, high-density lipoprotein; LDL, low-density lipoprotein; Pap, Papanicolaou

mologic toxicity which is relatively rare at the recommended low doses used to treat SLE (<6.5 mg/kg/day). However, current recommendations are to obtain an ophthalmologic examination before initiating treatment and every six to 12 months thereafter. Evaluation should include visual-acuity, slit-lamp, fundoscopic, and visual-field testing.

Antimalarials rarely have been associated with congenital defects in the developing fetus, and reports have been very encouraging with respect to hydroxychloroquine use during pregnancy (7). The decision to continue antimalarials during pregnancy should be made on an individual basis with consideration of both the fetal risk and the likelihood of flare in maternal disease activity.

Azathioprine

Azathioprine is a purine analogue that inhibits nucleic-acid synthesis and affects both cellular and humoral immune function. In SLE, this agent is used as an alternative to cyclophosphamide for treatment of nephritis or as a steroid-sparing agent for nonrenal manifestations. Azathioprine has fewer side effects than cyclophosphamide and may be con-

sidered for patients with focal proliferative nephritis (World Health Organization class III; see Table 17C-1) or those at low risk for progressive renal failure.

The most common side effects are bone-marrow and gastrointestinal toxicity. Regular monitoring of complete blood counts during therapy is recommended. Because of hepatic metabolism and urinary excretion, renal and liver function should be checked periodically. Dosage adjustments may be necessary in patients with renal or hepatic dysfunction. Azathioprine has been associated with a hypersensitivity syndrome that presents with fever, skin rash, and elevated hepatic transaminases. Toxicities typically are reversible with drug discontinuation. An increased risk of malignancy, such as non-Hodgkin's lymphoma, has been reported following treatment with azathioprine.

Cyclophosphamide

Cyclophosphamide has been one of the most extensively studied immunosuppressive agents for the treatment of SLE in the past several decades (8). It remains the mainstay of treatment for severe organ-system disease, particularly lupus nephritis.

In a series of studies with more than 20 years of follow-up, treatment with corticosteroids plus cyclophosphamide (intravenous bolus regimens of 0.5–1.0 g/mm²) was superior to corticosteroids alone in preventing progressive scarring in the kidney, preserving renal function, and inducing renal remission (9). The best response rates for cyclophosphamide appear to occur in diffuse proliferative lupus nephritis (WHO class IV; see Table 17C-1). Other pathologic classes of lupus nephritis have not been studied as extensively. Trends in favor of improvement in membranous nephropathy (WHO class V) have been reported. The milder stages of lupus nephritis (WHO class II/III) often are treated with corticosteroids alone; intolerable side effects from corticosteroids or progression to more severe forms of lupus nephritis may warrant addition of another immunosuppressive agent. The nonrenal manifestations of SLE that have been treated effectively with cyclophosphamide include cytopenia, CNS disease, pulmonary hemorrhage, and vasculitis.

Nausea and vomiting are common side effects of cyclophosphamide treatment, but effective antiemetic regimens minimize the gastrointestinal toxicity. Hair loss, which occasionally can be significant, typically reverses with cessation of therapy. A dose-dependent leukopenia with nadir occurring about eight to 12 days after intravenous administration can be regulated by dose adjustment. Patients treated with cyclophosphamide are at increased risk of bacterial, fungal, and viral infections, with particular susceptibility to herpes zoster.

Gonadal toxicity from cyclophosphamide can result in ovarian failure or azoospermia (10). Older age and higher cumulative drug dose are two major factors associated with the risk of ovarian failure in women. Although many strategies have been suggested for preserving ovarian function, including administration of gonadotropin-releasing hormone or oral contraceptives, none have been proven effective in SLE.

Acrolein, a drug metabolite of cyclophosphamide, is a bladder irritant and has been incriminated in the hemorrhagic cystitis, fibrosis, and transitional squamous cell carcinoma seen in people on long-term cyclophosphamide therapy. Daily oral cyclophosphamide poses the highest risk and should be accompanied by generous daily fluid intake. In patients treated with intravenous bolus cyclophosphamide, adequate hydration and administration of mesna, an acrolein binder, used at 20% of the total cyclophosphamide dose, are common practices, particularly in patients with a history of cystitis. Patients treated with cyclophosphamide should be screened routinely for bladder carcinoma, which can develop years after discontinuation of therapy. Urinalysis, urine cytology, and cystoscopy in patients with gross or microscopic hematuria should be considered.

Methotrexate

Although there is much evidence to support the use of methotrexate (MTX) in rheumatoid arthritis, very few controlled clinical trials have examined its efficacy in lupus. Results from a double-blind, randomized, placebo-controlled trial of MTX in lupus showed that MTX in dosages of 15–20 mg/week for six months effectively controlled disease activity and permitted prednisone dose reduction (11). Cutaneous and articular manifestations were the most responsive to MTX. Side effects were common and included hepatic serum enzyme elevations, gastrointestinal complaints, infections, and oral ulcers, but these adverse reactions may be due to the relatively high doses of MTX used in the trial. Current trials are examining the efficacy of 7.5–15 mg/week of MTX, a dosage intended to reduce side effects. Until these trials are completed and more definitive guidelines are established for the use of MTX in lupus, this agent continues to be used most commonly as a steroid-sparing agent for milder manifestations of disease. The beneficial role of MTX in systemic vasculitis, such as polyarteritis nodosa and Wegener's granulomatosis, provides impetus to examine the utility of MTX in more severe manifestations of SLE.

Cyclosporine

Cyclosporine, unlike cyclophosphamide or azathioprine, primarily inhibits T-cell–mediated responses. Cyclosporine has had a major impact in the field of organ transplantation and has been used increasingly to treat autoimmune conditions. Evidence to support the use of cyclosporine in lupus has been derived from case series and open trials. A recently published review of the literature summarizes the findings from 12 studies involving 214 people with SLE who were treated with cyclosporine (12). Dosages of cyclosporine ranging from 2.5 to 5 mg/kg/day generally were well-tolerated, with improvements observed in proteinuria, cytopenia (white blood cell and platelet counts), immunologic parameters [C3, C4, and anti–double-stranded DNA (dsDNA) antibodies], and overall lupus disease activity measured by SLEDAI (Systemic Lupus Erythematosus Disease Activity Index) and SLAM (Systemic Lupus Activity Measurement) scores. Side effects (including hypertension, gingival hyperplasia, hypertrichosis, and mild elevations in serum creatinine) were common, but rarely required discontinuation of therapy. Cyclosporine seems to have its greatest effect in membranous nephritis (WHO class V) or in patients with refractory nephrotic syndrome; however, close monitoring of blood pressure and renal function are warranted.

Mycophenylate Mofetil

Mycophenylate mofetil (MMF) is a reversible inhibitor of inosine monophosphate dehydrogenase, a critical enzyme in purine synthesis. In vitro, MMF blocks proliferation of B and T cells and decreases expression of adhesion molecules. MMF has been approved for treatment of renal allograft rejection and, more recently, has shown promise as an effective treatment for lupus nephritis. MMF effectively reduced proteinuria and improved serum creatinine levels in 13 people with SLE and cyclophosphamide-resistant nephritis over a mean of 12.8 months (13). Common side effects include leukopenia, nausea, and diarrhea. A larger study followed 42 SLE patients with diffuse proliferative glomerulonephritis for 12 months (14). It was found that the combination of MMF and prednisolone was as effective as oral cyclophosphamide and prednisolone, followed by azathioprine and prednisolone, at inducing complete renal remission (81% versus 76%) and partial renal remission (14% versus 14%). MMF generally was well-tolerated at dosages ranging from 500 mg to 1000 mg, twice a day. This agent holds promise as an alternative to conventional therapy for lupus nephritis.

Hormone Therapy

Bromocriptine, which selectively inhibits anterior pituitary secretion of the immune-stimulatory hormone prolactin, has shown benefit in reducing disease activity in SLE patients with and without evidence of hyperprolactinemia (15). Dehydroepiandrosterone (DHEA), an adrenal hormone with androgenic properties, has shown some promise for the treatment of mild to moderate lupus disease activity in several controlled and uncontrolled clinical trials on more than 200 patients (16). Decreased corticosteroid requirements has been one of the major reported benefits. The role of DHEA as an "add on" therapy for more severe SLE manifestations, including nephritis, serositis, and hematological abnormalities, remains unclear (17). Danazol, a synthetic corticosteroid with weak androgenic activity, generally has been well-tolerated and effective at dosages between 400 and 1200 mg/day in controlling autoimmune cytopenia, particularly thrombocytopenia and hemolytic anemia (18).

Miscellaneous Therapies

Thalidomide can be effective for the treatment of discoid lupus. Maintenance doses of 25–50 mg/day resulted in partial remission in 30% and complete remission in 60% of 30 lupus patients with discoid lesions refractory to corticosteroid and antimalarial therapy (19). On discontinuation, 75% of the patients relapsed. Peripheral neuropathy occurred in 27% of the patients, which is similar to the frequency reported in other series (20%–50%). The well-recognized risk of teratogenicity prohibits the use of this agent in women planning pregnancy. Dapsone is a sulfone that is effective in controlling some cutaneous eruptions, including discoid lupus. Retinoids, which have anti-inflammatory and immunosuppressive effects, have been used with success, both orally and topically, for the treatment of chronic cutaneous lupus.

Plasmapheresis

The original intent of plasmapheresis in the treatment of SLE was to remove circulating immune complexes and autoantibodies. The role of plasmapheresis with synchronized immunosuppressive therapy in lupus nephritis remains controversial. Heightened risk for infection and anaphylaxis, coupled with the high cost of the procedure,

has reduced the utility of this treatment modality. The most accepted indications for plasmapheresis in lupus include cryoglobulinemia, hyperviscosity syndrome, and thrombotic thrombocytopenia purpura (20). There may be a role for plasmapheresis in certain other life-threatening complications of lupus that are refractory to conventional approaches. The potential use of plasmapheresis for pregnancy complications related to anti-Ro antibody with congenital heart block and antiphospholipid antibodies remains unclear.

Intravenous Immunoglobulin

Intravenous immunoglobulin (IVIgG) is an immunomodulatory agent used in the treatment of some forms of SLE. The mechanisms of action of IVIgG are diverse and include Fc receptor blockade, complement regulation, and T-cell regulation. Whereas immunosuppressive therapies used in lupus may contribute to infection susceptibility, IVIgG provides a defense against infection. At dosages of 400 mg/kg/day for five consecutive days, improvement in thrombocytopenia, arthritis, nephritis, fever, mucocutaneous manifestations, and immunologic parameters have been reported (21). IVIgG is used most widely to treat refractory thrombocytopenia and can result in rapid rises in platelet counts within hours of administration. Adverse reactions of IVIgG include fever, myalgia, headache, arthralgia, and in rare instances, aseptic meningitis. Its use is contraindicated in people with SLE and IgA deficiency.

Dialysis and Kidney Transplantation

The availability of renal dialysis and kidney transplantation has improved the longevity and quality of life of people with SLE. However, patients on dialysis are at increased risk for infections and should be monitored closely. A recent study showed that graft failure and mortality following renal transplantation in patients with end-stage renal disease from SLE were similar to that found in patients with end-stage renal disease from other causes (22).

New Experimental Therapies

Drawbacks of traditional drug therapies include "global" suppressive effects on the immune system, common toxicities, and lack of specificity for the immune dysregulation unique to lupus. Several of the newer biologic agents currently under investigation for the treatment of SLE are designed to inhibit costimulatory pathways necessary for T-cell–B-cell activation, production of anti-dsDNA antibodies, and cytokine activation. One such agent is a monoclonal antibody to CD40 ligand (CD40LmAb). B-cell responses to T-cell–dependent antigens are inhibited when the CD40 (B cell)–CD40L (T cell) interaction is blocked. Trials examining the efficacy of CD40LmAb in the treatment of active lupus currently are underway. LJP 394 is a B-cell tolerogen that binds to anti-dsDNA on the B-cell surface and down-regulates production of anti-dsDNA antibodies. In a recent trial designed to examine whether LJP 394 could prevent renal flares, patients with a history of nephritis and high-affinity antibodies to the oligonucleotide epitope of LJP 394 had delayed onset of renal flare (23), and the drug was well-tolerated. A larger Phase III trial is underway to confirm these preliminary results.

Immune suppression followed by autologous hematopoietic stem-cell infusion has been proposed for the treatment of refractory and life-threatening lupus. Seven people with SLE who underwent stem-cell transplantation were free from active lupus at a median follow-up of 25 months (24). Durability of remission remains unknown. Other investigators have proposed immunoablative high-dose cyclophosphamide without stem-cell rescue for the treatment of severe autoimmune diseases, including lupus (25). These novel approaches for the treatment of SLE require further investigation regarding long-term safety and efficacy before they can be broadly incorporated into disease management.

SUSAN MANZI, MD, MPH

References

1. MacLeod JM. Lupus erythematosus: its nature and treatment. Lancet 1908;ii:1271–1275.
2. Ostensen M, Villiger PM. Nonsteroidal anti-inflammatory drugs in systemic lupus erythematosus. Lupus 2000;9:566–572.
3. Boumpas DT, Chrousos GP, Wilder RL, Cupps TR, Balow JE. Glucocorticoid therapy for immune-mediated diseases: basic and clinical correlates. Ann Intern Med 1993;119:1198–1208.
4. Toubi E, Rosner I, Rozenbaum M, Kessel A, Golan TD. The benefit of combining hydroxychloroquine with quinacrine in the treatment of SLE patients. Lupus 2000;9:92–95.
5. The Canadian Hydroxychloroquine Study Group. A randomized study of the effect of withdrawing hydroxychloroquine sulfate in systemic lupus erythematosus. N Engl J Med 1991;324:150–154.
6. Tsakonas E, Joseph L, Esdaile JM, et al. A long-term study of hydroxychloroquine withdrawal on exacerbations in systemic lupus erythematosus. The Canadian Hydroxychloroquine Study Group. Lupus 1998;7:80–85.
7. Parke A, West B. Hydroxychloroquine in pregnant patients with systemic lupus erythematosus. J Rheumatol 1996;23:1715–1718.
8. Ortmann RA, Klippel JH. Update on cyclophosphamide for systemic lupus erythematosus. Rheum Dis Clin North Am 2000;26:363–375.
9. Gourley MF, Austin HA III, Scott D, et al. Methylprednisolone and cyclophosphamide, alone or in combination, in patients with lupus nephritis. A randomized, controlled trial. Ann Intern Med 1996;125:549–557.
10. Slater CA, Liang MH, McCune JW, Christman GM, Laufer MR. Preserving ovarian function in patients receiving cyclophosphamide. Lupus 1999;8:3–10.
11. Carneiro JR, Sato EI. Double blind, randomized, placebo controlled clinical trial of methotrexate in systemic lupus erythematosus. J Rheumatol 1999;26:1275–1279.
12. Hallegua D, Wallace DJ, Metzger AL, Rinaldi RZ, Klinenberg JR. Cyclosporine for lupus membranous nephritis: experience with ten patients and review of the literature. Lupus 2000;9:241–251.
13. Dooley MA, Cosio FG, Nachman PH, et al. Mycophenolate mofetil therapy in lupus nephritis: clinical observations. J Am Soc Nephrol 1999;10:833–839.
14. Chan TM, Li FK, Tang CS, et al. Efficacy of mycophenolate mofetil in patients with diffuse proliferative lupus nephritis. Hong Kong-Guangzhou Nephrology Study Group. N Engl J Med 2000;343:1156–1162.
15. Alvarez-Nemegyei J, Cobarrubias-Cobos A, Escalante-Triay F, Sosa-Munoz J, Miranda JM, Jara LJ. Bromocriptine in systemic lupus erythematosus: a double-blind, randomized, placebo-controlled study. Lupus 1998;7:414–419.
16. Van Vollenhoven RF. Dehydroepiandrosterone in systemic lupus erythematosus. Rheum Dis Clin North Am 2000;26:349–362.
17. Van Vollenhoven RF, Park JL, Genovese MC, West JP, McGuire JL. A double-blind, placebo-controlled, clinical trial of dehydroepiandrosterone in severe systemic lupus erythematosus. Lupus 1999;8:181–187.
18. Cervera H, Jara LJ, Pizarro S, et al. Danazol for systemic lupus erythematosus with refractory autoimmune thrombocytopenia or Evans' syndrome. J Rheumatol 1995;22:1867–1871.
19. Godfrey T, Khamashta MA, Hughes GR. Therapeutic advances in systemic lupus erythematosus. Curr Opin Rheumatol 1998;10:435–441.
20. Wallace DJ. Apheresis for lupus erythematosus. Lupus 1999;8:174–180.
21. Levy Y, Sherer Y, Ahmed A, et al. A study of 20 SLE patients with intravenous immunoglobulin – clinical and serologic response. Lupus 1999;8:705–712.
22. Ward MM. Outcomes of renal transplantation among patients with end-stage renal disease caused by lupus nephritis. Kidney Int 2000;57:2136–2143.
23. Alarcon-Segovia D, Tumlin J, Furie R, et al. SLE trial shows fewer renal flares in LJP 394-treated patients with high-affinity antibodies to LJP 394: 90-95 trial results. Arthritis Rheum 2000;43:S272.
24. Traynor AE, Schroeder J, Rosa RM, et al. Treatment of severe systemic lupus erythematosus with high-dose chemotherapy and haemopoietic stem-cell transplantation: a phase I study. Lancet 2000;356:701–707.
25. Brodsky RA, Petri M, Smith BD, et al. Immunoablative high-dose cyclophosphamide without stem-cell rescue for refractory, severe autoimmune disease. Ann Intern Med 1998;129:1031–1035.

18 SYSTEMIC SCLEROSIS AND RELATED SYNDROMES
A. Epidemiology, Pathology and Pathogenesis

Systemic sclerosis (SSc), also called scleroderma (*skleros* hard, *derma* skin), is a multisystem disease characterized by functional and structural abnormalities of small blood vessels, fibrosis of the skin and internal organs, immune system activation, and autoimmunity. Localized scleroderma includes fibrotic diseases restricted to the skin, such as morphea and linear scleroderma, and are not discussed in this chapter.

Epidemiology

Systemic sclerosis is an acquired, noncontagious, rare disease of unknown etiology that occurs sporadically worldwide. Its incidence in the United States is about 19 cases per million per year, with a prevalence of 19–75 cases per 100,000 (1). Although it's estimated that 40,000–165,000 people in the United States have SSc, prevalence figures rise threefold to fourfold when they include patients who have mild SSc-like illnesses (1), but do not meet classification criteria (see Appendix I) (2).

Age, gender, and genetic background are host factors that modify disease susceptibility (3). SSc is rare in children, with peak occurrence in individuals aged 35–65 years. Female predominance is most pronounced during mid- and late-childbearing years, when ratios of women to men may reach 7–12:1. Families with more than one case of SSc have been reported, including reports of twins with SSc. A family history of other autoimmune illnesses is elicited more frequently than expected. Choctaw Native Americans in Oklahoma have the highest prevalence of SSc reported: 469 cases per 100,000 people. A 2-cM haplotype on chromosome 15q that contains the fibrillin-1 gene is associated with SSc in this group (4). This haplotype may be inherited from common ancestors of approximately 10 generations ago (4). Of note, a mutation of the fibrillarin-1 gene in an animal model of fibrosis, the tight skin mouse 1 (TSK1), duplicates a region that binds transforming growth factor β (TGF-β). The resultant fibrillarin chain is structurally abnormal and may lead to increased proteolysis (5). A Native American human leukocyte antigen (HLA)-DR2 haplotype that includes HLA class I and III regions also is associated with SSc in this Choctaw population, but TGF-β1 and platelet-derived growth factor (PDGF) gene families are not. In other populations, weak associations have been noted between SSc and HLA-DQA2, the C4A null allele, an allele of the Cγ2 T-cell antigen receptor gene, and low activity of P-450 enzymes. There are no associations of SSc with mutants of the fibronectin gene; alleles of proα$_1$(I), proα$_2$(II), or proα$_1$(III) collagen genes; or allotypes of α1 antitrypsin.

Ethnic background influences survival and disease manifestation. Progressive pulmonary interstitial fibrosis occurs less frequently and survival rates are better in Caucasian patients, compared with African-American and Japanese patients (6). Different ethnic groups also have different disease-specific antibody profiles. Caucasians are more likely to have anticentromere antibodies, and African Americans are more likely to have antitopoisomerase I (Scl-70) antibodies (6). Autoantibody specificities are associated with particular HLA alleles, and the HLA alleles associated with a given autoantibody may differ from one group to another. For example, in American Caucasians, the production of anticentromere antibodies is associated with HLA-DQB1 molecules with a polar glycine or tyrosine at position 26 (7). The HLA-DRB1 alleles associated with anti-DNA topoisomerase I antibodies vary across different ethnic groups: DRB1*1101-*1104 in Caucasians and African Americans, DRB1*1502 in Japanese, and DRB1*1602 in Choctaws (6).

Similar concordance rates for SSc in monozygotic and dizygotic twins, and the occurrence of SSc in conjugal pairs suggest the importance of environmental factors in disease development. Although there is no direct evidence for a viral etiology of SSc, human parvovirus B19 infection has been detected in bone marrow, and antibodies to human cytomegalovirus are increased. Homologies exist between SSc autoantigens and viruses. For example, there is homology between DNA topoisomerase 1 and the p30^{gag} protein from feline sarcoma virus and cytomegalovirus. Regions of the PM-Scl antigen are homologous to SV-40 large T antigen and HIV tat protein. U$_1$ ribonucleoprotein (RNP) shares an amino acid segment with herpes simplex virus type I ICP4 protein. There also are homologies between fibrillarin and a capsid protein encoded by herpes simplex virus type 1 and Epstein-Barr virus nuclear antigen 1.

Noninfectious environmental agents have been implicated in the development of SSc. Occupational exposure to silica dust is associated with a relative risk of 25, and frank silicosis with a relative risk of 110. Cases of SSc have been reported in individuals exposed to organic solvents; biogenic amines, including appetite suppressants; and urea formaldehyde. Fibrosing illnesses with SSc-like features occur after exposure to vinyl chloride, bleomycin, tainted rapeseed oil, and L-tryptophan. However, several retrospective studies have not found an increased incidence of silicone implants in women with SSc.

Pathology

Widespread small-vessel vasculopathy and fibrosis, which occur in the setting of immune system activation and autoimmunity, distinguish SSc from other connective-tissue diseases. The vasculopathy of SSc affects small arteries, arterioles, and capillaries and causes tissue ischemia, including recurrent episodes of ischemia-reperfusion. Patients have hypersensitivity of α_2 adrenergic receptors on vascular smooth-muscle cells, obliterative structural changes in the vessel wall, and failure to replace damaged vessels. Invasion of vessel walls by mononuclear cells is uncommon, and the vascular disease is not considered a vasculitis. Heightened sensitivity of α_2 adrenergic receptors to vasoconstricting stimuli is an early event and can be demonstrated when the endothelium of the vessel still is functionally intact (8). This increased sensitivity to vasoconstricting stimuli, such as cold and stress, causes Raynaud's phenomenon, which occurs in about 95% of patients. Structural damage appears to start with activation and apoptosis in the endothelium, (9). Activation is indicated by increased endothelial cell surface expression of HLA class II molecules, β_1 integrins, intercellular adhesion molecule 1 (ICAM-1), endothelial cell adhesion molecule 1 (ELAM-1), and P-selectin. Some endothelial cells show an active biosynthetic state, suggesting attempts at repair, but the net outcome is endothelial cell loss.

Smooth-muscle cells within the intima of small vessels, called myointimal cells, proliferate (9). Luminal narrowing develops and is exacerbated when the damaged endothelium induces platelet activation and thrombosis (9). Activated platelets release PDGF and thromboxane A_2, which can induce vasoconstriction and stimulate growth of endothelial cells and fibroblasts. Basement membranes thicken and reduplicate. Fibrin is deposited within and around the vessels. These events reduce transfusion of nutrients through the vessels. Similar obliterative and proliferative changes can be seen in pulmonary arteries of some patients, causing pulmonary artery hypertension (see Fig. 18A-1).

A striking lack of digital vessels often is seen on arteriograms of the hands or feet of patients with late-stage disease, indicating structurally damaged vessels and lack of new vessel growth to replace the damaged vessels. Levels of endostatin, an angiogenesis inhibitor, are increased.

Fibrosis in SSc is caused by increased production of collagen, fibronectin, and glycosaminoglycans. Synthesis of collagen types I, III, V, and VI messenger RNAs and proteins is increased, and normal ratios of type I to type III collagen are maintained. Limited studies suggest that degradation of extracellular matrix remains unchanged, with normal collagenase activity. The excessive production of collagen by dermal fibroblasts persists during in vitro passage. Myofibroblasts, which are smooth-muscle, α-actin–positive, fibroblast-like cells, may contribute to the excessive extracellular matrix produced in the skin and lungs. Myofibroblasts from the lungs of people with SSc show high expression of collagen type I mRNAs, and their proliferation is enhanced by exposure to PDGF and TGF-β1 (10,11). The excessive production of extracellular matrix causes thickening of the skin (see Fig. 18A-2) and fibrosis of internal organs.

Cellular infiltrates are found in biopsies of involved skin and lungs. In the skin, the infiltrates occur in perivascular regions and are scattered throughout the dermis and subcutaneous fat, especially in early disease (9). The dermal infiltrate consists of T cells (more CD4+ than CD8+), with some pericytes, Langerhans cells, plasma cells, macrophages, and rarely, B cells. The T cells show increased expression of β_1 and β_2 integrins, including leukocyte function-associated antigen (LFA)-1, and SSc fibroblasts have increased expression of ICAM-1. Lung biopsies may show inflammation, with patchy lymphocyte and plasma-cell infiltration of the alveolar walls, occasional focal lymphoid hyperplasia, interstitial fibrosis, increased macrophages, and occasional polymorphonuclear cells

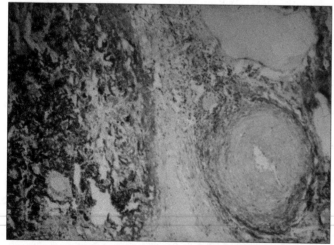

Fig. 18A-1. Pulmonary hypertension. Proliferative, obliterative changes that occur in pulmonary arteries cause pulmonary hypertension in some people with systemic sclerosis.

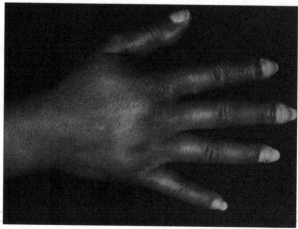

Fig. 18A-2. Dermal fibrosis. The skin on the hand of this patient with diffuse cutaneous systemic sclerosis is thickened due to dermal fibrosis. Hypo- and hyperpigmentation of the skin is common. The loss of digital pulp is associated with chronic ischemia of the digits.

and lymphocytes in the alveolar spaces (12). For example, Fig. 18A-3 shows thickened alveolar walls seen on an autopsy specimen. Memory T cells are increased in lung biopsies (13), and CD8⁺ T cells are increased selectively in bronchoalveolar lavage fluids from people with SSc (14). The alveolar macrophages are activated, with increased expression of adhesion receptors and receptors involved in signal transduction and/or inflammation. Fibronectin is released in higher amounts by scleroderma alveolar macrophages than by normal macrophages. Mast cells can be observed in close contact with interstitial fibroblasts. There is no evidence of immune complex deposition. Alveolar macrophages, bronchial epithelium, and hyperplastic type II pneumocytes express intracellular TGF-β1, and extracellular TGF-β1 can be found in the fibrous tissue immediately beneath the bronchial and hyperplastic alveolar epithelium.

Abnormalities of humoral immunity in people with SSc include hypergammaglobulinemia, with polyclonal increases in IgG, IgA, IgM, and IgE, autoantibody production, and immune complex formation. Antinuclear antibodies (ANA) are present at clinical presentation in 95% of SSc patients. The isotype of the ANA usually is IgG, especially the IgG3 subclass. Some autoantibody systems are quite specific for SSc, including the topoisomerase 1, centromere, RNA polymerase I, RNA polymerase III, and U₃ RNP systems.

Pathogenesis

Any model of the pathogenesis of SSc must account for small-vessel vasculopathy, fibrosis, and immune system activation with autoimmunity. One possible model is presented in Fig. 18A-4. A susceptible host, usually a middle-aged woman with a permissive genetic background, develops illness in response to external events or exposures. Inciting events remain unknown and may be different in different individuals. Early in the course of disease, immune system activation, endothelial cell activation and damage, and fibroblast activation all occur. Each of these processes probably augments the others, and if left unchecked, end-stage tissue damage occurs. The end-stage damage includes structural changes in small blood vessels and tissue fibrosis.

Activated T cells contribute to the disease by producing such profibrotic cytokines as interleukin (IL)-4 or TGF-β; cytolytic mediators; and help for autoantibody production. Oligoclonal expansion of Vδ1⁺ T cells in the blood and CD8⁺ T cells in the lungs provides evidence of some antigen-specific activation of T cells in vivo in people with SSc. The antigens that stimulate the T cells in vivo are unknown, but peripheral blood mononuclear cells from people with SSc proliferate in response to skin extracts and purified type I and type IV collagen, or they kill in response to cellular antigens on fibroblasts, epithelial cells, and muscle cells. Increased numbers of memory T cells in the lungs are associated with greater fibrosis in lung biopsies (13). Increased production of type 2 cytokines (IL-4 and IL-5) by CD8⁺ T

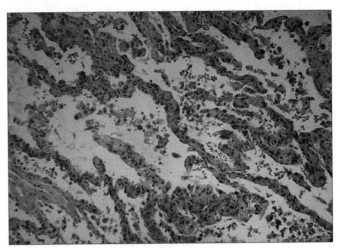

Fig. 18A-3. Interstitial fibrosis of the lung. This autopsy specimen shows mild to moderate thickening of the alveolar walls.

cells in bronchoalveolar lavage fluids is associated with greater subsequent decline in lung function (14).

SSc-specific autoantigens share the ability to be cleaved into novel fragments by metal-dependent, nonenzymatic mechanisms (15) or by granzyme B, a serine esterase found in cytolytic granules (16). Repeated episodes of ischemia reperfusion might lead to generation of oxygen radicals that facilitate the metal-dependent nonenzymatic cleavage of these autoantigens, promoting autoantibody formation (15). Alternatively, tissue damage caused by activated cytolytic CD8⁺ T cells might initiate autoantibody formation (16). It is unknown whether autoantibodies contribute to tissue damage in SSc. In vitro, anti-DNA topoisomerase I, anticentromere, and antimyenteric neuronal antibodies can inhibit function of their target antigens, and antiendothelial cell antibodies can induce endothelial cell apoptosis. However, many autoantibodies in SSc sera

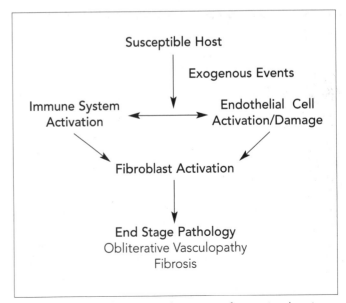

Fig. 18A-4. Model of immunopathogenesis of systemic sclerosis.

do not activate the complement cascade, and serum complement levels are normal. Immune complexes may be present in the sera of people with SSc, but there is scant evidence of tissue deposition.

Microchimerism, causing a graft-versus-host reaction, may be one of multiple factors involved in the development of SSc. During parturition, there is intermingling of maternal and fetal circulations. Both mother and baby have engraftment with allogeneic cells, which can persist for years. Microengrafted allogeneic cells are detected in peripheral blood mononuclear cells (PBMC) in a higher percentage of people with SSc (about 45%–65% of patients versus 5%–35% of controls) (17). The engrafted cells include $CD34^+CD38^+$ stem cells and CD3, CD19, CD14, and CD56/16 subsets (17). Engrafted cells have been found in involved skin from patients (18). HLA compatibility is not a requirement for persistent microchimerism in PBMC subsets, but does occur more commonly in systemic sclerosis patients than in controls (17). In both patients and controls, fetal microchimerism among T lymphocytes is strongly associated with HLA DQA1*0501 of the mother, and even more strongly with DQA1*0501 of a son (19). It is speculated that microengraftment leads to graft-versus-host disease, which shares clinical characteristics with SSc. However, no data have addressed what role these microengrafted cells play, if any, in the development of SSc.

Soluble immune mediators and antiendothelial cell antibodies may alter endothelial cell function in SSc. IL-1, IL-2, IL-4, IL-6, IL-8, lymphotoxin, tumor necrosis factor (TNF)-α, TGF-β, and PDGF reportedly increase in SSc sera or tissues, and all these agents regulate endothelial cell function. Other circulating factors that may damage or alter function of small vessels in people with SSc include granzyme 1, a lysosomal protein released by cytotoxic T cells; leukotriene B_4; and endothelin 1.

The endothelial cell itself is likely to contribute to activation of cells of the immune system and fibroblasts. Dermal endothelial cells of people with SSc have increased expression of ELAM-1, which is involved in the homing of T cells to the skin. Endothelin-1 and TGF-β, which can be produced by endothelial cells, stimulate extracellular matrix production by fibroblasts.

Increased production of extracellular matrix in SSc results from at least two events: stimulation of extracellular matrix production by cytokines, and outgrowth of fibroblasts that produce higher basal amounts of extracellular matrix. Soluble mediators that stimulate extracellular matrix production or fibroblast proliferation include IL-6, IL-4, TGF-β, PDGF, fibroblast growth factor, and endothelin 1. Of note, deletion of IL-4, STAT 6, or TGF-β curtails developing fibrosis in an animal model of SSc, the TSK1 mouse. Decreased production of interferon γ, which reduces collagen synthesis, may contribute to the profibrotic milieu. Potential cellular sources of the profibrotic factors include T cells, macrophages, and endothelial cells. Increased levels of TGF-β mRNA and proα1(I) collagen mRNA co-localize within inflammatory infiltrates in skin during the early

phase of disease. Scleroderma fibroblasts may be inherently abnormal in their responsiveness to cytokine stimulation. In vivo experiments suggest that the collagen promoter is more active in response to TGF-β in scleroderma fibroblasts than in control fibroblasts (20). Finally, autocrine regulation of collagen production by fibroblast-derived cytokines, including TGF-β, IL-6, and intracellular IL-1α, appears to contribute to the fibrotic process (21).

Only a subset of fibroblasts appears to contribute to fibrosis in SSc. In situ hybridization studies of scleroderma skin show that only some fibroblasts actively produce procollagen mRNA. A higher percentage of fibroblasts cloned from people with SSc produce large amounts of collagen, compared with fibroblasts cloned from controls.

The end result of these initial processes – smooth-muscle hyper-responsiveness to vasoconstrictors, endothelial cell activation and apoptosis, fibroblast activation, immune system activation, and autoimmunity – is the obliterative, proliferative small-vessel vasculopathy and fibrosis called SSc. Because structural changes in blood vessel walls and accompanying fibrosis are less likely to be reversible than the earlier pathologic processes, the hope of the future is that therapeutic interventions will target earlier steps in disease pathogenesis and disrupt the cycle of interacting events that lead to end-stage damage.

BARBARA WHITE, MD

References

1. Maricq HR, Weinrich MC, Keil JE, et al. Prevalence of scleroderma spectrum disorders in the general population of South Carolina. Arthritis Rheum 1989;32:998-1006.

2. Subcommittee for Scleroderma Criteria of the American Rheumatism Association Diagnostic and Therapeutic Criteria Committee. Preliminary criteria for classification of systemic sclerosis (scleroderma). Arthritis Rheum 1980;23:581-590.

3. Silmon AJ. Scleroderma – demographics and survival. J Rheumatol Suppl 1997;48:58-61.

4. Tan FK, Stivers DN, Foster MW, et al. Association of microsatellite markers near the fibrillin 1 gene on human chromosome 15q with scleroderma in a Native American population. Arthritis Rheum 1998;41:1729-1737.

5. Gayraud B, Keene DR, Sakai LY, Ramirez F. New insights into the assembly of extracellular microfibrils from the analysis of the fibrillin 1 mutation in the tight skin mouse. J Cell Biol 2000;150:667-680.

6. Kuwana M, Kaburaki J, Arnett FC, Howard RF, Medsger TA Jr, Wright TM. Influence of ethnic background on clinical and serologic features in patients with systemic sclerosis and anti-DNA topoisomerase I antibody. Arthritis Rheum 1999;42:465-474.

7. Reveille JD, Owerbach D, Goldstein R, Moreda R, Isern RA, Arnett FC. Association of polar amino acids at position 26 of the HLA-DQB1 first domain with the anticentromere autoantibody response in systemic sclerosis (scleroderma). J Clin Invest 1992;89:1209-1213.

8. Flavahan NA, Flavahan S, Liu Q, Wu S, Tidmore W, Wiener

CM, Spence RJ, Wigley FM. *Increased alpha2-adrenergic constriction of isolated arterioles in diffuse scleroderma. Arthritis Rheum* 2000;43:1886-1890.

9. Prescott RJ, Freemont AJ, Jones CJP, Hoyland J, Fielding P. *Sequential dermal microvascular and perivascular changes in the development of scleroderma. J Pathol* 1992;166:255-263.

10. Kirk TZ, Mark ME, Chua CC, Chua BH, Mayes MD. *Myofibroblasts from scleroderma skin synthesize elevated levels of collagen and tissue inhibitor of metalloproteinase (TIMP-1) with two forms of TIMP-1. J Biol Chem* 1995;270:3423-3428.

11. Ludwicka A, Ohba T, Trojanowska M, et al. *Elevated levels of platelet derived growth factor and transforming growth factor-beta 1 in bronchoalveolar lavage fluid from patients with scleroderma. J Rheumatol* 1995;22:1876-1883.

12. Harrison NK, Myers AR, Corrin B,. *Structural features of interstitial lung disease in systemic sclerosis. Am Rev Respir Dis* 1991;144:706-713.

13. Wells AU, Lorimer S, Majumdar S,. *Fibrosing alveolitis in systemic sclerosis: increase in memory T-cells in lung interstitium. Eur Respir J* 1995;8:266-271.

14. Atamas SP, Yurovsky VV, Wise R, et al. *Type 2 cytokines made by CD8+ lung cells predict decline in pulmonary function in patients with systemic sclerosis. Arthritis Rheum* 1999;142:1168-1178.

15. Casciola-Rosen L, Wigley F, Rosen A. *Scleroderma autoantigens are uniquely fragmented by metal-catalyzed oxidation reactions: implications for pathogenesis. J Exp Med* 1997;185: 71-79.

16. Casciola-Rosen L, Andrade F, Ulanet D, Wong WB, Rosen A. *Cleavage by granzyme B is strongly predictive of autoantigen status: implications for initiation of autoimmunity. J Exp Med* 1999;190:815-826.

17. Evans PC, Lambert N, Maloney S, Furst DE, Moore JM, Nelson JL. *Long-term fetal microchimerism in peripheral blood mononuclear cell subsets in healthy women and women with scleroderma. Blood* 1999;93:2033-2037.

18. Artlett CM, Smith JB, Jimenez SA. *Identification of fetal DNA and cells in skin lesions from women with systemic sclerosis. N Engl J Med* 1998;338:1186-1191.

19. Lambert NC, Evans PC, Hashizumi TL. *Cutting edge: persistent fetal microchimerism in T lymphocytes is associated with HLA-DQA1*0501: implications in autoimmunity. J Immunol* 2000;164:5545-5548.

20. Hitraya EG, Varga J, Artlett CM, Jimenez SA. *Identification of elements in the promoter region of the alpha1(I) procollagen gene involved in its up-regulated expression in systemic sclerosis. Arthritis Rheum* 1998;41:2048-2058.

21. Kawaguchi Y, Hara M, Wright TM. *Endogenous IL-1alpha from systemic sclerosis fibroblasts induces IL-6 and PDGF-A. J Clin Invest* 1999;103:1253-1260.

SYSTEMIC SCLEROSIS
B. Clinical Features

Systemic sclerosis (SSc) is a chronic multisystem disease (1). The initial symptoms typically are nonspecific and include Raynaud's phenomenon, fatigue or lack of energy, and musculoskeletal complaints. These symptoms may persist for weeks or months before other signs emerge. The first specific clinical clue to suggest a diagnosis of SSc is skin thickening that begins as swelling or "puffiness" of the fingers and hands. The subsequent course of clinical events is highly variable, but significant skin, pulmonary, cardiac, gastrointestinal, or renal disease can occur.

Systemic sclerosis is classified into subsets of disease defined by the degree of clinically involved skin (Table 18B-1). People with limited SSc have cutaneous thickening of the distal limbs without truncal involvement. The CREST syndrome of Calcinosis, Raynaud's phenomenon, Esophageal dysmotility, Sclerodactyly, and Telangiectasia falls within the limited subset of SSc. People with diffuse SSc have skin thickening over distal and proximal limb sites and/or the trunk. Established criteria for a diagnosis of SSc require skin thickening proximal to the metacarpophalangeal joints or signs of digital ischemia and pulmonary fibrosis (see Appendix I). The criteria are designed to be specific, and are relatively insensitive. Patients without skin changes (SSc sine scleroderma) and many patients with lim-

ited skin changes or the CREST syndrome do not meet these criteria, although they clearly have SSc. Some health care professionals advocate expanding the SSc spectrum to include patients with definite Raynaud's phenomenon and other features of SSc, including SSc nail-fold capillary changes and/or SSc-specific autoantibodies.

Patients with limited SSc usually have Raynaud's phenomenon for years, often one to 10 years, before other signs of the disease become evident. They are less likely than people with diffuse disease to develop severe lung, heart, or kidney disease, although all of these diseases can occur. Most patients with limited SSc gradually develop features of the CREST syndrome. Subcutaneous calcinosis presents as small, localized, hard masses on fingers, forearms, or other pressure points (Fig. 18B-1). Telangiectasias frequently become numerous, particularly on the face, mucous membranes, and hands. Serious manifestations of limited SSc include pulmonary hypertension, typically in the absence of severe pulmonary fibrosis, and arterial occlusive disease, indicated by digital ischemia and the need for amputation (2).

In contrast to limited SSc, diffuse SSc develops with only a short interval between the onset of Raynaud's phenomenon and significant organ involvement. Inflammatory signs that

TABLE 18B-1
Subsets of Systemic Sclerosis

Diffuse cutaneous systemic sclerosis
- Proximal skin thickening involving face/neck, trunk, and symmetrically, the fingers, hands, arms, and legs
- Rapid onset of disease following appearance of Raynaud's phenomenon
- Significant visceral disease: lung, heart, gastrointestinal, or kidney
- Associated with antinuclear antibodies and absence of anticentromere antibody
- Variable disease course but overall poor prognosis: survival 40%–60% at 10 years

Limited cutaneous systemic sclerosis
- Skin thickening limited to symmetrical change of fingers, distal arms, legs, and face/neck
- Progression of disease after onset of Raynaud's phenomenon
- Late visceral disease with prominent hypertension and digital amputation
- CREST syndrome
- Association with anticentromere antibody
- Relatively good prognosis: survival ≥70% at 10 years

Overlap syndromes
- Diffuse or limited systemic sclerosis with typical features of one or more of the other connective-tissue diseases
- Mixed connective-tissue disease: features of systemic lupus erythematosus, systemic sclerosis, polymyositis, rheumatoid arthritis, and presence of anti-U_1 RNP

Undefined connective-tissue disease
- Patients with features of systemic sclerosis who do not have definite clinical or laboratory findings to make a diagnosis

Localized scleroderma
- Morphea: plaques of fibrotic skin and subcutaneous tissue without systemic disease
- Linear scleroderma: longitudinal fibrotic bands that occur predominantly on extremities and involve skin and deeper tissues

appear in the early stages include edematous skin, painful joints and muscles, and in some cases, tendon friction rubs. Rapidly progressive skin changes appear during the first months of disease and continue for approximately two to three years, after which the skin tends to soften and either thin or return toward normal texture. Severe fibrosis of the skin causes irreversible atrophic changes and tethering to deeper tissue. This particularly is a problem in the fingers and hands and causes significant disability (Fig. 18B-2).

The overall course of SSc is highly variable, and disease activity is difficult to measure. However, once a remission occurs, relapse is uncommon. The diffuse form of the disease generally has a worse prognosis, with a 10-year survival rate of approximately 40%–60%, compared with a ≥70% 10-year survival rate in the limited form (3). Cardiopulmonary disease is the leading cause of death. Factors suggesting a poor prognosis include diffuse skin involvement, late age of disease onset, African- or Native-American race, the presence of tendon rubs, a diffusing capacity <40% of predicted values, the presence of a large pericardial effusion, proteinuria, hematuria, renal failure, low hemoglobin, elevated erythrocyte sedimentation rate, and abnormal electrocardiogram (4).

Serologic studies can help predict clinical features and survival. People with SSc and anticentromere antibodies (associated with the CREST syndrome) have relatively good prognoses, but may develop pulmonary hypertension or primary biliary cirrhosis, and may require digital amputation. Anti-RNA polymerase antibodies increase the risk of cardiac or renal disease, and antifibrillarin antibodies are associated with heart and lung involvement; the presence of either of these antibodies predicts a poor prognosis. Patients with antitopoisomerase and anti-U_1 RNP antibodies have intermediate survival rates and high risks of pulmonary disease.

Raynaud's Phenomenon

Patients with Raynaud's phenomenon complain of cold hands and feet associated with color changes of the skin of the digits (5). These symptoms appear suddenly as attacks that are triggered by cold temperature or emotional stress. Closure of the muscular digital arteries, precapillary arterioles, and arteriovenous shunts of the skin in response to temperature and neural signals cause skin pallor, followed by cyanosis. Reversal of the vasospastic period (rewarming) generally occurs 10 to 15 minutes after the stimulus has ended; the digits then return to normal color, have a blushed appearance, or appear mottled. The diagnosis of Raynaud's phenomenon usually is based on a compelling history of these features.

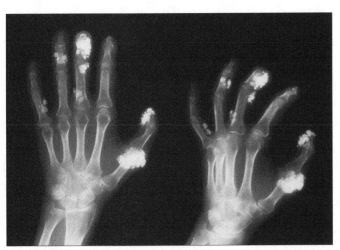

Fig. 18B-1. Radiograph demonstrating subcutaneous calcinosis on the fingers of a person with CREST syndrome.

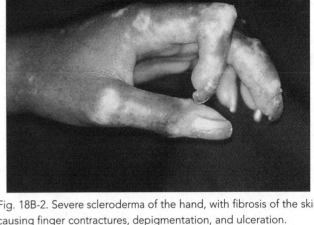

Fig. 18B-2. Severe scleroderma of the hand, with fibrosis of the skin causing finger contractures, depigmentation, and ulceration.

Surveys indicate that 4%–15% of the general population have symptoms of Raynaud's phenomenon (6). However, in most instances, symptoms are mild and not associated with either structural vascular changes or ischemic tissue damage. When there is no defined underlying cause and the physical examination and laboratory results are normal, *primary* Raynaud's phenomenon is the appropriate term. Onset of primary Raynaud's phenomenon typically occurs between the ages of 15 and 25 years. When the attacks are intense or begin after the age of 20, there is a greater likelihood that Raynaud's phenomenon is secondary to an underlying medical condition (Table 18B-2). Enlarged capillary loops and loss of normal capillaries in the nail fold of the digits are physical signs that help distinguish SSc from primary Raynaud's phenomenon.

More than 90% of people with SSc have Raynaud's phenomenon associated with tissue fibrosis of the fingers, loss of the digital pads (sclerodactyly), digital ulceration, and on occasion, ischemic demarcation and the need for digital amputation. In addition to the vasospasm of Raynaud's phenomenon, vascular occlusion occurs because of fibrosis of the intimal layer of the vessel, platelet activation, perturbation of the clotting cascade, and fibrin deposition. In SSc, strong evidence suggests the presence of "systemic" Raynaud's phenomenon, a generalized vasospastic disorder involving vasculopathy of the terminal arterial circulation of the lungs, kidneys, and heart.

Skin

In the earliest ("edematous") stage of disease, the skin appears mildly inflamed with nonpitting edema and, in some cases, erythema. Pruritus and swelling are associated with lymphocyte infiltration of the skin, fibroblast and mast cell activation, and local release of cytokines into the skin. Collagen deposition from activated fibroblasts thickens the dermis, with gradual damage to the normal skin and its appendages. The patient feels progressive tightening of

the skin and decreased flexibility. In diffuse SSc, the skin changes are widespread, and varying degrees of hypo- and hyperpigmentary changes may occur, giving the skin a tanned or "salt and pepper" appearance.

As SSc progresses into the fibrotic stage, the skin becomes more thickened, and severe drying of the surface provokes pruritus. This stage may persist and worsen over a period of one to three years or longer. Finally, inflammation and further fibrosis seem to cease as the atrophic stage begins. The skin then becomes atrophic and thinned, with tethering secondary to the binding of fibrotic tissue to underlying structures. Painful ulcerations can occur at sites of flexion contractures (e.g., the proximal interphalangeal joints) (Fig. 18B-2). In this late stage, other areas of the skin gradually remodel and may appear clinically normal, especially the trunk and proximal limbs.

Subcutaneous calcinosis composed of amorphous calcium hydroxyapatite is more prominent in limited SSc (Fig. 18B-1). This crystalline material can ulcerate the skin or cause recurrent episodes of local inflammation that mimic infection. Digital lesions observed in SSc include fissures, paronychia, and ulcerations due to trauma, ischemia, or both. Dilated capillary loops and areas of the loss of capillaries in the skin of the nail fold are characteristic of SSc. Telangiectasias are prominent in the skin of people with the CREST syndrome, and they also are seen in late diffuse SSc, especially on the trunk and back.

Musculoskeletal

Nonspecific musculoskeletal complaints, such as arthralgias and myalgias, are one of the earliest symptoms of SSc. A rheumatoid-like polyarthritis occasionally is seen, but pain and stiffness over joints generally are out of proportion with objective inflammatory signs. Discomfort can extend along tendons and into muscles of the arms and legs. Pain on motion of the ankle, wrist, knee, or elbow may be accompanied by a coarse friction rub caused by inflamma-

TABLE 18B-2
Causes of Secondary Raynaud's Phenomenon

Connective-tissue diseases
 Polymyositis and dermatomyositis
 Systemic sclerosis
 Sjögren's syndrome
 Systemic lupus erythematosus
 Systemic vasculitis
 Undifferentiated connective-tissue disease

Drugs and toxins
 Amphetamines
 Clonidine
 Ergotamines
 Vinblastine and bleomycin
 Vinyl chloride exposure

Structural arterial disease
 Athero-emboli
 Atherosclerosis
 Thoracic outlet syndrome
 Thromboangiitis obliterans (Buerger's disease)

Occupational disorders
 Hand-arm vibration syndrome
 Hypothenar hammer syndrome

Hematologic Diseases
 Cold agglutinin disease
 Cryoglobulinemia
 Paraproteinemia

Other
 Hypothyroidism
 Paraneoplastic
 Post-frostbite
 Reflex sympathetic dystrophy

tion and fibrosis of the tendon sheath or adjacent tissues. These rubs almost always are seen in diffuse skin disease and may predict a worse overall clinical outcome.

The dominant musculoskeletal problem in late SSc is muscle atrophy and weakness (7). Disuse and deconditioning resulting from contractures of fibrotic skin, along with malnutrition, are the major causes. However, muscle inflammation associated with a mild elevation in serum creatine kinase also may occur. An "overlap" syndrome with an inflammatory myopathy typical of dermatomyositis or polymyositis frequently is overlooked because of the severity of other, more obvious causes of weakness. Myopathy secondary to medications used in the treatment of SSc (e.g., corticosteroids, D-penicillamine) can mimic inflammatory or SSc muscle disease.

Pulmonary

Lung impairment is the leading cause of mortality in SSc (8). The most common initial symptom is dyspnea on exertion, without cough or chest pain. Pulmonary function testing may detect significant reductions in lung volumes or diffusing capacity early in the disease process, when lung involvement usually is clinically silent. Cough, a late manifestation of SSc lung disease, can be confused with gastrointestinal reflux or bronchitis. Chest pain generally is not caused by SSc lung disease, but may occur secondary to another process, such as musculoskeletal pain, esophageal reflux disease, or pericarditis.

Breathlessness results from a reduction in normal gas transfer from the alveolar space into the pulmonary circulation. This reduction may be caused by a fibrosing alveolitis that progresses to interstitial fibrosis and loss of lung volume (i.e., a restrictive ventilatory defect) or a pulmonary vasculopathy characterized by endothelial cell dysfunction and intimal fibrosis. Most patients have evidence of both interstitial fibrosis and pulmonary vascular disease. However, severe pulmonary fibrosis is more common among patients with diffuse skin disease, African American or Native American patients, and patients with antitopoisomerase antibodies. In contrast, isolated pulmonary hypertension without fibrosis is associated with the CREST syndrome.

Early detection of active lung disease is important, and periodic pulmonary function testing and 2D-echocardiography (2D-ECHO) are the most effective methods of detection. Physical examination and chest radiographs are relatively insensitive, but in advanced disease, lower-lobe fibrosis is found. Pulmonary function testing usually detects low lung volumes consistent with a restrictive ventilatory defect. An isolated, low diffusing capacity suggests either early restrictive lung disease or incipient pulmonary vascular disease. Active alveolitis can be detected by high-resolution computed tomography and/or bronchoalveolar lavage (BAL) studies. An abnormally high percentage of neutrophils in the BAL fluid predicts progressive interstitial lung disease. Approximately 35% of people with SSc will have pulmonary hypertension, as defined by a 2D-ECHO study. Clinical signs of pulmonary hypertension, an elevated right ventricular pressure, and a low diffusing capacity of less than 40% of predicted are all associated with a high mortality rate.

The disease process in the lung follows a highly variable course. The majority of patients have early, but modest, declines in lung function tests and then follow stable courses reflecting inactive lung disease (9). Approximately 20% of patients have an insidious decline that may lead to severe impairment of lung function and physical capacity in months. Less common problems of the lung include aspiration secondary to esophageal dysfunction or pharyngeal disease, chronic cough, respiratory distress associated with muscle disease, pulmonary hemorrhage, and pneumothorax. An increased prevalence of lung cancer exists among people with SSc.

Gastrointestinal

Gastrointestinal tract dysfunction is one of the most common problems encountered in SSc, and is found in diffuse and limited disease (10). A small oral aperture (Fig. 18B-3), dry mucosal membranes, and periodontal disease can lead to problems with chewing foods, loss of teeth, and poor nutrition. Dysphagia and heartburn are the most common gastrointestinal symptoms found in SSc, but severe esophageal reflux and esophagitis also can occur, with few symptoms. Studies with esophageal manometry have correlated loss of secondary peristalsis in the distal esophagus with loss of normal esophageal clearance and serious reflux. Untreated or persistent esophagitis can lead to erosions and bleeding, stricture, Barrett's metaplasia, and possibly adenocarcinoma. Other uncommonly recognized complications of esophageal disease include aspiration, unexplained coughing, hoarseness, and atypical chest pain.

In the early stages of SSc, abnormal function of the smooth muscle in the distal two-thirds of the esophagus likely is secondary to neuromuscular dysfunction. Later, there is smooth-muscle atrophy and fibrosis, as well as excess collagen deposition in the lamina propria and submucosa. Esophageal disease is associated with decreased pressures in the lower esophageal sphincter and poor gastric emptying. Delayed emptying of the stomach, associated with retention of solid foods, aggravates reflux and causes early satiety, bloating, nausea, and vomiting.

Dysmotility of the small intestine may be asymptomatic, or it can cause serious chronic pseudo-obstruction of the intestine, which presents with severe distension, abdominal pain, and vomiting. Mild abdominal distension, crampy abdominal pain, diarrhea, weight loss, and malnutrition also can be consequences of malabsorption caused by bacterial overgrowth in stagnant intestinal fluids. Occasionally, patients with advanced bowel disease have pneumatosis cystoides intestinalis caused by the dissection of intestinal gas into the bowel wall. Pneumatosis cystoides intestinalis may mimic a ruptured bowel if gas leaks into the peritoneal cavity. Although the presence of pneumatosis cystoides intestinalis is a poor prognostic sign, no medical (or surgical) intervention is required.

SSc also affects the large intestine and rectum. As a consequence of muscular atrophy of the large bowel wall, asymptomatic wide-mouth diverticula unique to SSc commonly are found in the transverse and descending colon (Fig. 18B-4). Fecal incontinence that is difficult to manage can be a consequence of fibrosis of the rectal sphincters.

Cardiac

The clinical manifestations of SSc heart disease are quite variable, usually subtle in expression, and often not seen until late in the course of the disease (11). Symptoms include dyspnea on exertion, palpitations, and less frequently, chest discomfort. Pathologic studies of the SSc heart and sensitive diagnostic testing have documented that

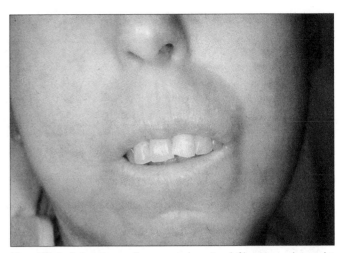

Fig. 18B-3. Scleroderma has caused perioral fibrosis and a tight pursed-lip appearance, with small oral aperture. Facial telangiectasia also is present.

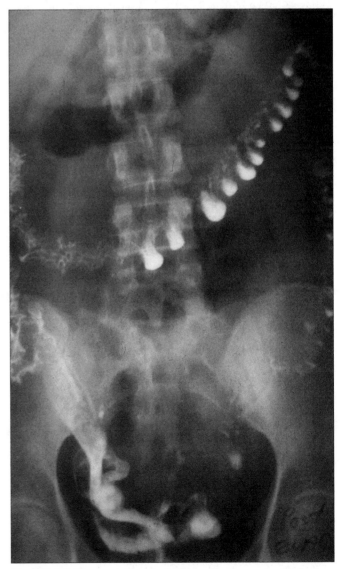

Fig. 18B-4. Wide-mouth diverticuli of the colon is seen on this barium study of a person with systemic sclerosis.

the myocardium, myocardial blood vessels, and the pericardium commonly are involved – particularly in patients with diffuse disease. Overt clinical signs of any cardiac disease correlate with a poor prognosis.

Patchy fibrosis throughout the entire myocardium unrelated to extramural coronary artery disease is characteristic of SSc. Areas of contraction-band necrosis are thought to occur as a consequence of hypoxia/reperfusion injury due to vasospasm of distal coronary vessels. Supporting this theory of vascular heart disease is the finding on thallium scintigraphy of perfusion defects that increase in number during cold provocation of Raynaud's attacks. Echocardiographic studies demonstrate that diastolic dysfunction occurs frequently. Decline in the left ventricular ejection fraction is a late clinical manifestation. Cardiomyopathy also can be a consequence of an associated inflammatory autoimmune myocarditis.

Small or large pericardial effusions can be demonstrated by echocardiography in 30%–40% of primarily asymptomatic SSc patients. Clinically overt pericarditis is uncommon, and cardiac tamponade is rare. Electrocardiograms often demonstrate asymptomatic conduction-system disease.

Renal

Although pathologic disease of the kidney almost always is present in SSc, the most important clinical manifestation is the SSc renal crisis, characterized by accelerated hypertension and/or rapidly progressive renal failure (12). Approximately 80% of cases of renal crisis occur within the first four or five years of disease, usually in patients with diffuse disease. The patient's blood pressure usually is abnormal (>150/90 mm Hg), but occasionally, normotensive crises occur. Laboratory data associated with SSc renal crisis include a high creatinine level, proteinuria, and microscopic hematuria. In severe cases, anemia and thrombocytopenia occur secondary to a microangiopathic process within the constricted renal vessels.

Poorer outcomes are more likely in men, patients with an older age of onset, and those who present with creatinine levels greater than 3 mg/dL. Risk factors for renal crisis include diffuse skin disease, new unexplained anemia, use of corticosteroids, pregnancy, and the presence of anti-RNA polymerase III antibodies. SSc patients may have reduced creatinine clearance, proteinuria, microscopic hematuria, and nonmalignant hypertension, but other causes for these abnormalities often are discovered.

Other Signs

Nearly 50% of people with SSc have symptoms of depression, often major depression that is responsive to treatment (13). Sexual dysfunction also is common. Impotence among male patients usually is secondary to organic neurovascular disease. The sicca complex is a frequent problem, with associated Sjögren's syndrome accounting for the majority of cases. Aggressive dental care and frequent use of topical natural tears to protect the cornea are important. Neuropathy

from carpal tunnel syndrome may require surgical release. Trigeminal neuralgia has been reported and may respond to tricyclic antidepressants or a neuroleptic drug. Hypothyroidism secondary to thyroid fibrosis or autoimmune thyroiditis is a common problem. Liver disease is infrequent, but primary biliary cirrhosis and autoimmune hepatitis have been associated with the CREST syndrome.

SSc-Like Disorders

Localized Scleroderma

Localized scleroderma denotes a condition characterized by circumscribed fibrotic areas involving different levels of the skin and, sometimes, the underlying soft tissue, muscle, and bone (14). It is seen more commonly in children and young women (15). The clinical course usually is benign, with the fibrosis limited to the skin and no internal organ disease. Localized scleroderma is divided into several subtypes: isolated morphea (a 1–15-cm plaque); generalized morphea (multiple lesions); linear scleroderma; nodular (keloid) scleroderma; and rarely, localized bullous lesions. A patient may have both linear scleroderma and morphea lesions. Adults can present with generalized morphea that follows a linear pattern on the body.

Localized scleroderma usually presents as a nonspecific area of erythema and pain that then expands, with an ivory-like fibrotic center surrounded by a margin of hyperpigmentation that is lilac in appearance. The lesion is characterized by infiltration of lymphocytes, mast cells, plasma cells, and eosinophils, with excess collagen deposition extending into the dermis, the subcutaneous fat and, in some forms, deeper structures. Lesions are distributed asymmetrically or become confluent in generalized morphea. Morphea lesions remain active for weeks to several years, but spontaneous softening that leaves a pigmented area is the rule.

Linear scleroderma is more common on the lower extremities. It appears as a nondermatomal fibrotic band that infiltrates skin, subcutaneous fat, fascia, and muscle. The fibrotic band disrupts normal bone growth and can cause disabling joint contractures. Midline facial involvement has been termed "en coup de sabre" to describe a deformity similar to the wound of a sword. This lesion may progress over years, causing severe facial hemiatrophy and linear hair loss

The cause of localized scleroderma is unknown, but genetic, infectious, and autoimmune mechanisms have been suggested. Autoantibodies, usually antinuclear antibodies and antibodies to single-stranded DNA and histone, frequently are detected in localized scleroderma. No treatment clearly alters the natural course of localized scleroderma, but moderate doses of systemic or locally injected corticosteroids, oral or topical vitamin D, weekly oral methotrexate, D-penicillamine, and photochemotherapy with 8-methoxypsoralen have been reported helpful.

Environment-Associated Disorders

Although various occupations and environmental exposures are suggested to cause SSc, there is no definitive evidence on the biologic importance of these associations (16). The most impressive finding is the association between SSc and silica dust (quartz) exposure in males who are stone masons or miners. Although exposure to silica dust increases the risk of developing typical diffuse SSc, this does not explain most male SSc cases. The role of solvent exposure (e.g., trichlorethylene, perchlorethylene) as a risk factor for SSc is debated. Mercury exposure, postmenopausal estrogen replacement, pesticides, and amines in epoxy resins also have been implicated in triggering SSc. Occupational acroosteolysis is an SSc-like illness that is associated with industrial exposure to vinyl chloride.

The association of silicone (a synthetic polymer containing silicon) and SSc or another connective-tissue disease has been suggested by anecdotal case reports of autoimmune disease in women who were exposed to silicone following breast augmentation. However, epidemiologic studies, including case-control investigations of large populations of women with and without SSc, have found no association between breast implants and SSc or other connective-tissue diseases (17).

Diffuse Fasciitis With Eosinophilia

Diffuse fasciitis with eosinophilia (DFE; also called eosinophilic fasciitis and Shulman's syndrome) occurs sporadically and mimics SSc, with swelling, stiffness, and decreased flexibility of the limbs associated with thickening of the subcutaneous tissue (18). Although it can be widespread and involve the trunk and limbs, in contrast to SSc, DFE usually spares the fingers, hands, and face. Raynaud's phenomenon, visceral involvement, and microvascular disease are absent, distinguishing DFE from SSc. Fibrosis puckers the overlying tissues ("peau d'orange" skin) and entraps subcutaneous veins, but the overlying skin still wrinkles. A diagnosis of DFE depends on histologic findings from a deep biopsy that includes skin, subcutaneous tissue, and muscle. Inflammation in subcutaneous tissue is characterized by mononuclear cell infiltration and, in some cases, striking tissue eosinophilia. Autoantibodies usually are absent, but peripheral eosinophilia and hypergammaglobulinemia are typical.

The cause of DFE is unknown, although approximately 30% of case series report the onset of DFE following vigorous exercise. There has been a temporal association with various hematologic conditions, including aplastic anemia, myelomonocytic and chronic lymphocytic leukemia, thrombocytopenia, monoclonal gammopathy, myeloproliferative syndrome, and lymphomas. DFE has been seen in late graft-versus-host disease and in association with some solid tumors. Toxin(s) and drug exposure also have been suggested as triggers.

The natural course of DFE is not well-defined, but patients seem to spontaneously regress or remain unchanged for years. Approximately 70% of cases appear to respond to corticosteroids. Physical therapy and monitoring for associated hematologic problems are highly recommended.

Epidemic Forms of SSc-Like Symptoms

Eosinophilia myalgia syndrome (EMS) and toxic oil syndrome (TOS) are toxin-induced disorders that mimic SSc and provide indirect evidence that environmental toxins could cause idiopathic SSc (19). Both syndromes are associated with subcutaneous tissue fibrosis. EMS was first reported in 1989, in association with the use of the amino acid L-tryptophan for such conditions as insomnia and depression. Certain batches of the L-tryptophan were contaminated with several potential toxins, including 1,1′-ethylidenebis(L-tryptophan) (EBT) and 3-(phenyl-amino)alanine. EMS presented as a multisystem disease with intense myalgias, arthralgias, fever, and a papular rash associated with eosinophilia. Subcutaneous edema with woody induration occurred, similar to DFE and mimicking SSc. A chronic phase of EMS is characterized by SSc-like skin changes, recurrent myalgias, paresthesias with peripheral neuropathy, neurocognitive dysfunction, and chronic fatigue. Treatment with corticosteroids appears to help in the acute inflammatory phase, but it is not clear that any agent alters the course or the chronic phase of EMS. A variety of agents, including nonsteroidal anti-inflammatory drugs, D-penicillamine, methotrexate, cyclophosphamide, azathioprine, and cyclosporine, have been used to treat EMS.

A TOS epidemic occurred in 1981, following individuals' ingestion of rapeseed oil denatured with aniline. TOS causes a widespread vasculopathy, characterized by inflammatory cells in the vessel wall and subintimal fibrosis in almost every organ. After an acute illness characterized by pulmonary infiltrates and myalgias, patients develop a chronic disease with Raynaud's phenomenon, muscle atrophy, fatigue, and musculoskeletal pain. Biopsy material from EMS and TOS patients demonstrates the presence of the profibrotic cytokines transforming growth factor β and platelet-derived growth factor AA, which suggests that toxins can induce production of these mediators of fibrosis. Although corticosteroids appear to help the acute phase of TOS, no therapy has been proven to alter the course of the disease.

Other SSc-Like Disorders

Scleredema can be either a transient illness of unknown cause or a fibrotic condition of the skin associated with insulin-dependent diabetes. Scleredema typically affects the neck, shoulder girdle, and upper back, with relative sparing of the hands and no symptoms of Raynaud's phenomenon. Sclerodactyly and fibrosis of the palmar fascia can occur in insulin-dependent diabetes, particularly the juvenile-onset type. SSc-like skin changes have been reported in other disorders, including the carcinoid syndrome, myeloma or paraproteinemia, scleromyxedema (papular mucinosis), chronic graft-versus-host disease, porphyria cutanea tarda, Werner's syndrome, progeria, phenylketonuria, bleomycin exposure, local lipodystrophies, and POEMS syndrome (*P*lasma cell dyscrasia, *P*olyneuropathy, *O*rganomegaly, *E*ndocrinopathy, *M*onoclonal spikes, and *S*Sc-like skin changes)(20).

FREDRICK M. WIGLEY, MD

References

1. Clements PJ, Furst DE (eds). Systemic Sclerosis. Baltimore: Williams & Wilkins, 1996.
2. Wigley FM, Wise RA, Miller R, Needleman BW, Spence RJ. Anticentromere antibody as a predictor of digital ischemic loss in patients with systemic sclerosis. Arthritis Rheum 1992;35: 688–693.
3. Mayes MD. Scleroderma epidemiology. Rheum Dis Clin North Am 1996;22:751–764.
4. Bryan C, Knight C, Black CM, Silman AJ. Prediction of five-year survival following presentation with scleroderma: development of a simplet model using three disease factors at first visit. Arthritis Rheum 1999;42:2660–2665.
5. Wigley FM, Flavahan NA. Raynaud's phenomenon. Rheum Dis Clin North Am 1996;22:765–782.
6. Maricq HR, Carpentier PH, Weinrich MC, et al. Geographic variation in the prevalence of Raynaud's phenomenon: Charleston, SC, USA, vs. Tarentaise, Savoie, France. J Rheumatol 1993;20:70–76.
7. Clements PJ, Furst DE, Campion DS, et al. Muscle disease in systemic sclerosis. Diagnostic and therapeutic considerations. Arthritis Rheum 1978;21:62–71.
8. Black CM, DuBois RM. Organ involvement: pulmonary. In: Clements PJ, Furst DE (eds). Systemic Sclerosis. Baltimore: Williams & Wilkins, 1996; pp 299–331.
9. Schneider PD, Wise RA, Hochberg MC, Wigley FM. Serial pulmonary function test in systemic sclerosis. Am J Med 1982; 73:385–394.
10. Sjögren RW. Gastrointestinal motility in scleroderma. Arthritis Rheum 1994;37:1265–1282.
11. Deswal A, Follansbee WP. Cardiac involvement in scleroderma. Rheum Dis Clin North Am 1996;22:841–860.
12. Steen VD. Scleroderma renal crisis. Rheum Dis Clin North Am 1996;22:861–878.
13. Roca RP, Wigley FM. Psychosocial aspects in systemic sclerosis. In: Clements PJ, Furst DE (eds). Systemic Sclerosis. Baltimore: Williams & Wilkins, 1996; pp 501–511.
14. Peterson LS, Nelson AM, Su WP. Classification of morphea (localized SSc). Mayo Clin Proc 1995;70:1068–1076.
15. Uziel Y, Krafchik B, Silverman ED, Thorner PS, Laxer RM. Localized scleroderma in childhood: a report of 30 cases. Semin Arthritis Rheum 1994;23:328–340.
16. Silman AJ, Hochberg MC. Occupational and environmental influences on scleroderma. Rheum Dis Clin North Am 1996; 22:737–749.
17. Gabriel SE, O'Fallon WM, Kurland LT, Beard CM, Woods JE, Melton LJ III. Risk of connective tissue diseases and other diseases after breast implantation. N Engl J Med 1994;330: 1697–1702.
18. Lakhanpal S, Ginsburg WW, Michet CJ, Doyle JA, Moore SB. Eosinophilia fasciitis: clinical spectrum and therapeutic response in 52 cases. Semin Arth Rheum 1988;17:221–231.
19. Varga J, Kahari VM. Eosinophilia-myalgia syndrome, eosinophilic fasciitis and related fibrosing syndromes. Curr Opin Rheumatol 1997;9:562–570.
20. Jablonska S, Blaszczyk. Differential diagnosis of SSc-like disorders. In: Clements PJ, Furst DE (eds). Systemic Sclerosis. Baltimore: Williams & Wilkins, 1996; pp 99–120.

SYSTEMIC SCLEROSIS
C. Treatment

Systemic sclerosis (SSc) has a wide spectrum of clinical manifestations and severity, as well as a variable course. Spontaneous improvement occurs frequently, rendering interpretation of therapeutic interventions difficult without comparison groups. Therapy can be divided into two categories: disease-modifying and symptomatic (organ-specific). Treatment that prolongs life or prevents heart, lung, or kidney damage can be considered disease-modifying. Guidelines for evaluating possible disease-modifying interventions have been published (1), but only the use of angiotensin-converting enzyme (ACE) inhibitors in patients with renal crisis meet that definition. Conversely, numerous symptomatic (organ-specific) therapies, almost all borrowed from other fields of medicine, have improved the management of organ complications in SSc. Evaluation of treatments as disease-modifying or symptomatic has been aided by the development of measures that quantify changes in the disease, including skin thickness, lung function, cardiac contractility, functional ability, and renal function) (1,2).

Disease-Modifying Interventions

Treatment of SSc can be based on a model of its pathogenesis (see Fig. 18A-4). This model posits a genetic background upon which external stimuli act, resulting in immune activation, vascular injury, fibroblast proliferation, and collagen deposition (3). Collagen, in turn, increases immune activation, resulting in perpetuation of the activation/injury cycle. If this pathogenetic model holds true, intervention can occur at the level of preventing vascular injury, forestalling fibrosis, or immunosuppression.

Several treatments previously considered disease-modifying have undergone evaluations in randomized, controlled trials. The effectiveness of penicillamine (4), chlorambucil, ketanserin, interferon (IFN)-α (5), and photopheresis was not supported in these trials. Methotrexate was the subject of two randomized, controlled trials. One study showed trends favoring methotrexate over placebo for skin-softening and general well-being, but a larger trial was reported as negative, in abstract form (6,7).

Although the immunosuppressive agents cyclosporine and IFN-γ have shown promise for improving skin-thickening in small, uncontrolled series, both drugs have substantial toxicity, including hypertension and renal impairment (8,9). One very small, randomized, controlled trial of IFN-γ failed to show efficacy, compared with placebo (10). The clinical usefulness of cyclosporine and IFN-γ has yet to be demonstrated.

A 24-week, randomized, placebo-controlled trial showed that the subcutaneous infusion of recombinant human relaxin in doses (25 μg/kg/day) that produce serum levels three to five times those of pregnancy decreased skin-thickening in patients with diffuse cutaneous scleroderma to a greater extent than did placebo (11). Unfortunately, a larger, placebo-controlled trial failed to show that the course of skin-thickening or other clinical variables in the two drug groups was significantly different from that of the placebo group (unpublished observations).

Minocycline, oral bovine collagen type I, immunoablation with peripheral-blood stem-cell rescue, and halofuginone have shown promise, but their clinical efficacy awaits confirmation in controlled studies.

Symptomatic (Organ-Specific)
Skin
Because the skin's natural ability to moisturize is impaired in SSc, local skin care with topical moisturizers is essential. Pruritus can be very troublesome, especially early in diffuse scleroderma. Oral antihistamines, topical analgesics (e.g., lidocaine and dibucaine), and topical corticosteroids are worth trying, but often are incompletely effective. Fortunately, pruritus usually subsides with time.

Skin ulcers should be kept clean with mild soap and water. Topical antibiotic ointments (especially ointments with local analgesics) can be applied. Analgesics are important for pain control. Infected ulcers should be treated with antistaphylococcal antibiotics.

No treatment has been shown to prevent subcutaneous calcinosis. However, a short course of oral colchicine may reduce the inflammatory response to hydroxyapatite crystals. When calcinosis leads to skin breakdown and drainage, surgical debridement may be indicated, with the expectation of good healing by primary or secondary intention.

Raynaud's Phenomenon and Ischemia
Raynaud's phenomenon affects the vast majority of people with SSc. Its management should be appropriate to its level of severity. All patients should be cautioned to avoid cold exposure when possible; to use layers of warm, loose-fitting clothing (including warm socks, headgear, and mittens/gloves) when in the cold; and to stop smoking. Raynaud's that interferes with daily activities or is complicated by digital-tip ulcers may require vasodilator therapy (particularly oral nifedipine or other calcium-channel blockers, prazosin, or topical nitroglycerin paste) and oral analgesics (often containing narcotics). In a recent, randomized, controlled trial, extended-release nifedipine diminished Raynaud's attacks. In the same trial, biofeedback was ineffective (12).

Fingers and toes that are frankly necrotic or constantly blue/purple and painful are truly ischemic and require more aggressive treatment. Intravenous prostaglandin (PGE$_1$; i.e., alprostadil) and prostacyclin (PGI$_2$; i.e., epoprostenol) may be infused continuously in hospital or by daily, six- to eight-hour outpatient infusions over three to five days (13). Medical lumbar or cervical sympathetic blocks may be used as primary treatment or as a way to determine the potential for reversal of vasospasm prior to performing permanent sympathectomies. Surgical micro-arteriolysis (digital sympathectomy) and vascular reconstruction also can be considered. Amputation is a last resort.

Gastrointestinal
Smooth-muscle hypomotility is the primary pathophysiologic abnormality that underlies gastrointestinal involvement (14). Reflux esophagitis and dysphagia are the most common clinical manifestations of esophageal involvement. Ideally, treatment should correct predisposing conditions, suppress acid production, and improve motility. Nonpharmacologic treatments include elevating the head of the bed (by four to six inches), eating frequent small meals (five to six per day), avoiding lying down within three or four hours of eating, and abstaining from caffeine-containing beverages and cigarette smoking.

Pharmacologic therapies, such as oral antacids and H$_2$ blockers, may control minor reflux symptoms, but proton-pump inhibitors (e.g., omeprazole and lansoprazole) are the drugs of choice for more severe complaints, such as esophageal strictures and recalcitrant reflux (14). Proton-pump inhibitors help control gastrointestinal side effects of calcium-channel blockers and nonsteroidal anti-inflammatory drugs, and are used in the management of bleeding from the upper gastrointestinal tract (e.g., watermelon stomach and erosive esophagitis). Esophageal strictures usually respond to periodic dilatation and proton-pump inhibition. Surgical procedures to prevent reflux have not met with general acceptance.

Gastroparesis frequently aggravates reflux and often underlies the symptoms of early satiety, nausea, and vomiting. Promotility agents (i.e., metoclopramide) may be helpful. Small intestinal dysmotility may cause postprandial bloating, diarrhea, malabsorption, weight loss, and pseudo-obstruction (14). Broad-spectrum antibiotics (e.g., amoxicillin, metronidazole, doxycycline, vancomycin, trimethoprim-sulfamethoxazole, and ciprofloxacin) given in rotating, two-week courses may improve symptoms dramatically. Promotility agents, such as metoclopramide, erythromycin, and octreotide, also may help. Supplementation with fat-soluble vitamins, calcium, vitamin B$_{12}$, and medium-chain triglycerides may be required for patients with malabsorption. Pseudo-obstruction should be managed medically with nasogastric suction, bowel rest, and parenteral alimentation. Cachexia and recalcitrant pseudo-obstruction are reasons to consider long-term, home-based, total parenteral hyperalimentation.

Constipation can be managed with increased fluid intake, increased dietary bulk, and stool softeners. Recalcitrant constipation may benefit from judicious amounts of oral osmotic colon cleansers containing polyethylene glycol and electrolytes (e.g., Nulytely and Golytely). Conversely, fecal incontinence may require control of diarrhea, which often is caused by small-bowel bacterial overgrowth, with rotating antibiotics, low-residue diet, antidiarrheal medications, bile-acid binding resins (e.g., cholestyramine), and biofeedback.

Cardiopulmonary

Interstitial pulmonary fibrosis and obstructive pulmonary vasculopathy are the two primary manifestations of pulmonary involvement in SSc. In their most severe forms, these complications can be fatal. Available data suggest that interstitial fibrosis usually is preceded by inflammatory alveolitis. Results from an uncontrolled series of 18 patients suggest that cyclophosphamide or azathioprine combined with low doses of corticosteroids may stabilize or improve lung function in patients with alveolitis (15). IFN-γ, proven effective in a small randomized trial of people with idiopathic pulmonary fibrosis (16), also holds promise in SSc. Although lung transplantation is reasonable for patients with end-stage disease, few such procedures have been performed for SSc. Periodic *Pneumococcal* pneumonia vaccines and annual flu shots are indicated.

In the past, severe pulmonary artery hypertension was uniformly fatal within five years of diagnosis. Conventional management of pulmonary artery hypertension includes low-flow nasal oxygen (especially at night), rigorous management of right-sided heart failure, smoking cessation, and possibly, anticoagulation therapy. Until the recent approval by the Food and Drug Administration of continuous ambulatory intravenous epoprostenol for SSc-related pulmonary hypertension, pharmacologic strategies (e.g., vasodilators, anti-inflammatory agents, and immunosuppressive agents) had been unsatisfactory. Intravenous epoprostenol was shown in a randomized, controlled trial to improve exercise capacity, hemodynamics, and dyspnea in SSc patients with pulmonary hypertension (13). Combined heart-lung or single-lung transplantation procedures are reasonable in severe cases, but few have been performed in people with SSc.

Pericarditis, congestive heart failure, and serious arrhythmias are the major cardiac complications of SSc. All are treated as they would be in any patient. Large pericardial effusions usually are not hemodynamically compromising and usually do not require pericardiocentesis. They are, however, a harbinger of renal crisis and should be viewed as an early warning sign.

Kidneys

Renal crisis (acute oliguric renal failure, usually associated with malignant hypertension) once was the most feared complication of SSc. With the introduction of ACE inhibitors, which reverse the hyper-reninemia and hypertension characteristic of renal crisis, the one-year survival rate has increased from 15% to 76% (17). Although angiotensin-II receptor inhibitors have been used in renal crisis, their benefit has not been as consistent. This finding may be related to a major difference in action between the two classes of drugs. Although both classes diminish the effects of angiotensin II, only ACE inhibitors increase levels of bradykinin and angiotensin 1-7, two potent renal vasodilators. ACE inhibitors remain the drugs of first choice for management of acute renal crisis. Once renal crisis is controlled, the angiotensin II receptor inhibitors may help maintain renal function and control hypertension. The ACE inhibitors or angiotensin II receptor inhibitors should be continued indefinitely.

The keys to successfully managing renal crisis are early detection (patients should take their blood pressure at home several times a week) and early introduction of ACE inhibitors and normalization of blood pressure. Other antihypertensives may be added, as needed. Despite these interventions, some patients will need dialysis, at least temporarily. As long as the ACE inhibitors are continued, approximately 50% of patients will have enough improvement in renal function to stop dialysis in six to 18 months. If dialysis is required after 18 months, renal transplantation should be considered.

Musculoskeletal

Musculoskeletal pain, arthritis, tendinitis (often with tendon friction rubs), muscle weakness, and joint contractures are common, especially in people with early diffuse cutaneous scleroderma. Treatment should include measures to relieve pain, to stretch contractures, and to strengthen weak muscles. Nonsteroidal anti-inflammatory drugs (NSAIDs) may reduce pain and stiffness and improve joint function. If gastrointestinal intolerance or complications occur, proton pump inhibitors may protect the esophagus and stomach. Cyclooxygenase-2 inhibitors may be useful in patients at risk for gastrointestinal bleeding. Pure analgesics, such as acetaminophen, propoxyphene, and tramadol, also may be useful. When these measures are inadequate, narcotic analgesics and low-dose corticosteroids (<10 mg/day of prednisone) may be added.

Physical therapy should be instituted early and aggressively in patients with rapidly progressive diffuse SSc and joint contractures. Patients and caregivers alike should be taught a home program of physical therapy. Because joint stretching may be painful, such prophylactic pain measures as NSAIDs, analgesics, and heat may be required before each stretching session. Dynamic splinting is not effective.

Muscle weakness is very common in SSc. Inflammatory myositis is not frequent but should be considered in the differential diagnosis of weakness, especially in the presence of significant elevations of serum creatine kinase. Corticosteroids and methotrexate are the drugs of choice for inflammatory myositis. More common causes of weakness in SSc are a noninflammatory myopathy (with mildly elevated creatine kinase levels) and deconditioning. These conditions should be approached by muscle strengthening exercises. If exercising is painful, pain-control modalities can be used prophylactically.

Carpal tunnel syndrome occasionally is an early event in SSc, often preceding the diagnosis of SSc. A combination of wrist splints and carpal tunnel injections of corticosteroids often suffice. Occasionally, surgical release of the carpal tunnel is indicated.

PHILIP J. CLEMENTS, MD

References

1. White B, Bauer EA, Goldsmith LA, et al. Guidelines for clinical trials in systemic sclerosis (scleroderma). I. Disease-modifying interventions. The American College of Rheumatology Committee on Design and Outcomes in Clinical Trials in Systemic Sclerosis. Arthritis Rheum 1995;38:351–360.
2. Clements P, Lachenbruch P, Seibold J, et al. Inter and intraobserver variability of total skin thickness score (modified Rodnan TSS) in systemic sclerosis. J Rheumatol 1995;22:1281–1285.
3. Furst DE, Clements PJ. Pathogenesis, fusion (summary). In: Clements PJ, Furst DE (eds). Systemic Sclerosis. Baltimore: Williams & Wilkins, 1996; pp 275–286.
4. Clements PJ, Furst DE, Wong WK, et al. High-dose versus low-dose D-penicillamine in early diffuse systemic sclerosis: analysis of a two-year, double-blind, randomized, controlled clinical trial. Arthritis Rheum 1999;42:1194–1203.
5. Black CM, Silman AJ, Herrick AI, et al. Interferon-alpha does not improve outcome at one year in patients with diffuse cutaneous scleroderma: results of a randomized, double-blind, placebo-controlled trial. Arthritis Rheum 1999;42:299–305.
6. van den Hoogen FH, Boerbooms AM, Swaak AJ, Rasker JJ, van Lier HJ, van de Putte LB. Comparison of methotrexate with placebo in the treatment of systemic sclerosis: a 24 week randomized double-blind trial, followed by a 24 week observational trial. Br J Rheumatol 1996;35:364–372.
7. Pope J, Bellamy N, Seibold J, et al. A randomized, controlled trial of methotrexate versus placebo in early diffuse scleroderma – a preliminary analysis. Arthritis Rheum 1998;41:S102.
8. Zachariae H, Halkier-Sorenson L, Heickendorff L, Zachariae E, Hansen HE. Cyclosporin A treatment of systemic sclerosis. Br J Dermatol 1990;122:677–681.
9. Freundlich B, Jimenez SA, Steen VD, Medsger TA Jr, Szkolnicki M, Jaffe HS. Treatment of systemic sclerosis with recombinant interferon gamma. A phase I/II clinical trial. Arthritis Rheum 1992;35:1134–1142.
10. Luk AJ, Wong M, Lambert EL, et al. Treatment of scleroderma with interferon-gamma. Arthritis Rheum 1996;39:S152.
11. Seibold JR, Korn JH, Simons R, et al. Recombinant human relaxin in the treatment of scleroderma. Ann Intern Med 2000;132:871–879.
12. Thompson B, Geller NL, Hunsberger S, et al. Behavioral and pharmacologic interventions: the Raynaud's Treatment Study. Control Clin Trials 1999;20:52–63.
13. Badesch DB, Tapson VF, McGoon MD, et al. Continuous intravenous epoprostenol for pulmonary hypertension due to the scleroderma spectrum of disease. A randomized, controlled trial. Ann Intern Med 2000;132:425–434.
14. Sjögren RW. Gastrointestinal motility disorders in scleroderma. Arthritis Rheum 1994;37:1265–1282.
15. Silver RM, Miller KS, Kinsella MB, Smith EA, Schabel SI. Evaluation and management of scleroderma lung disease using bronchoalveolar lavage. Am J Med 1990;88:470–476.
16. Ziesche R, Hofbauer E, Wittman K, Petkov V, Block LH. A preliminary study of long-term treatment with interferon gamma-1b and low-dose prednisolone in patients with idiopathic pulmonary fibrosis. N Engl J Med 1999;341:1264–1269.
17. Steen VD. Organ involvement: renal. In: Clements PJ, Furst DE (eds). Systemic Sclerosis. Baltimore: Williams & Wilkins, 1996; pp 425–440.

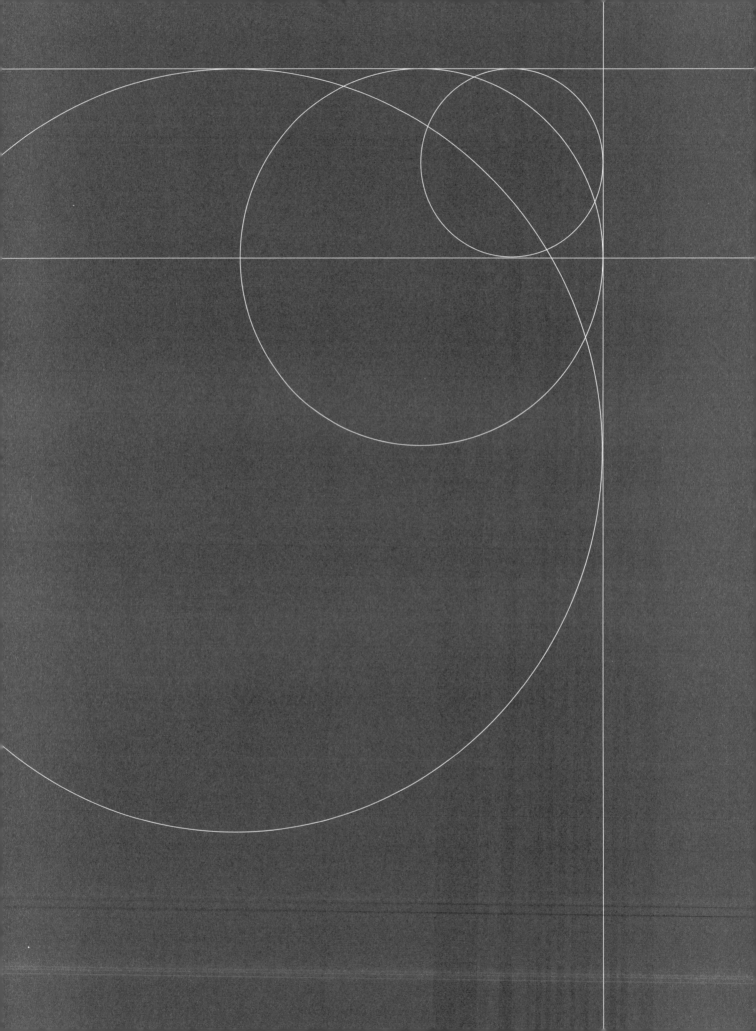

19 INFLAMMATORY AND METABOLIC DISEASES OF MUSCLE

Idiopathic Inflammatory Myopathies

The idiopathic inflammatory myopathies are a heterogeneous group of disorders characterized by proximal muscle weakness and nonsuppurative inflammation of skeletal muscle (Table 19-1). Generally accepted criteria for the diagnosis of an idiopathic inflammatory myopathy include 1) proximal muscle weakness; 2) elevated serum levels of enzymes derived from skeletal muscle; 3) myopathic changes demonstrated by electromyography; and 4) muscle biopsy evidence of inflammation. The addition of a skin rash (criterion 5) allows the diagnosis of dermatomyositis (1) (see Appendix I). A more specific disease designation can be assigned based on the patient's age, additional findings, or the coexistence of another disease (2). More recently, circulating myositis-specific autoantibodies have been identified in some patients with idiopathic inflammatory myopathies (3) (Table 19-2).

Epidemiology

Accurate estimates of the prevalence of the idiopathic inflammatory myopathies are difficult to obtain because the diseases are rare and lack universally accepted specific diagnostic criteria (1,4–6). Estimates of incidence range from 0.5 to 8.4 cases per million. The incidence appears to be increasing, although this may reflect increased awareness and more accurate diagnosis.

Overall, the age at onset for the idiopathic inflammatory myopathies has a bimodal distribution, with peaks between ages 10 and 15 years in children, and between 45 and 60 years in adults. However, the mean ages for specific groups differ. The age at onset for myositis associated with another

TABLE 19-1
Clinical Classification of the Idiopathic Inflammatory Myopathies

Polymyositis
Dermatomyositis
Juvenile dermatomyositis
Myositis associated with neoplasia
Myositis associated with collagen vascular disease
Inclusion body myositis

collagen vascular disease is similar to that for the associated condition, but myositis associated with malignancy and inclusion body myositis are more common after age 50. In general, women are affected twice as often as men by idiopathic inflammatory myopathies; however, inclusion body myositis affects men twice as often. Racial differences are apparent. In adults, the lowest rates are reported in the Japanese and the highest in African Americans.

Pathogenesis

The idiopathic inflammatory myopathies are immune-mediated processes, believed to be triggered by environmental factors in genetically susceptible individuals. Two observations provide strong support for the hypothesis that the idiopathic inflammatory myopathies are disorders of autoimmunity. First is the recognized association with other autoimmune diseases, including Hashimoto's thyroiditis, Graves' disease, myasthenia gravis, type I diabetes mellitus, primary biliary cirrhosis, and connective tissue diseases. Second is the high prevalence of circulating autoantibodies (3). The autoantibodies associated with polymyositis and dermatomyositis include the myositis-specific autoantibodies (MSAs) found almost exclusively in these diseases. Other autoantibodies that occur commonly in myositis, but are not specific for these disorders, are called myositis-*associated* autoantibodies and typically are found in patients with overlap syndromes.

The specific causes or triggering events of idiopathic inflammatory myopathies remain unknown, but viruses have been strongly implicated. The seasonal variation in the onset of disease among different MSA subsets (first half of the year for antisynthetase syndrome and latter half for anti-SRP) suggests that infectious agents may play a role. The most striking evidence of a viral cause for the idiopathic inflammatory myopathies is found in animal models. Chronic myositis develops following infection with a picornavirus and persists long after the virus can no longer be detected in the tissue. The best-described model is produced by injecting coxsackievirus 131 into neonatal Swiss mice. Infection of adult BALB/C mice with encephalomyocarditis virus-221A also produces a "dose-dependent" viral model of polymyositis.

The importance of genetic factors is evident in mouse models of disease and in studies of class II immunohistocompatibility antigens. Individuals with HLA-DR3 are at increased risk for developing inflammatory muscle disease, including polymyositis and juvenile dermatomyositis. All patients with anti-Jo-1 antibodies have the HLA antigen

TABLE 19-2
Syndromes Associated With Myositis-Specific Autoantibodies

Autoantibody	Clinical features	Treatment response

Antisynthetase[a]	Polymyositis or dermatomyositis with
	  Relatively acute onset
	  Fever
	  Arthritis
	  Raynaud's phenomenon
		Moderate with disease persistence

Anti-SRP[b]	Polymyositis with
	  Very acute onset
	  Often in fall
	  Severe weakness
	  Palpitations
		Poor

Anti-Mi2	Dermatomyositis with
	  V sign and shawl disease
	  Cuticular overgrowth
		Good

[a] Anti-Jo-1 is the most common myositis-specific antibody. Other antisynthetase antibodies include anti-PL-7, anti-PL-12, anti-EJ, and anti-OJ.
[b] SRP, signal recognition particle.

DR52. Caucasian patients also have a high prevalence of HLA-138, HLA-DR3, and DR6. Associations with HLA-DR1, DR6, and DQ1 have been determined for inclusion body myositis.

The pathologic changes in muscle provide the strongest evidence that these diseases have an immune-mediated pathogenesis (7,8). The changes in polymyositis and inclusion body myositis appear to result from cell-mediated antigen-specific cytotoxicity. Non-necrotic muscle fibers are seen surrounded and invaded by CD8+ mononuclear cells, with cytotoxic cells outnumbering suppressor cells by a ratio of 3:1 in the CD8+ cell population. B cells and natural killer cells do not appear to play a significant role in polymyositis or inclusion body myositis. The fibers invaded by T cells show increased major histocompatibility complex (MHC) class I expression, a necessary condition for T-cell–mediated cytotoxicity. ICAM-1 adhesion molecules are identified on muscle fiber membranes. These findings suggest that the pathology of polymyositis and inclusion body myositis involves recognition of an antigen on the surface of muscle fibers by antigen-specific T cells.

In contrast to polymyositis, humoral immune mechanisms appear to play a greater role in dermatomyositis. Invasion of non-necrotic fibers is universal, and the cellular infiltrates are predominantly perivascular in location. ICAM-1 molecules are expressed on the walls of small blood vessels, and B cells outnumber T cells. Among T lymphocytes, CD4+ cells are common, whereas CD8+ cells and activated T cells are rare. The vasculopathy that is so prominent in juvenile dermatomyositis and occasionally present in the adult form of the disease also appears to be mediated by the immune system through humoral mechanisms. Immunoglobulins and complement components, including the C5-9 membrane attack complex, are deposited in the capillaries and small arterioles in this disease, but not in polymyositis.

Although the immune mechanisms involved in polymyositis and inclusion body myositis are similar, there are differences in pathology. The rimmed vacuoles, which are seen only in inclusion body myositis, indicate unique pathogenetic mechanisms for this group. Amyloid deposits have been identified in the vacuolated muscle fibers in inclusion body myositis, and abnormal accumulation of ubiquitin, beta-amyloid protein, beta-amyloid precursor protein, and prion protein have been found in the rimmed vacuoles. An increased number of ragged-red fibers are seen in muscle from patients with this disorder, suggesting a possible connection with mitochondrial myopathies.

Clinical Features
The dominant clinical feature of the idiopathic inflammatory myopathies is symmetrical proximal muscle weakness. The weakness can be accompanied by systemic symptoms of fatigue, morning stiffness, and anorexia. Laboratory investigation reveals elevated levels of serum enzymes derived from skeletal muscle, especially creatine kinase (CK). Electromyography (EMG) demonstrates myopathic changes consistent with inflammation, and muscle histology shows inflammatory changes. These manifestations can occur in a variety of combinations or patterns, and no single feature is specific or diagnostic.

Polymyositis
The clinical features of polymyositis in the adult are representative of all the inflammatory myopathies (2,7). Adult-

onset polymyositis begins insidiously over three to six months, with no identifiable precipitant. The shoulder and pelvic girdle muscles are affected most severely. Weakness of neck muscles, particularly the flexors, occurs in about one-half of all patients, but ocular and facial muscles are virtually never involved. Dysphagia may develop secondary to esophageal dysfunction or cricopharyngeal obstruction. Pharyngeal muscle weakness may cause dysphonia and swallowing difficulty. Myalgias and arthralgias are not uncommon, but severe tenderness and frank synovitis are unusual. Raynaud's phenomenon sometimes is present, and periorbital edema may occur.

Pulmonary and cardiac manifestations may develop at any time during the course of disease. "Velcro-like" crackles may be heard on chest auscultation with interstitial fibrosis or interstitial pneumonitis. Aspiration pneumonia may complicate the disease course in patients with swallowing difficulties. Cardiac involvement usually is restricted to asymptomatic electrocardiographic abnormalities, although supraventricular arrhythmia, cardiomyopathy, and congestive heart failure may develop.

The CK level is elevated at some time during the course of disease. Normal CK levels may be found very early in the course of disease, in advanced cases with significant muscle atrophy, or as a result of circulating inhibitors of CK-level activity. Elevation of serum CK levels is a reasonable indicator of disease severity in most patients. Other muscle enzymes, including aldolase, aspartate aminotransferase (AST), alanine aminotransferase (ALT), and lactate dehydrogenase (LDH), are elevated in most cases. The erythrocyte sedimentation rate is normal in 50% of patients with polymyositis, and is elevated above 50 mm/hour in only 20%.

Electromyography classically reveals the following triad: 1) increased insertional activity, fibrillations, and sharp positive waves; 2) spontaneous, bizarre, high-frequency discharges; and 3) polyphasic motor-unit potentials of low amplitude and short duration. This triad is characteristic, but not diagnostic. The complete triad is seen in approximately 40% of patients. In contrast, 10%–15% of patients may have completely normal EMGs. In a small number of patients, abnormalities are limited to the paraspinal muscles.

In classic polymyositis, muscle biopsy demonstrates varying stages of necrosis and regeneration of muscle fibers. The inflammatory cell infiltrate is predominantly focal and endomysial. T lymphocytes, especially CD8[+] cytotoxic cells accompanied by a smaller number of macrophages, are found surrounding and invading the initially non-necrotic fibers. In other cases, degeneration is seen in the absence of inflammatory cells in the immediate area. Intact fibers may vary in size. Destroyed fibers are replaced by fibrous connective tissue and fat. However, in some cases, no fiber necrosis is observed, and the only recognized change is type II fiber atrophy.

Dermatomyositis in Adults
The clinical features of dermatomyositis include all those described for polymyositis, plus a variety of cutaneous manifestations. Rashes may antedate the onset of muscle weakness by a year or more. Skin involvement varies widely from person to person. Gottron's papules – lacy, pink or violaceous areas (raised or macular) found symmetrically on the dorsal aspect of interphalangeal joints, elbows, patellae, and medial malleoli – are considered pathognomonic. Characteristic changes include heliotrope (violaceous) discoloration of the eyelids, often with associated periorbital edema; macular erythema of the posterior shoulders and neck (shawl sign), anterior neck and upper chest (V-sign), face, and forehead; and dystrophic cuticles. Periungual telangiectasias and nail-fold capillary changes similar to those observed in people with scleroderma or systemic lupus erythematosus and Raynaud's phenomenon may be seen.

The muscle histopathology of classic adult dermatomyositis may be like that of polomyositis, but more commonly, it shows a perivascular infiltration of inflammatory cells composed of higher percentages of B lymphocytes and CD4[+] T-helper lymphocytes. Biopsies reveal perifascicular atrophy, which may be diagnostic of dermatomyositis.

Some people with biopsy-confirmed, classic cutaneous findings of dermatomyositis have no clinical evidence of muscle disease. The terms *amyotrophic dermatomyositis* and *dermatomyositis sine myositis* have been used to describe this condition. About 10% of all dermatomyositis cases may fall into this category. Although overt muscle weakness is not demonstrable, fatigue may be a dominant complaint, and analysis of energy-containing compounds (such as ATP) by magnetic resonance spectroscopy reveals abnormal muscle energy metabolism and altered exercise capacities (9). Some of these patients become weak over time. There may be an increased prevalence of neoplasia associated with this presentation.

Juvenile Dermatomyositis
The inflammatory myopathic process usually observed in children has a highly characteristic pattern, although a disease similar to adult polymyositis occasionally occurs (10). Juvenile dermatomyositis differs from the adult form because of the coexistence of vasculitis, ectopic calcification, lipodystrophy, and muscle weakness. In juvenile dermatomyositis, the skin lesions and weakness almost always are coincidental, but the severity and progression of each symptom varies greatly from patient to patient. In some patients, remission is complete with little or no therapy. However, in dermatomyositis accompanied by vasculitis, progression may be devastating, despite therapy. Gastrointestinal ulcerations resulting from vasculitis may cause hemorrhage or perforation of a viscus. Ectopic calcifications can occur in the subcutaneous tissues or in the muscles.

The histologic changes found in juvenile dermatomyositis essentially are the same as those for the adult form, although perifascicular atrophy is much more prevalent (7). Endothelial hyperplasia and deposition of immunoglobulin (Ig)G, IgM, and complement within the vessel wall are prominent.

Myositis and Other Collagen Vascular Diseases

Muscle weakness is a common finding in people with collagen vascular diseases. The features of idiopathic inflammatory myopathy may dominate the clinical picture in some patients with scleroderma, systemic lupus erythematosus, mixed connective tissue disease, and Sjögren's syndrome. In other cases, weakness may be accompanied by normal enzyme levels and an absence of EMG abnormalities. The full picture of polymyositis is less common but can occur in rheumatoid arthritis, adult-onset Still's disease, Wegener's granulomatosis, and polyarteritis nodosa. In vasculitic syndromes, muscle weakness more commonly is related to arteritis and nerve involvement than to nonsuppurative inflammatory changes of muscles.

Myositis and Malignancy

A subset of patients with inflammatory myopathies develops muscle weakness with an underlying malignancy. The true incidence of this relationship is not clear (11). Malignancy may precede or follow the onset of muscle weakness, and associated malignancy may be more common with dermatomyositis. The association is rare in childhood but has occurred in patients of all ages in all subsets of disease. It appears that the sites or types of malignancy that occur in association with myositis are those expected for the patient's age and gender. Ovarian cancer occurs with a higher frequency than expected in women with dermatomyositis.

Inclusion Body Myositis

Inclusion body myositis mainly affects older individuals (4,12). The symptoms begin insidiously and progress slowly. Symptoms often are present for five to six years before diagnosis. The clinical picture in some patients differs from that of typical polymyositis in that it may include focal, distal, or asymmetric weakness, as well as neurogenic or mixed neurogenic/myopathic changes on EMG. Dysphagia is noted in more than 20% of patients. As the muscle weakness becomes severe, it is accompanied by atrophy and diminished deep-tendon reflexes. In some patients, the disease continues a slow, steady progression; in others, it seems to plateau, leaving the individual with fixed weakness and atrophy of the involved musculature.

The characteristic change in inclusion body myositis is the presence of intracellular vacuoles (4,7). On paraffin sections, the vacuoles appear lined with eosinophilic material, but on frozen preparations, basophilic granules lining the vacuoles are evident. Lined vacuoles are not specific for inclusion body myositis. Electron microscopy reveals either intracytoplasmic or intranuclear inclusions, which may be tubular or filamentous. These structures are straight and rigid-appearing, with periodic transverse and longitudinal striations. Myelin figures (also called myeloid bodies) and membranous whorls are common.

Myositis-Specific Autoantibodies

Several autoantibodies are found almost exclusively in people with idiopathic inflammatory myopathies (5) (Table 19-2).

Although these MSAs are found in fewer than 50% of patients, the presence of a particular MSA identifies a relatively homogeneous group of patients, with regard to clinical manifestations and prognosis. With extremely rare exceptions, individual patients have only one MSA.

The MSAs can be categorized as those directed at aminoacyl-tRNA synthetases, nonsynthetase cytoplasmic antigens, and nuclear antigens. The antisynthetases show immunochemical properties characteristic of autoantibodies. They immunoprecipitate transfer RNA, inhibit enzyme function, and react with conformational epitopes. The antisynthetases do not cross-react or occur together.

The most common MSAs are directed against amino acyl-tRNA synthetase activities. The most common MSA, directed against anti-histidyl-tRNA synthetase, is called the anti-Jo-1 antibody. Anti-Jo-1 antibodies are present in up to 20% of patients and are more common in polymyositis than in dermatomyositis. Patients with these autoantibodies typically demonstrate myositis and several extramuscular features including interstitial lung disease, arthritis, Raynaud's phenomenon, and mechanic's hands (darkened or dirty-appearing horizontal lines and fissures that are seen across the lateral and palmar aspects of the fingers). This combination of disorders is referred to as the antisynthetase syndrome. These patients are difficult to treat because they usually do not sustain complete remissions.

Anti-Mi-2 antibodies are directed against helicase activities. These antibodies are found almost exclusively in people with dermatomyositis, and are markers for a high likelihood of good treatment response. In contrast, patients with anti-SRP (signal recognition particle) antibodies develop polymyositis of rapid onset and are relatively treatment-resistant. These patients also may develop cardiomyopathy and distal muscle weakness.

Treatment

Treatment of the inflammatory myopathies is largely empirical (2,13). Before initiating treatment, the patient's clinical status should be evaluated as objectively as possible. Pretreatment testing of the strength of individual muscle groups provides valuable information, and these baseline measures can be compared with those obtained after therapy is initiated. Chest radiography, pulmonary function studies, and swallowing studies may be indicated. Muscle enzymes, including CK, aldolase, AST, ALT, and LDH, should be measured, as should other laboratory values that might be affected by therapy. Cancer screening tests indicated by the patient's age and gender should be performed.

Physical therapy plays an important role in treatment. However, bed rest may be required during intervals of severe inflammation. Passive range-of-motion exercises are encouraged during these intervals to maintain movement and prevent contractures. With improvement, therapy should progress from active-assisted to active exercises.

Corticosteroids are the standard first-line medication for any idiopathic inflammatory myopathy. Initially, prednisone is given in a single dose of 1 mg/kg/day, but in severe cases, the daily dose can be divided or intravenous methylprednisolone used. Clinical improvement may be noted in the first weeks or gradually, over three to six months. Generally, the earlier in the disease course prednisone is started, the faster and more effectively it works. As many as 90% of patients improve at least partially with corticosteroid therapy, and 50%–75% of those patients achieve complete remission.

If a patient does not respond to corticosteroid therapy, another agent is added, usually methotrexate or azathioprine. Methotrexate generally is given on a weekly schedule at doses of 5–15 mg orally or 15–50 mg intravenously; the typical dosage of azathioprine is 2–3 mg/kg/day (maximum of 150 mg/day). Other agents that have been used in steroid-resistant cases include cyclophosphamide, 6-mercaptopurine, chlorambucil, cyclosporine, plasmapheresis, lymphapheresis, total-body (or total-nodal) irradiation, and intravenous immunoglobulin. Hydroxychloroquine can be used to treat the cutaneous lesions of dermatomyositis, although it has no recognized effect on the myositis.

Metabolic Myopathies

Metabolic myopathies are a heterogeneous group of conditions that share abnormalities in muscle energy metabolism, leading to skeletal muscle dysfunction (13). Some metabolic myopathies should be considered primary because they are associated with known or postulated biochemical defects that affect the ability of the muscle fibers to maintain adequate levels of ATP. The prevalence of these disorders appears to be greater than previously thought. Secondary metabolic myopathies may be caused by such endocrine disorders as thyroid or adrenal diseases or electrolyte abnormalities.

Primary Metabolic Myopathies
Disorders of Glycogen Metabolism
Myophosphorylase deficiency (McArdle's disease) is one of nine diseases that share an underlying defect in glycogen synthesis, glycogenolysis, or glycolysis. These disorders often are referred to as the glycogen storage diseases, because each defect results in abnormal deposition and accumulation of glycogen in skeletal muscle (13,14). The classic clinical manifestation of a glycogen storage disease is exercise intolerance, which may be experienced as pain, fatigue, stiffness, weakness, or intense cramping. Most affected persons are asymptomatic at rest and can function without difficulty at low levels of exercise. Symptoms tend to develop when carbohydrates provide the majority of energy for muscular work, that is, activities of high intensity and short duration or activities of less intensity for longer intervals. Some patients experience a "second wind" phenomenon; although they must stop an activity because of symptoms, they often are able to resume the exercise after resting.

Symptoms develop during childhood in most patients, but significant problems, including severe cramping and exercise-induced rhabdomyolysis and myoglobinuria with renal failure, may not develop until adolescence or adulthood. A subset of patients develops progressive proximal muscle weakness in adulthood that may be difficult to differentiate from polymyositis, because patients with glycogen storage disease have elevated CK levels and myopathic changes on EMG. The diagnosis of glycogen storage diseases may be suggested by finding the classic changes of glycogen deposition on muscle biopsy. The forearm ischemic exercise test is a useful method of screening for glycogen storage disease (Table 19-3). The suspected diagnosis should be confirmed by specific enzyme analysis of muscle tissue, using histology or ischemic exercise testing.

Inherited deficiency of acid maltase includes infantile, childhood, and adult forms. Because acid maltase activity, localized to lysosomes, does not affect cytosolic glycogen metabolism, the results of ischemic exercise testing are normal. The diagnosis of adult acid maltase deficiency should be suspected when characteristic electromyographic changes are seen. These changes include an unusually intense electrical irritability in response to movement of the needle electrode, and myotonic discharges in the absence of clinical myotonia.

Mitochondrial Myopathies
The recognized disorders of lipid metabolism that cause myopathic problems are due to abnormalities in the transport and processing of fatty acids for energy in mitochondria. A large number of abnormalities involving these activities have been recognized.

Carnitine palmityltransferase (CPT) activity is necessary for the transport of long-chain fatty acids into mitochondria. Deficiency of CPT is an autosomal recessive disorder that causes attacks of myalgia and myoglobinuria. These attacks typically are associated with vigorous physical activity but may occur with fasting, infection, or cold exposure. Serum CK levels, EMG, and muscle histology are normal, except during episodes of rhabdomyolysis. The diagnosis is made by assaying muscle tissue for activity of the CPT enzyme.

TABLE 19-3
Forearm Ischemic Exercise Test[a]

1. Venous blood is drawn without a tourniquet for baseline levels of lactate and ammonia.
2. A sphygmomanometer is placed around the upper arm and inflated to 20–30 mm Hg above systolic pressure.
3. The subject vigorously exercises the hand by squeezing until reaching complete fatigue or for a minimum of 2 minutes with the cuff inflated.
4. At the completion of exercise, the cuff is deflated and venous blood samples for lactate and ammonia are collected 2 minutes later.

[a] In normal subjects, both lactate and ammonia levels increase at least threefold above baseline. The major reason for a false-positive result is insufficient exercise effort. A positive result should always be confirmed by analysis of the putative enzyme activity in skeletal muscle.

Carnitine is an essential intermediate that acts as a carrier of long-chain fatty acids into mitochondria, where beta-oxidation occurs. Carnitine deficiency causes abnormal lipid deposition in skeletal muscle and can result from inherited or acquired causes. Primary carnitine deficiencies can be divided into systemic and muscle types. Patients with muscle carnitine deficiency present with chronic muscle weakness in late childhood, adolescence, or early adulthood. The process mainly affects proximal muscles but may involve facial and pharyngeal musculature. Muscle carnitine deficiency may be confused with polymyositis because serum CK levels are elevated in more than half the patients, and EMG often reveals myopathic changes. Acquired carnitine deficiencies have been reported with pregnancy, renal failure requiring long-term hemodialysis, end-stage cirrhosis, myxedema, adrenal insufficiency, and therapy with valproate or pivampicillin.

Other mitochondrial myopathies are clinically heterogeneous disorders that cause morphologic abnormalities in the number, size, or structure of mitochondria (15,16). The metabolic abnormalities described in these conditions are numerous and can be attributed to defects in pyruvate and acyl-CoA processing, beta-oxidation, the respiratory chain, or energy conservation. Many mitochondrial myopathies are inherited through maternal transmission and are caused by defects in mitochondrial DNA. The clinical spectrum of these conditions is quite diverse and includes progressive muscle weakness, external ophthalmoplegia with or without proximal myopathy, progressive exercise intolerance, and multisystem disease. More than 25 specific enzyme abnormalities have been described, and at least six of them may present with exercise intolerance or progressive muscle weakness in adults. Ragged-red fibers are the histologic hallmark of these diseases. Depending on the defect, treatment with L-carnitine, riboflavin, ascorbate, coenzyme Q10, or a combination of these substances may be beneficial.

Myoadenylate Deaminase Deficiency

The primary form of myoadenylate deaminase deficiency is inherited in an autosomal recessive pattern. The primary deficiency is due to a nonsense mutation at codon 12 of the adenosine monophosphate deaminase 1 gene, which has been identified in 22% of normal individuals. Thus, 2% of the population is homozygous for this deficiency. No clinical abnormalities have been associated with this deficiency, and individuals will have normal serum CK levels, EMGs, and muscle histology. However, results of the forearm ischemic exercise test are abnormal because people with this condition are unable to generate ammonia under those conditions (17).

Other Causes of Muscle Weakness

Although inflammatory and metabolic myopathies are relatively rare, many diseases can cause myopathic symptoms that lead patients to seek medical attention (Table 19-4).

Neurologic diseases generally can be differentiated because they cause asymmetric weakness, distal extremity involvement, altered sensorium, or abnormal cranial nerve function. In con-

trast, myopathies tend to cause proximal and symmetric weakness. Exceptions include some mitochondrial myopathies, which may be accompanied by ocular problems, and inclusion body myositis, which may have neuropathic features.

Cancer must be considered in the evaluation of patients with myopathic symptoms. Weakness and fatigue suggestive of myopathy can occur in neoplastic disease, due to systemic effects of cytokines released by tumor cells or immune response to the malignancy, and prominent neuromuscular changes also can develop as features of paraneoplastic syndromes.

Numerous drugs can cause myopathic changes by a variety of mechanisms. Some, such as D-penicillamine and procainamide, are immune-mediated. Others, such as alcohol, may have direct toxic effects. Drugs that may cause metabolic or electrolyte abnormalities include clofibrate, lovastatin, gemfibrozil, and other lipid-lowering agents, which probably alter muscle fiber energetics; thiazide diuretics, which can cause weakness, myalgias, and cramps by inducing hypokalemia; and zidovudine (AZT), which can induce a mitochondrial myopathy.

Numerous infections can cause a myopathy, with viruses being the most common. Children with influenza A and B viral infections can experience severe myalgias associated with very high CK levels. Weakness is a common finding in people with acquired immune deficiency syndrome and may be due to cachexia, central or peripheral nervous system diseases, polymyositis emerging as a consequence of altered immune function, AZT toxicity, or opportunistic infections (e.g., cytomegalovirus, *Mycobacterium avium intracellulare*, *Cryptococcus*, *Trichinella*, *Toxoplasma*, pyomyositis).

Testing for Muscle Disease
Chemistries

Elevated serum enzymes derived from skeletal muscle, including CK, aldolase, AST, ALT, and LDH, help confirm the presence of a myopathic process (18). High levels of these enzymes are found in the inflammatory diseases of muscle but are not specific for those diagnoses. Creatine kinase generally is the most useful enzyme to follow because elevated serum levels result from muscle necrosis or leaking membranes. Trauma is a well-recognized cause of high CK levels, as are isometric and aerobic exercise (especially in poorly conditioned individuals). Occasionally, elevated CK levels are observed in asymptomatic individuals. Racial differences in normal CK levels must be considered in this context because healthy African American males have higher CK levels than do whites or Hispanics, with the majority of their values appearing abnormal by usual laboratory values.

Electromyography

Electromyography is valuable for determining the classification, distribution, and severity of diseases affecting skeletal muscle (19). Although the changes identified are not specific, EMG can allow differentiation between myopathic and neuropathic conditions and can localize the site of

TABLE 19-4
Differential Diagnosis of Muscle Weakness[a]

Neuropathic diseases	Infections
Muscular dystrophies	Viral
Denervating conditions	Advenovirus
Neuromuscular junction disorders	Coxsackievirus
Proximal neuropathies	Cytomegalovirus
Myotonic diseases	Echovirus
Neoplasm	Epstein-Barr virus
Paraneoplastic syndromes	Human immunodeficiency virus (HIV)
Eaton-Lambert syndrome	Influenza viruses
Drug-related conditions	Rubella virus
Alcohol	Bacterial
Amiodarone	*Clostridium welchii*
Clofibrate	*Mycobacterium tuberculosis*
Cocaine	Spirochetal
Colchicine	*Borrelia burgdorferi* (Lyme spirochete)
Cyclosporine	Fungal
Enalapril	*Cryptococcus*
Fenofibrate	Parasitic
Gemfibrozil	*Toxoplasma gondii*
Corticosteroids	Helminthic
Heroin	*Trichinella*
Hydroxychloroquine	Inborn errors of metabolism
Ketoconazole	Nutritional-toxic
Levodopa	Endocrine disorders
Lovastatin	Miscellaneous causes
Nicotine acid	Sarcoidosis
D-Penicillamine	Atherosclerotic emboli
Phenytoin	Behçet's disease
Valproic acid	Fibromyalgia
Zidovudine (AZT)	Psychosomatic

[a] Does not include inflammatory or metabolic causes described in the text.

the neurologic abnormality to the central nervous system, spinal cord anterior horn cell, peripheral nerves, or neuromuscular junction. In addition, knowledge of the distribution and severity of abnormalities can guide selection of the most appropriate site on which to perform a biopsy.

Forearm Ischemic Exercise Testing
During vigorous ischemic exercise, skeletal muscle functions anaerobically, generating lactate and ammonia. Lactate is the product of glycolysis, and ammonia is a coproduct of myoadenylate deaminase activity. The forearm ischemic exercise test takes advantage of this physiology and has been standardized for use in screening glycogen storage diseases (except acid maltase deficiency) and myoadenylate deaminase deficiency (Table 19-3). In individuals with a glycogen storage disease, the ammonia level increases normally, but lactate levels remain at baseline. In contrast, in myoadenylate deaminase deficiency, lactate levels increase but ammonia levels do not.

Imaging Techniques
Neither conventional radiography nor radionuclide imaging has proved particularly useful in patients with muscle diseases. However, computer-based image analysis using ultrasonography, computed tomography, and magnetic resonance imaging (MRI) provide useful images. Of these methods, MRI offers the best imaging of soft tissue and muscle. Because MRI can detect early or subtle disease changes and show patchy muscle involvement, it may prove superior to EMG in determining the site for muscle biopsy. Magnetic resonance imaging can be used to grade muscle involvement semiquantitatively, and therefore can be used to follow the response to therapy of several muscle diseases (9) (Fig 19-1).

Muscle Biopsy
Four types of evaluation can be performed on skeletal muscle: histology, histochemistry, electron microscopy, and assays of enzyme activities or other constituents. Hematoxylin–eosin and modified Gomori's trichrome stains are used for most

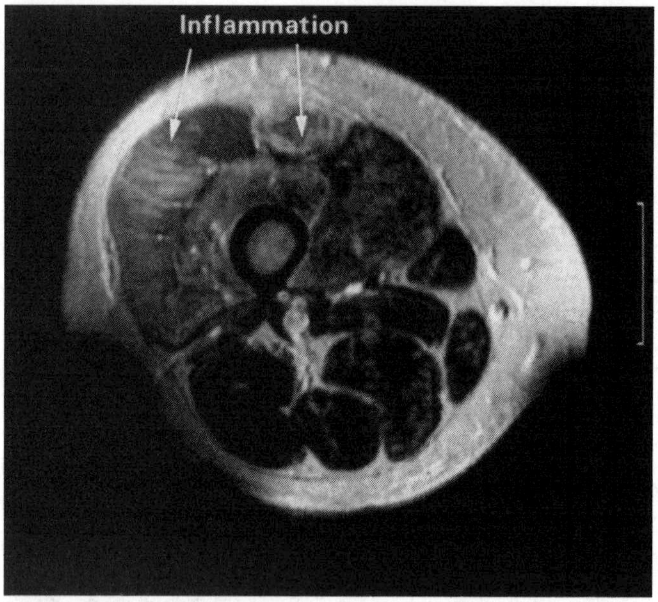

Fig. 19-1. T2-weighted image of upper leg muscle from a person with dermatomyositis revealing inflammatory changes (8).

histology. The latter stain is useful in identifying ragged-red fibers, typical findings in many mitochondrial myopathies. A wide variety of stains is used for histochemistry: ATPase stains determine fiber type, NADH and succinic dehydrogenases reflect the mitochondria, periodic acid-Schiff stains are used for glycogen, and oil red for lipid.

A combination of histologic and histochemical analyses can be useful in differentiating myopathic from neuropathic processes. Myopathic changes include rounding and variation of fiber size, presence of internal nuclei, fiber atrophy, degeneration and regeneration, fibrosis, and fatty replacement. Neuropathic conditions that cause denervation produce small, atrophic, angular fibers and target fibers. Reinnervation causes fiber-type grouping, i.e., aggregation of fibers of the same type.

Enzyme deficiency states may be identified with appropriate histochemical stains, but are best diagnosed by assays for the specific enzyme activity. Ultrastructural analysis shows characteristic changes in cases of inclusion body myositis, increased numbers of mitochondria with altered morphology in mitochondrial myopathies, and abnormal glycogen or lipid deposition.

ROBERT L. WORTMANN, MD

References

1. Bohan A, Peter JB. Polymyositis and dermatomyositis: first of two parts. N Engl J Med 1975;292:344–347.
2. Oddis CV. Idiopathic inflammatory myopathies. In: Wortmann RL (ed). Diseases of Skeletal Muscle, 1st ed. Philadelphia: Lippincott Williams & Wilkins, 2000; pp 45–86.
3. Targoff IN. Autoantibodies and muscle disease. In: Wortmann RL (ed). Diseases of Skeletal Muscle, 1st ed. Philadelphia: Lippincott Williams & Wilkins, 2000; pp 267–292.
4. Calabrese LH, Mitsumoto J, Chou SM. Inclusion body myositis presenting as treatment-resistant polymyositis. Arthritis Rheum 1987;30:397–403.
5. Tanimoto K, Nakano K, KanoS, et al. Classification criteria for polymyositis and dermatomyositis. J Rheumatol 1995;22:668–674.
6. Targoff IN, Miller FW, Medsger TA Jr, Oddis CV. Classification criteria for the idiopathic inflammatory myopathies. Curr Opin Rheumatol 1997;9:527–535.
7. Engel AG, Hohfeld R, Banker BQ. The polymyositis and dermatomyositis syndromes. In: Engel AG, Franzini-Armstrong C (eds). Myology, 2nd ed. New York: McGraw-Hill, 1994; pp 1335–1383.
8. Messner RP. Pathogenesis of idiopathic inflammatory myopathies. In: Wortmann RL (ed). Diseases of Skeletal Muscle, 1st ed. Philadelphia: Lippincott Williams & Wilkins, 2000; pp 129–146.
9. Park JFL Vital TZ, Ryder NM, et al. Magnetic resonance imaging and P-31 magnetic resonance spectroscopy provide unique quantitative data useful in the longitudinal management of patients with dermatomyositis. Arthritis Rheum 1994;37:736–746.
10. Pachman LM. Inflammatory myopathies in children. In: Wortmann RL (ed). Diseases of Skeletal Muscle, 1st ed. Philadelphia: Lippincott Williams & Wilkins, 2000; pp 87–110.
11. Airic, A, Puklaala E, Isomaki A. Elevated cancer incidence in patients with dermatomyositis: a population based study. J Rheumatol 1995;22:1300–1303.
12. Leff RL, Miller FW, Hicks J, et al. The treatment of inclusion body myositis: a retrospective review and a randomized, prospective trial of immunosuppressive therapy. Medicine 1993;72:225–235.
13. Wortmann RL. Metabolic diseases of muscle. In: Wortmann RL (ed). Diseases of Skeletal Muscle, 1st ed. Philadelphia: Lippincott Williams & Wilkins, 2000; pp 157–188.
14. DiMauro S, Tsujino S. Nonlysosomal glycogenoses. In: Engel AE, Franzini-Armstrong C (eds). Myology, 2nd ed. New York: McGraw-Hill, 1994; pp 1554–1576.
15. Johns JR. Mitochondrial DNA and disease. N Engl J Med 1995;333:638–644.
16. Vladutiu G. The molecular diagnosis of metabolic myopathies. Neurol Clinics 2000;18;53–104.
17. Morisake T, Gross M, Morisaki H, et al. Molecular basis of AMP deaminase deficiency in skeletal muscle. Proc Natl Acad Sci USA 1992;89:6457–6461.
18. Bohlmeyer T, Wu ALL, Perryman MB. Evaluation of laboratory tests as a guide to diagnosis and therapy of myositis. Rheum Dis Clin North Am 1994;22:845–856.
19. Mahowald ML, David WS. Electrophysiologic evaluation of muscle disease. In: Wortmann RL (ed). Diseases of Skeletal Muscle, 1st ed. Philadelphia: Lippincott Williams & Wilkins, 2000; pp 313–322.

20 SJÖGREN'S SYNDROME

Sjögren's syndrome (SS) is a debilitating autoimmune disorder that has been described as a form of "epitheliitis" or an exocrinopathy. Salivary and lacrimal gland involvement is prominent and associated with decreased production of saliva and tears. Other epithelial components of the body that commonly are involved include the skin and the urogenital, respiratory, and gastrointestinal tracts. Other systemic autoimmune manifestations include synovitis, neuropathy, vasculitis, and presence of autoantibodies, particularly antinuclear antibodies (anti-SSA/Ro and anti-SSB/La) and rheumatoid factor (RF). Immunoglobulin levels frequently are elevated. SS may be associated with malignancies, especially non-Hodgkin's lymphoma. In secondary SS, the disorder coexists with other autoimmune diseases, such as rheumatoid arthritis, systemic lupus erythematosus, scleroderma, polymyositis, and polyarteritis nodosa.

Epidemiology

Reported prevalences of primary SS vary widely, from 0.05% to 4.8% of the population (1–5), and SS frequency appears to increase with age. The diagnosis usually is made in midlife, but SS may occur at any age. The onset most often is insidious, and diagnosis may be delayed for a number of years. The female:male ratio is about 9:1. Differences in classification criteria may complicate the interpretation of epidemiologic data.

Classification Criteria and Diagnosis

Various classification criteria, which have included the requirement of keratoconjunctivitis sicca, xerostomia, and autoantibodies, have been proposed for SS. Preliminary criteria proposed by the European Community are the most widely accepted (6). The European criteria had been criticized because it was possible for individuals without evidence of autoimmunity (negative labial salivary gland biopsy and negative serology) to meet them. However, the criteria have been revised by the American-European Consensus Group (Table 20-1). The rules for applying the criteria and the exclusions are shown in Table 20-2. For practical purposes, individuals satisfying the Revised International Classification Criteria may be diagnosed as having SS. A valid alternative method for classifying cases of SS is the classification tree procedure shown in Fig. 20-1. The differential diagnosis for SS includes the disorders listed as exclusions in Table 20-2.

Pathogenesis

The pathogenesis of SS remains unknown (7). It is speculated that an as-yet-unidentified environmental agent (for example, a virus) may trigger a cascade of events in genetically susceptible hosts, resulting in the development of SS. A number of viruses have a predilection for causing disease in salivary glands (8). Organisms that have been investigated include herpesviruses such as Epstein-Barr virus, cytomegalovirus, human herpesvirus (HHV)-6 and -8, retroviruses that include human T-cell lymphotropic virus-1, human immunodeficiency virus-1, and human retrovirus 5. Hepatitis C virus also may produce salivary gland swelling and may mimic SS. To date, however, no specific organism has emerged as the cause of SS.

Due to the striking preponderance of SS in women, it has been postulated that hormonal factors have a role in disease pathogenesis. In addition, there is evidence to suggest hypofunction of the hypothalamic–pituitary–adrenal axis in SS, a phenomenon that occurs in other autoimmune rheumatic diseases.

Genetic factors also may have a role in SS. Family members may have an increased prevalence of SS and autoantibodies, particularly anti-SSA/Ro. The human leukocyte antigen (HLA)-DR3 and HLA-DQ2 alleles are more common among Caucasian patients with primary SS, whereas different alleles are more common among African American and Japanese patients. A subset of patients has shown an increased frequency of alleles for peptide transporter genes TAP1 (0101) and TAP2 (0101) in addition to microsatellite a2 alleles (9).

Focal mononuclear cell infiltration of exocrine tissues and the presence of autoantibodies (especially anti-SSA/Ro, anti-SSB/La, and RF) are hallmarks of SS. The infiltrates in such exocrine tissues as the salivary and tear glands consist mainly of T cells (with relatively few B cells), macrophages, and mast cells. Most of the T cells are CD4$^+$ helper cells, which bear the memory phenotype CD45RO$^+$. They express the α/β T-cell receptor and lymphocyte function-associated antigen type 1 (LFA-1), and may contribute significantly to the B-cell hyperactivity observed in SS. Adhesion molecules and LFA-1 promote homing to exocrine tissue. The infiltrating periductal lymphocytes appear to be resistant to apoptosis despite their increased expression of Fas, allowing autoreactive cells to persist in the exocrine tissues. Apoptosis may be blocked by the suppressor proto-oncogene Bcl-2 (10).

Salivary and lacrimal gland epithelial cells in SS express HLA-DR antigens, which allow these epithelial

TABLE 20-1
Revised International Classification Criteria for Sjögren's Syndrome

I.   Ocular symptoms: a positive response to at least one of the following questions:
    a. Have you had daily, persistent, troublesome dry eyes for more than three months?
    b. Do you have a recurrent sensation of sand or gravel in the eyes?
    c. Do you use tear substitutes more than three times a day?

II. Oral symptoms: a positive response to at least one of the following questions:
    a. Have you had a daily feeling of dry mouth for more than three months?
    b. Have you had recurrently or persistently swollen salivary glands as an adult?
    c. Do you frequently drink liquids to aid in swallowing dry food?

III. Ocular signs: objective evidence of ocular involvement defined as a positive result for at least one of the following two tests:
    a. Schirmer's test, performed without anesthesia (≤5 mm in 5 minutes)
    b. Rose bengal score or other ocular dye score (≥4 according to van Bijsterveld's scoring system).

IV. Histopathology: In minor salivary glands (obtained through normal-appearing mucosa) focal lymphocytic sialoadenitis, evaluated by an expert histopathologist, with a focus score ≥1, defined as a number of lymphocytic foci that are adjacent to normal-appearing mucous acini and contain more than 50 lymphocytes per 4 mm^2 of glandular tissue.

V.   Salivary gland involvement: objective evidence of salivary gland involvement defined by a positive result for at least one of the following diagnostic tests:
    a. Unstimulated whole salivary flow (≤1.5 ml in 15 minutes)
    b. Parotid sialography showing the presence of diffuse sialectasias (punctate, cavitary or destructive pattern), without evidence of obstruction in the major ducts.
    c. Salivary scintigraphy showing delayed uptake, reduced concentration and/or delayed excretion of tracer.

VI. Autoantibodies: presence in the serum of the following autoantibodies:
    a. Antibodies to SSA/Ro or SSB/La antigens, or both

cells to present exogenous antigens and autoantigens to the CD4$^+$ T cells (10). Interactions between these cells may result in production of cytokines and stimulation of B-cell proliferation and differentiation. Furthermore, B-cell activation is usual in SS and may progress toward B-cell lymphoid malignancy (10). In addition, proinflammatory cytokines, interleukin (IL)-1β, IL-6, and tumor necrosis factor α are produced by epithelial cells, and IL-10 and interferon (IFN)-γ are produced mainly by infiltrating T cells. IL-10 may have a role in B-cell proliferation; IFN-γ increases HLA-DR and SSB/La expression by glandular epithelial cells.

Activated B cells in SS produce increased amounts of immunoglobulins with autoantibody reactivity for IgG (rheumatoid factor), SSA/Ro, and SSB/La (10). Evidence has emerged that the B cells also produce antibodies targeting the muscarinic M3 receptor (10,11). In this respect, SS may be analogous to myasthenia gravis, an autoimmune disease in which the autoantigenic target is a postsynaptic receptor for acetylcholine at the neuromuscular junction. In SS, the blockade of the muscarinic (acetylcholine) receptor in exocrine tissue would inhibit secretions.

Several other possible explanations exist for decreased production of exocrine secretions. For example, cytokines may interact directly with epithelial cells. Alternatively, autoantibodies may interfere with the nerve supply of exocrine tissue, resulting in a decrease in secretions disproportionate to tissue destruction. Tissue destruction may result in insufficient tissue to produce secretions. Evidence suggests that about half of the ducts and acini have been destroyed in individuals who report substantial dryness (9). Complete destruction of the salivary tissue rarely is seen in salivary gland biopsies of people with SS.

Research into the pathogenesis and genetic factors contributing to the development of SS involves a number of mouse models, including the nonobese diabetic (NOD) mice and the NOD.B10, NOD.SCID, and MRL/lpr mice. The NOD mouse displays a similar immunologic profile to that seen in human disease associated with decreased saliva production. In addition, the transforming growth factor β (TGF-β) knockout mouse develops salivary and lacrimal gland exocrinopathy, highlighting the potential role of that cytokine in SS. TGF-β dampens immune responses, has a role in acinar cell differentiation, and may be important early in the course of SS (10).

TABLE 20-2
Revised Rules for Classification of Sjögren's Syndrome

For primary SS
In patients without any potentially associated disease, primary SS may be defined as follows:
a. the presence of *any four of the six items* is indicative of primary SS, as long as either item IV (Histopathology) or VI (Serology) is positive.
b. the presence of *any three of the four objective criteria items* (i.e., items III, IV, V, VI)
c. *the classification tree procedure* represents a valid alternative method for classification, although it should be more properly used in clinical-epidemiological surveys (see Fig. 20-2).

For secondary SS
In patients with a potentially associated disease (for example, another well-defined connective tissue disease), the presence of *item I or item II plus any two from among items III, IV, and V* may be considered as indicative of secondary SS.

Exclusion criteria
Past history of head and neck radiation therapy, hepatitis C infection, acquired immunodeficiency disease (AIDS), pre-existing lymphoma, sarcoidosis, graft-versus-host disease, use of anticholinergic drugs (within four half-lives of the drug).

Cardinal Manifestations

The cardinal manifestations of SS are oral and ocular symptoms and signs of dryness, the presence of autoantibodies, and a positive labial salivary gland biopsy.

Ocular Manifestations

Precorneal tear film usually is described as having three distinct layers; moving outward from the corneal surface, these layers are mucus, water, and oil (12). Precorneal tear fluid consists of a complex biochemical mixture that includes water, electrolytes, mucins, antimicrobial proteins (such as lactoferrin and lysozyme), immunoglobulins, and growth factors (such as TGF-α). The precorneal mucus, protein, and aqueous components form a hydrated gel. When the gel is removed experimentally, changes similar to those in keratoconjunctivitis sicca occur: the barrier to fluorescein dye decreases, contrast sensitivity declines, and irregularity of the corneal surface increases. The outermost layer of the precorneal tear film, which covers the hydrated gel produced by the meibomian gland, is composed of a complex mixture of nonpolar and polar lipids.

A classification scheme for dry eyes is shown in Fig. 20-2. The dry eyes of SS are due to aqueous tear deficiency (ATD).

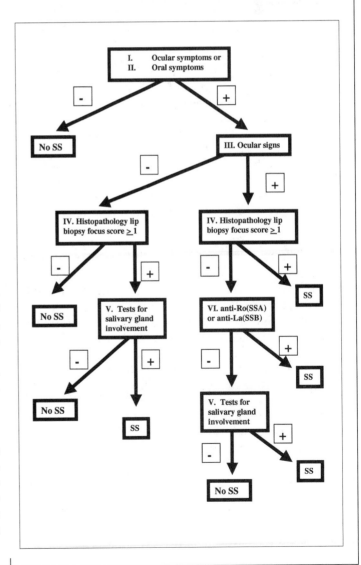

Fig. 20-1. Classification tree for primary Sjögren's syndrome (SS). Patients with symptoms of dry eyes or dry mouth may be classified as having SS with 96% sensitivity and 94% specificity by following the scheme below. Negative results are indicated by "−" and positive results by "+." The variables used at each step are assigned the same roman numerals as in the criteria listed in Table 20-1. The variables in classification tree are applied from the top. Variables at the top of the tree give the highest yield of cases, compared with noncases.

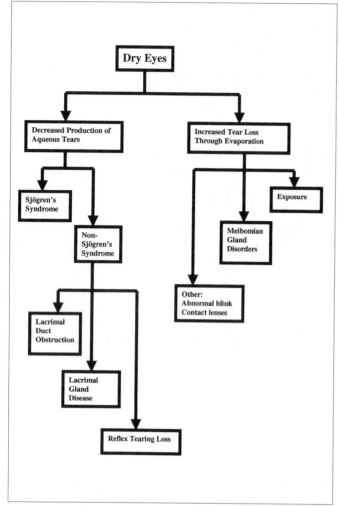

Fig. 20-2. A classification scheme for dry eyes. This shows that Sjögren's syndrome (SS) may be classified as a form of aqueous tear deficiency and must be distinguished from non-SS causes of aqueous tear deficiency, as well as from tear loss due to evaporation.

However, ATD may be due to other lacrimal gland diseases, lacrimal duct obstruction, and loss of reflex tearing in the absence of SS. The differential diagnosis of dry eyes includes problems that result in evaporative tear deficiency, such as meibomian gland disease, contact lenses, and blink abnormality. People with SS often report a sensation of sand or grit in the eyes.

The eyes may be evaluated by performing a Schirmer's test, which defines abnormal tear production as 5 mm or less of wetting of a standard rectangular strip of filter paper in five minutes. A fluorescein tear film breakup time of less than 10 seconds (observed on slit lamp examination) also suggests dry eyes. Staining of rose bengal or other vital dyes on the ocular surface may be scored according to the van Bijsterveld system (13). It should be noted that in the United States and United Kingdom, ophthalmologists tend to use lissamine green rather than rose bengal, because it is much less irritating to the eye. Evaluation of keratinization also may be used to evaluate dryness of the ocular surface.

In addition, histopathologic studies based on surface cytology and on lacrimal gland biopsy may be used. Finally, analyses of tear composition have been performed in research studies.

Oral Manifestations

Common oral symptoms of SS include a sensation of decreased saliva, oral dryness when eating, the need to drink liquids when swallowing dry foods, intolerance of spicy foods, altered taste, and a chronic burning sensation (14). Difficulties with speech may make social and business interactions more difficult. It is important to ask patients about their current and past medications as well history of radiation exposure. More than 400 medications have been associated with dry mouth symptoms, including a number of drugs commonly prescribed for hypertension, depression, and insomnia. Radiation therapy for head and neck tumors may result in profound symptoms of oral dryness. Radioactive iodine for thyroid disorders concentrates in exocrine glands, particularly the salivary glands, and patients who receive this treatment may later present with oral dryness. An oral examination commonly reveals tooth erosions and caries, especially at the gingival margins and on the incisal edges of the teeth. Soft-tissue changes are particularly common on the tongue, which may become furrowed, and the mucosa may become dry and sticky. At times, the mucosa may have the typical erythema and white patches associated with candidiasis, which occurs commonly in this disorder. Examination often reveals decreased or absent salivary pooling. Swallowing difficulties may be evaluated by barium swallows or ultrasound studies, which may demonstrate esophageal dysmotility.

Visible enlargement of the major salivary glands may occur. The parotid gland may be seen as a swelling that displaces the earlobe and extends downward over the angle of the jaw (Fig. 20-3). Medial to the angle of the jaw, submandibular salivary gland swelling may be seen or, more often, palpated. The glands may or may not be tender; swelling may be transient or chronic, and often is recurrent, thus distinguishing it from mumps.

Laboratory Features

Hypergammaglobulinemia is common in SS, and a majority of cases are associated with the presence of RF (90%), or anti-SSA/Ro or anti-SSB/La (50%–90%) (15). Antinuclear antibodies are present in about 80% of cases. Antibodies to the 52-kDa Ro antigen are more often associated with SS, whereas antibodies to the 60-kDa Ro antigen appear to be more frequent in systemic lupus erythematosus. Autoantibodies that precipitate anti-SSA/Ro are associated with systemic manifestations of the disease, including anemia, leukopenia, thrombocytopenia, purpura, cryoglobulinemia, hypocomplementemia, lymphadenopathy, and vasculitis.

Autoantibodies directed against other antigenic targets that have been recognized in SS, include carbonic anhydrase, pancreatic antigen, α fodrin, 97-kDa Golgi complex, mitotic spindle apparatus, M3 muscarinic acetylcholine receptors,

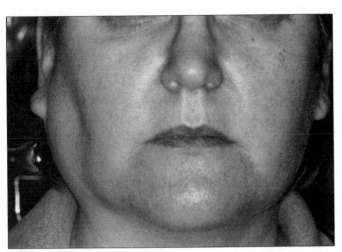

Fig. 20-3. Parotid gland enlargement seen as a swelling that displaces the earlobe and extends downward over the angle of the jaw.

and Fc γ receptors. However, presence of these autoantibodies currently is not used to diagnose or monitor the disease.

Other Manifestations
Cutaneous
Dry skin may occur in about half of people affected with SS. Sweating and responses to pilocarpine may be decreased. Pruritus may be associated with dry skin and, in some cases, with peripheral neuropathy. Repeated scratching may result in hyperpigmentation, excoriations, and lichenification of the skin. In addition, palpable or nonpalpable purpura and petechiae may occur in some patients, most frequently on the legs, in showers of lesions lasting up to four days. These lesions are histologically consistent with either leukocytoclastic vasculitis (typically associated with anti-SSA/Ro and anti-SSB/La antibodies, RF, antinuclear antibodies, cryoglobulins, hypocomplementemia, hypergammaglobulenemia, and circulating immune complexes) or mononuclear inflammatory vasculopathy (usually not associated with seroreactivity and hypocomplementemia). Vasculitic lesions may also have the appearance of urticaria, erythema multiforme, erythematous macules, patches or nodules, and digital ulcers. The presence of erythema nodosum should raise the suspicion of sarcoidosis.

Thyroid
Thyroid disease, particularly hypothyroidism, is common in people with SS. This has led to the impression that autoimmune thyroiditis may be a manifestation of SS. However, the evidence for a true association is unconvincing. Ramos-Casals and colleagues found no significant differences in the prevalence of thyroid disease among SS patients, compared with individuals of similar age and gender who did not have SS (16).

Respiratory
Nonproductive cough occurs frequently in SS, probably because of tracheal dryness and a diminution in mucus pro-

duction. Progressive pulmonary disease, however, is unusual. Mucosal biopsies and bronchoalveolar lavage reveal increased submucosal CD4+ T lymphocytes. The cough also may be related to hyper-reactive airways in both primary and secondary SS. Smaller airways may be obstructed, leading to minor abnormalities on pulmonary function testing, and lymphocytic infiltrates may be observed in bronchiolar walls. In addition, interstitial pulmonary disease may occur in SS, but generally is mild. Rheumatoid-like pulmonary nodules may occur in SS. It is important to consider metastatic carcinoma, such granulomatous lesions as sarcoidosis, and other causes in the differential diagnosis. Sarcoidosis is associated with hilar adenopathy, and granulomatous lesions on salivary gland biopsy. There is evidence that pleural effusions can occur in primary SS. The effusions may contain lymphocytes and antibodies to the SSA/Ro and SSB/La antigens (17).

Musculoskeletal
Musculoskeletal features of SS may include myalgias, arthralgias, and arthritis. Patients may develop a symmetrical polyarthritis that resembles rheumatoid arthritis, but is nondeforming and tends to respond well to standard treatments used in rheumatoid arthritis. Rheumatoid arthritis itself may begin before or after the onset of SS. Although an increased frequency of sicca symptoms has been described in fibromyalgia, it is unclear if fibromyalgia occurs more frequently in people with SS.

Neurologic
Peripheral neuropathy is not uncommon in SS. It is most prominent in the lower limbs, and most often is sensory, with numbness, tingling, and burning as the principal symptoms. Autonomic neuropathy also has been described. Involvement of the central nervous system has been described, but the prevalence of central nervous system disease probably has been overestimated in some studies because of selection bias.

Hematologic
The most important hematologic complication of SS is lymphoid malignancy. There is a 44-fold increase in the frequency of B-cell lymphomas among people with SS (18). These growths usually are non-Hodgkin's lymphomas of mucosa-associated lymphoid tissues (19). Often, cervical lymph nodes and salivary glands are involved. Although not malignant, glandular swelling with reactive changes occur more often, and it is important to rule out malignancy in significantly or prominently swollen salivary glands or nodes in the neck. Diagnostic imaging, such as computerized tomographic scans, fine-needle aspirates for cytologic and flow cytometric analyses, and biopsies must be considered.

Reproductive
Obstetrical complications in SS may be related to concomitant autoimmune disease, particularly systemic lupus erythematosus. The risks include prematurity, preeclampsia,

intrauterine growth retardation, and fetal loss. However, these problems do not appear to be increased in primary SS. Because anti-SSA/Ro antibodies occur in SS, there is a risk of congenital heart block, although the frequency is low (20). Women with SS also experience vaginal dryness, which commonly is associated with dyspareunia.

Urinary Tract

Urinary tract symptoms consistent with irritable bladder are not uncommon (21). Increased urinary frequency may relate to increased fluid intake to alleviate oral dryness. In SS, renal abnormalities include diminished ability to concentrate urine in about half of all cases, distal renal tubular acidosis (RTA) in about 15%, nephrocalcinosis, renal stones, and less often, interstitial nephritis and glomerular disease. Urine pH generally is above 5.5 in RTA. RTA is associated with systemic acidosis, resulting in the mobilization of calcium from bone, promoting osteoporosis and resulting in hypercalciuria. In addition, urinary citrate, which normally complexes a substantial proportion of urine calcium, is low. The risk of calcium phosphate stones is increased. Tubular proteinuria may occur in about half of SS cases. Glomerular disease may occur in about 2% of the patients, especially in those with longer disease duration, and tends to be associated with cryoglobulins (21). Patients with glomerulonephritis tend to have mixed cryoglobulinemia and low C4 levels in the serum.

Treatment of Sjögren's Syndrome

Patient Education and Self-Care

As in any chronic disease, it is important to help patients develop strategies for self-management and coping with physical, mental, and social challenges associated with their condition. Patient education on the manifestations, course, prognosis, complications, self-help mechanisms, and treatment of the disease minimizes complications (15). Because there often is a lag of years before the diagnosis is made, acknowledging the patient's concerns is helpful in establishing confidence in the physician or other caregivers.

Sicca Symptoms

Keratoconjunctivitis Sicca

Treatment of dry eyes includes tear replacement and conservation, as well as topical ocular and systemic medications (22). Artificial tears, which are derivatives of cellulose, are instilled as drops into the eyes frequently to ameliorate symptoms. Because preservatives may irritate or damage the ocular surface, and because patients may become allergic to them, preservative-free preparations are superior. Artificial tears in small dispensers minimize the risk of bacterial growth and infection. Rubbing the eyes and rinsing the ocular surface with tap water is discouraged, because this may inoculate an already compromised eye with infectious organisms.

When the benefit of artificial tears is of insufficient duration, more concentrated, viscous solutions or hydroxypropylcellulose pellets inserted under the lower eyelids may be used. These pellets dissolve by absorbing water, usually from concomitantly administered artificial tears, and prolong the retention of moisture in the eye. Ointments typically are used only at night, since they are viscous and may interfere with vision. Tear preparations may dry, leaving crusts on the eyelashes, and excessive use of ointments may block the meibomian glands. These residual materials may be removed by gentle washing of the lashes with baby shampoo, which will treat and help prevent blepharitis. There is growing evidence to suggest that topical corticosteroids, cyclosporine, and intraocular androgens may be beneficial in the treatment of keratoconjunctivitis sicca. Systemic pilocarpine, which has been approved for the treatment of dry mouth, probably also improves ocular symptoms. The role of systemic treatment for the ocular manifestations of SS remains unclear.

In refractory cases, punctal plugs may be inserted. Collagen plugs dissolve and last about two days. Silicon plugs are durable and may be removed if there are excessive tears after the plugs are inserted. If the condition of the eye surface is improved by the use of punctal plugs without resulting in excessive tears, permanent punctal occlusion can be performed.

Xerostomia

Frequent dental care is important for people with SS (14). Daily topical fluoride use and antimicrobial mouth rinse may help prevent caries in patients with reduced salivary flow. Medications that promote oral dryness or its complications may be replaced by ones that do not. Artificial saliva and lubricants may ameliorate symptoms in some patients. Sugar-free chewing gum or candies may stimulate sufficient salivary secretions to ameliorate oral dryness. Patients should be counseled on the appropriate diet and the importance of limiting sugar intake. Problems with swallowing may be treated with oral moisturizers and lubricants, and through dietary modifications. Use of humidifiers also may decrease sicca symptoms.

Secretagogues, such as pilocarpine, may increase secretions in patients with sufficient exocrine tissue (23). Typically, pilocarpine is given in a dosage of 5 mg orally four times a day, and the total daily dose usually does not exceed 30 mg. Adverse effects include increased perspiration, feeling hot and flushed, as well as symptoms associated with increased bowel and bladder motility. Caution must be exercised in the presence of bronchospasm. Some patients who experience adverse effects may benefit from one to three 5-mg doses per day to ameliorate symptoms at the most troublesome times of day. A new secretagogue, cevimeline has recently been approved for the treatment of dry mouth in SS in a dosage of 30 mg orally three times daily. Like pilocarpine, it is a muscarinic agonist that increases production of saliva, and possibly tears and other secretions. The drug is contraindicated for individuals with uncontrolled asthma, iritis, and narrow-angle glaucoma.

Oral candidiasis, which is a common complication of dry mouth in SS, is treated by sucking oral troches or vaginal suppositories of antifungal agents, such as nystatin or clotrimazole. Angular cheilitis may require topical antifungal agents (14). Bacterial parotitis should be treated with warm compresses, massage of the parotid gland, and if necessary, antibiotics.

Systemic Manifestations

The exocrine or systemic autoimmune and inflammatory manifestations may be treated by various immunomodulatory drugs. Hydroxychloroquine commonly is used for milder systemic manifestations of autoimmune disorders, such as fever, rashes, and arthritis. Whether or not hydroxychloroquine is effective for the exocrine manifestations is unclear, although serologic measures improve in people with SS on this medication. Drugs such as methotrexate, prednisone, azathioprine, and other immunomodulatory drugs tend to be used in patients with prominent systemic manifestations in an approach similar to that used to treat systemic lupus erythematosus. However, few randomized, double-blind clinical trials have been performed to demonstrate whether or not these agents are beneficial in SS.

Special attention is needed in treating certain organ complications in SS. In patients with RTA, oral alkaline preparations containing sodium and potassium citrate in a dose of 1–2 mEq/kg/day are used to correct the acidosis and decrease the risk of stones. In addition, urine calcium levels should be monitored and patients should receive potassium supplements. Patients with RTA have increased mobilization of calcium from bone, which requires appropriate monitoring and treatment. Bronchodilators may be useful in patients with a chronic cough, since SS is associated with increased airway reactivity. The management of thyroid disorders in people with SS is no different than that for others of similar age and sex (16). The arthritis of SS tends to respond well to standard treatments for rheumatoid arthritis. Cutaneous dryness is treated with decreased frequency of bathing and increased use of lubricants. Pruritis may be treated with mentholated lotions. Superficial vasculitis and dermatitis are treated with steroids. Vaginal dryness and dyspareunia may respond to water-soluble lubricants, and vaginal estrogen preparations may be beneficial in postmenopausal women.

Conclusion

Although advances continue in our understanding of SS, only symptomatic treatments have been approved specifically for the treatment of this debilitating disorder. Immunomodulatory treatments, replacement of destroyed salivary gland tissue by artificial salivary glands, and the possibilities for gene therapies are under active investigation.

STANLEY R. PILLIMER, MD

References

1. Drosos AA, Andonopoulos AP, Costopoulos JS, Papadimitriou CS, Moutsopoulos HM. *Prevalence of primary Sjogren's syndrome in an elderly population.* Br J Rheumatol 1988; 27(2):123–127.

2. Sjögren H. *Zur Kenntnis der Keratoconjunktivitis Sicca (Keratitis Filiformis bei Hypofunktion der Tränedrusen).* Acta Ophtalmol 1933;11:1–151.

3. Jacobsson LT, Axell TE, Hansen BU, et al. *Dry eyes or mouth — an epidemiological study in Swedish adults, with special reference to primary Sjogren's syndrome.* J Autoimmun 1989; 2:521–527.

4. Zhang NZ, Shi CS, Yao QP, et al. *Prevalence of primary Sjogren's syndrome in China.* J Rheumatol 1995;22:659–661.

5. Thomas E, Hay EM, Hajeer A, Silman AJ. *Sjogren's syndrome: a community-based study of prevalence and impact.* Br J Rheumatol 1998;37:1069–1076.

6. Vitali C, Bombardieri S, Moutsopoulos HM, et al. *Preliminary criteria for the classification of Sjogren's syndrome. Results of a prospective concerted action supported by the European Community.* Arthritis Rheum 1993;36:340–347.

7. Fox RI, Maruyama T. *Pathogenesis and treatment of Sjogren's syndrome.* Curr Opin Rheumatol 1997;9:393–399.

8. Venables PJ, Rigby SP. *Viruses in the etiopathogenesis of Sjogren's syndrome.* J Rheumatol 1997;24(Suppl 50):3–5.

9. Fox RI, Tornwall J, Michelson P. *Current issues in the diagnosis and treatment of Sjogren's syndrome.* Curr Opin Rheumatol 1999;11:364–371.

10. Anaya JM, Talal N. *Sjogren's syndrome comes of age.* Semin Arthritis Rheum 1999;28:355–359.

11. Waterman SA, Gordon TP, Rischmueller M. *Inhibitory effects of muscarinic receptor autoantibodies on parasympathetic neurotransmission in Sjogren's syndrome.* Arthritis Rheum 2000;43:1647–1654.

12. Pflugfelder SC. *Advances in the diagnosis and management of keratoconjunctivitis sicca.* Curr Opin Ophthalmol 1998;9: 50–53.

13. van Bijsterveld OP. *Diagnostic tests in the sicca syndrome.* Arch Ophthalmol 1969;82:10–14.

14. Daniels TE, Fox PC. *Salivary and oral components of Sjogren's syndrome.* Rheum Dis Clin North Am 1992;18:571–589.

15. Bell M, Askari A, Bookman A, et al. *Sjogren's syndrome: a critical review of clinical management.* J Rheumatol 1999;26: 2051–2061.

16. Ramos-Casals M, Garcia-Carrasco M, Cervera R, et al. *Thyroid disease in primary Sjogren syndrome. Study in a series of 160 patients.* Medicine (Baltimore) 2000;79:103–108.

17. Kawamata K, Haraoka H, Hirohata S, Hashimoto T, Jenkins RN, Lipsky PE. *Pleurisy in primary Sjogren's syndrome: T cell receptor beta-chain variable region gene bias and local autoantibody production in the pleural effusion.* Clin Exp Rheumatol 1997;15:193–196.

18. Kassan SS, Thomas TL, Moutsopoulos HM, et al. *Increased risk of lymphoma in sicca syndrome.* Ann Intern Med 1978; 89:888–892.

19. Voulgarelis M, Dafni UG, Isenberg DA, Moutsopoulos HM. *Malignant lymphoma in primary Sjogren's syndrome: a multicenter, retrospective, clinical study by the European Concerted Action on Sjogren's Syndrome.* Arthritis Rheum 1999;42: 1765–1772.

20. Julkunen H, Siren MK, Kaaja R, Kurki P, Friman C, Koskimies S. Maternal HLA antigens and antibodies to SS-A/Ro and SS-B/La. Comparison with systemic lupus erythematosus and primary Sjogren's syndrome. Br J Rheumatol 1995;34:901–907.

21. Goules A, Masouridi S, Tzioufas AG, Ioannidis JP, Skopouli FN, Moutsopoulos HM. Clinically significant and biopsy-documented renal involvement in primary Sjogren syndrome. Medicine (Baltimore) 2000;79:241–249.

22. Pflugfelder SC, Solomon A, Stern ME. The diagnosis and management of dry eye: a twenty-five-year review. Cornea 2000;19:644–649.

23. Vivino FB, Al Hashimi I, Khan Z, et al. Pilocarpine tablets for the treatment of dry mouth and dry eye symptoms in patients with Sjogren syndrome: a randomized, placebo-controlled, fixed-dose, multicenter trial. P92-01 Study Group. Arch Intern Med 1999;159:174–181.

21

VASCULITIDES
A. Polyarteritis Nodosa, Microscopic Polyangiitis, and the Small-Vessel Vasculitides

The medium- and small-vessel vasculitides are a complex, heterogeneous group of disorders that involve the destruction of blood vessel walls by a diverse array of inflammatory mediators (1). Because the pathophysiology of most of these disorders remains incompletely understood, classification of the vasculitides is organized according to several principles: 1) the size of the blood vessel involved; 2) current knowledge of disease pathophysiology; and 3) the pattern of organ involvement.

Polyarteritis nodosa (PAN), the first form of vasculitis described (2), is the prime example of a medium-vessel vasculitis (MVV). MVVs involve arteries that contain muscular walls, corresponding in size to vessel diameters of approximately 50 to 150 μm. The disorders comprising the small vessel vasculitides (SVVs) are more numerous and their classification more complex (Table 21A-1). SVVs tend to affect blood vessels that are <50 μm in diameter, i.e., capillaries, glomeruli (which may be viewed as differentiated capillaries), post-capillary venules, and nonmuscular arterioles. In reality, however, clinical distinctions between MVVs and SVVs are imprecise. Overlap in the size of vessels affected is common among the vasculitic disorders, even in conditions termed "pure" MVV or SVV.

After they've been classified by vessel size, vasculitides may be subclassified on the basis of certain pathophysiologic features, e.g., evidence that immune complexes participate in disease biology; association with characteristic autoantibodies, such as antineutrophil cytoplasmic antibodies (ANCA); or the presence or absence of granulomatous inflammation. Finally, some forms of vasculitis are distinguished further by their tropisms for particular organs. For example, both microscopic polyangiitis (MPA) and cutaneous leukocytoclastic angiitis (CLA) cause syndromes of cutaneous vasculitis that are clinically and pathologically indistinguishable. Although MPA may affect the kidneys, lungs, peripheral nerves, skin, and other organs, CLA is confined to the skin.

In this chapter, PAN, MPA, and the major forms of SVV are reviewed. Specific pathophysiologic features, epidemiologic characteristics, clinical findings, and treatment guidelines for the individual disorders are discussed in context.

TABLE 21A-1
Small Vessel Vasculitides

Immune-complex mediated
Cutaneous leukocytoclastic angiitis ("hypersensitivity" vasculitis)
Henoch-Schönlein purpura
Urticarial vasculitis
Cryoglobulinemia
Connective tissue disorders

ANCA-associated disorders
Wegener's granulomatosis
Microscopic polyangiitis
Churg-Strauss syndrome
Drug-induced ANCA-associated vasculitis

Miscellaneous small vessel vasculitides
Behçet's disease
Erythema elevatum diutinum
Paraneoplastic
Bacterial, viral, or fungal infections
Inflammatory bowel disease

Polyarteritis Nodosa

In 1866, Kussmaul and Maier (2) described the case of a 27-year-old journeyman tailor whose illness was characterized by fever, weight loss, abdominal pain, and polyneuropathy. The patient's condition led to paralysis and death within several weeks of onset. At autopsy, the nodular swellings found along the course of muscular arteries inspired the name "periarteritis nodosa," subsequently revised to "*poly*arteritis nodosa" to reflect more accurately the panarteritic nature of this disease. The 1994 Chapel Hill Consensus Conference (CHCC) on the nomenclature of systemic vasculitides defined classic PAN as necrotizing inflammation of medium-sized or small arteries that spares the smallest blood vessels (arterioles, venules, and capillaries) and is not associated with glomerulonephritis (GN)(3). Under this narrow definition, classic PAN as described by Kussmaul and Maier is believed to be a rare condition. During a six-year period, no cases of classic PAN were reported in the region of the Norwich Health Authority (U.K.), an area including a population of more than 400,000 people (4). Other reported annual incidence rates have ranged from two to nine cases per million people per year (5–7).

The pathologic changes in PAN are limited to the arterial circulation. In gross specimens, aneurysmal bulges of the arterial wall may be visible. Histologic sections reveal infiltration and destruction of the blood vessel wall by inflammatory cells, accompanied by fibrinoid necrosis (Fig. 21A-1).

Neutrophils are the principal component of the acute inflammatory infiltrate, but mononuclear cells predominate in later stages. Varying degrees of intimal proliferation and thrombosis occur. The lesions of PAN are segmental and favor the branch points of arteries. A critical pathologic feature of PAN is the absence of granulomas or granulomatous inflammation. A minority of PAN cases are associated with hepatitis B virus (HBV) infections (8). Other microbial pathogens may contribute to many of the remaining cases, but no definitive links with other infectious agents have been established. An association between PAN and hairy-cell leukemia has been observed. No genetic susceptibility to PAN has been identified, and familial PAN is rare.

Clinical Features

Polyarteritis nodosa usually begins with nonspecific symptoms that may include malaise, fatigue, fever, myalgias, and arthralgias. Overt signs of vasculitis may not occur until weeks or months after onset of the first symptoms. Though protean in its manifestations, PAN demonstrates a striking

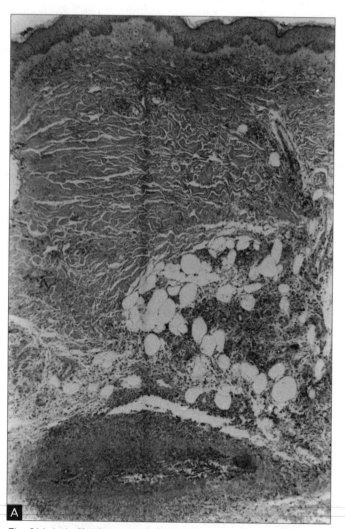

predilection for certain organs, particularly the skin, peripheral nerves, gastrointestinal (GI) tract, and kidneys (the medium-sized renal and intrarenal arteries). Skin lesions of PAN include livedo reticularis, subcutaneous nodules, ulcers, and digital gangrene. Cutaneous PAN is a variant of PAN, consisting of MVV limited to the skin.

A majority of people with PAN (>80% in some series) have vasculitic neuropathy, typically in the pattern of a mononeuritis multiplex (MM) (8). MM affects "named" nerves, most often the peroneal, tibial, ulnar, median, and radial nerves, leading to symptoms and signs in the distal extremities, such as foot or wrist drop. MM almost always causes sensory abnormalities, particularly painful dysesthesias; motor involvement occurs in one-third of patients. Electrodiagnostic testing (nerve-conduction studies) may unmask the presence of multiple axonal neuropathies. Central nervous system (CNS) disease in PAN usually results from hypertension rather than intracranial vasculitis, but CNS vasculitis sometimes occurs (9).

The classic manifestation of "intestinal angina" associated with PAN is postprandial periumbilical pain. Perforation of an ischemic bowel or rupture of a mesenteric microaneurysm are life-threatening complications of PAN. PAN also can affect individual GI tract organs such as the gallbladder or appendix, presenting as cholecystitis or appendicitis. Renal involvement, nearly universal at autopsy, produces few clinical symptoms during life, except for renin-mediated hypertension caused by vasculitis of the interlobar renal vessels (10). Cardiac lesions may lead to myocardial infarction or congestive heart failure, but usually remain subclinical. For reasons that are not understood, PAN usually spares the lungs.

Laboratory Features

The laboratory features of PAN, often strikingly abnormal, are nonspecific. Anemia, thrombocytosis, elevation of the

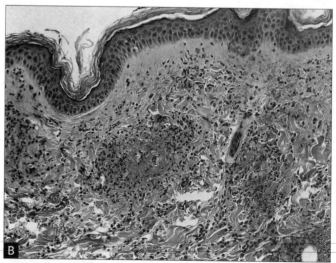

Fig. 21A-1. **A:** Skin biopsy with fibrinoid necrosis of a medium-sized muscular artery located in the deep dermis of a patient with polyarteritis nodosa. **B:** Skin biopsy revealing leukocytoclasis and fibrinoid necrosis of a small artery in the superficial dermis of a patient with microscopic polyangiitis.

erythrocyte sedimentation rate, and microscopic hematuria (in the absence of GN) are common. The diagnosis of PAN requires a tissue biopsy or an angiogram demonstrating microaneurysms (11). Simultaneous nerve and muscle biopsies (e.g., of the sural nerve and gastrocnemius muscle) are of high yield if there is a clinical suspicion of MM. Even in patients without GI symptoms, mesenteric angiography may demonstrate telltale microaneurysms. However, blind biopsies of asymptomatic organs (e.g., the testicle) rarely are diagnostic.

Treatment

For people with idiopathic PAN, prolonged immunosuppression is the cornerstone of therapy. Approximately one-half of people with PAN achieve remissions or cures with high dosages of corticosteroids (12). In most cases, treatment should begin with a minimum of 60 mg of prednisone per day, or approximately 1 mg/kg/day. The most severely ill patients may receive "pulse" therapy with methylprednisolone (1 gram/day for 3 days) at the start of treatment. Cyclophosphamide is indicated for patients whose disease is refractory to corticosteroids or who have serious involvement of major organs. Frequent monitoring of the white blood cell count (e.g., every two weeks) to avoid neutropenia is essential to prevent opportunistic infections. Prophylaxis against *Pneumocystis carinii* pneumonia with trimethoprim/sulfamethoxazole also is advisable.

In recent years, antiviral agents have improved the treatment of HBV-associated PAN substantially. One effective strategy involves the initial use of prednisone (1 mg/kg/day) to suppress the inflammation (8). Patients begin six-week courses of plasma exchange (approximately three exchanges/week) simultaneously with the start of prednisone. The corticosteroids are tapered rapidly (total course of approximately two weeks), followed by the initiation of antiviral therapy (e.g., lamivudine 100 mg/day).

Microscopic Polyangiitis

In 1948, Davson (13) suggested the division of PAN into two groups based on the presence or absence of GN. One group, later called classic PAN, demonstrated renal vasculitis only in medium-sized vessels of the kidneys, sparing the glomeruli. In contrast, patients in the other group had GN (i.e., SVV), with or without the involvement of medium-sized vessels. Davson designated this subset of patients with SVV of the kidney as having microscopic PAN. More recently, the term microscopic poly*angiitis* has been preferred in recognition of the disorder's tendency to involve not only arterioles and arteries, but also capillaries, venules, and veins. The 1994 CHCC defined MPA as a process that: 1) involves necrotizing vasculitis with few or no immune deposits (i.e., is "pauci-immune"); 2) affects the smallest blood vessels (capillaries, venules, and arterioles); 3) may affect medium-sized vessels; and 4) demonstrates tropisms for the kidneys (GN) and lungs (pulmonary capillaritis) (3).

Clinical Features

Disease characteristics of MPA are compared to those of classic PAN in Table 21A-2. Distinction between these two disorders is appropriate for several reasons. In contrast to PAN, MPA often involves the lung, may involve veins as well as arteries, rarely causes severe hypertension, commonly is associated with ANCA, nearly always requires cyclophosphamide to induce remission, and is more likely to flare following remissions. Epidemiologic data suggest that MPA is more common than classic PAN, with an annual incidence of 2.4 cases per million (4).

Pauci-immune, necrotizing GN is a dominant feature of MPA, occurring in nearly four-fifths of all patients (14). Glomerular damage leads to crescent formation and red blood cell casts in the renal tubules and urinary sediment (Fig. 21A-2). Pulmonary capillaritis may lead rapidly to life-threatening alveolar hemorrhage and hemoptysis. Approximately 12% of people with MPA develop this complication (14). In one MPA series, the most common disease manifestations were GN (79%), weight loss (73%), MM (58%), and fever (55%) (14). Upper-respiratory tract symptoms in MPA are much milder than those associated with Wegener's granulomatosis and are not associated with erosion of the bony sinuses, scarring of the subglottic region,

TABLE 21A-2
Microscopic Polyangiitis Versus Polyarteritis Nodosa

Feature	Microscopic polyangiitis	Polyarteritis nodosa
Granulomatous inflammation	No	No
Size of involved vessels	Small (and medium)	Medium
Renovascular hypertension	Yes	No
Glomerulonephritis	Yes	No
Lung involvement	Alveolar hemorrhage	No
Mononeuritis multiplex	Yes	Yes
ANCA positive	P-ANCA (anti-myeloperoxidase)	Rare
Hepatitis B association	No	Sometimes (10%)
Vascular aneurysms	Occasionally	Commonly

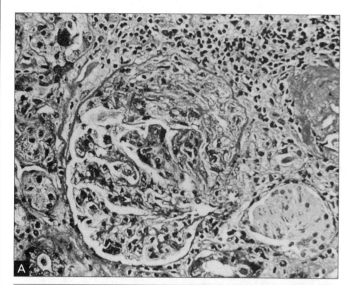

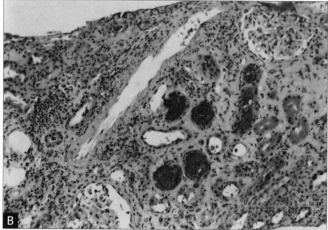

Fig. 21A-2. **A:** Glomerular crescent in a patient with glomerulonephritis associated with microscopic polyangiitis. **B:** Red blood cell casts within the tubules of the same patient.

or saddle-nose deformities. The essential difference between the two diseases, however, is the absence of granulomatous inflammation in MPA.

Seventy percent of people with MPA are positive for ANCA. In MPA, the most common staining pattern on immunofluorescence testing for ANCA is perinuclear (P-ANCA), which usually corresponds to the presence of antimyeloperoxidase antibodies.

Treatment

In MPA patients with GN, alveolar hemorrhage, MM, or other severe manifestations, treatment with a combination of cyclophosphamide and corticosteroids is indicated. People with MPA may achieve adequate response with intravenous cyclophosphamide (750 mg/m^2 of body surface area, once a month, for six treatments) combined with high doses of corticosteroids. With regard to efficacy and safety, however, the optimal route of cyclophosphamide administration (i.e., monthly intravenous or daily oral) in MPA remains unresolved.

Cutaneous Leukocytoclastic Angiitis

In the first classification scheme ever devised for the vasculitides, Zeek (15) coined the term hypersensitivity vasculitis (HSV) to describe a form of necrotizing SVV distinct from PAN, the only form of vasculitis recognized until that time. Use of the word "hypersensitivity" stemmed from animal models of vasculitis induced by the administration of horse serum, sulfonamides, and other drugs. Since Zeek's work, HSV has been defined further as a form of SVV confined to the skin and *not* associated with any other primary form of vasculitis. The American College of Rheumatology (ACR) formulated criteria for the classification of HSV in 1990 (16), and in 1994, the CHCC proposed a preferred alternative term for the disorder: cutaneous leukocytoclastic angiitis. The new designation emphasizes that the identification of an inciting antigen is not a prerequisite for the diagnosis of CLA, because no such precipitant is found in many of the people whose clinical and pathologic features are compatible with this disorder.

Clinical Features

The syndrome of CLA has several characteristic features. First, lesions typically occur initially in dependent regions, i.e., the lower extremities or buttocks. Second, the skin lesions occur in crops – groups of lesions similar in age – because of simultaneous exposure to the inciting antigen. Third, the lesions may be asymptomatic, but usually are accompanied by a burning or tingling sensation. A wide array of skin lesions may occur in CLA (and all other forms of SVV with cutaneous involvement), including palpable purpura, papules, urticaria, erythema multiforme, vesicles, pustules, superficial ulcers, and necrosis. The presence of livedo reticularis or the development of deep ulcers usually indicates the involvement of medium-sized arteries as well.

The pleomorphic presentation of CLA and the large number of vasculitis mimickers make it essential to confirm the diagnosis by skin biopsy. In addition to analysis by light microscopy, direct immunofluorescence (DIF) studies should be performed on skin biopsies. Biopsies of active lesions (<48 hours old, if possible) usually demonstrate leukocytoclastic vasculitis in the postcapillary venules. On DIF, the variable patterns of immunoglobulin and complement deposition suggest an immune complex-mediated pathogenesis, but are not distinctive (unlike in Henoch-Schönlein purpura, urticarial vasculitis, and cryoglobulinemia).

Treatment

There are two keys to the diagnosis and management of CLA: 1) exclusion of systemic involvement by a careful history, physical examination, and selected laboratory tests; and 2) identification and removal of the offending agent. For cases in which a precipitant can be identified (e.g., CLA induced by a medication), removal of the offending agent usually leads to resolution within days to weeks. Mild cases may be treated with leg elevation and the administration of nonsteroidal anti-inflammatory agents (NSAIDs) and/or H_1 antihistamines. For persistent disease not associated with cutaneous gangrene, colchicine, hydroxychloroquine, or dapsone may be effective. For refractory or more severe disease, immunosuppressive agents may be indicated, beginning with corticosteroids. However, excessive corticosteroid requirements dictate the use of an additional immunosuppressive agent, such as azathioprine (2–2.5 mg/kg/day).

Henoch-Schönlein Purpura

Henoch-Schönlein purpura (HSP) is characterized by the clinical tetrad of purpura, arthritis, abdominal pain, and GN. The defining histopathologic feature of this disease is the deposition of immunoglobulin (Ig)A in and around blood vessel walls. Most patients also have increased levels of IgA and IgA-containing immune complexes in the serum. Although there are two subclasses of IgA, HSP is associated only with increases of IgA1. The reasons for this remain obscure.

Henoch-Schönlein purpura can develop at any age, but occurs most frequently in children. More than 90% of children affected are less than 10 years of age (17). Among children, the incidence of HSP is 135 cases/million/year (18). In adults, the incidence is far lower, estimated in one study to be 1.2 cases/million/year (4). The incidence of HSP in adults may be underestimated because of the common failure to perform DIF studies on skin biopsies. Two-thirds of people with HSP report antecedent upper respiratory illnesses, suggesting an infectious trigger for the disease.

Clinical Features

People with HSP typically present with the acute onset of fever, palpable purpura on the lower extremities and buttocks, abdominal pain, arthritis, and hematuria. The purpura may be extensive and confluent, and occasionally involves the arms and trunk as well as dependent areas. The abdominal pain, caused by either bowel edema or frank mesenteric ischemia, often is colicky and may worsen after meals. Some patients experience nausea, vomiting, and upper or lower GI bleeding. The joint disease in HSP manifests itself as arthralgias or arthritis in large joints, especially the knees and ankles and, to a lesser degree, the wrists and elbows, often in a migratory pattern. The clinical hallmark of GN in HSP is microscopic hematuria accompanied by proteinuria. GN almost always follows the appearance of cutaneous lesions in HSP, in contrast to the GI disease and arthritis, which may precede the onset of purpura. HSP rarely involves organs other than the skin, joints, GI tract, and kidneys, but pulmonary involvement (hemoptysis) has been reported.

The manifestations of HSP vary with age. Among children with HSP, infants have milder disease. Children under the age of two are less likely than older children to develop GN or abdominal complications. As a group, children with HSP have more frequent GI involvement (particularly ileoileal intussusception) but less renal disease than do adults. GN in adults is more likely to lead to renal insufficiency (13% of adult cases) (17).

HSP must be distinguished from CLA, cryoglobulinemia, ANCA-associated vasculitides, connective-tissue disorders associated with vasculitis, and infections (e.g., endocarditis). Classification criteria for HSP have been established by the ACR (19). Because cutaneous purpura is the *sine qua non* of HSP, skin biopsy provides a means for definitive diagnosis through the demonstration of IgA deposition in blood vessel walls. Leukocytoclastic vasculitis is the dominant finding on light microscopy in most affected organs, including the skin and GI tract. Renal lesions range from minimal disease to focal or diffuse proliferative GN with crescents. Immunofluorescence studies of renal biopsies show mesangial IgA deposition. Medium-sized blood vessels rarely are involved in HSP except in patients with IgA monoclonal gammopathies.

Treatment

With the exception of patients with severe renal disease, HSP is a self-limited condition lasting an average of only four weeks (range: three days to two years)(17). Treatment of HSP has not been studied extensively. NSAIDs may alleviate arthralgias (at the risk of exacerbating GI symptoms) but should be avoided in patients with GN. Corticosteroids ameliorate the joint and GI symptoms, but their effectiveness in renal disease is controversial (17). Uncontrolled trials suggest that the combination of high-dose corticosteroids and a cytotoxic agent help patients with severe GN. Chronic renal failure is rare, except in adults with more than 50% crescents on renal biopsy.

Urticarial Vasculitis

At least three subtypes of urticarial vasculitis (UV) are known: 1) a normocomplementemic form that generally is idiopathic, self-limited, and benign (and which may be viewed as a form of CLA); 2) a hypocomplementemic form, which often is associated with a systemic inflammatory disease; and, finally 3) the hypocomplementemic urticarial vasculitis syndrome (HUVS), a potentially severe systemic lupus erythematosus (SLE)-like condition usually associated with autoantibodies to the collagen-like region of C1q (20). Most people with UV have the hypocomplementemic subtype and demonstrate low C3, C4, and CH50 during periods of active disease.

Clinical Features

The lesions of UV must be distinguished from chronic idiopathic urticaria. Only about 10% of people with chronic urticaria have UV. In contrast to common urticaria, the lesions of UV last more than 48 hours, often have a purpuric (nonblanchable) component, are associated with sensations of stinging and burning rather than pruritus, and often leave postinflammatory hyperpigmentation. Normocomplementemic UV also must be distinguished (by skin biopsy) from neutrophilic urticaria, a refractory form of hives not associated with vasculitis.

A small number of people with hypocomplementemic UV have HUVS, a disorder resembling SLE (21). Like SLE,

HUVS has a striking female predominance, with a female:male ratio of 8:1. However, SLE-specific antibodies (e.g., those to double-stranded DNA and the Sm antigen) do not occur in HUVS, and several clinical features distinguish these two disorders. For example, HUVS may be associated with angioedema, uveitis, and chronic obstructive pulmonary disease, all of which are highly atypical of SLE. As in SLE, kidney biopsies in people with HUVS may reveal mesangial inflammation or membranoproliferative GN, but progression to end-stage renal disease in HUVS is unusual.

Most people with HUVS make C1q precipitins, i.e., IgG autoantibodies to the collagen-like region of C1q. Assays for these antibodies are not available widely, and their true role in the pathogenesis of HUVS remains unclear. Anti-C1q antibodies also are detected in up to one-third of people with SLE (and more than 80% of those with GN). Despite the prevalence of these antibodies in SLE, few people with SLE and anti-C1q antibodies develop urticarial lesions. However, glomeruli from people with lupus nephritis contain large quantities of anti-C1q antibodies. Theoretically, these antibodies may amplify tissue injury by rendering dsDNA immune complexes less soluble and more inflammatory (22).

Treatment
The natural history of UV is difficult to predict. The normocomplementemic form usually requires little therapy. In the hypocomplementemic form of UV limited to the skin, hydroxychloroquine, dapsone, and low doses of corticosteroids may be useful. HUVS may cause life-threatening involvement of the lungs or other organs and sometimes requires periods of intensive immunosuppression. These regimens must be tailored to the disease characteristics of individual patients.

Cryoglobulinemic Vasculitis

Cryoglobulins (CGs) are antibodies that precipitate from serum under conditions of cold and resolubilize upon warming (23). Isolation of these proteins in the laboratory may require refrigeration at 4°C for several days. CGs occur in association with a number of systemic conditions (e.g., autoimmune diseases and malignancies) and may lead to clinical complications that include vasculitis and hyperviscosity. CGs are classified into Types I, II, or III based on the presence or absence of monoclonality and rheumatoid factor (RF) activity (24). Type I CGs, which are monoclonal and lack RF activity, are associated with certain hematopoietic malignancies and often lead to hyperviscosity, rather than vasculitis. In contrast, Type II and Type III CGs may be associated with systemic vasculitis involving small-sized (and often medium-sized) blood vessels. In these conditions, vasculitis results from the deposition of CG-containing immune complexes in blood vessel walls and the activation of complement.

Cryoglobulin Types II and III are called "mixed" CGs because they consist of both IgG and IgM antibodies. The IgM components in Type II and III CGs possess RF activity.

Although the IgM component in Type II CG is monoclonal, the IgM in Type III is polyclonal. Ninety percent of patients with vasculitis secondary to mixed cryoglobulinemia are hypocomplementemic, with C4 levels characteristically more depressed than C3 levels (23). The presence of RF and depressed levels of C4 in the serum, and the occurrence of clinical features similar to those of rheumatoid arthritis or SLE, often lead to misdiagnoses.

Clinical Features
The most common manifestations of cryoglobulinemic vasculitis are recurrent crops of palpable purpura on the legs (Fig. 21A-3). MVV may be associated with large, painful ulcerations. In addition to leukocytoclastic vasculitis, skin biopsies (with DIF) show granular IgM and C3 deposits in and around small and medium-sized blood vessels. Other common manifestations are vasculitic neuropathy, GN, arthralgias, malaise, and fatigue. Some patients develop mesenteric vasculitis, Raynaud's phenomenon, livedo reticularis, or secondary Sjögren's syndrome. The features of Type II and III cryoglobulinemia are virtually indistinguishable, except that GN almost always is associated with Type II CGs (23). CNS vasculitis occurs in a small minority of people with CG.

Infection with the hepatitis C virus (HCV) accounts for at least 80% of the vasculitis cases associated with mixed CGs. Compared to serum levels, anti-HCV antibodies and HCV RNA in CG precipitates are concentrated 1000-fold. Because of the burgeoning HCV epidemic, an increasing number of cryoglobulinemic vasculitis cases are anticipated. However, vasculitis occurs in only a minority of people with HCV, although 50% of patients infected with HCV have demonstrable CGs. This finding probably relates both to host genetic factors and to specific features of the infecting HCV quasi-species.

Treatment
For CG patients with relatively mild disease (e.g., frequent purpuric lesions, shallow cutaneous ulcers), interferon α (3 × 10⁶ units three times per week) alone or combined with

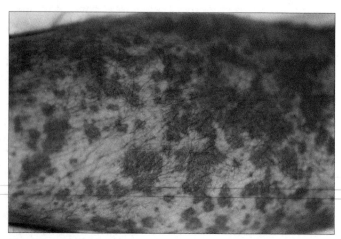

Fig. 21A-3. Palpable purpura.

ribavirin (1000–1200 mg/day) may be effective. If antiviral therapy is initiated prior to control of the inflammatory process with immunosuppression, temporary exacerbations of the vasculitic process may result from unfavorable alterations of the antigen:antibody ratio. For patients with MM or other manifestations of severe disease, corticosteroids and cyclophosphamide are required, and plasmapheresis may be a useful adjunctive therapy. In such cases, antiviral therapy may begin after control of the inflammatory process with traditional immunosuppressive agents.

JOHN H. STONE, MD, MPH

References

1. Nowack R, Flores-Suarez L, van der Woude F. New developments in pathogenesis of systemic vasculitis. Curr Opin Rheum 1998;10:3–11.
2. Kussmaul A, Maier R. Ueber eine bisher nicht beschriebene eigenthumliche arterienerkrankung (periarteritis nodosa), die mit morbus brightii und rapid fortschreitender allgemeiner muskellahmung einhergeht. Dtsch Arch Klin Med 1866;1:484–518.
3. Jennette J, Falk R, Andrassy K, et al. Nomenclature of systemic vasculitides. Proposal of an international consensus conference. Arthritis Rheum 1994;37:187–192.
4. Watts RA, Carruthers DM, Scott DG. Epidemiology of systemic vasculitis: changing incidence or definition? Semin Arthritis Rheum 1995;25:28–34.
5. Scott D, Bacon P, Elliott P, et al. Systemic vasculitis in district general hospital 1972-1980: clinical and laboratory features, classification and prognosis of cases. Q J Med 1982;51:292–311.
6. Kurland L, Chuang T, Hunder G. The epidemiology of systemic arteritis. In: Lawrence R, Shulman L (eds). The Epidemiology of the Rheumatic Diseases. New York: Gower, 1984; pp 196–205.
7. Sack M, Cassidy J, Bole C. Prognostic factors in polyarteritis. J Rheumatol 1975;2:411–420.
8. Guillevin L, Lhote F, Cohen P, et al. Polyarteritis nodosa related to hepatitis B virus. A prospective study with long-term observation of 41 patients. Medicine 1995;74:238–253.
9. Guillevin L, Huong L, Godeau P, Jais P, Wechsler B. Clinical findings and prognosis of polyarteritis nodosa and Churg-Strauss angiitis: a study in 165 patients. Br J Rheum 1988;27:258–264.
10. Heptinstall RH. Polyarteritis (periarteritis) nodosa, Wegener's syndrome, and other forms of vasculitis. In: Heptinstall RH. Pathology of the Kidney, 4th edition. Boston: Little, Brown, 1992; pp 1097-1102.
11. Ewald E, Griffin D, McCune W. Correlation of angiographic abnormalities with disease manifestations and disease severity in polyarteritis nodosa. J Rheumatol 1987;14:952–956.
12. Guillevin L, Lhote F. Treatment of polyarteritis nodosa and microscopic polyangiitis. Arthritis Rheum 1998;41:2100–2105.
13. Davson J, Ball J, Platt R. The kidney in periarteritis nodosa. QJM 1948;17:175–192.
14. Guillevin L, Durand-Gasselin B, Cevallos R, et al. Microscopic polyangiitis: clinical and laboratory findings in eighty-five patients. Arthritis Rheum 1999;42:421–430.
15. Zeek P. Periarteritis nodosa: a critical review. Am J Clin Pathol 1952;221:777–790.
16. Calabrese L, Michel B, Bloch D, et al. The American College of Rheumatology 1990 criteria for the classification of hypersensitivity vasculitis. Arthritis Rheum 1990;33:1108–1113.
17. Saulsbury F. Henoch-Schonlein purpura in children. Medicine (Baltimore) 1999;78:395–409.
18. Stewart M, Savage J, Bell B, McCord B. Long term renal prognosis of Henoch-Schonlein purpura in an unselected childhood population. Eur J Pediatr 1988;147:113–115.
19. Mills J, Michel B, Bloch D, et al. The American College of Rheumatology 1990 criteria for classification of Henoch-Schonlein purpura. Arthritis Rheum 1990;33:1114–1121.
20. Wisnieski J. Urticarial vasculitis. Curr Opin Rheum 2000;12:24–31.
21. Wisnieski J, Baer A, Christensen J, et al. Hypocomplementemic urticarial vasculitis syndrome: clinical and serological findings in 18 patients. Medicine (Baltimore) 1995;74:24–41.
22. Mannik M, Wener M. Deposition of antibodies to the collagen-like region of C1q in renal glomeruli of patients with proliferative lupus glomerulonephritis. Arthritis Rheum 1997;40:1504–1511.
23. Lamprecht P, Gause A, Gross W. Cryoglobulinemic vasculitis. Arthritis Rheum 1999;42:2507–2516.
24. Brouet J, Clauvel J, Danon F, Klein M, Seligmann M. Biologic and clinical significance of cryoglobulins. A report of 86 cases. Am J Med 1974;57:775–778.

VASCULITIDES
B. Wegener's Granulomatosis and Churg-Strauss Vasculitis

Within the heterogenous group of inflammatory blood vessel diseases, Wegener's granulomatosis (WG) and Churg-Strauss Syndrome (CSS) share several pathologic features that set them apart from other vasculitides. In classic cases of WG and CSS, medium-sized and small vessels are affected. The inflammatory infiltrate can be granulomatous in character and may be necrotizing. Granuloma formation and tissue necrosis are present in blood vessels and outside of vascular structures. Both syndromes can be associated with the production of antibodies to neutrophil cytoplasmic antigens, but only CSS is associated with eosinophilia, atopy, and asthma.

Wegener's Granulomatosis

Disease manifestations in WG are the result of tissue injury from aseptic inflammation, which may be nonspecific (e.g., pleomorphic infiltrates and necrosis), or may include more characteristic features, such as granuloma formation and vasculitis. Sites most commonly affected are the upper and lower respiratory tract and the kidneys (glomerulonephritis). Vascular injury is most evident in small and medium-sized vessels (vasculitis). Musculoskeletal features are common and may be quite painful. Pain often is disproportionate to signs of inflammation. Joint deformity or destruction, although reported, is very unusual. Approximately 25% of cases have peripheral or central nervous system disease (Table 21B-1). Morbidity is related most often to airway, renal, auditory, and ocular damage. Immunosuppressive therapy has been very effective in controlling disease progression, but may not produce sustained remissions and often is associated with serious complications (1,2).

Epidemiology

Wegener's granulomatosis affects approximately one in 20,000–30,000 people (3). The majority of patients are adults, although individuals of all ages can be affected. There are no significant preferences in regard to gender (1,4,5). WG is recognized predominantly in Caucasians. African Americans are underrepresented (2%–3% of WG patients), relative to their population in the United States (11%). Nonetheless, WG can occur in persons of all ethnic and racial backgrounds (3–5).

Clinical Features

At initial presentation, most patients do not have renal involvement or overt lung disease. However, during the course of illness, approximately 70%–80% will develop pulmonary and/or renal disease (1,2). Most patients initially seek medical care because of upper or lower airway symptoms. Nasal, sinus, tracheal, and ear abnormalities are responsible for presenting complaints in >70% of patients. More than 90% of patients eventually will develop upper airway and/or ear abnormalities. Prior to the diagnosis of WG, these problems often are considered to be secondary to allergy or infection. Symptomatic treatment, followed by such persistent symptoms and complications as recurrent epistaxis, mucosal ulcerations, nasal septal perforation, and nasal deformity, usually leads to more extensive evaluation. Otolaryngeal symptoms, especially in conjunction with an active urine sediment (regardless of serum creatinine value), pulmonary abnormalities, elevated erythrocyte sedimentation rate (ESR), or unexplained anemia, may prompt an antineutrophil cytoplasmic antibodies (ANCA) test. ANCA are positive in the majority of people with active WG. However, because ANCA may be negative in a significant minority of cases, especially in mild forms of disease (up to

TABLE 21B-1
Wegener's Granulomatosis: Clinical Profile[a]

Abnormality	Frequency at presentation (%)	Frequency during disease course (%)
Upper airways	73->93	92–99
Lower airways	48–55	66–85
Kidneys	18–54	70–75
Joint	32–61	67–77
Eye	15–40	52–61
Skin	13–23	30–46
Nerve	1–21	20–40

[a] Data adapted from Hoffman et al. Ann Intern Med 1992;116:488–498 and Reinhold-Keller et al. (1).

40%), a biopsy of an involved site may be required to support a definitive diagnosis (5).

Pulmonary infiltrates or nodules initially are present in approximately 50% of patients (Fig. 21B-1). Symptoms may include cough, hemoptysis, pleuritis, and dyspnea. Approximately 85% of these patients eventually will develop WG lung disease. About one-third of people with WG have asymptomatic pulmonary involvement, an important point to consider in initial and longitudinal selection of diagnostic studies (5).

Although a minority of patients have features of glomerulonephritis at presentation, approximately 75% of people with WG eventually will develop glomerulonephritis. In almost all cases, until the point of advanced uremia, renal disease is asymptomatic. This observation indicates the need for episodic evaluation of the urine to detect glomerulonephritis as early as possible. Some authorities advocate teaching patients to perform biweekly dipstick analyses to detect the first signs of renal involvement (1,5), but this approach is not useful if glomerulonephritis already is present and the urine contains blood.

Prognosis

A diagnosis of WG once was considered a death sentence. Prior to the 1970s, only 50% of patients survived five months from the time of diagnosis, and 82% of patients died within one year (2). In 1967, Hollander and Manning (6) reported a mean survival of 12.5 months in 26 patients treated with corticosteroids. In 1973, Fauci and Wolff (7) noted 13 remissions among 15 people with WG who received daily low-dose cyclophosphamide (14 patients) or azathioprine (one patient). As of 1991, the outcome of the extended WG National Institutes of Health (NIH) experience had included 158 patients followed for six months to 24 years (mean duration of follow up, eight years) (5). Among all patients treated with daily cyclophosphamide and corticosteroids, 91% had marked improvement and 75% achieved remission. Among 99 patients followed for

>5 years, 44% had remissions of >5 years' duration. Unfortunately, 50% of remissions later were associated with one or more relapses. Over a mean follow-up period of eight years, mortality from disease or treatment was 13%, a dramatic improvement over historical series, in which 50% mortality occurred over five months.

Treatment

The NIH protocol for WG has become the standard for other severe forms of vasculitis, such as CSS, microscopic polyangiitis (MPA), and polyarteritis nodosa (PAN), when critical organ involvement is present. The qualified success of this protocol requires review of its application in practice.

In severe forms of vasculitis, initial therapy consists of cyclophosphamide (2 mg/kg/day, orally) in combination with prednisone (1 mg/kg/day, orally). In patients with fulminant and rapidly progressive disease, cyclophosphamide therapy may be started at 3–5 mg/kg/day, for two to three days, using the leukocyte count to guide subsequent dosage adjustments. Under these circumstances, prednisone (or a soluble parenteral equivalent) usually is given at a dose that varies from 2 to 15 mg/kg/day for the first few days, followed by a return to 1 mg/kg/day. The latter dose is continued for approximately four weeks. If marked improvement occurs, prednisone is tapered gradually; in the setting of sustained remission, it is discontinued over three to six months.

In the past, cyclophosphamide would have been continued for at least one full year after sustained remission. However, increased awareness of cyclophosphamide's long-term toxicity has led to alternative strategies for care. Long-term daily cyclophosphamide therapy may be associated with bladder cystitis (50%), bladder cancer (5% at 10-year follow up and, 16% at 15-year follow up), and myelodysplasia (2%). The rate of malignancy in people with WG in the NIH series, compared with controls in the National Cancer Institute Registry, showed 2.4-fold increase in all malignancies, 33-fold increase in bladder cancer, and 11-fold increase in lymphomas (5,8). Almost all patients who had cyclophosphamide-associated bladder cancer previously had either microscopic or gross hematuria. This led Hoffman and colleagues to recommend cytoscopic examination of the bladder if hematuria was not clearly due to glomerulonephritis, as demonstrated by an active urine sediment with or without a rise in serum creatinine. However, although atypical cells on a urine cytology examination may warn of the possibility of bladder cancer, urine cytology is a relatively insensitive test in this setting (5,8).

Fifty percent of patients in the NIH series experienced severe infections, one of the most serious and common complications of intense immunosuppressive therapy. Eleven of 180 patients (6%) developed *Pneumocystis carinii* pneumonia, and one of these 11 died from the infection. All of the *Pneumocystis*-infected patients had been receiving corticosteroids plus a cytotoxic agent, were in the earliest phase of treatment for disease exacerbations, and were lymphopenic (mean lymphocyte count = 303 cells/mm^3). These observations have led to the recommendation for *Pneumocystis*

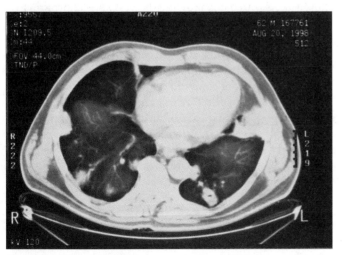

Fig. 21B-1. Wegener's granulomatosis. Lung disease may take the form of diffuse or focal infiltrates or nodules, which may cavitate.

chemoprophylaxis during the period of immunosuppressive therapy when treatment is most intense (9).

Alternatives to Long-Term Cyclophosphamide

Several prospective studies have evaluated intermittent high-dose intravenous (pulse) cyclophosphamide; trimethoprim/sulfamethoxazole therapy for non–life-threatening manifestations of WG; and corticosteroids plus intermittent (weekly) low-dose (15–25 mg) methotrexate (MTX) therapy.

Cyclophosphamide pulse therapy and daily corticosteroids may provide substantial initial improvement, but pulse therapy is not as effective as daily low-dose cyclophosphamide in maintaining the improvement (10,11). This conclusion has provoked much controversy and continued study.

MTX has been under study at the NIH for more than 12 years. It has been used in patients not judged to have immediately life-threatening disease, which is defined as severe diffuse pulmonary infiltrates and potential or actual ventilator dependency, or rapidly progressive glomerulonephritis with a serum creatinine in excess of 2.5 mg/dL. This protocol initiates treatment with MTX at 0.3 mg/kg/week, followed by a gradual increase in dose to the maximum tolerated, not to exceed 25 mg/week. (Lower doses are used for mild to moderate renal impairment.) Seventy-one percent of patients in this study achieved remission within a mean period of 4.2 months. An additional 12% had substantial improvement, but not complete remission. Thirty-six percent of patients subsequently relapsed over a mean period of 29 months and required retreatment. Initiating and maintaining therapy with MTX clearly is a reasonable alternative to cyclophosphamide in a select group of people with WG (12).

The most promising among the new approaches is induction therapy with daily cyclophosphamide, followed in three to six months with maintenance MTX (13,14) or azathioprine (15). This strategy has led to induction and maintenance of remission in approximately 80% of patients in three groups that were followed for periods of 18 months to two years. Other studies are exploring whether etanercept, leflunomide, and mycophenolate mofetil can help maintain remission in WG.

Principles for Monitoring Cytotoxic Therapy

Peripheral leukocyte counts can guide adjustment of cyclophosphamide, MTX, and azathioprine doses. To avoid undue risks of toxicity, the leukocyte count should not be allowed to drop below 3500 cells/mm³, nor the neutrophil count to below 1000–1500 cells/mm³. Observing the leukocyte count's slope of decrease is essential to the proper adjustment of dosage (5,7). If the leukocyte count approaches neutropenic levels, dosages should be reduced. When using cyclophosphamide in the early induction phase of treatment, it is advisable to monitor the leukocyte count approximately every three days and, after the leukocyte count stabilizes, check the counts at intervals no longer than every two weeks. Because elderly patients are more prone to drug toxicity, renal insufficiency, and opportunistic infections, these

patients may need to be monitored more frequently (16). It cannot be overemphasized that therapeutic benefits do not depend on the production of leukopenia or neutropenia. These end points are not an inherent goal of therapy.

Churg-Strauss Syndrome

Epidemiology

Churg-Strauss syndrome (allergic granulomatosis and angiitis) is extremely rare. Epidemiologic analyses are scant. In one study from the United Kingdom, the annual incidence was estimated to be about three per million people (17). There is no clear sexual preference, and people of any age may be affected.

Clinical Features

This syndrome differs clinically from PAN, MPA, and WG in that systemic vasculitis occurs in the setting of asthma, eosinophilia, pulmonary infiltrates, and allergic rhinitis. Pathologic studies reveal intra- and/or extravascular granulomas and inflammatory lesions rich in eosinophils (18). CSS affects small and medium-sized vessels, but there is a predilection for smaller arteries, arterioles, capillaries, and venules.

Asthma usually precedes evidence of vasculitis by months to many years. In up to 20% of cases, both processes may begin simultaneously. The presence of rhinitis, sinusitis, and occasionally pulmonary nodules can lead to confusion with WG. However, the allergic nasal and sinus disease of CSS generally is not a destructive process, pulmonary nodules are less common than fleeting infiltrates, and if nodules do occur, they generally do not cavitate (as often occurs in WG). Coronary arteritis, myocarditis, and gut involvement are more frequent in CSS (Table 21B-2).

Treatment

Churg-Strauss syndrome generally is more responsive to corticosteroid therapy than are MPA, PAN, or WG. Response to high-dose prednisone (1 mg/kg/day) often is prompt. Cytotoxic agents, such as cyclophosphamide, should be reserved for individuals with severe, progressive disease, which includes involvement of the kidneys, gut, heart, and in cases of diffuse pulmonary hemorrhage, lungs (19). In one preliminary study, interferon α (7.5–63 million units per week) led to improvement or remission in four patients treated over a period of 14–25 months (20).

During the past three years, questions have been raised about the possible role of leukotriene antagonists in precipitating CSS. It is uncertain whether these agents cause CSS in uniquely susceptible people or whether established subclinical CSS becomes apparent in the course of corticosteroid withdrawal facilitated by leukotriene antagonists.

Antineutrophil Cytoplasmic Antibodies

Since 1985, ANCA studies have achieved popularity as an adjunct to diagnosis of WG, MPA, glomerulonephritis

TABLE 21B-2
Churg-Strauss Syndrome: Clinical Profile[a]

Abnormality	Frequency (%)
Pulmonary	
Asthma	100
Pulmonary infiltrates	30–70
Pleural effusion	0–30
Allergic rhinitis	~75
Sinusitis	~75
Cardiovasular	85
Congestive heart failure	25–50
Pericarditis	10–30
Hypertension	30–75
Cutaneous	66
Purpura	~50
Erythema/urticaria	35–56
Nodules	10–30
Nervous system	
Mononeuritis multiplex	35–75
Central nervous system	25–60
Gastrointestinal	~90
Abdominal pain	20–60
Diarrhea	~30
Bleeding	~20
Renal	
Glomerulonephritis	40–85
Renal failure	~10
Musculoskeletal	20–70
Myalgias	40
Arthralgias/arthritis	30–50

[a] Data adapted from Lanham et al. Medicine 1984;63:65–81.
Chumbley et al. Mayo Clin Proc 1977;52:477–484. 1977.
Churg J, Strauss L. Am J Pathol 1951;27:277–301.

with scant or absent immune complexes (pauci-immune), and to a lesser extent, CSS. By indirect immunofluorescent techniques, two principal ANCA patterns are recognized: cytoplasmic and perinuclear. Current terminology that distinguishes between c-ANCA and p-ANCA is based on the fluorescence appearance on ethanol-fixed neutrophil cytospin preparations: c-ANCA indicates cytoplasmic staining and refers to the coarse, granular, centrally accentuated, cytoplasmic fluorescence pattern. The characteristic c-ANCA pattern usually is caused by antibodies against proteinase 3 (PR3), a neutral serine protease present in the azurophil granules of neutrophils (21).

Clearly distinct from the c-ANCA is the perinuclear (p-ANCA) fluorescence pattern on ethanol-fixed neutrophils. Perinuclear fluorescence is due in part to an artifact of ethanol fixation of polymorphonuclear leukocytes. Ethanol alters neutrophil cytoplasmic granule integrity, causing release of constituents. Positively charged granule proteins are displaced to the negatively charged nuclear membrane. The use of cross-linking fixatives, such as formalin, during the preparation of the neutrophil substrates prevents the perinuclear rearrangement of charged antigens, allowing true p-ANCA to be distinguished from antinuclear antibody (ANA). On formalin-fixed neutrophils, a true p-ANCA will display diffuse granular cytoplasmic staining, whereas an ANA-containing serum sample will display nuclear staining (21).

Enzyme-linked immunosorbent assay (ELISA) techniques enable identification of many target antigens that are associated with autoantibodies causing c- or p-ANCA fluorescence. Myeloperoxidase (MPO) is the p-ANCA target antigen with the greatest clinical utility because of the frequent association of MPO-ANCA with MPA and pauci-immune glomerulonephritis. However, autoantibodies against elastase, cathepsin G, lactoferrin, lysozyme, and azurocidin have been identified as causing the p-ANCA phenomenon. In a significant proportion of p-ANCA–positive sera, the target antigens have not been characterized. Ideally, immunofluorescence results should be corroborated with antigen-specific testing for PR3 and MPO (21).

The most clear-cut association of a disease in which ANCA is directed against a specific target antigen is WG, for which the antigen usually is PR3 (50%–90% sensitivity). Eighty percent to 95% of all ANCA found in WG are c-ANCA. An estimated 5%–20% of ANCA in WG may be p-ANCA that are directed mostly against MPO, and directed only rarely against other known target antigens. The sensitivity of c-ANCA/PR3-ANCA for WG generally, albeit not always, is related to the extent, severity, and activity of disease.

ANCA have been detected with variable frequency in people with CSS. Both PR3 and MPO have been described as target antigens. In one study, only four of eight people with CSS had ANCA by immunofluorescence (all p-ANCA), but six had MPO-ANCA detectable by ELISA. In another report, eight of 12 people with CSS were ANCA-positive by immunofluorescence, half had a cytoplasmic pattern, half had a perinuclear pattern, and four of eight were reactive to MPO by ELISA. In another series, only five of 25 patients with CSS were ANCA-positive, and all had a cytoplasmic pattern. Consequently, the diagnostic utility and pathologic significance of ANCA in CSS is uncertain (21).

Utility of Sequential ANCA Studies

Should ANCA play a role in treatment decisions for people with established diagnoses of vasculitis? Persistent high titers or rising titers of ANCA (anti-MPO or anti-PR3) often are associated with relapse from remission in MPA or WG. However, up to one-third or more of patients with such ANCA profiles may not relapse during one or more years of follow-up. Certainly, if treatment for these diseases were free of risk, lifelong therapy or therapy tailored to even imperfect correlations of disease activity and ANCA titer could be endorsed. However, aggressive treatment with corticosteroids and cytotoxic agents carries substantial risk. It is clear that good outcomes are compromised by either unrecognized disease relapses or injudiciously applied potent and toxic therapies. The prognostic value of a rise in ANCA titer is imperfect. Its use as the sole parameter to justify immunosuppressive therapy puts about one-third of patients at risk of overtreatment and unnecessary toxicity, and cannot be endorsed. Such therapy should be instituted only on unequivocal evidence of relapse. What role sequential ANCA studies should play in patient care after diagnosis is unclear (21).

GARY S. HOFFMAN, MD

References

1. Reinhold-Keller E, Beuge N, Latza U, et al. An interdisciplinary approach to the care of patients with Wegener's granulomatosis. Long-term outcome in 155 patients. Arthritis Rheum 2000;43:1021–1032.

2. Walton EW. Giant cell granuloma of the respiratory tract (Wegener's granulomatosis). Br Med J 1958;2:265–270.

3. Cotch MF, Hoffman GS, Yerg DE, Kaufman GI, Targonski P, Kaslow RA. The epidemiology of Wegener's granulomatosis. Arthritis Rheum 1996;39:87–92.

4. Bajema IM, Hagen EC, van der Woude FJ, Bruijn JA. Wegener's granulomatosis: a meta-analysis of 349 literary case reports. J Lab Clin Med 1997;129:17–22.

5. Hoffman GS, Kerr GS, Leavitt RY, et al. Wegener granulomatosis: an analysis of 158 patients. Ann Intern Med 1992;116:488–498.

6. Hollander D, Manning RT. The use of alkylating agents in the treatment of Wegener's granulomatosis. Ann Intern Med 1967;67:393–398.

7. Fauci AS, Wolff SM. Wegener's granulomatosis: studies in eighteen patients and a review of the literature. Medicine (Baltimore) 1973;52:535–561.

8. Talar-Williams C, Hijazi YM, Walther MM, et al. Cyclophosphamide-induced cystitis and bladder cancer in patients with Wegener's granulomatosis. Ann Intern Med 1996;124:477–484.

9. Ognibene FP, Shelhamer JH, Hoffman GS, et al. Pneumocystis carinii pneumonia: a major complication of immunosuppressive therapy in patients with Wegener's granulomatosis. Am J Respir Crit Care Med 1995;151:795–799.

10. Hoffman GS, Leavitt RY, Fleisher TA, Minor JR, Fauci AS. Treatment of Wegener's granulomatosis with intermittent high-dose intravenous cyclophosphamide. Am J Med 1990;89:403–410.

11. Guillevin L, Cordier JF, Lhote F, et al. A prospective, multicenter, randomized trial comparing steroids and pulse cyclophosphamide versus steroids and oral cyclophosphamide in the treatment of generalized Wegener's granulomatosis. Arthritis Rheum 1997;40:2187–2198.

12. Sneller MC, Hoffman GS, Talar-Williams C, Kerr GS, Hallahan CE, Fauci AS. An analysis of 42 Wegener's granulomatosis patients treated with methotrexate and prednisone. Arthritis Rheum 1995;38:608–613.

13. De Groot K, Reinhold-Keller E, Tatsis E, et al. Therapy for the maintenance of remission in 65 patients with generalized Wegener's granulomatosis: methotrexate versus trimethoprim/sulfamethoxazole. Arthritis Rheum 1996;39:2052–2061.

14. Langford CA, Talar-Williams C, Barron KS, Sneller MC. A staged approach to the treatment of Wegener's granulomatosis. Arthritis Rheum 1999;42:2666–2673.

15. Luqmani R, Jayne D, EUVAS (European Vasculitis Study Group). A multicenter randomized trial of cyclophosphamide versus azathioprine during remission in ANCA-associated systemic vasculitis. Arthritis Rheum 1999;42(S):928.

16. Krafcik SS, Covin RB, Lynch JP III, Sitrin RG. Wegener's granulomatosis in the elderly. Chest 1996;109:430–437.

17. Reid AJ, Scott DG, Watts RA, et al. Churg Strauss syndrome in the United Kingdom. A 13 year experience. Sarcoidosis Vasc Diffuse Lung Dis 1996;13:271.

18. Lanham JG, Elkon KB, Pusey CD, Hughes GR. Systemic vasculitis with asthma and eosinophilia: a clinical approach to Churg-Strauss syndrome. Medicine 1984;63:65–81.

19. Gayraud M, Guillevin L, Cohen P, et al. Treatment of good-prognosis polyarteritis nodosa and Churg Strauss syndrome: comparison of steroids and oral or pulse cyclophosphamide in 25 patients. Br J Rheumatol 1997;36:1290–1297.

20. Tatsis E, Schnabel A, Gross WL. Interferon-α treatment of four patients with Churg Strauss syndrome. Ann Intern Med 1998;129:370–374.

21. Hoffman GS, Specks U. Antineutrophil cytoplasmic antibodies. Arthritis Rheum 1998;41:1521–1537.10.

VASCULITIDES
C. Giant Cell Arteritis, Polymyalgia Rheumatica, and Takayasu's Arteritis

Despite the spatial closeness of blood vessels and inflammatory cells, blood vessel walls infrequently are the site of inflammation. The walls of capillaries and small blood vessels consist of only a few cell layers, and inflammatory destruction essentially is caused by a perivasculitis. In contrast, the medium-sized and large arteries have walls sizeable enough to be sites for inflammatory infiltrates. Two syndromes, giant cell arteritis (GCA) and Takayasu's arteritis (TA), are characterized by an inflammatory attack on vessel walls. GCA and TA display tissue tropism and preferentially affect defined vascular territories. GCA predominantly manifests in the second- to fifth-order branches of the aorta, often in the extracranial arteries of the head, and less frequently, in the aorta itself. The aorta and its major branches are the prime targets of TA.

Clinical symptoms of vascular inflammation and vascular insufficiency usually are accompanied or preceded by manifestations of systemic inflammation in both diseases. Systemic inflammation also is characteristic of polymyalgia rheumatica (PMR), a syndrome of muscle pain and stiffness in the neck, shoulders, and hips. PMR can accompany, precede, or follow GCA, but it may occur independently. In at least one subset of patients, PMR is a forme fruste of GCA, with a vasculitic component that is present but remains subclinical.

Giant Cell Arteritis

Epidemiology
Giant cell arteritis occurs almost exclusively in individuals older than 50 years, with disease incidence increasing progressively with age (1). Women are more likely than men to be affected. The prevalence is highest in Scandinavian countries and in regions settled by people of Northern European descent, with incidence rates reaching 15–25 cases per 100,000 persons aged 50 years and older. GCA occurs much less frequently in Southern Europeans (six cases per 100,000 individuals), and is rare in blacks and Hispanics (one to two cases per 100,000 individuals).

Etiology and Pathogenesis
The Lesion
The histologic hallmark of GCA is a mononuclear cell infiltrate dominated by T lymphocytes and macrophages that penetrate all layers of the wall of a mid-sized artery (Fig. 21C-1). The infiltrates can be granulomatous, with accumulation of histiocytes and multinucleated giant cells. Granuloma formation is most likely encountered in the media. Although the presence of multinucleated giant cells inspired the name of the disease, these cells often are absent, and the mononuclear infiltrates lack a complex

organization. If present, giant cells have a tendency to lie in close proximity to the fragmented internal elastic lamina. The presence of multinucleated giant cells has been correlated with increased risk for ischemic complications. GCA also can present with perivascular cuffing of vasa vasorum or T-cell–macrophage infiltrates in the adventitia, sometimes arranged along the external elastic lamina, consistent with studies that suggest the adventitia is a critical site in the disease process.

The inflammation causes a series of structural changes to the arterial wall. Fibrinoid necrosis is explicitly rare, but the medial smooth-muscle cell layer loses thickness. The intima often is hyperplastic, compromising or occluding the arterial lumen; luminal thrombosis is uncommon. Hyperplasia of the intimal layer with scarring in the media and fragmentation of the elastic laminae are irreversible changes that persist beyond the stages of active arterial inflammation.

Immune Response in the Arterial Wall
All experimental evidence supports a T-cell–mediated immunopathology of GCA (2). B cells essentially are absent from the vascular lesions; pathognomonic antibodies have not been identified and hypergammaglobulinemia is absent, suggesting that humoral immunity is not important. The emerging concept of immune stimulation and recognition in the vascular wall has benefited from a chimeric animal model generated by implanting human temporal arteries into severe combined immunodeficiency (SCID) mice.

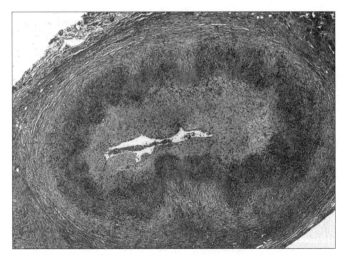

Fig. 21C-1. Histomorphology of giant cell arteritis. A typical temporal artery biopsy specimen is shown. Characteristic changes include a panmural mononuclear infiltrate, destruction of the internal and external elastic laminae, and concentric intimal hyperplasia.

Depletion of T cells from the implanted vascular lesions disrupts the inflammatory response with subsequent clearing of the inflammatory infiltrate. The T-cell cytokine interferon (IFN)-γ has been identified as a key player in the inflammatory response. IFN-γ derives from CD4 T cells located in the adventitia, assigning critical regulatory control to this region of the artery. Vasa vasorum currently are considered to be the site of entrance for tissue-invading T cells and macrophages, refuting the previous belief that inflammatory cells enter from the major lumen of the artery. This disease model has de-emphasized the role of the macroendothelium in GCA and has, instead, focused attention on the small capillaries in the arterial wall itself.

Just as T-cell function is linked closely to precise regions in the arterial wall, macrophage function is multifaceted, with a close correlation between topographical arrangement and commitment (3).

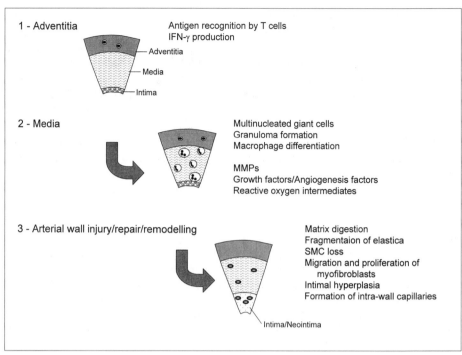

Fig. 21C-2. Schematic diagram of the sequence of pathogenetic events in giant cell arteritis. 1) Mononuclear cells enter the adventitia via the vasa vasorum, where T cells recognize antigen and produce interferon γ. 2) The infiltrate advances to the media, where macrophages and giant cells undergo differentiation and exert tissue-injurious effector functions. 3) The artery responds with neoangiogenesis and intimal hyperplasia.

Macrophages in the adventitia, intermingling with activated T cells, produce interleukin (IL)-1, IL-6, and transforming growth factor (TGF)-β. Macrophages in the medial layer are specialized in their production of metalloproteinases and contribute to oxidative damage. End products of lipid peroxidation, a cell injury mechanism driven by oxygen radicals, typically are found on medial smooth-muscle cells (4). Macrophages recruited to the intimal layer are committed to the production of nitric oxide synthase 2; nitric oxide is suspected to be involved in tissue injury, cellular activation, and vascular remodeling. Multinucleated giant cells, previously assumed to function in the removal of indigestible debris, now are believed to be active secretory cells that produce molecular mediators relevant to structural changes in the arterial wall. The presence of giant cells in GCA corresponds with the presence of high adventitial levels of IFN-γ (5), which explains why these particular cells are not seen in all cases of GCA.

The Artery: Active Collaborator in Arteritis
The assumption that all pathogenic mechanisms in inflamed arteries are mediated by tissue-infiltrating immune cells does not take into account that T cells and macrophages in the arterial wall do not live and function in isolation (6). The amazing compartmentalization of immune pathways in the wall indicates a close interaction between immune cells and stromal components of the blood vessel. Vascular abnormalities leading to clinical disease are related to nonthrom-

botic luminal occlusion, caused by rapid and concentric growth of the intima. These structural alterations result from the response to injury elicited in arterial cells (Fig. 21C-2). Intimal hyperplasia is generated by the mobilization of smooth-muscle cells, their directed migration toward the lumen, and their proliferation and matrix deposition. This process is under the control of growth factors. Platelet-derived growth factor (PDGF), which can support the outgrowth of the hyperplastic intima, is present in inflamed arteries. It derives from macrophages and multinucleated giant cells. Patients with low PDGF production have minimal or no lumen-occlusive intimal proliferation, whereas patients with excessive PDGF production are at risk for ischemic complications (7).

A second pathway of the arterial injury response process relates to formation of new capillaries. The media and intima of normal arteries are avascular, but intense neoangiogenesis is induced in GCA (8). Vascular endothelial growth factor (VEGF) is critical in driving the generation of neovessels in the media and intima. VEGF, like PDGF, originates from macrophages and multinucleated giant cells. The arterial response pattern initiated by the production of PDGF and VEGF leads to profound structural arterial abnormalities with subsequent stenosis and tissue ischemia, emphasizing that the immune system succeeds in coercing the artery towards a nonbeneficial reaction pattern. However, the inflammation also induces protective response patterns that are aimed at healing and tissue repair. An example is the up-regulation of the enzyme aldose reductase (9), which metabolizes and detoxifies end products of oxidative damage.

The Systemic Inflammatory Response

Inflammation and immune activation are not limited to vascular lesions. Circulating monocytes in people with GCA are highly activated and produce IL-1 and IL-6. IL-6 is a potent inducer of acute-phase responses, characteristically seen in patients with GCA. Release of this key player from circulating monocytes has led to the belief that the systemic component of GCA is an independent dimension of the disease process, rather than a spillover from vessel-wall inflammation.

Genetic Risk Factors

The high incidence rates of GCA in regions settled by people of Scandinavian ethnicity strongly suggests inherited risk factors. The best available information is for human leukocyte antigen (HLA) genes. HLA-DR4 haplotypes are associated with increased disease risk, and several allelic variants of HLA-DR4 are enriched among patients. Selective binding of antigenic peptides has been proposed as the mechanism underlying this genetic association. In contrast to other HLA-DR4–associated diseases, such as rheumatoid arthritis, HLA polymorphisms in GCA are not correlated with clinical patterning and disease severity. Other genetic risk factors have not been unequivocally defined.

Clinical Features

The diagnostic category of GCA encompasses multiple variants (Fig. 21C-3). Each of these subtypes has characteristic clinical features; however, it is important to note that the clinical manifestations of the different subtypes partially overlap and that none of the clinical symptoms is unique for any one of the variants. Increased awareness of GCA, a growing population of individuals older than 50 years, and optimized diagnostic procedures have led to increased detection of cases formerly considered to be atypical presentations.

In essence, GCA presents with two major symptomatic complexes: signs of vascular insufficiency resulting from impaired blood flow and signs of systemic inflammation. Notably, vascular changes are those of occlusion; arterial-wall dilation occurs only when the aorta is involved.

Cranial GCA

Giant cell arteritis also is known as temporal arteritis because extracranial branches of the carotid arteries are targeted preferentially. In 80%–90% of patients, histomorphologic evidence for vasculitis is detected in the extracranial arterial tree, most often in the superficial temporal, vertebral, ophthalmic, and posterior ciliary arteries, and less frequently, the internal and external carotid and central retinal arteries. Patients complain of throbbing, sharp or dull headaches, usually severe enough to prompt clinical evaluation; these headaches may or may not be associated with scalp tenderness. In typical cases, the patients notice temporal tenderness when wearing glasses, grooming, or lying on a pillow. Headaches may be temporary and subside without treatment, but in most cases, they cease promptly in response to corticosteroid therapy.

On physical examination, involved vessels are thickened, tender, and nodular; pulses are reduced or absent. Abnormalities are most frequent in the temporal arterial branches, but they can be detected in the occipital arteries or other superficial scalp vessels. In one-third of patients, temporal arteries appear normal.

Focal arteritic lesions in the ophthalmic artery produce the most feared complication of GCA, vision loss. The disease has been ranked as the prime ophthalmic emergency because prompt recognition and treatment can prevent blindness. Ischemia anywhere along the visual pathway can lead to vision loss, but ischemic optic neuropathy is the most common cause. Loss of vision is sudden, painless, and usually permanent. *Amaurosis fugax*, reported as fleeting visual blurring with heat or exercise, or posture-related visual blurring and diplopia, may precede partial or complete blindness. On ophthalmologic examination, anterior ischemic optic neuropathy is recognized by optic-disc edema, eventually followed by sectoral or generalized optic atrophy with optic-disc cupping. In addition to

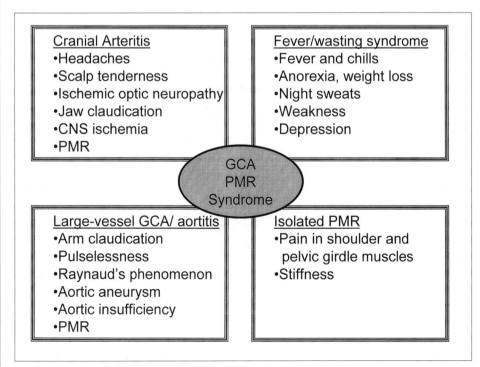

Fig. 21C-3. Clinical spectrum of the giant cell arteritis/polymyalgia rheumatica syndrome.

optic neuropathy, the spectrum of ophthalmic complications is wide-ranging, from pupillary defects to orbital ischemia, and ocular motor ischemia to anterior- and posterior-segment ischemia.

A relatively disease-specific manifestation of GCA present in about one-half of patients is intermittent claudication of the masseter and temporalis muscles caused by compromised blood flow in the extracranial branches of the carotid artery. Prolonged talking and chewing produce jaw claudication, and cases of trismus have been described. Claudication of the tongue and painful dysphagia are less frequent. Facial pain and neck or throat soreness are more likely to be seen in TA than in GCA. Vasoocclusive disease of the carotid and vertebrobasilar arteries results in ischemia of the central nervous system, manifesting as transient ischemic attacks or infarcts. Neurologic manifestations are being recognized and can be expected in 20%–30% of patients.

Vasculitis of the pulmonary artery branches is suspected as the pathomechanism underlying such respiratory symptoms as cough, hoarseness, and chest pain. Rarely, frank pulmonary infiltrates develop. Chronic, nonproductive cough can be an initial presentation.

GCA Manifesting as Fever of Unknown Origin
Symptoms related to systemic inflammation are frequent, and laboratory abnormalities are detected in more than 90% of patients. In a subset of patients, the disease process is dominated by the manifestation of a systemwide inflammatory syndrome. Fever of unknown origin, with spiking temperatures and chills, usually leads to a diagnostic work-up to exclude malignancy. In less dramatic cases, malaise, anorexia, weight loss, low-grade fever, and fatigue are severe enough to prompt medical attention. Physical examination of the scalp arteries often is negative and symptoms of vascular insufficiency can be absent. However, even in the setting of normal findings on clinical examination, temporal artery biopsy is the procedure of choice in making the diagnosis.

Large-Vessel GCA
In 10%–15% of patients, GCA targets the large arteries. Preferred vascular beds are the carotid, subclavian, and axillary arteries. Vasculitis of the femoral arteries is infrequent. The major clinical presentation is that of aortic arch syndrome, producing claudication of the arms, absent or asymmetrical pulses, paresthesias, Raynaud's phenomenon, and occasionally, peripheral gangrene. Patients with the large-vessel variant of GCA often lack evidence of cranial involvement: They do not complain about headaches, temporal arteries appear normal on examination, and almost 50% of temporal artery biopsies are negative for vasculitis (10). The diagnostic procedure of choice is angiography. Stenotic vascular lesions typically are located at the subclavian axillary junction and can be unilateral. The high rate of negative temporal artery biopsies in this subset of GCA patients emphasizes the need to consider aortic arch syndrome, even in the absence of temporal lesions.

Aortitis in GCA can coexist with cranial arteritis. Whether the patient subset with subclavian-axillary GCA is distinct from the subset that progresses to aortic involvement is not known. Overall, people with GCA have a 17-fold increase in the risk of developing thoracic aortic aneurysm. The elastic membranes supporting the aortic wall are destroyed and replaced by fibrotic tissue. The resulting histomorphology can be indistinguishable from that of TA. Most cases of aortitis have been diagnosed several years after the initial diagnosis of GCA, raising the possibility that smoldering aortitis is more common than previously believed (11). The spectrum of clinical manifestations ranges from silent aneurysm to aortic dissection and fatal rupture.

Laboratory Features
A pathognomonic laboratory test for GCA does not exist, and specific autoantibodies have not been identified. Highly elevated acute-phase responses are typical for GCA, but are not present in all patients. Traditionally, a high erythrocyte sedimentation rate (ESR) has prompted consideration of GCA. In a recent study, 25% of all patients with a positive temporal artery biopsy had a normal ESR prior to corticosteroid therapy (12). Other markers of acute-phase response, particularly C-reactive protein (CRP), may be more sensitive than ESR. The marker with the highest sensitivity for detecting ongoing systemic inflammation is the level of serum IL-6, both before and after corticosteroid therapy. IL-6 is a strong inducer of acute-phase reactants and probably functions upstream in the disease process. Patients often have mild to moderate normochromic or hypochromic anemia. Elevated platelet counts are common. Liver function tests, particularly alkaline phosphatase, can be abnormal.

Diagnosis
The diagnosis of GCA should be considered in people aged 50 years and older with recent onset of unexplained headache, signs of tissue ischemia in the extracranial vascular territory, loss of vision, or PMR and laboratory evidence for acute-phase responses. Prompt histologic proof of arteritis should be sought, with preference given to clinically abnormal arteries. Because of its easy accessibility, the superficial temporal artery usually is the site of tissue collection. The rate of false-negative biopsies can be minimized by taking a sufficient length of biopsy, examining serial sections, and removing the contralateral temporal artery in cases in which the first biopsy is free of arteritis. Vasoocclusive disease of the large arteries needs to be documented by angiography. Computed tomography (CT) and magnetic resonance imaging (MRI) are sensitive enough to detect wall abnormalities of the aorta and its primary branches. Noninvasive vascular studies, including fluorescein angiography, transcranial Doppler flow studies, and Doppler ultrasonography have been applied, but they likely identify only cases with pronounced, lumen-stenosing disease.

Treatment
Corticosteroids are effective in suppressing clinical manifestations of GCA. Since the introduction of corticosteroids,

the rate of GCA-related blindness has declined, documenting the effectiveness of this immunosuppressive approach. In almost all patients, corticosteroids induce complete relief within 12–48 hours. The excellent response of the disease to this therapy has been suggested as a diagnostic criterion.

In view of the severity of GCA-related morbidity, initial dosages of 60 mg/day prednisone or an equivalent have been recommended. Steroids cannot reverse intimal hyperplasia, but may help reduce ischemic insult by reducing tissue edema, and may contribute to improved vision. Initial doses should be maintained until reversible manifestations of the disease have responded and the systemic inflammatory syndrome is suppressed. With close monitoring for clinical signs of disease reactivation, the dose of prednisone generally can be tapered by 10% every one to two weeks.

Recent evidence suggests that the concept of GCA as a self-limited inflammatory disease probably is incorrect (11). In a prospective study of 25 patients with biopsy-proven GCA, clinical signs of the disease in all disappeared in response to 60 mg/day prednisone (12). However, disease relapses occurred in 60% of patients throughout the course of treatment. Disease reactivation typically produced symptoms of systemic inflammation, but no vascular complications were seen. Serum IL-6 levels were more sensitive than CRP and ESR measurements in detecting inflammation prior to and during corticosteroid therapy. Serum IL-6 levels remained elevated after discontinuation of therapy, indicating smoldering continuation of the disease process. Given the high rate of clinical response, the advisability of more intense immunosuppression, aimed at eradicating systemic inflammation, should be studied.

So far, none of the immunosuppressants used to manage other rheumatic disease has proved useful in treating GCA (13). Methotrexate, for example, has been shown to lack steroid-sparing activity in the treatment of GCA. Identifying molecular pathways of arterial-wall injury and systemic inflammation will provide new targets for future therapy, e.g., suppressing the outgrowth of hyperplastic intima or counteracting oxidative damage.

Prognosis

The most significant morbidity of GCA relates to reduced blood flow to the eye and optic nerve, as well as malperfusion of the brain. Progression of the downstream effects of arterial-wall inflammation, particularly lumen occlusion with tissue ischemia, can be prevented if diagnosed and treated promptly. Histologic or angiographic verification of vasculitis should be pursued because the side effects of high-dose corticosteroids given over a prolonged period of time can be serious, especially in patients older than 50 years.

The systemic component of GCA, the origin of which remains unexplained but appears to be closely related to activation of circulating monocytes, can be treated effectively with corticosteroids. Although sensitive to the immunosuppressive effect of corticosteroids, this manifestation of GCA may not permanently remit, but may require chronic monitoring and management. Chronic smoldering of the disease may be more relevant than previously thought.

Polymyalgia Rheumatica

Polymyalgia rheumatica is diagnosed in people presenting with pain and stiffness of at least four weeks duration in the muscles of the neck, shoulder girdle, and pelvic girdle. The myalgias are combined with such signs of systemic inflammation as malaise, weight loss, sweats, and low-grade fever. Most patients have laboratory abnormalities, such as elevated ESR, elevated CRP, and anemia, which are indicative of a systemic inflammatory syndrome. Up-regulation of acute-phase reactants is important in distinguishing PMR from other pain syndromes. A pathognomonic test for PMR is not available, and it is critical to rule out other diseases with similar clinical presentation. The systemic inflammatory syndrome associated with PMR is sensitive to corticosteroid therapy, to the extent that prompt improvement of clinical symptoms with corticosteroid therapy has been proposed as a diagnostic criterion.

Pathomechanisms in PMR are related closely to those in GCA. PMR often is considered to be a form of GCA that lacks fully developed vasculitis. Findings of blood vessel wall inflammation overrule the diagnosis of PMR and establish the diagnosis of GCA.

Epidemiology

Because PMR is a clinical diagnosis, epidemiologic studies are difficult. PMR affects the same patient population as GCA and occurs approximately twofold to threefold more frequently (1). Women are affected more frequently than men are, and the diagnosis is extremely unlikely in individuals younger than 50 years. In high-risk populations, such as Scandinavians and people of Northern European descent, annual incidence rates have been estimated at 20–53 per 100,000 persons older than 50 years. In low-risk populations, such as Italians, about 10 cases per 100,000 individuals 50 years and older are found each year.

Etiology and Pathogenesis

Although the sudden onset of intense inflammation suggests an infectious etiology, no causative agent has been identified. Most pathogenic abnormalities in people with PMR are reminiscent of those in GCA, supporting the emerging concept that PMR is a GCA variant that is characterized by dominance of the systemic inflammatory syndrome over the vascular component.

HLA polymorphisms that are genetic risk factors for GCA also are associated with PMR. There is no evidence that the HLA has a role in determining whether the disease process will remain limited to the polymyalgic syndrome or will progress to fully developed vasculitis.

One source of inflammation in PMR appears to lie in the circulating blood, where monocytes are highly activated and spontaneously produce IL-1 and IL-6. The triggering of circulating monocytes/macrophages is a feature common to PMR and GCA. Additional sites of inflammation may exist. Whether synovitis of shoulder and hip joints is a consistent feature of PMR is not clear. It is possible that such patients have seronegative RA, which sometimes presents with prominent proximal pain.

In situ transcription of proinflammatory cytokines, presumably derived from macrophages and T cells, can be demonstrated in temporal artery biopsies from people with PMR in whom standard histomorphology does not identify a typical infiltrate (14). Arteries from people with PMR typically lack tissue production of IFN-γ, which may be the critical event in transforming subclinical vasculitis into fully developed arteritis. The detection of vessel-wall inflammation by highly sensitive imaging techniques has been cited as demonstrating vascular involvement in PMR.

Clinical Features

People with PMR have aching and pain in the muscles of the neck, shoulders, low back, hips, thighs, and occasionally, the trunk. In typical cases, the onset is abrupt and the myalgias are symmetrical and initially affect the shoulders. Often, patients have pain during the night and have difficulties arising and dressing themselves. Weight loss, anorexia, malaise, and depression are common. Pyrexia and chills should raise the suspicion of fully developed GCA. Men, in particular, can present with diffuse edema of the hands and feet. Joint inflammation has been described, but usually requires sensitive diagnostic tests to be detected.

Polymyalgia rheumatica is a heterogeneous syndrome and includes mild disease that responds promptly to therapy and remits within a few months (15). Myalgias frequently are reactivated when corticosteroid doses are tapered. It is possible that the monophasic and remittive types of PMR are distinct diseases. A third subset of patients requires higher initial doses of steroids than are required by typical PMR patients.

Patients with PMR must be evaluated carefully for possible GCA. A negative temporal artery biopsy does not exclude the possibility of large-vessel vasculitis targeting primarily the subclavian and axillary arteries and the aorta. Signs of vascular insufficiency, including claudication in the extremities, bruits over arteries, and discrepant blood pressure readings should alert the physician to the possibility of frank GCA (10).

Clinical symptoms of PMR can be mimicked by other arthropathies, shoulder disorders, inflammatory myopathies, hypothyroidism, and Parkinson's disease. The differential diagnosis also includes malignancies and infections. No clear guidelines have been developed to determine whether patients with PMR should be screened for occult malignancies. Lack of typical and impressive improvement upon initiation of therapy should prompt reevaluation of the diagnosis of PMR.

Treatment

Polymyalgia rheumatica is explicitly responsive to corticosteroid therapy. Currently there are no data documenting steroid-sparing effects of other medications. However, almost all cases of PMR can be managed safely with steroids because dosages for long-term treatment are low and unlikely to cause serious side effects.

A critical issue in treating PMR is the dosage of corticosteroids required for successful suppression of symptoms and inflammation. The steroid requirements may differ quite markedly among patients. Two-thirds of patients can be expected to respond with remission of pain and stiffness when started on 20 mg prednisone per day (15). Some patients will need dosages as high as 40 mg/day for complete clinical control. Such patients have continuously elevated inflammatory markers, such as serum IL-6, while treated with prednisone at 20 mg per day. It is possible that such patients are at higher risk to progress to full-blown GCA. Patients reporting resolution of polymyalgias on 20 mg prednisone per day usually can taper the dosage by 2.5 mg every 10–15 days. More careful tapering may be necessary when daily doses of 7–8 mg prednisone are attained. Dose adjustments should be based mainly on clinical evaluation, not exclusively on laboratory abnormalities. In many patients, PMR can go into long-term remission and prednisone can be discontinued. Occasionally, successful suppression of recurrent myalgias and stiffness may be achieved only by giving very low doses of prednisone over an extended period. Patients should be warned about the potential of PMR progressing to GCA and should be monitored for vascular complications, particularly when discontinuing corticosteroid therapy.

Prognosis

The prognosis of people with PMR is good. In the majority of patients, the condition is self-limiting. A proportion of patients eventually will present with typical symmetrical polyarthritis, fulfilling criteria for the diagnosis of seronegative rheumatoid arthritis. Such patients may require disease-modifying antirheumatic drug therapy.

Takayasu's Arteritis

Takayasu's arteritis is a vasculitis of the large elastic arteries, specifically the aorta and its main branches, but it also may affect the coronary and pulmonary arteries (16). Inflammatory injury of the vessel wall leads to patchy disappearance of the elastic smooth-muscle layer, resulting in stenosis or aneurysm. Complete occlusion of the upper-extremity arteries results in loss of pulse, hence the name "pulseless disease." The preference for the aorta and its primary branches is signified in the name aortic arch syndrome. The American College of Rheumatology has developed a set of criteria to distinguish TA from other vasculitic syndromes (see Appendix I).

Epidemiology

Takayasu's arteritis is a rare disease that affects primarily adolescent girls and young women. The diagnostic criteria include an age of less than 40 years at disease onset; however, TA can start later in life, particularly in Asians (17). Incidence rates are highest in Asia (Japan, Korea, China, India, and Thailand) with estimates of approximately one case per 1 million persons annually. TA can occur in all

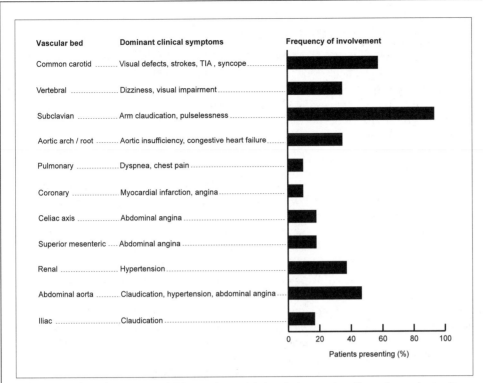

Vascular bed	Dominant clinical symptoms	Frequency of involvement
Common carotid	Visual defects, strokes, TIA, syncope	
Vertebral	Dizziness, visual impairment	
Subclavian	Arm claudication, pulselessness	
Aortic arch / root	Aortic insufficiency, congestive heart failure	
Pulmonary	Dyspnea, chest pain	
Coronary	Myocardial infarction, angina	
Celiac axis	Abdominal angina	
Superior mesenteric	Abdominal angina	
Renal	Hypertension	
Abdominal aorta	Claudication, hypertension, abdominal angina	
Iliac	Claudication	

Patients presenting (%)

Fig. 21C-4. Clinical spectrum of Takayasu's arteritis in relation to the affected vascular territory. Data from Kerr et al (20).

races and geographic regions, but South American countries have been recognized as areas of relatively high incidence. An international survey among 20 countries has indicated differences in the clinical spectrum of TA in different ethnic groups.

Etiology and Pathogenesis

Takayasu's arteritis is a granulomatous polyarteritis. The adventitia is characterized by striking thickening, often with intense perivascular infiltrates around the vasa vasorum. Granuloma formation and giant cells are found predominantly in the media of the large elastic arteries. The medial elastic smooth-muscle cell layer is destroyed in a centripetal direction and replaced by fibrotic tissue, providing the conditions for vessel-wall dilatation and aneurysm formation. Smooth tapering, narrowing, or complete occlusion of the vascular lumen results from proliferation of the intima, occasionally with thrombosis.

The etiology of TA remains unknown. In view of the systemic features of the syndrome, microbial infections have been implicated, but no conclusive evidence for infectious organisms has been provided. In aortic-wall lesions, CD8 T cells have been identified as a major cell type distinguishing the vascular infiltrates in TA from those in GCA. Cytotoxic capabilities of tissue-infiltrating CD8 T cells, mediated by release of the pore-forming enzymes perforin and granzyme B, have been suspected to contribute to damage of smooth-muscle cells (18).

Support for a role of CD8 T-cell mediated cytolytic tissue injury has come from the observation that selected HLA class I molecules, specifically HLA-B52, are over-represented

in people with TA (19). CD8 T cells recognize antigens when bound to HLA class I molecules. The role of CD4 T-cell responses and the contribution of macrophage effector functions in the vascular lesions are not understood. The focus of lymphocytic infiltrates on the adventitia and accumulation of T cells around vasa vasorum make it less likely that the macroendothelium has major involvement in the pathogenesis of TA.

Clinical Features

Clinical manifestations of TA are caused by two major components of the disease that can be dissociated in time and intensity. A syndrome of generalized inflammation can produce fever, night sweats, malaise, anorexia, weight loss, and diffuse myalgias. Because of the age of typical patients, these symptoms often are misdiagnosed as infection. More specific are manifestations of vascular insufficiency that may be preceded by complaints of pain over involved arteries, specifically the more superficial neck vessels.

The clinical pattern of ischemic complication directly reflects the vascular territory targeted by the disease (Fig. 21C-4). Involvement of the carotid and vertebral arteries leads to neurologic and ophthalmologic symptoms, including dizziness, tinnitus, headaches, syncope, stroke, and visual disturbances. Atrophy of facial muscles and jaw claudication mostly are late manifestations. Inflammatory occlusion of the subclavian arteries impairs or disrupts blood flow to the upper extremities, presenting as arm claudication, pulselessness, and discrepant blood pressures. Bruits over the subclavian vessels can be helpful diagnostically.

Cardiac disease, including ischemic coronary disease, arrhythmia, and congestive heart failure can be related to aortitis of the ascending aorta or to severe hypertension. Aortic regurgitation, a serious complication that requires prompt clinical attention, is a consequence of arterial-wall dilation. Coronary arteries can be directly or indirectly involved, producing classic symptoms of myocardial ischemia. Progressively enlarging aneurysms and possible rupture are of major concern in patients with TA of the aortic arch and the descending thoracic aorta. Lesions in the abdominal aorta, including the renal arteries, cause renovascular hypertension as a lead symptom and are found more frequently in some ethnic groups, such as Indians, Chinese, and Koreans. The proximal ends of mesenteric arteries are affected less frequently, but such gastrointestinal symptoms as nausea, vomiting, and ischemic bowel disease are common in patients with TA.

Diagnosis

A combination of vasoocclusive disease and systemic inflammation in a young patient should raise immediate suspicion for TA. Typically, the diagnosis is made by characteristic findings on vascular imaging; tissue rarely is available. Angiography provides the best information about the vessel lumen and can be combined with angioplasty, if indicated. A complete aortic arteriography can help determine the distribution and degree of involvement. Noninvasive vascular imaging techniques with CT, MRI, and magnetic resonance angiography allow evaluation of the arterial wall and can help estimate the extent of wall inflammation. These techniques are particularly important in monitoring the effect of therapy and monitoring the diameter of the aortic root.

Treatment

Corticosteroids remain the therapy of choice for management of TA. Recommendations for initial doses vary, but 40–60 mg of prednisone per day may be necessary to sufficiently control vascular and systemic inflammation. Unfortunately, monitoring of acute-phase reactants (ESR, CRP) is helpful in only a subset of patients. In an NIH cohort, 50% of patients had active, progressive disease, despite nonelevated acute-phase reactants (20). Vascular imaging can help guide immunosuppression by adding information beyond laboratory parameters, which typically reflect only the systemic component of the disease. Prednisone doses are tapered as clinically indicated and tolerated, usually by 5 mg/day every two weeks, until a maintenance dose of 10 mg/day is reached. Further dose reductions must be tailored to the individual patient. Low-dose aspirin or other antiplatelet agents should complement corticosteroid therapy. Methotrexate, given in weekly doses of up to 25 mg, has shown some promise in sparing steroids (21). Overall, cytotoxic agents do not have impressive therapeutic benefit in this inflammatory vasculopathy.

Aggressive surgical and angioplastic management has gained importance in the management of TA and may be one reason for improved outcomes. Ideally, arterial-wall inflammation should be treated prior to intervention, but that option may not always be practical.

Prognosis

Historically, TA was a devastating disease, but early diagnosis, immunosuppression, and aggressive surgical management have led to improved prognosis. Long-term follow-up of almost 1,000 Japanese patients found stable clinical conditions in two-thirds and serious complications in only 25%. Cardiac complications, including congestive heart failure and ischemic heart disease, have become the most common cause of death in Japanese patients with TA. Acceleration of atherosclerotic disease is a critical factor in long-term outcome.

CORNELIA M. WEYAND, MD
JÖRG J. GORONZY, MD

References

1. Hunder GG. Giant cell arteritis and polymyalgia rheumatica. Med Clin North Am 1997;81:195-219.
2. Weyand CM. The Dunlop-Dottridge Lecture: The pathogenesis of giant cell arteritis. J Rheumatol 2000;27:517-522.
3. Weyand CM, Wagner AD, Bjornsson J, Goronzy JJ. Correlation of the topographical arrangement and the functional pattern of tissue-infiltrating macrophages in giant cell arteritis. J Clin Invest 1996;98:1642-1649.
4. Rittner HL, Kaiser M, Brack A, Szweda LI, Goronzy JJ, Weyand CM. Tissue-destructive macrophages in giant cell arteritis. Circ Res 1999;84:1050-1058.
5. Weyand CM, Tetzlaff N, Bjornsson J, Brack A, Younge B, Goronzy JJ. Disease patterns and tissue cytokine profiles in giant cell arteritis. Arthritis Rheum 1997;40:19-26.
6. Weyand CM, Goronzy JJ. Arterial wall injury in giant cell arteritis. Arthritis Rheum 1999;42:844-853.
7. Kaiser M, Weyand CM, Bjornsson J, Goronzy JJ. Platelet-derived growth factor, intimal hyperplasia, and ischemic complications in giant cell arteritis. Arthritis Rheum 1998;41:623-633.
8. Kaiser M, Younge B, Bjornsson J, Goronzy JJ, Weyand CM: Formation of new vasa vasorum in vasculitis. Production of angiogenic cytokines by multinucleated giant cells. Am J Pathol 1999;155:765-774.
9. Rittner HL, Hafner V, Klimiuk PA, Szweda LI, Goronzy JJ, Weyand CM. Aldose reductase functions as a detoxification system for lipid peroxidation products in vasculitis. J Clin Invest 1999;103:1007-1013.
10. Brack A, Martinez-Taboada V, Stanson A, Goronzy JJ, Weyand CM. Disease pattern in cranial and large-vessel giant cell arteritis. Arthritis Rheum 1999;42:311-317.
11. Evans JM, O'Fallon WM, Hunder GG. Increased incidence of aortic aneurysm and dissection in giant cell (temporal) arteritis. A population-based study. Ann Intern Med 1995;122:502-507.
12. Weyand CM, Fulbright JW, Hunder GG, Evans JM, Goronzy JJ. Treatment of giant cell arteritis: interleukin-6 as a biologic marker of disease activity. Arthritis Rheum 2000;43:1041-1048.
13. Hoffman GS, Cid M, Hellman D, et al. A multicenter placebo-controlled study of methotrexate (MTX) in giant cell arteritis (GCA). Arthritis Rheum 2000;43:S115.
14. Weyand CM, Hicok KC, Hunder GG, Goronzy JJ. Tissue cytokine patterns in patients with polymyalgia rheumatica and giant cell arteritis. Ann Intern Med 1994;121:484-491.
15. Weyand CM, Fulbright JW, Evans JM, Hunder GG, Goronzy JJ. Corticosteroid requirements in polymyalgia rheumatica. Arch Intern Med 1999;159:577-584.
16. Kerr GS. Takayasu's arteritis. Rheum Dis Clin North Am 1995;21:1041-1058.
17. Numano F. Differences in clinical presentation and outcome in different countries for Takayasu's arteritis. Curr Opin Rheumatol 1997;9:12-15.
18. Seko Y. Takayasu arteritis: insights into immunopathology. Jpn Heart J 2000;41:15-26.

19. Kimura A, Kitamura H, Date Y, Numano F. Comprehensive analysis of HLA genes in Takayasu arteritis in Japan. Int J Cardiol 1996;54:S61-S69.

20. Kerr GS, Hallahan CW, Giordano J, Leavitt RY, Fauci AS, Rottem M, Hoffman GS: Takayasu arteritis. Ann Intern Med 1994;120:919-929.

21. Langford CA, Sneller MC, Hoffman GS: Methotrexate use in systemic vasculitis. Rheum Dis Clin North Am 1997;23: 841-853.

VASCULITIDES
D. Vasculitis of the Central Nervous System

Vasculitis affecting the central nervous system (CNS) remains one of the most poorly understood forms of vascular inflammatory disease (1). Reasons for such clinical uncertainty include the rarity of these disorders, the inaccessibility of the brain and spinal cord for pathologic analysis, and the lack of efficient noninvasive diagnostic tests.

Vasculitis of the CNS can be divided into primary and secondary forms. The primary form of CNS vasculitis, called primary angiitis of the central nervous system (PACNS), is far more challenging clinically and less well-understood. Secondary vasculitis of the CNS refers to conditions, including infectious diseases, drug exposures, malignancies, systemic vasculitides, and connective-tissue diseases, that may involve the CNS.

Primary Angiitis of the Central Nervous System

Until the mid-1980s, PACNS was considered a distinctly rare disorder, uniformly fatal, and relatively homogeneous in terms of its clinicopathologic features. Since that time, the view of PACNS has evolved, and it now is recognized as not nearly as rare, more treatable, and highly heterogeneous. PACNS still is defined according to the criteria of Calabrese and Malek (2). It requires the presence of an acquired neurologic deficit that remains unexplained after a thorough initial basic evaluation; classic angiographic evidence consistent with vasculitis or histopathologic demonstration of angiitis within the CNS; no evidence of systemic vasculitis or any other condition to which the angiographic and pathologic features could be secondary (Table 21D-1).

Using these criteria, a diverse group of disorders can be defined. Among these disorders are a few homogeneous subsets that deserve nosologic distinction, such as granulomatous angiitis of the central nervous system (GACNS) and a less pernicious variant known as benign angiopathy of the central nervous system (BACNS) or reversible vasoconstrictive disorder (1). Unfortunately, the majority of cases fulfilling the working definition of PACNS do not fall neatly into either of these disease categories, and must be defined descriptively.

Granulomatous Angiitis of the Central Nervous System

Approximately 20% of cases with PACNS fit the descrip-

tion of GACNS (1,3). GACNS is a slowly progressive disorder characterized by a prodrome of six or more months, associated with additive focal and diffuse neurologic deficits, and virtually always associated with spinal-fluid findings that are consistent with chronic meningitis. Biopsy of involved tissues, particularly the leptomeninges and underlying cortex, reveals a necrotizing granulomatous angiitis with or without giant cells. It is regarded as highly fatal and progressive, but will respond to aggressive immunosuppressive therapy.

The most frequently encountered clinical findings are chronic headache, focal neurologic defects, alterations in higher cortical function, cerebrospinal fluid (CSF) abnormalities consistent with chronic meningitis, and inflammatory spinal cord lesions (3). Rarely, people may present with only focal neurologic dysfunction or even pure dementia, but these presentations are uncommon. Isolated stroke virtually is never a presenting manifestation of GACNS. People with GACNS have minimal or no signs of systemic vasculitis, and traditional screening tests for systemic vasculitis, such as elevated acute-phase reactants and anemia, generally are absent.

If GACNS is suspected, a lumbar puncture should be performed. More than 90% of patients with this diagnosis will have abnormal spinal fluids characterized by a mononuclear cell pleocytosis and elevated protein with normal glucose. Neuroradiographic studies, such as computed tomography or the more sensitive magnetic resonance imaging (MRI), almost always are abnormal. There are no specific neuroradiographic findings of PACNS, but the most common findings reflect multifocal vascular insults that evolve over time. Enhancement of the leptomeninges on MRI can increase the diagnostic accuracy of biopsy, but is neither highly sensitive nor specific for GACNS. Normal lumbar puncture and normal MRI results virtually rule out the possibility of GACNS. Cerebral angiography, often considered a gold standard for diagnosis of CNS vasculitis, is woefully inefficient in securing the diagnosis of GACNS (1,3,4). Although such characteristic findings as multifocal areas of stenosis and ectasia can be seen in up to 40% of these patients, the cerebral angiograph may be normal in 40% of these patients, and highly nonspecific in the remaining 20% (5). When GACNS is the suspected diagnosis, particularly in the setting of CSF consistent with chronic meningitis, biopsy of CNS tissues is the diagnostic modality of choice. Biopsy of the leptomeninges and underlying cortex increases the yield of the procedure, but unfortunately, results may be falsely negative in up to one-fifth of patients, due to the skip-lesion nature of the underlying disease and the small amount of tissue obtained.

Benign Angiopathy of the Central Nervous System

A review of the literature on PACNS reveals numerous isolated case reports, diagnosed solely on angiographic grounds, that differ considerably from cases of GACNS. It has been noted by several groups (5,6) that such patients tend to be young women who have acute onset of a severe headache or focal neurologic deficit, relatively normal CSF analyses, and highly abnormal angiograms. The clinical course for these patients frequently has been described as monophasic and relatively benign. Such patients appear not to require aggressive therapy with long-term glucocorticoids and cyclophosphamide. Based upon these clinical features, the diagnostic term benign angiopathy of the central nervous system (BACNS) has been proposed (7).

Diagnosis of cerebral angiitis on the basis of an angiogram is insufficient to label a person as having BACNS, because 40% of people with GACNS also have highly abnormal angiograms. Some patients who have this type of presentation (i.e., acute focal presentations with normal CSF and highly abnormal angiograms) do not have a benign outcome, and significant neurologic sequelae and fatal cerebral hemorrhage have been reported. The diagnosis of BACNS typically is based on both clinical and radiographic findings, and requires further analysis to differentiate it from more progressive forms of PACNS, which require more aggressive therapy.

Some people diagnosed with BACNS may not have angiitis at all, but a form of reversible vasoconstriction. Evidence supporting this finding is the similarity of BACNS to several other conditions with similar clinical and angiographic pictures, including angiopathy in the postpartum state, pheochromocytoma, complex headaches – particularly effort-induced headache – and a syndrome of "arteritis" associated with sympathomimetic drugs (1,8,9). Based on these observations, the fact that many such patients have a better prognosis, and that they may avoid prolonged and intense immunosuppressive therapy, we believe reversible vasoconstriction deserves distinction.

Other Forms of PACNS

More than 50% of cases do not fit neatly into GACNS or BACNS variants. This heterogeneity is defined by nongranulomatous pathology, including both lymphocytic and leukocytoclastic variants, and atypical clinical and neuroradiographic features. Some people may present with all the clinical features of GACNS, but have normal spinal fluids. Another subset of people with PACNS, up to 15%, present with a mass lesion. These patients always must be approached as having a potentially neoplastic or infectious

TABLE 21D-1
Conditions Resembling PACNS To Be Excluded

Systemic vasculitides
Polyarteritis nodosa
Allergic granulomatosis
Hypersensitivity vasculitis
Vasculitis with connective-tissue disease
Wegener's granulomatosis
Temporal arteritis
Takayasu's arteritis
Behçet's disease
Lymphomatoid granulomatosis
Cogan's syndrome
Infections
Viral: HIV, HCV, VZV
Bacterial
Fungal
Rickettsial
Spirochetal
Neoplasm
Angioimmunoproliferative disorders
Carcinomatous meningitis
Infiltrating glioma
Malignant angioendotheliomatosis
Drug use
Amphetamines
Ephedrine
Phenylpropanolamine
Cocaine
Ergotamine
Vasospastic disorders
Postpartum angiopathy
Eclampsia
Pheochromocytoma
Subarachnoid hemorrhage
Migraine and exertional headache
Other vasculopathies and mimicking conditions
Atherosclerosis
Fibromuscular dysplasia
Moyamoya disease
Thrombotic thrombocytopenic purpura
Sickle cell anemia
Neurofibromatosis
Cerebrovascular atherosclerosis
Demyelinating disease
Sarcoidosis
Emboli (i.e., SBE, cardiac myxoma, paradoxical emboli)
Acute posterior placoid pigment epitheliopathy and cerebral vasculitis
Antiphospholipid antibody syndrome and other hypercoagulable states
Others

HIV, human immunodeficiency virus; HCV, hepatitis C virus; VZV, varicella-zoster virus; SBE, subacute bacterial endocarditis.

disease until proved otherwise. A smaller subset of people present with disease limited to the spinal cord. These cases present diagnostic challenges in the absence of other signs of vasculitis, and the majority have granulomatous pathology on biopsy.

Diagnosis of PACNS

A useful principle for guiding the diagnostic search for PACNS is that clinicians statistically are more likely to encounter other conditions that explain the neurologic problem. A recent study (10) reviewed the records of 30 patients referred for evaluation of PACNS who ultimately required biopsy or cerebral angiography. In this study, only seven patients had documented PACNS, with the other 23 having a variety of disorders.

In every case of suspected cerebral angiitis, it is essential to perform a thorough search for conditions capable of causing secondary forms of cerebral arteritis or producing noninflammatory vascular disease that may mimic cerebral arteritis (Table 21D-1). Infectious disorders are the most important conditions to rule out because they not only may cause angiographic abnormalities similar to angiitis, but also may cause an angiocentric inflammatory disease with similar histologic appearance to PACNS upon biopsy. A search for systemic infection, culture, special stains, and molecular diagnostic techniques applied to spinal fluid and biopsy tissue are critically important. Other diagnostic considerations include a wide variety of sterile inflammatory diseases, including carcinomatous meningitis and sarcoidosis.

When GACNS is suspected, particularly in the setting of a CSF finding of chronic meningitis, biopsy of CNS tissues is the diagnostic modality of choice. Biopsy of the leptomeninges and underlying cortex increases the yield of the procedure. Enhancement of the leptomeninges on MRI can increase the diagnostic accuracy of biopsy, but is neither highly sensitive nor specific for GACNS. If prolonged immunosuppressive therapy is contemplated, biopsy generally is warranted. It probably is equally important to perform a biopsy of CNS tissues to rule out mimicking conditions, such as infections and neoplasms, as it is to secure the diagnosis of angiitis. A recent study has demonstrated a superior predictive value of brain biopsy over angiography in a large cohort of patients with suspected CNS angiitis (4).

In people with acute presentations, such as severe headache with or without stroke or transient ischemic attacks, accompanied by normal CSF, it is important to make a detailed search for emboli and hypercoagulable states. It is also important to determine patient use of such drugs as sympathomimetics and cocaine, and to consider other conditions associated with this presentation, such as postpartum state and pheochromocytoma. In this setting, it is reasonable to perform angiography initially, since this may support the diagnosis of BACNS, which requires less aggressive therapy. It cannot be overemphasized that this diagnosis should be based on both clinical and angiographic findings, requiring a diffusely abnormal angiogram consistent with vasoconstriction or spasm (Fig. 21D-1), associated

with an acute illness that initially appears nonprogressive. Lesser degrees of angiographic abnormalities, such as focal cut-off and isolated areas of irregularity, are not suggestive of this syndrome. For people with clinical presentations representing admixtures of GACNS and BACNS or for those with atypical features, both angiography and biopsy may be required.

A team approach to the diagnosis of CNS vasculitis is essential. No clinician is completely expert in the myriad disorders that can present with the clinical angiographic or pathologic presentation of cerebral angiitis. The ideal team includes a competent and interested neurosurgeon, neuroradiologist, neuropathologist, neurologist, and a clinician expert in the diagnosis and treatment of systemic vasculitides.

Treatment

Although no controlled trials of any therapy for PACNS or BACNS exist, reports have suggested that if patients are diagnosed and treated promptly, the majority can achieve clinical remission (1). For people with GACNS, high-dose prednisone (e.g., 1 mg/kg/day) and cyclophosphamide (2 mg/kg/day) are indicated. After convincing improvement has occurred or progression has been arrested, the corticosteroids are tapered. Cyclophosphamide therapy is continued for approximately six to 12 months after the disease has been controlled. Essential in the treatment plan is the serial evaluation of disease activity. For patients with GACNS, repeat lumbar puncture to ensure a dramatic improvement or normalization of the CSF is essential. MRI lesions frequently do not resolve completely, but serial studies can ensure that no silent progression is occurring. For

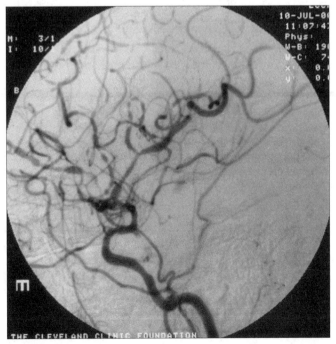

Fig. 21D-1. Cerebral angiogram in primary angiitis of the central nervous system. Multiple areas of stenosis, ectasia, and luminal irregularities in a person with primary angiitis of the central nervous system.

patients with a highly abnormal angiogram, a repeat study in 12 weeks should show dramatic improvement.

For people presenting with BACNS or reversible vaso-constrictive disease, a short course of high-dose corticosteroids (e.g., 1 mg/kg/day prednisone) for a period of two to three months with taper is given. Calcium-channel blockers also may be used in such patients, based on a presumed role of vasoconstriction, although evidence for efficacy of both of these agents is anecdotal.

For patients who do not fall neatly into the GACNS or BACNS categories, an empirically derived therapy based on the severity of disease manifestations and the rate of illness progression is justified. For patients with mild to moderate disease, high-dose corticosteroids may be used alone. Patients with rapidly progressive and profound disease may require a regimen similar to that outlined for GACNS.

Secondary Forms of CNS Vasculitis

Secondary forms of CNS vasculitis include those due to infections, drugs, neoplasms, and a number of systemic diseases (1). Diagnosing these conditions is important because many of these vasculitides have specific therapies, and some conditions, such as CNS vasculitis due to infections, may be affected adversely by immunosuppressive drug therapy.

Infections

Infection-related blood-vessel inflammation is the most important secondary form of CNS vasculitis to exclude. A variety of infectious agents, including bacteria, fungi, mycobacteria, viruses, spirochetes and other atypical agents, are capable of inducing a vascular inflammatory disease within the CNS (11). These agents may manifest with an angiographic picture indistinguishable from idiopathic PACNS or, histologically, by the presence of a necrotizing and, at times, granulomatous vasculitis. Although culture and special stains often are effective for identifying traditional infectious agents, other agents are more elusive. In all people with suspected CNS vasculitis, a detailed history of epidemiologic risk for infectious agents is essential. Culture of all available bodily fluids, including CSF, is standard, and molecular analysis for viruses and atypical pathogens should be performed when indicated. CNS biopsy should include special stains and culture for infectious agents. Certain pathogens deserve special mention because of their capacity to induce or be associated with CNS vasculitis. Herpes zoster and human immunodeficiency virus should be routinely considered in all patients with suspected CNS vasculitis, especially in patients with compromised immune systems (11,12).

Drugs

The most commonly implicated drugs with CNS vasculitis are cocaine, amphetamines, ephedrine, phenylpropanolamine, and other sympathomimetic agents, but the clinical and epidemiologic data supporting a true association is less than clear (9). Some of these agents are capable of inducing vasospasm and may cause cerebral angiopathy rather than true vasculitis, but others have been associated with rare, histologically documented, cases of CNS angiitis (9). Patients should be questioned about current or previous use of these agents. Additional therapies, similar to those used in the treatment of BACNS, may be of benefit.

Neoplasms

Vasculitis of the CNS has been associated with a variety of neoplasms, but most frequently with lymphoproliferative diseases, especially Hodgkin's and non-Hodgkin's lymphoma. The vasculitis often is indistinguishable from idiopathic GACNS. Optimal therapy is unclear, aside from aggressive treatment of the underlying malignancy. Overall, the prognosis is poor, with a three-year mortality rate of 90% (11).

Connective-Tissue Disease and Systemic Vasculitis

Vasculitis of the CNS is encountered in the setting of a variety of connective-tissue diseases and vasculitic syndromes, but occurs with greater frequency in some and is rare in others (13). Systemic lupus erythematosus (SLE) and Sjögren's syndrome are two well-recognized associations, although in patients with either disorder, developing CNS dysfunction is much more likely due to other factors (including noninflammatory CNS vascular disease, drug effects, or infection). CNS dysfunction in SLE is quite common, but frank vasculitis accounts for less than 7% of cases. Among the systemic vasculitides, CNS vasculitis is encountered most often with polyarteritis nodosa, ANCA-associated diseases, and Behçet's disease. When CNS symptoms develop in the setting of connective-tissue disease, it is imperative to rule out other causes first, such as infection in the immunocompromised host.

LEONARD H. CALABRESE, DO

References

1. Calabrese LH, Duna GF, Lie JT. Vasculitis in the central nervous system. Arthritis Rheum 1997;40:1189-1201.
2. Calabrese LH, Malek JA. Primary angiitis of the central nervous system. Report of eight new cases, review of the literature and proposal for diagnostic criteria. Medicine 1994;67:20-40.
3. Younger DS, Calabrese LH, Hays AP. Granulomatous angiitis of the nervous system. Neurol Clin 1997;15:821-834.
4. Chu CT, Gray L, Goldstein LB, Hulette CM. Diagnosis of intracranial vasculitis: a multidisciplinary approach. J Neuropathol Exp Neurol 1998;57:30-38.
5. Calabrese LH, Furlan AJ, Gragg LA, Ropos TJ. Primary angiitis of the central nervous system. Diagnostic criteria and clinical approach. Cleve Clin J Med 1992;59:293-306.
6. Hankey GJ. Isolated angiitis/angiopathy of the central nervous system. Cerebrovasc Dis 1991;1:2–15.
7. Calabrese LH, Gragg LA, Furlan AJ. Benign angiopathy: a distinct subset of angiographically defined primary angiitis of the central nervous system. J Rheumatol 1993;20:2046-2050.

8. Call GK, Fleming MC, Sealfon S, Levine H, Kistler JP, Fisher CM. *Reversible cerebral segmental vasoconstriction.* Stroke 1988;19:1159-1170.

9. Calabrese LH, Duna GF. *Drug-induced vasculitis.* Curr Opin Rheumatol 1996;8:34-40.

10. Duna GF, Calabrese L. *Limitations in the diagnostic modalities in the diagnosis of primary angiitis of the central nervous system (PACNS).* J Rheumatol 1995;22:662-667.

11. Giang DW. *Central nervous system vasculitis secondary to infections, toxins, and neoplasms.* Semin Neurol 1994;14:313-319.

12. Gilden DH, Kleinschmidt-DeMasters BK, LaGuardia JJ, Mahalingam R, Cohrs RJ. *Neurologic complications of the reactivation of varicella-zoster virus.* N Engl J Med 2000;342: 635-645.

13. Moore PM, Calabrese LH. *Neurologic manifestations of systemic vasculitides.* Semin Neurol 1994;14:300-306.

VASCULITIDES
E. Kawasaki Syndrome

Kawasaki syndrome (KS), an acute vasculitis of childhood, is the primary cause of acquired heart disease in children in the United States and Japan. Initially described by Dr. Tomisaku Kawasaki in 1967 (1), the syndrome was thought to be a benign, self-limited febrile illness. It now is known to be a systemic vasculitis that occurs predominantly in small and medium-sized muscular arteries, especially the coronary arteries. Morbidity and mortality of the disease most often are due to cardiac sequelae, and treatment is based on preventing aneurysm formation. Although many infectious agents and toxins have been implicated in the disease etiology, none has been identified. Activation of the immune system is known to occur in the acute stage of the disease and plays an important role in its pathogenesis.

Epidemiology

Kawasaki syndrome is a disease of infants and young children. Eighty percent of cases occur in children younger than 5 years. The peak incidence is in children aged 2 years and younger, with boys affected 1.5 times as often as girls. Although all racial groups are represented, children of Asian ancestry predominate. The syndrome recurs in 2% to 4% of cases. The occurrence in siblings is rare. In North America, cases occur throughout the year, with larger numbers appearing in late winter to early spring. Time-space clusters of cases and community-wide outbreaks with wavelike spread often develop over a two- to four-year period, both in Japan and the United States.

Etiology

The age-restricted susceptible population, the seasonal variation, the well-defined epidemics, and the acute, self-limited clinical illness all suggest a widespread infectious agent that produces disease or immunity early in life. Many organisms and toxins have been reported as possible agents, including *Staphylococcus, Streptococcus, Candida,* and *Rickettsia* species; retroviruses; and Epstein-Barr virus. Enterotoxins and exotoxins of staphylococci and streptococci have been identified in cultures, predominantly of the rectum and oral pharynx, in a small cohort of children with KS. While some

investigators speculate that these toxins may act as superantigens in the disease process (2), others have failed to confirm this association (3,4).

Pathogenesis

Immune activation and cytokine production appear to play a major role in KS pathogenesis. Alterations in T cells, B cells, monocytes, and macrophages have been described. Increased levels of serum interleukin (IL)-1, IL-2, soluble IL-2 receptors, IL-4, IL-6, IL-10, tumor necrosis factor α, interferon γ, and soluble CD30 serum antigen have been

TABLE 21E-1
Diagnostic Guidelines for Kawasaki Syndrome[a]

Fever lasting for ≥5 days plus four of the following five criteria:

1. Polymorphous rash

2. Bilateral conjunctival injection

3. One or more of the following mucous membrane changes:
   a. Diffuse injection of oral and pharyngeal mucosa
   b. Erythema or fissuring of the lips
   c. Strawberry tongue

4. Acute, nonpurulent cervical lymphadenopathy (usually a single lymph node, 1.5 cm)

5. One or more of the following extremity changes:
   a. Erythema of the palms or soles
   b. Indurative edema of the hands or feet
   c. Membranous desquamation of the fingertips
   d. Beau's lines

Other illness with similar clinical signs must be excluded

[a] Based on the Centers for Disease Control and Prevention case definition.

reported (5–10). The pathologic consequences of immune system activation consist primarily of vasculitis that affects small and medium-sized blood vessels.

Diagnostic Criteria

The Japanese Kawasaki Research Committee established diagnostic criteria for KS based on Dr. Kawasaki's first report. The Centers for Disease Control and Prevention adopted these same criteria for case definition in the United States (11) (Table 21E-1). Fever lasting five days and four of five other criteria must be present. "Atypical" cases may require fewer criteria for diagnosis when coronary artery aneurysms are noted by echocardiography or angiography.

TABLE 21E-2
Differential Diagnosis of Kawasaki Syndrome

Infection
  Bacterial
    Streptococcus species
    Staphylococcus species
    Propionibacterium acnes
    Mycoplasma infection
  Viral
    Rubella
    Roseola
    Rubeola
    Adenovirus
    Parainfluenza
    Epstein-Barr virus
    Cytomegalovirus
    Retroviruses
    Enterovirus
  Spirochetal
    Leptospira species
  Rickettsial
    Rocky Mountain spotted fever
    Typhus
  Fungal
    Candida species

Toxicosis
  Mercury (acrodynia)

Allergic/autoimmune
  Drug reactions (antibiotics, antifungals, anticonvulsants)
  Stevens-Johnson syndrome
  Systemic-onset juvenile rheumatoid arthritis
  Other vasculitides

Malignancies
  Leukemia
  Lymphoma

The clinical features of KS mimic many childhood illnesses, and the differential diagnosis includes infections, toxicosis, drug reactions, and connective-tissue diseases, as summarized in Table 21E-2.

Clinical Manifestations

Kawasaki syndrome begins acutely with fever that is high (100°–104° F), prolonged (1–2 weeks), and remittent in untreated patients. Within one to three days, a rash, conjunctival injection, and oral mucosal changes typically appear. The rash does not have a distinct morphologic pattern. Most commonly noted are irregular, nonpruritic erythematous plaques or a morbilliform rash (Fig. 21E-1). Some patients, however, may exhibit a scarlatiniform rash, erythema marginatum, or even pustules. Diffuse erythema, crusting, petechiae, purpura, and vesicle formation are not characteristic of KS and should suggest other diagnoses. Erythema of the perineum, which evolves into desquamation within 48 hours, also is common.

Early in the disease, there may be brawny induration of the hands and feet. The swelling may be painful and must

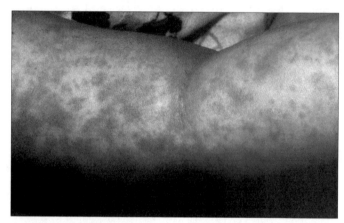

Fig. 21E-1. A polymorphous rash, consisting here of nonpruritic, erythematous plaques, occurs early in patients with Kawasaki syndrome.

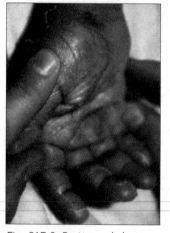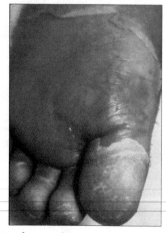

Fig. 21E-2. Periungual desquamation frequently occurs in the convalescent stage of Kawasaki syndrome, and may involve the palm of the hand and sole of the foot.

be distinguished from the arthritis that also occurs in people with KS. In the convalescent state of the disease (10–14 days after the onset of fever), characteristic periungual desquamation occurs and may involve the entire hand and foot (Fig. 21E-2).

Beau's lines (transverse grooves) of the nails occur several months later as a testament to the acute illness. Ocular findings range from inflammatory, nonpurulent conjunctival injection to anterior uveitis. Oral mucosal findings of ulcers, petechiae, and exudates typical of other febrile exanthems are not features of KS.

Ninety percent or more of children with KS experience a rash, conjunctival injection, and changes of the peripheral extremities. Cervical adenopathy (>1.5 cm) occurs in 50%–75% and usually is unilateral. The nodes are firm, variably tender, and nonpurulent.

Kawasaki syndrome is a systemic illness, and abnormalities have been described in all organ systems. Central nervous system disease includes aseptic meningitis, facial palsy, subdural effusion, and symptomatic and asymptomatic cerebral infarction. Sensorineural hearing loss has been reported, albeit in conjunction with aspirin therapy. Pulmonary infiltrates and pleural effusions may be present. Gastrointestinal manifestations include hepatomegaly (which is sometimes associated with jaundice), hydrops of the gallbladder, diarrhea, and pancreatitis. Renal manifestations may include sterile pyuria (most likely secondary to urethral inflammation), proteinuria, or rarely, acute renal insufficiency from interstitial nephritis.

Cardiac abnormalities are numerous and varied. Acute-stage manifestations include pericardial effusions in approximately 30% of cases. Myocarditis also is common in the acute phase and manifests with frequent tachycardia and gallop rhythms that are disproportionate to the degree of fever and anemia. Congestive heart failure and atrial and ventricular arrhythmias can occur. Electrocardiogram findings include decreased R-wave voltage, ST-segment depression, and T-wave flattening or inversion. Slowed conduction also can occur with PR or QT prolongation. Mitral regurgitation develops in approximately 30% of patients.

Coronary artery lesions are responsible for most of the morbidity and mortality of the disease. Coronary artery ectasia or aneurysms develop in 15% to 25% of affected children without treatment with high-dose intravenous immune globulin (IVIgG) (12). Administration of IVIgG in the acute phase of the disease reduces the prevalence of coronary dilation to fewer than 5%, and that of giant coronary aneurysms to fewer than 1% (13). Boys, children younger than one year, and children with prolonged fever or a persistently elevated erythrocyte sedimentation rate are more likely to develop aneurysms. Aneurysms usually appear one to four weeks after the onset of fever and, rarely, after six weeks of illness (Fig. 21E-3). Aneurysms are detected most easily by transthoracic two-dimensional echocardiography, are described as small (4 mm), medium (4 to 8 mm), or giant (>8 mm), and are located proximal more commonly than distal. Ectasia of the vessels (vessel size larg-

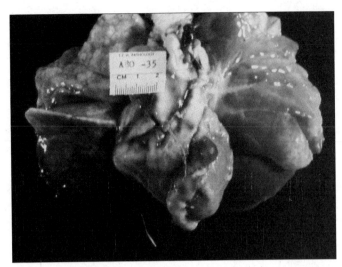

Fig. 21E-3. Coronary artery aneurysms in a pathologic specimen from a child with Kawasaki syndrome.

er than age-matched controls) is a common finding. Small and medium-sized aneurysms generally regress radiographically within five years; however, these vessels most likely remain abnormal because response to pharmacologic dilation may remain impaired (14). Factors positively associated with regression of aneurysms are smaller size and fusiform morphology of the aneurysms, female sex, and age less than one year. Children with giant aneurysms have the worst prognosis. Giant aneurysms rarely regress and frequently develop complicating thromboses, stenoses, or total occlusion. Myocardial infarction, when it occurs, is most likely to appear in the first year, with 40% occurring in the first three months of illness. There are, however, case reports of young adults suffering myocardial infarctions more than a decade after their initial disease and others with coronary artery aneurysms who were not known to have KS as children.

Other vessels may be involved, including the abdominal aorta, and the superior mesenteric, axillary, subclavian, brachial, iliac, and renal arteries, with resultant distal ischemia and necrosis. Peripheral-extremity ischemia occurs infrequently, but may result in gangrene of the affected area. Vasculitis with resultant vessel spasm is thought to be responsible.

Laboratory Findings

Laboratory studies are not diagnostic in KS, but may help the clinician make the diagnosis and identify patients at highest risk for coronary involvement. Laboratory findings in acute KS reflect the marked degree of systemic inflammation. Common findings at presentation include a leukocytosis with a left shift, normochromic, normocytic anemia; elevated acute-phase reactants; elevated liver transaminase levels; and depressed albumin. In the second week of illness, there is a profound lymphocytosis, with a marked expansion of the B-cell subset (15). Increased platelet turnover and marked hypercoagulability occur in the acute phase, and thrombocytosis (often greater than 1 million) usually peaks in the third to fourth week after onset of fever. Urinalysis may reveal mild proteinuria or sterile pyuria from urethritis, but creatinine rarely is elevated. In children with meningeal signs, cerebrospinal fluid may reveal a non-specific pleocytosis, with normal protein and glucose. Complement levels are normal or increased. Tests for antinuclear antibodies and rheumatoid factor are negative. Antineutrophil cytoplasmic antibodies and antiendothelial antibodies have been detected in some patients but are of no diagnostic significance (16).

An electrocardiogram is recommended in the first week of illness. A two-dimensional echocardiogram with careful attention to the coronary arteries should be obtained at diagnosis, within two to three weeks of illness onset, and about one month later. If results of these studies are abnormal, additional studies may be needed (12).

Treatment

Treatment in the acute phase of the disease is aimed at limiting inflammation. Aspirin has been the most widely used therapeutic agent for KS, given at a dosage of 80–100 mg/kg/day, orally, until the fever has subsided. The dosage then is reduced to 3–5 mg/kg/day, which is sufficient for the antiplatelet effect, and continued until the platelet count and indicators of inflammation (sedimentation rate, etc.) have returned to normal. There is no convincing evidence that aspirin, used alone, affects the incidence of coronary artery abnormalities (13).

Treatment with IVIgG in various regimens has been shown to decrease significantly the incidence of coronary artery aneurysm formation, lessen the fever, and reduce myocardial inflammation (17–19). In the United States, the standard of care is 2 g/kg IVIgG as a single infusion. Aspirin is given concurrently. Approximately 10% of children treated with IVIgG have persistent, recurrent fever, despite treatment (19). If the fever persists, a second dose of IVIgG may result in defervescence, although it is unknown whether retreatment prevents the development of coronary artery lesions (20,21). A subgroup of patients who are resistant to IVIgG therapy are at greatest risk of developing coronary artery aneurysms and long-term sequelae of the disease. In preliminary studies, some patients with IVIgG-resistant KS reportedly respond to treatment with corticosteroid therapy (22).

The mechanism of action of IVIgG in KS is unknown. The recommended dose and duration of treatment for both IVIgG and aspirin may change as additional study results become available. More specific therapy awaits the discovery of causative agents.

Long-Term Follow-Up

The duration, frequency, and best imaging methods for long-term follow-up are a matter of debate. Of greatest concern are children with initial coronary artery aneurysms, because

thrombosis or segmental stenosis may occur in the chronic phase of the disease. The American Heart Association has recommended guidelines for long-term follow-up (11). Children with multiple aneurysms, giant aneurysms, or known coronary artery obstruction require close follow-up and possible long-term anticoagulation therapy. Stress testing in the adolescent years is important, especially in patients with a history of coronary artery involvement, because abnormalities may require limitations in physical activity and may indicate the need for angiography to assess the degree of coronary artery stenosis or obstruction.

KARYL S. BARRON, MD

References

1. Kawasaki T. Acute febrile mucocutaneous lymph node syndrome with lymph node involvement with specific desquamation of the fingers and toes in children [in Japanese]. Jpn J Allerg 1967;16:178–222.
2. Leung D, Meissner H, Fulton D, Murray DL, Kotzin B, Schlievert P. Toxic shock syndrome-secreting Staphylococcus aureus in Kawasaki syndrome. Lancet 1993;342:1385–1388.
3. Terai M, Miwa K, Williams T, et al. Failure to confirm involvement of staphylococcal toxin in the pathogenesis of Kawasaki disease. In: Kato H (ed). Kawasaki Disease. New York: Elsevier, 1995; pp 144–148.
4. Marchette NJ, Cao X, Kihara S, Martin J, Melish ME. Staphylococcal toxic shock syndrome toxin-1, one possible cause of Kawasaki syndrome? In: Kato H (ed). Kawasaki Disease. New York: Elsevier, 1995; pp 149–155.
5. Maury C, Salo E, Pelkonen P. Circulating interleukin-1 beta in patients with Kawasaki disease [letter]. N Engl J Med 1988;319:1670–1671.
6. Lin CY, Lin CC, Hwang B, Chiang BN. The changes of interleukin-2, tumour necrotic factor and gamma-interferon production among patients with Kawasaki disease. Eur J Pediatr 1991;150:179–182.
7. Barron K, Montalvo J, Joseph A, et al. Soluble interleukin-2 receptors in children with Kawasaki disease. Arthritis Rheum 1990;33:1371–1377.
8. Hirao H, Hibi S, Andoh T, Ichimura T. High levels of circulating interleukin-4 and interleukin-10 in Kawasaki disease. Int Arch Allergy Immunol 1997;112:152–156.
9. Ueno Y, Takano N, Kanegane H, et al. The acute phase nature of interleukin-6: studies in Kawasaki disease and other febrile illnesses. Clin Exp Immunol 1989;76:337–342.
10. Vagliasindi C, Spinozzi F, Sensi L, et al. Soluble CD30 serum antigen in Kawasaki disease. Acta Pediatr 1997;86:317–318.
11. Morens DM, O'Brien RJ. Kawasaki disease in the United States. J Infect Dis 1978;137:91–93.
12. Dajani AS, Taubert KA, Takahashi M, et al. Guidelines for long-term management of patients with Kawasaki disease. Report from the Committee on Rheumatic Fever, Endocarditis, and Kawasaki Disease, Council on Cardiovascular Disease in the Young, American Heart Association. Circulation 1994;89:916–922.

13. *Duronpisitkul K, Gururaj VJ, Park JM, Martin CF. The prevention of coronary artery aneurysms in Kawasaki disease: a meta-analysis on the efficacy of aspirin and immunoglobulin treatment. Pediatrics 1995;96:1057–1061.*

14. *Sugimura T, Kato H, Inoue O, Takagi J, Fukuda T, Sato N. Vasodilatory response of the coronary arteries after Kawasaki disease: evaluation by intracoronary injection of isosorbide dinitrate. J Pediatr 1992;121:684–688.*

15. *Barron K. Immune abnormalities in Kawasaki disease: prognostic implications and insight into pathogenesis. Cardiol Young 1991;1:206–211.*

16. *Guzman J, Fung M, Petty RE. Diagnostic value of anti-neutrophil cytoplasmic antibodies and anti-endothelial cell antibodies in early Kawasaki disease. J Pediatr 1994;124:917–920.*

17. *Newburger J, Takahashi M, Burns J, et al. Treatment of Kawasaki syndrome with intravenous gamma globulin. N Eng J Med 1986;315:341–347.*

18. *Barron K, Murphy D, Silverman E, et al. Treatment of Kawasaki syndrome: a comparison of two dosage regimes of intravenously administered immune globulin. J Pediatr 1990; 117:638–644.*

19. *Newburger J, Takahashi M, Beiser A, et al. A single intravenous infusion of gamma globulin as compared with four infusions in the treatment of acute Kawasaki syndrome. N Engl J Med 1991;324:1633–1639.*

20. *Sundel RP, Burns JC, Baker A, Beiser A, Newburger JW. Gamma globulin retreatment in Kawasaki disease. J Pediatr 1993;123:657–659.*

21. *Burns JC, Capparelli EV, Brown JA, Newburger JW. Intravenous gamma globulin treatment and retreatment in Kawasaki disease. US/Canadian Kawasaki Syndrome Study Group. Pediatr Infect Dis J 1998;17:1144–1148.*

22. *Wright DA, Newburger JW, Baker A, Sundel RP. Treatment of immune globulin-resistant Kawasaki disease with pulsed doses of corticosteroids. J Pediatr 1996;128:146–149.*

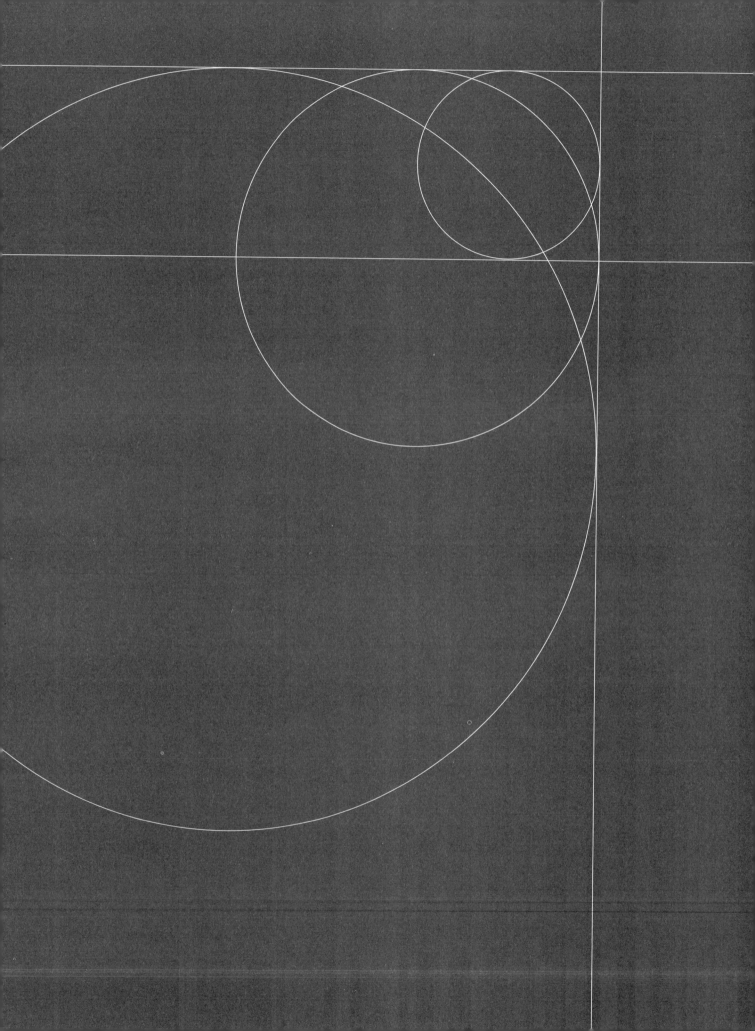

22 BEHÇET'S DISEASE

Behçet's disease (BD) is a chronic inflammatory vascular disorder of unknown etiology (1). Although the disease is recognized worldwide, the prevalence is highest in countries of the eastern Mediterranean, the Middle East, and East Asia, thus the name "Silk Road disease." Behçet's disease occurs primarily in young adults; the mean age at onset is 25–30 years, and juvenile cases are infrequent. The male-to-female ratio is almost 1:1 along the Silk Road, but in Japan, Korea, and Western countries, females predominate. Prevalence rates are increasing worldwide, probably because of increased awareness and recognition of the disease.

Pathogenesis

Genetic studies have shown a strong association with human leukocyte antigen (HLA)-B51, but the role of this gene in the development of BD is uncertain. An association with HLA-DRB1*04 has been reported in Caucasian patients (2). Evidence exists for neutrophil hyperreactivity (3) and for antigen-driven immune mechanisms in pathogenesis. The MICA gene (major histocompatibility complex class I chain-related gene A), found in linkage dysequilibrium with HLA-B51, is another candidate gene. MICA gene products are expressed on fibroblasts and endothelial cells, and may have a role in the presentation of antigen to natural killer cells or $\gamma\delta^+$ T cells (4). Activated $\gamma\delta^+$ T cells are increased in the circulation and in mucosal lesions, but the exact role of these cells in pathogenesis is uncertain. Cytokine analysis and cellular characterization suggest a T-helper 1 (Th1) response by lymphocytes. Molecular techniques have identified herpes simplex viral RNA and DNA in cells from people with BD, and streptococcal antigens are suspected to trigger disease activity. Peptides from mycobacterial heat shock proteins (HSP) and homologous human peptides have been found to specifically stimulate $\gamma\delta^+$ T cells from people with BD (5). It is postulated that crossreactivity and molecular mimicry between peptides from streptococcal or viral HSP, homologous human HSP, and mucosal antigens result in selection of autoreactive T cells (6).

Clinical Features

Aphthous oral ulcers usually are the first and most persistent clinical feature of BD. Aphthae occur as 2–12-mm, discrete, painful, round or oval, red-rimmed lesions that affect mainly the nonkeratinized mucosa of the cheeks, tongue, palate, and pharynx (Fig. 22-1). Oral ulcers are identical to the lesions of recurrent aphthous stomatitis; however, six or

more ulcers of variable size, with surrounding erythema, that involve the soft palate and oropharynx should increase the suspicion for BD.

Genital ulcers occur on the vulva, in the vagina, or on the scrotum and penis. Although vulvar lesions are painful and may result in scarring, vaginal ulcers may be asymptomatic or produce a discharge. Scrotal lesions may be superficial or deep and may heal with scarring (Fig. 22-2). Perianal ulcers also may be present.

Skin lesions are common, and include erythema nodosum, pseudofolliculitis, papulopustular lesions, or acneiform nodules. Erythema nodosum lesions must be differentiated from superficial thrombophlebitis. Occasionally, intense neutrophilic inflammation results in lesions similar to those seen in Sweet's syndrome. Pyoderma gangrenosum-like lesions or cutaneous aphthosis may occur, and a patient may have more than one type of skin lesion.

A positive skin test for pathergy test (an excessive skin response to trauma as a result of neutrophil hyperreactivity) is considered highly specific for BD. To perform the test, a sterile, sharp, 20-gauge needle is inserted perpendicularly to

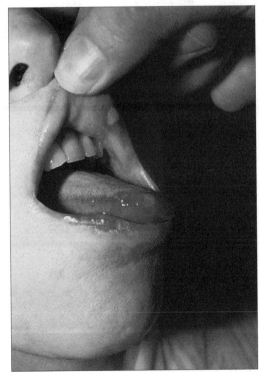

Fig. 22-1. Aphthous lesions of the tongue and buccal mucosa in Behçet's disease. (Photograph provided by J. D. O'Duffy, M.B.)

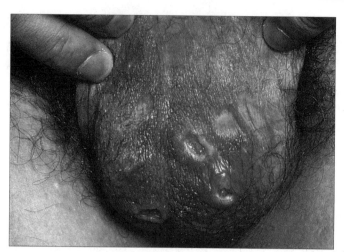

Fig. 22-2. Active ulcers and scarring of the scrotum in Behçet's disease. (Photograph provided by J. D. O'Duffy, M.B.)

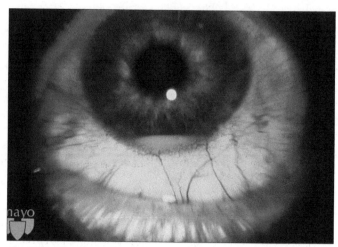

Fig. 22-3. Hypopyon uveitis in Behçet's disease.

the skin and subcutaneous tissue of the volar forearm to a depth of about 0.5 cm, rotated briefly on its axis, and then removed. After 48 hours, the appearance of an erythematous papule or pustule (>2 mm in diameter) at the puncture site constitutes a positive test. The positivity of the test may vary during the course of the disease, and test results are more likely to be positive at times of active disease. Pathergy equivalents may occur in the form of sterile abscesses or pustules after therapeutic injections, at intravenous injection sites, or after skin trauma.

Ocular inflammation typically follows mucocutaneous symptoms by a few years, but it often progresses with a chronic, relapsing course that affects both eyes. The ocular finding in Behçet's original patients was hypopyon uveitis (Fig. 22-3), which is seen infrequently among patients in Western countries. In addition to anterior uveitis, panuveitis with posterior chamber involvement and retinal vasculitis may occur and lead to visual impairments. Vasculitis leads to episodes of retinal occlusion and areas of ischemia, which may be followed by neovascularization, vitreous hemorrhage and contraction, glaucoma, and retinal detachment. Isolated optic disk edema suggests cerebral venous thrombosis rather than ocular disease, but papillitis may occur with ocular inflammation and central nervous system disease. Cranial nerve palsies may result from brain-stem lesions, and visual-field defects may occur with intracranial lesions.

Large-vessel involvement of both arterial and venous systems is common, and it is a major cause of morbidity and mortality (7). Deep venous thrombosis is the most common vascular complication, and patients with recurrences are at risk for chronic stasis changes in the legs. Occlusion of the vena cava is associated with a high risk of mortality. Additional thrombotic complications include Budd-Chiari syndrome, cerebral venous thromboses, cavernous transformation of the portal vein, and chest-wall, abdominal, and esophageal varices.

Arterial lesions may occur in the systemic circulation or the pulmonary arterial bed; stenoses, occlusions, and

aneurysms frequently coexist (8). Arterial aneurysms of the aorta or its branches are at high risk for rupture. Pulmonary artery aneurysms often lead to the development of pulmonary artery-bronchial fistula and hemoptysis. Coronary vascular disease and myocardial infarction are uncommon.

Central nervous system disease in BD appears to be more common in Europe and the United States than in Asia, affecting about 30% of patients in Western countries (9). The clinical combination of stroke, aseptic meningitis with cerebrospinal fluid pleocytosis, and mucocutaneous lesions can be diagnostic of BD. Focal or multifocal nervous system involvement reflects the predilection of the disease for small vessels in the brain stem and periventricular white matter. Magnetic resonance imaging is the most sensitive imaging technique for demonstrating these lesions.

Gastrointestinal symptoms include melena or abdominal pain, and lesions consist of single or multiple ulcerations involving primarily the distal ileum and cecum. Gastrointestinal lesions have a tendency to perforate or bleed and may recur postoperatively. The lesions in BD must be differentiated from those of inflammatory bowel disease and mucosal changes induced by nonsteroidal antiinflammatory drugs.

An intermittent, symmetric oligoarthritis of the knees, ankles, hands, or wrists affects one-half of the patients with BD; arthralgia also is common. Destructive arthropathy is unusual. Synovial fluid findings include increased white blood cell counts, primarily neutrophils. Synovial biopsies reveal superficial neutrophilic infiltration. In some studies, an increased frequency of ankylosing spondylitis or radiographic sacroiliitis has been reported (10).

Glomerulonephritis and peripheralneuropathy are much less frequent in BD than might be expected in a systemic vasculitis. AA-type amyloidosis, presenting as nephrotic syndrome, has been reported primarily in patients in Mediterranean countries. Epididymitis occurs in about 5% of patients. Mouth and genital ulcers with inflamed cartilage

TABLE 22-1
International Study Group Criteria for Behçet's Disease

Recurrent oral ulceration	Minor aphthous, major aphthous, or herpetiform ulceration observed by physician or patient, which recurred at least three times in one 12-month period[a]
Plus 2 of:	
Recurrent genital ulceration	Aphthous ulceration or scarring, observed by physician or patient[a]
Eye lesions	Anterior uveitis, posterior uveitis, or cells in vitreous on slit lamp examination; or retinal vasculitis observed by ophthalmologist
Skin lesions	Erythema nodosum observed by physician or patient, pseudofolliculitis, or papulopustular lesions; or acneiform nodules observed by physician in postadolescent patients not receiving corticosteroid treatment[a]
Positive pathergy test	Read by physician at 24–48 hours

[a] Findings applicable only in the absence of other clinical explanations.

(MAGIC) syndrome is diagnosed in patients who have features of both BD and relapsing polychondritis (11).

Acute-phase reactants may be increased, especially in patients with large-vessel vasculitis, but they may be normal with active eye disease. Measurements of rheumatoid factor, cryoglobulins, and complement components usually are normal or negative. The histocompatibility antigen HLA-B51 is associated with BD in areas of high prevalence and in patients with ocular disease.

Diagnosis

The International Study Group criteria for the classification of BD (Table 22-1) are not meant to replace clinical judgment in individual cases (12). For patients in Western countries, large-vessel disease or acute central nervous system infarction in the setting of aphthosis should suggest the diagnosis (13). The multiple manifestations of BD may occur simultaneously or may be separated in time, occasionally by several years. For definitive diagnosis, the manifestations must be documented or witnessed by a physician.

The prevalence of recurrent aphthous stomatitis is greater than that of BD, and the diagnosis of "possible BD" in patients who only have aphthae is inappropriate. Ulcers in BD often fit the description of "complex aphthosis," which typically consists of multiple recurrent or persisting lesions that may include perianal or genital ulceration. The diagnosis of BD in patients with complex aphthosis requires the presence of other characteristic lesions and the exclusion of other systemic disorders associated with mucocutaneous involvement. Sprue, hematologic disorders, herpes simplex infection, inflammatory bowel disease, cyclic neutropenia, and acquired immunodeficiency syndrome may cause similar lesions. Other disorders responsible for oral-genital-ocular syndromes include erythema multiforme, reactive arthritis, mucous membrane pemphigoid, and the vulvovaginal-gingival form of erosive lichen planus. Differential diagnosis often requires evaluation by an experienced dermatologist as well as biopsy of the lesions. In reactive arthritis, mucocutaneous lesions are nonulcerative and painless, and the uveitis is usually limited to the anterior chamber.

Disease Activity

For mucocutaneous manifestations, disease activity is recognized and monitored by recording the number, size, and location of lesions and the percentage of time that the lesions have been present since the patient's last evaluation. Frequent ophthalmologic examinations are essential for people with ocular disease, and periodic monitoring of the eyes is recommended for patients at risk. A careful history and examination, with attention to the vascular and neurologic systems, should be part of the physician's assessment. Standardized forms for scoring disease activity and ocular inflammation have been developed for use in clinical trials and the care of individual patients (14).

Treatment

Aphthous lesions are treated with topical or intralesional corticosteriods or dapsone. Colchicine is used in the treatment of mucocutaneous manifestations and as an adjunct in the treatment of more serious manifestations (15).

Thalidomide can be used for the prevention and treatment of mucosal and follicular lesions in males, but toxicity is a concern (16). Methotrexate can be effective in the treatment of mucocutaneous disease (17).

Azathioprine has been reported to have a beneficial effect on the development and progression of ocular disease, mucosal ulcers, arthritis, deep venous thrombosis, and to improve long-term prognosis (18). Because young males are at greatest risk of eye complications, especially uveitis, expectant and more aggressive treatment generally is warranted. Cyclosporine has a role in the management of uveitis. In open trials, interferon α has been found useful for treating mucocutaneous lesions and arthritis, and is emerging as an effective treatment for ocular disease (19). Combination treatment with cyclosporine and azathioprine has been used when single-agent treatment has failed (20). Immunosuppression with chlorambucil or cyclophosphamide may be used for uncontrolled ocular disease, central nervous system disease, and large-vessel vasculitis, including recurrent deep venous thrombosis. Corticosteroids are useful for suppressing inflammation in acute phases of the disease, but have a limited role in chronic management of central nervous system or ocular complications.

Surgical treatment usually is indicated for systemic arterial aneurysms, which are at risk for rupture. Pulmonary arterial aneurysms with uncontrolled bleeding require surgical treatment or percutaneous embolization. Arterial vasculitis with aneurysms of the systemic or pulmonary circulation should be treated with alkylating agents. If surgery is required, these agents also are necessary to minimize the high risk of anastomotic recurrences or continued disease (8).

Cerebral venous thrombosis responds well to treatment with heparin, colchicine, and corticosteroids (21). Venous thrombosis may be progressive or recurrent in spite of warfarin treatment. Because inflammation underlies the thrombosis, corticosteroids and immunosuppressive agents should be considered in these cases. The treatment of Budd-Chiari syndrome has included anticoagulants, colchicine, and corticosteriods or a combination of antiaggregants. Portocaval shunting is recommended if the inferior vena cava is patent.

KENNETH T. CALAMIA, MD

References

1. Sakane T, Takeno M, Suzuki N, Inaba G. Behçet's disease. N Engl J Med 1999;341:1284–1291.
2. O'Duffy JD, Tirzaman O, Weyand CM, Goronzy JJ. HLA-DRB1 alleles in Behçet's disease (A). Proceedings of the Eighth International Congress on Behçet's disease, Reggio-Emilia, Italy 1998, p 113.
3. Takeno M, Kariyone A, Yamashita N, et al. Excessive function of peripheral blood neutrophils from patients with Behçet's disease and from HLA-B51 transgenic mice. Arthritis Rheum 1995;38:426–433.
4. Mizuki N, Ohno S, Sato T, et al. Microsatellite polymorphism between the tumor necrosis factor and HLA-B genes in Behçet's disease. Hum Immunol 1995;43:129–135.
5. Hasan A, Fortune F, Wilson A, et al. Role of gamma delta T cells in pathogenesis and diagnosis of Behçet's disease. Lancet 1996;347:789–794.
6. Lehner T. The role of heat shock protein, microbial and autoimmune agents in the aetiology of Behçet's disease. Int Rev Immunol 1997;14:21–32.
7. Koç Y, Gullu I, Akpek G, et al. Vascular involvement in Behçet's disease. J Rheumatol 1992;19:402–410.
8. Le Thi Huong D, Wechsler B, Papo T, et al. Arterial lesions in Behçet's disease. A study in 25 patients. J Rheumatol 1995;22:2103–2113.
9. O'Duffy JD, Goldstein NP. Neurologic involvement in seven patients with Behçet's disease. Am J Med 1976;61:170–178.
10. Olivieri I, Salvarani C, Cantini F. Is Behçet's disease part of the spondyloarthritis complex? [editorial]. J Rheumatol 1997;24:1870–1872.
11. Firestein GS, Gruber HE, Weisman MH, Zvaifler NJ, Barber J, O'Duffy JD. Mouth and genital ulcers with inflamed cartilage: MAGIC syndrome. Five patients with features of relapsing polychondritis and Behçet's disease. Am J Med 1985;79:65–72.
12. International Study Group for Behçet's Disease. Criteria for diagnosis of Behçet's disease. Lancet 1990;335:1078–1080.
13. Schirmer M, Calamia KT, O'Duffy JD. Is there a place for large vessel disease in the diagnostic criteria for Behçet's disease. J Rheumatol 1999;26:2511–2512.
14. Kaklamani VG, Vaiopoulos G, Kaklamanis PG. Behçet's Disease. Semin Arthritis Rheum 1998;27:197–217.
15. Yurdakul S, Mat C, Özyazgan Y, et al. A double blind study of colchicine in Behçet's syndrome (BS). Arthritis Rheum 1998;41:S356.
16. Hamuryudan V, Mat C, Saip S, et al. Thalidomide in the treatment of the mucocutaneous lesions of the Behçet syndrome. A randomized, double-blind, placebo-controlled trial. Ann Intern Med 1998;128:443–450.
17. Jorizzo JL, White WL, Wise CM, Zanolli MD, Sherertz EF. Low-dose weekly methotrexate for unusual neutrophilic vascular reactions: cutaneous polyarteritis nodosa and Behçet's disease. J Am Acad Dermatol 1991;24:973–978.
18. Hamuryudan V, Özyazgan Y, Hizli N, et al. Azathioprine in Behçet's syndrome: effects on long-term prognosis. Arthritis Rheum 1997;40:769–774.
19. Kotter I, Eckstein AK, Stubiger N, Zierhut M. Treatment of ocular symptoms of Behçet's disease with interferon alpha 2a: a pilot study. Br J Ophthalmol 1998;82:488–494.
20. Hamuryudan V, Ozdogan H, Yazici H. Other forms of vasculitis and pseudovasculitis. Baillieres Clin Rheumatol 1997;11:335–355.
21. Wechsler B, Vidailhet M, Piette JC, et al. Cerebral venous thrombosis in Behçet's disease: clinical study and long-term follow-up of 25 cases. Neurology 1992;42:614–618.

23 RELAPSING POLYCHONDRITIS

Relapsing polychondritis is an uncommon disorder characterized by widespread and progressive inflammation of cartilagenous structures that leads to tissue destruction. Common clinical features are auricular, nasal, and respiratory tract chondritis with involvement of organs of special sense, such as the eyes and audiovestibular apparatus. Polyarthritis and vascular involvement also are common (1–3). Pearson et al (4) first used the term *relapsing polychondritis* to describe the episodic nature of the disease, and it is the widely accepted terminology. The etiology is unknown. It is considered to be an autoimmune disorder with evidence of cellular and humoral response to cartilagenous structures, including collagen types II, IX, and XI (5). A 60% increase in frequency of human leukocyte antigen (HLA)-DR4, compared with 25% in normal controls has been reported (2). About 20% of HLA-DR4–positive patients also have disease associated with rheumatoid arthritis (2). The disease occurs in all age groups, with peaks between 40 and 50 years. Both genders are affected equally (6,7), but women more often have serious airway involvement (8). Although relapsing polychondritis is well-described, it is frequently unrecognized, resulting in a mean delay in diagnosis of 2.9 years (3).

Clinical Features

The clinical features of relapsing polychondritis are summarized in Table 23-1. Auricular chondritis is the most common presenting symptom. It is characterized by sudden onset of pain and swelling, with redness and warmth, involving the cartilaginous portion of the external ear, with sparing of the lobule (Fig. 23-1). The inflammation may subside spontaneously or with treatment. With repeated attacks, the involved external ear becomes soft and floppy

TABLE 23-1
Clinical Manifestations of Relapsing Polychondritis

Manifestation	Frequency %[a]	
	At onset	Cumulative
Auricular chondritis	62	91
Nasal chondritis	29	53
Saddle nose deformity	9	25
Arthritis	34	63
Ocular symptoms	25	53
Laryngotracheal-bronchial symptoms	26	49
Laryngotracheal stricture	15	23
Hearing loss	9	29
Vestibular dysfunction (vertigo)	6	30
Systemic vasculitis	1.5	11
Valvular dysfunction	0	6
Cardiovascular involvement	2	23
Aneurysm	0	4
Cutaneous lesions	6	30
Renal involvement	2	7
Central nervous system involvement	0	10

[a] Data modified from Michet (1), Zeuner et al. (2), and Trentham and Le (3).

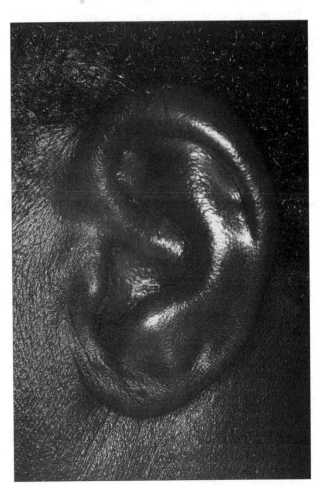

Fig. 23-1. Erythematous, swollen external ear with sparing of ear lobule.

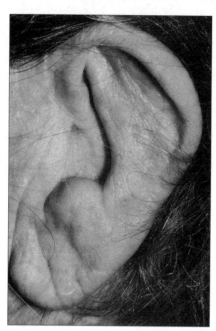

Fig. 23-2. Floppy appearance of external ear due to chronic chondritis.

(Fig. 23-2). Sudden onset of hearing loss and vertigo may occur due to involvement of the audiovestibular structures or vasculitis of the internal auditory artery.

Polyarthritis is the second most common presenting symptom at onset in most reported series, except in the group of patients described by Zeuner et al. (2). The joint pattern usually is migratory, asymmetric, episodic, nonerosive, and nondeforming polyarthritis involving large and small joints of the peripheral and/or axial skeleton (1).

Chondritis of the respiratory tract may result in collapse of the nasal cartilage, causing saddle nose deformity. Involvement of the laryngeal and tracheobronchial tract may result in hoarseness, a choking sensation, tenderness over the thyroid cartilage, cough, stridor, wheezes, and dyspnea (1,9). Tracheobronchial wall thickening and stenosis are frequent in patients with respiratory tract involvement and can be asymptomatic (1,9). Involvement of upper and lower respiratory tract in asymptomatic patients may be recognized only when there are associated secondary infections, such as bronchitis or pneumonia (1). Major airway collapse causes acute respiratory obstruction, with high morbidity and mortality, requiring emergency recognition and treatment (8).

Ocular inflammation is a frequent manifestation. Common presentations are scleritis/episcleritis (Fig. 23-3), conjunctivitis, iritis/chorioretinitis, and keratitis. Less common are optic neuritis, scleromalacia, retinal detachment, proptosis, exophthalmos, extraocular muscle palsy, and glaucoma (10).

Cardiovascular involvements in relapsing polychondritis include aortic regurgitation, mitral regurgitation, atrioventricular block, pericarditis, and cardiac ischemia (11). Acute aortic valve cusp rupture can occur early in the course of the disease (12). Aortic and mitral valve replace-

ment have limited success, with about 24% of patients requiring repeat valvuloplasty due to periprosthetic leak or aortic aneurysm, and about 50% mortality during the first four post-operative years (13). Vascular involvement of large vessels may present as aortic aneurysms, which can occur in multiple sites (1). Sudden heart-valve rupture or aneurysm can occur in patients without active disease; periodic evaluation of the cardiovascular system is recommended (11). Arterial thrombosis of major vessels may be due to vasculitis or coagulopathy. Medium-vessel disease presents as polyarteritis; leukocytoclastic vasculitis indicates small-vessel involvement (1).

Various mucocutaneous manifestations are seen, including erythema nodosum, panniculitis, livedo reticularis, urticaria, cutaneous polyarteritis nodosa, and aphthous ulcers. Renal involvement is uncommon but can occur as segmental, proliferative, and crescenteric glomerulonephritis (14).

Nervous system involvement occurs infrequently, with acute or subacute disorders of cranial nerves II, III, IV, VI, VII, and VIII causing ocular palsy, optic neuritis, facial palsy, hearing loss, and vertigo. Other neurologic complications are hemiplegia, chronic headache, ataxia, seizure, confusion, dementia (15), and meningoencephalitis (16).

Associated Disorders

Approximately 40% of patients with relapsing polychondritis have other autoimmune, rheumatologic, inflammatory or hematologic disorders (1–3,7). Diseases that have been associated with relapsing polychondritis are systemic vasculitis, systemic lupus erythematosus (SLE), rheumatoid arthritis, Sjögren's syndrome, systemic sclerosis, overlap connective tissue disease, Behçet's disease, essential mixed cryoglobulinemia, thyroid disease, inflammatory bowel disease, spondyloarthropathies, myelodysplastic syndrome, and malignancy (1–3,7). Bone marrow pathology in relapsing polychondritis shows a high frequency of myelodysplasia (17); transformation to or concurrent findings of leukemia or myeloma also have been reported (18, 19). In most

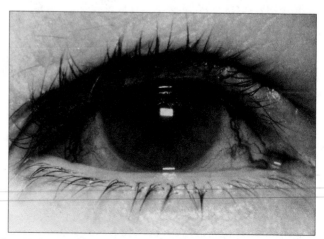

Fig. 23-3. Episcleritis and scleritis with engorged, tortuous blood vessels.

instances, polychondritis follows the associated disorders by several months to years (3,7).

Diagnosis

Abnormal results of laboratory tests generally are nonspecific. Most patients have anemia typical of chronic disease, mild leukocytosis, or thrombocytosis. Elevated erythrocyte sedimentation rate and hypergammaglobulinemia are common (6). Urinalysis typically is normal, but proteinuria or cellular sediments may be seen in patients with renal involvement. Rheumatoid factor is found in 10%–20% of patients, and antinuclear antibodies are found in 15%–25% of patients. Antinative DNA has been reported, but these patients may have had coexisting SLE. Serum complement levels usually are normal or high. Cryoglobulins can be found in a small number of patients, and autoantibodies to collagen type II, IX, and XI have been reported (5). Antineutrophil cytoplasmic antibodies (ANCA) are found in about 25% of patients during active disease, but there is no association of cytoplasmic ANCA with Wegener's granulomatosis or perinuclear ANCA with microscopic polyarteritis (20).

The diagnosis of relapsing polychondritis is based on clinical features – biopsy is not always necessary. McAdam et al. (6) proposed the following diagnostic criteria: bilateral auricular chondritis, nonerosive and seronegative inflammatory polyarthritis, nasal chondritis, ocular inflammation, respiratory tract chondritis, and cochlear or vestibular dysfunction. To make a definite diagnosis of relapsing polychondritis, a person must have at least three of these signs (6). If clinical presentation is uncertain, other causes of chondritis must be excluded, especially infectious diseases. Biopsy and cultures or other tests are necessary to exclude fungal disease, syphilis, leprosy, and other bacterial infections.

All patients with relapsing polychondritis should be evaluated for airway involvement to detect potential silent disease (1). Abnormal pulmonary function tests show an obstructive pattern (9,21). Tracheobronchial tract narrowing or stricture can be identified with computed tomography (CT) scan (9,22). A CT scan is safe, rapid, and accurate, and is the procedure of choice. Typical findings are lumen narrowing by wall thickening and collapse of the supporting cartilagenous structures.

Echocardiography, cardiac catherization, and angiography should be done in patients with prominent symptoms and signs of cardiovascular involvement. Echocardiography has been suggested as a routine test to detect silent disease (1).

Treatment

Nonsteroidal anti-inflammatory drugs may be adequate for patients with mild polychondritis limited to arthralgia and nasal or auricular chondritis. Corticosteroid treatment is used in patients with more severe disease, i.e., scleritis/uveitis and systemic symptoms. Dosages of 30–60 mg/day of prednisone (or an equivalent drug) and an immunosuppressive agent, such as azathioprine or cyclophosphamide, should be initiated. The corticosteroid dosage should be tapered soon after the observation of clinical improvement. Methotrexate has been used successfully as a steroid-sparing agent (3). In patients refractory to conventional treatment, cyclosporin A has been used with good response (1).

Acute airway obstruction unresponsive to oral corticosteroids has been treated successfully with intravenous pulse methylprednisolone (23). Improvement of renal function has been reported in a patient after six months of monthly treatment with pulse intravenous cyclophosphamide (24). A combination of oral prednisone, dapsone, and cyclophosphamide has been used, with variable response. Acute airway obstruction may require tracheostomy, and stents are necessary in patients with airway collapse (25). Surgical intervention is indicated for patients with severe cardiac valvular involvement (13) or with large-vessel aneurysms. Infections during corticosteroid and immunosuppressive therapy demand aggressive measures to identify the infectious agent and to initiate prompt treatment.

Prognosis and Survival

The survival rate for people with relapsing polychondritis is 74% at five years and 55% at 10 years (7). More recent studies by Trentham and Le show improved survival rates of 94% (3). Improved medical and surgical management of the respiratory and cardiovascular complications have contributed to the better survival rate during the past decade (3). Infection is the most common cause of death (7). Cardiovascular disease (with systemic vasculitis, rupture of large-vessel aneurysms, or cardiac valvular disease) is the second most common cause of death (6,7). Airway obstruction is the cause of death in 10% (7), and airway obstruction with superimposed infection is the cause of death in 28% of cases (6). Only 48% of the fatalities were considered to be related to relapsing polychondritis in the study by Michet et al (7), compared with 86% in an earlier study by McAdam et al (6). This difference was thought to be due to age because patients in the Michet study were older and were more likely to die from other unrelated causes. Malignancy is an uncommon cause of death.

VALEE HARISDANGKUL, MD, PhD

References

1. Michet CJ Jr. Relapsing polychondritis. In: Koopman WJ. (ed). Arthritis and Allied Conditions. A Textbook of Rheumatology, 13th edition, volume 2. Baltimore: Williams and Wilkins, 1997; pp 1595–1603.
2. Zeuner M, Straub RH, Rauh G, Albert ED, Scholmerich J, Lang B. Relapsing polychondritis: clinical and immunogenetic analysis of 62 patients. J Rheumatol 1997;24:96–101.
3. Trentham DE, Le CH. Relapsing polychondritis. Ann Intern Med 1998;129:114–122.
4. Pearson CM, Kline HM, Newcomer VD. Relapsing polychondritis. N Engl J Med 1960;263:51–58.

5. Alsalameh S, Mollenhauer J, Scheuplein F, et al. Preferential cellular and humoral immune reactivities to native and denatured collagen types IX and XI in a patient with fatal relapsing polychondritis. J Rheumatol 1993;20:1419–1424.

6. McAdam LP, O'Hanlan MA, Bluestone R, Pearson CM. Relapsing polychondritis: prospective study of 23 patients and a review of the literature. Medicine 1976;55:193–215.

7. Michet CJ, McKenna CH, Luthra HS, O'Fallon WM. Relapsing polychondritis. Survival and predictive role of early disease manifestations. Ann Intern Med 1986;104:74–78.

8. Eng J, Sabanathan S. Airway complications in relapsing polychondritis. Ann Thorac Surg 1991;51:686–692.

9. Tillie-Leblond I, Wallaert B, Leblond D, et al. Respiratory involvement in relapsing polychondritis. Clinical, functional, endoscopic and radiographic evaluations. Medicine (Baltimore) 1998;77:168–176.

10. Chen CJ, Harisdangkul V, Parker JL. Transient glaucoma associated with anterior diffuse scleritis in relapsing polychondritis. Glaucoma 1982;4:109–111.

11. Del Rosso A, Petix NR, Pratesi M, Bini A. Cardiovascular involvement in relapsing polychondritis. Semin Arthritis Rheum 1997;26:840–844.

12. Marshall DA, Jackson R, Rae AP, Capell HA. Early aortic valve cusp rupture in relapsing polychondritis. Ann Rheum Dis 1992;51:413–415.

13. Lang-Lazdunski L, Hvass U, Paillole C, Pansard Y, Langlois J. Cardiac valve replacement in relapsing polychondritis. A review. J Heart Valve Dis 1995;4:227–235.

14. Chang-Miller A, Okamura M, Torres VE, et al. Renal involvement in relapsing polychondritis. Medicine (Baltimore) 1987;66:207–217.

15. Sundaram MB, Rajput AH. Nervous system complications of relapsing polychondritis. Neurology 1983;33:513–515.

16. Hanslik T, Wechsler B, Piette JC, Vidailhet M, Robin PM, Godeau P. Central nervous system involvement in relapsing polychondritis. Clin Exp Rheumatol 1994;12:539–541.

17. Diebold J, Rauh G, Jager K, Lohrs U. Bone marrow pathology in relapsing polychondritis: high frequency of myelodysplastic syndromes. Br J Haematol 1995;89:820–830.

18. Shirota T, Hayashi O, Uchida H, Tonozuka N, Sakai N, Itoh H. Myelodysplastic syndrome associated with relapsing polychondritis: unusual transformation from refractory anemia to chronic myelomonocytic leukemia. Ann Hematol 1993;67:45–47.

19. Hall R, Hopkinson N, Hamblin T. Relapsing polychondritis, smouldering non-secretory myeloma and early myelodysplastic syndrome in the same patient: three difficult diagnoses produce a life threatening illness. Leuk Res 2000;24:91–93.

20. Papo T, Piette JC, Huong Du LT, et al. Antineutrophil cytoplasmic antibodies in polychondritis. Ann Rheum Dis 1993;52:384–385.

21. Krell WS, Staats BA, Hyatt RE. Pulmonary function in relapsing polychondritis. Am Rev Respir Dis 1986;133:1120–1123.

22. Port JL, Khan A, Barbu RR. Computed tomography of relapsing polychondritis. Comput Med Imaging Graphics 1993;17:119–123.

23. Lipnick RN, Fink CW. Acute airway obstruction in relapsing polychondritis: treatment with pulse methylprednisolone. J Rheumatol 1991;18:98–99.

24. Stewart KA, Mazanec DJ. Pulse intravenous cyclophosphamide for kidney disease in relapsing polychondritis. J Rheumatol 1992;19:498–500.

25. Sarodia BD, Dasgupta A, Mehta AC. Management of airway manifestations of relapsing polychondritis: case reports and review of literature. Chest 1999;116:1669–1675.

24 ANTIPHOSPHOLIPID SYNDROME

The major clinical features of the antiphospholipid syndrome (APS) include recurrent arterial or venous thromboses and pregnancy morbidity, including fetal losses, associated with the persistent presence of anticardiolipin antibodies or the lupus anticoagulant (Table 24-1). A number of minor clinical features also are seen, including thrombocytopenia, hemolytic anemia, livedo reticularis, cardiac valve disease, transient cerebral ischemia, transverse myelopathy, multiple sclerosis-like syndromes, chorea, and migraine. The syndrome may be primary or secondary to systemic lupus erythematosus and other autoimmune diseases. The clinical and laboratory features are similar in both primary and secondary APS (1).

The syndrome has been described most frequently in adults, but children occasionally are affected. APS is reported more frequently in women than men, which may reflect the fact that pregnancy morbidity is a prominent feature of the disorder. Although APS in more than one family member is unusual, relatives of affected patients often have anticardiolipin antibodies or the lupus anticoagulant without clinical complications (2). There probably is an association of APS with the major histocompatibility complex alleles, especially at the human leukocyte antigen (HLA)-DQB locus (3).

Etiology and Pathogenesis

Not all people with antiphospholipid antibodies experience clinical complications, suggesting that other factors related to antibody specificity or host susceptibility may be involved. A number of studies in animals suggest that these antibodies may be involved in disease pathogenesis. For example, mice passively immunized with human anticardiolipin antibodies suffer pregnancy wastage or fetal resorption

TABLE 24-1
Clinical Criteria of the Antiphospholipid Syndrome

Vascular thrombosis
- a) One or more clinical episodes of arterial, venous or small-vessel thrombosis in any tissue or organ and
- b) Thrombosis confirmed by imaging or Doppler studies or histopathology, with the exception of superficial venous thrombosis and
- c) Histopathologic confirmation with thrombosis in the absence of evidence of inflammation in the vessel wall.

Pregnancy morbidity
- a) One or more unexplained deaths of a morphologically normal fetus at or beyond the 10th week of gestation, with normal fetal morphology documented by ultrasound or by direct examination of the fetus or
- b) One or more premature births of a morphologically normal neonate at or before the 34th week of gestation because of severe preeclampsia or severe placental insufficiency or
- c) Three or more unexplained consecutive spontaneous abortions before the 10th week of gestation, with maternal anatomic or hormonal abnormalities and paternal and maternal chromosomal causes excluded.

Laboratory criteria
- a) Anticardiolipin antibody of IgG and/or IgM isotype in blood, present in medium or high titer on two or more occasions at least six weeks apart, measured by standard enzyme linked immunosorbent assay for β_2-glycoprotein 1 dependent anticardiolipin antibodies or
- b) Lupus anticoagulant present in plasma on two or more occasions at least six weeks apart, detected according to the guidelines of the International Society on Thrombosis and Hemostasis.

Definite APS is considered to be present if at least one of the clinical and one of the laboratory criteria are met.

Adapted from Wilson et al (14). Ig, immunoglobulin

(4,5). In other studies, mice infused with either purified immunoglobulins or affinity-purified anticardiolipin antibodies from people with APS developed increased thrombus size and delayed thrombus disappearance (6). The mechanisms by which antiphospholipid antibodies induce thrombosis remain unknown. These antibodies are heterogenous, with specificities for proteins, such as β_2-glycoprotein 1 (β_2GP1) and prothrombin; phospholipids, such as cardiolipin and phosphatidylserine; and phosphatidylethanolamine and protein–phospholipid complexes. Antiphospholipid antibodies have been shown to activate endothelial cells both in vitro (7) and in vivo (8), resulting in up-regulation of adhesion molecules. Other possibilities include antibody-mediated platelet activation (9) or selective inhibition of the protein C anticoagulant pathway (10).

The role of β_2GP1 in antiphospholipid antibody-mediated thrombosis is of considerable interest (11). β_2GP1, a plasma protein, binds negatively charged molecules and is a "natural anticoagulant" that inhibits coagulation reactions catalyzed by negatively charged phospholipids, such as the prothrombin–thrombin conversion. β_2GP1 markedly enhances binding of antiphospholipid antibodies from people with APS to cardiolipin in enzyme-linked immunosorbent assays (ELISA), a reaction attributed to the binding of anticardiolipin antibodies to β_2GP1 directly, a β_2GP1–phospholipid complex, or to epitopes on phospholipids in phospholipid–β_2GP1 complexes (11,12). Immunization of mice with β_2GP1 results in production of antibodies specific for both β_2GP1 and cardiolipin (13). It is possible that antiphospholipid antibodies induce thrombosis by neutralizing the anticoagulant effects of β_2GP1 (11,12).

Clinical Features

The major clinical features of APS are thrombosis and recurrent pregnancy morbidity. Preliminary classification criteria have been established to facilitate clinical studies (Table 24-1) (14).

Thrombosis

Venous and arterial thromboses may occur anywhere in the body, leading to a variety of clinical presentations. These events usually are sporadic and appear to be unrelated to antibody levels, which can remain high for several years. In the majority of patients, recurrent events are confined to either the arterial or the venous circulation, suggesting that factors influencing arterial and venous thromboses may differ. The deep veins of the leg are the sites most frequently affected in the venous circulation, but thrombosis also has been described in the pulmonary vessels, inferior vena cava, renal, hepatic (Budd–Chiari syndrome), axillary, and sagittal veins. Strokes or transient ischemic attacks are the most common presentations of arterial thrombosis, but myocardial, adrenal, and gastrointestinal infarction, and gangrene of the extremities also may occur.

Some patients experience severe widespread thromboses with life-threatening consequences, a presentation called the catastrophic antiphospholipid syndrome (15). In this situation, thrombotic thrombocytopenic purpura and diffuse intravascular coagulation must be excluded.

Pregnancy Morbidity

Although fetal death in the second or third trimester is characteristic of APS, recurrent pregnancy loss can occur at any stage of gestation. The cause of fetal death is believed to be thrombosis of the placental vessels, resulting in infarction. An intriguing hypothesis is that antiphospholipid antibodies may displace the protein annexin V from the surfaces of trophoblasts and vascular endothelial cells in the placenta, resulting in placental vessel thrombosis (16). Annexin V is an anticoagulant protein believed to play a thromboregulatory role at the vascular–blood interface in the placenta by shielding anionic phospholipids. These phospholipids, when exposed to coagulation proteins in the blood, would induce thrombus formation.

The aborted fetus usually is small for its gestational period, but often is otherwise normal. Other complications, such as preeclampsia, placental insufficiency, preterm birth, and maternal thrombosis contribute to pregnancy morbidity in women with antiphospholipid antibodies (17).

Other Features

Patients with APS occasionally present with thrombocytopenia alone. More frequently, however, mild-to-moderate thrombocytopenia (platelet counts in the range of 100,000–150,000 cells/mm³) accompanies other clinical complications. Unfortunately, thrombocytopenia in APS does not necessarily protect patients from thrombosis, but anticoagulation as part of therapy for the syndrome may increase the risk of hemorrhage.

Other clinical and laboratory features reported in APS include livedo reticularis, cardiac valvular vegetations (Libman–Sacks endocarditis), valvular insufficiency, pulmonary hypertension, leg ulcers, migraine headaches, and a variety of neurologic complications, including chorea, memory loss, dementia, multiple sclerosis-like syndromes, and transverse myelopathy. Some patients have positive Coombs' tests that occasionally are associated with hemolytic anemia.

Differential Diagnosis

None of the clinical or laboratory features of APS are confined to this disorder. A diagnosis of APS should be considered in the following circumstances: unexplained arterial or venous thrombosis, thrombosis at unusual sites (e.g., renal or adrenal veins), thrombosis in a person younger than 50 years, recurrent thrombotic events, second- or third-trimester losses, and more than one clinical feature in the same individual. In these settings, the diagnosis is confirmed by the finding of an unequivocally positive test for lupus anticoagulant or medium-to-high titers of anticardiolipin antibodies (preferably the immunoglobulin G isotype) persisting for more than six weeks (Table 24-1).

Other diagnoses that should be considered in people with unexplained venous thrombosis include factor V Leiden (activated protein-C resistance); protein-C, protein-S, or antithrombin III deficiency; dysfibrinogenemias; abnormalities of fibrinolysis; nephrotic syndrome; polycythemia vera; Behçet's disease; paroxysmal nocturnal hemoglobinuria; and thrombosis associated with oral contraceptives. In patients with arterial occlusions, the differential diagnosis includes hyperlipidemias, diabetes mellitus, hypertension, vasculitis, sickle cell disease, homocystinuria, and Buerger's disease.

APS accounts for only a small fraction of pregnancy losses. Other causes of pregnancy wastage include fetal chromosomal abnormalities, anatomic anomalies of the maternal reproductive tract, and maternal disorders, such as endocrine, infectious, autoimmune, and drug-induced disease (17).

Laboratory Tests

Both anticardiolipin antibody and lupus anticoagulant tests should be requested for people suspected of having APS, since one test can be positive without the other. Anticardiolipin tests use a standardized ELISA technique (18). Results are reported according to isotype (IgG, IgM, or IgA) and level of positivity (18). Because of variations among laboratories, anticardiolipin antibody levels also should be reported semiquantitatively as high (>80 units), medium (20–80 units), or low (10–20 units). A medium-to-high positive IgG, IgM, or rarely, IgA anticardiolipin assay is most specific for the diagnosis of APS, but the clinical features of APS have been observed with low titers of IgG or IgM anticardiolipin antibodies.

The lupus anticoagulant test is attributable to prolongation of clotting times by antiphospholipid antibodies in vitro (19). However, deficiencies of coagulation factors and clotting factor inhibitors (e.g., antiprothrombin, antifactor VIII) also may prolong clotting times. The lupus anticoagulant is identified by the following criteria: 1) demonstration of an abnormal phospholipid-dependent screening test of hemostasis (e.g., the activated prothrombin time, Russell viper venom time, kaolin clotting time, dilute prothrombin time, or textarin time); 2) failure to correct the prolonged screening coagulation test value upon mixing with normal platelet-poor plasma; 3) shortening or correction of the prolonged screening test value upon the addition of excess phospholipids or hexagonal-phase phospholipids (a phenomenon seen only with the lupus anticoagulant); and 4) exclusion of other coagulopathies (e.g., factor VIII inhibitors and the presence of heparin) (19). Lupus anticoagulant tests cannot be performed reliably in patients on oral anticoagulants or heparin.

Treatment

Thrombosis

People who have APS with venous or arterial thrombosis have a high risk of recurrence, and prophylaxis with oral anticoagulants is necessary. Recent studies suggest that a target international normalized ratio of 3.0 usually is effective in preventing thrombosis (20). Patients who suffer thrombotic recurrences despite adequate anticoagulation with warfarin may be treated with twice-daily subcutaneous heparin at doses sufficient to achieve a partial thromboplastin time of 1.5 to two times normal, although the evidence for this is anecdotal. Immunosuppressive therapy has little or no role in the treatment of this syndrome. In patients with catastrophic APS, high doses of prednisone (tapered over a few months), intravenous cyclophosphamide pulses, plasma exchange, and heparin followed by warfarin have been employed, but these treatments remain unproved (15).

Pregnancy Morbidity

Pregnancy outcome can be markedly improved in women with APS and previous pregnancy losses by using subcutaneous heparin at doses of 5000 to 10,000 units twice a day, plus one low-dose daily aspirin (60–80 mg) (17,21). Because osteoporosis may be a consequence of prolonged heparin therapy, calcium and vitamin D supplements should be considered. Thrombocytopenia and, rarely, thrombosis are idiosyncratic side effects of heparin therapy. If pregnancy loss occurs despite heparin, four-day or five-day pulses of intravenous gamma globulin (0.4 gm/kg/day) given monthly, plus one low-dose daily aspirin, may be an effective, safe, but expensive alternative (22). Although, high-dose corticosteroid therapy may be effective in reducing the risk of pregnancy loss, the side effects associated with its use make it an unsatisfactory therapeutic option (17). Children born to mothers with APS have developed normally, and their risk of developing APS is low.

Prognosis

The occurrence of one clinical complication of APS need not necessarily mean that the patient will be subject to others. For example, some women with recurrent pregnancy losses never have thrombosis, and vice versa. Some patients, however, experience all the major complications of the syndrome.

The risks of thrombosis are unknown in women who have only a history of pregnancy losses and in people with anticardiolipin or lupus anticoagulant antibodies but no clinical symptoms. Prolonged follow-up studies in these patients, however, suggest an increased risk of developing one or more clinical features of the syndrome (23). The risk of recurrent thrombosis in people treated appropriately with oral anticoagulants is small, but prolonged anticoagulation is associated with a significant risk of hemorrhage (20).

E. NIGEL HARRIS, MD

References

1. Vianna JL, Khamashta MA, Ordi-Ros J, et al. Comparison of the primary and secondary antiphospholipid syndrome: a European multicenter study of 114 patients. Am J Med 1994;96:3–9.

2. Goldberg SN, Conti-Kelly AM, Greco TP. *A family study of anticardiolipin antibodies and associated clinical correlations.* Am J Med 1995;99:473–479.

3. Wilson WA, Gharavi AE. *Genetic risk factors for aPL syndrome.* Lupus 1996;5:398–403.

4. Branch DW, Dudley DJ, Mitchell MD, et al. *Immunoglobulin G fractions from patients with antiphospholipid antibodies cause fetal death in BALB/c mice: a model for autoimmune fetal loss.* Am J Obstet Gynecol 1990;163:210-216.

5. Blank M, Tincani A, Shoenfeld Y. *Induction of experimental antiphospholipid syndrome in naive mice with purified IgG antiphosphatidylserine antibodies.* J Rheumatol 1994;21: 100–104.

6. Pierangeli SS, Liu XW, Barker JH, Anderson G, Harris EN. *Induction of thrombosis in a mouse model by IgG, IgM and IgA immunoglobulins from patients with the antiphospholipid syndrome.* Thromb Haemost 1995;74:1361–1367.

7. Del Papa N, Guidali L, Sala L, et al. *Endothelial cells as target for antiphospholipid antibodies. Human polyclonal and monoclonal anti-$\beta_2$glycoprotein 1 antibodies react in vivo with endothelial cells through adherent $\beta_2$glycoprotein and induce endothelial cell activation.* Arthritis Rheum 1997;40:551–561.

8. Pierangeli SS, Colden-Stanfield M, Liu X, Barker JH, Anderson GL, Harris EN. *Antiphospholipid antibodies from antiphospholipid syndrome patients activate endothelial cells in vitro and in vivo.* Circulation 1999;99:1997–2002.

9. Joseph JE, Harrison P, Mackie IJ, Machin SJ. *Platelet activation markers and the primary antiphospholipid syndrome (PAPS)* Lupus 1998;7:S48–S51.

10. Smirnov MD, Triplett DT, Comp PC, Esmon NL, Esmon CT. *On the role of phosphatidylethanolamine in the inhibition of activated protein C activity by antiphospholipid antibodies.* J Clin Invest 1995;95:309–316.

11. Roubey RAS. *Autoantibodies to phospholipid-binding plasma proteins: a new view of lupus anticoagulants and other "antiphospholipid" autoantibodies.* Blood 1994;84:2854–2867.

12. Reddel SW, Wang YX, Sheng YH, Krilis S. *Epitope studies with anti-β_2-glycoprotein 1 antibodies from autoantibody and immunized sources.* J Autoimmun 2000;15:91–96.

13. Gharavi AE, Sammaritano LR, Wen J, Elkon KB. *Induction of antiphospholipid autoantibodies by immunization with beta 2 glycoprotein 1 (apolipoprotein H).* J Clin Invest 1992; 90:1105–1109.

14. Wilson WA, Gharavi AE, Koike T, et al. *International consensus statement on preliminary classification criteria for definite antiphospholipid syndrome. Report of an International Workshop.* Arthritis Rheum 1999;42:1309–1311.

15. Asherson RA. *The catastrophic syndrome, 1998. A review of the clinical features, possible pathogenesis and treatment.* Lupus 1998;7:S55–S62.

16. Rand JH. *Antiphospholipid antibody-mediated disruption of the annexin V antithrombotic sheild: a thrombogenic mechanism for the antiphospholipid syndrome.* J Autoimmn 2000; 15:107–111.

17 Porter TF, Silver RM, Branch DW. *Pregnancy loss and antiphospholipid antibodies.* In: Khamashta MA (ed). Hughes Syndrome, Antiphospholipid Syndrome. London: Springer, 2000; pp 179–194.

18. Harris EN, Pierangeli SS, Birch D. *Anticardiolipin wet workshop report: 5th International Symposium on Antiphospholipid Antibodies.* Am J Clin Pathol 1994;101:616–624.

19. Triplett DA. *Use of the dilute Russell viper venom time (dRVVT): its importance and pitfalls.* J Autoimmunity 2000; 15:173–178.

20. Khamashta MA, Cuadrado MJ, Mujic F, Taub NA, Hunt BJ, Hughes GR. *The management of thrombosis in the antiphospholipid-antibody syndrome.* N Engl J Med 1995;332: 993–997.

21. Rai R, Cohen H, Dave M, Regan L. *Randomised controlled trial of aspirin and aspirin plus heparin in pregnant women with recurrent miscarriage associated with phospholipid antibodies (or antiphospholipid antibodies)* BMJ 1997;314: 253–257.

22. Spinnatto JA, Clark AL, Pierangeli SS, Harris EN. *Intravenous immunoglobulin therapy for the antiphospholipid syndrome in pregnancy.* Am J Obstet Gynecol 1995; 172:690–694.

23. Shah NM, Khamashta MA, Atsumi T, Hughes GR. *Outcome of patients with anticardiolipin antibodies: a 10 year follow up of 52 patients.* Lupus 1998;7:3–6.

25 ADULT STILL'S DISEASE

The clinical features of adult Still's disease resemble the systemic form of juvenile rheumatoid arthritis. The disorder is rare, affects both genders equally, and exists worldwide. The majority of people with adult Still's disease present at age 16–35 years (1).

Pathogenesis

The etiology of adult Still's disease is unknown. Studies of linkage to HLA antigens have been inconclusive (2,3). It has been suggested that immune complexes may play a pathogenic role (3), but this suspicion has not been confirmed (2). The principal hypothesis is that Still's disease results from a virus or other infectious agent, but study results lack consistency (4). Pregnancy and use of female hormones have not been associated with the development of Still's disease (5). The possible role of stress as an inducing phenomenon has been raised, but lacks confirmation (5).

Clinical, Laboratory, and Radiographic Findings

The clinical manifestations and laboratory findings of adult Still's disease (2,6) are summarized in Table 25-1. The initial symptom usually is the sudden onset of a high, spiking fever. The fever spikes once daily (rarely, twice daily), usually in the evening, and the temperature returns to normal in 80% of patients untreated with antipyretics. Arthralgia and severe myalgia are universal. Arthritis is almost universal but may be mild and overlooked by a physician whose attention is drawn to more dramatic manifestations. Initially, the arthritis affects only a few joints but may then evolve into polyarticular disease. The most commonly affected joints are the knee (84%) and wrist (74%). The ankle, shoulder, elbow, and proximal interphalangeal joints are involved in one-half of patients and the metacarpophalangeals in one-third. Involvement of the distal interphalangeal joints in one-fifth of patients is notable (2,3,7).

Still's rash, present in more than 85% of patients, is almost pathognomonic. The rash is salmon pink, macular or maculopapular, frequently evanescent, and often occurs with the evening fever spike. Because the patient may not notice the rash, a check during evening rounds can lead to the detection of this near-diagnostic finding. The rash is most common on the trunk and proximal extremities, but is present on the face in 15% of patients. It can be precipitated by mechanical irritation from clothing, rubbing (Koebner's phenomenon), or a hot bath. The rash may be mildly pruritic.

An elevated erythrocyte sedimentation rate is universal. Leukocytosis is present in 90% of cases, and in 80%, the white blood cell count is 15,000/mm³ or more. The liver function tests may be elevated in up to three-quarters of patients (2,8,9). Anemia, sometimes profound, is common. Tests for rheumatoid factor and antinuclear antibody generally give negative results or, when present, show low titer. Synovial and serosal fluids are inflammatory, with a predominance of neutrophils (2).

Radiographic findings at presentation are nonspecific. Early in the disease course, soft-tissue swelling and periarticular osteoporosis may be found. With time, cartilage narrowing or erosion develops in most patients. Characteristic radiographic findings typically are found in the wrist, including nonerosive narrowing of the carpometacarpal and intercarpal joints, which progresses to bony ankylosis (2,3,10,11).

Diagnosis

Although several sets of diagnostic criteria have been proposed (7,12,13), the criteria of Cush et al (7) are a practical guide (Table 25-2). It is important to note that most patients do not present with the full-blown syndrome. Fever is the most common initial manifestation, and other features develop over a period of weeks or, occasionally, months. A patient with high, daily fever spikes, severe myalgia, arthralgia, arthritis, Still's rash, and leukocytosis (frequently in combination with other manifestations outlined in Table 25-1) is unlikely to have anything other than adult Still's disease. Thus, this diagnosis should top the differential diagnosis list (Table 25-3). Most other diagnoses can be excluded on clinical grounds or by simple diagnostic tests. It has been proposed that a markedly elevated serum ferritin is highly suggestive of Still's disease (12,14).

Disease Course and Outcome

Approximately one-fifth of people with Still's disease experience long-term remission within one year. One-third of patients have a complete remission, followed by one or more relapses. The timing of relapse is unpredictable, although relapse tends to be less severe and of shorter duration than the initial episode (2,3,7). The remaining patients have a chronic disease course. The principal problem is chronic arthritis, and some patients with severe involve-

TABLE 25-1
Clinical Manifestations and Laboratory Tests in Adult Still's Disease[a]

Characteristic[b]	Patients positive/patients total	Percentage
Clinical manifestations		
Female	145/283	51
Childhood episode (≤15 years)	38/236	16
Onset 16–35 years	178/233	76
Arthralgia	282/283	100
Arthritis	249/265	94
Fever ≥39°C	258/266	97
Fever ≥39.5°C	54/62	87
Sore throat	57/62	92
JRA rash	248/281	88
Myalgia	52/62	84
Weight loss ≥10%	41/54	76
Lymphadenopathy	167/264	63
Splenomegaly	138/265	52
Abdominal pain	30/62	48
Hepatomegaly	108/258	42
Pleuritis	79/259	31
Pericarditis	75/254	30
Pneumonitis	17/62	27
Alopecia	15/62	24
Laboratory tests		
Elevated ESR	265/267	99
WBC ≥10,000 cells/mm³	228/248	92
WBC ≥15,000 cells/mm³	50/62	81
Neutrophils ≥80%	55/62	88
Serum albumin <3.5 g/dl	143/177	81
Elevated hepatic enzymes[c]	169/232	73
Anemia (hemoglobin ≤10 g/dl)	159/233	68
Platelets ≥400,000/mm³	37/60	62
Negative antinuclear antibody test	256/278	92
Negative rheumatoid factor	259/280	93

[a] Data from Pouchot et al. (2), including patients reviewed by Ohta et al. (J Rheumatol 1987;14:1139–1146). Data for fever ≥39.5°C, sore throat, myalgia, weight loss, abdominal pain, pneumonitis, alopecia, WBC ≥15,000 cells/mm³, neutrophils, and platelets are from Pouchot et al (2) only, as these data were likely underreported in early studies.

[b] JRA, juvenile rheumatoid arthritis; ESR, erythrocyte sedimentation rate; WBC, white blood cell.

[c] Any elevated liver function test.

ment of the hips and, to a lesser extent, the knees have required total joint replacement (2,7,9).

The presence of polyarthritis (four or more joints involved) or root joint involvement (shoulders or hips) has been identified as markers for a chronic disease course in a number of studies (2,7,9). A childhood episode, which occurs in about one of six patients, and a need for more than two years of therapy with systemic corticosteroids may be poor prognostic markers (7).

A controlled study noted that 10 years after diagnosis, on average, people with adult Still's disease had significantly higher levels of pain, physical disability, and psychologic disability than their unaffected siblings of the same gender. However, the levels of pain and disability in people with adult Still's disease were lower than in people with other chronic rheumatic diseases. Educational attainment, occupational prestige, social functioning, and family income did not differ between the Still's patients and the controls (15). The results suggest that patients with Still's disease are remarkably resilient in overcoming handicaps. However, premature death may be slightly increased above that expected. Causes of fatality include hepatic failure, disseminated intravascular coagulation, amyloidosis, and sepsis, all of which likely were due to Still's disease (2,6,7,9).

TABLE 25-2
Criteria for the Diagnosis of Adult Still's Disease

A diagnosis of adult Still's disease requires the presence of all of the following:
  Fever ≥39°C (102.2°F)
  Arthralgia or arthritis
  Rheumatoid factor <1:80
  Antinuclear antibody <1:100

In addition, any two of the following are required:
  White blood cell count ≥15,000 cells/mm³
  Still's rash
  Pleuritis or pericarditis
  Hepatomegaly or splenomegaly or generalized lymphadenopathy

From Cush et al (4).

TABLE 25-3
Differential Diagnosis of Adult Still's Disease

Granulomatous disorders
  Sarcoidosis
  Idiopathic granulomatosis hepatitis
  Crohn's disease

Vasculitis
  Serum sickness
  Polyarteritis nodosa
  Wegener's granulomatosis
  Thrombotic thrombocytopenic purpura
  Takayasu's arteritis

Infection
  Viral infection (e.g., hepatitis B, rubella, parvovirus, Coxsackie virus, Epstein-Barr, cytomegalovirus, HIV)
  Subacute bacterial endocarditis
  Chronic meningococcemia
  Gonococcemia
  Tuberculosis
  Lyme disease
  Syphilis
  Rheumatic fever

Malignancy
  Leukemia
  Lymphoma
  Angioblastic lymphadenopathy

Connective tissue disease
  Systemic lupus erythematosus
  Mixed connective tissue disease

Treatment

Acute Disease

Approximately one-fourth of patients respond to nonsteroidal anti-inflammatory drugs (NSAIDs), and this group of patients usually has a good prognosis. High-dose enteric-coated aspirin (to achieve a serum salicylate level of 15–25 mg/dL), sometimes combined with indomethacin, commonly has been used. Data are not available on selective cyclooxygenase-2 (COX-2) NSAIDs in adult Still's disease, but these drugs are likely to prove useful. However, response to NSAIDs may be slow (2).

A major concern with NSAID therapy has been hepatotoxicity. Liver function test abnormalities, a common finding on presentation, likely are an integral part of the disease and usually return to normal despite continued NSAID therapy (2). However, frequent monitoring of liver function, even after hospital discharge, is mandatory for patients receiving NSAIDs. NSAIDs also may increase the risk of intravascular coagulopathy.

Patients whose disease fails to respond to NSAIDs, and those with severe disease, require systemic corticosteroids. Severe disease includes pericardial tamponade, myocarditis, severe pneumonitis, intravascular coagulopathy, and rising values on liver function tests during NSAID treatment. Generally, prednisone in a dose of 0.5–1.0 mg/kg/day is needed initially, but relapse can occur with tapering (2). Intravenous pulse methylprednisolone has been used for life-threatening acute disease (16).

Chronic Disease

No controlled studies of second-line agents for the treatment of Still's disease have been published. Arthritis is the most common cause of chronicity. Intramuscular gold, hydroxychloroquine, sulfasalazine, and penicillamine have been used to control the arthritis, and anecdotal reports suggest these drugs are beneficial (2). Increased toxicity may occur with sulfasalazine (17). Weekly methotrexate in low doses, similar to doses used in adult rheumatoid arthritis, has been used to control both chronic arthritis and chronic systemic disease (18,19). Although methotrexate is potentially hepatotoxic, it seems likely that use of this agent will become more common. Mild, chronic systemic disease (e.g., fatigue, fever, rash, and serositis) also may respond to hydroxychloroquine.

Immunosuppressive agents, including azathioprine, cyclophosphamide, and cyclosporine (20), have been used in resistant cases. Intravenous immunoglobulin (21) has been used, but its use is controversial. Tumor necrosis factor (TNF)-α is elevated in Still's disease (22) and anti-TNF therapies likely will be studied increasingly in the next few years (23). A decade after disease onset, approximately one-half of patients still require second-line agents, and one-third of these patients require low-dose corticosteroids (15).

Adult Still's disease can be particularly devastating because it affects primarily young adults at a time when they are completing their education, establishing a career, or starting a family. Physiotherapists, occupational therapists, psychologists, and arthritis support groups may be needed to care for individual patients. A knowledgeable, caring physician can make a tremendous difference. It is important to realize that Still's disease can remit even years after onset, and that the vast majority of patients continue to lead remarkably full lives a decade after disease onset.

JOHN M. ESDAILE, MD, MPH

References

1. Magadur-Joly G, Billaud E, Barrier JH, et al. Epidemiology of adult Still's disease: estimate of the incidence by a retrospective study in west France. Ann Rheum Dis 1995;54:587–590.
2. Pouchot J, Esdaile JM, Beaudet F, et al. Adult Still's disease: manifestations, disease course, and outcome in 62 patients. Medicine (Baltimore) 1991;70:118–136.
3. Elkon KB, Hughes GR, Bywaters EG, et al. Adult-onset Still's disease. Twenty-year followup and further studies of patients with active disease. Arthritis Rheum 1982;25:647–654.
4. Newkirk MM, Lemmo A, Commerford K, Esdaile JM, Brandwein S. Aberrant cellular localization of rubella viral genome in patients with adult Still's disease – a pilot study. Autoimmunity 1993;16:39–43.
5. Sampalis JS, Medsger TA Jr, Fries JF, et al. Risk factors for adult Still's disease. J Rheumatol 1996;23:2049–2054.
6. Ohta A, Yamaguchi M, Tsunematsu T, et al. Adult Still's disease: a multicenter survey of Japanese patients. J Rheumatol 1990;17:1058–1063.
7. Cush JJ, Medsger TA Jr, Christy WC, Herbert DC, Cooperstein LA. Adult-onset Still's disease. Clinical course and outcome. Arthritis Rheum 1987;30:186–194.
8. Esdaile JM, Tannenbaum H, Lough J, Hawkins D. Hepatic abnormalities in adult Still's disease. J Rheumatol 1979;6:673–679.
9. Wouters JM, van de Putte LB. Adult-onset Still's disease: clinical and laboratory features, treatment and progress of 45 cases. Q J Med 1986;61:1055–1065.
10. Medsger TA Jr, Christy WC. Carpal arthritis with ankylosis in late onset Still's disease. Arthritis Rheum 1976;19:232–242.
11. Bjorkengren AG, Pathria MN, Sartoris DJ, et al. Carpal alterations in adult-onset Still disease, juvenile chronic arthritis and adult-onset rheumatoid arthritis: comparative study. Radiology 1987;165:545–548.
12. Yamaguchi M, Ohta A, Tsunematsu T, et al. Preliminary criteria for classification of adult Still's disease. J Rheumatol 1992;19:424–430.
13. Masson C, Le Loet X, Liote F, et al. Comparative study of 6 types of criteria in adult Still's disease. J Rheumatol 1996;23:495–497.
14. Van Reeth C, Le Moel G, Lasne Y, et al. Serum ferritin and isoferritins are tools for diagnosis of active adult Still's disease. J Rheumatol 1994;21:890–895.
15. Sampalis JS, Esdaile JM, Medsger TA Jr, et al. A controlled study of the long-term prognosis of adult Still's disease. Am J Med 1995;98:384–388.
16. Khraishi M, Fam AG. Treatment of fulminant adult Still's disease with intravenous pulse methylprednisolone therapy. J Rheumatol 1991;18:1088–1090.
17. Jung JH, Jun JB, Yoo DH, et al. High toxicity of sulfasalazine in adult-onset Still's disease. Clin Exp Rheumatol 2000;18:245–248.
18. Fujii T, Akizuki M, Kameda H, et al. Methotrexate treatment in patients with adult onset Still's disease – retrospective study of 13 Japanese cases. Ann Rheum Dis 1997;56:144–148.
19. Fautrel B, Borget C, Rozenberg S, et al. Corticosteroid sparing effect of low dose methotrexate treatment in adult Still's disease. J Rheumatol 1999;26:373–378.
20. Marchesoni A, Ceravolo GP, Battafarano N, Rossetti A, Tosi S, Fantini F. Cyclosporin A in the treatment of adult onset Still's disease. J Rheumatol 1997;24:1582–1587.
21. Vignes S, Wechsler B, Amoura Z, et al. Intravenous immunoglobulin in adult Still's disease refractory to non-steroidal anti-inflammatory drugs. Clin Exp Rheumatol 1998;16:295–298.
22. Stambe C, Wicks IP. TNF-alpha and response of treatment-resistant adult-onset Still's disease to thalidomide. Lancet 1998;352:544–548.
23. Weinblatt ME, Maier A, Overman SS, Mease PJ, Fraser PA, Gravallese EM. Etanercept in Still's disease in the adult. Arthritis Rheum 2000;43:S391.

26 LESS COMMON ARTHROPATHIES
A. Hematologic and Malignant Disorders

Hemophilic Arthropathy

Hemophilia is an inherited X-linked, recessive disorder of blood coagulation found almost exclusively in males. Female heterozygotes generally are asymptomatic carriers of the disease. Hemophilia A (classic hemophilia) is caused by factor VIII deficiency, and Hemophilia B (Christmas disease) is caused by factor IX deficiency.

Epidemiology and Pathology

Factor VIII is a 265-kDa protein that circulates bound to von Willebrand factor and activates factor X via proteases in the intrinsic coagulation pathway. The gene for factor VIII has been mapped to the X chromosome, facilitating prenatal diagnosis and carrier detection. Approximately one in 10,000 males is born with deficiency of factor VIII, which results in the disorder characterized by bleeding into soft tissues, muscles, and joints. Factor VIII levels of 5% or less virtually always are associated with spontaneous hemarthrosis. Factor levels of greater than 5% generally require trauma to produce bleeding.

Infrequently, female heterozygotes have low factor VIII levels, due to random inactivation of X chromosomes in factor VIII-producing tissues. These carriers may have abnormal bleeding with major surgery, menses, or trauma. Rarely, true female hemophilia may occur as a result of consanguinity within hemophilia A families. Spontaneous bleeding into muscle or soft tissues may result in large collections of blood or pseudotumors, producing muscle necrosis and compartment syndromes. Compressive femoral neuropathy may result from retroperitoneal hematomas.

Factor IX is a 55-kDa proenzyme that is converted to an active protease by factor IXa or by the tissue–factor VIIa complex. Factor IX subsequently activates factor X, in combination with activated factor VIII. The factor IX gene has been cloned and localized to the X chromosome. Deficiency of factor IX occurs in approximately one in 100,000 male births, producing a clinical picture indistinguishable from factor VIII deficiency. Other factor deficiencies, such as those of factors II, V, VII, X, and XI, rarely are associated with hemarthrosis.

Pathogenesis

The pathogenesis of hemophilic arthropathy is incompletely understood, but it may result from excessive iron deposition in the synovial membrane and cartilage. Because prothrombin and fibrinogen are absent within joints, blood remains as a liquid. Plasma gradually is reabsorbed, and the remaining red blood cells are phagocytized by synovial lining cells and macrophages. Hemosiderin, found in synovial lining cells, can be toxic and lead to chronic proliferation of synovium or pannus comprised of few lymphocytes, but primarily fibrous tissue (Fig. 26A-1). Although circulating immune complexes and decreased total serum complement have been found in some patients, a specific immune response does not appear to be involved, and no single HLA haplotype appears to relate to either the presence of hemophilia or hemophilic arthropathy (1). In a rabbit model of hemophilic arthropathy, the resulting destructive arthritis showed macroscopic and microscopic changes similar to those described in hemophilic arthritis, with synovial evidence of cartilage iron load (2).

Clinical Features

Hemarthrosis, the most common bleeding manifestation in hemophilia, occurs in up to two-thirds of patients (3). Hemarthrosis occurs spontaneously or with minor trauma, and is heralded by the onset of stiffness, pain, warmth, and swelling. The age of onset and frequency of hemarthrosis is

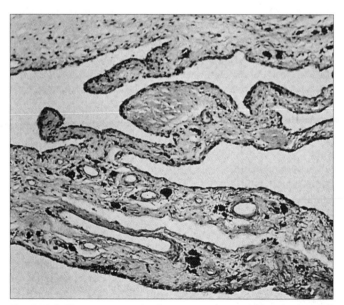

Fig. 26A-1. Photomicrograph of synovium obtained from the knee of a 76-year-old man with classic hemophilia (factor VIII deficiency) who had repeated episodes of hemarthrosis and developed severe osteoarthritis. Note heavy deposits of iron-containing pigment (hemosiderin) in lining cells and deeper portions of the synovium. Reprinted from Koopman WJ (ed): Arthritis and Allied Conditions. Philadelphia: Lea & Febiger, 1993, with permission.

determined by the level of factor deficiency. The knee, elbow, and ankle are the joints most frequently affected. Subacute and chronic arthropathy develop, with persistent synovial thickening, pain, and deformity. Late manifestations also include chronic joint contracture and degenerative joint disease, particularly of the knees (4). Septic arthritis is a rare complication of hemophilic arthropathy, although it may become more prevalent with the high incidence of human immunodeficiency virus (HIV) infection in people with hemophilia (5). Chronic arthritis appears to be more frequent in classic hemophilia than in Christmas disease, although hemarthrosis is equally prevalent (3).

Radiographic findings in hemophilic arthropathy include findings typical of degenerative arthritis: joint-space narrowing, subchondral sclerosis, and subchondral cyst formation. The extensive iron deposition in synovium leads to increased soft-tissue density around joints. In children, radiographic features include epiphyseal irregularities, widening of the femoral intracondylar notch, squaring of the interior patella, and enlargement of the proximal radius in the elbow. Magnetic resonance imaging may be useful, even in late-stage joints, to detect synovial hypertrophy amenable to synovectomy (6).

Treatment

Since the 1960s, the widespread availability of plasma products concentrated with factor VIII has revolutionized the care of people with hemophilia, reducing the severity of bleeding episodes and joint deformity and permitting surgical procedures. Tragically, these products also led to the proliferation of HIV infection, viral hepatitis, and chronic liver disease among people with hemophilia. Currently, more hemophiliacs die of acquired immunodeficiency syndrome than any other cause. Increased morbidity with concomitant HIV infection also may result from reduced muscle tone and bulk (7). Purification of factor VIII concentrates with monoclonal antifactor VIII antibody and heat lyophilization has markedly increased the safety of factor VIII therapy. Furthermore, recombinant factor VIII now is available and should eliminate the risk of infectious complications. People with hemophilia who have received multiple transfusions may develop inhibitors of (antibodies to) factor VIII, which prevent effective replacement therapy. These individuals may require specialized transfusion therapy or plasmapheresis.

Treatment of acute hemarthrosis includes prompt administration of factor VIII concentrate or its recombinant form. Adjunctive therapy includes rest, ice packs, analgesics, and eventually, physiotherapy. Aspiration generally is avoided, unless the joint is unusually tense, or sepsis is suspected. If necessary, aspiration should be accomplished after factor VIII replacement. Corticosteroids (either intra-articular or systemic) are not effective. The subacute synovitis that develops later may be treated (cautiously) with nonsteroidal anti-inflammatory drugs. D-penicillamine appears to be effective in a rabbit model of hemophilia and in human hemophilic arthropathy. Surgical or radiation synovectomy may reduce the frequency of hemarthrosis

(8,9). Joint replacement arthropathy appears to be an effective approach for end-stage disease (10–12).

Hemoglobinopathy-Associated Arthropathy

The hemoglobinopathies that produce musculoskeletal complications include sickle cell anemia (S-S) and the compound heterozygous states, including sickle β-thalassemia, sickle C disease (S-C), and sickle D disease (S-D). With deoxygenation, hemoglobin S (Hb S) polymerizes, and red blood cells containing Hb S change from a biconcave disc to an elongated, crescent-shaped cell. Sickle cells lack the deformability of normal red cells and may cause obstruction in the microcirculation, leading to tissue hypoxia and further sickling. The musculoskeletal complications of the sickle cell hemoglobinopathies include painful crises, dactylitis, osteonecrosis, gout, and osteomyelitis.

Painful crises are the most common musculoskeletal complication of sickle cell disease. Recurrent painful crises particularly affect the abdomen, chest, back, and joints. Precipitants include viral or bacterial infection, dehydration, and acidosis. Juxta-articular areas of long bones are the most frequent sites of involvement. Localized swelling may occur, especially in the anterior tibial area. The duration of painful crises varies, but longer than two weeks is rare. Supportive therapy includes intravenous hydration, oxygen, folate supplementation, and analgesics.

Joints may be involved directly in sickle cell crises, producing a painful arthritis of large joints, with small effusions. The synovial fluid typically is noninflammatory, with a predominance of mononuclear cells. The mechanism of sickle cell arthropathy may be a reaction to juxta-articular bone infarctions or synovial ischemia and infarction. In one unusual case of inflammatory arthritis, electron microscopy of synovial fluid revealed crystal-like arrays of sickled hemoglobin tactoids in erythrocytes that were enfolded and phagocytized by the cells of the synovial fluid, suggesting that sickled cells sometimes may provoke an inflammatory response (13). Treatment of arthritis associated with sickle cell disease is identical to that of painful crises.

Osteonecrosis of the femoral head occurs in up to 33% of patients with S-S, and osteonecrosis of the humeral head in up to 26%. Osteonecrosis generally is thought to result from local hypoxia due to veno-occlusion by sickled cells, although one recent study suggested that it may be due to a septic process involving the presence of bacteria in necrotic bone (14). In the spine, bony infarcts result in the characteristic biconcave or "fishmouth" vertebrae. Radiographic findings may include juxta-articular osteopenia and bone infarcts (Fig. 26A-2). Treatment of osteonecrosis of the hip consists of total hip arthroplasty, but a relatively high failure rate (particularly due to acetabular loosening) may result from marrow hyperplasia and intramedullary sclerosis (15).

Dactylitis may occur in children with sickle cell disease (either S-S, S-C, or S-thalassemia) and is due to vaso-occlusions in the bones of the hands and feet (the so-called "hand-foot syndrome"). The syndrome is characterized by an acute, painful, nonpitting swelling of the hands and feet. The average age at the time of diagnosis is 18 months, and hand-foot syndrome may be the presenting manifestation (16). Fever and leukocytosis are frequent and may cause diagnostic confusion. Radiographic features include periosteal new bone formation or intramedullary densities in the phalanges, metacarpals, and metatarsals (Fig. 26A-3). Usually, symptoms resolve within a week, but recurrences are common. Epiphyseal necrosis may lead to digital shortening.

Osteomyelitis is increased in frequency by as much as 300-fold in individuals with S-S, probably due to the combination of bone infarction and impaired host defenses. *Salmonella* osteomyelitis accounts for approximately 50% of the cases; the reason for the predominance of this organism is unclear.

Gout, a rare complication of sickle cell disease, presumably results from the increased synthesis of nucleic acids associated with the erythropoietic response to hemolysis, and the subsequent catabolism of the nucleic acid to urate. Renal damage during the third decade resulting from infarction and/or ischemia also leads to sustained hyperuricemia (17).

Thalassemia

The thalassemias are a group of congenital disorders characterized by defects in the synthesis of one or more of the Hb subunits. Only β-thalassemia is associated with musculoskeletal complications. Patients with β-thalassemia minor have qualitatively normal β chains of Hb, but the chains are produced in reduced or sometimes undetectable amounts. By contrast, β-thalassemia major (also known as Cooley's anemia) is one of the most severe forms of congenital hemolytic anemia. Individuals with this form of the disease typically are transfusion-dependent and survive into adulthood.

A variety of musculoskeletal complications of β-thalassemia major, including osteoporosis, pathologic fractures, and epiphyseal deformities, may result from expansion of the erythroid marrow. Thalassemia minor has been associated with recurrent asymmetrical arthritis, with episodes lasting less than a week (18). A more persistent, nonerosive synovitis without joint effusions also has been described. Synovial fluid is noninflammatory in thalassemia minor (19). Synovial biopsy, in one case, revealed no light microscopy abnormalities, but electron microscopy showed multilamination of vascular basement membrane and large amounts of thin fibrils surrounding connective-tissue cells (20). Similar to the bone abnormalities associated with thalassemia major, the arthritis associated with thalassemia minor may be due to para-articular bone thinning caused by chronic marrow expansion.

Myeloma-Associated Bone and Joint Disorders

Multiple myeloma, one of the most common plasma-cell dyscrasias, frequently is associated with lytic bone lesions, osteoporosis, and pathologic fractures. Approximately 15%

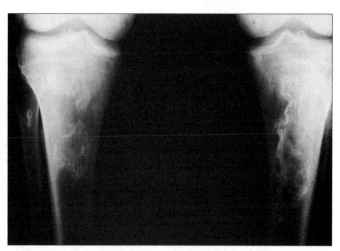

Fig. 26A-2. Knees of a person with sickle cell anemia. This posteroanterior projection of both knees demonstrates moderate osteopenia and coarse trabeculae. The medullary cavity is widened throughout, with atrophy of the cortices. Small-bone infarcts are seen in the femoral shafts. The joints are normal. Reprinted from Lally EV, Buckley WM, Claster S. Diaphyseal bone infarctions in a patient with sickle cell trait. J Rheumatol 1983;10:813–6.

of patients have associated amyloidosis of the light-chain type, which sometimes is associated with a symmetrical small-joint arthropathy that mimics rheumatoid arthritis. More commonly, amyloid infiltration in the synovium of the shoulders produces the so-called "shoulder pad sign." Bone pain, particularly in the back or chest wall, occurs in as many as 60% of patients with multiple myeloma. Up to one-third of patients can present with generalized bone loss due to the combined activity of cytokines secreted by myeloma cells (e.g., interleukin 1, tumor necrosis factor, and lymphotoxin). Distinguishing between idiopathic osteoporosis may be difficult initially, but serum protein electrophoresis, immunoelectrophoresis, and determination of Bence-Jones proteinuria usually allow detection of multiple myeloma. Because the bone lesions are lytic rather than blastic, radioisotope bone scans may fail to demonstrate lesions due to myeloma. Plain radiographs are the study of choice.

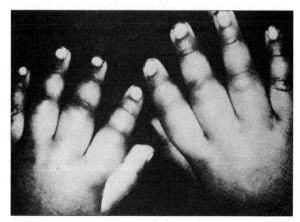

Fig. 26A-3. Sickle cell dactylitis or "hand-foot" syndrome.

Osteosclerotic myeloma is a rare form of the disease associated with sclerotic, rather than lytic, bone lesions and a more indolent course. A severe neuropathy is a frequent accompaniment. POEMS syndrome is a rare condition characterized by the combination of *p*olyneuropathy, *o*rganomegaly, *e*ndocrinopathy, *M*-protein, and *s*kin changes (21). The dermatologic findings consist of thickening, abnormal pigmentation, and in some cases, a scleroderma-like appearance. Fever, weight loss, and thrombocytosis are frequently observed.

Waldenstrom's Macroglobulinemia

Waldenstrom's macroglobulinemia (WM) is a lymphoproliferative disorder associated with monoclonal IgM in the serum. In contrast to myeloma, WM is associated with lymphadenopathy, hepatosplenomegaly, and symptoms of hyperviscosity, and is not associated with bone lesions or hypercalcemia. Infrequently, purpuric skin lesions may be seen, and associated light-chain amyloidosis may occur.

Cancer and Arthritis

Associations between a number of connective-tissue diseases and malignancies have been observed, notably dermatomyositis and various solid tumors; Sjögren's syndrome and lymphoma; scleroderma and adenocarcinoma of the lung. Treatment with cytotoxic agents is associated with an increased risk of certain cancers. These conditions and hypertrophic pulmonary osteoarthropathy (a syndrome associated with solid tumors) are discussed in other chapters. The remainder of this section will discuss hematologic malignancies and malignancies associated with diffuse articular symptoms.

Carcinoma Polyarthritis

Rarely, metastatic cancer or an occult malignancy may be associated with arthritis. In the case of metastatic disease, the arthritis usually is monarticular, and often is the result of metastasis to the joint or periarticular bone. Polyarthritis has been associated with occult malignancy of the breast and lung. The abrupt onset of a seronegative arthritis that spares the small joints of the hands and wrists serves to distinguish lung malignancies from rheumatoid arthritis, although polymyalgia rheumatica sometimes is misdiagnosed in this setting.

Leukemia

The leukemias are neoplasms of hematopoietic cells that develop initially in the bone marrow, then spread to peripheral blood, spleen, lymph nodes, and other tissues. The acute leukemias are characterized by the clonal proliferation of immature hematopoietic cells. Although joint symptoms are uncommon in adults with acute leukemia, up to 60% of children with acute lymphoblastic leukemia develop arthralgias and arthritis; these conditions may be a presenting feature of the disease in children (22). The arthritis typically is an asymmetric polyarthritis involving large joints, such as the knees, shoulders, and ankles, and may predate abnormalities of the peripheral blood (22). The occasional presence of rheumatoid factor and antinuclear antibodies can be a source of confusion. Nocturnal bone pain, hematologic abnormalities, and occasional radiographic abnormalities, such as periosteal elevation, should suggest the possibility of leukemia.

Leukemic arthropathy can be due to direct infiltration of the synovium, para-articular periostitis, intra-articular hemorrhage, or rarely, crystal-induced synovitis. Immunocytologic analysis of joint fluids can establish the diagnosis of leukemic arthritis in the early stages (23,24). Occasionally, no definite cause can be determined. Treatment of the underlying malignancy generally results in resolution of the arthritis.

Lymphoma

Symptomatic skeletal involvement is uncommon with the lymphomas, but bone lesions are detected in up to 50% of cases at autopsy. Polyarthralgia may be associated with lymphoma but rarely is a presenting manifestation. Cutaneous T-cell lymphoma has been associated with polyarthritis simulating rheumatoid arthritis.

Angioimmunoblastic Lymphadenopathy

Angioimmunoblastic lymphadenopathy (AILD) is a lymphoproliferative disorder characterized by lymphadenopathy, hepatosplenomegaly, urticaria or maculopapular skin eruptions, and constitutional signs of fever and weight loss. Coombs-positive hemolytic anemia and polyclonal hypergammaglobulinemia are other common features. Serositis (pleural and pericardial) and polyarthritis occur less frequently. The polyarthritis typically is noninflammatory and nonerosive. The condition may be confused with such autoimmune diseases as rheumatoid arthritis, adult Still's disease, or systemic lupus erythematosus, although serum rheumatoid factor and antinuclear antibodies generally are absent. The diagnosis is confirmed by lymph-node biopsy. The distinctive histopathology consists of a proliferation of small blood vessels and replacement of normal lymph-node architecture by a combination of plasma-cell immunoblasts and eosinophils. Treatment consists of combinations of corticosteroids and cytotoxic agents, but approximately 35% of patients with AILD will develop B-cell lymphoma, despite therapy.

ROBERT W. SIMMS, MD

References

1. *Steven MM, Sturrock RD, Forbes CD, Dick HM. HLA antigens in haemophilic arthritis: a family study. Dis Markers 1986;4:239–242.*
2. *Madhok R, Bennett D, Sturrock RD, Forbes CD. Mechanisms of joint damage in an experimental model of hemophilic arthritis. Arthritis Rheum 1988;31:1148–1155.*

3. Steven MM, Yogarajah S, Madhok R, Forbes CD, Sturrock RD. Haemophilic arthritis. Q J Med 1986;58:181–197.

4. Arnold WD, Hilgartner MW. Hemophilic arthropathy. Current concepts of pathogenesis and management. J Bone Joint Surg Am 1977;59:287–305.

5. Gregg-Smith S, Pattison R, Dodd C, Giangrande P, Duthie R. Septic arthritis in hemophilia. J Bone Joint Surg Br 1993;75:368–370.

6. Nuss R, Kilcoyne RF, Geraghty S, Wiedel J, Manco-Johnson M. Utility of magnetic resonance imaging for management of hemophilic arthropathy in children. J Pediatr 1993;123:388–392.

7. Bale J, Contant C, Garg B, Tilton A, Kaufman D, Wasiewski W. Neurologic history and examination results and their relationship to human immunodeficiency virus type I serostatus in hemophilic subjects: results from the hemophilia growth and development study. Pediatrics 1993;91:736–741.

8. van Kasteren ME, Novakova IR, Boerbooms AM, Lemmens JA. Long term follow up of radiosynovectomy with yttrium-90 silicate in hemophilic hemarthrosis. Ann Rheum Dis 1993;52:548–550.

9. Mannucci PM, De Franchis R, Torri G, Pietrogrande V. Role of synovectomy in hemophilic arthropathy. Isr J Med Sci 1977;13:983–987.

10. Nelson IW, Sivamurugan S, Latham PD, Matthews J, Bulstrode CJ. Total hip arthroplasty for hemophilic arthropathy. Clin Orthop 1992;276:210–213.

11. Teigland JC, Tjonnfjord GE, Evensen SA, Charania B. Knee arthroplasty in hemophilia. 5-12 year follow-up of 15 patients. Acta Orthop Scand 1993;64:153–156.

12. Hofmann P, Menge M, Brackmann HH: Reconstructive surgery in the lower limb in hemophiliacs. Isr J Med Sci 1977;13:988–994.

13. Mann D, Schumacher HR Jr. Pseudoseptic inflammatory knee effusion caused by phagocytosis of sickled erythrocytes after fracture into the knee joint. Arthritis Rheum 1995;38:284–287.

14. Shah A, Mukherjee A, Moreau PG. 9 knee arthroplasties for sickle cell disease. Acta Orthop Scand 1993;64:150–152.

15. Moran MC, Huo MH, Garvin KL, Pellicci PM, Salvati EA. Total hip arthroplasty in sickle cell hemoglobinopathy. Clin Orthop 1993;294:140–148.

16. Worrall VT, Butera V. Sickle-cell dactylitis. J Bone Joint Surg Am 1976;58:1161–1163.

17. Reynolds MD. Gout and hyperuricemia associated with sickle-cell anemia. Semin Arthritis Rheum 1983;12:404–413.

18. Gerster JC, Dardel R, Guggi S. Recurrent episodes of arthritis in thalassemia minor. J Rheumatol 1984;11:352–354.

19. Schlumpf U, Gerber N, Bunzli H, Elsasser U, Pestalozzi A, Boni A. Arthritis in thalassemia minor. J Suisse de Med 1977;107:1156–1162.

20. Schumacher HR, Dorwart BB, Bond J, Alavi A, Miller W. Chronic synovitis with early cartilage destruction in sickle cell disease. Ann Rheum Dis 1977;36:413–419.

21. Fam A, Rubenstein J, Cowan D. POEMS Syndrome. Arthritis Rheum 1986;29:233–241.

22. Saulsbury FT, Sabio H. Acute leukemia presenting as arthritis in children. Clin Pediatr (Phila) 1985;24:625–628.

23. Brooks PM. Rheumatic manifestations of neoplasia. Curr Opin Rheumatol 1992;4:90–93.

24. Harden EA, Moore JO, Haynes BF. Leukemia-associated arthritis: identification of leukemic cells in synovial fluid using monoclonal and polyclonal antibodies. Arthritis Rheum 1984;27:1306–1308.

LESS COMMON ARTHROPATHIES
B. Rheumatic Disease and Endocrinopathies

Most endocrine disorders are associated with systemic manifestations caused by changes in the quantity or activity of various hormones. Musculoskeletal signs and symptoms are among the more frequent clinical sequelae of endocrinopathies. In some cases, the first clinical sign or symptom of endocrine disease will be rheumatic. Some rheumatic symptoms, such as myalgias, can be seen in a variety of different endocrinopathies; other rheumatic manifestations, such as Raynaud's phenomenon, are indicative of only one or two certain diseases. Various endocrinopathies also may be associated with specific rheumatic diseases.

Understanding the associations between endocrine and rheumatic diseases is important for several reasons. First, appreciating these clinical connections will help clinicians avoid misdiagnoses of primary rheumatic disease and can lead to prompt treatment of a primary endocrine disorder. Second, many of these rheumatic syndromes respond, in full or in part, to treatment of the underlying endocrinopathy. Third, some of the associations are sufficiently common or striking to justify screening for specific endocrine diseases when patients manifest certain rheumatic symptoms or signs. Finally, endocrine disorders may affect the disease activity of established autoimmune diseases. Such findings have led to the investigation of pathophysiologic links between autoimmune and endocrine diseases.

Rheumatic Sequelae of Specific Endocrine Diseases
Diabetes Mellitus
Diabetes mellitus is associated with a wide variety of musculoskeletal problems, some of which are unique to the disease (1,2). The spectrum of rheumatologic syndromes seen in people with diabetes is outlined in Table 26B-1. The

nomenclature of these conditions can be confusing, with some having more than one name in the medical literature. Some of these manifestations are secondary to the microvascular disease, neuropathic complications, or proliferation of connective tissue seen in diabetes. These rheumatic syndromes affect people with either type I or type II diabetes, especially those with evidence of organ damage.

A number of syndromes of limited joint mobility occur in people with diabetes (3). *Diabetic hand syndrome* (diabetic cheiroarthropathy) is a condition stemming from alterations in the soft tissue of the hands and fingers, resulting in stiff, waxy skin and joint contractures. This condition can be confused with arthritis and the sclerodactyly seen in systemic sclerosis. Cheiroarthropathy is demonstrated when patients are asked to oppose the palmar surfaces of their hands and fingers (the prayer sign), and they are unable to fully touch these surfaces. *Adhesive capsulitis* (frozen shoulder, periarthritis) is a similar condition that leads to shoulder-joint contractures, which often are severe. This condition frequently is bilateral and sometimes is accompanied by calcific deposits in the surrounding soft tissues (4). Physical therapy appears to be helpful, and spontaneous resolution may occur over months to years. *Dupuytren's contractures* and *trigger finger* (flexor tenosynovitis) are frequent, annoying, and potentially disabling conditions that are more common among people with diabetes. These finger problems may respond to glucocorticoid injection or surgical correction.

Two other common musculoskeletal diseases with an increased prevalence and generally younger age of presentation in people with diabetes are *osteoporosis* and *diffuse idiopathic skeletal hyperostosis* (DISH syndrome). Insulin-like growth factors are thought to play a pathogenic role in these diseases. Although the association between diabetes and osteoporosis has been questioned, the link between hyperostosis and diabetes is established more firmly. DISH is accompanied by ossification and calcification of spinal ligaments, but does not necessarily cause significant clinical problems.

Patients with diabetes mellitus may encounter several types of neuropathies that result in musculoskeletal symptoms or that may mimic rheumatic diseases. *Neuropathic arthritis* (Charcot joints, diabetic osteoarthropathy), a destructive bone and joint condition that is the consequence of peripheral neuropathy, most commonly affects the foot (5). Despite the resulting joint obliteration, ankylosis, and deformities, patients usually have little or no pain, and the diagnosis is based on radiographic appearance. Plain radiography, bone scintigraphy, and magnetic resonance imaging are useful imaging modalities for diagnosing diabetic osteoarthropathy and documenting the extent of disease. Similarly, the peripheral neuropathy of diabetes increases the incidence of foot infections and foreign-body reactions, in which patients may be unaware of injury due to anesthetic feet; both of these conditions may lead to septic arthritis.

The incidence of *carpal tunnel syndrome*, a median nerve neuropathy, is increased in people with diabetes and may occur bilaterally. Similarly, *reflex sympathetic dystrophy* (causalgia) is more common among people with diabetes. *Diabetic amyotrophy* is characterized by painless, often bilateral, muscle weakness resulting from a mononeuropathy with noninflammatory atrophy of type II muscle fibers (6). Spontaneous improvement may occur. Other neuropathies that can occur among people with diabetes may be central or peripheral, and include such conditions as mononeuritis multiplex and radiculopathies that mimic other musculoskeletal conditions.

Diabetic muscle infarction is a rare but increasingly recognized syndrome of acute infarction of multiple muscle areas in people with diabetes and organ damage (7). This condition usually occurs with severe pain in one extremity. Diabetic muscle infarction can be confused with pyomyositis or venous thrombosis. MRI can be diagnostic, although biopsy may be needed in some cases. Although self-limited, this condition can recur. The etiology of diabetic muscle infarction is unclear but may be related to microvasculopathy and microthrombosis.

Improved glycemic control may not reverse the conditions outlined in Table 26B-1, but may help prevent future episodes. When these syndromes are present without an obvious explanation, it is appropriate to consider screening patients for undiagnosed diabetes mellitus by testing fasting glucose and glycosylated hemoglobin levels.

TABLE 26B-1
Rheumatologic Manifestations of Diabetes Mellitus

Syndromes of limited joint mobility
  Diabetic hand syndrome (diabetic cheiroarthropathy)
  Adhesive capsulitis (frozen shoulder, periarthritis)
  Trigger finger (flexor tenosynovitis)
  Dupuytren's contractures

Osteoporosis

Diffuse idiopathic skeletal hyperostosis (DISH)

Neuropathies
  Neuropathic arthritis (Charcot joints, diabetic osteoarthropathy)
  Carpal tunnel syndrome
  Diabetic amyotrophy
  Reflex sympathetic dystrophy (multiple synonyms)
  Various other neuropathies

Diabetic muscle infarction

Thyroid Disease

Thyroid disease frequently is accompanied by various musculoskeletal problems (Table 26B-2) (8,9). Hyperthyroidism, hypothyroidism, and thyroxine replacement therapy, in particular, are associated with rheumatic disease. Some studies report that thyroid abnormalities are more common among people with various autoimmune syndromes, including rheumatoid arthritis, systemic lupus erythematosus, and systemic sclerosis. However, these associations have been questioned, and the perceived increased prevalence of thyroid disorders among patients with these autoimmune diseases may be confounded by the fact that thyroid diseases are common among women, and women account for 75%–90% of people with these autoimmune diseases. Musculoskeletal problems may be the first, and sometimes only, clinical sign of thyroid disease.

Because thyroid diseases are easily diagnosed and highly responsive to treatment, screening for thyroid dysfunction among people with various rheumatic symptoms is essential. Achieving a euthyroid status improves many, but not all, of these conditions.

Hyperthyroidism

Hyperthyroidism is an important, reversible, and easily detected cause of *osteoporosis*. Administration of levothyroxine as replacement therapy or for suppression of thyroid nodules may lead to osteoporosis (10).

Thyrotoxicosis often causes a proximal *myopathy* that may be severe. Most patients with this myopathy do not have elevated creatinine kinase levels but do have electromyographic abnormalities. This myopathy almost always is reversible upon attainment of a euthyroid state. All patients presenting with weakness must be screened for thyrotoxicosis.

A shoulder *periarthritis* (often bilateral) may be seen in people with hyperthyroidism.

Thyroid acropachy, an unusual late manifestation of Graves' disease, involves painful soft-tissue swelling of hands, fingers, and toes, with clubbing and periostitis. Although similar to hypertrophic osteoarthropathy, most patients with acropachy already have established exophthalmos, pretibial myxedema, and measurable levels of long-acting thyroid stimulator in the serum. Acropachy usually presents after treatment of hyperthyroidism and is thought to have an immunologic basis.

Although many drugs have been associated with vasculitis, some of these associations are poorly supported by the literature. However, the evidence is compelling that propylthiouracil and related thionamides used in the treatment of hyperthyroidism can cause vasculitis syndromes associated with antineutrophil cytoplasmic antibodies.(11)

Hypothyroidism

Hypothyroidism in children or fetuses results in multiple skeletal abnormalities, as well as severe developmental problems. In adults, hypothyroidism can cause a series of musculoskeletal problems. Given the high prevalence of hypothyroidism in adults, this diagnosis must be considered in all patients presenting with the syndromes described in this section. The discovery of previously undiagnosed thyroid deficiency among people presenting with rheumatic symptoms is common.

Joint symptoms are extremely common among patients with hypothyroidism, and range from vague *arthralgias* to a *symmetric polyarthritis* that may be confused with rheumatoid arthritis. The joint effusions seen in hypothyroidism are noninflammatory. Additionally, an increased incidence of *joint laxity* has been noted among people with myxedema. *Carpal tunnel syndrome* is associated with hypothyroidism and may be bilateral. When a euthyroid state is attained, these rheumatologic symptoms often remit fully.

There is an increased incidence of hypothyroidism among patients with crystal-induced arthritis. In particular, asymptomatic *chondrocalcinosis* and clinical *pseudogout* are associated with hypothyroidism. Similarly, there are reports linking hypothyroidism to asymptomatic *hyperuricemia* and *gout*.

Myopathy is a common feature of hypothyroidism and can include myalgias and weakness (especially proximally). The weakness usually is mild to moderate in severity and is accompanied by abnormal findings on electromyography. In contrast to the myopathy seen in hyperthyroidism, serum creatinine kinase levels are elevated in most patients with muscle disease associated with hypothyroidism. Muscle bulk is not changed appreciably, and biopsy specimens may demonstrate evidence of degeneration and regeneration of muscle fibers without inflammation. The myopathy reverses with treatment of the underlying thyroid disorder.

Parathyroid Disease

Table 26B-3 outlines the rheumatologic manifestations of parathyroid disease.

Hyperparathyroidism

A wide variety of bone and joint abnormalities have been associated with hyperparathyroidism. Some of these conditions have become less common, due to the earlier detection

TABLE 26B-2
Rheumatologic Manifestations of Thyroid Disease

Hyperthyroidism
  Osteoporosis
  Myopathy
  Periarthritis
  Acropachy

Hypothyroidism
  Arthralgias
  Symmetrical polyarthritis
  Joint laxity
  Carpal tunnel syndrome
  Chondrocalcinosis and pseudogout
  Hyperuricemia and gout
  Myopathy

TABLE 26B-3
Rheumatologic Manifestations of Parathyroid Disease

Hyperparathyroidism
Osteoporosis
Osteitis fibrosa cystica
Erosive arthritis
Joint laxity
Chondrocalcinosis and pseudogout
Hyperuricemia and gout
Myopathy

Hypoparathyroidism
Ectopic calcification
Myopathy

and treatment of hyperparathyroidism. Nevertheless, rheumatologic manifestations of hyperparathyroidism commonly are the presenting features of disease. This section outlines the rheumatologic problems encountered in primary hyperparathyroidism. A series of similar disorders can result from secondary hyperparathyroidism associated with renal failure or malabsorption.

Osteoporosis is a direct consequence of excess parathormone and can cause severe, irreversible bone loss. Bone loss

TABLE 26B-4
Rheumatologic Manifestations of Acromegaly

Articular
Arthralgias
Bursal enlargement
Osteoarthritis
Joint laxity
Cartilage hypertrophy and degeneration
Pseudogout (possibly)
Tendinous and capsular calcification

Bone
Back pain
Osteoporosis
Bone hypertrophy and resorption

Neuromuscular
Myopathy and muscle hypertrophy
Compression neuropathy, especially carpal tunnel syndrome
Ischemic neuropathy

Miscellaneous
Raynaud's phenomenon

associated with hyperparathyroidism is greater in cortical than in cancellous regions.

Osteitis fibrosa cystica is a syndrome of multiple bony abnormalities associated with severe hyperparathyroidism. Due to earlier detection, this disorder is rarely seen in areas with comprehensive medical care. Osteitis fibrosis cystica involves unique radiographic findings, including bone cysts and subperiosteal erosions. Diffuse bone pain can be present, and an erosive, noneffusive arthritis has been reported. Increased *joint laxity*, tendon laxity and ruptures, and ectopic calcifications also are associated with hyperparathyroidism.

Chondrocalcinosis and *pseudogout* commonly occur in people with hyperparathyroidism and may be presenting features of disease (12). A noninflammatory polyarthritis also has been reported. An increased prevalence of *hyperuricemia* and *gout* is seen among people with hyperparathyroidism secondary to nephrocalcinosis. These crystal-induced diseases persist even after correction of excess parathormone production.

Although people with hyperparathyroidism commonly report vague myalgias and malaise, a reversible proximal *myopathy* is unusual and is associated only with severe disease. Ectopic calcifications, including intravascular lesions, occasionally may result in various neuropathies.

Hypoparathyroidism
Hypoparathyroidism and the related disorders of pseudohypoparathyroidism and pseudopseudohypoparathyroidism are associated with unusual bony abnormalities and *ectopic calcification* of subcutaneous tissue and paraspinal ligaments. *Myopathies* also have been reported.

Acromegaly
Acromegaly, a rare disorder of pituitary hypersecretion of growth hormone, usually is caused by an adenoma and is associated with a large variety of musculoskeletal abnormalities. The syndrome illustrates the protean effects of growth hormone on human physiology (13). In children whose epiphyses have not yet closed, growth hormone excess causes *gigantism* and presents a set of problems different from those seen in adults with acromegaly. Growth hormone exerts many of its actions via the production of insulin-like growth factors (IGF or somatomedins). In particular, IGF-I and growth hormone itself promote proliferation of soft tissues and bone. Tissues affected by acromegaly include synovium, cartilage, bursae, and muscle.

Table 26B-4 outlines the rheumatic manifestations of acromegaly and categorizes them as articular, bone, neuromuscular, or miscellaneous problems.

The musculoskeletal manifestations of acromegaly usually are present long before the underlying endocrinopathy is diagnosed. Treatment, through a combination of surgical resection of the adenoma and administration of octreotide, can prevent worsening of some aspects of the disease and a few of its complications. In view of the potential for this disease to cause significant deformities, morbidity, and mortality, early detection is a key factor to improving the lives of people with acromegaly.

Articular problems that occur in acromegaly are due to a combination of cartilage hypertrophy, synovial proliferation, and osteophytosis. Vague *arthralgias*, joint-space widening, *joint laxity*, and noninflammatory effusions may be followed by degenerative joint disease and clinical osteoarthritis. Whether chondrocalcinosis and pseudogout are associated with acromegaly remains a controversial issue.

Back pain is quite common and may be due to hypertrophy of the vertebral bodies and discs. Patients often exhibit spinal hypermobility. *Osteoporosis* may develop secondary to the hypogonadism that often occurs. Because increased bone thickness can occur, bone-density measurements can be difficult to interpret.

Many of the articular, soft-tissue, and bone abnormalities in acromegaly result in characteristic radiographic features, including joint-space widening, heel-pad hypertrophy, and terminal phalanx enlargement. Once bone and joint problems occur, treatment of acromegaly does not appear to reverse musculoskeletal manifestations and may not prevent damage progression.

The neuromuscular problems seen in acromegaly also are secondary to tissue hypertrophy, including *compression* and *ischemic neuropathies*. Carpal tunnel syndrome is especially common and often is bilateral. This complication of acromegaly usually remits with proper treatment of the endocrinopathy. Although *muscle hypertrophy* can occur, some patients develop proximal muscle weakness and fatigue. The myopathy may not remit with treatment of the growth hormone excess.

Raynaud's phenomenon occurs in some patients with acromegaly. The etiology of this complication is not clear.

Octreotide, a somatostatin analog used to treat acromegaly, occasionally causes neuromuscular weakness. Octreotide also may cause hypothyroidism, leading to the rheumatic problems discussed previously.

Miscellaneous Endocrine Disorders

Glucocorticoid excess (Cushing's syndrome) from primary adrenal hyperproduction, pituitary stimulation (Cushing's disease), or exogenous administration can cause a variety of musculoskeletal problems. Osteoporosis is a particular problem with these disorders and can lead to pathologic fractures. Osteonecrosis can occur in Cushing's disease but is associated more commonly with exogenous corticosteroid administration (14). The so-called "steroid myopathy" can occur with any form of glucocorticoid excess. This proximal muscle weakness is noninflammatory, not associated with elevated serum creatinine kinase levels, and resolves with correction of the hormone imbalance.

Glucocorticoid deficiency (Addison's disease) can cause myalgias, arthralgias, and flexion contractures. These problems are responsive to glucocorticoid replacement therapy.

Reported rheumatologic manifestations of the carcinoid syndrome include arthralgias, muscle wasting, bony erosions, and retroperitoneal fibrosis (15).

PETER A. MERKEL, MD, MPH

References

1. Pastan RS, Cohen AS. The rheumatologic manifestations of diabetes mellitus. Med Clin North Am 1978;62:829–839.
2. Crisp AJ, Heathcote JG. Connective tissue abnormalities in diabetes mellitus. J R Coll Physicians Lond 1984;18:132–141.
3. Schulte L, Roberts MS, Zimmerman C, Ketler J, Simon LS. A quantitative assessment of limited joint mobility in patients with diabetes. Goniometric analysis of upper extremity passive range of motion. Arthritis Rheum 1993;36:1429–1443.
4. Mavrikakis ME, Drimis S, Kontoyannis DA, Rasidakis A, Moulopoulou ES, Kontoyannis S. Calcific shoulder periarthritis (tendinitis) in adult onset diabetes mellitus: a controlled study. Ann Rheum Dis 1989;48:211–214.
5. Sinha S, Munichoodappa CS, Kozak GP. Neuro-arthropathy (Charcot joints) in diabetes mellitus (clinical study of 101 cases). Medicine (Baltimore) 1972;51:191–210.
6. Krendel DA, Costigan DA, Hopkins LC. Successful treatment of neuropathies in patients with diabetes mellitus [see comments]. Arch Neurol 1995;52:1053–1061.
7. Grigoriadis E, Fam AG, Starok M, Ang LC. Skeletal muscle infarction in diabetes mellitus. J Rheumatol 2000;27: 1063–1068.
8. Bland JH, Frymoyer JW. Rheumatic syndromes of myxedema. N Engl J Med 1970;282:1171–1174.
9. Bland JH, Frymoyer JW, Newberg AH, Revers R, Norman RJ. Rheumatic syndromes in endocrine disease. Semin Arthritis Rheum 1979;9:23–65.
10. Wartofsky L. Levothyroxine therapy and osteoporosis. An end to the controversy? Arch Intern Med 1995; 155:1130-1.
11. Merkel P. Drugs Associated with Vasculitis. Curr Opin Rheumatol 1998; 10:45-50
12. Alexander GM, Dieppe PA, Doherty M, Scott DG. Pyrophosphate arthropathy: a study of metabolic associations and laboratory data. Ann Rheum Dis 1982;41:377–381.
13. Bluestone R, Bywaters EG, Hartog M, Holt PJ, Hyde S. Acromegalic arthropathy. Ann Rheum Dis 1971;30:243–258.
14. Phillips KA, Nance EP Jr, Rodriguez RM, Kaye JJ. Avascular necrosis of bone: a manifestation of Cushing's disease. South Med J 1986;79:825–829.
15. Plonk JW, Feldman JM. Carcinoid arthropathy. Arch Intern Med 1974;134:651–654.

LESS COMMON ARTHROPATHIES
C. Hyperlipoproteinemia and Arthritis

Musculoskeletal problems can occur in association with hyperlipoproteinemia, a condition in which an underlying genetic defect leads to overproduction and/or impaired removal of lipoproteins. The abnormality, which can be of the lipoprotein or its receptor, results in elevated, measurable lipoprotein levels that can lead to premature atherosclerosis. Recognition of these syndromes facilitates proper diagnosis and management of the musculoskeletal complaint and appropriate diagnosis of a treatable condition that could have significant cardiovascular consequences.

Several recognized heritable disorders of lipid metabolism result in a number of clinical phenotypes (1) (Table 26C-1), and these disorders can be associated with distinct musculoskeletal manifestations. Hyperlipidemia also can occur secondary to another disorder (for example, nephrosis or primary biliary cirrhosis) or cause (e.g., cigarette smoking). Concurrent arthritis and hyperlipidemia also may be the result of a common risk factor (for example, obesity as a risk factor for secondary hyperlipidemia and osteoarthritis). In this section, we will focus on musculoskeletal syndromes believed to be directly related to the hyperlipidemia.

Xanthomas

Xanthomas can occur in any of the inherited hyperlipoproteinemias. Tendinous xanthomas are associated most notably with type II (familial hypercholesterolemia) and type III (familial dysbetalipoproteinemia) hyperlipoproteinemias (1). Tendinous xanthomas characteristically occur on the dorsum of the hands over the digit extensor tendons, or on the heels at the Achilles tendon insertions (2). They have been described at other extensor surfaces as well, including the triceps, olecranon, or quadriceps insertions. Achilles tendon xanthomas are more strongly associated with type III hyperlipidemia (1). Although patients with polygenic hypercholesterolemia can have similar lipid profiles, xanthomata are not seen in these patients.

Tendinous xanthomas often are noticeable but not necessarily symptomatic. Tendinitis or tenosynovitis can occur, however, particularly in the Achilles tendon, where the mass effect of the xanthoma contributes to local irritation by overlying footwear. Radiographic findings can include calcifications within the xanthomas, or even periarticular cortical erosions, presumably secondary to pressure effects of the enlarged tendons (3). Tendinitis preceding xanthoma formation or even spontaneous tendon ruptures are rare, but have been described in type IIa hyperlipoproteinemia (4,5). The tendinous xanthomas reside within the tendon fibers and move in conjunction with the tendon. Pathologic examination of such xanthomas reveals infiltrates of foam cells that seem to be macrophages congested with remnants of ingested (endocytosed) circulating lipoproteins.

Osseous xanthomas can be seen in type III hyperlipoproteinemia and can predispose to pathologic fractures,

TABLE 26C-1
Classification of Hyperlipidemia

Phenotype	Lipoprotein abnormality	Lipid abnormality	Musculoskeletal manifestations
Type I	Chylomicrons increased	Markedly increased triglycerides	Eruptive xanthomas
Type IIa	LDL increased	Increased cholesterol	Tendinous, tuberous xanthomas; migratory, episodic polyarthritis; Achilles tendinitis
Type IIb	LDL and VLDL increased	Increased cholesterol and triglycerides	Tendinous, tuberous xanthomas; migratory, episodic polyarthritis; Achilles tendinitis
Type III	Chylomicrons and VLDL remnants increased	Increased cholesterol; increased- to markedly increased triglycerides	Tendinous, tuberous, and plane xanthomas
Type IV	VLDL increased	Increased triglycerides	Eruptive tendinous and tuberous xanthomas; arthralgias
Type V	Chylomicrons and VLDL increased	Increased cholesterol, markedly increased triglycerides	Eruptive xanthomas

Modified from Fredrickson et al (13) with permission. LDL, low-density lipoprotein; VLDL, very low-density lipoprotein.

particularly if present in long bones, such as the femur or humerus. Other locations include the small bones of the hands, skull, spine, and pelvis. Radiographically, such xanthomas appear as well-defined, round or oval lucencies (6). In a patient with type V hyperlipidemia, pathologic evaluation of a cystic femoral lesion revealed foamy histiocytes with granulomatous reaction around cholesterol clefts (7).

Tuberous xanthomas are subcutaneous masses, generally found over extensor surfaces, including the elbows, knees, and hands, or on the buttocks. They can be observed in types II, III, and IV hyperlipoproteinemias. Xanthomas on the palmar surfaces (xanthoma striata palmaris) can be seen in type III hyperlipoproteinemia and are the result of lipid deposition in that location (1).

Although xanthomas generally are associated with heritable disorders of lipid metabolism, other, rarer causes have been recognized. Cerebrotendinous xanthomatosis is a rare autosomal recessive disorder in which accumulation of cholestanol or dihydrocholesterol in neural tissue or tendons results in clinical manifestations of disease, including ataxia, paresis, dementia, and tendon xanthomas (8). These manifestations can appear as early as the second decade. Another disorder associated with tendinous xanthomas is beta-sitosterolemia, an autosomal recessive disorder in which there is hyperabsorption of cholesterol and plant sterols from the intestine (9). These disorders should be considered when a patient presents with tendinous xanthomas, particularly at a young age, in the absence of marked elevation of serum cholesterol. Xanthomata also can be seen in the secondary hypercholesterolemia associated with cholestatic liver disease, such as primary biliary cirrhosis.

Articular Disease

There is some controversy about the association of articular disease with familial hyperlipoproteinemias. Some of the proposed associated arthropathies were based on descriptive case series (5,10,11) that have not necessarily been borne out in controlled studies (12,13), although other controlled series have supported the association (14,15). Certain musculoskeletal presentations, however, are well-recognized. An episodic, acute, migratory inflammatory arthritis has been well-described and occurs in up to 50% of homozygotes with type II hyperlipoproteinemia (16,17). This condition primarily affects large peripheral joints, such as knees and ankles, but the small joints of the hands and feet can be involved. The joints are erythematous, warm, and swollen, and acute-phase reactants, such as sedimentation rate and plasma fibrinogen, are elevated. The distinction from acute rheumatic fever can be difficult, particularly because some of those patients may have atherosclerotic valvular disease. The presence of tendinous xanthomas and markedly elevated cholesterol, and the absence of antecedent *Streptococcal* infection helps distinguish the entities. Generally, the episodes are self-limited and resolve within two weeks. This pattern of arthritis is seen much less commonly (approximately 4%) in heterozygotes.

Self-limited episodes of acute mono- or oligoarthritis, often of the knee or ankle, can be seen in familial hypercholesterolemia. In type IV hyperlipoproteinemia, a more chronic arthritis can occur. Patients complain of morning stiffness and a bland, often asymmetric, polyarticular arthritis. Both large and small joints may be involved, including proximal interphalangeal joints, metacarpophalangeal joints, wrists, knees, shoulders, and tarsophalangeal and metatarsophalangeal joints (18). Synovial fluid analysis reveals minimally inflammatory or noninflammatory fluid, without crystals. Synovial biopsy has been described as revealing moderate synovial hyperplasia, with a modest infiltrate of mononuclear cells and foam cells. There may be a relationship between serum triglyceride level and joint complaints.

Even xanthomata, the hallmark physical finding in hyperlipoproteinemias, can be mistaken for other entities, such as gouty tophi in a person with oligoarthritis, or rheumatoid nodules in a person with polyarthritis. It is important, therefore, that the clinician caring for people with musculoskeletal complaints be aware of these hyperlipoproteinemia-related musculoskeletal syndromes and distinguish them from other, more common arthropathies.

Crystal Disease

Hyperuricemia and gout can be associated with hypertriglyceridemia in type I, IV, and V hyperlipoproteinemia. It is important to recognize this very treatable cause of acute monarthritis or oligoarthritis by examining the synovial fluid for crystals when possible. Interestingly, the presence of cholesterol crystals has been associated with a worse outcome for a joint affected by degenerative or inflammatory arthritis, and has been shown to maintain the inflammatory reaction in experimental animals (19). In people with primary hyperlipoproteinemia, however, cholesterol crystals have not been specifically implicated in the associated acute or chronic arthritides. Crystals were found in a retrocalcaneal bursa adjacent to a xanthoma in a patient with type II hyperlipoproteinemia, but the significance of these crystals has not been determined (20).

Management

The acute migratory polyarthritis or oligoarthritis associated with type II hyperlipoproteinemia tends to be self-limited. Nonsteroidal anti-inflammatory drugs can be helpful. Treating the underlying dyslipidemia can lead to regression of tendinous xanthomas. Surgical excision also can be beneficial, particularly in the Achilles tendon, where mechanical irritation by footwear can cause pain and debility. Recurrences can occur. The arthropathy associated with type IV hyperlipidemia seems to wane with improved control of serum lipid levels.

ROBERT F. SPIERA, MD

References

1. Fredrickson DS, Levy RI, Lees RS. Fat transport in lipoproteins: an integrated approach to mechanisms and disorders. N Engl J Med 1967;276:34–42, 94–103, 148–156, 215–225, 273–281.

2. Fahey JJ, Stark HH, Donovan WF, Drennan DB. Xanthoma of the Achilles tendon. J Bone Joint Surg 1973;55A:1197–1211.

3. Yaghami I. Intra- and extraosseous xanthomata associated with hyperlipidemia. Radiology 1978;128:49–54.

4. Shapiro JR, Fallat RW, Tsang RC, Glueck CJ. Achilles tendinitis and tenosynovitis. Am J Dis Child 1974;128:486–490.

5. Glueck CJ, Levy R, Fredrickson DS. Acute tendinitis and arthritis. A presenting symptom of familial type II hyperlipoproteinemia. JAMA 1968;206:2895–2897.

6. Bardin T, Kuntz D. Primary hyperlipidemias and xanthomatosis. In: Klippel JH, Dieppe P (eds). Rheumatology. London: Times Mirror International Publishers Limited, 1994; pp 7:27.1–4.

7. Siegelman SS, Schlossberg I, Becker NH, Sachs BA. Hyperlipoproteinemia with skeletal lesions. Clin Orthop 1972;87:228–232.

8. Truswell AS, Pfister PJ. Cerebrotendinous xanthomatosis. Br Med J 1972;1:353–354.

9. Shulman RS, Bhattacharyya AK, Connor WE, Fredrickson DS. Beta-sitosterolemia and xanthomatosis. N Engl J Med 1976;294:482–483.

10. Rooney PJ, Third J, Madkour MM, Spencer D, Dick WC. Transient polyarthritis associated with familial hyperbetalipoproteinemia. Q J Med 1978;47:249–259.

11. Mathon G, Gagne C, Brun D, Lupien PJ, Moorjani S. Articular manifestations of familial hypercholesterolemia. Ann Rheum Dis 1985;44:599–602.

12. Welin L, Larsson B, Svardsudd K, Tibblin G. Serum lipids, lipoproteins and musculoskeletal disorders among 50- and 60-year-old men. Scand J Rheumatol 1977;7:7–12.

13. Struthers GR, Scott DL, Bacon PA, Walton KW. Musculoskeletal disorders in patients with hyperlipidemia. Ann Rheum Dis 1983;42:519–523.

14. Wysenbeek AJ, Shani E, Beigel Y. Musculoskeletal manifestations in patients with hypercholesterolemia. J Rheumatol 1989;16:643–645.

15. Klemp P, Halland AM, Majoos FL, Steyn K. Musculoskeletal manifestations in hyperlipidemia: a controlled study. Ann Rheum Dis 1993;52:44–48.

16. Khachadurian AK. Migratory polyarthritis in familial hypercholesterolemia (type II hyperlipoproteinemia). Arthritis Rheum 1968;11:385–393.

17. Rimon D, Cohen L. Hypercholesterolemic (type II hyperlipoproteinemic) arthritis. J Rheumatol 1989;16:703–705.

18. Buckingham RB, Bole GG, Bassett DR. Polyarthritis associated with type IV hyperlipoproteinemia. Arch Intern Med 1975;135:286–290.

19. Lazarevic MB, Skosey JL, Vitic J, et al. Cholesterol crystals in synovial and bursal fluid. Semin Arthritis Rheum 1993;23:99–103.

20. Schumacher HR, Michaels R: Recurrent tendinits and Achilles tendon nodule with positively birefringent crystals in a patient with hyperlipoprotenemia. J Rheumatol 1989;16:1387–1389.

LESS COMMON ARTHROPATHIES
D. Neuropathic Arthropathy

Neuropathic arthropathy is a destructive arthritis characterized by fracture, subluxation, and dislocation of articular structures in the setting of neurologic damage to the involved joint or limb. The concept of an association between neurologic lesions and arthritis was elegantly described by Jean-Martin Charcot in 1868 (1). Consequently, the terms Charcot's arthropathy, as well as the terms neurotrophic arthropathy and neuroarthropathy are used synonymously with neuropathic arthropathy.

Epidemiology

It is difficult to determine accurate figures for the incidence and prevalence of neuropathic arthropathy in the general population. The presence of sensory neuropathy is the only established risk factor for neuropathic arthropathy. Although motor function usually is preserved in the affected limb, neuropathic arthropathy has been reported after vigorous physical therapy in patients with severe weakness (2). Central (upper motor neuron) and peripheral (lower motor neuron) lesions may produce neuropathic arthropathy.

The neurologic diseases associated with neuropathic arthropathy have changed with time (Table 26D-1). In the pre-penicillin era, neuropathic arthropathy was seen most commonly in the setting of tabes dorsalis from tertiary syphilis. Diabetic neuropathy currently is the most common cause of neuropathic arthropathy, and is seen in 0.15% to 2.5% of people with diabetes (3). Syringomyelia, spina bifida, and spinal cord injuries also are frequently associated with neuropathic arthropathy. Less commonly encountered causes of neuropathic arthropathy include inflammatory or neoplastic lesions of the spinal cord or peripheral nerves, congenital neurologic abnormalities, and alcoholism. Rarely, cases occur in which no neurologic abnormality is identifiable (2).

Pathology

The pathologic changes in neuropathic arthropathy are similar to those of advanced osteoarthritis, with cartilage destruction, bone eburnation, osteophytosis, and loose-body formation. The presence of "detritic synovium," defined as fragments of cartilage and bone embedded in the synovium, is characteristic of neuropathic arthropathy, but also is seen in severe osteoarthritis and other conditions (2). As reflected radiographically, neuropathic arthropathy can cause exuberant bone and cartilage overgrowth, as well as joint destruction. Usually both processes are seen, but one process often predominates.

Pathophysiology

Two major theories have been proposed to explain the development of neuropathic arthropathy. The neurovascular theory postulates that joint denervation produces physiologic changes, such as increased blood flow from the loss of sympathetic regulation; these changes promote an imbalance between bone resorption and formation, resulting in osteopenia. The neurotraumatic theory proposes that repeated episodes of minor trauma to joints unprotected by the usual response to pain facilitate damage through further trauma and inadequate repair. The neurovascular hypothesis is supported by two findings: clinical reports of neuropathic arthropathy in patients at bedrest who could not have sustained trauma, and the finding that demineralization of the affected limb may precede the development of neuropathic arthropathy (3). In contrast, the observation that injury often accelerates or initiates neuropathic arthropathy supports the neurotraumatic hypothesis (4,5). Elements of both theories probably are correct.

Clinical Features

Neuropathic arthropathy typically presents as an acute or subacute monarthritis with swelling, erythema, and variable amounts of pain in the affected joint. The two most constant clinical features of neuropathic arthropathy are the presence of a significant sensory deficit and a degree of pain that is less than would be expected, considering the amount of joint destruction evident on radiographs. Abnormal sensation can be detected accurately with the Semmes-Weinstein monofilament test (6). There is variability in the speed of onset, the rate of progression, and the balance between bone destruction and bony overgrowth. When slowly progressive, neuropathic arthropathy often resembles osteoarthritis. When rapidly progressive and acute in onset, it mimics osteomyelitis.

Initial examinations show swelling, erythema, effusions, and variable amounts of tenderness. With time, the neuropathic joint becomes deformed, with large effusions, palpable osteophytes, and loss of range of motion. Eichenholtz described three clinical stages of neuropathic arthropathy (7). The early or destructive phase is characterized by signs of inflammation, followed by a quiescent or healing phase; remodeling occurs in the final phase.

The pattern of joint involvement in neuropathic arthropathy depends on the location of the neurologic impairment and may involve small as well as large joints. In diabetes, the foot is most commonly involved. In tabes dorsalis and spina bifida, the knee, hip, ankle, and lumbar

TABLE 26D-1
Neurologic Conditions Associated With Neuropathic Arthropathy

Diabetes mellitus
Syringomyelia
Spina bifida
Brain or spinal cord trauma
Peripheral nerve trauma
Syphilis
Multiple sclerosis
Charcot-Marie-Tooth disease
Riley-Day syndrome
Pernicious anemia
Congenital insensitivity to pain
Alcoholism
Amyloidosis
Thalidomide exposure
Polyneuropathy of Dejerine-Sottas disease
Leprosy
Yaws
Neurofibromatosis

spine are affected. Patients with syringomyelia typically develop neuropathic arthropathy of upper-extremity joints.

Neuropathic Arthropathy in the Diabetic Foot
Neuropathic arthropathy of the diabetic foot is particularly common and deserves special consideration (8). Sixty percent of patients have involvement of the tarsometatarsal joint, 30% the metatarsophalangeal joints, and 10% have involvement of the tibiotalar joint (9). Patients present with a swollen foot or ankle and variable amounts of erythema, warmth, and pain. Skin temperature on the affected foot is elevated and concurrent skin ulcers are common. A history of minor trauma is common. The onset of symptoms and rate of destruction may be acute and dramatic, with radiographic evidence of joint dissolution occurring within weeks (4). Involvement of the midfoot may result in reversal of the curve of the metatarsal arch and "rocker-bottom" deformity. The possibility of osteomyelitis or soft-tissue infection in the feet always must be considered in people with diabetes.

Diagnosis

The diagnosis of neuropathic arthropathy can be made clinically. Helpful diagnostic tests include plain radiographs, bone scans, indium 111-labeled white blood cell (WBC) scans, and synovial fluid analysis. The differential diagnosis of neuropathic arthropathy includes osteomyelitis and other deep-tissue infections, gout, calcium pyrophosphate dihydrate (CPPD) deposition disease, Milwaukee shoulder/knee syn-

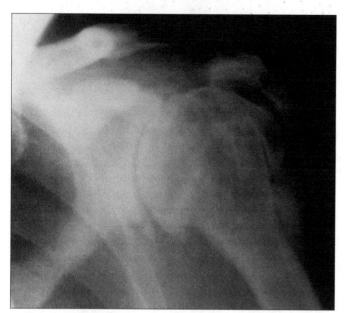

Fig. 26D-1. Neuropathic arthropathy in a shoulder of a patient with syringomyelia. Note the demineralization, bone fragmentation, loose-body formation, and joint space narrowing.

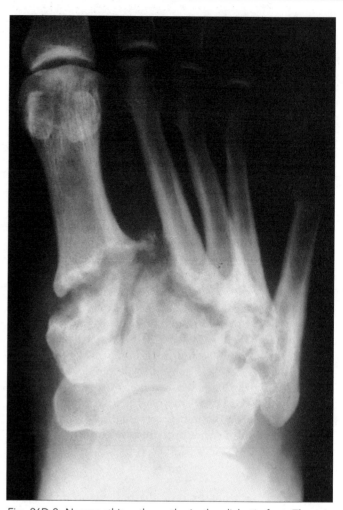

Fig. 26D-2. Neuropathic arthropathy in the diabetic foot. There is involvement of both the metatarsophalangeal joints and the midfoot. The typical combination of resorptive and reparative processes results in a disorganized appearance.

drome, osteonecrosis, and post-traumatic osteoarthritis. The differentiation between osteomyelitis and acute neuropathic arthropathy in the diabetic foot often is a challenge.

Plain radiographs are extremely helpful in making the diagnosis of neuropathic arthropathy (2). Early features include demineralization, joint-space narrowing, and osteophyte formation. Later features are bone fragmentation, periarticular debris formation, and joint subluxation (Fig. 26D-1). Bone absorption, bone shattering, sclerosis, and massive soft-tissue swelling are seen in some patients. Neuropathic joints often are described radiographically as "disorganized," with features of chaotic bone destruction and repair. The presence of sharply defined articular surfaces in neuropathic arthropathy is helpful in differentiating radiographic changes of neuropathic arthropathy from those of infection, where involved bone surfaces are indistinct. In neuropathic arthropathy of the diabetic foot, destruction with prominent fragmentation and loose-body formation typically occurs in the tarsal bones, whereas absorptive changes may predominate in the metatarsals and forefoot (Fig. 26D-2). In the spine, multilevel thoracic and lumbar involvement is common. Ankylosis occurs rarely in neuropathic arthropathy.

Bone scintigraphy with technetium 99m-MDP and indium 111-labeled WBC scans may be useful diagnostic tests (10). Increased uptake of radiolabeled technetium and gallium occurs in neuropathic arthropathy. Unfortunately, uncomplicated neuropathy and infection also are associated with increased blood flow to the affected area on bone scan. In contrast, increased uptake of indium 111-labeled WBC occurs more commonly in osteomyelitis than neuropathic arthropathy. Preliminary evidence supports the use of nuclear medicine techniques to differentiate the marrow uptake seen in neuropathic arthropathy from the bone uptake seen with osteomyelitis (11). Magnetic resonance imaging also can be useful (10). A combined approach using multiple imaging techniques with or without bone cultures often is necessary to differentiate infection from neuropathic arthropathy.

Synovial fluid typically is noninflammatory in neuropathic arthropathy. Fifty percent of synovial fluids from affected joints are hemorrhagic or xanthochromic. Effusions may be very large. CPPD crystals and basic calcium phosphate crystals have been identified in these joint effusions, but whether these crystals are markers of severe joint destruction or contribute to the pathogenesis of neuropathic arthropathy remains to be determined.

Treatment

There are no specific therapies for neuropathic arthropathy. The prognosis of affected people is variable and depends on the severity of the condition and the response to treatment.

Standard management strategies for the early active phase of neuropathic arthropathy include joint immobilization (usually achieved by casts, braces, and orthotics) and restricted weight-bearing. On average, it takes 5.7 ± 3.5 months of immobilization for neuropathic arthropathy of the diabetic foot to heal (3). Better control of blood glucose levels and amitryptilene may improve neuropathic pain in people with diabetes. There is some preliminary evidence for the efficacy of bisphosphonates in the early destructive phase of the disease (12).

Surgical treatments are another mainstay of therapy, but are recommended after healing of the active phase. Goals are to improve pain, joint stability, and alignment, and to prevent or treat overlying skin ulceration from bony deformities. Arthrodesis is useful in the spine, foot, ankle, and knee (13). Exostectomy may restore some motion and decrease joint pain in people with severe rocker-bottom deformities of the foot (14). Traditionally, total joint replacement was considered risky because of a high rate of prosthesis failure. With current techniques, however, joint replacement may be effective for selected patients (15). Unfortunately, amputation of the affected joint still is required far too frequently (3).

Prevention is perhaps the best therapy. Prompt attention to any minor trauma to the diabetic foot or ankle may prevent the development of neuropathic arthropathy. Good control of blood glucose levels in people with diabetes decreases the incidence of neuropathy and thereby reduces the risk of neuropathic arthropathy.

ANN ROSENTHAL, MD

References

1. Gupta R. A short history of neuropathic arthropathy. Clin Orthop 1993;296:43–49.
2. Resnick D. Neuropathic osteoarthropathy. In: Resnick D (ed). Diagnosis of Bone and Joint Disorders, 3rd edition. Philadelphia: W.B. Saunders Company 1995; pp 3413–3442.
3. Sinacore DR, Withrington NC. Recognition and management of acute neuropathic (Charcot) arthropathies of the foot and ankle. J Orthop Sports Phys Ther 1999;29:736–746.
4. Slowman-Kovacs SD, Braunstein EM, Brandt KD. Rapidly progressive Charcot arthropathy following minor joint trauma in patients with diabetic neuropathy. Arthritis Rheum 1990;33:412–417.
5. Johnson JT. Neuropathic fractures and joint injuries: pathogenesis and rationale of prevention and treatment. J Bone Joint Surg Am 1967;49:1–30.
6. Birke JA, Sims DS. Plantar sensory threshold in the ulcerated foot. Lepr Rev 1986;57:261–267.
7. Eichenholtz SN. Charcot Joints. Springfield: Charles C. Thomas, 1966.
8. Schon LC, Easley ME, Weinfeld SB. Charcot neuroarthropathy of the foot and ankle. Clin Orthop 1998;349:116–131.
9. Armstrong DG, Todd WF, Lavery LA, Harkless LB, Bushman TR. The natural history of acute Charcot's arthropathy in a diabetic foot specialty clinic. Diabetic Med 1997;14:357–363.
10. Lipman BT, Collier BD, Carrera GF, et al. Detection of osteomyelitis in the neuropathic foot: nuclear medicine, MRI and conventional radiography. Clin Nucl Med 1998;23:77–82.
11. Palestro CJ, Mehta HH, Patel M, et al. Marrow versus infection in the Charcot joint: Indium-111 leukocyte and technetium-99m sulfur colloid scintigraphy. J Nucl Med 1998;39:346–350.
12. Selby PL, Young MJ, Boulton AJ. Bisphosphonates: a new treatment for diabetic Charcot neuroarthropathy? Diabet Med 1994;11:28–31.
13. Drennan DB, Fahey JJ, Maylahn DJ. Important factors in achieving arthrodesis of the Charcot knee. J Bone Joint Surg Am 1971;53:1180–1193.
14. Brodsky JW, Rouse AM. Exostectomy for symptomatic bony prominences in diabetic Charcot feet. Clin Orthop 1993;296:21–26.
15. Soudry M, Binazzi R, Johanson NA, Bullough PG, Insall JN. Total knee arthroplasty in Charcot and Charcot-like joints. Clin Orthop 1986;208:199–204.

LESS COMMON ARTHROPATHIES
E. Miscellaneous Syndromes Involving Skin and Joints

Panniculitides

The term "panniculitis" indicates inflammation of the subcutaneous fat. Several inflammatory, infectious, and lymphoproliferative disorders may be associated with panniculitis. The histological classification of panniculitis into "septal" and "lobular" forms, with or without vasculitis, is practical, but oversimplified. In most cases of panniculitis, the inflammatory pattern is mixed, i.e., there are components of both septal and lobular inflammation, with variable degrees of vascular or perivascular infiltration.

Erythema Nodosum
The classic septal-dominant panniculitis not associated with significant vascular or perivascular infiltrates, erythema nodosum typically presents as extremely painful nodules that tend to appear on pretibial areas (1). Although most cases of erythema nodosum are idiopathic, some have iden-

tifiable associations, including sarcoidosis, inflammatory bowel disease, infections (e.g., *Streptococcus*, *Yersinia*, tuberculosis, and deep fungal infections), and medications (e.g., oral contraceptives and sulfa medications). Constitutional symptoms, mild polyarticular synovitis, and elevated acute-phase reactants commonly are observed in people with erythema nodosum. These cutaneous lesions usually resolve within a few weeks, even without treatment, and they respond dramatically to systemic corticosteroids or potassium iodide (2). Nonsteroidal anti-inflammatory agents also are therapeutically effective. For secondary erythema nodosum, treatment is directed against the underlying condition.

Recurrent lesions almost always are associated with an identifiable underlying disease or trigger, especially when they affect atypical areas (e.g., the trunk or upper extremities). The most important disorder in the differential diagnosis of erythema nodosum is cutaneous polyarteritis nodosa. This vasculitis, which affects medium-sized blood vessels, should be considered in the setting of ulcerative lesions or when nodules favoring the region of the medial malleoli display a significant underlying synovitis. Deep-skin biopsies are essential in the diagnostic evaluation of people with these signs and symptoms.

Erythema Induratum of Bazin

Historically, the term erythema induratum of Bazin described a lobular-dominant panniculitis associated with a significant degree of vasculitis, occurring in the setting of tuberculosis. In people without evidence of tuberculosis, this condition has been called "nodular vasculitis" (3). However, the principal clinical and histopathologic features of this disorder are indistinguishable from those observed in cutaneous polyarteritis nodosa (4,5). The most common clinical findings are painful, ulcerative nodules that favor the calves (6). Systemic corticosteroids, antimetabolite agents (e.g., azathioprine, mycophenolate mofetil), and alkylating agents are effective treatments.

Panniculitis Associated With Connective-Tissue Disease

The most common cutaneous lesion in the group of lobular-dominant panniculitides without significant septal vasculopathy is "lupus profundus." Generalized lupus profundus frequently is associated with complement deficiencies and extensive discoid lesions (7). Similar lesions can be observed in dermatomyositis or overlap syndromes (8,9).

The typical clinical lesions of panniculitis associated with connective-tissue disease are indurated, erythematous plaques on regions rich in subcutaneous fat, such as the cheeks, upper arms, breasts, abdomen, and thighs. After treatment, the lesions resolve with lipodystrophy. Lobular-dominant lymphoplasmocytic infiltrates accompanied by hyaline degeneration of the fat lobules are characteristic features of this condition, but are not pathognomonic (10).

Systemic corticosteroids, antimalarials, antimetabolite agents (e.g., azathioprine and mycophenolate mofetil), and thalidomide are effective therapies. Intralesional corticosteroids should be used cautiously because this therapy can provoke a superimposed iatrogenic lipodystrophy.

Weber-Christian Disease

Although long regarded as a unique entity, "Weber-Christian disease" is comprised of numerous independent disorders. Most cases labeled "Weber-Christian disease" in the past probably represented erythema nodosum, cutaneous lymphomas, panniculitis associated with α-1 antitrypsin deficiency, the viral hemophagocytic syndrome, panniculitis caused by pancreatic disease, and panniculitis associated with connective-tissue disease (11). Indurated and suppurative plaques on the extremities and gluteal areas are the most common clinical findings. Patients almost invariably experience significant constitutional symptoms.

The typical histologic features are a lobular-dominant lymphocytic panniculitis and fat necrosis, often with a variable degree of atypia and hemophagocytosis. Subcutaneous T-cell lymphoma always should be excluded in the setting of a lobular-dominant panniculitis with atypical cells or hemophagocytic syndrome (12).

Thrombotic Disorders

Atrophie Blanche

The term "atrophie blanche" denotes a syndrome of painful ulcerative lesions that tend to form on the ankles and heal with atrophic, white, stellate scars (13). The entity also is referred to in the medical literature as "livedoid vasculitis." The typical histologic feature is a thrombotic vasculopathy of the dermal blood vessels. The disorder may mimic clinically the cutaneous lesions of polyarteritis nodosa, but the conditions usually are distinguishable by other disease features and properly interpreted skin biopsies.

The treatment of atrophie blanche, though largely empiric, is based on anticoagulation, beginning with strategies least likely to cause harm and advancing to warfarin for more refractory cases. Aspirin, persantine, and warfarin have all been used successfully. There is no role for immunosuppression in the treatment of atrophie blanche.

Degos' Disease (Malignant Atrophic Papulosis)

Extremely rare, Degos' disease is characterized by multiple ulcerations of the skin that heal with atrophic, porcelain-white scars. It usually is associated with severe gastrointestinal involvement, such as bleeding and perforation, and vasoocclusive disease of the central nervous system. The characteristic histologic feature is a wedge-shaped area of dermal necrosis overlying dermal/subcutaneous vessels with a pauci-inflammatory occlusive vasculopathy. This entity must be distinguished from thrombotic disorders (e.g., the antiphospholipid syndrome) or vasculitides affecting medium-sized blood vessels (e.g., polyarteritis nodosa and vasculitis associated with connective-tissue disease) (14–16).

Neutrophilic Dermatoses

The neutrophilic dermatoses include several clinically distinct dermatoses that share a common histology: interstitial neutrophilic dermal infiltrates without vasculitis.

Sweet's Syndrome

Painful, erythematous, and edematous plaques on the head, neck, and upper extremities (Fig. 26E-1) (17) characterize Sweet's syndrome, also known as "benign febrile neutrophilic dermatosis." This disorder often affects middle-aged women and is associated with significant constitutional symptoms. Extracutaneous involvement of the lungs and joints has been described (18). Most cases are idiopathic, but disorders that have been associated with Sweet's syndrome include malignancies, inflammatory bowel disease, and drug reactions (e.g., oral contraceptives, sulfa medications, and granulocyte colony-stimulating factors). A dramatic response to moderate doses of systemic corticosteroids is typical of this disease. Alternative therapeutic agents are dapsone and potassium iodide.

Pyoderma Gangrenosum

The disorder called pyoderma gangrenosum is characterized by ulcers with clean, granulating centers and overhanging, violaceous borders (Fig. 26E-2). These lesions tend to favor the lower extremities. Regional lymphadenopathy and constitutional symptoms occasionally occur. Most cases have no known disease association. However, multiple chronic, refractory lesions have been observed in some patients with underlying disorders, such as inflammatory bowel disease, rheumatoid arthritis, IgA monoclonal gammopathy, and Behçet's disease (19). Systemic corticosteroids and immunosuppressive agents, particularly calcineurin inhibitors (e.g., cyclosporine and tacrolimus), are effective (20).

Others

Erythema Elevatum Diutinum

An unusual form of cutaneous vasculitis, erythema elevatum diutinum presents with erythematous nodules and plaques on the extensor surfaces, especially on the dorsum of the hands (21). Constitutional symptoms usually are absent (22). Histologic features vary with the stage of disease. Early lesions may show leukocytoclastic vasculitis with eosinophilic infiltrates. In contrast, fully developed lesions show lymphocytic vasculitis and significant perivascular fibroplasia. Associated disorders are rheumatoid arthritis, connective-tissue disorders, acquired immunodeficiency syndrome, and IgA monoclonal gammopathy. Dapsone (100 mg/day) is an effective treatment for erythema elevatum diutinum.

Multicentric Reticulohistiocytosis

Multicentric reticulohistiocytosis is a rare, non-Langerhans-cell histiocytosis that presents with asymptomatic, infiltrative, yellowish nodules on the extensor surfaces of the extremities (Fig. 26E-3) and along the rim of the nose and eyelids. It usually is associated with a severe, deforming arthritis (23). Histologic examination of the lesions reveals a benign proliferation of foamy histiocytes and multinucleated giant cells. An association with monoclonal gammopathies has been described. There is no effective treatment for this condition.

Superficial Ulcerative Rheumatoid Necrobiosis

Superficial ulcerative rheumatoid necrobiosis is an unusual skin disorder that sometimes complicates the course of rheumatoid arthritis. The disease manifests with superficial lower-extremity ulcerations. Histopathologic examination of these lesions demonstrates palisading granulomatous infiltration of the dermis and subcutaneous fat (24). These findings are indistinguishable from those of Churg-Strauss or cutaneous extravascular necrotizing granulomas (Fig. 26E-4).

Acne Fulminans

A severe form of acne, acne fulminans is characterized by the acute onset of nodulocystic inflammatory lesions on the trunk and face, fever, a nondeforming oligoarthritis, and aseptic osteolytic lesions (25). Acne fulminans is observed in white male adolescents who have a history of nodulocystic

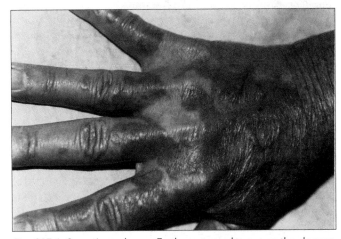

Fig. 26E-1. Sweet's syndrome. Erythematous plaques on the dorsum of the hand of a person with myelodysplastic syndrome.

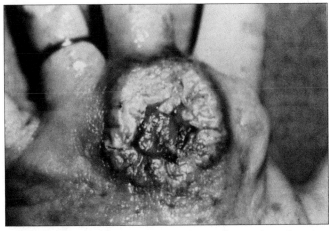

Fig. 26E-2. Pyoderma gangrenosum. Ulcer with typical overhanging borders on the dorsum of a hand.

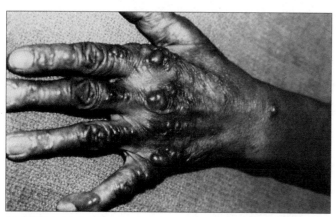

Fig. 26E-3. Multicentric reticulohistiocytosis. Indurated papules on the dorsum of the hand of a person with severe, deforming arthritis.

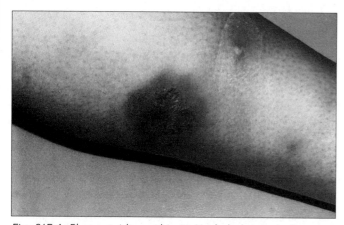

Fig. 26E-4. Rheumatoid necrobiosis. Healed ulcerated plaque on the leg of a person with seronegative rheumatoid arthritis.

acne of the trunk, and it often is triggered by exercise, viral illness, and full doses of isotretinoin therapy. Systemic corticosteroids are recommended as the first-line therapy, with subsequent therapy consisting of low-dose isotretinoin.

HOSSEIN CARLOS NOUSARI, MD

References

1. Psychos DN, Voulgari PV, Skopouli FN, Drosos AA, Moutsopoulos HM. Erythema nodosum: the underlying conditions. Clin Rheumatol 2000;19:212–216.
2. Sterling JB, Heymann WR. Potassium iodide in dermatology: a 19th century drug for the 21st century-uses, pharmacology, adverse effects, and contraindications. J Am Acad Dermatol 2000;43:691–697.
3. Malcic I, Buljevic AD, Vucinic D, Carin R. [Polyarteritis nodosa – cutaneous or systemic form? Possible role of bacterial superantigens in the onset of systemic disease]. Reumatizam 1996;43:16–24.
4. Cho KH, Kim YG, Yang SG, Lee DY, Chung JH. Inflammatory nodules of the lower legs: a clinical and histological analysis of 134 cases in Korea. J Dermatol 1997;24:522–529.
5. Sams WM Jr. Necrotizing vasculitis. J Am Acad Dermatol 1980;3:1–13.
6. Rockl H. [The significance of histopathology for the diagnosis of nodular leg dermatoses. Also a contribution on the question of existence of erythema induratum Bazin]. Hautarzt 1968;19: 540–547.
7. Nousari HC, Kimyai-Asadi A, Provost TT. Generalized lupus erythematosus profundus in a patient with genetic partial deficiency of C4. J Am Acad Dermatol 1999;41:362–364.
8. Chao YY, Yang LJ. Dermatomyositis presenting as panniculitis. Int J Dermatol 2000;39:141–144.
9. Ghali FE, Reed AM, Groben PA, McCauliffe DP. Panniculitis in juvenile dermatomyositis. Pediatr Dermatol 1999;16:270–272.
10. Martens PB, Moder KG, Ahmed I. Lupus panniculitis: clinical perspectives from a case series. J Rheumatol 1999;26:68–72.
11. White JW Jr, Winkelmann RK. Weber-Christian panniculitis: a review of 30 cases with this diagnosis. J Am Acad Dermatol 1998;39:56–62.
12. Marzano AV, Berti E, Paulli M, Caputo R. Cytophagic histiocytic panniculitis and subcutaneous panniculitis-like T-cell lymphoma: report of 7 cases. Arch Dermatol 2000;136:889–896.
13. Acland KM, Darvay A, Wakelin SH, Russell-Jones R. Livedoid vasculitis: a manifestation of the antiphospholipid syndrome? Br J Dermatol 1999;140:131–135.
14. Grattan CE, Burton JL. Antiphospholipid syndrome and cutaneous vasoocclusive disorders. Semin Dermatol 1991;10: 152–159.
15. Tsao H, Busam K, Barnhill RL, Haynes HA. Lesions resembling malignant atrophic papulosis in a patient with dermatomyositis. J Am Acad Dermatol 1997;36:317–319.
16. Castanet J, Lacour JP, Perrin C, Rodot S, Ortonne JP. Cutaneous vasculitis with lesions mimicking Degos' disease and revealing Crohn's disease. Acta Derm Venereol 1995;75:408–409.
17. Hensley CD, Caughman SW. Neutrophilic dermatoses associated with hematologic disorders. Clin Dermatol 2000;18: 355–367.
18. Vignon-Pennamen MD. The extracutaneous involvement in the neutrophilic dermatoses. Clin Dermatol 2000;18:339–347.
19. Callen JP. Pyoderma gangrenosum. Lancet 1998;351:581–585.
20. Nousari HC, Lynch W, Anhalt GJ, Petri M. The effectiveness of mycophenolate mofetil in refractory pyoderma gangrenosum. Arch Dermatol 1998;134:1509–1511.
21. Stone JH, Nousari HC. "Essential" cutaneous vasculitis: what every rheumatologist should know about vasculitis of the skin. Curr Opin Rheumatol 2001;13:23–34.
22. Gibson LE, el-Azhary RA. Erythema elevatum diutinum. Clin Dermatol 2000;18:295–299.
23. Gorman JD, Danning C, Schumacher HR, Klippel JH, Davis JC Jr. Multicentric reticulohistiocytosis: case report with immunohistochemical analysis and literature review. Arthritis Rheum 2000;43:930–938.
24. Jorizzo JL, Olansky AJ, Stanley RJ. Superficial ulcerating necrobiosis in rheumatoid arthritis. A variant of the necrobiosis lipoidica-rheumatoid nodule spectrum? Arch Dermatol 1982;118:255–259.
25. Seukeran DC, Cunliffe WJ. The treatment of acne fulminans: a review of 25 cases. Br J Dermatol 1999;141:307–309.

LESS COMMON ARTHROPATHIES
F. Foreign Body Synovitis

Foreign material may be introduced into joints, tendon sheaths, or periarticular tissues, and may induce a chronic noninfectious monarthritis, tenosynovitis, or dactylitis (1–5). The most common types of material associated with foreign body synovitis are plant thorns, wood splinters, and sea urchin spines. Among the many types of plant thorns described are the date palm, sentinel palm, blackthorn, rose thorn, and cactus (6). Such materials as glass (7), plastic (7), lead (8), and starch (9) may be introduced by penetrating injury and cause chronic inflammation. Metal (10), silicone (11), and polyethylene (12) detritus formed from breakdown products of joint prostheses also may induce a chronic granulomatous synovitis.

Clinical Features

A prolonged delay between injury and diagnosis is common in foreign body synovitis. When obtaining a history from a patient with monarticular synovitis or tenosynovitis, it is essential to ask about recent or past trauma to the joint or surrounding tissue. Although most patients will have local pain and inflammation at the time of a penetrating injury, this initial reaction often is followed by an asymptomatic period that lasts days, weeks, or months (3). The intensity and duration of the initial inflammatory reaction may depend on the type of foreign body, toxic protein coating or charge, degree of bacterial contamination, and concomitant treatment with antibiotics and anti-inflammatory agents. As a result of the time lapse between injury and the development of chronic synovitis, patients and physicians might not associate the current problem with the past injury, leading to further diagnostic delay. After the latent period that follows injury, the synovitis often becomes subacute or chronic, with variable degrees of inflammation, synovial thickening, and effusion. Fever characteristically is absent, except when due to sea urchin spines (2). In such a case, patients may present with fever, myalgias, regional lymph node enlargement, and even synovitis of surrounding joints.

Although any joint can be involved, the joints most commonly affected are those typically unprotected by clothing, such as the hands, wrists, and knees. Children are affected most often (4), followed by adults with an occupational proclivity toward trauma, such as construction workers, farmers, and gardeners (3). Swimmers and people involved in other marine recreational activities (2) are at risk for penetrating injury to the feet and hands from sea urchins.

Differential diagnosis includes other forms of acute and chronic monarticular arthritis, such as septic arthritis, tuberculous or fungal arthritis, osteomyelitis, and juvenile rheumatoid arthritis. The differential diagnosis of dactylitis would include sarcoidosis, psoriasis, erysipeloid, sporotrichosis, and atypical mycobacteria.

Laboratory, Radiologic, and Pathologic Findings

Results of blood tests, such as erythrocyte sedimentation rate and white blood cell count with differential, usually are normal and help differentiate foreign body synovitis from acute bacterial infection. Synovial fluid obtained by aspiration is inflammatory, with cell counts ranging up to 100,000 cells/mm^3 (3). The predominant type of cell in the synovial fluid is the polymorphonuclear leukocyte. Bacterial and fungal cultures are sterile, except in the rare instance where a contaminating agent has been introduced along with the foreign body. Plant thorns and other particulate matter most often are embedded in the synovium and not visible in synovial fluid. The exception occurs in detritic synovitis, in which fragments of metal, polyethylene, or methylmethacrylate may be found in synovial fluid (11).

Radiographs may detect metallic foreign bodies; sea urchin spines, which are composed of calcium carbonate (Fig. 26F-1); and glass, especially if it is leaded or pigmented. Plant thorns and wood are not visualized on radiograph. Nonspecific acute radiographic changes include soft-tissue swelling and periostitis in nonarticular lesions, and joint effusion in articular involvement. In the case of primary bone involvement, a well-circumscribed osteolytic lesion or pseudotumor may be found.

For the purposes of diagnosis and perioperative localization, ultrasound may be used to detect wood or plastic foreign bodies (13). In a review of date palm injuries (4), the sensitivity of ultrasound (83%) was found to be superior to that of computerized tomography (25%) when identifying retained fragments. Magnetic resonance imaging (MRI) can demonstrate characteristic features in silicone synovitis (14), and

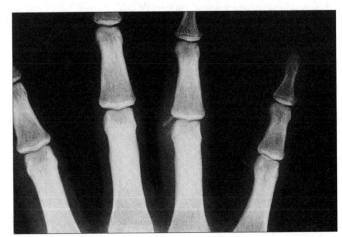

Fig. 26F-1. Soft-tissue swelling surrounds a radiopaque sea urchin spine (composed of calcium carbonate) in a person with foreign body synovitis.

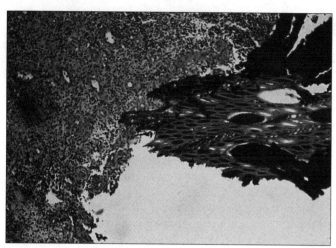

Fig. 26F-2. Photomicrograph of synovium revealing a wood fragment surrounded by a diffuse chronic mononuclear cell infiltrate. The birefringent multiple cell walls separated by thin fibrous septae are characteristic of vegetable material, such as wood and plant thorns. This patient's knee was punctured by a toothpick.

may be useful when characteristic radiographic features of silicone synovitis (i.e., nodular soft-tissue swelling, well-defined subchondral lytic defects, and erosions with preservation of joint space). The role of MRI in other types of foreign body synovitis has not been clearly delineated.

Accurate diagnosis requires surgical removal of the foreign body and pathologic and microbiologic studies. Pathologic examination of the synovium reveals lining-cell proliferation, hyperemia, and cellular infiltration (4). Lymphocytes are the predominant cells in the synovium, with focal collections of polymorphonuclear cells. Variable numbers of plasma cells and eosinophils also have been described. These features contrast with the marked diffuse polymorphonuclear infiltrates seen in acute septic arthritis. Giant cell formation, prominent in patients with foreign body synovitis (3), is another feature distinguishing this disorder from acute septic arthritis. Polarized light microscopy should be performed on synovial tissue and may reveal intensely birefringent plant thorn material (Fig. 26F-2).

Treatment

Although anti-inflammatory agents may provide symptomatic relief, excisional biopsy with synovectomy usually is necessary for definitive treatment of chronic foreign body synovitis (3,5). Excision can be performed through an arthroscope if preoperative localization of the foreign body has been accomplished and if adequate arthroscopic synovectomy is possible. However, because foreign bodies often are fragmented and poorly detectable by radiologic means, an open biopsy and extensive synovectomy often is required.

MICHAEL MARICIC, MD

References

1. Sugarman M, Stobie DG, Quismorio FP, Terry R, Hanson V. Plant thorn synovitis. Arthritis Rheum 1977;20:1125–1128.
2. Cracchiolo A, Goldberg L. Local and systemic reactions to puncture injuries by the sea urchin spine and date palm thorn. Arthritis Rheum 1977;20:1206–1212.
3. Reginato AJ, Ferreiro JL, O'Connor CR, et al. Clinical and pathologic studies of twenty-six patients with penetrating foreign body injury to the joints, bursae, and tendon sheaths. Arthritis Rheum 1990;33:1753–1762.
4. Adams CD, Timms FJ, Hanlon M. Phoenix date palm injuries: a review of injuries from the Phoenix date palm treated at the Starship Children's Hospital. Aust N Z J Surg 2000;70:355–357.
5. Olenginski TP, Bush DC, Harrington TM. Plant thorn synovitis: an uncommon cause of monoarthritis. Semin Arthritis Rheum 1991;21:40–46.
6. Lindsey D, Lindsey W. Cactus spine injuries. Am J Emerg Med 1988;6:362–369.
7. Goodnough CP, Frymoyer JW. Synovitis secondary to nonmetallic foreign bodies. J Trauma 1975;15:960–965.
8. Farber JM, Rafii M, Schwartz D. Lead arthropathy and elevated serum levels of lead after gunshot wound of the shoulder. AJR Am J Roentgenol 1994;162:385–386.
9. Freemont AJ, Porter ML, Tomlinson I, Clague RB, Jayson MI. Starch synovitis. J Clin Pathol 1984;37:990–992.
10. Kitridou RC, Schumacher HR Jr, Sbarbaro JL, Hollander JL. Recurrent hemarthrosis after prosthetic knee arthroplasty: identification of metal particles in the synovial fluid. Arthritis Rheum 1969;12:520–528.
11. Christie AJ, Pierret G, Levitan J. Silicone synovitis. Semin Arthritis Rheum 1989;19:166–171.
12. Kaufman RL, Tong I, Beardmore TD. Prosthetic synovitis: clinical and histologic characteristics. J Rheumatol 1985;12:1066–1074.
13. Little CM, Parker MG, Callowich MC, Sartori JC. The ultrasonic detection of soft tissue foreign bodies. Invest Radiol 1986;21:275–277.
14. Chan M, Chowchuen P, Workman T, Eilenberg S, Schweitzer M, Resnick D. Silicone synovitis: MR imaging in five patients. Skeletal Radiol 1998;27:13–17.

27 REFLEX SYMPATHETIC DYSTROPHY AND TRANSIENT REGIONAL OSTEOPOROSIS

Reflex Sympathetic Dystrophy

The symptom complex of reflex sympathetic dystrophy (RSD) is characterized by severe pain, swelling, and autonomic dysfunction in an extremity. American physician and author S. Weir Mitchell first described this condition in 1864 after observing that some soldiers recovering from gunshot wounds complained of persistent burning pain in their limbs (1). Weir called the syndrome *causalgia,* and several other designations have been applied to it, including Sudeck's atrophy, algodystrophy, and shoulder-hand syndrome. Controversy over the role of the sympathetic nervous system in disease pathogenesis led to the development of a new appellation: complex regional pain syndrome (CRPS) (2). There are two subtypes of CRPS: type 1 is RSD in the setting of no associated nerve lesion, and type 2 is RSD that occurs with a definable nerve lesion. This terminology, however, has not been adopted widely in clinical practice or the medical literature, and reflex sympathetic dystrophy remains the preferred term.

Epidemiology

Reflex sympathetic dystrophy has been observed in every race and all geographic locations, but the lack of uniform diagnostic criteria makes accurate epidemiologic analysis difficult. Although seen most commonly in people 40–60 years old, RSD can occur in children and the elderly. Trauma (sometimes as minor as stubbing a toe) is the most common precipitating factor, followed by peripheral nerve injury, including entrapment neuropathies. RSD also is associated with radiculopathies, stroke, hemiplegia, arthroscopy, neoplasm, arterial or venous thrombosis, and use of such medications as antituberculous drugs and barbiturates.

Pathogenesis

The mechanisms that lead to the development of RSD are not well understood, but numerous theories have been proposed. Current hypotheses are based on two different mechanisms: altered sympathetic outflow and regional inflammation (3).

Speculation that altered sympathetic outflow may mediate at least some RSD features is based on the presence of vasomotor instability and reports of dramatic improvement following sympathetic nerve blockade. A study documented that cutaneous sympathetic vasoconstrictor reflexes are impaired markedly in the early stages of RSD (4). Abnormal synapses between damaged afferent sensory nerves and efferent sympathetic nerves may permit mechanical and chemical cross-talk, resulting in sympathetic overactivity. Peripheral–central mechanisms also have been proposed; in one model, mechanoreceptors stimulated at the site of injury trigger excessive repetitive excitation of the internuncial neurons in the spinal column. Activation of adjacent motor and sympathetic efferent nerves promotes increased blood flow and vasomotor abnormalities in the affected extremity, resulting in hyperalgesia, edema, color changes, and patchy osteopenia. Continued sensory input from the periphery promotes additional excitation in the spinal column, setting up a reverberating circuit of pain and response. This sequence, which may be amplified by sympathetic fibers, has been labeled "sympathetically mediated pain" (5).

The view that sympathetic dysfunction is responsible for RSD has been challenged (6). Some evidence suggests that sympathetic nerve blocks can produce a significant placebo response, and controlled studies demonstrating efficacy with this intervention have not been published. Drummond et al (7) demonstrated that plasma levels of norepinephrine in people with RSD are lower on the affected side than in the uninvolved limb, which suggests that autonomic disturbances are not related to sympathetic overactivity.

Alternatively, it has been proposed that RSD is a regional inflammatory response modulated by the peripheral and central nervous system (neurogenic inflammation) (8). In this model, injured nerve endings release such mediators as substance P and calcitonin gene-related peptide, which have proinflammatory actions and may interfere with neural pathways. Other authors have suggested that RSD is not a single syndrome but a heterogeneous group of disorders with multiple etiologies and pathogenic mechanisms (9).

Clinical Features

The predominant and most disabling feature of RSD is pain. It is an intense, deep, chronic burning sensation exacerbated by movement, dependent posture, and emotional stress. The pain does not follow a dermatomal pattern or specific nerve distribution, and it is out of proportion with the inciting injury or event. Typically, patients complain of allodynia (pain induced by a non-noxious stimulus) and hyperalgesia (lowered pain threshold and enhanced pain perception). Most patients guard the affected limb from any stimulus and resist even the slightest movement, making physical examination difficult. Hand or foot involvement is most common, but RSD can affect more proximal portions of the limb, such as the knee or shoulder. Some patients have recurrent episodes.

Local edema and vasomotor changes often accompany the pain. Initially, the extremity often is warm, red, and dry, but can become cyanotic, cool, pale, and hyperhidrotic. Cyanosis, mottling, and livedo reticularis may be observed in the contralateral extremity. Some patients develop motor abnormalities such as weakness, muscular incoordination, tremor, and muscle spasms. Dystrophic changes produce shiny, thin skin, and the nails may become brittle and exhibit altered growth patterns. Contractures can develop, especially in the palmar fascia and tendon sheaths of the hands.

Steinbrocker and Argyros described three clinical stages of RSD (10). Stage 1 (acute) lasts three to six months and is characterized by pain, hypersensitivity, swelling, and vasomotor changes that lower (or raise) the temperature in the extremity, giving it a dusky purple appearance and causing dependent rubor. Sudomotor changes frequently occur, manifesting as hyperhidrosis and hypertrichosis. Stage 2 (dystrophic) is characterized by persistent pain, disability, and atrophic skin changes. Stage 3 (atrophic) is marked by atrophy of subcutaneous tissues and, often, contractures. However, not all patients follow this pattern of clinical progression (11).

Diagnosis

The diagnosis is based on recognition of the distinctive array of signs and symptoms in the setting of preceding trauma or an associated medical condition. It is essential to exclude other conditions (Table 27-1). Accurate diagnosis of RSD may be complicated by the diversity of clinical manifestations, which are atypical and incomplete in many patients. Although there are no defining laboratory abnormalities, diagnostic studies can help support the diagnosis. Plain radiographs of the involved extremity may show patchy osteopenia, called Sudeck's atrophy. Unfortunately, this is an inconsistent finding that also can occur following disuse or immobilization of a limb. Three-phase bone scan is specific for RSD, but estimates of sensitivity vary from 50% to 90% (12,13). The first two phases may demonstrate asymmetric blood flow and pooling, but the delayed image (third phase) is more typically abnormal, with enhanced uptake in the periarticular structures of the involved extremity (Fig. 27-1). Thermography can detect slight temperature differences between the involved and contralateral extremity (Fig. 27-2), but the test lacks specificity. The results of autonomic function studies (resting sweat output and quantitative sudomotor axon reflex test) may be abnormal in people with RSD (14).

Treatment

A variety of modalities, often administered in combination, have been used to treat RSD. It is essential to initiate therapy early, because the changes that occur in the later stages of RSD often are irreversible. Unfortunately, with the exception of corticosteroids, controlled trials have not demonstrated efficacy over placebo (15). Nevertheless, a multidisciplinary

TABLE 27-1
Differential Diagnosis of RSD

Chronic arterial insufficiency
Raynaud's phenomenon
Thromboembolism
Infection: osteomyelitis, cellulitis
Crystalline arthropathies: gout, pseudogout
Erythromelalgia
Vasculitis
Fractures
Inflammatory or infectious arthritis
Osteonecrosis
Malingering
Peripherial neuropathy

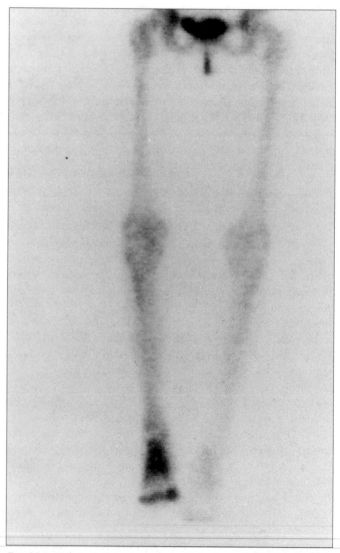

Fig. 27-1. Delayed-phase bone scan of the lower limbs in a 70-year-old woman with reflex sympathetic dystrophy of the right foot (anterior view). Increased radionuclide uptake is present in the right leg and is highest in the periarticular tissues of the right foot.

approach involving rheumatology, orthopedics, neurology, and pain treatment that incorporates basic elements of pain management, supportive care, and rehabilitation can be remarkably effective in some patients (16). The major goals of therapy are adequate pain control, early joint mobilization, prevention of contractures, and treatment of associated depression or anxiety (17).

Pain control is an essential component of therapy and frequently requires the use of narcotic analgesics. Antidepressant medications provide pain relief and improve depressive symptoms. Physiotherapy should be initiated promptly to mobilize the affected extremity and lessen local edema. Passive and active range-of-motion exercises, tissue massage, contrast baths (alternating temperatures), and in some cases, transcutaneous electrical nerve stimulation (TENS) can be helpful. Other conditions (carpal tunnel syndrome) or biomechanical problems (metatarsalgia resulting from altered gait) may be additional sources of discomfort and should be addressed with the use of splints or assistive devices. Modification of the home or work environment may lessen pain and permit maximum function.

Oral corticosteroids have proved very effective in the treatment of RSD, especially in patients with abnormal findings on bone scan (18). The initial dose of prednisone is 1 mg/kg/day, given in four divided doses for two weeks, then tapered and discontinued by the third or fourth week. Occasionally, patients require long-term, low-dose prednisone (5–10 mg/day) to control symptoms. Calcitonin,

TABLE 27-2
Treatment of RSD

Pain control
Early mobilization
Physical therapy
Oral corticosteroids
Calcitonin, IV alendronate
Gabapentin
Antidepressant medications
Sympathetic blockade

intravenous alendronate, or regional ketanserin have been reported to provide sustained pain relief in uncontrolled trials (16). Gabapentin can be effective in patients with refractory symptoms (19). In one report, only 7% of wrist-fracture patients given 500 mg of vitamin C developed RSD, compared with 22% of patients given a placebo (20).

Sympathetic nerve blockade has long been a popular treatment for RSD, although controlled studies demonstrating long-term efficacy have not been performed (15). Therapeutic blocks are performed by injecting a local anesthetic into the lumbar sympathetic ganglia for lower-extremity RSD and into the cervical sympathetic ganglia for upper-extremity involvement. Regional blocks can be performed with the Bier block technique, which involves isolating the affected limb with a pneumatic tourniquet, injecting guanethidine, reserpine, or bretylium, and then releasing the tourniquet after 10–20 minutes. Usually a series of blocks are performed and the therapeutic effects monitored. If the response to regional block is transient, surgical sympathectomy can be performed. In rare instances, amputation has been performed to control pain, eradicate infection, or improve function; however, recurrence of RSD in the stump is common (21).

Transient Regional Osteoporosis

The syndrome of transient regional osteoporosis, seen primarily in young and middle-aged individuals, manifests as monarticular or oligoarticular pain accompanied by striking osteopenia of the involved joint (22). Histologic changes observed in biopsies of osteopenic sites include bone-marrow edema, osteoclastic bone resorption, and reactive bone formation (23). Some health professionals consider this entity a variant of RSD, but there are several distinguishing features. Neuropathic pain, upper extremity involvement, and preceding trauma are unusual in transient regional osteoporosis. Furthermore, vasomotor instability and dystrophic changes are not associated features, and there is a predilection for hip joint involvement. Transient regional osteoporosis is more common in men, although it does occur in women, particularly during the second and third trimester of pregnancy (24).

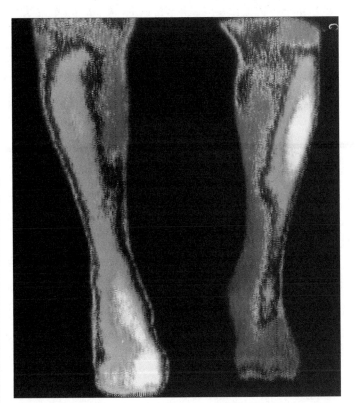

Fig. 27-2. Thermography of the same patient in Fig. 27-1 (anterior view). Note intense hyperthermia in the right foot, with the highest temperatures occurring dorsomedially.

A diagnosis of transient regional osteoporosis is based on the presence of joint pain, diminished joint mobility, and localized osteopenia on plain radiographs. Bone scans reveal increased radionuclide uptake in the involved joint, and transient bone marrow edema has been documented by magnetic resonance imaging (25). Treatment is conservative and consists of avoiding weight-bearing and taking analgesics. In contrast to RSD, this syndrome does not benefit from corticosteroids. Most patients recover completely in several weeks, and permanent joint damage is rare. However, a significant percentage of patients have recurrent episodes.

CHRISTOPHER T. RITCHLIN, MD

References

1. Mitchell SW, Morehouse GR, Keen WW. Gunshot wounds and other injuries of nerves. Clin Orthop 1982;163:2-7.
2. Mersky H, Bogduk N. Classification of Chronic Pain: Descriptions of Chronic Pain Syndromes and Definitions of Pain Terms. Seattle: IASP Press, 1994.
3. Bonica JJ. Causalgia and other reflex dystrophies. In: Bonica JJ (ed). The Management of Pain, 2nd edition. Philadelphia: Lee & Febiger, 1990; pp 220–243.
4. Wasner G, Heckmann K, Maier C, Baron R. Vascular abnormalities in acute reflex sympathetic dystrophy (CRPS 1): complete inhibition of sympathetic nerve activity with recovery. Arch Neurol 1999;56:613–620.
5. Roberts J. A hypothesis on the physiologic basis for causalgia and related pains. Pain 1986;24:297–311.
6. Oyen WJG, Arntz IE, Claessens RM, Van der Meer JW, Corstens FH, Goris RJ. Reflex sympathetic dystrophy of the hand: an excessive inflammatory response. Pain 1993;55:151–157.
7. Drummond PD, Finch PM, Smythe GA. Reflex sympathetic dystrophy: the significance of differing plasma catecholamine concentrations in affected and unaffected limbs. Brain 1991;114:2025–2036.
8. Schott GC. An unsympathetic view of pain. Lancet 1995;245:634–636.
9. Ochoa JL, Verdugo RJ. Reflex sympathetic dystrophy: a common clinical avenue for somatoform expression. Neurologic Clin 1995;13:351–363.
10. Steinbrocker O, Argyros TG. The shoulder–hand syndrome: present status as a diagnostic and therapeutic entity. Med Clin North Am 1958;42:1533–1553.
11. Veldman PH, Reynen HM, Arntz IE, Goris RJ. Signs and symptoms of reflex sympathetic dystrophy: prospective study of 829 patients. Lancet 1993;342:1012–1016.
12. Kozin F, Genant HK, Bekerman C, McCarty D. The reflex sympathetic dystrophy syndrome: II. Recognition and scintographic evidence of biraterality and of periarticular accentuation. Am J Med 1976;60:332–338.
13. Werner R, Davidoff G, Jackson MD, Cremer S, Ventocilla C, Wolf L. Factors affecting the sensitivity and specificity of the three-phase technetium bone scan in the diagnosis of reflex sympathetic dystrophy syndrome in the upper extremity. J Hand Surg 1989;14A:520–523.
14. Chelimsky TC, Low PA, Naessens JM, Wilson PR, Amadio PC, O'Brien PC. Value of autonomic testing in reflex sympathetic dystrophy. Mayo Clin Proc 1995;70:1029–1040.
15. Kingery WS. A critical review of controlled clinical trials for peripheral neuropathic pain and complex regional pain syndromes. Pain 1997;73:123–139.
16. Wasner G, Backonja MM, Baron R. Traumatic neuralgias: complex regional pain syndromes (reflex sympathetic dystrophy and causalgia): clinical characteristics, pathophysiologic mechanisms and therapy. Neurol Clin 1998;16:851–868.
17. Doury P, Dequeker J. Algodystrophy/reflex sympathetic dystrophy syndrome. In: Klippel JH, Dieppe PA (eds). Rheumatology. London: Mosby, 1994; pp 7.38.1–7.38.6.
18. Kozin F, Ryan LM, Carerra GF, Soin JS, Wortmann RL. The reflex sympathetic dystrophy syndrome: III. Scintigraphic studies, further evidence for the therapeutic efficacy of systemic corticosteroids and proposed diagnostic criteria. Am J Med 1981;20:23–30.
19. Mellick GA, Mellick LB. Reflex sympathetic dystrophy treated with gabapentin. Arch Phys Med Rehabil 1997;78:98–105.
20. Zollinger PE, Tuinebreijer WE, Kreis R, Breederveld RS: Effect of vitamin C on frequency of reflex sympathetic dystrophy in wrist fractures: a randomized trial. Lancet 1999;354:2025–2028.
21. Dielissen PW, Claassen A, Veldman PH, Goris RJ. Amputation for reflex sympathetic dystrophy. J Bone Joint Surg 1995;77:270–273.
22. Lakhanpal S, Ginsburg WW, Luthra HS, Hunder GG. Transient regional osteoporosis: a study of 56 cases and review of the literature. Ann Intern Med 1987;106:444–450.
23. McCarthy EF. The pathology of transient regional osteoporosis. Iowa Orthop J 1998;18:35–42.
24. Brodell JD, Burns JE, Heiple KG. Transient osteoporosis of the hip of pregnancy. J Bone Joint Surg 1989;71:1252–1257.
25. Fertakos RJ, Swayne LC, Colston WC. Three phase bone imaging in bone marrow edema of the knee. Clin Nucl Med 1995;20:587–590.

28 SARCOIDOSIS

Sarcoidosis is a systemic, chronic, granulomatous disease of unknown etiology that chiefly strikes young adults in their 20s and 30s (1–4). The disease occurs in all ethnic groups, but it is most common in the United States and tends to be more severe in African Americans (2,4). Although it involves the lungs most notably, sarcoidosis can affect nearly any organ system and mimic rheumatic diseases capable of causing fever, arthritis, uveitis, myositis, rash, or neurologic deficits.

Pathogenesis

Although the cause of sarcoidosis is unknown, the immune response clearly plays a central role in pathogenesis (5–7). The disease is characterized by disseminated, noncaseating granulomas. The sarcoid granuloma contains a central follicle of tightly packed epithelioid cells and multinucleated giant cells surrounded by lymphocytes, macrophages, monocytes, and fibroblasts. In the lung, the initial inflammation is an alveolitis composed chiefly of activated CD4 T-helper cells whose cytokines recruit other cells to help form the granulomas (5,8). Alveolar T cells also preferentially express specific antigen receptors, which suggests T-cell response to a specific stimulus, such as an organism or self-antigen (7,9). The character and intensity of the alveolitis is reflected in bronchoalveolar lavage fluid, which typically shows an increase in the lymphocytes and a high CD4/CD8 T-cell ratio.

Granulomas are widely distributed in sarcoidosis, occurring in the lung (86% of patients), lymph nodes (86%), liver (86%), spleen (63%), heart (20%), kidney (19%), bone marrow (17%), and pancreas (6%) (1–4). Granulomas compress tissues and mediate disease by secreting cytokines that provoke constitutional symptoms, recruiting inflammatory cells whose products injure local tissues, and elaborating growth factors that cause fibrosis (2,4,6–8). In addition, activated monocytes in granulomas convert vitamin D precursors to 1,25-dihydroxyvitamin D, which can increase intestinal absorption of calcium and cause hypercalcemia (10).

Peripheral blood reveals the dichotomy of depressed cellular immunity and enhanced humoral immunity (8). Depressed cellular immunity is evidenced by lymphopenia, a low helper/suppressor T-cell ratio (0.8:1 in sarcoidosis patients versus 1.8:1 in healthy controls), and cutaneous anergy (affecting 70% of patients). In contrast, activated humoral immunity is manifested by polyclonal gammopathy and autoantibody production. Approximately 20%–30% of patients have rheumatoid factor or antinuclear antibodies.

Clinical Features

Sarcoidosis is most common in African Americans and Caucasians of northern European descent. The prevalence among African Americans (40 per 100,000) is eight times higher than that among Caucasian Americans (2,4). Women develop the disease with a slightly higher frequency than men do.

People with sarcoidosis commonly present with one of four problems: pulmonary symptoms (40%–45%), asymptomatic hilar adenopathy detected on chest roentgenogram (5%–10%), constitutional symptoms (25%), or extrathoracic inflammation (25%), which may include rheumatic manifestations (2,4).

Pulmonary Involvement

Respiratory symptoms are the most common presenting complaints and include dry cough, dyspnea, and nonspecific chest pain. Hemoptysis, rare at initial presentation, may become recurrent, massive, and even fatal in patients who develop mycetomas in pulmonary cysts (2,4). Pleural effusions are rare in sarcoidosis.

Regardless of initial symptoms, 90% of people with sarcoidosis have abnormal findings on chest radiographs. Four types are recognized (4): type 0 shows no abnormalities and occurs in 10% of patients; type I is most common (43%) and shows enlargement of hilar, mediastinal, and, often, right paratracheal lymph nodes; type II (34%) exhibits the adenopathy found in type I plus pulmonary infiltrates, and is most common in patients presenting with symptomatic respiratory disease; and type III (13%) demonstrates infiltrates without adenopathy. This classification has prognostic significance. Approximately 80% of patients with type I chest films remit within two years (4). In contrast, only 30%–50% of patients with type II and fewer than 20% of patients with type III remit.

Constitutional Symptoms

Fever, weight loss, fatigue, and malaise are the presenting symptoms in 25% of patients. Fever frequently is associated with hepatic granulomas.

Rheumatologic Manifestations

Arthritis occurs in 10%–15% of patients with sarcoidosis (2,11–15). Two patterns of joint disease are recognized, classified by whether the arthritis occurs early (within the first six months of disease onset) or late in the course. The first form, in which arthritis is part of the initial presentation, is most common. The arthritis often begins suddenly in one or both feet and ankles. Periarticular swelling is more common than frank joint effusion, although when effusions occur, synovial fluid usually is noninflammatory. The pain often is periarticular and much more severe than the few objective signs of inflammation would suggest. Tenosynovitis and heel pain also may occur. The arthritis occasionally spreads in additive fashion to involve the knees, proximal interphalangeal joints, metacarpophalangeal joints, wrists, and elbows. The axial skeleton is spared. Typically, two to six joints are involved, and monarthritis is unusual in this early phase. Erythema nodosum is strikingly associated with early arthritis, occurring in 66% of patients.

The syndrome of acute arthritis, erythema nodosum, and bilateral hilar adenopathy (Löfgren's syndrome) has an excellent prognosis, with a 90% remission rate. Radiographs of sarcoidosis patients with acute arthritis almost never show bony or cartilaginous changes. The duration of acute arthritis averages several weeks, but may be as short as a few days, or as long as three months. Few patients have repeated attacks of arthritis. The pain and swelling of lower extremities in early arthritis may suggest thrombophlebitis, especially if the patient has multiple lesions of erythema nodosum that have coalesced along a linear streak. The prominent heel pain seen in some patients may suggest ankylosing spondylitis or another spondyloarthropathy. Migratory arthritis of sarcoidosis may mimic rheumatic fever. Because hyperuricemia is common in sarcoidosis, patients with foot and ankle pain from early arthritis of sarcoidosis may be misdiagnosed as having gout.

The second form of arthritis begins six months or more after the onset of sarcoidosis (11). Late joint disease generally is less severe and less widespread. The knees are the joints most commonly involved, followed by the ankles and

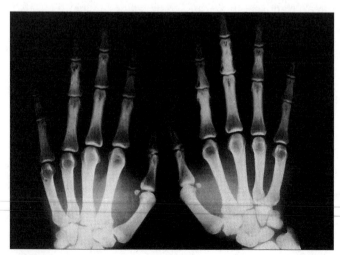

Fig. 28-1. Radiograph of hands of a patient with chronic sarcoidosis. Note punched-out lesions on phalanges and soft-tissue swelling.

proximal interphalangeal joints. The average number of joints involved is two or three, but monarthritis can occur. Synovial effusions are noninflammatory or mildly inflammatory, as evidenced by synovial-fluid white blood cell (WBC) counts of 250–6200 cells/mm^3 with 56%–100% mononuclear cells (15). Synovial histology often is less inflammatory than it is in rheumatoid arthritis, and occasionally reveals granulomas. In contrast to early arthritis, late disease is associated with chronic cutaneous sarcoidosis, but not with erythema nodosum.

Late arthritis can be transient or chronic. The chronic form often manifests itself by dactylitis, a sausage-like swelling of a digit, frequently accompanied by overlying cutaneous sarcoidosis. Typically, activities of daily living are not greatly impaired, and pain is not intense. Radiographic changes are uncommon, but destructive and cystic changes can occur and are noted most often in the middle and distal phalanges of the hand (Fig. 28-1). Cystic lytic lesions in the middle portion of the phalanx are typical. Less obvious, but also characteristic, are diffuse trabecular changes that give the bone a honeycomb appearance. These radiographic findings occur most frequently in patients with dactylitis, but occasionally, they occur in patients without arthritis. Lytic lesions resembling metastatic lesions may occur in the vertebrae (2).

Several other rheumatologic manifestations may accompany sarcoidosis (Table 28-1). Sarcoidosis of the larynx, nasal turbinates, and nasal cartilage resembles Wegener's granulomatosis. Eye disease, most commonly uveitis, eventually develops in 22% of people with sarcoidosis (2,4). Patients may develop lachrymal gland enlargement, conjunctival nodules, keratoconjunctivitis (similar to that seen in Sjögren's syndrome), and proptosis (similar to that seen in Wegener's granulomatosis). Clinically evident sarcoidosis of the skeletal muscles resembles polymyositis, characterized by slowly progressive proximal weakness, elevated creatine phosphokinase, and a myopathic pattern on electromyography. Muscle biopsy may reveal granulomatous myositis. Muscle involvement also can present as mass-like lesions (16). Mononeuritis multiplex, facial nerve palsy, and parotid gland enlargement are other signs common to both sarcoidosis and other rheumatic diseases (Table 28-1).

Other Extrathoracic Manifestations

Peripheral lymphadenopathy, one of the most common manifestations of sarcoidosis, occurs in 75% of patients. Typically, the lymph nodes are not tender, range in size from 1 cm to 5 cm, and involve at least the cervical and often the axillary, epitrochlear, and inguinal regions (1–4). Skin involvement occurs in one-third of patients and serves as a marker for prognosis (2,4). Erythema nodosum appears early and is associated with an excellent prognosis. Potentially disfiguring papules, nodules, plaques, and scaling lesions are associated with chronic sarcoidosis. Sarcoidosis causing violaceous plaques over the cheeks, nose, and ears is called *lupus pernio*. Most patients (86%) have hepatic granulomas, but only 20% have hepatomegaly or elevated

TABLE 28-1
Rheumatic Manifestations of Sarcoidosis

Manifestation	Frequency in sarcoidosis (% of patients)	Differential diagnosis
Arthritis	15	Rheumatoid arthritis, rheumatic fever, systemic lupus erythematosus, gonococcal arthritis, gout, spondyloarthropathies
Parotid gland enlargement	5	Sjögren's syndrome
Upper airway disease (sinusitis, laryngeal inflammation, saddle-nose deformity)	3	Wegener's granulomatosis
Uveitis		
Anterior	18	Spondyloarthropathies
Posterior	7	Behçet's disease
Keratoconjunctivitis	5	Sjögren's syndrome
Proptosis	1	Wegener's granulomatosis
Myositis	4	Polymyositis
Mononeuritis multiplex	1	Systemic vasculitis
Facial nerve palsy	2	Lyme disease

liver enzymes (especially alkaline phosphatase). Jaundice, intrahepatic cholestasis, postnecrotic cirrhosis, and portal hypertension without cirrhosis have been reported. Neurosarcoidosis, which occurs in 5% of patients, rarely is the sole presenting sign (2,4,17). Central nervous system manifestations include basilar meningitis, hydrocephalus, intracranial mass lesions, seizures, and neuroendocrine disorders, such as hypopituitarism and diabetes insipidus. Heart involvement leads to tachyarrhythmias, cardiomyopathy, or sudden death. Cor pulmonale complicates severe pulmonary disease. Renal manifestations of sarcoidosis include membranous glomerulonephritis, nephrocalcinosis, renal calculi, and renal insufficiency, with or without hypercalcemia (3). In the absence of massive hemoptysis, anemia is not a prominent feature of sarcoidosis. Leukopenia (WBC <4000/mm^3) occurs in 28% of patients, mild eosinophilia (>5% eosinophils) in 34%, and hypercalcemia in 19%. Serum angiotensin-converting enzyme (ACE) is elevated in 60% of people with sarcoidosis, as it is in tuberculosis, lymphoma, diabetes, hyperthyroidism, Whipple's disease, Gaucher's disease, and other disorders (2,4,18).

Diagnosis and Management

No single finding or laboratory test establishes the diagnosis of sarcoidosis. Therefore, the diagnosis depends on a compatible clinical picture involving at least two organ systems, histologic evidence of noncaseating granulomas, and exclusion of other possible causes (2). Biopsy is not necessary for an asymptomatic patient 20–40 years old with classic radiographic findings of paratracheal and bilateral symmetric hilar lymphadenopathy; such a patient is exceedingly unlikely to have any other disorder. In symptomatic patients, however, other causes must be excluded, especially infections or lymphoma. When a patient does not have specific skin or conjunctival lesions, transbronchial lung biopsy usually is the preferred diagnostic test. Biopsy results are positive in nearly 90% of sarcoidosis patients with abnormal findings on chest radiographs and in two-thirds of those with normal findings.

Skin anergy is typical but not diagnostic. The Kveim-Siltzbach test is performed by intradermal injection of a heat-treated suspension of sarcoidosis spleen extract, followed by a biopsy four to six weeks later. In approximately three-fourths of people with sarcoidosis, evidence of a granulomatous inflammatory reaction is detected. However, the biopsy results may have a 5% false-positive rate, and due to concern about human immunodeficiency virus and other transmissible diseases, most centers no longer have valid and approved test material (2). Cells in the sarcoid granuloma produce angiotensin-converting enzyme (ACE) and 1,25-dihydroxyvitamin D. Accordingly, up to two-thirds of patients have elevated serum ACE levels, and the vast majority have hypercalcemia or hypercalciuria.

The prognosis is good for most people with sarcoidosis. Many, especially those with a type I chest film, remit spontaneously. However, 25% of patients develop pulmonary disability, and 10% die from progressive sarcoidosis.

African Americans tend to have more severe disease (2). Other markers for chronic symptomatic disease are advanced disease on radiograph, lupus pernio, and cardiac or neurologic involvement.

Treatment depends on the specific manifestations. Asymptomatic hilar adenopathy requires no therapy. Many patients with early or late sarcoid arthritis respond to nonsteroidal anti-inflammatory drugs, including salicylates (2,11,14,15). Colchicine can be effective, especially for acute sarcoidosis arthropathy. Mucocutaneous sarcoidosis often improves with chloroquine or hydroxychloroquine (2,4).

Corticosteroids are indicated for severe lung disease, liver disease, hypercalcemia, cardiac inflammation, posterior uveitis, neurosarcoidosis, and severe sarcoidosis of other organs (2,4,19). The initial prednisone dose is 0.5 mg/kg/day (2). Single, daily doses are preferred, unless divided doses are required to control fever. The dose then is tapered by 5 mg every two weeks to a 0.25 mg/kg/day dose, which is maintained for four to eight months to make certain the improvement has plateaued. If possible, prednisone then can be tapered off completely (2,19,20). Inhaled corticosteroids have not been consistently effective for pulmonary sarcoidosis (2).

The efficacy of immunosuppressive drugs is not established. Methotrexate may be corticosteroid-sparing in patients with chronic disease (20). Cyclosporine has been ineffective in treating central nervous system disease (2).

Assessing treatment response depends chiefly on careful clinical examination, supplemented by changes in key tests, such as chest radiographs and pulmonary function tests. Bronchoalveolar lavage fluid analysis, serum ACE levels, and gallium lung scanning have been useful in research, but have not yet altered patient management (2,4).

DAVID B. HELLMANN, MD

References

1. Longcope WT, Freiman DG. A study of sarcoidosis based on a combined investigation of 160 cases including 30 autopsies from the Johns Hopkins Hospital and Massachusetts General Hospital. Medicine 1952;31:1–132.
2. Johns CJ, Michele TM. The clinical management of sarcoidosis. A 50-year experience at the Johns Hopkins Hospital. Medicine 1999;78:65–111.
3. Mayock RL, Bertrand P, Morrison CE, Scott JH. Manifestations of sarcoidosis: analysis of 145 patients, with a review of nine series selected from the literature. Am J Med 1963;35:67–89.
4. Bascom RA, Johns CJ. The natural history and management of sarcoidosis. In: Stollerman GH, Harrington WJ, Lamont JT, Leonard JJ, Siperstein MD (eds). Advances in Internal Medicine, Volume 31. Chicago: Yearbook Medical Publishers, 1986; pp 213–241.
5. Keogh BA, Hunninghake GW, Line BR, Crystal RG. The alveolitis of pulmonary sarcoidosis: evaluation of natural history and alveolitis-dependent changes in lung function. Am Rev Respir Dis 1983;128:256–265.
6. Crystal RG, Roberts WC, Hunninghake GW, Gadek JE, Fulmer JD, Line BR. Pulmonary sarcoidosis: a disease characterized and perpetuated by activated lung T-lymphocytes. Ann Intern Med 1981;94:73–94.
7. Moller DR. Etiology of sarcoidosis. Clin Chest Med 1997;18:695–706.
8. Kataria YP, Holter JF. Immunology of sarcoidosis. Clin Chest Med 1997;18:719–739.
9. Forman JD, Klein JT, Silver RF, Liu MC, Greenlee BM, Moller DR. Selective activation and accumulation of oligoclonal Vβ-specific T cells in active pulmonary sarcoidosis. J Clin Invest 1994;94:1533–1542.
10. Mason RS, Frankel T, Chan Y, Lissner D, Posen S. Vitamin D conversion by sarcoid lymph node homogenate. Ann Intern Med 1984;100:59–61.
11. Gumpel JM, Johns CJ, Shulman LE. The joint disease of sarcoidosis. Ann Rheum Dis 1967;26:194–205.
12. Spilberg I, Siltzbach LE, McEwen C. The arthritis of sarcoidosis. Arthritis Rheum 1969;12:126–137.
13. Kaplan H. Sarcoid arthritis: a review. Arch Intern Med 1963;112:924–935.
14. Glennas A, Kvien TK, Melby K, et al. Acute sarcoid arthritis: occurrence, seasonal onset, clinical features and outcome. Br J Rheumatol 1995;34:45–50.
15. Palmer DG, Schumacher HR. Synovitis with non-specific histological changes in synovium in chronic sarcoidosis. Ann Rheum Dis 1984;43:778–782.
16. Zisman DA, Biermann JS, Martinez FJ, Devaney KO, Lynch JP. Sarcoidosis presenting as a tumorlike muscular lesion. Case report and review of the literature. Medicine (Baltimore) 1999;78:112–122.
17. Chapelon C, Ziza JM, Piette JC, et al. Neurosarcoidosis: signs, course and treatment of 35 confirmed cases. Medicine (Baltimore) 1990;69:261–276.
18. Ainslie GM, Benatar SR. Serum angiotensin converting enzyme in sarcoidosis: sensitivity and specificity in diagnosis: correlations with disease activity, duration, extra-thoracic involvement, radiographic type and therapy. Q J Med 1985;55:253–270.
19. Hunninghake GW, Gilbert S, Pueringer R, et al. Outcome of the treatment for sarcoidosis. Am J Respir Crit Care Med 1994;149:893–898.
20. Baughman RP, Lower EE. Steroid-sparing alternative treatments for sarcoidosis. Clin Chest Med 1997;18:853–864.

29 STORAGE AND DEPOSITION DISEASES

This chapter covers a number of unusual arthropathies that are caused by deposition of normal material, such as metal ions, or storage of abnormal material, such as lipids (1). Hemochromatosis, ochronosis, and Wilson's disease are characterized by cellular deposition of normal metal ions: iron, calcium, and copper, respectively. In the case of Gaucher's disease, Fabry's disease, Farber's disease, and multicentric reticulohistiocytosis, rheumatic manifestations result from cellular storage of abnormal lipids. In hemochromatosis, arthralgias may be the first indication of a systemic disorder, but in ochronosis, Gaucher's disease, and multicentric reticulohistiocytosis, arthritis evolves as a predominant feature.

Hemochromatosis

Hemochromatosis is a common, inherited, autosomal recessive disorder that affects as many as five per 1000 Caucasians of European extraction. It is characterized by excessive body-iron stores and the deposition of hemosiderin, which cause tissue damage and organ dysfunction (2). The disorder rarely appears before age 40 unless there is a family history, and men are affected 10 times more frequently than women, who are protected by menstruation. Increased intestinal iron absorption and visceral deposition can lead to the phenotypic features of hepatic cirrhosis, cardiomyopathy, diabetes mellitus, pituitary dysfunction (including hypogonadism), sicca syndrome, and abnormal skin pigmentation (mostly of melanin) (2).

In a survey of 2851 patients with hemochromatosis, symptoms had been present for an average of 10 years before the diagnosis was made. Arthralgia (44%) was among the most common and troublesome complaints (3).

The gene for hemochromatosis (*HFE, HLA-H*) was discovered in 1996 by positional cloning methods near the HLA-A locus on chromosome 6 (4). More than 90% of patients typically possess the C282Y mutation of the *HFE* gene. Homozygous and heterozygous genotypes correlate with major and minor disease expression, respectively. The association of hemochromatosis with arthritis is most common in homozygotes with the heaviest iron overload. Another mutation of *HFE*, H63D, although not associated with iron overload, may act synergistically with C3824 in a small percentage of patients with hemochromatosis. Iron overload in the absence of the C282Y mutation has been reported in some European populations (5).

Prolonged excessive iron ingestion and repeated blood transfusion in chronic hypoproliferative anemia and tha-

lassemia may result in iron deposition. If iron overload occurs without tissue damage, the disorder is known as *hemosiderosis*. With tissue damage, it is called secondary hemochromatosis. The iron deposition in macrophages in secondary hemochromatosis is associated with less tissue damage and end-organ dysfunction compared with the idiopathic form.

Yersinia septic arthritis or septicemia is an unusual complication that may occur in people with hemochromatosis because of a microbial requirement for an iron-rich environment. Hepatitis B and C viral infections may accelerate liver damage in people with hemochromatosis (6).

Clinical Features
Chronic progressive arthritis, predominantly affecting the second and third metacarpophalangeal (MCP) and proximal interphalangeal (PIP) joints, is the presenting feature in about one-half of cases (Fig. 29-1). Involvement of the MCP joints is the most common rheumatologic feature at the time of diagnosis (7). The dominant hand may be solely or more severely affected. The finger joints and wrists are mildly tender and limited in motion. Larger joints, such as

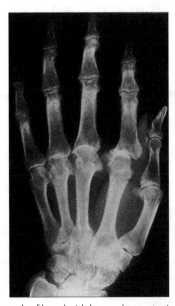

Fig. 29-1. Radiograph of hand with hemochromatosis. Note the joint-space narrowing, cystic subchondral lesions, joint-space irregularity, mild subluxation, bony sclerosis, and small osteophytes in the metacarpophalangeal joints. Chondrocalcinosis is present in the ulnar carpal joint, and soft tissue has calcified around the interphalangeal joint of the thumb. Courtesy of Dr. HR Schumacher, Jr.

the shoulders, hips, and knees, also may be affected. Hemochromatotic arthropathy of the hips or shoulders may, at times, be rapidly progressive. True morning stiffness is not a feature of hemochromatosis.

The detection of an osteoarthritis-like disease that involves MCP and wrist joints, particularly in men during the fourth and fifth decade of life, should signal the possibility of underlying hemochromatosis. Arthropathy has been reported in individuals as young as 26 years, before any other manifestations of the disease develop.

Radiographic Features

The radiologic changes of hemochromatosis resemble osteoarthritis, except that in hemochromatosis, there is less osteophytosis. Ulnar styloid erosion may suggest rheumatoid diseases, but the irregular joint narrowing and sclerotic cyst formation are more indicative of a degenerative process. Although the distal interphalangeal joints may be affected, the carpometacarpal joint changes of generalized osteoarthritis are not a feature. Somewhat similar MCP changes can occur in calcium pyrophosphate dihydrate (CPPD) crystal deposition without hemochromatosis. Some degree of diffuse osteoporosis may be present, presumably due to hypogonadism, but a direct effect of iron on bone also is possible.

Chondrocalcinosis is characteristic of the arthropathy and is a late complication in about 50% of patients; it may be the sole abnormality (7). The hyaline cartilage of the shoulder, wrist, hip, and knee, and the fibrocartilage of the triangular ligament of the wrist and symphysis pubis may be affected. Superimposed attacks of CPPD crystal synovitis occur in these cases. The finding of chondrocalcinosis should suggest the possibility of hemochromatosis.

Laboratory Features

Synovial fluid has good viscosity, with leukocyte counts below 1000 cells/mm^3. During acute episodes of pseudogout, synovial-fluid leukocytosis with calcium pyrophosphate crystals can be found. Except for such episodes, the erythrocyte sedimentation rate usually is normal. In patients with chronic liver disease, rheumatoid factor tests may be positive.

The diagnosis may be suspected by a raised serum iron and high ferritin concentration with increased saturation of the plasma iron-binding protein transferrin (5). The latter, however, is more specific and should be regarded as the cornerstone test for diagnosis (5). For population screening, the simpler unbound iron binding capacity (UIBC) showed higher sensitivity and fewer false-positives (5). Needle biopsy of the liver provides definitive evidence of iron overload in hemochromatosis, but this procedure usually is reserved for cases in diagnostic doubt or, more often, to assess the severity of liver damage associated with fibrosis, cirrhosis, or hepatoma.

In idiopathic hemochromatosis, iron deposits affect parenchymal hepatic cells, whereas in secondary forms, reticuloendothelial cells are most affected. In hemochromatosis, synovial biopsy shows iron deposition in the type B synthetic lining cells of synovium. In rheumatoid arthritis, traumatic hemarthrosis, hemophilia, and villonodular synovitis, synovial biopsy shows deposits in the deeper layers or in the phagocyte type A lining cells. Hemosiderin deposits may be found in the chondrocytes. Further evidence of iron may be found in biopsies of skin and intestinal mucosa, or in bone marrow, buffy coat, or urine sediment. The amount of iron excreted in the urine after administration of the iron-chelating agent deferoxamine correlates with the presence of parenchymal hepatic iron in hemochromatosis. Where available, direct noninvasive magnetic measurements of hepatic iron stores provide a quantitative method for early detection of iron overload and rapid evaluation of treatment.

The pathogenesis of the arthritis is unknown, as degenerative joint changes do not necessarily develop in relation to synovial iron. The low frequency of chondrocalcinosis in people with hemophilia and rheumatoid arthritis weighs against synovial hemosiderin as a cause of chondrocalcinosis. It is speculated that ionic iron might inhibit pyrophosphatase activity and lead to a local concentration of calcium pyrophosphate in the joint. The deposition of calcium in cartilage appears to predispose to inflammatory and degenerative joint disease (2).

Treatment

Following the diagnosis of hemochromatosis in any patient, it is imperative for medical preventive reasons to obtain biochemical screening of at least first-degree relatives. Screening may be done by measuring serum iron-binding transferrin or by performing the UIBC test. Genotyping for the C282Y mutation of the *HFE* gene is a useful diagnostic aid and helpful in counseling and predicting the risk of disease in healthy relatives (5). However, it gives no indication of iron stores or prognosis.

Aggressive phlebotomy therapy promotes longevity and can prevent or reverse much organ damage. Weekly phlebotomies generally are needed until iron is depleted and mild anemia is present. Venesection may not prevent the progression of arthritis in hemochromatosis, but in some cases, arthritis may improve after this therapy. It has been suggested that prophylactic phlebotomy should be considered on the basis of genetic predisposition. Iron-chelating therapy with intravenous deferoxamine generally is effective but impractical because of the expense and the need for intravenous administration.

Arthritis symptoms may be difficult to control, even with nonsteroidal anti-inflammatory drugs. Agents requiring hepatic metabolism, such as diclofenac or nabumetone, should be avoided. Prosthetic hip, knee, and shoulder arthroplasties can be performed when required.

Alkaptonuria (Ochronosis)

Alkaptonuria (AKU), a rare autosomal recessive disorder, results from a complete deficiency of the enzyme homogentisic acid oxidase (HGO) (8). In six reported pedigrees, the

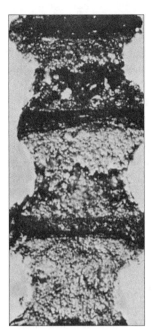

Fig. 29-2. Part of a lumbar vertebral column of a 49-year-old woman with alkaptonuria who died of renal failure (ochronotic nephrosis). Blackened intervertebral discs are thin and focally calcified. This patient had incapacitating pain since age 36, with progressive limitation of back motion. Microscopic examination of the discs, which splintered easily, revealed nonrefractile granular pigment. Reprinted with permission from Cooper J, Moran TJ. Studies on ochronosis. I. Report of case with death from ochronotic nephrosis. Arch Pathol 1957;61:46–53.

gene was mapped to chromosome 3q2. Since then, a Spanish group has reported the cloning of the human *HGO* gene and established that it is the gene responsible for AKU (9). The *HGO* gene harbors misuse mutations that represent a loss of function. This defect causes accumulation of homogentisic acid, a normal intermediate in the metabolism of phenylalanine and tyrosine. Alkalization and oxidation of this acid, which usually is excreted in the urine, cause the urine to turn black. The homogentisic acid retained in the body is deposited as a pigmented polymer in the cartilage and, to a lesser degree, in skin and sclerae. The darkening of tissues by this pigment is designated *ochronosis*.

The pigment, which is found in the deeper layers of the articular cartilage, is bound to collagen fibers, causing this tissue to lose its normal resiliency and become brittle and fibrillated. The erosion of this abnormal cartilage leads to denuding of subchondral bone and the penetration of tiny shards of pigmented cartilage into the bone, synovium, and joint cavity (10). It is likely that these pigmented cartilage fragments become a nidus for the formation of osteochondral bodies.

Clinical Features

A progressive degenerative arthropathy develops, with symptoms usually beginning in the fourth decade of life. Features include arthritis of the spine (ochronotic spondylosis) and larger peripheral joints, with chondrocalcinosis,

formation of osteochondral bodies, and synovial effusions (ochronotic peripheral arthropathy). Initially, the spinal column is affected, with pigment found in the annulus fibrosus and nucleus pulposus of the intervertebral discs (Fig. 29-2). Later, the knees, shoulders, and hips deteriorate; the small peripheral joints are spared. In adults, the first sign of spondylosis may be an acute disc syndrome. Eventually, it clinically resembles ankylosing spondylitis, with progressive lumbar rigidity and loss of stature.

Stiffness and loss of joint mobility are the predominant complaints, with pain less prominent. Knee effusions, crepitus, and flexion contractures are common, but other signs of articular inflammation ordinarily are lacking. Fragments of darkly pigmented cartilage occasionally can be found floating in the joint fluid. Osteochondral bodies, which form in response to the deposition of cartilaginous fragments in the synovium, often are palpable in and around the knee joint and may reach several centimeters in diameter.

Nonarticular features of ochronosis include bluish discoloration and calcification of the ear pinnae, triangular pigmentation of the sclera, and pigmentation over the nose, axillae, and groin. Prostatic calculi are common in men, and cardiac murmurs may develop from valvular pigment deposits.

Radiographic Features

The earliest features visible on radiographs are multiple vacuum discs of the spine. Eventually, the entire spine shows ossification of the discs, with narrowing, collapse, and fusion. Chondrocalcinosis may affect the symphysis pubis, costal cartilage, and ear helix. In contrast to ankylosing spondylitis, the sacroiliac and apophyseal joints are not affected. The roentgenographic appearance of the peripheral joints resembles that found in primary osteoarthritis, with loss of cartilage space, marginal osteophytes, and eburnation of the subchondral bone. In contrast to primary osteoarthritis, however, degeneration of the shoulders and hips is more severe, and osteochondral bodies are seen.

Laboratory Features

The diagnosis of AKU is suspected when the patient gives a history of passing dark urine, or when fresh urine turns black on standing or on alkalinization. In individuals lacking this history, the diagnosis is made only after the detection of a false-positive test for diabetes mellitus or the onset of arthritis. Darkly pigmented synovium may be seen on arthroscopy. A specific enzymatic method permits quantitation of homogentisic acid in urine and blood, and molecular cloning of the HGO gene enables detection of heterozygotic carriers (9).

Synovial fluid usually is clear, yellow, and viscous and does not darken with alkalinization. At times, the fluid may be speckled with many particles of debris resembling ground pepper (Fig. 29-3). Leukocyte counts of a few hundred cells are predominantly mononuclear. Occasionally, the cytoplasm of mononuclear and polymorphonuclear

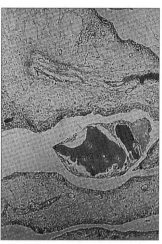

Fig. 29-3. Ochronosis: synovial fluid and synovium (gross and microscopic). On the left, the synovial fluid reveals numerous dark particles and shards having the appearance of ground pepper. On the right, a low-power microscopic view of the synovium shows fragments of darkly pigmented cartilage (H&E). Reprinted with permission from Hunter T, Gordon DA, Ogryzlo MA. The ground pepper sign of synovial fluid: a new diagnostic feature of ochronosis. J Rheumatol 1974;1:45–53.

cells contains dark inclusions of phagocytosed ochronotic pigment. Centrifugation and microscopic examination of synovial-fluid sediment may show fragments of pigmented cartilage. Effusions may contain CPPD crystals and show no inflammation. Pigmented cartilage fragments are embedded in synovium and often are surrounded by giant cells (8,10).

Treatment

No effective treatment is available for the underlying metabolic disorder. Large amounts of ascorbic acid might prevent deposition of ochronotic pigment, but long-term effects of this therapy are unknown. Surgical removal of osteochondral loose bodies from the knee joint is warranted when they interfere with motion. Prosthetic joint replacement may be helpful.

Wilson's Disease

Wilson's disease (hepatolenticular degeneration) is a rare metabolic disorder in which deposition of copper leads to dysfunction of the liver, brain, and kidneys. It is inherited as an autosomal recessive trait, affecting about 1 in 30,000 persons in most populations. It becomes symptomatic for individuals aged six to 40 years. A defective gene and related mutations provide some explanation for the wide phenotypic variation seen in Wilson's disease (11).

Clinical Features

Total body copper is increased. The accumulation of copper in the liver leads to cirrhosis; in the cornea, characteristic Kayser-Fleischer rings; in the basal ganglia, lenticular degeneration and movement disorders; in the kidneys, renal tubular damage (11). An arthropathy may develop in as many as 50% of affected adults, but arthritis is rare in children (12). Patients usually develop hepatic or neurologic symptoms in childhood or adolescence. Liver disease is the most common presentation between ages eight and 16, with symptoms of jaundice, nausea, vomiting, and malaise. Acute hepatic failure may develop, but rarely. Neurologic symptoms are rare before age 12. Dysarthria and decreased coordination of voluntary movements are the most common complaints. Other presenting symptoms include acute hemolytic anemia, arthralgias, renal stones, and renal tubular acidosis.

The arthropathy is characterized by mild premature osteoarthritis of the wrists, MCP joints, knees, or spine. Occasionally, joint hypermobility may be found (12). Ossified bodies of the wrists may be associated with subchondral cysts. Chondromalacia patellae, osteochondritis dissecans, or chondrocalcinosis of the knee may be associated with mild knee effusions. Arthropathy tends to be mild in patients treated early in life, but it may be more severe in patients with untreated disease of longer duration. A few patients show acute or subacute polyarthritis that resembles rheumatoid arthritis and may be associated with a positive rheumatoid factor. These seropositive cases could be the result of penicillamine therapy.

The pathogenesis of the arthropathy is unclear, and its presence does not correlate with neurologic, hepatic, or renal disease. Although chondrocalcinosis has been observed in patients with Wilson's disease, light and transmission electron microscopy have failed to detect crystals containing calcium in synovial fluids or in biopsies of cartilage and synovium. Copper has been found in the articular cartilage by elemental analysis of a few patients with Wilson's disease and theoretically could cause tissue damage mediated by oxygen-derived free radicals (12). Although the arthropathy generally is milder than that seen in hemochromatosis, its cause may be similar and it may involve deposition of CPPD crystals and the development of chronic arthritis.

Radiographic Features

Radiologic features may include subchondral cysts, joint-space narrowing, sclerosis, marked osteophyte formation, and multiple calcified loose bodies, especially at the wrist. Involvement of the hip and MCP joints is uncommon. Periostitis at the femoral trochanters and other tendinous insertions, periarticular calcifications, and chondrocalcinosis have been reported. Changes in the spine are seen mainly in the midthoracic to lumbar areas and include squaring of the vertebral bodies, intervertebral joint-space narrowing, osteophytes, and osteochondritis.

Skeletal manifestations of Wilson's disease include generalized osteoporosis in as many as 50% of patients. The osteoporosis usually is asymptomatic, but spontaneous fractures may occur (12). Osteomalacia, milkman pseudofractures, and renal rickets have been reported. Some cases are from geographic areas where nutritional deficiencies may contribute to skeletal abnormalities.

Laboratory Features

Although Kayser-Fleischer corneal rings are pathognomonic of Wilson's disease, laboratory investigations establish the diagnosis. Low serum copper and decreased serum ceruloplasmin levels occur in most cases, and in symptomatic patients, urinary copper excretion is increased. Biliary excretion of copper is decreased markedly. Microchemical evidence of copper deposition may be obtained from needle biopsy of the liver, but histochemical methods are unreliable. In doubtful cases, specialized studies with radioactive copper may be necessary.

Synovial biopsies show hyperplasia of synovial lining cells with mild inflammation. Neither calcium pyrophosphate nor copper are seen by standard methods. Limited data are available concerning morphologic changes in joints. Microvilli formation, initial cell hyperplasia, chronic inflammatory infiltrates, and vascular changes have been reported in synovium. Joint fluids have had low leukocyte counts.

Treatment

Copper chelation with penicillamine in conjunction with dietary copper restriction is the treatment of choice. Whether penicillamine can control the arthropathy is unclear, but contemporary series suggest that earlier diagnosis with more intensive chelation therapy lessen the arthropathy. Rarely, side effects from penicillamine are reported, including acute polyarthritis, polymyositis, or a syndrome resembling systemic lupus erythematosus. Trientine is a chelating agent available for patients intolerant of penicillamine. Liver transplantation is the only treatment option available for acute hepatic failure or long-standing cirrhosis where penicillamine or trientine are not options. Otherwise, symptomatic measures suffice to control arthritis symptoms.

Gaucher's Disease

Gaucher's disease is a lysosomal glycolipid storage disease in which glucocerebroside accumulates in the reticuloendothelial cells of the spleen, liver, and bone marrow (13). It is an autosomal recessive disorder caused by subnormal activity of the hydrolytic enzyme glucocerebrosidase. The gene for Gaucher's disease is located on chromosome 1 in the q21 region. Modern DNA technology has led to cloning of glucocerebroside genes and identification of their mutations. In Gaucher's disease, all cells are deficient in glucocerebroside activity, but it is the glycolipid-engorged macrophages that account for the disease's non-neurologic features.

Fortunately, the most severe forms of Gaucher's disease are extremely rare, but milder forms are encountered frequently, particularly in the Jewish population. Gaucher's disease has been classified into clinical subdivisions. Type 1, the most common form, is the adult or chronic type, which accounts for more than 99% of cases. It occurs primarily in Ashkenazi Jews, whereas other types occur in all ethnic groups. It is defined by the lack of neurologic involvement, and affected adults present with accumulation of glucocerebroside in the reticuloendothelial system, causing organomegaly, hypersplenism, conjunctival pingueculae, skin pigmentation, and osteoarticular disease. Type 1 has the best prognosis, but may be mistaken for juvenile rheumatoid arthritis.

Clinical Features

Some patients with type 1 disease have few or no clinical manifestations. In these cases, the condition may be discovered only when bone marrow is examined for some other reason, or if mild thrombocytopenia is investigated.

Type 2, infantile Gaucher's disease, is a fulminating disorder with severe brain involvement; death occurs within the first 18 months of life. Type 3, the intermediate or juvenile form, begins in early childhood and shows many features of the chronic form, with or without central nervous system dysfunction.

Skeletal involvement is characteristic of type 1 and, to a lesser extent, type 3, but not type-2 disease. Musculoskeletal involvement occurs in the adult and juvenile forms, but it rarely is the first symptom. Patients usually present with lymphadenopathy, hepatosplenomegaly, or signs and symptoms of hypersplenism, but rheumatic complaints may appear early in the disease course. Pain in the hip, knee, or shoulder is caused by disease of adjacent bone. In young individuals, the most common complaint is chronic aching around the hip or proximal tibia. This may last only a few days, but usually is recurrent. Another complaint is excruciating pain (bone crisis) involving the femur and tibia, with tenderness, swelling, and erythema. Monarticular hip or knee degeneration is typical, and unexplained migratory polyarthritis sometimes occurs. Bone pain tends to lessen with age.

Other skeletal features include pathologic long-bone fractures, vertebral compression, and osteonecrosis of the femoral or humeral heads or proximal tibia. The osteonecrosis can develop slowly, or rapidly with bone crisis. These crises usually affect only one bone area at a time. Because acute-phase reactants and bone scans usually are positive, the clinical picture of acute osteomyelitis is mimicked (pseudo-osteomyelitis). Surgical drainage in these cases commonly leads to infection and chronic osteomyelitis. Due to this increased susceptibility to infection, conservative management of bony lesions is recommended.

Radiographic Features

Asymptomatic radiologic areas of rarefaction, patchy sclerosis, and cortical thickening are common. Osteonecrosis of bone, particularly of the hips, and pathologic fractures of the femur and vertebrae are the most serious and deforming features of Gaucher's disease. Involvement of the femur is thought to be a "barometer" of bone symptoms. Widening of the distal femur with the radiologic appearance of an Erlenmeyer flask is a frequent finding, but flaring of the bones can occur in the tibia and humerus as well.

Laboratory Features

When bone pain or other articular symptoms appear, serum acid phosphatase and angiotensin-converting enzymes usually are elevated. However, the most reliable method for diagnosing Gaucher's disease is the determination of leukocyte β-glucosidase. Diagnosis has been confirmed by examination of bone marrow aspirate for the Gaucher cell, a large lipid-storage histiocyte. This cell should be differentiated from globoid cells of another lysosomal storage disorder, Krabbe's disease (galactocerebrosidosis). However, histologic diagnosis of Gaucher's disease is unnecessary and can be misleading. Bone biopsy is not recommended because of the risk of secondary infection. Needle biopsy of the liver for assay of glucocerebroside may be performed, but washed leukocytes and extracts of cultured skin fibroblasts are easily obtained for glucocerebrosidase testing. These assays also may be used to detect heterozygous carriers. Amniocentesis has been used for the prenatal detection of diseased fetuses. When the diagnosis is established, genetic counseling for family members or prospective parents is recommended. Although enzyme assays are useful for genetic screening, DNA analysis using the polymerase chain reaction are much more precise (13).

Treatment

Historically, therapy for Gaucher's disease was mostly symptomatic, aimed at controlling pain and infection. Bisphosphonates have been used to treat accompanying bone disease, and intermittent intravenous pamidronate with oral calcium has effectively treated a few patients with type-1 disease and severe bone involvement. In adults, splenectomy may control hypersplenism, but bone disease may then accelerate. Partial splenectomy has been recommended as protection against postsplenectomy infection, and for its hepatic- and bone-sparing effect. Arthroplasty and complete joint replacement often are necessary, but loosening of prostheses occurs more often than in other disorders. Bleeding can be an operative problem.

Replacement enzyme, a modified form of glucocerebroside (Ceredase), is a relatively new option that provides costly but effective treatment of Gaucher's disease (14). Periodic intravenous infusions of the enzyme over many months result in regression of the disease's symptoms (13,14). For type-1 disease, oral treatment with N-butyl-doxynojirimycin has shown promise in decreasing glucocerebroside substrate (15). This agent reduced visceromegaly and may have value as monotherapy or in combination with intravenous enzyme replacement. Allogeneic bone marrow transplantation may be an option in advanced disease if an HLA-identical donor is available. Gene-transfer therapy using retroviral vector constructs also shows promise for coding the gene for glucocerebrosidase into hematopoietic progenitors.

Fabry's Disease

Fabry's disease, a slowly progressive disorder predominantly affecting males, is a lysosomal lipid-storage disease in which glycosphingolipids accumulate widely in nerves, viscera, skin, and osteoarticular tissues. It is a sex-linked inherited disease caused by a deficiency of the enzyme α-galactosidase A. The gene and its mutations responsible for expression of this enzyme have been localized to the middle of the long arm of the X chromosome.

Clinical Features

Clinical features are widespread and nonspecific, and diagnosis often is missed or delayed. In childhood, the deposition is particularly marked in and around blood vessels, giving rise to the characteristic rash of dark blue or red angiokeratomas or angiectases around the buttocks, thighs, and lower abdomen. When diffuse, it is referred to as *angiokeratoma corporis diffusum* and almost always is associated with hypohydrosis.

The kidneys are the main target organs, and proteinuria gradually develops in childhood or adolescence, with abnormal urinary sediments that include birefringent lipid crystals (Maltese crosses). Progressive renal disease leads to renal failure. Cardiovascular and cerebrovascular deposition of the sphingolipid parallels the renal disease, with vascular insufficiencies or sudden death. Ocular changes are severe. A characteristic corneal opacity seen by slit-lamp examination occurs early and can be helpful in diagnosis, even in heterozygous women.

Some patients experience the insidious development of polyarthritis with degenerative changes and flexion contractures of the fingers, particularly of the distal interphalageal joints. Foam cells have been described in the synovial vessels and connective tissues. Radiographs may show infarct-like opacities of bone and osteoporosis of the spine. Osteonecrosis of the hip and talus have been described. Eighty percent of children or young adults undergo painful crises of burning paresthesias of the hands and feet and, later, of whole extremities. These attacks are associated with fever and elevations of the erythrocyte sedimentation rate.

Genetic counseling should be offered to affected families. Measurement of α-galactosidase to α-galactosidase activity ratios in leukocytes and fibroblasts provides reasonable discrimination between carriers and noncarriers. Identification by DNA studies is reserved for subjects showing equivocal results.

Treatment

Treatment has not been satisfactory. However, the prospect of gene therapy using recombinant adenovirus AxCAGα-gal to provide enzyme replacement may provide better outcomes (16). Antiplatelet medication may suppress vascular damage. Burning paresthesias may benefit from phenytoin or carbamazepine. Without dialysis or transplantation, most affected males succumb to renal failure before age 50.

Farber's Disease

Farber's disease is a lysosomal lipid-storage disease in which a glycolipid ceramide accumulates in many tissues, including the skin and musculoskeletal system (17). It is an autosomal recessive disorder caused by a deficiency of the enzyme acid ceramidase. Affected children show disease manifestations by the age of four months and die before the age of four years.

A hoarse cry from thickened vocal cords or swollen, painful joints may be the first features. The appearance of tender, subcutaneous nodules follows, and the early occurrence of nodules correlates with shortened survival. All the extremities may be swollen and tender, but this condition gives way to more localized joint swelling, with nodules appearing on the fingers, wrists, elbows, and knees. Joint contractures, especially affecting the fingers and wrists, develop later. The gastrointestinal, cardiovascular, and nervous systems gradually become involved, and death results from respiratory disease. Diagnosis can be confirmed by demonstrating a deficiency of ceramidase in leukocytes and fibroblasts.

Lipochrome Histiocytosis

Lipochrome histiocytosis is an extremely rare lysosomal storage disease associated with pulmonary infiltrates, splenomegaly, hypergammaglobulinemia, polyarthritis, and increased susceptibility to infection (18). The disorder is familial. Histiocytes show lipochrome pigment granulation, and peripheral blood leukocytes exhibit impaired activity.

Multicentric Reticulohistiocytosis

Multicentric reticulohistiocytosis is a rare dermatoarthritis of unknown cause or familial association. It is characterized by the cellular accumulation of glycolipid-laden histiocytes and multinucleated giant cells in skin and joints (19). The most common presentation is a painful destructive polyarthritis resembling rheumatoid arthritis, for which affected persons mistakenly may be treated. The joint manifestations precede the appearance of skin lesions in most patients, but the appearance and location of the skin nodules are not entirely characteristic of rheumatoid arthritis (Fig. 29-4). Although a self-limited form may be seen in childhood, adult multicentric reticulohistiocytosis predominantly affects middle-aged women.

Clinical Features

Disease onset is insidious and is characterized by polyarthritis, skin nodules, and in many cases, xanthelasma. Small papules and bead-like clusters around the nail folds are characteristic, with skin nodulation of the face and hands. Skin nodules vary in size, are yellowish or purple, and occur over the hands (Fig. 29-4), elbows, face, and ears. Oral, nasal, and pharyngeal mucosa involvement, sometimes with ulceration, is seen in one-fourth of patients. Various visceral sites may be affected.

Symmetric polyarthritis resembles rheumatoid disease when PIP joints are affected, and psoriatic arthritis when distal interphalangeal joint involvement predominates. Tenosynovial involvement may occur. Remission of polyarthritis may be seen after many years of progressive disease.

Early radiographs show "punched out" bony lesions resembling gouty tophi. Severe joint destruction will be seen in later radiographs. Spinal involvement with erosions and subluxations, including atlantoaxial damage, may occur.

Laboratory Features

No specific laboratory abnormality has been demonstrated, and the diagnosis is established by examining biopsies of affected tissues. Large, multinucleated giant cells infiltrate the skin and synovium (Fig. 29-5). The cytoplasm has a ground-glass appearance and stains positively for lipids and glycoproteins with periodic acid-Schiff stain (PAS-positive). Definitive analysis of these cell contents has not been made, but the contents probably are glycolipids. Triglycerides, cholesterol, and phosphate esters appear to be present in the lesion, suggesting that histiocytes are stimulated to produce these substances or that this is a form of lipid storage disease. A lymphocytic origin for the giant cells has been proposed because of the presence of T-cell markers, but multicentric reticulocytosis cells also stain for macrophage markers (19). A monocyte/macrophage origin for these cells has been suggested because of the detection of macrophage-activated cytokines of interleukin (IL)-1β, IL-12, and tumor necrosis factor α (TNF-α). The distribution of TNF-α appears similar to that for rheumatoid synovial cell proliferation. Synovial-fluid leukocyte counts range from 220 to 79,000 cells/mm^3, with mononuclear cells predominating. Scanning the synovial-fluid, Wright-stained smear or wet preparation may reveal giant cells or large, bizarre macrophages.

This histologic picture of multicentric reticulohistiocytosis is quite different from the arrangement of myofibroblast cells in a collagen matrix that is characteristic of the cutaneous nodules and polyarthritis of fibroblastic rheumatism (20).

Although the pathogenesis is unknown, hidden malignancy and tuberculosis have been implicated. Rheumatoid

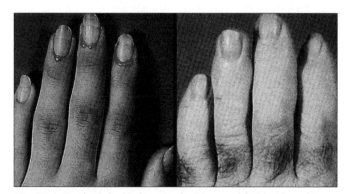

Fig. 29-4. On the left, the fingers of a 16-year-old girl with multicentric reticulohistiocytosis reveal multiple, reddish-brown, tender papulonodules that are periungual in distribution. On the right is another patient with multiple nodules in the fingers. These nodules are firm, can fluctuate in size, and may disappear spontaneously. Reprinted from the Revised Clinical Slide Collection on the Rheumatic Diseases, with permission of the American College of Rheumatology.

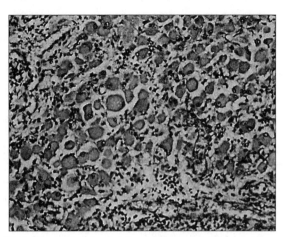

Fig. 29-5. Photomicrograph of synovium (knee) from a 54-year-old woman with multicentric reticulohistiocytosis shows numerous histiocytes and multinucleated giant cells that contain large amounts of periodic acid-Schiff (PAS)-positive material. Reprinted with permission from McCarty DJ, Koopman WJ. Arthritis and Allied Conditions. Philadelphia: Lea & Febiger, 1993.

factor does not occur. Some patients develop positive reactions to tuberculin (PPD-positive). There are case descriptions with associated Sjögren's syndrome and polymyositis. Multicentric reticulohistiocytosis also has been identified with a variety of malignancies (19). Death due to the disease itself has not been reported, but patients may be left with severe joint disability.

Treatment

Spontaneous remission of skin disease and arthritis occurs in some cases, especially in childhood. In the remainder, corticosteroids or topical nitrogen mustard may improve the skin lesions. In cases with severe skin and joint disease, combinations of corticosteroid, methotrexate, plus cyclophosphamide or cyclosporine have been effective. Low-dose methotrexate alone has shown prolonged effect, and methotrexate plus hydroxychloroquine has been beneficial. The presence of synovial TNF-α in the disease suggests that there might be a therapeutic role for one of the newer TNF-α inhibitors.

DUNCAN A. GORDON, MD

References

1. Rooney PJ. Hyperlipidemias, lipid storage disorders, metal storage disorders and ochronosis. Curr Opin Rheumatol 1991;3:166–171.
2. Mendlein J, Cogswell ME, McDonnell SM, Franks AL, Black M. Iron overload, public health and genetics. Ann Intern Med 1998;129:S921–S996.
3. McDonnell SM, Preston BL, Jewell SA, et al. A survey of 2,851 patients with hemochromatosis: symptoms and response to treatment. Am J Med 1999;106:619–624.
4. Feder JN, Gnirke A, Thomas W, et al. A novel MHC class I-like gene is mutated in patients with hereditary hemochromatosis. Nat Genet 1996;13:399–408.
5. Adams PC, Kertesz AE, McLaren CE, Barr R, Bamford A, Chakrabarti S. Population screening for hemochromatosis: a comparison of unbound iron-binding capacity, transferrin saturation, and C282Y genotyping in 5,211 voluntary blood donors. Hepatology 2000;31:1160–1164.
6. Piperno A, Fargion S, D'Alba R, et al. Liver damage in Italian patients with hereditary hemochromatosis is highly influenced by hepatitis B and C virus infection. J Hepatol 1992;16: 364–368.
7. Mathews JL, Williams HJ. Arthritis in hereditary hemochromatosis. Arthritis Rheum 1987;30:1137–1141.
8. Schumacher HR, Holdsmith DE. Ochronotic arthropathy. I. Clinicopathologic studies. Semin Arthritis Rheum 1977;6:207–246.
9. Fernandez-Canon JM, Granadino B, Beltran-Valero de Bernabe D, et al. The molecular basis of alkaptonuria. Nat Genet 1996;14:19–24.
10. Gaines JJ Jr, Tom GD, Khankhanian N. The ultrastructural and light microscopic study of the synovium in ochronotic arthropathy. Hum Pathol 1987;18:1160–1164.
11. Gow PJ, Smallwood RA, Angus PW, Smith AL, Wall AJ, Sewell RB. Diagnosis of Wilson's disease: an experience over three decades. Gut 2000;46:415–419.
12. Menerey KA, Eider W, Brewer GJ, Brauenstein EM, Schumacher HR, Fox IH. The arthropathy of Wilson's disease: clinical and pathologic features. J Rheumatol 1988;15:331–337.
13. Zimran A. Gaucher's disease. Baillieres Clinical Hematology 1997;10:621–846.
14. Grabowski GA, Barton NW, Pastores G, et al. Enzyme therapy in Type 1 Gaucher disease: comparative efficacy of mannose-terminated glucocerebrosidase from natural and recombinant sources. Ann Intern Med 1995;122:33–39.
15. Cox T, Lachmann R, Hollak C, et al. Novel oral treatment of Gaucher's disease with N-butyldeoxynojirimycin (OGT918) to decrease substrate biosynthesis. Lancet 2000;355:1481–1485.
16. Ohsugi K, Kobayashi K, Itoh K, Sakuraba H, Sakuragawa N. Enzymatic corrections for cells derived from Fabry disease patients by a recombinant adenovirus vector. J Hum Genet 2000;45:1-5.
17. Chanoki M, Ishii M, Fukaik, et al. Farber's lipogranulomatosis in siblings: light and electron microscopic studies. Br J Dermatol 1989;121:779–785.
18. Rodey GE, Park BH, Ford DK, Gray BH, Good RA. Defective bacteriocidal activity of peripheral blood leukocytes in lipochrome histiocytosis. Am J Med 1970;49:322–327.
19. Gorman JD, Danning C, Schumacher HR, Klippel JH, Davis JC Jr. Multicentric reticulohistiocytosis: case report with immunochemical analysis and literature review. Arthritis Rheum 2000;43:930–938.
20. Romas E, Finlay M, Woodruff T. The arthropathy of fibroblastic rheumatism. Arthritis Rheum 1997;40:183–187.

30 AMYLOIDOSES

For more than a century and a half, pathologists have described organs infiltrated with a homogeneous eosinophilic material that stains with iodine. Virchow designated this material "amyloid." During the past 30 years, a body of data showing there are many amyloidoses has replaced the notion that a single amyloid substance appears during the course of multiple diseases. Each amyloid is derived from a different protein and is disease-specific, with the resulting organ compromise related to the location, quantity, and rate of deposition. The amyloidoses represent the extracellular subset of a larger disease group related to tissue dysfunction occurring as the result of aberrant protein conformation. The disorders, which include, among others, Parkinson's and Huntington's diseases, reflect the loss of protein solubility under physiologic conditions. The insoluble products, α-synuclein in Parkinson's and huntingtin in Huntington's, serve as both mediator and harbinger of the diseases.

The amyloidoses entered the domain of rheumatology because of the historic association of long-standing inflammatory joint disease with amyloid deposition in the kidneys, liver, and spleen. However, arthropathy as the major clinical presentation of amyloid is infrequent. It is found in three forms of amyloidosis: AL, the amyloid associated with immunoglobulin L-chain deposition; $A\beta_2m$, the amyloid derived from β_2-microglobulin in patients with chronic renal failure; and ATTR, the transthyretin (TTR) associated familial disease.

Pathology and Pathogenesis

All amyloidoses appear as homogeneous, hyaline, eosinophilic material on hematoxylin and eosin staining. They bind Congo red, demonstrate apple-green–positive birefringence under polarized light, have a fibrillar structure on electron microscopy, and stain positively with antibody specific for P-component. These features distinguish the amyloidoses from the other disorders of protein conformation. So far, 20 discrete fibril precursors have been identified in human diseases (Table 30-1).

What makes any protein amyloidogenic is uncertain. The fibrils all display a crossed, β-pleated sheet structure. However, not all the precursors contain such elements in their soluble precursor form; some adopt the beta secondary structure only in the course of fibril formation. To date, with one possible exception, the fibril subunits are derived from precursors that are 3.5–30 kDa. It may be that in vivo fibrillogenesis involves certain size constraints. Various pathogenic modes are involved. Increased production of a precursor, either locally or systemically, as a result of a prolonged normal stimulus to the synthesizing cell (amyloid protein AA), or monoclonal proliferation of a cell producing the amyloidogenic protein (amyloid protein AL), may be responsible. There may be decreased excretion of the precursor, as in $A\beta_2m$ deposition. Aberrant, inappropriate, or incomplete proteolytic cleavage may lead to increased amounts of profibrillogenic precursor (amyloid proteins AβPP, AA). Structural abnormalities of a normal protein, secondary to a germline mutation, also may predispose to fibril formation (amyloid protein TTR). Finally, it is possible that a defect may exist in an as-yet undefined process responsible for the normal degradation and disposition of single proteins or a group of proteins that have amyloidogenic properties at physiologic or slightly higher concentrations.

Amyloidosis is diagnosed by demonstrating the characteristic staining in biopsies from clinically affected organs. Sampling of readily accessible tissues, notably the rectum, other regions of the gastrointestinal tract, and subcutaneous fat, also have a good return with lower risk (Table 30-2) (1). Because each form of amyloid is defined by the chemical nature of the fibril protein, pathologic specimens from any site can be stained with antibodies specific for the precursors to establish the character of the responsible disease (2).

Several nonfibril molecules are found in all amyloid deposits. The P-component is a salt-soluble molecule with the electron microscopic appearance of a pentagon. It is derived from a serum precursor, serum amyloid P-component (SAP), that behaves as an acute-phase reactant in mice, but not in humans. It shares structural features with C-reactive protein and several other proteins that are members of the pentraxin (five subunit) family. The role of the P-component in the pathogenesis of amyloid deposition has not been defined, but intravenously injected purified radiolabeled P-component binds to deposited fibrils in tissues and can be used in gamma scanning to determine the presence and extent of deposits in some tissues of people with clinical disease (3).

A second molecule, common to all amyloids, is apolipoprotein E (Apo E). Its role also is unclear, but an allele, Apo E4, is in statistically significant linkage dysequilibrium with sporadic cases of Alzheimer's disease (4). It has not been determined if the Apo E found in the brain deposits of people with Alzheimer's actually is E4 or another allele. Studies in people with familial Mediterranean fever (FMF) who have AA amyloid or familial amyloidotic polyneuropathy (FAP) with TTR amyloid indicate that the degree of deposition is not related to the presence of the Apo E4 allele. Thus it is possible that Apo E4 does not

TABLE 30-1
Amyloid Fibril Proteins and Their Precursors in Humans

Amyloid protein	Precursor	Systemic (S) or localized (L)	Syndrome or involved tissues
AL	Immunoglobulin light chain	S, L	Primary Myeloma-associated
AH	Immunoglobulin heavy chain	S, L	Primary Myeloma-associated
ATTR	Transthyretin	S	Familial (prototype Portuguese, Japanese, Swedish) polyneuropathy Senile systemic
		L?	Tenosynovium
AA	(Apo)serum AA	S	Secondary, reactive
Aβ_2m	β_2-microglobulin	S	Chronic hemodialysis
		L?	Joints
AApoAI	Apolipoprotein AI	S	Familial
		L	Aortic (atherosclerotic plaques)
AGel	Gelsolin	S	Familial (prototype Finish)
ALys	Lysozyme	S	Familial
AFib	Fibrinogen β-chain	S	Familial
ACys	Cystatin C	S	Familial (prototype Icelandic)
Aβ	Aβ protein precursor (AβPP)	L	Alzheimer's Disease, aging Familial (prototype Dutch)
APrP	Prion protein	L	Spongiform encephalopathies
ACal	(Pro)calcitonin	L	C-cell thyroid tumors
AIAPP	Islet amyloid polypeptide	L	Islets of Langerhans Insulinomas
AANF	Atrial natriuretic factor	L	Cardiac atria
APro	Prolactin	L	Aging pituitary Prolactinomas
AIns	Insulin	L	Iatrogenic
ALac[a]	Lactoferrin	L	Cornea
Amedin[a]	Lactadherin	L	Aorta-media
Aker	Keratin	L	Cutaneous
AKE	Keratoepithelin	L	Cornea

[a] Preliminary, awaiting confirmation
Reprinted with permission from Westermark P, Araki S, Benson MD, et al. Amyloid: Int J Exp Clin Invest 1999;6:64.

impart an increased risk for any form of amyloid deposition other than Alzheimer's disease.

A third common component of amyloids is the heparan sulfate proteoglycan (HSPG) perlecan, a normal constituent of basement membranes. Its role in the process of fibrillogenesis or deposition is unknown. However, the administration of low–molecular-weight analogs of HSPGs inhibits the development of experimental murine AA amyloid produced in the course of an inflammatory response. These compounds are being investigated as potential therapeutic agents for all forms of amyloid. Other basement membrane components, such as laminin, have been found in some amyloid deposits, but their universality and specificity have not been established beyond doubt.

Clinical Features
Amyloid L (AL) Disease
The systemic disorder most likely to come to the attention of rheumatologists in the United States is AL disease, either

TABLE 30-2
Diagnostic Yield of Tissue Sampling Procedures in the Major Amyloidoses

Tissue	AL	AA	ATTR
Subcutaneous fat aspiration[a]	112/145 (77%)	44/69[b] (64%)	26/27 (96%)
Rectal biopsy[a]	146/194 (75%)	54/65 (85%)	–
Bone marrow biopsy	221/394 (56%)	12/26 (46%)	–
Stomach and small bowel biopsy[c]	19/23 (83%)	15/16 (94%)	–
Labial salivary gland biopsy[c]	13/16 (81%)	13/14 (93%)	–

[a] Neither subcutaneous fat aspiration nor rectal biopsy is useful in $A\beta_2$-microglobulinemia.

[b] The results of subcutaneous fat aspiration in AA amyloid do not include patients with familial Mediterranean fever who are generally not positive from this site.

[c] Not broadly utilized; need confirmation by other clinical groups.

AL, amyloid L disease; AA, amyloid A disease; ATTR, transthyretin-associated familial disease.

Reprinted with permission from Buxbaum (1).

in the form of primary amyloidosis or in the course of multiple myeloma (5). The usual presentation is nephropathy with proteinuria or renal failure. The renal disease may be severe, occurring as full-blown nephrotic syndrome, or relatively mild. True nephropathic proteinuria must be distinguished from the excretion of large amounts of free monoclonal L-chains, sometimes seen in light-chain myeloma, which may have no pathogenic effect or may form massive tubular casts with resultant renal failure (myeloma kidney). In AL urine, the monoclonal component usually is minor in the glomerular-leakage pattern of proteinuria. The amount of urinary protein may diminish with the onset of renal insufficiency. Occasionally, renal tubular disorders precede renal failure, and both concentration and acidification defects have been described. Hypertension can occur, and the kidneys may be normal in size, small, or enlarged. As in all forms of proteinuric nephropathy, intravenous urography should be carried out with care, if at all.

The second most common presentation of AL disease is cardiomyopathy. The earliest echocardiographic abnormality appears to be diastolic dysfunction, with a change in the flow patterns to a state in which the atrial component to ventricular filling is increasingly important. This change also occurs during the course of normal aging, and may not be diagnostic in elderly patients. In advanced disease, there are noncompliant hemodynamics, thickening of the interventricular septum and valve leaflets, and the presence of "sparkling" of the ventricular echoes. Ultimately, a restrictive cardiomyopathy picture emerges. The presence of cardiac amyloid can be established by endomyocardial biopsy, followed by staining with the appropriate immunohistochemical reagents to identify deposition of monoclonal L-chain or other forms of amyloid. Radioactive technetium scanning has been advocated as a diagnostic screen for cardiac amyloid deposition, but the results have been inconsistent (6). Coronary deposition of AL and AA has been noted, but myocardial deposits of AA are less common. Digoxin

and nifedipine toxicity have been reported in people with cardiac amyloid deposition. Evidence suggests that these drugs are bound to the fibrils, and their effective concentrations disproportionately increase in the myocardial deposits.

About 20% of people with AL amyloid have a dominant neuropathic presentation. Symptoms are sensorimotor, with the first manifestation frequently being carpal tunnel syndrome. The lower extremities may be involved. Biopsy of an involved nerve may reveal amyloid deposition, but examination of an asymptomatic sural nerve is not a high-yield procedure. Carpal tunnel syndrome is only rarely associated with AL disease in the absence of other symptoms, although it may be the presenting complaint and precede other manifestations by a significant time period. Amyloid deposits have been found in some people with carpal tunnel syndrome who have no other signs of systemic disease, even after long periods of observation (7). TTR amyloid is the most common form of isolated carpal tunnel amyloid deposition and may occur in the absence of other clinically significant organ involvement. However, only 2%–3% of people requiring carpal tunnel release due to symptomatic median nerve compression, in the absence of systemic disease, have any form of amyloid in the tissue (8).

Periarticular amyloid deposition, presenting as pseudoarthrosis, has been reported in AL disease. Joint effusions may be present, with amyloid fibrils found in fluid obtained by arthrocentesis. A soft-tissue "shoulder pad sign" may be the major physical finding.

A potentially fatal complication of AL disease is an acquired deficiency of clotting factor X. In vivo studies suggest the factor may be bound to the fibrils in the deposits in some patients.

Organ failure produced by extensive amyloid deposition is treated by supportive measures. Patients with end-stage renal disease have undergone dialysis and renal transplantation, with reasonable responses (9). If precursor synthesis is not abrogated, however, the transplanted organ will show evidence of recurrent disease within four years.

Randomized prospective trials of melphalan and prednisone in regimens similar to those used in the treatment of multiple myeloma have shown enhanced survival (10). Colchicine alone or added to the regimen had no effect. The data suggest that, in the absence of contraindications, all AL patients should be offered treatment with these agents. Preliminary studies have shown promising results from more intensive chemotherapy in AL disease (11). However, it is apparent that individuals with significant cardiac involvement do not tolerate the high-intensity treatment regimen. Some anthracycline compounds may inhibit the process of fibrillogenesis without affecting the proliferative capacity of the immunoglobulin-producing cells (12,13). The mechanism of the inhibition is unknown. Although the initial trials seemed promising, toxicity has been problematic, and data demonstrating statistically significant prolonged survival have not been published.

In most people with AL disease, serum and/or urine immunoelectrophoresis reveals the monoclonal immunoglobulin (Ig) precursor. The chemical features of Ig light chains that render them amyloidogenic have been under intense investigation from the time they were identified as amyloid precursors. Fibrils from the deposits of 60 people with AL have been obtained in sufficient quantity to establish the subunit size, L-chain class and subclass, and in many cases, partial or full amino-acid sequence (14). Lambda chains are the precursor more than twice as frequently as are kappa chains. Fibrils belonging to all L-chain, V-region subclasses have been identified. In comparison with all human L-chains that have been sequenced, serum and urine L-chains and fibrils from patients with AL disease have shown statistically significant increases in the proportion of proteins belonging to the $V_\lambda 6$ and $V_\kappa 1$ subclasses. Most deposits contain L-chain fragments that begin with a normal amino terminus. Fewer than 10% contain only intact L-chains. About one-quarter contain both intact chains and one or more fragments, whereas 10% contain fragments 12 kDa or smaller. The last observation suggests why 10%–15% of AL tissue deposits may not stain with commercially available antisera specific for L-chain constant region determinants. These data are most consistent with some form of proteolysis playing a major role in the pathogenesis of disease; however, biosynthetic experiments suggest a possible role for the synthesis of abnormal chains. Marrow cells from all patients, including the 10%–20% who show no monoclonal L-chains in the serum or urine, synthesize excess, free L-chains. The aberrant products may be smaller, as a result of fragment synthesis or intracellular degradation, or larger, as a result of glycosylation. Analyses comparing amyloidogenic and nonamyloidogenic L-chains suggest that certain substitutions at particular positions may result in more amyloidogenic structures (15).

A second, related condition called light chain (or light and heavy chain) deposition disease shares many of the clinical features of AL (16). Renal and cardiac deposition of IgL or L- and H-chain–related molecules that do not bind Congo red have been reported in approximately 5% of people with multiple myeloma and in some people without clinical evidence of myeloma. In the absence of Congo-red staining, the diagnosis can be made by immunofluorescent or immunohistochemical demonstration of the monoclonal deposits, accompanied by the characteristic electron microscopic appearance.

Amyloid ß₂-Microglobulin (Aß₂m) Disease

The second form of amyloid deposition associated with a significant articular presentation is the deposition of β_2-microglobulin–related fibrils in patients with chronic renal disease (17). Originally, in all reported cases, people presenting with joint pain, carpal tunnel syndrome, and osteonecrosis had been on dialysis, usually for periods longer than seven years. More recently, the condition has been reported after shorter periods of renal support, and at least one case has been identified in which the patient had not been dialyzed. In each case, the deposited fibril protein was found to be $\beta_2 m$, the 12.5-kDa polypeptide component of class I proteins of the major histocompatibility complex. The subunit is an intact polypeptide with a normal amino-acid sequence. It may be deposited either as a monomer or as dimers; it sometimes shows evidence of nonenzymatic glycation (18). It has been suggested that there is active monocyte/macrophage participation in the pathogenesis of deposition, rather than deposition being a result of decreased renal clearance. Subcutaneous fat aspiration is not useful in this form of systemic deposition.

Amyloid A (AA) Disease

The third rheumatologically associated form of amyloidosis is AA, which is found in people with such chronic infectious diseases as tuberculosis and osteomyelitis, and such noninfectious inflammatory diseases as rheumatoid arthritis (RA) and FMF. The AA protein was unknown before its discovery as the main component in inflammation-associated amyloid deposits (19). The fibril has a serum precursor called serum amyloid A (SAA), which has a polypeptide weight of 12.5 kDa. The precursor circulates as an apoprotein of high-density lipoprotein (HDL) in a molecular complex of about 250 kDa. It appears to play a role in cholesterol metabolism during the inflammatory process and behaves as an acute-phase reactant in all species in which it has been studied (20). Serum AA is synthesized primarily in the liver in response to elevated levels of the cytokine interleukin-6. The deposited fibril subunit has a normal sequence, with a molecular size of 7.5 kDa, although a range of polypeptides has been found in various preparations.

In much of the world, AA is the most common form of amyloidosis, largely related to the frequency of such chronic infectious diseases as leprosy, tuberculosis, and osteomyelitis. In the United States, AL is the most common systemic amyloidosis and AA usually occurs in the context of chronic, noninfectious, inflammatory disease. Older autopsy studies indicate that as many as 25% of patients with RA had significant tissue amyloid deposits, with the severity of the deposition correlated with the extent and duration of disease. More recent analyses by rectal biopsy or subcutaneous fat aspiration in the United States and the United Kingdom have shown that about 5% of people with RA have detectable deposits, with perhaps one-third of these people displaying clinical disease, usually related to renal or hepatic deposition. Frequencies from some countries appear to be somewhat higher. It is not clear whether this reflects environmental factors, genetic background, or less adequate control of the inflammatory disease. Amyloid renal disease was the cause of 10% of the deaths in people with RA during a 10-year period when 35% of the initial 1000 patients died from all causes (21).

Amyloid A has been associated with virtually every form of inflammatory arthropathy. One possible exception is systemic lupus erythematosus, in which reports of amyloid deposition are rare. The frequency in the course of juvenile rheumatoid arthritis is higher in Europe (5%–10%) than it is in the United States (1%). Polymorphisms in the SAA gene may be associated with the propensity for certain individuals to develop AA amyloidosis in the course of chronic inflammatory disease (22,23).

Investigations of the genetic predisposition toward AA deposition have been encouraged by the discovery that AA protein was the amyloid found in some well-defined groups of patients with the autosomal recessive disorder FMF. Virtually all Sephardic Jews and many Turks who display the clinical features of the disease (i.e., episodes of fever, arthralgias, and abdominal or pleuritic inflammation) develop renal amyloidosis, usually by the end of their second decade. Ashkenazi Jews, Armenians, and other groups display the episodic inflammatory disease but do not develop amyloid as readily. The inflammatory disease is caused by mutations in the MEFV gene on chromosome 16, which encodes the protein pyrin/marenostrin; this gene's function has not been determined. It is unclear whether the dichotomy in the occurrence of amyloid is related to ethnic variation in the distribution of the mutations within MEFV, an inability to process the SAA produced in the course of the inflammation, or the production of a dominant amyloidogenic isoform. It has been established that daily colchicine administration can abort acute episodes and the development of amyloid in susceptible individuals, if the colchicine is administered before renal disease develops (24).

Aging and Amyloid

Five different anatomic sites of amyloid deposition have been associated with aging, apparently without predisposing disease. The fibril precursors have been identified in all of them: the beta protein of Alzheimer's disease (brain), islet-associated polypeptide (pancreas) associated with type II diabetes mellitus, atrial natriuretic factor (isolated atrial amyloid), and transthyretin [senile systemic (cardiac) amyloid]. The aorta is the fifth site where amyloids related to two precursors are seen. Medin, a fragment of the milk-fat globule protein lactadherin, has been identified as a precursor of human

aortic medial amyloid, while the amyloid associated with atherosclerotic plaques is derived from APO A1. All precursors appear to be of the wild-type protein structure, although the aortic deposits are composed of fragments.

Mutant forms of the Aβ protein, TTR and Apo A1 have been associated with more severe, autosomal dominant forms of amyloid deposition. Abnormal accumulation of the Aβ protein and the amyloid precursor protein (AβPP) have been identified in the rimmed vacuoles in muscle from patients with inclusion body myositis. The mutant TTRs produce severe sensorimotor and autonomic neuropathy, vitreopathy, cardiomyopathy, and nephropathy. Some people with FAP related to TTR mutations have come to the attention of rheumatologists when they present with Charcot joints.

Familial Amyloidosis

Other rare, familial, autosomal dominant forms of amyloidosis have been associated with the deposition of a mutant form of gelsolin, an actin-binding protein found in the Finnish form of amyloidotic neuropathy and lattice corneal dystrophy; and with a mutation in the gene encoding cystatin C, a lysosomal proteinase inhibitor deposited in the cerebral blood vessels of Icelandic kindreds with hereditary cerebral hemorrhage with amyloid.

Three familial forms of amyloid are nephropathic. One is associated with a mutation in the Aα chain of fibrinogen, one with mutant APO A1, and one, the Ostertag form of renal amyloidosis, is caused by mutations in lysozyme (25).

Summary

What may one conclude after inspecting the family of amyloid fibrils, their precursors, and the diseases in which they occur? Data have suggested that many proteins have the capacity to form amyloid fibrils under the appropriate conditions. Study of the amyloidoses has allowed the identification of these molecules by the diseases they produce in humans. It is likely, but not certain, that the propensity to form amyloid is the price paid for selection of certain structural features of proteins that have proved useful in carrying out their physiologic functions in the course of evolution. Alternatively, it is possible that amyloidogenicity of some proteins, notably those that exhibit the prion-like property of self-replication, serves some as-yet undefined, evolutionary function.

JOEL BUXBAUM, MD

References

1. Buxbaum J. The Amyloidoses. In: Dieppe P, Klippel JH (eds). Textbook of Rheumatology, 2nd edition. London: Mosby, 1998; pp 27.1–27.10.
2. Gallo GR, Feiner HD, Chuba JV, Beneck D, Marion P, Cohen DH. Characterization of tissue amyloid by immunofluorescence microscopy. Clin Immunol Immunopathol 1986;39: 479–490.

3. Hawkins PN, Lavender JP, Pepys MB. Evaluation of systemic amyloidosis by scintigraphy with ^{125}I-labeled serum amyloid P component. N Engl J Med 1990;323:508–513.

4. Corder EH, Saunders AM, Strittmatter WJ, et al. Gene dose of apolipoprotein E type 4 allele and the risk of Alzheimer's disease in late onset families. Science 1993;261:921–923.

5. Kyle RA, Gertz MA. Primary systemic amyloidosis: clinical and laboratory features in 474 cases. Sem Hemat 1995;32:45-59.

6. Simons M, Isner JM. Assessment of relative sensitivities of noninvasive tests for cardiac amyloidosis in documented cardiac amyloidosis. Am J Cardiol 1992;68:425–427.

7. Kyle RA, Gertz MA, Linke RP. Amyloid localized to tenosynovium at carpal tunnel release. Immunohistochemical identification of amyloid type. Am J Clin Pathol 1992;97:250–253.

8. Bjerrum OW, Rygaard-Olsen C, Dahlerup B, et al. The carpal tunnel syndrome and amyloidosis. A clinical and histological study. Clin Neurol Neurosurg 1984;86:29–32.

9. Brown JH, Doherty CC. Renal replacement therapy in multiple myeloma and systemic amyloidosis. Postgrad Med J 1993;69:672–678.

10. Kyle RA, Gertz MA, Greipp PR, et al. A trial of three regimens for primary amyloidosis: colchicine alone, melphalan and prednisone, and melphalan, prednisone, and colchicine. N Engl J Med 1997;336:1202–1207.

11. Comenzo RL, Sanchorawala V, Fisher C, et al. Intermediate-dose intravenous melphalan and blood stem cells mobilized with sequential GMCSF or G-CSF alone to treat AL (amyloid light chain) amyloidosis. Br J Haematol 1999;104:553–559.

12. Merlini G, Anesi E, Garini P, et al. Treatment of AL amyloidosis with 4'-Iodo-4'-deoxydoxorubicin: an update [letter]. Blood 1999;93:1112–1113.

13. Gianni L, Bellotti V, Gianni AM, Merlini G. New drug therapy of amyloidoses: resorption of AL-type deposits with 4'-iodo-4'-deoxydoxorubicin. Blood 1995;86:855–861.

14. Buxbaum J. Mechanisms of disease: monoclonal immunoglobulin deposition. Amyloidosis, light chain deposition disease, and light and heavy chain deposition disease.. Hematol Oncol Clin North Am 1992;6:323–346.

15. Raffen R, Dieckman LJ, Szpunar M, et al. Physicochemical consequences of amino acid variations that contribute to fibril formation by immunoglobulin light chains. Protein Science 1999;8:509–517.

16. Buxbaum J, Gallo G. Nonamyloidotic monoclonal immunoglobulin deposition disease. Light-chain, heavy-chain, and light- and heavy-chain deposition diseases. Hematol Oncol Clin North Am 1999;13:1235–1248.

17. Gejyo F, Yamada T, Odani S, et al. A new form of amyloid protein associated with chronic hemodialysis was identified as β_2-microglobulin. Biochem Biophys Res Commun 1985;129:701–706.

18. Miyata T, Hori O, Zhang J, et al. The receptor for advanced glycation end products (RAGE) is a central mediator of the interaction of AGE-beta2microglobulin with human mononuclear phagocytes via an oxidant-sensitive pathway. Implications for the pathogenesis of dialysis-related amyloidosis. J Clin Invest 1996;98:1088–1094.

19. Levin M, Franklin EC, Frangione B, Pras M. The amino acid sequence of a major nonimmunoglobulin component of some amyloid fibrils. J Clin Invest 1972;51:2773–2776.

20. Artl A, Marsche G, Lestavel S, Sattler W, Malle E. Role of serum amyloid A during metabolism of acute-phase HDL by macrophages. Arterioscler Thromb Vasc Biol 2000;20: 763–772.

21. Mutru O, Laakso M, Isomaki H, Koota K. Ten year mortality and causes of death in patients with rheumatoid arthritis. Br Med J 1985;290:1797–1799.

22. Moriguchi M, Terai C, Koseki Y, et al. Influence of genotypes at SAA1 and SAA2 loci on the development and the length of latent period of secondary AA-amyloidosis in patients with rheumatoid arthritis. Human Genetics 1999;105:360–366.

23. Booth DR, Booth SE, Gillmore JD, Hawkins PN, Pepys MB. SAA1 alleles as risk factors in reactive systemic AA amyloidosis. Amyloid 1998;5:262–265.

24. Zemer D, Revach M, Pras M, et al. A controlled trial of colchicine in preventing attacks of familial Mediterranean fever. N Engl J Med 1974;291:932–934.

25. Buxbaum JN, Tagoe CE. The genetics of the amyloidoses. Ann Rev Med 2000;51:543–569.

31 NEOPLASMS OF THE JOINT

Although some neoplasms originate in the joint, others penetrate or metastasize to it. Pigmented villonodular synovitis and synovial chondromatosis are the most common proliferative disorders arising from within the joint. Other primary lesions are rare and include lipoma arborescens, synovial hemangiomas, intracapsular chondromas, and synovial chondrosarcomas. Synovial sarcoma and giant cell tumors are neoplasms that tend to extend into the joint. The malignancies that metastasize to bone also may metastasize to the joint.

Primary Joint Neoplasms

Pigmented Villonodular Synovitis

Pigmented villonodular synovitis (PVNS) is a rare proliferative disorder of unknown etiology that affects the synovial lining. It occurs in three forms: an isolated lesion involving the tendon sheaths (giant cell tumor of the tendon sheath); a solitary intra-articular nodule (localized PVNS); and a diffuse villous and pigmented lesion involving synovial tissue (diffuse PVNS) (1,2). This section focuses on the latter two forms.

The typical presentation is a 20–40-year-old patient who complains of a traumatic swelling of a single joint (3–8). The knee is involved 80% of the time. Some patients may experience pain, warmth, and stiffness in the joint (6,7,9). Mechanical symptoms, such as locking and instability, may develop, particularly if the joint contains a large pedunculated nodule (10). The symptoms typically are episodic or slowly progressive (6).

Results of laboratory studies, such as a complete blood count and erythrocyte sedimentation rate, are within normal limits and can help exclude infection and rheumatoid arthritis. Aspiration of the joint reveals a brown, red, or yellow fluid (6,8,11).

During the initial stages, plain radiographs reveal periarticular synovial swelling, absence of synovial calcification, normal bone density, and preservation of the cartilage space (12). Bone changes develop in the later stages. In joints with small synovial volumes (e.g., the hip), the villi will abut the bone and cause subtle erosions. As the villi grow, pressure within the joint capsule increases. The villi then invade the bone and juxta-articular cysts appear (13,14). If the disorder is not diagnosed and treated, joint destruction can ensue.

Due to deposition of hemosiderin, a magnetic resonance image (MRI) typically will show nodular foci of decreased signal on both T1 and T2 images (11). In cases of localized PVNS, the MRI will show the single nodular mass (5). It

also may show the extent of the disease, which helps the surgeon plan appropriate treatment.

If the diagnosis remains in question, an arthroscopic exam can show the gross appearance of the lesion. In its localized form, PVNS appears as a solitary, yellow, pedunculated nodule. The surface often is lobulated and cuts with a "buttery" feel. It often occurs on the anterior aspect of the knee and is similar in appearance to giant cell tumor of the tendon sheath (5,7).

In the diffuse form, the thickened synovium contains folds of villi and sessile or pedunculated nodules. The entire joint appears to be covered with brown and orange seaweed. The nodules have been described as "grape-like masses" protruding into the joint cavity. They typically are friable and bleed with minimal trauma. Some of the villi contain bulbous ends and give the appearance of a "straggly

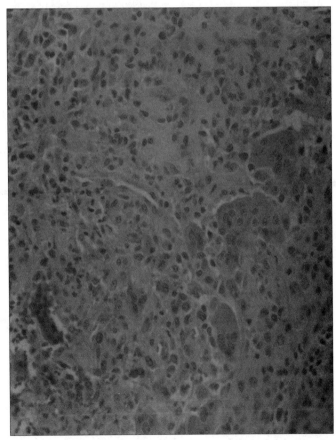

Fig. 31-1. Histology of pigmented villonodular synovitis. Giant cells, polyhedral cells with pale nuclei, foam cells (upper right), and hemosiderin deposits are seen.

beard." Other villi possess fine points and look like "ferns." The villi may invade bone or, less commonly, extend beyond the joint capsule and into the extra-articular soft tissue (3–5,15).

A biopsy can confirm the diagnosis of PVNS. All three forms of PVNS share a similar histology, characterized by hypercellular subsynovial connective tissue (16). The synovial lining is one to three layers thick and outlines the nodules and villi. In some areas, the ends of the villi fuse to form clefts.

The subsynovial stroma contains collagen-producing fibroblasts and phagocytic histiocytes. These cells are polyhedral and contain pale nuclei and abundant cytoplasm. They tend to proliferate and may be visualized in their mitotic stage. Some histiocytes will phagocytize hemosiderin; some will fuse to form multinucleated cells; and others will form foam cells. The hemosiderin-laden macrophages give PVNS its rusty brown color and are more common in the diffuse form. The lipid-filled foam cells account for the yellow color that dominates the localized form. The foam cells and hemosiderin-laden macrophages tend to localize to the periphery, and giant cells tend to be scattered throughout the areolar tissue (16) (Fig. 31-1).

Good results can be obtained with local excision of a solitary nodule (5). However, once diffuse pigmented villonodular synovitis (DPVNS) is diagnosed in a young patient, a total synovectomy is recommended (8,11).

If the MRI shows the lesion to be accessible by arthroscopy, arthroscopic resection may be worthwhile, as it is associated with relatively low morbidity (11). However, an open synovectomy may be necessary because lesions typically extend beyond the reach of the arthroscope (1,2,8).

In the past, synovectomy has been associated with recurrence rates as high as 40%. An incomplete synovectomy has been cited consistently as the main cause (1,6,8,14). Following open synovectomies via an anterior and posterior approach in knees with PVNS, an 8% recurrence rate and minimal morbidity was noted (8).

If DPVNS is diagnosed in an older patient with degenerative joint disease, an arthroplasty can give excellent results. In a young patient, arthrodesis may be considered as a salvage procedure.

Intra-articular injection of yttrium 90 has been used to treat DPVNS. Studies regarding its effectiveness are inconclusive, and its use remains experimental. It may prove useful as an adjunct to subtotal excision in extensive lesions in which complete excision would result in unacceptable morbidity. Prior to its use, patients ought to be informed that it can impair tissue healing, exacerbate stiffness, and possibly cause sarcomatous degeneration (6,8).

Synovial Chondromatosis

Synovial chondromatosis is a benign metaplastic disorder that occurs when subsynovial mesenchymal cells mature into chondroblasts instead of fibroblasts. Rather than producing collagen, these cells form nodules of cartilage. These nodules initially expand within the loose areolar tissue, then protrude into the joint cavity that is covered only by the synovial lining. Eventually, the cartilaginous nests are extruded and form loose bodies. Nourished by the synovial fluid, the chondroblasts continue to multiply. As the loose body enlarges, its central portion loses contact with the nutritional source and dies. The necrotic area then calcifies (17).

On gross exam, the synovial lining appears swollen because it contains multiple nodules of hyaline cartilage. These masses are of various sizes and are of a translucent, whitish-gray color (Fig. 31-2). The microscope shows the cartilage nests to be in different stages of maturity. Occasionally, a capillary may invade some of these areas and allow endochondral ossification to occur (17).

Synovial chondromatosis occurrs in three phases (18). During the initial phase, there are no loose bodies, but metaplastic activity occurs within the synovium. Loose bodies appear during the intermediate phase. During the final phase, metaplastic activity ceases, but multiple loose bodies persist.

The disease most often afflicts those in their third or fourth decade and occurs twice as often in men. It is almost always monarticular, and only rarely is it isolated to a bursa or tendon sheath. It affects the knee joint more than 50% of the time, although the hip, elbow, shoulder, ankle, and other joints may be involved (17,19). Swelling, discomfort, and decreased range of motion are the most common symptoms. As the disease progresses, such mechanical symptoms as locking and giving way may develop (19,20). Eventually, the pedunculated cartilaginous masses and loose bodies can destroy the joint surfaces and lead to more severe symptoms.

During the early stages, plain radiographs may show a nonspecific soft-tissue mass, due to the presence of nonmineralized cartilage. Bony erosions may be seen, secondary to focal pressure. During the second and third stages, multiple juxta-articular calcifications or loose bodies are seen (Fig. 31-3). These nodules typically are of a similar size

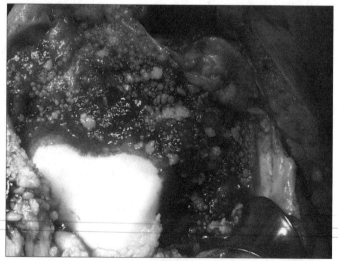

Fig. 31-2. Gross photograph of synovial chondromatosis showing calcified deposits in the knee joint.

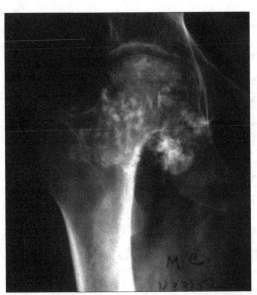

Fig. 31-3. Plain radiograph of synovial chondromatosis showing calcified cartilage in the hip joint.

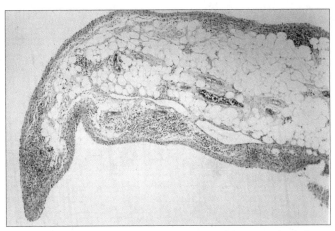

Fig. 31-4. Histology of lipoma arborescens showing multiple large adipose cells.

and uniformly scattered. Joint-space narrowing, osteophytes, sclerosis, and abundant, calcified loose bodies represent end-stage disease (21).

If osteonecrosis, rheumatoid arthritis, or post-traumatic or degenerative arthritis is noted, a diagnosis of secondary synovial chondromatosis must be considered. This diagnosis is especially likely if the presence of the disorder preceded the diagnosis of chondromatosis. In contrast to the primary form, secondary synovial chondromatosis shows fewer osteochondral bodies, which vary more in size, and does not recur or show histologic atypia (10,21,22).

Magnetic resonance imaging can help define the location of the cartilaginous nodules and is the best noninvasive study to confirm a diagnosis of synovial chondromatosis. An intermediate density on T1 sequences and an intermediate to high density on T2 sequences characterize the immature nodules. Calcified and ossified areas appear hypointense on both T1 and T2 images. The exception occurs when a loose body contains marrow fat, which appears as a hyperintense area on T1 (21,23).

Synovial chondromatosis is treated by removal of the loose bodies and excision of all abnormal synovium. Stiffness may occur, and recurrence rates have been reported as high as 11% after this treatment. In rare cases, the lesion may transform into a chondrosarcoma (20–22).

Other Primary Joint Tumors

A solitary intra-articular lipoma may occur but is extremely rare. More commonly, excessive intra-articular adipose tissue is due to lipoma arborescens (Fig. 31-4). This entity involves fatty synovial villi and often is associated with osteoarthritis, rheumatoid arthritis, and trauma. It usually occurs in the knee and causes joint swelling and pain (23). Synovectomy often is curative.

Synovial hemangioma usually occurs in children and

young adults and almost exclusively involves the knee. Plain films often show the pathognomonic phleboliths. Histologically, it is identical to the soft-tissue hemangiomas. Both the localized and diffuse forms can cause pain and hemarthrosis. This benign vascular neoplasm is treated by surgical excision (23,24).

Intracapsular solitary chondromas, like extra-articular chondromas, are benign cartilaginous neoplasms that may calcify. They may present as a firm intra-articular mass.

Synovial chondrosarcoma is exceptionally rare and may be primary or secondary to synovial chondromatosis. Treatment is wide surgical resection (22).

Secondary Joint Neoplasms

Synovial Sarcoma

Synovial sarcoma is an uncommon, highly malignant tumor involving synovial cells. It typically occurs near tendon and fascial planes, although on rare occasions, it may arise within or adjacent to a joint (17,25). The lower extremities are affected most frequently and the incidence is highest among those between the ages of 15 and 40 years (24).

Patients typically present complaining of a slowly growing soft-tissue mass. Approximately 50% of the time, the lesion is described as painful. Plain radiographs often reveal a large, lobulated, juxta-articular mass. Calcification is seen in up to one-third of cases and often has a diffuse speckled appearance. MRI shows nonspecific characteristics, but can narrow the diagnosis and define the lesion's anatomic location (23).

A biopsy often is required to confirm the diagnosis and will show the sarcoma to be one of three types. The biphasic form is the most common and involves obvious epithelial and mesenchymal differentiation. The plump cuboidal or tall columnar epithelial cells line mucin-filled clefts and cyst-like spaces. The round and oval epithelial cells form nests and cords. The fibroblasts are spindle-shaped and may be arranged in a manner similar to that seen in fibrosarcoma. Sometimes, the field is dominated largely by either the

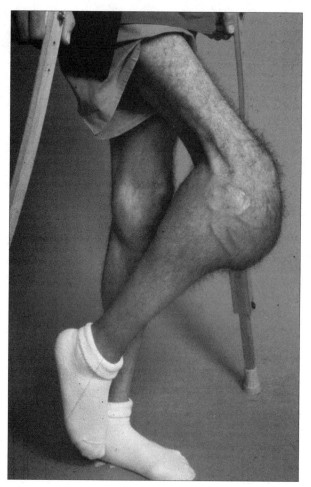

Fig. 31-5. Young man with giant cell tumor of the proximal tibia extending into the joint.

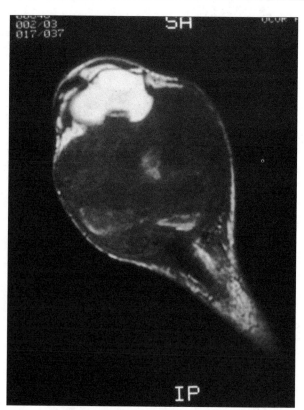

Fig. 31-6. Computed tomography scan of the giant cell tumor shown in Fig. 31-5. The tumor has completely eroded into the joint such that the tibia cannot be seen on this image.

epithelial cell (rarely) or the fibroblast (more commonly). The lesion then is categorized as monophasic. The monophasic form can be confused with other neoplasms of fibrous or epithelial origin and is thought by some to carry a worse prognosis. A rare, poorly differentiated type, represented histologically by numerous mitotic round cells, also has been described. Rapid growth and a very poor prognosis characterize this form (17,24,26).

Once synovial sarcoma is diagnosed, wide surgical resection with removal of any affected lymph nodes is indicated (24). Although adjuvant radiation and chemotherapy have improved the overall prognosis, the risk of regional and pulmonary metastasis remains high. Reports have shown the five- and 10-year survival rates to be 55% and 40%, respectively (27). Increased age, tumor size greater than 5 cm, and 10 or more mitotic figures per 10 high-powered fields are thought to increase the risk of metastasis and/or death (25).

Giant Cell Tumor

Giant cell tumor is a benign, but locally aggressive, tumor of unknown origin that most commonly affects 20–40 year olds. This lesion involves the knee (distal femur and proxi-

mal tibia) 50% of the time (24), and the distal radius and proximal humerus are the next most common sites. Plain radiographs show a purely lytic lesion that begins in the epiphysis and abuts the articular surface (17). It frequently extends into the joint (Figs. 31-5 and 31-6), tends to recur, and 1%–2% of the time, it will become malignant and metastasize to the lungs. The addition of phenol, bone graft, and methyl methacrylate to marginal resection can decrease the recurrence rate and allow the joint to be preserved. The use of a high-speed burr also can decrease the rate of recurrence. Radiation therapy should be reserved for inoperable tumors, as it is associated with malignant transformation (24).

TODD ATKINSON, MD
SEAN P. SCULLY, MD, PhD

References

1. *Rao AS, Vigorita VJ. Pigmented villonodular synovitis (giant cell tumor of the tendon sheath and synovial membrane): a review of eighty-one cases. J Bone Joint Surg Am 1984;66: 76–94.*

2. *Granowitz SP, D'Antonio J, Mankin HL. The pathogenesis and long term end results of pigmented villonodular synovitis. Clin Orthop 1976;114:335–351.*

3. *Docken WP. Pigmented villonodular synovitis: a review with illustrative case reports. Semin Arthritis Rheum 1979;9:1–22.*

4. Dorwart RH, Genant HK, Johnston WH, Morris JM. Pigmented villonodular synovitis of synovial joints: clinical, pathologic, and radiologic features. Am J Roentgenol 1984;143:877–885.

5. Bravo SM, Winalski CS, Weissman BN. Pigmented villonodular synovitis. Radiol Clin North Am 1996;34:311–326.

6. Byers PD, Cotton RE, Deacon OW, et al. The diagnosis and treatment of pigmented villonodular synovitis. J Bone Joint Surg Br 1968;50:290–305.

7. Flandry F, Hughston JC. Pigmented villonodular synovitis. J Bone Joint Surg Am 1987;69:942–949.

8. Flandry F, Hughston JC, Jacobson KE, Barrack RL, McCann SB, Kurtz DM. Surgical treatment of diffuse pigmented villonodular synovitis of the knee. Clin Orthop 1994;300:183–192.

9. Wu KK, Ross PM, Guise ER. Pigmented villonodular synovitis: a clinical analysis of twenty-four cases treated at Henry Ford Hospital. Orthopedics 1980;3:751–758.

10. Jaffe HL. Tumors and Tumorous Conditions of the Bone and Joints. Philadelphia: Lea & Febiger, 1958.

11. Michael RH. Pigmented villonodular synovitis. Orthop Nurs 1997;16(3):66–68.

12. Lewis RW. Roentgen diagnosis of pigmented villonodular synovitis and synovial sarcoma of knee joint. Radiology 1947;49:26.

13. Schwartz HS, Unni KK, Pritchard DJ. Pigmented villonodular synovitis. A retrospective review of affected large joints. Clin Orthop 1989;247:243–255.

14. Scott PM. Bone lesions in pigmented villonodular synovitis. J Bone Joint Surg Br 1968;50:306–311.

15. Goldman AB, DiCarlo EF. Pigmented villonodular synovitis: diagnosis and differential diagnosis. Radiol Clin North Am 1988;26:1327–1347.

16. Jaffe HL, Lichtenstein L, Sutro CJ. Pigmented villonodular synovitis, bursitis and tenosynovitis. Arch Pathol 1941;31:731–765.

17. Enneking WF. Clinical Musculoskeletal Pathology, 3rd ed. Gainesville, FL: University of Florida Press, 1990; pp 243–250, 255–259, 312–317, 439–441.

18. Milgram JW. Synovial osteochondromatosis. J Bone Joint Surg Am 1977;59:792–801.

19. Trias A, Quintana O. Synovial chondrometaplasia: review of world literature and a study of 18 Canadian cases. Can J Surg 1976;19:151-158.

20. Coles MJ, Tara HH. Synovial chondromatosis: a case study and brief review. Am J Orthop 1997;26:37–40.

21. Crotty JM, Monu JU, Pope TL. Synovial osteochondromatosis. Radiol Clin North Am 1996;34:327–342.

22. Wuisman PI, Noorda RJ, Jutte PC. Chondrosarcoma secondary to chondromatosis. Report of two cases and a review of the literature. Arch Orthop Trauma Surg 1997;116:307–311.

23. Laorr A, Helms CA. MRI of Musculoskeletal Masses. A Practical Text and Atlas. New York: Igaku-Shoin, 1997; pp 159–161, 275–280, 329–345.

24. Campanacci M. Bone and Soft Tissue Tumors. New York: Springer-Verlag, 1981; pp 99–135, 1109–1126, 1243–1252, 1289–1306.

25. Kaakaji Y, Valle DE, McCarthy KE, Nietzschman HR. Case of the day. Case 4: Synovial sarcoma. Am J Roent 1998;171: 868–870.

26. Machen KS, Easley KA, Goldblum JR. Synovial sarcoma of the extremities. A clinicopathologic study of 34 cases, including semi-quantitative analysis of spindled, epithelial, and poorly differentiated areas. Am J Surg Pathol 1999;23: 268–275.

27. Enzinger FM, Weiss SW. Soft Tissue Tumors, 2nd ed. St. Louis: Mosby, 1988; pp 638–688, 861–881.

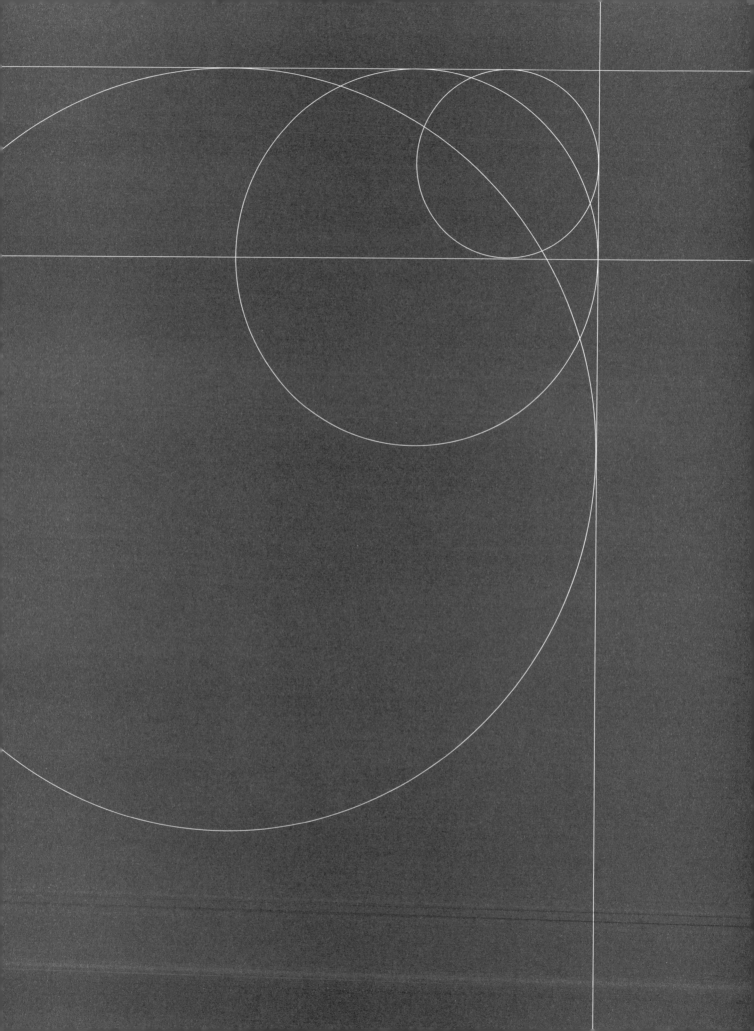

32 MUSCULOSKELETAL PROBLEMS IN DIALYSIS PATIENTS

People treated with prolonged hemodialysis now survive longer and, increasingly, develop musculoskeletal problems. Renal osteodystrophy, crystal deposition, and β_2-microglobulin amyloidosis are the major clinical entities.

Renal Osteodystrophy

Secondary Hyperparathyroidism

Hyperparathyroid disease is the most frequent form of osteodystrophy in hemodialysis patients (1). The predominant causes of uremic hyperparathyroidism are hyperphosphatemia, deficient generation of 1,25-dihydroxyvitamin D by the kidney, and low calcium intake and absorption (2). Monoclonal proliferation of parathyroid cells may be one explanation for the failure of medical management (3).

Preventive treatments include the use of high calcium concentrations in the dialysate and control of phosphatemia by dietary phosphorus restriction and the use of phosphorus binders, such as calcium carbonate with meals. Further enrichment of the diet with calcium supplements between meals and with vitamin-D derivatives may be necessary. The use of aluminum-containing phosphate binders is restricted drastically because of the risk of aluminum intoxication. Serum immunoreactive 1-84 parathyroid hormone (PTH) should be maintained at a concentration of 1.5 to three times the upper value of normal, to avoid adynamic bone disease.

Secondary hyperparathyroidism usually is asymptomatic, but may be the source of bone pain, polyarthralgia, or enthesopathy. Serum alkaline-phosphatase activity, pyridinoline, osteocalcin, and immunoreactive 1-84 PTH concentrations are increased. Serum phosphate levels usually are elevated, but the level of serum calcium varies. The most characteristic radiologic feature is subperiosteal resorption of bone, which is seen most clearly on the radial border of the middle phalanges (Fig. 32-1). Bone resorption may lead to acroosteolysis of the phalangeal tufts, widening of the acromioclavicular and sacroiliac joints or of the pubic symphysis, and small, articular erosions. The frequency of these erosions increases with dialysis duration (4), but they do not correlate with symptoms (5) and are not always related to hyperparathyroidism. More advanced hyperparathyroidism may be responsible for painful erosions at the sites of tendon attachment, which bear a high risk of tendon rupture. The skull may be affected and exhibit a "pepper pot" appearance. Osteosclerosis of the spine may be observed, with vertebral bodies showing a "rugger-jersey" appearance, due to resorption of bone from the central por-

tion. Brown tumors are rare and must be differentiated from amyloid erosions. Extraskeletal calcifications can develop, particularly in the eye, periarticular tissues, and small blood vessels or skin, leading to pruritus.

Secondary hyperparathyroidism can be treated by 1α hydroxylated vitamin-D derivatives, provided that calcium and phosphorus serum levels can be controlled and that no extensive soft-tissue or vascular calcifications develop. Pulse intravenous administration of these sterols has been reported as particularly effective, due to direct negative effect on PTH secretion obtained by high concentrations. The effect of calcimimetic compounds aimed at decreasing PTH secretion by acting on calcium-sensing receptors is under investigation (6). When hyperparathyroidism is too

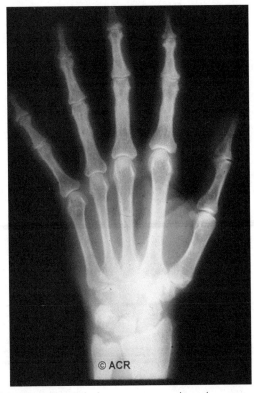

© ACR

Fig. 32-1. This radiograph demonstrates moderately severe osteopenia in the hand of a person with hyperparathyroidism. Subperiosteal bone resorption is marked at the radial aspect of the middle phalanges (the index and middle fingers typically are involved). Note that the distal phalanges of the thumb and index finger exhibit subperiosteal bone resorption and acrolysis. Reprinted from the Revised Clinical Slide Collection on the Rheumatic Diseases, with permission of the American College of Rheumatology.

advanced or resists medical management, subtotal parathyroidectomy is indicated.

Aluminum-Induced Bone Disease

Aluminum-induced bone disease follows intoxication with high aluminum content in the dialysate solution and/or prolonged ingestion of aluminum-containing phosphate binders. It has become very rare because these two factors usually are prevented. Affected patients typically experience bone pain, proximal muscle weakness, and pathologic fractures, particularly of first ribs (7). Serum calcium levels are normal or elevated, especially if the patient is treated with vitamin D. Serum alkaline phosphatase activity and intact PTH concentrations are normal or low. Aluminum serum levels are elevated spontaneously or after deferoxamine mesylate infusion. Bone histology demonstrates heavy staining for aluminum of the mineralization front and decreased cellular activity. Osteoid levels correlate with the two histologic forms of the disease; with increased osteid in osteomalacia, and normal osteid in adynamic bone disease. Elimination of the source of aluminum and treatment with deferoxamine mesylate can cure this disabling osteopathy.

Adynamic Bone Disease

Adynamic bone histology may develop in the absence of aluminum intoxication (1). It is the most frequent type of osteodystrophy in continuous ambulatory peritoneal dialysis patients. The major cause appears to be overtreatment of hyperparathyroidism. The condition may be associated with osteopenia and increased incidence of fractures.

Muscle Involvement

Muscle cramps are common during hemodialysis and are thought to be due to extracellular volume contraction (8). A proximal myopathy may affect dialysis patients, due to aluminum intoxication or abnormal vitamin D metabolism and, very rarely, to excessive phosphorus binding causing hypophosphatemia. Hyperparathyroidism may be responsible for arterial calcification and muscle infarctions.

Disorders of Microcrystalline Origin

Periarticular calcifications are common and are related to hyperphosphatemia, high serum calcium-phosphorus products, and secondary hyperparathyroidism. Such calcifications are composed of calcium phosphate (mainly apatite) crystals. They usually are asymptomatic, but apatite can induce acute articular or, more frequently, periarticular inflammatory episodes. Despite careful search for crystals and infectious agents, some acute joint and bursal effusions remain unexplained. Occasionally, calcium deposits grow into pseudotumor masses. Apatite deposition in dialysis patients may lead to joint erosions (9) and contribute to a destructive arthropathy of the spine (10).

Calcium oxalate crystal deposition can occur at various sites, including bone, synovium, and cartilage, and is one cause of synovial calcification or chondrocalcinosis in dialysis patients. This condition has been observed mainly in patients whose diets are supplemented with vitamin C, a precursor of oxalate (11). Gout and calcium pyrophosphate crystal deposition disease are rare, despite the frequency of hyperuricemia and gout before dialysis (5) and the presence of secondary hyperparathyroidism.

Bone and Joint Infections

Bone and joint infections are well-documented complications of hemodialysis and require urgent management with appropriate antibiotics (12). Immune defenses of patients treated with hemodialysis are impaired, and the arteriovenous fistula is a potential source of hematogenous spread. Intra- or periarticular corticosteroid injections also are an important source of infection and should be avoided. Unusual infections can include listeriosis associated with secondary iron overload after transfusions.

Dialysis Arthropathy and β_2-Microglobulin Amyloid

The deposition of β_2-microglobulin amyloid in articular and periarticular tissues of dialysis patients has been well-documented (12–14). Carpal tunnel syndrome, a prominent feature, usually is bilateral and severe enough to require surgery. A chronic, grossly symmetric arthropathy frequently is observed and includes chronic arthralgias, particularly of the shoulders, chronic joint swelling with noninflammatory effusions, recurrent hemarthrosis, Baker's cysts, and finger tendon tenosynovitis. Large subchondral bone erosions, predominantly of the wrist and hip at sites of synovium attachment or reflexion, may lead to pathologic fracture of the femoral neck. Shoulder pain may be related to amyloid thickening of the rotator cuff tendons or subacromial bursa, which can lead to a chronic impingement syndrome. Destructive arthropathy may involve the spine – and may lead to spinal cord or nerve root compromise – and large joints of the limbs. Some patients may develop a pseudorheumatoid arthropathy, with grossly symmetric amyloid infiltration and morning stiffness of short duration. The diagnosis can be suspected on the presence of multiple subchondral bone erosions or ultrasound demonstration of thickening of the rotator cuff tendon (15) and is established by examination of synovial fluid (16), as well as by biopsy. Systemic deposits are rare but may be responsible for intestinal hemorrhage or cardiac dysfunction.

Lack of β_2-microglobulin catabolism by the kidney and unsatisfactory elimination of the molecule through dialysis membranes are important in the pathogenesis of the disorder. β_2-microglobulin modified with advanced glycation products has been identified in deposits and shown to stimulate monocyte chemotaxis and macrophage secretion of tumor necrosis factor and interleukin 1 (17). β_2-microglobulin amyloid deposits have been observed even before the start of dialysis therapy (18), but the frequency of dialysis arthropathy increases with the patient age and length of survival, affecting up to 65% of individuals who have received 10 or more years of maintenance hemodialysis using standard cuprophane membranes, which are impermeable to β_2-microglobulin. The use of more permeable membranes may delay the onset of the disease, but does not prevent its development. Kidney transplantation halts disease progression, even though deposits persist, and improves the joint symptoms dramatically, probably as a consequence of steroid treatment (19).

THOMAS BARDIN, MD

References

1. Sherrard DJ, Hercz G, Pei Y, et al. The spectrum of bone disease in end-stage renal failure. An evolving disorder. Kidney Int 1993;43:436–442.

2. Hruska KA, Teitelbaum SL. Renal osteodystrophy. N Engl J Med 1995;333:166–174.

3. Arnold A, Brown MF, Urena P, Gaz RD, Sarfati E, Druëke T. Monoclonality of parathyroid tumors in chronic renal failure and in parathyroid hyperplasia. J Clin Invest 1995;95:2047–2053.

4. Rubin LA, Fam AG, Rubinstein J, Campbell J, Saiphoo C. Erosive azotemic osteoarthropathy. Arthritis Rheum 1984;27:1086–1094.

5. Chou CT, Wasserstein A, Schumacher HR Jr, Fernandez P. Musculoskeletal manifestations in hemodialysis patients. J Rheumatol 1985;12:1149–1153.

6. Coburn JW, Elangovan L, Goodman WG, Frazaô JM. Calcium-sensing receptor and calcimimetic agents. Kidney Int 1999;53(suppl 73):S52–S58.

7. Kriegshauser JS, Swee RG, McCarty JT, Hauser MF. Aluminum toxicity in patients undergoing dialysis: radiological findings and prediction of bone biopsy results. Radiology 1987;164:399–403.

8. Milutinovitch J, Graefe U, Follete WC, Scribner BH. Effect of hypertonic glucose on the muscular cramps of hemodialysis. Ann Intern Med 1979;90:926–928.

9. Schumacher HR, Miller JL, Ludivico C, Jessar RA. Erosive arthritis associated with apatite crystal deposition. Arthritis Rheum 1981;24:31–37.

10. Kuntz D, Naveau B, Bardin T, Drueke T, Treves R, Dryll A. Destructive spondylarthropathy in hemodialyzed patients: a new syndrome. Arthritis Rheum 1984;27:369–375.

11. Reginato AJ, Kurnik B. Calcium oxalate and other crystals associated with kidney diseases and arthritis. Semin Arthritis Rheum 1989;18:198–224.

12. Kay J, Bardin T. Osteoarticular problems of renal origin: disease related and iatrogenic. Baillière's Best Pract Res Clin Rheumatol 2000;14:285–305.

13. Bardin T, Drüeke T, Kuntz D: β_2-microglobulin amyloidosis. Rev Rhum Engl Ed 1994;61(suppl):1S–104S.

14. van Ypersele C, Drüeke T (eds). Dialysis Amyloid. New York: Oxford University Press, 1996.

15. Kay J, Benson CB, Lester S, et al. Utility of high-resolution ultrasound for the diagnosis of dialysis-related amyloidosis. Arthritis Rheum 1992;35:926–932.

16. Munoz-Gomez J, Gomez-Pérez R, Solé-Arques M, Llopart-Buisan E. Synovial fluid examination for the diagnosis of synovial amyloidosis in patients with chronic renal failure undergoing haemodialysis. Ann Rheum Dis 1987;46:324–326.

17. Miyata T, Inagi R, Iida Y, et al. Involvement of β_2-microglobulin modified with advanced glycation end products in the pathogenesis of hemodialysis-associated amyloidosis. J Clin Invest 1994;93:521–528.

18. Zingraff JJ, Noel LH, Bardin T, et al. Beta-2 microglobulin amyloidosis in chronic renal failure (letter). N Engl J Med 1990;323:1070–1071.

19. Bardin T, Lebail-Darné JL, Zingraff J, et al. Dialysis arthropathy: outcome after renal transplantation. Am J Med 1995;99:243–248.

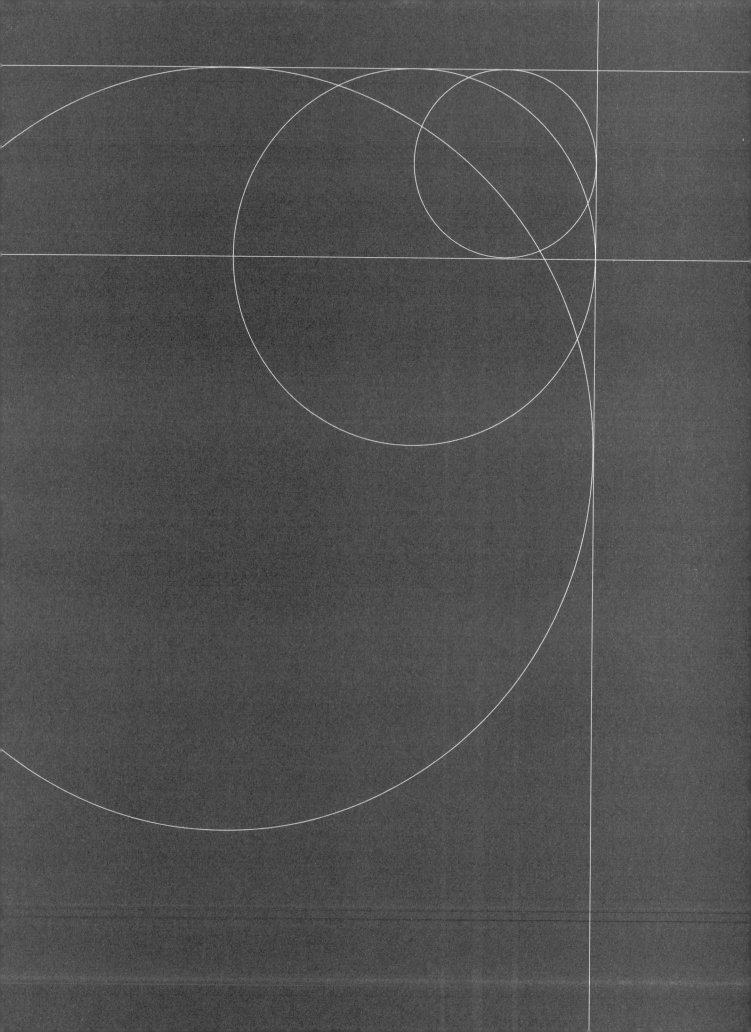

33 HERITABLE DISORDERS OF CONNECTIVE TISSUE

The molecular composition and organization of connective tissue, known as the extracellular matrix, are extraordinarily complex. Much remains unknown about the number, structure, map location, and regulation of genes that control synthesis, organization, and metabolism of this ubiquitous tissue. However, the genes that specify more than 195 proteins involved in connective-tissue metabolism and skeletal development have been mapped (1). Mutations in the genes for these proteins cause a variety of disorders. The heritable disorders of connective tissue (HDCT) follow Mendel's laws, but like many such disorders, show both considerable variability within and among families and genetic heterogeneity (2,3).

Some common disorders, such as osteoarthritis, osteoporosis, and aortic aneurysms, involve predominantly connective tissue and are mendelian in occasional families. For the majority of cases, however, multiple genes and other factors likely are important in cause and pathogenesis (4).

The phenotypic characterization of the HDCT, crude as it sometimes is, still outstrips biochemical or genetic understanding (5). More than 200 conditions are called HDCT. The more familiar ones have prevalences of 1 in 3000 to 1 in 50,000; many are less prevalent. More refined classification of the HDCT is unsatisfactory, and ultimately must be based on pathobiology. But several phenotypic groupings traditionally are used: 1) disorders of fibrous elements, such as osteogenesis imperfecta; 2) disorders of proteoglycan metabolism, including the mucopolysaccharidoses; 3) dysostoses and osteochondrodysplasias, such as achondroplasia (see Chapter 35); and 4) inborn errors of metabolism that secondarily affect connective tissue, such as homocystinuria and alkaptonuria.

Marfan Syndrome

People with Marfan syndrome (MFS) have abnormalities in multiple organs and tissues, especially the skeletal, ocular, cardiovascular, pulmonary, and central nervous systems. Diagnosis is based primarily on clinical features and the autosomal dominant inheritance pattern (6). The basic defect in all cases studied is in fibrillin 1, the principal constituent of extracellular microfibrils (7). The locus (FBN1) for this protein maps to 15q21. Microfibrils are ubiquitous, 10–14 nm structures that, in conjunction with tropoelastin, form elastic fibers. Thus, fibrillin is a functionally important molecule in any organ containing elastic fibers, such as arteries, ligaments, and lung parenchyma. In other tissues, such as the zonular fibers of the eye, at the epidermal-der-mal junction and in the perichondrium, microfibrils are not associated with elastin. Thus, defective fibrillin is consistent with the pleiotropic manifestations of the MFS.

The current challenges are to understand the molecular and cellular pathogenesis of each manifestation in MFS, and to understand the range of expression of fibrillin mutations, in MFS and other disorders distinct from MFS. Autosomal dominant ectopia lentis, autosomal dominant aortic aneurysm, and autosomal dominant tall stature are caused by mutations in FBN1 in the absence of MFS (8). Some patients with the Shprintzen-Goldberg syndrome have mutations in FBN1. Congenital contractural arachnodactyly is due to mutations in FBN2 on chromosome 5, a locus that specifies the other member of the fibrillin family of proteins.

Skeletal manifestations of MFS include excessive stature; abnormal body proportions with a long arm span and an abnormally low ratio of the upper segment to the lower segment (dolichostenomelia); elongated digits (arachnodactyly); anterior thoracic deformity (pectus excavatum, carinatum, or an asymmetric combination); abnormal vertebral column curvature (loss of thoracic kyphos resulting in "straight back" and scoliosis); hyperextensibility or, less often, congenital contractures of appendicular joints; protrusio acetabulae; and pes planus with a long, narrow foot. Most patients have myopia, and approximately half have subluxation of the lenses (ectopia lentis). The ascending aorta, beginning in the sinuses of Valsalva, gradually dilates in association with fragmentation of the medial elastic fibers; aortic regurgitation and dissection result and are the main causes of death. Mitral valve prolapse occurs in a majority and leads to severe mitral regurgitation in some, occasionally in childhood. Hernias are frequent; apical bullae lead to pneumothorax in 5%; and striae atrophicae over the pectoral, deltoid, and lumbar areas are a helpful diagnostic sign. Dural ectasia producing erosion of lower lumbar and sacral vertebrae usually is an incidental finding on computed tomography or magnetic resonance imaging, but may lead to pelvic meningoceles or radicular problems (9,10).

Management is both palliative and preventive. The size of the ascending aorta should be followed by echocardiography. β-adrenergic blockade is advisable to reduce stress on the aortic wall, and repair of the aortic root should be undertaken when the aortic diameter is greater than twice expected (about 55 mm in the adult) (11). Scoliosis should be managed aggressively with bracing in the child and adolescent; when curvature exceeds about 40°, surgical stabilization should be considered (12). Hormonal advancement of pubarche can modulate excessive stature and reduce the time when vertebral curvature can worsen; this therapy has been used occasionally in young girls, but rarely in boys. Most patients do not dislocate joints, but in those who do, the patella is the most common dislocation. People with MFS may be predisposed to develop degenerative arthropathy and osteoporosis in middle age. Women with MFS are at increased risk of aortic dissection and rupture during pregnancy; an aortic-root diameter greater than 40 mm is a contraindication to pregnancy.

Homocystinuria

Homocystinuria usually refers to an inborn error in the metabolism of methionine due to deficient activity of the enzyme cystathionine β-synthase. Clinical features are similar superficially to those of MFS and include ectopia lentis, tall stature, dolichostenomelia, arachnodactyly, and anterior chest and spinal deformity (13). Generalized osteoporosis, "tight" joints, arterial and venous thrombosis, malar flush, mental retardation, and autosomal recessive inheritance are features of homocystinuria not consistent with MFS, whereas aortic aneurysm and mitral prolapse are not features of homocystinuria. Back pain and vertebral collapse due to osteoporosis occur in some patients. Most patients have no specific arthropathy.

The pathogeneses of the three cardinal manifestations – mental retardation, connective tissue disorder, and thrombosis – are not understood. One hypothesis holds that sulfhydryl groups of homocysteine and methionine interfere with collagen cross-linking. If true, this is a form of thiolism such as occurs from prolonged administration of penicillamine, a compound structurally similar to homocysteine. Fibrillin is rich in cysteine, and intra- and interchain disulfide bonds are crucial to the formation and function of microfibrils. Some of the phenotypic resemblance of homocystinuria to MFS may be due to disruption of microfibrils by the reactive sulfhydryl moiety of homocysteine (14).

Approximately one-half of patients respond biochemically and clinically to large doses of vitamin B_6 (usually more than 50 mg pyridoxine per day), an obligate cofactor for cystathionine β-synthase. Adequate levels of folate and vitamin B_{12} are required for therapeutic and biochemical response. Pre-existing mental retardation and ectopia lentis are not reversed by pyridoxine treatment in patients who show biochemical correction, emphasizing the need for early diagnosis and therapy. Early diagnosis is feasible because many states include testing for elevated blood methionine as part of newborn screening. Unfortunately, some pyridoxine-responders may escape detection in the typical screening protocols. In pyridoxine-nonresponders, a low methionine diet and oral betaine therapy (to stimulate remethylation of homocysteine to methionine) are the usual treatments; this approach can be successful if the diet and vitamin are tolerated.

Stickler Syndrome

Stickler syndrome is a relatively common, autosomal dominant condition with severe, progressive myopia; vitreal degeneration; retinal detachment; progressive sensorineural hearing loss; cleft palate; mandibular hypoplasia; hyper- and hypomobility of joints; epiphyseal dysplasia; and potential disability from joint pain, dislocation, or degeneration (15). This condition, also called progressive arthroophthalmopathy, is underdiagnosed, in part due to patients often not having the full syndrome and in part due to the clinician's failure to obtain a detailed family history that might suggest a hereditary condition. The diagnosis should be strongly considered in any infant with congenitally enlarged ("swollen") wrists, knees, or ankles, particularly when associated with the Robin anomalad (hypognathia, cleft palate, and glossoptosis); any young adult with degenerative hip disease; and anyone suspected of MFS who has hearing loss, degenerative arthritis, or retinal detachment. The Stickler syndrome can be caused by mutations in at least four genes, three of which have been identified (16). Mutations in the α1(II) or the α1(XI) procollagen loci (COL2A1 and COL11A2, respectively) cause classic Stickler syndrome. These two genes are expressed in cartilage and the vitreous, in which both types II and XI collagen are prominent. A form of Stickler syndrome in which ocular features are absent is due to mutations in α2(XI) procollagen (COL11A2); this protein is a component of type XI collagen only in cartilage and not in the vitreous. Some families show genetic linkage to none of these three genes. Variability in clinical features among families is much more extensive than within a family, which likely reflects the genetic heterogeneity (17).

Ehlers-Danlos Syndromes

The Ehlers-Danlos syndromes (EDS) are a group of disorders whose wide phenotypic variability is due largely to extensive genetic heterogeneity. The cardinal features relate to the joints and skin: hyperextensibility of skin, easy bruisability, increased joint mobility, and abnormal tissue fragility (18,19). Internal manifestations tend to occur only in specific types of EDS. Six main EDS types are accepted, based on phenotypic and inheritance characteristics (Table 33-1), but numerous other clinical types occur (20). Within individual types, however, biochemical studies have demonstrated considerable heterogeneity. Extensive phenotypic and biochemical characterization nonetheless fails the clinician as often as it helps; approximately one-half of patients who have at least one "cardinal" feature defy categorization.

Ehlers-Danlos, Classical Type

People with classical type EDS (formerly, types I and II) have generalized hyperextensibility of joints and skin; bruisability and fragility of the skin, with gaping wounds from minor trauma; and poor retention of sutures. Congenital dislocation of the hips in the newborn, habitual dislocation of joints in later life, joint effusions, clubfoot, and spondylolisthesis are all consequences of loose-jointedness. Hemarthrosis and "hemarthritic disability" have been described and are analogous to the bruisability of the skin

TABLE 33-1
Ehlers-Danlos Syndromes

Type	Former name	Clinical features[a]	Inheritance	OMIM #(s)[b]	Molecular defect
Classical	EDS I and II	Joint hypermobility; skin hyperextensibility; atrophic scars; smooth, velvety skin; subcutaneous spheroids	AD	130000 (EDS I)	Structure of type V collagen (EDS I)
Hypermobility	EDS III	Joint hypermobility; some skin hyperextensibility; ± smooth and velvety skin	AD	130010 (EDS II) 130020	? COL5A1, COL5A2 (EDS II) ?
Vascular	EDS IV	Thin skin; easy bruising; pinched nose; acrogeria; rupture of large and medium caliber arteries, uterus, and large bowel	AD	130050 (225350) (225360)	Deficient type III collagen
Kyphoscoliotic	EDS VI	Joint hypermobility; congenital, progressive scoliosis; scleral fragility with globe rupture; tissue fragility; aortic dilatation; MVP	AR	225400	
Arthrochalasia	EDS VIIA and VIIB	Joint hypermobility, severe, with subluxations;congenital hip dislocation; skin hyperextensibility; tissue fragility	AD	130060	No cleavage of N-terminus of type I procollagen 2° mutations in COL1A1 or COL1A2
Dermatosparaxis	EDS VIIC	Severe skin fragility; decreased skin elasticity; easy brusing; nernias; premature rupture of fetal membranes	AR	225410	No cleavage of N-terminus of type I procollagen 2° deficiency of peptidase
Unclassified types	EDS V	Classic features	XL	305200	?
	EDS VIII	Classic features and peridontal disease	AD	130080	?
	EDS X	Mild classic features, MVP	?	225310	?
	EDS XI	Joint instability	AD	147900	?
	EDS IX	Classic features; occiptial horns	XL	309400	allelic to Menkes syndrome

[a] Listed in order of diagnostic importance.
[b] Entries in Online Mendelian Inheritance in Man (1).
   AD, autosomal dominant; AR, autosomal recessive; XL, X-linked; MVP, mitral valve prolapse; OMIM, Online Mendelian Inheritance in Man; ?, unknown.

in this syndrome. Scoliosis sometimes is severe. This type of EDS is inherited as an autosomal dominant trait with wide variability. Management of classical EDS stresses prevention of trauma and great care in treating wounds. Pregnancies of fetuses with EDS are prone to premature rupture of membranes. This form of EDS is genetically heterogenous, with mutations in *COL1A1*, *COL5A1*, and *COL5A2* all causing the phenotype (21).

Ehlers-Danlos, Hypermobility Type

Hypermobility type EDS (formerly type III) has less marked skin involvement than the classical form; joint hyperextensibility ranges from extreme to moderate. Many people with mild joint laxity and without joint instability, are labeled as having this type, particularly if relatives show a similar manifestation (22). In some cases, such labeling does more harm than good, unless it is made quite clear that little disability, if any, is likely.

Ehlers-Danlos, Vascular Type

Vascular-type EDS (formerly type IV) is by far the most serious type because of a propensity for spontaneous rupture of arteries and bowel (23). The unifying pathogenetic theme is abnormal production of type III collagen. A variety of mutations have been described in the *COL3A1* gene. Skin involvement is variable: thin, nearly translucent skin is present in some, and mildly hyperextensible skin is the only feature in others. Joint laxity also varies, but may be limited to the digits. Inheritance usually is autosomal dominant, and many cases are sporadic occurrences in their pedigree, suggesting they are heterozygous for a new mutation. The majority of patients with the vascular type of EDS have a relative deficiency of type III collagen, compared with type I collagen, and this deficiency is detectable in cultured dermal fibroblasts. Because this test is relatively straightforward to conduct, and because the results are highly specific for this condition, the diagnosis often is confirmed biochemically (23).

Ehlers-Danlos, Kyphoscoliosis Type

Kyphoscoliosis-type EDS (formerly type VI) is characterized by fragility of the ocular globe, marked joint and skin hyperextensibility, a propensity to severe scoliosis, and autosomal recessive inheritance. Collagen in skin contains little hydroxylysine because of a deficiency of the enzyme that hydroxylates selected lysyl residues in the nascent collagen chains. Vitamin C is a necessary cofactor of lysyl hydroxylase, and pharmacologic doses may be beneficial.

Ehlers-Danlos, Arthrochalasia Type

Arthrochalasia-type EDS (formerly type VIIA and VIIB) is typified by profound loose-jointedness, congenital dislocations, moderately short stature, and variable skin involvement. The underlying defect is an inability to cleave the N-propeptide from type I procollagen, a process that is necessary for conversion to mature collagen. Mutations at the cleavage site of α1(I) and α2(I) procollagens can cause this phenotype; the procollagen defects behave as dominant traits.

Ehlers-Danlos, Dermatosparaxis Type

Dermatosparaxis-type EDS (formerly type VIIC) is a recessive condition due to deficiency of the N-propeptidase that cleaves type I procollagen. The disorder affects primarily skin and fascia, and joints are affected little.

Joint Instability Syndromes

The cardinal manifestation of *familial joint instability*, which once was classified as an Ehlers-Danlos type, is instability of numerous appendicular joints. Recurrent dislocation is the usual presenting complaint (24). Joint hyperextensibility is variable but usually mild, and skin involvement is uncommon. This syndrome is not rare and often is associated with considerable disability. Autosomal dominant inheritance with marked variability within a family is the rule, emphasizing the need for a comprehensive family history, including examination of close relatives if possible. The biochemical defect is unknown.

Larsen syndrome is characterized by congenital dislocations; a characteristic facies of prominent forehead, depressed nasal bridge, and widely spaced eyes; joint dislocations; and skeletal dysplasia (25,26). Dislocation occurs at the knees (characteristically, anterior displacement of the tibia on the femur), hips, and elbows. The metacarpals are short, with cylindrical fingers that lack the usual tapering. Cleft palate, hydrocephalus, abnormalities of spinal segmentation, and moderate to severe short stature have occurred in some. Several instances of multiple affected siblings with normal parents are known, suggesting autosomal recessive inheritance; however, parent–child involvement also occurs, consistent with dominant inheritance. The recessive form is associated more often with severe short stature and neurologic complications of spinal deformity. The gene for the dominant form has been mapped to chromosome 3p21.1-p14.1.

Osteogenesis Imperfecta Syndromes

Several phenotypically distinct osteogenesis imperfecta (OI) syndromes exist (2,5,27). The disorders share osseous, ocular, dental, aural, and cardiovascular involvement. Classification is based on inheritance pattern and clinical criteria (Table 33-2).

Type I Osteogenesis Imperfecta

Type I is the most common form of OI. It is autosomal dominant and is associated with considerable intrafamilial variability. One patient might be markedly short of stature, with frequent fractures and much disability, while an affected relative leads an unencumbered, vigorous life. Defects in the genes for both α1(I) and α2(I) procollagen can cause this syndrome.

Type II Osteogenesis Imperfecta

Type II encompasses the classic congenital variants, near-

TABLE 33-2
Osteogenesis Imperfecta Syndromes

Type	Clinical features	Inheritance	OMIM #[a]	Basic defects
I	Fractures variable in number; little deformity; stature normal or nearly so; blue sclerae; hearing loss common but not always present; DI uncommon	AD	166200	Typically, one nonfunctional *COL1A1* allele
II	Lethal in utero or shortly after birth; many fractures at birth involving ribs (may appear beaded) and other long bones; little mineralization of calvarium; pulmonary hypertension	AD	166210	*COL1A1* or *COL1A2*: typically substitution of glycyl residues; occasionally deletions of a portion of the triple-helical domain
		AR	259400	Deletion in *COL1A2* plus nonfunctional allele
III	Fractures common, but long bones progressively deform starting in utero; stature markedly reduced; sclerae often blue but become lighter with age; ID and hearing loss common	AD	259420	One (single amino acid substitution) or rarely two mutations in *COL1A1* and/or *COL1A2*
		AR (rare)	259440	
IV	Fractures common; stature usually reduced; bone deformity common but rarely severe; scleral hue normal to grayish; hearing loss variable; DI common	AD	166220; 166240	Point mutations in *COL1A1* or *COL1A2*; exon skipping mutations in *COL1A2*

[a] Entry in Online Mendelian Inheritance in Man (OMIM; 1)
DI, dentinogenesis imperfecta; AD, autosomal dominant; AR, autosomal recessive

ly all of which are lethal in infancy, if not in utero. Most cases arise as the result of a new mutation (the phenotype being dominant transmissable, if the patient lived and reproduced) in either α1(I) or α2(I) procollagen. A "dominant-negative" model explains the severe phenotype produced by a heterozygous mutation. Rare patients have affected siblings and normal parents; in some of these cases, a parent has been shown to have the mutation at low level in the gonads, resulting in the potential for multiple affected offspring.

Type III Osteogenesis Imperfecta
Type III comprises severe skeletal deformity, kyphoscoliosis, short stature, and variable fractures. It usually occurs sporadically, suggesting new mutations or autosomal recessive inheritance.

Type IV Osteogenesis Imperfecta
Type IV is similar phenotypically and genetically to type I, only less common, not associated with blue sclerae, and having fewer fractures, on average.

Natural History
The natural histories of skeletal involvement among these types bear similarities. "Brittle bones" are a unifying theme; sometimes fractures occur in utero, particularly in type II, and permit radiographic antenatal diagnosis. In such cases, the limbs are likely to be short and bent at birth, and multiple rib fractures give a characteristic "beaded" appearance on radiographs. Other patients with types I or IV have few or no fractures, although the presence of blue sclerae, opalescent teeth, or hearing loss indicates the presence of the mutant gene. Brittleness and deformability result from a defect in the collagenous matrix of bone. The skeletal aspect of OI is, therefore, a hereditary form of osteoporosis. "Codfish vertebrae" (scalloping of the superior and inferior vertebral bodies by pressure from the expansile intervertebral disc) or flat vertebrae are observed, particularly in older patients in whom senile or postmenopausal changes exaggerate the change, or in young patients who are immobilized after fractures or orthopedic surgery.

Frequency of fractures usually decreases at puberty for

TABLE 33-3
Mucopolysaccharidoses

Disorder OMIM #[a] Eponym	Clinical manifestations	Genetics	Urinary MPS	Enzyme deficiency	Locus
MPS I 252800		AR	Dermatan sulfate; heparan sulfate	α-L-iduronidase; *IDUA*	4p16.3
MPS IH Hurler	Coarse facies, severe DM, clouding of cornea, progressive MR death usually before 10 years				
MPS IS Scheie	Stiff joints, cloudy cornea, aortic valve disease, normal intelligence and survival to adulthood				
MPS IH/S Hurler-Scheie	Intermediate phenotype				
MPS II 309900		XL	Dermatan sulfate; heparan sulfate	Iduronate 2-sulfatase; *IDS*	Xq28
Hunter, severe	No corneal clouding, otherwise similar to MPS IH, death before 15 years				
Hunter, mild	Stiff joints, survival to 30s–60s, fair intelligence				
MPS IIIA 252900 Sanfilippo A	Mild physical features and DM, severe progressive MR	AR	Heparan sulfate	Heparan N-sulfatase (sulfamidase)	17q25.3
MPS IIIB 252920 Sanfilippo B	Indistinguishable from MPS IIIA	AR	Heparan sulfate	N-acetyl-α-D-glucosa-minidase; *NAGLU*	*SGSH* 17q21
MPS IIIC 252930 Sanfilippo C	Indistinguishable from MPS IIIA	AR	Heparan sulfate	Acetyl-CoA-α-glucosa-minide; N-acetyltrans-ferase; *MPS3C*	14
MPS IIID 252940 Sanfilippo D	Indistinguishable from MPS IIIA	AR	Heparan sulfate	N-acetylglucosamine-6-sulfate sulfatase; *GNS*	12q14

patients with types I, III, and IV. Pseudoarthrosis occurs in some patients due to nonunion of fractures. Hypertrophic callus occurs frequently in patients with OI and may be difficult to distinguish from osteosarcoma. Debate continues as to whether the risk of true osteosarcoma is increased in any form of OI; regardless, the risk is not great, but worthy of consideration whenever skeletal pain occurs in the absence of fracture, particularly in an older patient. Joint laxity sometimes is striking in type I; dislocation of joints can result from deformity secondary to repeated fractures, lax ligaments, or rupture of tendons.

The differential diagnosis of OI includes idiopathic juvenile osteoporosis, Hajdu-Cheney syndrome (osteoporosis, multiple wormian bones, acroosteolysis), pycnodysostosis

Disorder OMIM #[a] Eponym	Clinical manifestations	Genetics	Urinary MPS	Enzyme deficiency	Locus
MPS IVA 253000 Morquio A	Severe, distinctive bone changes; cloudy cornea; aortic regurgitation; thin enamel	AR	Keratan sulfate	Galactosamine-6-sulfate sulfatase; *GALNS*	16q24.3
MPS IVB 253010 Morquio B (O'Brien-Arbisser)	Mild bone changes; cloudy cornea; hypoplastic odontoid; normal enamel	AR	Keratan sulfate	β_1-galactosidase; *GLB1*	3p21.33
MPS V	No longer used				
MPS VI 253200 Maroteaux-Lamy		AR	Dermatan sulfate	Arylsulfatase B (N-acetyl-galactosamine 4-sulfatase); *ARSB*	5q11-q13
Severe	Severe DM and corneal clouding; valvular heart disease; striking WBC inclusions; normal intellect; survival to 20s				
Intermediate	Same spectrum as severe, but milder				
Mild	Same spectrum as severe, but mild				
MPS VII 253230 Sly	DM; progressive MR; WBC inclusions, hepatosplenomegaly	AR	Dermatan sulfate; heparan sulfate	β_1-glucuronidase; *GUSB*	7q21.11
MPS VIII 253230	No longer used				
MPS IX 601492	Short stature, progressive soft tissue and periarticular accumulations of hyaluronan	AR	Hyaluroran	Hyaluronidase; *HYAL1*	3p21.3-p21.2

[a] Entry in Online Mendelian Inheritance in Man (1).
AD, autosomal dominant; AR, autosomal recessive; XL, X-linked; DM, dysostosis multiplex; MR, mental retardation; WBC, white blood cell.

(dwarfism, brittle bones, absent mandibular ramus, persistent cranial fontanelles, acroosteolysis), and hypophosphatasia. In one family, susceptibility to osteoporosis was found to be due to a mutation in type I collagen. This emphasizes that the ability to identify mutations in a particular gene does not necessarily facilitate clinical diagnosis. Furthermore, common problems that are not thought to be

syndromic may be due to defects in one or another of the components of the extracellular matrix.

Pseudoxanthoma Elasticum

The cardinal features of pseudoxanthoma elasticum occur in the eyes, blood vessels, and skin (28). Although the most easily recognized finding in the ocular fundus is the angioid streak, due to a break in Bruch's membrane, progressive visual loss occurs from retinal hemorrhages. The media of muscular arteries develops degeneration of the elastic fibers and a histologic pattern similar to Mönckeberg arteriolosclerosis. Peripheral pulses gradually are lost, and intermittent claudication is common. Myocardial infarction, stroke, and gastrointestinal hemorrhage are complications of vascular involvement and the leading causes of death. The condition gets its name from characteristic skin lesions that develop in regions of flexural stress and resemble plucked chicken skin. The skeleton and joints usually are not involved. Elastic fibers throughout the body show calcification. Genetic heterogeneity is evident by both autosomal recessive (the most common form) and autosomal dominant inheritance. Both forms are due to mutations in the same gene, *ABCC6*, which encodes a membrane protein of unclear function (29).

Fibrodysplasia Ossificans Progressiva

Fibrodysplasia ossificans progressiva (FOP) is characterized by progressive ossification of ligaments, tendons, and aponeuroses (30). An inexorable course begins in the first year or so of life, usually with a seemingly inflammatory process and nodule formation on the back of the thorax, neck, or scalp. Local heat, leukocytosis, and elevated sedimentation rate are observed at this stage, and acute rheumatic fever sometimes is diagnosed. A valuable clue to the correct diagnosis is a short great toe with or without a short thumb; FOP is the leading cause of congenital hallux valgus. Most cases of this autosomal dominant disorder are the consequence of new mutation. Life expectancy is reduced considerably, with progressive restriction in lung capacity contributing to respiratory insufficiency and terminal pneumonia. The cause of FOP remains unclear, although the gene has been mapped to 4q27-q31 and bone morphogenic protein 4 has been found to be overexpressed in cells from FOP lesions (31).

Mucopolysaccharidoses

The mucopolysaccharidoses (MPS) are the result of inborn errors of proteoglycan catabolism (32). Although phenotypically diverse, the individual disorders share mucopolysacchariduria and deposition of catabolites of proteoglycan in various tissues. Numerous distinct types of MPS can be distinguished, based on combined phenotypic, genetic, and biochemical analysis (Table 33-3). Relative short stature is the rule in all forms of MPS, and can be profound in types IH (Hurler syndrome), II (Hunter syndrome), IV (Morquio syndrome, a prototype of short-trunk dwarfism), and VI (Maroteaux-Lamy syndrome). Radiologically, the skeletal dysplasia is quite similar in character in all but MPS IV, differing among the others largely in severity (25). Although the term *dysostosis mul-*

tiplex has been used, it is not specific for the MPS, because similar changes occur in a variety of storage disorders. The chief radiologic features are a thick calvaria; an enlarged, J-shaped sella turcica; a short and wide mandible; biconvex vertebral bodies; hypoplasia of the odontoid; broad ribs; short and thick clavicles; coxa valga; metacarpals with widened diaphyses and pointed proximal ends; and short phalanges.

Survival to adulthood without severe retardation occurs with types IS (Scheie's syndrome), II mild, IV, and VI. In these forms, progressive arthropathy and transverse myelopathy secondary to C1–C2 subluxation account for considerable disability. Joint replacement, particularly of the hips, has been beneficial in several forms, especially type IS. Cervical fusion should be considered whenever upper motor neuron signs appear, a particular concern in types IH, IV, and VI. Stiff joints are a more-or-less striking feature of all except type IV. Like other somatic features, such as coarse facies, reduced joint mobility is less striking in type III. In type IS, stiff hands, hip arthropathy, and clouding of the corneae produce the main disabilities. Carpal tunnel syndrome contributes to disability in all types. The major life-threatening problems in types II mild, IV, and VI are valvular heart disease and progressive narrowing of the middle and lower airways. The latter frequently presents as obstructive sleep apnea or complications with general anesthesia.

Genetic disturbances of mucopolysaccharide metabolism without mucopolysacchariduria include the mucolipidoses (33). Type II, a severe disorder similar to Hurler syndrome, also is called I-cell disease because of conspicuous inclusions in cultured cells. Type III, also called pseudo-Hurler polydystrophy, has stiff joints, cloudy corneae, carpal tunnel syndrome, short stature, coarse facies, and sometimes, mild mental retardation, and is compatible with survival to adulthood. Neither type shows mucopolysacchariduria, despite lysosomal storage of mucopolysaccharide and a demonstrable defect in degradation of mucopolysaccharides. Both are autosomal recessive and genetically heterogeneous. The basic biochemical defect is an enzyme responsible for post-translational modification of lysosomal enzymes. This defect results in multiple enzyme deficiencies and accumulation in tissues of both mucopolysaccharides and mucolipids.

Mucopolysacchariduria can be identified by one of several standard screening tests, at least one of which is part of the standard battery performed when a metabolic screen is ordered. Fractionation and characterization of the urinary mucopolysaccharides are useful in separating the several types of disorders, but enzymatic assay may be needed for diagnostic confirmation. Prenatal diagnosis by biochemical or molecular genetic methods is possible (34).

Like other lysosomal disorders, the mucopolysaccharide and mucolipid disorders have distinctive characteristics: 1) intracellular storage occurs; 2) storage material is heterogeneous because the degradative enzymes are not strictly specific; 3) deposition is vacuolar on electron microscopy; 4) many tissues are affected; and 5) the disorders are clinically progressive. Therapy by replacing the enzyme that is deficient is possible, but technically difficult and of transient benefit. Bone marrow transplant clearly is effective in the disorders lacking central nervous system involvement, and it is being investigated in patients with mental retardation (35).

REED EDWIN PYERITZ, MD, PhD

References

1. *Online Mendelian Inheritance in Man OMIM. McKusick-Nathans Institute for Genetic Medicine, Johns Hopkins University (Baltimore), and National Center for Biotechnology Information, National Library of Medicine (Bethesda, MD). Available at http://www.ncbi.nlm.nih.gov/omim*

2. *Royce PM, Steinmann B (eds): Connective Tissue and Its Heritable Disorders: Molecular, Genetic and Medical Aspects, 2nd edition. New York: Wiley-Liss, 2001.*

3. *Beighton P (ed): McKusick's Heritable Disorders of Connective Tissue, 5th edition. St. Louis: CV Mosby, 1993.*

4. *Pyeritz RE. Common structural disorders of connective tissue. In: King RA, Rotter JI, Motulsky AG (eds). The Genetic Basis of Common Diseases, 2nd edition. New York: Oxford University Press, 2001.*

5. *Beighton P, de Paepe A, Danks D, et al. International nosology of heritable disorders of connective tissue, Berlin, 1986. Am J Med Genet 1988;29:581–594.*

6. *DePaepe A, Deitz HC, Devereux RB, Hennekem R, Pyeritz RE. Revised diagnostic criteria for the Marfan syndrome. Am J Med Genet 1996;62:417–426.*

7. *Dietz HC, Pyeritz RE. Mutations in the human gene for fibrillin-1 (FBN1) in the Marfan syndrome and related disorders. Hum Mol Genet 1995;4:1799–1809.*

8. *Pyeritz RE. Marfan syndrome and other disorders of fibrillins. In: Rimoin DL, Connor JM, Pyeritz RE, Korf B (eds): Principles and Practice of Medical Genetics, 4th edition. New York: Churchill Livingstone, 2001.*

9. *Pyeritz RE, Fishman EK, Bernhardt BA, Siegelman SS. Dural ectasia is a common feature of the Marfan syndrome. Am J Hum Genet 1988;43:726–732.*

10. *Fattori R, Nienaber CA, Descovich B, et al. Importance of dural ectasia in phenotypic assessment of Marfan's syndrome. Lancet 1999;354:910–913.*

11. *Gott VL, Greene PS, Alejo DE, et al. Replacement of the aortic root in patient's with Marfan's syndrome. N Engl J Med 1999;340:1307–1313.*

12. *Sponseller PD, Hobbs W, Riley LH III, Pyeritz RE. The thoracolumbar spine in Marfan syndrome. J Bone Joint Surg Am 1995; 77:867–876.*

13. *Pyeritz RE. Homocystinuria. In: Beighton P (ed). McKusick's Heritable Disorders of Connective Tissue, 5th edition. St. Louis: CV Mosby, 1993; pp 137–178.*

14. *Majors A, Pyeritz RE. Deficiency of cysteine impairs deposition of fibrillin-1: implications for the pathogenesis of cys-*

tathionine β–synthase deficiency. Mol Genet Metab 2000; 70:252-260.

15. *Rai A, Wordsworth P, Coppock JS, Zaphiropoulos GC, Struthers GR. Hereditary arthro-ophthalmopathy (Stickler syndrome): a diagnosis to consider in familial premature osteoarthritis. Br J Rheumat 1994;33:1175–1180.*

16. *Snead MP, Yates JR. Clinical and molecular genetics of Stickler syndrome. J Med Genet 1999;36:353–359.*

17. *Zlotogora J, Sagi M, Schuper A, Leiba H, Merin S. Variability of Stickler syndrome. Am J Med Genet 1992;42:337–339.*

18. *Byers PH: The Ehlers-Danlos syndromes. In: Rimoin DL, Connor JM, Pyeritz RE, Korf B (eds). Principles and Practice of Medical Genetics, 4th edition. New York: Churchill Livingstone, 2001; S241-S286.*

19. *Byers PH. Disorders of collagen biosynthesis and structure. In: Scriver CR, Beaudet AL, Sly WS, Valle DZ (eds). Metabolic and Molecular Bases of Inherited Disease, 8th edition. New York: McGraw-Hill, 2001.*

20. *Beighton P, De Paepe A, Steinmann B, Tsipouras P, Wenstrup RJ. Ehlers-Danlos syndromes: revised nosology, Villefranche, 1997. Am J Med Genet 1998;77:31–37.*

21. *Michalickova K, Susic M, Willing MC, Wenstrup RJ, Cole WG. Mutations of the alpha-2(V) chain of type V collagen impair matrix assembly and produce Ehlers-Danlos syndrome type I. Hum Mol Genet 1998;7:249–255.*

22. *Beighton P, Grahame R, Bird H. Hypermobility of Joints, 2nd edition. New York: Springer-Verlag, 1989.*

23. *Pepin M, Schwarze U, Superti-Furga A, Byers PH. Clinical and genetic features of Ehlers-Danlos syndrome type IV, the vascular type. N Engl J Med 2000;342:673–680.*

24. *Horton WA, Collins DL, DeSmet AA, Kennedy JA, Schmike RN. Familial joint instability syndrome. Am J Med Genet 1980;6:221–228.*

25. *Wynne-Davies R, Hall CM, Apley AG. Atlas of Skeletal Dysplasias. Edinburgh: Churchill Livingstone, 1985.*

26. *Vujic M, Hallstensson K, Wahlstrom J, Lundberg A, Langmaack C, Martinson T. Localization of a gene for autosomal dominant Larsen syndrome to chromosome region 3p21.1-14.1 in the proximity of, but distinct from, the COL7A1 locus. Am J Hum Genet 1995;57:1104–1113.*

27. *Sillence D. Osteogenesis imperfecta. In: Rimoin DL, Connor JM, Pyeritz RE, Korf B (eds). Principles and Practice of Medical Genetics, 4th edition. New York: Churchill Livingstone, 2001.*

28. *Uitto J. Inherited abnormalities of elastic tissue. In: Rimoin DL, Connor JM, Pyeritz RE, Korf B (eds). Principles and Practice of Medical Genetics, 4th edition. New York: Churchill Livingstone, 2001.*

29. *Bergen AA, Plomp AS, Schuurman EJ, et al. Mutations in ABCC6 cause pseudoxanthoma elasticum. Nat Genet 2000; 25:228–231.*

30. *Smith R, Athanasou NA, Vipond SE. Fibrodysplasia (myositis) ossificans progressiva: clinicopathological features and natural history. QJM 1996;89:445–446.*

31. *Feldman G, Li M, Martin S, et al. Fibrodysplasia ossificans progressiva, a heritable disorder of severe heterotopic ossification, maps to human chromosome 4q27-31. Am J Hum Genet 2000;66:128–135.*

32. *Neufeld EF, Muenzer J. The mucopolysaccharidoses. In: Scriver CR, Beaudet AL, Sly WS, Valle D (eds). Metabolic Basis of Inherited Disease, 8th edition. New York: McGraw-Hill, 2001; pp 3421-3452.*

33. *Kornfield S, Sly WS. I-cell disease and pseudo-hurler polydystrophy: Disorders of lysosomal enzyme phosphorylation. In: Scriver CR, Beaudet AL, Sly WS, Valle D (eds). The Metabolic and Molecular Bases of Inherited Disease, 8th edition. New York: McGraw-Hill, 2001.*

34. *Burke LW, Pyeritz RE. Prenatal diagnosis of connective tissue disorders. In: Milunsky A (ed). Genetic Disorders and the Fetus: Diagnosis, Prevention and Treatment, 4th edition. Baltimore: Johns Hopkins Univ Press, 1998; pp 612–634.*

34 HYPERTROPHIC OSTEOARTHROPATHY

Hypertrophic osteoarthropathy (HOA) or *acropachy* is a syndrome characterized by excessive proliferation of skin and bone at the distal parts of the extremities. Its most conspicuous feature is a bulbous deformity of the tips of the digits, conventionally known as clubbing (Fig. 34-1). In advanced stages, periosteal proliferation of the tubular bones and synovial effusions become evident. The classification of HOA is shown in Table 34-1 (1). Any proposed scheme for the pathogenesis of HOA must explain how such diverse diseases could induce the same connective-tissue abnormalities of HOA. Primary HOA has a high male-to-female ratio of 9:1 and appears to be associated with a familial predisposition; one-third of these patients report a close relative with the same illness.

Pathology and Pathogenesis

The bulbous deformity of the digits develops as a result of edema and excessive collagen deposition. Endothelial cell activation and vascular hyperplasia are prominent features. At the tubular bone level, there is vascular hyperplasia, with proliferation of the periosteal layers (2).

Cyanotic heart diseases are an excellent model for studying the pathogenesis of HOA, because nearly all of these patients have lifelong clubbing, and more than one-third display the fully developed syndrome. Platelet abnormalities, a feature of cardiogenic HOA, may provide a clue to pathogenesis. Patients with cardiogenic HOA

TABLE 34-1
Classification of Hypertrophic Osteoarthropathy

Digital Clubbing

Hypertrophic Osteoarthropathy

Primary — Secondary

Secondary: Generalized — Localized

Localized: Hemiplegia | Aneurysm | Infective arteritis | Patent ductus arteriosus

Pulmonary	Cardiac	Hepatic	Intestinal	Mediastinal	Miscellaneous
Cystic fibrosis	Congenital cyanotic diseases	Cirrhosis	Crohn's disease	Esophageal carcinoma	Graves' disease
Pulmonary fibrosis		Carcinoma			Thalassemia
	Infective endocarditis		Ulcerative colitis	Thymoma	
Chronic infections				Achalasia	Diverse malignancies
			Chronic infections		
Cancer: primary or metastatic					POEMS syndrome
			Laxative abuse		
Arterio-venous fistulae					Others
			Polyposis		
Mesothelioma					
			Malignant tumors		

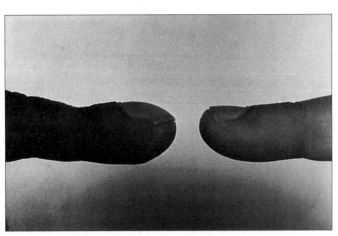

Fig. 34-1. A clubbed finger (left) is compared with a normal finger.

frequently have circulating macrothrombocytes, with distorted volume-distribution curves. Such abnormalities support the notion that under normal circumstances megakaryocytes rupture in the highly dichotomized pulmonary vascular bed. In patients with right-to-left shunts, large platelets gain direct access to the systemic circulation, reach its most distal sites on axial streams, and interact with endothelial cells, which subsequently release growth factor, inducing acropachy (3) (Fig. 34-2). The finding of elevated levels of von Willebrand factor antigen in people with cardiogenic acropachy or primary HOA further supports the notion that enhanced activation of platelets and endothelial cells is central to HOA (4).

Vascular endothelial growth factor (VEGF) may be involved in the pathogenesis of HOA. This growth factor, a potent angiogenic stimulus and osteoblast-differentiation agent, is derived from platelets and induced by hypoxia. A variety of malignant tumors also produce VEGF, fostering their uncontrolled growth. People with primary HOA and HOA associated with lung cancer have elevated levels of VEGF in their plasma (2). Overproduction of VEGF may explain how diverse hypoxic or neoplastic pathologies induce HOA. It also may explain how diseases with prominent endothelial cell involvement, such as infective endocarditis, Graves' disease, or mesothelioma, lead to acropachy. More studies are needed to elucidate the pathogenesis of HOA.

Clinical Features

Many people with HOA are asymptomatic and unaware of the deformity of their digits (Fig. 34-1). However, other patients, particularly those with pulmonary malignancies, suffer incapacitating bone pain (5). Characteristically, this pain is deep-seated and often more prominent in the legs.

Because the bulbous deformity of the digits is unique to HOA, diagnosis is based primarily on physical examination. The increased volume of soft tissue molds the fingernail into a "watch-crystal" convexity, and the nail bed (NB) rocks when palpated. Toes also are affected, but normal splaying makes early changes more difficult to discern. The digital index is a practical bedside method to measure clubbing. With a nonelastic string, the circumference of each finger is measured at the NB and at the distal interphalangeal joint (DIP). If the sum of the 10 NB/DIP ratios is more than 10, clubbing most likely is present (6).

When the complete features of HOA are evident, bone thickening may be detected in areas of the extremities not covered by muscles, such as ankles and wrists. These areas can be tender to palpation. Effusions in large joints are a common, but not universal, finding. On examination, there is no detectable synovial hypertrophy. Range of motion of the affected joint may be slightly decreased. Arthrocentesis yields a clear, viscous fluid with few inflammatory cells; the leukocyte count typically is less than 1000 cells/mm³. These findings indicate that HOA does not cause inflammatory or proliferative synovial disease, but rather, the effusions are most likely a sympathetic reaction to the adjacent periostosis (7).

People with primary HOA may display a generalized skin hypertrophy called *pachydermoperiostosis*. This skin overgrowth roughens the facial features and can reach the extreme of *cutis verticis gyrata*, which is the most advanced stage of cutaneous hypertrophy. These patients often demonstrate glandular dysfunction of the skin that is manifested as hyperhidrosis, seborrhea, or acne (7).

Particular types of HOA are associated with distinctive clinical findings. For example, thyroid acropachy is distinguished by an exuberant periosteal proliferation that principally involves the small tubular bones of the hands and feet; clubbing usually coexists with exophthalmos and pretibial myxedema.

Variant forms of HOA are localized to one or two extremities. Usually they occur as a response to prominent endothelial injury to the involved limb, such as damage caused by aneurysms or infective endarteritis. They also are associated with patent ductus arteriosus and reversal of blood flow.

Laboratory Features and Imaging

There are no distinctive clinical laboratory-test abnormalities associated with HOA. However, an array of biochemical alterations that reflect the underlying illness may be found. Plain radiographs of the extremities may reveal abnormalities in an asymptomatic patient. Radionuclide bone scanning is a sensitive method for demonstrating periosteal involvement. Long-standing clubbing produces a prominent bone remodeling of the distal phalanx.

Periostosis evolves in an orderly manner, with symmetrical bone changes. Initially, periostosis affects the distal parts of the lower extremities and then evolves in a centripetal fashion (8). When mild, it involves only a few bones, usually the tibia and fibula; periosteal apposition is limited to the diaphysis and has a monolayer configuration. In contrast, severe periostosis affects all tubular bones, spreads to the metaphyses and epiphyses, and generates irregular configurations. Typically, however, the joint space is preserved, and there are no erosions or periarticular osteopenia.

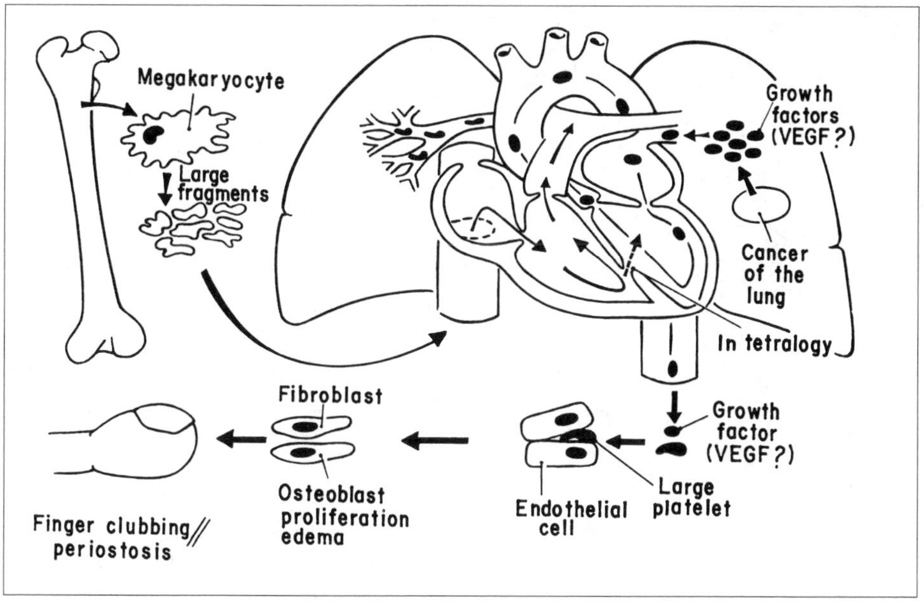

Fig. 34-2. The theoretical pathogenesis of hypertrophic osteoarthropathy. Under normal circumstances, megakaryocytes emerging from the bone marrow are fragmented in the lung microvasculature. In cases of cyanotic heart disease, the large fragments do not enter the pulmonary circulation, but rather, enter the systemic circulation directly. This aberration leads to effects at the most distal sites of circulation: activation of endothelial cells, release of growth factors (e.g., VEGF), and the induction of clubbing and periosteal proliferation. In cases of lung cancer, growth factors derived from the tumor enter the systemic circulation and induce hypertrophic osteoarthropathy.

Diagnosis

When HOA is fully expressed, the "drumstick" fingers are so unique that recognition poses no dilemma. However, the symptoms of HOA can be subtle. In some patients with lung cancer, painful arthropathy may be the initial manifestation, occurring before clubbing is detectable. Such patients could be misclassified as having an inflammatory arthritis. People with the exuberant skin hypertrophy of HOA may be misdiagnosed as having acromegaly.

The diagnosis of HOA requires the combined presence of clubbing and periostosis of the tubular bones (1). Synovial effusion is not essential for the diagnosis. Important features that distinguish HOA from inflammatory types of arthritis are that in HOA, the pain involves not only the joint but also the adjacent bones, the synovial fluid is not inflammatory, and rheumatoid factor is absent from the serum (5,7).

If a previously healthy individual develops any of the manifestations of HOA, a thorough search for underlying illness should be undertaken. Primary HOA should be diagnosed only after careful clinical scrutiny fails to disclose any of the internal illnesses listed in Table 34-1. In an individual with a previous diagnosis of pulmonary fibrosis, cystic fibrosis, or liver cirrhosis, the development of clubbing usually is a poor prognostic sign. Clubbing in a person with known rheumatic heart disease may indicate infective endocarditis. Similarly, clubbing in a patient with polyneuropathy of recent onset should lead to the suspicion of POEMS syndrome (polyneuropathy, organomegaly, endocrinopathy, M-protein, and skin changes) (9).

Treatment

Apart from disfigurement, clubbing usually is asymptomatic and does not require therapy. Painful osteoarthropathy generally responds to analgesics or nonsteroidal anti-inflammatory drugs. Correction of a heart defect, removal of a lung tumor, or successful treatment of endocarditis produce rapid regression of the syndrome.

MANUEL MARTÍNEZ-LAVÍN, MD

References

1. Martínez-Lavín M, Matucci-Cerinic M, Pineda C, et al. Hypertrophic osteoarthropathy: consensus on its definition, classification, assessment and diagnostic criteria. J Rheumatol 1993;20:1386–1387.
2. Silveira L, Martínez-Lavín M, Pineda C, Navarro C, Fonseca MC, Nava A. Vascular endothelial growth factor in hypertrophic osteoarthropathy. Clin Exp Rheumatol 2000;18:57–62.
3. Vazquez-Abad D, Martínez-Lavín M. Macrothrombocytes in the peripheral circulation of patients with cardiogenic hypertrophic osteoarthropathy. Clin Exp Rheumatol 1991;9:59–62.
4. Matucci-Cerinic M, Martínez-Lavín M, Rojo F, Fonseca MC, Kahaleh BM. von Willebrand factor antigen in hypertrophic osteoarthropathy. J Rheumatol 1992;19:765-767.
5. Schumacher HR. Articular manifestations of hypertrophic pulmonary osteoarthropathy in bronchogenic carcinoma. Arthritis Rheum 1976;19:629–636.
6. Vazquez-Abad D, Martínez-Lavín M. Digital clubbing: a numerical assessment of the deformity. J Rheumatol 1989;16:518–520.
7. Martínez-Lavín M, Pineda C, Valdéz T, et al. Primary hypertrophic osteoarthropathy. Semin Arthritis Rheum 1988;17:156–162.
8. Pineda C, Fonseca C, Martínez-Lavín M. The spectrum of soft tissue and skeletal abnormalities in hypertrophic osteoarthropathy. J Rheumatol 1990;17:626–632.
9. Martínez-Lavín M, Vargas AS, Cabré J, et al. Features of hypertrophic osteoarthropathy in patients with POEMS syndrome. A metaanalysis. J Rheumatol 1997;24:2267–2268.

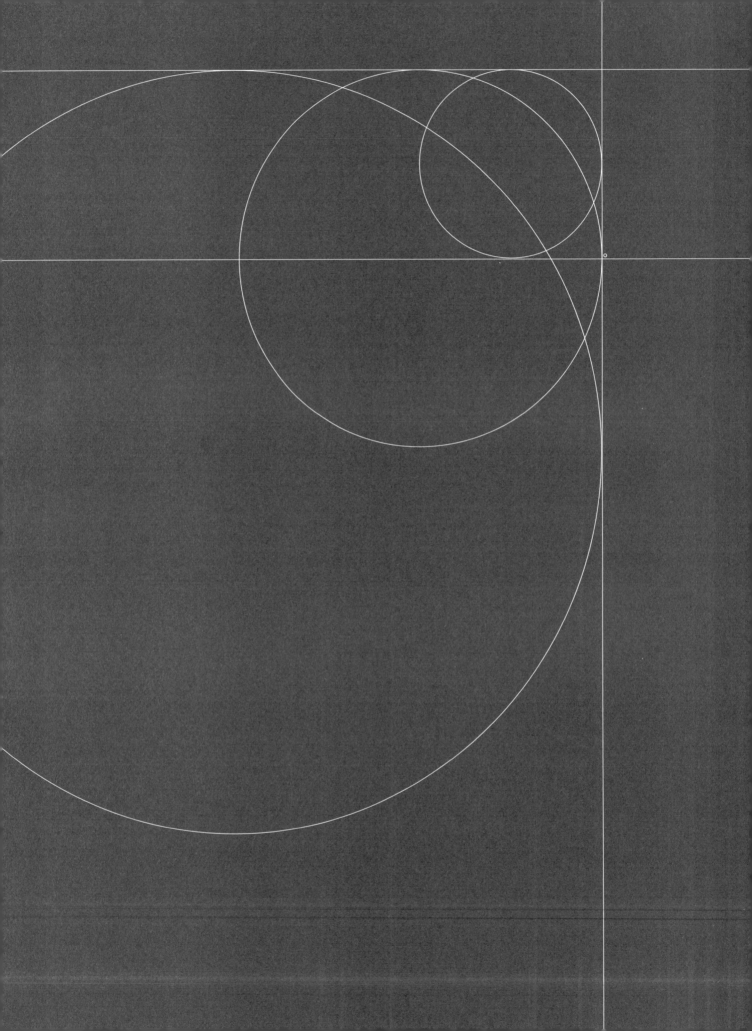

35 BONE AND JOINT DYSPLASIAS

Bone dysplasias are a broad group of conditions in which skeletal development and function are disturbed. These conditions include the chondrodysplasias and osteochondroses discussed in this chapter; osteodysplasias, such as osteogenesis imperfecta syndromes (discussed in Chapter 33); and many other conditions that are extremely rare or of little relevance to rheumatology.

Chondrodysplasias

The term chondrodysplasia – literally, abnormal (*dys*) cartilage (*chondro*) growth (*plasia*) – designates inherited disorders of cartilage that affect its function as a template for bone growth (1). The clinical picture typically is dominated by varying degrees of dwarfism and bone and joint deformities. Because the genes that harbor chondrodysplasia mutations often are not specific to bone growth, the clinical manifestations frequently extend to other cartilages, such as articular cartilage, and to other tissues (1–3).

Pathogenesis

Most bones develop and grow through the process of endochondral ossification, in which cartilage serves as a template for bone formation. In postembryonic, growing bone, ossification occurs in growth plates near the ends of bones (4). Growth plates have a leading and trailing edge. In essence, template cartilage is synthesized de novo at the leading edge and is degraded and replaced by an expanding front of bone at the trailing edge. Endochondral ossification accounts for linear bone growth from midgestation through the end of puberty.

The chondrodysplasias result from mutations in the genes that encode structural proteins of cartilage matrix and proteins that regulate growth-plate function, including growth factors, receptors, and transcription factors. These proteins, which contribute to different aspects of endochondral ossification, are required for normal bone growth (4,5). Although poorly understood, the different types of chondrodysplasias reflect functional consequences of disturbances in these proteins, with regard to bone growth and other clinical manifestations.

Classification

More than 100 clinical forms of chondrodysplasia currently are recognized. Based on their differences in clinical presentation, characteristic appearances of skeletal radiographs, growth plate histology, and pattern of inheritance, these disorders have been grouped over the past decade into classes that often correspond to a common mutated gene (1,6). A well-defined chondrodysplasia class, such as the achondroplasia or spondyloepiphyseal dysplasia (SED) classes, typically contains a group of disorders ranging in severity from lethal at or around birth to very mild, often blending into the normal population. The current classification scheme is based primarily on molecular genetics, but the genetic basis of many disorders has yet to be determined, and as a consequence, the scheme continues to evolve (see Table 35-1).

Achondroplasias

This class of autosomal dominant disorders includes thanatophoric dysplasia, the most common chondrodysplasia that is lethal in the perinatal period; achondroplasia, by far the most common nonlethal chondrodysplasia; and hypochondroplasia. Although the three differ substantially in severity, the features are qualitatively similar. Heterozygous mutations of the gene encoding fibroblast growth factor receptor 3 have been identified in all three conditions.

Achondroplasia: The prototype of short-limb dwarfism, achondroplasia is recognizable at birth by a long, narrow trunk, short limbs (especially proximally), and a large head, with prominent forehead and hypoplasia of the midface. Most joints are hyperextensible, especially the knees, but elbow mobility is limited. The most serious problems are related to a small spinal canal, especially at the foramen magnum level. This anomaly contributes to hypotonia, failure to thrive, developmental delay, apnea, and even quadriparesis and sudden death in some infants. Common childhood problems include middle-ear infections, dental crowding, and bowing of the legs.

Life span is normal in the absence of life-threatening neurologic problems in early life. In adulthood, men reach an average height of 132 cm (about 45 inches) and women, 124 cm (about 40 inches). Pain in weight-bearing joints is common, probably due to misalignment of bones aggravated by physical activity and obesity, which is common. However, people with achondroplasia rarely develop osteoarthritis. Stenosis of the lumbar spine may cause paresthesias, claudication, and numbness of the legs, and bowel and bladder dysfunction.

Pregnant women with achondroplasia need to be monitored carefully and delivered by cesarean section. Because of the high prevalence of heterozygous achondroplasia in the short-stature community, when people with this condition intermarry, their offspring have a 25% risk of inheriting the much more severe homozygous achondroplasia.

TABLE 35-1
Features of Selected Chondrodysplasias[a]

Class and disorder	OMIM	Inheritance	Gene Locus	Overall severity	Rheumatologic complications
Achondroplasia					
Thanatophoric dysplasia	187600/187610	AD	FGFR3	Lethal	
Achondroplasia	100800	AD	FGFR3	++/+++	Arthralgias
Hypochondroplasia	146000	AD	FGFR3	+	
Spondyloephipyseal dysplasia (SED)					
Achondrogenesis type II	200610	AD	COL2A1	Lethal	
Hypochondrogenesis	14600	AD	COL2A1	Lethal	
SED congenita	183900	AD	COL2A1	+++	Precocious OA
Kniest dysplasia	156550	AD	COL2A1	+++	Contractures, precocious OA
Stickler syndrome	108300	AD	COL2A1	++	Precocious OA
Stickler-like dysplasia	184840	AD	COL11A1	++	Precocious OA
Stickler-like dysplasia	184850	AR	COL11A2	++	Precocious OA
SED late onset		AD	COL2A1	+	Precocious OA
SED tarda	313400	XLR	SEDL	+	Precocious OA
Multiple epiphyesal dysplasia (MED)/pseudoachondroplasia					
MED	600969	AD	COMP	+++	Arthralgias, precocious OA
Pseudoachondroplasia	177170	AD	COMP	+++	Arthralgias, precocious OA
Diastrophic dysplasia					
Achondrogenesis type 1B	600972	AR	DTDST	Lethal	
Ateleosteogenesis type II	256050	AR	DTDST	Lethal	
Diastrophic dysplasia	222600	AR	DTDST	+++	Precocious OA, contractures
Metaphyseal chondrodysplasia					
Jansen type	156400	AD	PTHR1	+++	Contractures
Schmid type	156500	AD	COL10A1	++	
McKusick type	250250	AR	Unknown	+++	
Metatropic dysplasia					
Metatropic dysplasia	250600	AD	Unknown	+++	Contractures
Chondrodysplasia punctata					
Rhizomelic type	215100	AR	ACDPA	Lethal	Contractures
X-linked recessive type (CDPX1)	302950	XLR	ARSE	+++	
X-linked dominant type (CDPX2)	302960	XLD	EBP	++/+++	Contractures
Brachyolmia					
Hobaek type	271530	AR	Unknown	++	Arthralgia, stiffness in hip, back
Maroteaux type		AR	Unknown	++	Arthralgia, stiffness in hip, back
Autosomal dominant type	113500	AD	Unknown	++	Arthralgia, stiffness in hip, back

[a] AD, autosomal dominant; AR, autosomal recessive; XLD, X-linked dominant; XLR, X-linked recessive, FGFR3, fibroblast growth factor receptor 3; COL2A1, type II collagen αl chain; COL10A1, type X collagen αl chain; COL11A1, type XI collagen αl chain; COL11A2, type XI collagen α2 chain; COMP, cartilage oligomeric matrix protein; DTDST, diastrophic dysplasia sulfate transporter; PTHR1, parathyroid hormone-related protein receptor 1; ACDPA, acetyl-CoA dihydroxyacetone phosphate acetyltransferase; ARSE, arylsulfatase E; EBP, delta(8)-delta(7) sterol isomerase emopamil-binding protein; OA, osteoarthritis; OMIM, Online Mendelian Inheritance of Man (which provides extensive references at http://www.ncbi.nlm.nih.gov/omim).

Hypochondroplasia. Not usually recognized until mid to late childhood, people with hypochondroplasia appear to have "mild" achondroplasia, with short limbs (mostly the proximal segments), a stocky build, and a normal or slightly enlarged head. The natural history usually is unremarkable, other than short stature (approximately five feet or less). The true incidence of hypochondroplasia is unknown; because its features are mild, it often may escape detection.

Spondyloepiphyseal Dysplasias

Spondyloepiphyseal dysplasia (SED) is a large, diverse class of autosomal dominant disorders with clinical features that reflect varying degrees of dysfunction of type II collagen, the principal structural protein of cartilage. In severe forms, many types of cartilage and other tissues containing type II collagen are affected; in milder forms, only articular cartilage is involved.

SED Congenita. This form of dysplasia is a prototype of short-trunk dwarfism. Neonates with SED congenita have a short neck; a short, barrel-shaped trunk; and sometimes, cleft palate and clubfoot. The proximal limbs are short, but the hands, feet, head, and face appear to be normal in size. The shortening becomes more prominent with time. Scoliosis commonly develops in childhood and may cause respiratory compromise. Odontoid hypoplasia may predispose to cervicomedullary instability and spinal-cord compression, but sudden death is uncommon. Osteoarthritis, especially of the hips and knees, typically appears in the third decade. Severe myopia is common, and retinal detachment may occur in older children and adults. Adults range in height from 95 to 128 cm (about 35 to 50 inches).

Kniest dysplasia. At birth, infants with Kniest dysplasia have a short trunk and limbs, a flat face, and prominent eyes. Their fingers are long and knobby, and clubfoot and cleft palate are common. The most debilitating aspect is the progressive enlargement of joints during childhood, which is associated with painful contractures and, eventually, osteoarthritis. Hearing loss is common, as is severe myopia, which often is complicated by retinal detachment.

Stickler syndrome. The clinical picture of Stickler syndrome is dominated by ocular problems. Severe myopia usually is present at birth, as are cleft palate and a small jaw. Retinal detachment may occur during childhood, as may choroidoretinal and vitreous degeneration. Sensorineural hearing loss often develops during adolescence. Osteoarthritis typically begins during the second or third decade of life. Short stature is not a feature of Stickler syndrome; indeed, some patients exhibit a Marfan-type habitus and joint laxity. A dysplasia similar to Stickler syndrome may arise from mutations of genes that encode type XI collagen.

Late-onset SEDs. Some type II collagen mutations manifest primarily as precocious osteoarthritis of weight-bearing joints. Radiographs usually reveal subtle changes of SED, but many of these patients are of normal stature and have no other abnormalities. The term familial (or autosomal dominant) osteoarthritis sometimes is used to describe this syndrome. Recurrent mutations of the type II collagen gene have been observed in a few instances of familial osteoarthritis. Mutations of an X-linked gene that encodes a protein termed "sedlin" can produce a similar but distinct clinical picture in males, which is called SED tarda.

Multiple Epiphyseal Dysplasia and Pseudoachondroplasia

Multiple epiphyseal dysplasia (MED) and pseudoachondroplasia are classified together because mutations in the cartilage oligomeric matrix protein (COMP) gene have been found in both disorders.

The Fairbank type of MED usually is diagnosed in childhood because of moderately short limbs, a waddling gait, and painful joints. Radiographs show generalized epiphyseal involvement. The Ribbing type of MED may not be detected until adolescence. Because involvement typically is restricted to the proximal femurs, the Ribbing type often is confused with bilateral Legg–Calvé–Perthes disease. Both types of MED are associated with moderately short stature (145–170 cm) and osteoarthritis of weight-bearing joints.

Pseudoachondroplasia typically presents in the second or third year of life, with a dramatic slowing of bone growth accompanied by a waddling gait and generalized joint laxity. The head and face appear normal, but the hands are short and broad, and ulnar deviation occurs. The growth deficiency worsens with age. Major complications are related to excessive joint mobility, most notably involving the knees, where it produces various deformities. Osteoarthritis of the hips and knees is common.

Diastrophic Dysplasia

Diastrophic dysplasia usually is apparent at birth. Infants display very short extremities and distinctive hands, with short digits and proximal displacement of the thumb (hitchhiker thumb). There may be bony fusion of metacarpophalangeal joints, producing symphalangism and ulnar deviation of the hands. Cleft palate and clubfoot are common. The external ears often become inflamed soon after birth; healing results in small, fibrotic ears (cauliflower deformity). Scoliosis and multiple joint contractures usually begin during childhood and typically are progressive and severe. Adult height varies from 105 cm to 130 cm (40–44 inches).

Metaphyseal Chondrodysplasias

The metaphyseal chondrodysplasias (MCDs) are a heterogeneous group of disorders that share radiographic involvement of the metaphyses. However, studies have shown that they do not share a common genetic basis.

Jansen MCD. Severely shortened limbs, prominent forehead, and small jaw are present at birth. Some infants have clubfoot and hypercalcemia. Joints enlarge and become restricted during childhood. Flexion contractures at the hips and knees often result in a bent-over posture.

Schmid MCD. This disorder usually becomes apparent at age 2–3 years because of mild shortening of the limbs, especially the legs (which are bowed), a waddling gait, and sometimes hip pain. Adults are of mildly short stature and have few problems.

McKusick MCD. Also called cartilage-hair hypoplasia, the McKusick-type MCD manifests as growth deficiency at age 2–3 years. It is characterized by short limbs, bowed legs, and flaring of the lower ribcage. Hands and feet are short and broad, and fingers are short and stubby. Ligamentous laxity is marked. The hair tends to be blond and thin, and the skin is lightly pigmented. Some patients have associated problems, including immune deficiency, anemia, Hirschsprung's disease, and malabsorption. Adults exhibit marked dwarfism and are predisposed to certain infections and malignancies of the skin and lymphoid tissue.

Metatropic Dysplasia

Newborn infants with metatropic dysplasia have short limbs and a long, narrow trunk. Kyphoscoliosis, which starts during late infancy or early childhood, may cause cardiorespiratory problems. Odontoid hypoplasia is common. Most joints become large and have restricted mobility, and contractures often develop at the hips and knees.

Chondrodysplasia Punctata

Disorders classified as chondrodysplasia punctata (CDP) share the radiographic finding of stippled epiphyses, but specific features differ substantially.

Rhizomelic CDP. Rhizomelic CDP is evidenced at birth by severe and symmetric shortening of limbs, multiple joint contractures, cataracts, ichthyosiform rash, absent hair, microcephaly, and flat face, with hypoplasia of the nasal tip. These infants fail to thrive and usually die during the first year.

X-Linked CDP. CDP may be X-linked dominant or recessive. The recessive form, CDPX1, is symmetric and severe; the dominant form, CDPX2, is relatively mild and asymmetric in distribution. Varying degrees of contractures, cataracts, skin rash, and hair loss are found in CDPX2. The asymmetry may worsen and scoliosis may develop over time, but people with CDPX2 usually have a normal life span.

Brachyolmia

Three types of brachyolmia are recognized, all of which have similar clinical features (Table 35-1). They present in early to mid childhood, with mildly short stature, mainly involving the trunk. Back and hip pain typically arise during adolescence and continue into adulthood. Back stiffness is common and some patients develop scoliosis.

Diagnosis

A few conditions, such as achondroplasia, can be diagnosed simply by seeing a patient. However, diagnosis usually is based on recognizing a unique combination of clinical, radiographic, and genetic features (1–3, 7). Because the clinical features typically evolve over time, the natural history must be taken into account when patients are evaluated. The most useful information usually comes from skeletal radiographs; specific radiologic diagnostic criteria have been developed (7–10). Like the clinical picture, radiographic characteristics change with age. Films taken before puberty usually are more informative because the radiographic hallmarks of many disorders disappear after closure of the epiphyses. In fact, it often is difficult to make a specific diagnosis from postpubertal radiographs. Because many patients are the first and only known case in a family, a pedigree may be of little help because the inheritance pattern cannot be determined. Nevertheless, a family history sometimes provides critical clues toward a diagnosis.

TABLE 35-2
Juvenile Osteochondroses

Region affected	Eponym	Typical age at presentation	Sex predilection
Capital femoral epiphysis	Legg-Calvé-Perthes disease, coxa plana	3–12 years	Male
Tibial tubercle	Osgood–Schlatter disease	10–16 years	None
Os calcis	Sever's disease	6–10 years	None
Head of second metatarsal	Freiberg's disease	10–14 years	None
Vertebral bodies	Scheuermann's disease	Adolescence	Male
Medial aspect of proximal tibial epiphysis	Blount's disease, tibia vara	Infancy or adolescence	None
Subchondral areas of diarthroidal joints (particularly knee, hip, elbow, and ankle)	Osteochondritis dissecans	10–20 years	Male

Historically, laboratory tests have not been useful in diagnosing chondrodysplasias. However, as the mutations become better defined, genetic testing may be helpful in disorders caused by a recurrent mutation in the population, as is the case with achondroplasia and, perhaps, in some forms of late-onset SED associated with precocious osteoarthritis. Although histologic evaluations of growth-plate specimens often reveal characteristic changes, biopsy seldom is warranted because the diagnosis usually can be made by other means.

Salient features of the more common chondrodysplasias are summarized in Table 35-1 (6), and additional information can be found in several reviews (1,2,5,7,11). The most up-to-date information and references are available through the *Online Mendelian Inheritance in Man* (http://www.ncbi.nlm.nih.gov/omim/), developed by McKusick and colleagues.

Juvenile Osteochondroses

The juvenile osteochondroses, summarized in Table 35-2, are a heterogeneous group of disorders in which localized noninflammatory arthropathies result from regional disturbances of skeletal growth (12,13). Children may present with painless limitation of movement of affected joints (such as in Legg–Calvé–Perthes disease and Scheuermann's disease) or with local pain and, sometimes, tenderness and swelling (such as in Freiberg's disease, Osgood–Schlatter disease, and osteochondritis dissecans). Bone growth may be altered and produce deformities, such as bowing of the tibia in Blount's disease.

Diagnosis

The diagnosis of juvenile osteochondrosis usually can be confirmed radiographically, and magnetic resonance imaging sometimes is useful to define the lesions. The pathogenesis is thought to involve ischemic necrosis of primary or secondary endochondral ossification centers. Some cases may be related to stress and injury. Most of these disorders occur sporadically, but familial forms have been described.

Management

No definitive treatment is available to counter defective bone growth for any of the bone and joint dysplasias. Consequently, management is directed at preventing and correcting skeletal deformities and preventing nonskeletal complications. Management is guided by knowledge of the natural history of these disorders, so that disorder-specific problems can be anticipated and treated early.

Problems common to many chondrodysplasias include respiratory distress, osteoarthritis of weight-bearing joints, dental crowding, obesity, obstetrical difficulties, and psychologic problems related to short stature. General recommendations can be made to address these problems (1,3). For example, most patients with a chondrodysplasia should avoid contact sports and other activities that traumatize or stress joints. Joint replacement often is necessary for progressive osteoarthritis. Dietary control should be instituted during childhood to prevent obesity in adulthood. Dental care should be started in early childhood to manage crowding and misalignment. Because of their small pelvic bones, pregnant women with most chondrodysplasias should be managed in high-risk prenatal clinics and, in many instances, be delivered by cesarean section. Intelligence usually is normal in people with the nonlethal chondrodysplasias, but because patients are so easily recognized as being "different" from their peers, they and their families often benefit from nonclinical support. Such groups as the Little People of America and the Human Growth Foundation, publications directed to the lay population (11), and such web sites as http://www.lpaonline.org provide useful information.

WILLIAM A. HORTON, MD

References

1. *Horton WA, Hecht JT. Chondrodysplasias: part I. General concepts, diagnostic and management considerations. In: Royce P, Steinmann B (eds). Connective Tissue and Its Heritable Disorders. New York: Wiley-Liss, (In Press) 2001.*
2. *Rimoin DL, Lachman RS. Genetic disorders of the osseous skeleton. In: Beighton P (ed). McKusick's Heritable Disorders of Connective Tissue, 5th ed. St Louis: Mosby, 1993; pp 557–690.*
3. *Bassett GS. The osteochondrodysplasias. In: Morrissy RT, Weinstein SL (eds). Lovell & Winter's Pediatric Orthopaedics, 4th ed. Philadelphia: J.B. Lippincott, 1996; pp 203–254.*
4. *Morris N, Keene DR, Horton WA. Morphology of connective tissue: cartilage. In: Royce P, Steinmann B (eds). Connective Tissue and Its Heritable Disorders. New York: Wiley-Liss, (In Press) 2001.*
5. *Horton WA. Molecular genetic basis of the human chondrodysplasias. Endocrinol Metab Clin North Am 1996;25: 683–697.*
6. *Rimoin DL, Francomano CA, Giedion A, et al. International nomenclature and classification of the osteochondrodysplasias. Am J Med Genet 1998;79:376–382.*
7. *Spranger J, Maroteaux P. The lethal osteochondrodysplasias. Adv Hum Genet 1995;19:1–103.*
8. *Spranger JW, Langer LO, Wiedemann H-R. Bone Dysplasias, An Atlas of Constitutional Disorders of Skeletal Development. Philadelphia: W.B.Saunders Co., 1974.*
9. *Wynne-Davies R, Hall CM, Apley AG. Atlas of Skeletal Dysplasias. Edinburgh: Churchill Livingstone, 1985.*
10. *Tabyi H, Lachman RS. Radiology of Syndromes, Metabolic Disorders, and Skeletal Dysplasias, 4th ed. St. Louis: Mosby, 1996.*
11. *Scott CI Jr, Mayeux N, Crandall R, Weiss J. Dwarfism, the Family and Professional Guide. Irvine: Short Stature Foundation & Information Center, Inc., 1994.*
12. *Sharrard WJW. Abnormalities of the epiphyses and limb inequality. In: Paediatric Orthopaedics and Fracture, 3rd ed. Oxford: Blackwell Scientific Publications, 1993; pp 719–814.*
13. *Tachdjian MO. Osteochondroses and related disorders. In: Pediatric Orthopedics, 2nd ed. Philadelphia: W.B. Saunders, 1990; pp 932–1062.*

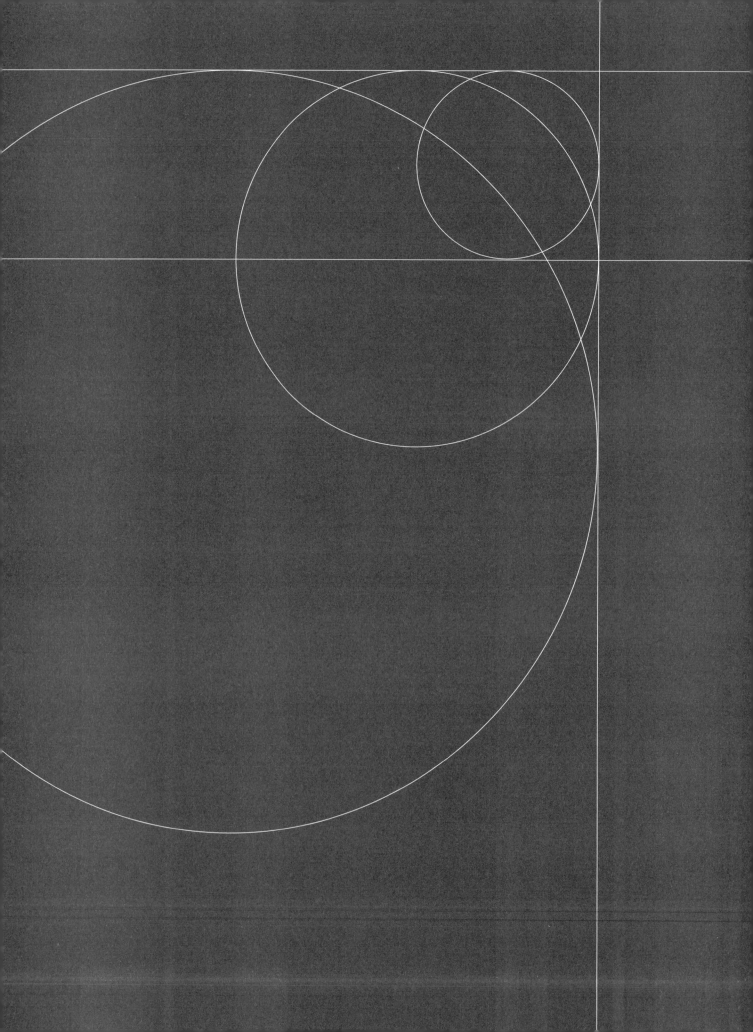

36 OSTEONECROSIS

Osteonecrosis is a generic term used to describe the death of all cellular elements of bone. Other terms for this condition are ischemic bone necrosis, avascular necrosis, and aseptic necrosis, but osteonecrosis is the preferred term. Osteonecrosis may occur in a variety of clinical settings in association with defined diseases (e.g., Gaucher's disease), medications (e.g., corticosteroids), physiologic or pathologic processes (e.g., pregnancy or thromboembolism), or no apparent predisposing factors (idiopathic). The disorder affects individuals of both genders and all age groups. For the most part, osteonecrosis involves the epiphyses of long bones, such as the femoral and humeral heads, but other bones (e.g., carpal and tarsal) also can be affected. More than one bone may be involved, either sequentially or simultaneously.

Pathogenesis

Bone death is the result of diminished arterial blood supply, an easily understood mechanism that can be reproduced in experimental animals. If blood flow is completely interrupted and not promptly restored, bone death inevitably ensues. The final outcome of the process depends on the size of the affected area and the success of reparative processes in which viable bone cells replace necrotic or nonviable bone. Failure to revitalize large, involved areas leads to bone collapse, joint incongruity, and eventually, secondary osteoarthritis. The characteristic histopathologic findings of osteonecrosis include marrow fibrosis, fat-cell necrosis, necrotic bone, and some evidence of attempts at repair.

Prolonged ischemia may occur as a result of intra- or extravascular pathology within the bone itself. Small-vessel vasculitis, arteriolar thrombosis, venous occlusion, and microembolism are well-recognized causes of ischemia. Infiltrative processes, such as Gaucher's disease, indirectly alter the vascular supply by compressing the sinusoids. The direct toxic effect of some substances on different cell populations of the bone also can lead to osteonecrosis. For example, even moderate amounts of alcohol are toxic to osteocytes. Corticosteroids (endogenous or exogenous) are toxic to lipocytes, yet promote the conversion of hematopoietic marrow into fat (1); whether or not this lipogenicity can be modified is being investigated (2).

Elevated intraosseous pressure (IOP) has been postulated as the common pathway of osteonecrosis (3). Increased pressure in bone – an organ that essentially is incapable of expanding – leads to ischemia and cell damage. The presence of increased IOP has been used in the past as a tool for early diagnosis of osteonecrosis. Although it is likely that increased IOP plays an important role in the pathogenesis of osteonecrosis, other factors, such as cytotoxicity, may be equally important.

Increased IOP is not the *sine qua non* of this disorder because it also occurs in other pathologic processes (e.g., osteoarthritis). Likewise, increased IOP has not been found in histologically proven, experimentally induced osteonecrosis in rabbits (4). Further insights into the pathogenesis of osteonecrosis may result from histopathologic and imaging investigations performed in early disease, before clinical signs or radiologic evidence of damage is present.

Clinical Features

The first clinical manifestation of osteonecrosis is the relatively abrupt onset of pain. Initially, pain is elicited only with movement (e.g., in hip involvement, during weight-bearing activities), but later escalates to pain at rest. In the early stages, decreased range of motion is related primarily to pain. Some patients experience severe pain as the disease progresses, but other patients with similar radiographic changes are comparatively asymptomatic. Bone remodeling allows some patients to remain functional for years, despite decreased range of motion. However, most patients have persistent and worsening pain, progressive range-of-motion losses, and significant loss of function. The time from onset of symptoms to development of an end-stage joint varies widely, from months to years.

A common clinical presentation encountered by rheumatologists is that of a young woman with systemic lupus erythematosus and cushingoid features secondary to prolonged treatment with corticosteroids. The average dosage, cumulative dosage, duration of use, and route of administration typically varies among people who develop osteonecrosis, but the greater the use of corticosteroids, the higher the likelihood of osteonecrosis. Table 36-1 lists other, less common conditions associated with osteonecrosis.

A preclinical stage has been demonstrated in magnetic resonance imaging (MRI) studies comparing symptomatic and asymptomatic joints in people at high risk for osteonecrosis (5). Abnormalities in asymptomatic joints may predate clinical symptoms by several weeks.

Diagnosis

For years, the diagnosis of osteonecrosis was based on plain radiographs, which identify advanced disease but do not detect early stages. Plain radiographs, such as neutral

TABLE 36-1
Diseases or Conditions Associated With Osteonecrosis

Trauma
  Hip dislocation
  Hip fracture
  Postarthroscopy
Connective-tissue disorders (CTDs)[a]
  Systemic lupus erythematosus
  Rheumatoid arthritis
  Systemic vasculitis
  Antiphospholipid antibody syndrome
  Other CTDs
Hematologic disorders
  Sickle cell disease
  Sickle cell-C disease
  Thalassemia minor
  Clotting disorders[b]
Infiltrative disorders
  Gaucher's disease
  Solid tumors
Metabolic disorders
  Gout
Disorders associated with fat necrosis
  Pancreatitis
  Pancreatic carcinoma
Embolism
  Decompression sickness
Corticosteroids (exogenous and endogenous)
  Asthma
  Aplastic anemia
  Leukemias and lymphomas
  Celiac disease
  Inflammatory bowel disease
  Cushing syndrome
  Organ transplantation
  Intra-articular, pulse intravenous, and enteral
    administration
Gastrointestinal disorders
  Inflammatory bowel disease[a]
Cytotoxic agents
  Vinblastine
  Vincristine
  Cisplatin (intra-arterial)
  Cyclophosphamide
  Methotrexate
  Bleomycin
  5-Fluorouracil
Alcohol
Radiation
Pregnancy
Idiopathic[c]

[a] May occur independent of corticosteroid use.
[b] Intravascular coagulation associated with infections, included.
[c] No associated disorders or precipitating factors recognized.

anteroposterior and frog views for detecting hip disease, still are useful, but MRI is the diagnostic tool of choice for identifying early disease.

Although several classification systems for osteonecrosis have been developed, the one most commonly used describes five stages of disease (6). A fifth stage, 0 (zero), has been added to include asymptomatic patients whose radiographs show no abnormalities, but for whom MRI studies confirm the presence of disease. These stages are defined in Table 36-2. Magnetic resonance evaluations demonstrate the extent of bone involvement, which helps predict patient outcomes (7).

There are no clear data on the sensitivity, specificity, or predictive values (positive and negative) of diagnostic procedures, including MRI, in osteonecrosis. Because histologically proven dead bone (the "gold standard" for diagnosis) is not obtained in all patients, these data may never be available. MRI permits distinction between normal bone and marrow; unrepaired, dead bone and marrow; unrepaired, dead bone, with marrow replaced by debris; and zones of repair. Necrotic bone and bone marrow produce a high-signal intensity in both T1 and T2 images, and subchondral bone appears as dark striations. The combined appearance of these signals gives the characteristic, well-described serpiginous pattern. Bone-marrow edema

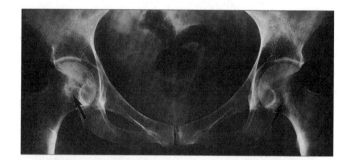

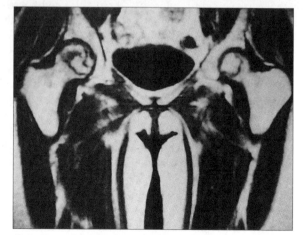

Fig. 43-1. Stage II osteonecrosis of both femoral heads. Top: Plain film of the pelvis and both hips shows patchy foci of increased density (arrows) characteristic of stage II osteonecrosis. The femoral heads are not collapsed. Bottom: T1-weighted coronal MRI shows curvilinear areas of low signal in both femoral heads typical of osteonecrosis. Courtesy of Wanda K. Bernreuter, MD.

without the other findings described is characteristic of transient osteoporosis, a reversible condition for which surgical interventions are contraindicated (8).

Treatment

Outcome criteria for the treatment of osteonecrosis have been developed (9). Stages 0, I, and II may be treated by conservative measures or by core decompression. Conservative treatment includes the following: judicious use of analgesics, physical therapy to maintain muscle strength and prevent contractures, and assistive devices to facilitate ambulation. Patients with osteonecrosis of non–weight-bearing joints may not require any intervention, because they may have only mild to moderate pain and limited, tolerable functional losses.

The rationale for core decompression is to reduce IOP, reestablish blood supply, and allow living bone adjacent to dead bone to contribute to the reparative process. Good to excellent results have been obtained in the majority of people with stages I and II osteonecrosis, and in a significant proportion of patients with stage III disease. The most convincing evidence of efficacy comes from a randomized, controlled study (9). Fifty hips from 31 patients with osteonecrosis staged I–III were randomized to undergo conservative (non–weight-bearing) or surgical (core decompression) treatment. In stage I and II patients, decompression reduced pain more reliably and led to less hip surgery in the follow-up period than did conservative treatment. Clinical stabilization was achieved by core decompression in 90% of stage I and II cases (9). In another study, core decompression and bone grafting halted disease progression in patients with early disease. In contrast, patients with advanced disease and large areas of bone involvement typically suffer clinical and radiographic evidence of disease progression. Smith et al (10) reported on 114 hips in 92 patients with osteonecrosis due to different causes (e.g., corticosteroid use, alcohol, and trauma). Clinical failure, which was defined as the need for more surgery, occurred in 16% of the hips in stage I, 53% in stage IIA, 80% in stage IIB, and 100% in stage IV. Combined experiences indicate that core decompression is a reasonable treatment alternative for patients in early stages of osteonecrosis, particularly stage I.

In contrast to these positive results, two separate studies have reported the failure of core decompression, even in patients in early-stage osteonecrosis (11, 12). In addition, these studies reported substantial morbidity, particularly the incidence of postsurgical subtrochanteric fractures, and strongly recommended the abandonment of this procedure.

Patients with persistent, intractable pain and progressive functional loss should be considered for arthroplasty. Ideally, patients with hip involvement should undergo arthroplasty before total collapse of the femoral head occurs. The relative utilities of cemented or uncemented prostheses is a matter of controversy. Regardless of the type of prosthesis, younger patients experience higher rates of mechanical failure than do

TABLE 36-2
Staging in Osteonecrosis[a]

Stage 0	Clinical manifestations absent; normal radiographs.[b]
Stage I	Clinical manifestations present; normal radiographs.[b]
Stage II	Areas of osteopenia and osteosclerosis in radiographs.
Stage III	Early bone collapse manifested as the "crescent sign" (translucent subcortical bone delineates the area of dead bone).
Stage IV	Late bone collapse manifested as flattening of the femoral head, with or without joint incongruity.

[a] Adapted from Arlet and Ficat (16).
[b] Diagnosis made by magnetic resonance imaging.

older patients (13). The indications for arthroplasty include not only evidence of radiographic progression but also worsening pain and incapacitation.

Over the past few years, significant data have accumulated about bone grafting as an alternative for the treatment of osteonecrosis. A follow-up study of 89 patients (103 affected hips), some with idiopathic osteonecrosis and some with histories of corticosteroid use, alcohol use, or trauma revealed a low incidence of failure following bone grafting (14). The probability of failure, defined as the need for arthroplasty, within five years varied from 11% for people in early-stage disease to nearly 30% for those with advanced osteonecrosis. All patients improved significantly, as measured by the standardized Harris questionnaire (14). Bone grafting may be a reasonable attempt to delay arthroplasty in relatively young patients.

Prognosis

Diagnosing very early osteonecrosis using MRI may lead to better outcomes. Conservative management may be the only treatment required for patients with stages 0 and I disease, although core decompression may offer some advantage in these cases. In more advanced disease, bone grafting can delay the need for arthroplasty and allow the patient to remain functional. A combination of factors (e.g., size of the necrotic area, degree of bone collapse, and presence of an underlying condition) likely explains the lower success rate of arthroplasty in osteonecrosis than in other disorders, particularly osteoarthritis.

GRACIELA S. ALARCÓN, MD, MPH

References

1. Vande Berg BC, Malghem J, Lecouvet FE, Devogelaer JP, Maldague B, Houssiau FA. Fat conversion of femoral marrow in glucocorticoid-treated patients: a cross-sectional and longitudinal study with magnetic resonance. Arthritis Rheum 1999; 42:1405–1411.

2. Wang GJ, Cui Q, Balian G. The pathogenesis and prevention of steroid induced osteonecrosis. Clin Orthop Rel Res 2000;370: 295–310.

3. Zizic TM, Marcoux C, Hungerford DS, Stevens MB. The early diagnosis of ischemic necrosis of bone. Arthritis Rheum 1986; 29:1177–1186.

4. Warner JJP, Philip JH, Brodsky GL, Thornhill TS. Studies of nontraumatic osteonecrosis. Manometric and histologic studies of the femoral head after chronic steroid treatment: an experimental study in rabbits. Clin Orthop 1987;225:128–140.

5. Shinoda S, Kawasaki S, Tagawa N. Magnetic resonance imaging of osteonecrosis in divers: comparison with plain radiographs. Skeletal Radiol 1997;26:354–359.

6. Arlet J, Ficat P. Diagnostic de l'osteonecrose femorocapitale primitive au stade I (stade preradiologic): [The diagnosis of primary femur head osteonecrosis at stage I (pre-radiologic stage)]. Rev Chir Orthop Reparatrice Appar Mot 1968;54: 637–648.

7. Sugano N, Ohzono K, Masuhara K, Takaoka K, Ono K. Prognostication of osteonecrosis of the femoral head in patients with systemic lupus erythematosus of magnetic resonance imaging. Clin Orthop 1994;305:190–199.

8. Alarcón GS, Sanders C, Daniel WW. Transient osteoporosis of the hip: magnetic resonance imaging. J Rheumatol 1987;14: 1184–1189.

9. Stulberg BN, Bauer TW, Belhobek GH. Making core decompression work. Clin Orthop 1990;261:186–195.

10. Smith SW, Fehring TK, Griffin WL, Beaver WB. Core decompression of the osteonecrotic femoral head. J Bone Joint Surg Am 1995;77:674–680.

11. Camp JF, Colwell CWJ. Core decompression of the femoral head for osteonecrosis. J Bone Joint Surg Am 1986;68: 1313–1319.

12. Hopson CN, Siverhus SW. Ischemic necrosis of the femoral head. Treatment by core decompression. J Bone Joint Surg Am 1988;70-A:1048–1051.

13. Ortiguera CJ, Pulliam IT, Cabanela ME. Total hip arthroplasty for osteonecrosis: matched-pair analysis of 188 hips with long-term follow-up. J Arthroplasty 1999;14:21–28.

14. Urbaniak JR, Coogan PG, Gunneson EB, Nunley JA. Treatment of osteonecrosis of the femoral head with free vascularized fibular grafting. A long-term follow-up study of one hundred and three hips. J Bone Joint Surg Am 1995;77: 681–694.

37 PAGET'S DISEASE

In 1877, the British physician Sir James Paget first described the disease that now bears his name (1). He observed that the disorder "begins in middle age or later (and) affects most frequently the long bones of the lower extremities and the skull. . . . The bones enlarge and soften, and those bearing weight yield and become unnaturally curved and misshapen." Paget's disease, as we now understand it, is a localized disorder of hyperactive bone remodeling, where abnormal osteoclasts accelerate the process of normal bone turnover. This process results in the production of bone that is disorganized, thickened, weakened, and often hypervascular. The clinical sequelae of these changes include bony pain, deformity, and fracture. Neurologic symptoms may develop, either from nerve impingement or vascular steal from hypervascular bone. Although Paget's disease typically does not affect joints, bony deformities may result in secondary joint disorders and a referral for rheumatologic evaluation (2).

Epidemiology

Because many people with asymptomatic Paget's disease remain undiagnosed, it has been difficult to determine disease prevalence. In a British study of 30,000 abdominal radiographs, the prevalence of Paget's disease among people over the age of 55 was 6.2% in men and 3.9% in women, with an overall prevalence of about 5%. Prevalence increased in an age-dependent manner, rising from a rate of 2% among men aged between 55 and 59 years to about 20% among men older than 85 (3). Paget's disease appears to be more common in Britain and among people of British and European descent. In the United States, the overall prevalence probably is approximately 2%. Paget's disease is reported less frequently among blacks, and appears to be even more rare in Asians. Interestingly, the prevalence of Paget's disease appears to be decreasing, although the reason for this trend is unclear.

Etiology

Paramyxovirus infection has been implicated in the development of Paget's disease. However, this hypothesis remains controversial. Several studies have demonstrated both measles virus and canine distemper virus in pagetic bone. However, these results have not been replicated universally (4). Furthermore, the lack of animal models for Paget's disease makes it difficult to apply Koch's postulates to this disorder. It also appears that genetic susceptibility may be necessary for the development of Paget's disease; 15%–30% of patients report a positive family history of the disease (5).

Clinical Features

Paget's disease is seen most commonly in the axial skeleton. The sites affected most frequently are the pelvis, spine, and femur. Involvement of the skull and tibia also is common (6). The bony abnormalities of Paget's disease appear to be driven by populations of abnormal osteoclasts. Large numbers of these highly multinucleated osteoclasts result in extensive bone resorption, with the subsequent recruitment of bone-forming osteoblasts. Although these osteoblasts appear to be normal, the hyperactivity of the remodeling process results in a disorganized mosaic of woven and lamellar bone. These microarchitectural abnormalities result in a weakened bone that is prone to fracture. Pagetic bone can be excessively vascular. This hypervascularity may lead to excessive bleeding (particularly in the setting of surgery) and vascular steal syndromes.

Because Paget's disease frequently is asymptomatic, the diagnosis often is made as an incidental finding. These patients typically have either pagetic findings on routine radiographic studies or elevated levels of alkaline phosphatase in the absence of liver dysfunction. In contrast, people with symptomatic Paget's disease usually present with pain, bony deformity, or neurologic manifestations (7).

Pain resulting from Paget's disease may have several etiologies, including hypervascularity (usually associated with warmth over the affected area), periosteal distortion due to thickened bone, or fractures (including stress and full fractures). Although Paget's disease classically spares joints, periarticular disease may result in significant pain at the hips, knees, or spine. In these cases, radiographs of the affected joint often reveal classic signs of Paget's disease in the adjacent bones. Paget's disease also may involve the proximal femur or the pelvis near the acetabulum. In these settings, hip pain may be a direct result of pagetic involvement (2).

Back pain is common in patients with Paget's disease. Possible etiologies include vertebral enlargement with loss of lumbar lordosis, vertebral fracture, nerve-root impingement, and gait changes secondary to Paget's disease at other sites. Hypervascular vertebral bone may result in a spinal artery steal syndrome. Because Paget's disease may coexist with other causes of back pain, such as osteoarthritis, it often is difficult to determine the role of Paget's disease when evaluating people with back pain.

Bony deformities are less common, but highly specific for Paget's disease. These changes typically are asymmetric. Deformities of the femur and tibia may result in the classically described finding of a bowed leg. Skull abnormalities may include frontal bossing or an enlarged maxilla, and may lead to neurologic sequelae. The most common of these neurologic findings is hearing loss. The etiology appears to multifactorial, including cochlear dysfunction (secondary to temporal bone involvement) and compression of cranial nerve VIII. Involvement of the basilar skull may result in obstructive hydrocephalus or long-tract signs secondary to pressure on the brain stem. In these settings, skull radiographs commonly reveal pagetic bony changes (4).

In addition to the clinical manifestations, people with Paget's disease are at risk for two potentially serious complications: excessive bleeding after a fracture through hypervascular pagetic bone and the development of bony malignancy (8). The former can be seen in both spontaneous fractures and during orthopedic procedures, such as internal fixation and joint replacement. Most authorities suggest that Paget's disease be well-controlled with bisphosphonate therapy before elective orthopedic surgery. It also has been suggested that bisphosphonate therapy, particularly intravenous pamidronate, may be a valuable intervention before urgent or emergent surgery.

Neoplastic degeneration is quite rare, and probably occurs in fewer than 1% of people with Paget's disease. It typically presents with a severe and rapid worsening of pain in an area of long-standing pagetic bone. Pathologic fracture also may occur. Patients with a sudden worsening of pagetic symptoms should have radiographic studies of the affected area.

Radiographic and Laboratory Features

The diagnosis of Paget's disease is made by radiographs, routine laboratory testing, or both. The classic radiographic finding is mixed areas of bony lysis (reflecting osteoclast activity) and sclerosis (reflecting osteoblast activity). Bone thickening is highly characteristic of Paget's disease, as is a flame-shaped lytic lesion seen in long bones. Radiographs are useful in assessing the status of nearby joints and determining if there are any fractures through pagetic bone.

Bone scans can help determine the extent of bony involvement, but should not be used to make the diagnosis of Paget's disease. Although about 20% of people with Paget's disease will have involvement of only one bone, the presence of monostotic disease on bone scan should raise suspicion for other lesions, including fracture, infection, and malignancy. Because the sites of pagetic involvement tend to be stable, an initial bone scan can be quite useful for long-term follow-up and for assessing new symptoms that may (or may not) be related to Paget's disease.

Biochemical testing is useful in the diagnosis of Paget's disease, ruling out other causes of metabolic bone disease, and determining the effectiveness of medical therapy (9).

Because Paget's disease affects bone resorption and formation, markers of these processes typically are elevated. Measurements of bone resorption include urinary hydroxyproline and collagen cross-links (e.g., N-telopeptides and C-telopeptides). Bone formation is reflected in total or fractionated measurements of bone alkaline phosphatase, but if total measurements are used, liver disease may complicate interpretation of the assay results. Approximately 85% of people with Paget's disease will have an elevated alkaline phosphatase, and levels greater than 10 times normal often are associated with skull involvement (4,9). Testing alkaline phosphatase levels probably is the most effective method for monitoring disease activity and assessing the effectiveness of antipagetic therapy.

Results from other tests commonly used to evaluate metabolic bone disease typically are normal in Paget's disease (7). These tests include serum calcium, phosphorous, parathyroid hormone (PTH), vitamin D, and osteocalcin levels. An elevated calcium level should raise suspicion for malignancy or primary hyperparathyroidism. It is also worth noting that secondary hyperparathyroidism (i.e., an elevated PTH in the setting of normal calcium levels) may sometimes be seen in active Paget's disease.

Treatment

There has been significant progress in the availability and effectiveness of therapy for Paget's disease (10). Current first-line therapy for Paget's disease is one of the later-generation bisphosphonates. In the United States, alendronate, pamidronate, risedronate, and tiludronate are approved for the treatment of Paget's disease (11). These agents generally have replaced the use of calcitonin and etidronate (an earlier bisphosphonate), due to their greater effectiveness in reducing disease activity and the prolonged duration of response after short courses of therapy. There are no specific guidelines for identifying which patients should be treated for Paget's disease. However, given the excellent effectiveness, good tolerability, and short duration (two to three months) of bisphosphonate therapy, it appears reasonable to treat patients who are symptomatic, at risk for complications, and with markedly elevated levels of alkaline phosphatase (4,7). Most studies suggest that bisphosphonate therapy will normalize alkaline phosphatase in one-half to two-thirds of affected patients. Alkaline phosphatase levels should be monitored during bisphosphonate therapy, and subsequently, at three- to six-month intervals. If alkaline phosphatase levels rise, an additional course of bisphosphonates often is effective in reducing pagetic activity.

Bisphosphonates tend to be poorly absorbed and may cause erosive disease of the upper gastrointestinal tract. Typical guidelines for their administration include taking the medication on an empty stomach with 6–8 oz of water; ingesting no other food, beverage, or medication for the next 30 minutes; and maintaining an upright posture (sitting or standing) during that time. Although unusual in the treatment of Paget's disease, bisphosphonates may reduce serum calcium levels, and patients must receive adequate amounts of calcium and vitamin D (4).

Summary

In summary, Paget's disease of bone is a complex disorder affecting bone, joints, neurologic structures, and the vascular system. The etiology remains unclear, although paramyxovirus infection may be involved. Most patients probably remain asymptomatic. However, a minority may develop pain, bony deformities, joint disease, and neurologic manifestations. Rarely, patients may have excessive bleeding after fracture through pagetic bone or malignant degeneration of affected sites. The diagnosis usually is made clinically and confirmed with radiologic and biochemical studies. Bisphosphonate therapy has proven effective in relieving symptoms and reducing disease activity, but it does not result in remission of the disease. Patients with Paget's require ongoing monitoring of their disease, including prompt evaluation and management of its clinical sequelae.

ROBERT LASH, MD

References

1. Smith R. Paget's disease of bone: past and present. Bone 1999; 24:S1-S2.
2. Altman RD. Paget's disease of bone: rheumatologic complications. Bone 1999;24:S47-S48.
3. Cooper C, Dennison E, Schafheutle K, Kellingray S, Guyer P, Barker D. Epidemiology of paget's disease of bone. Bone 1999; 24:S3-S5.
4. Siris ES. Paget's disease of bone. In: Fauvus MJ (ed). Primer on the Metabolic Bone Diseases and Disorders of Mineral Metabolism, 4th edition. Philadelphia: Lippincott-Raven, 1999; pp 415-425.
5. Siris ES, Canfield RE, Jacobs TP. Paget's disease of bone. Bull NY Acad Med 1980;56:285-304.
6. Davie M, Davies M, Francis R, Fraser W, Hosking D, Tansley R. Paget's disease of bone: a review of 889 patients. Bone 1999;24: S11-S12.
7. Hosking D, Meunier PJ, Ringe JD, Reginster JY, Gennari C. Paget's disease of bone: diagnosis and management. BMJ 1996; 312:491-494.
8. Kaplan FS. Severe orthopaedic complications of Paget's disease. Bone 1999;24:S43-S46.
9. Eastell R. Biochemical markers of bone turnover in paget's disease of bone. Bone 1999;24:49-50.
10. Reginster JY, Lecart MP. Efficacy and safety of drugs for Paget's disease of bone. Bone 1995;17:S485-S488.
11. Hines SE. Paget's disease of bone: a new philosophy of treatment. Patient Care 1999;33:40-60.

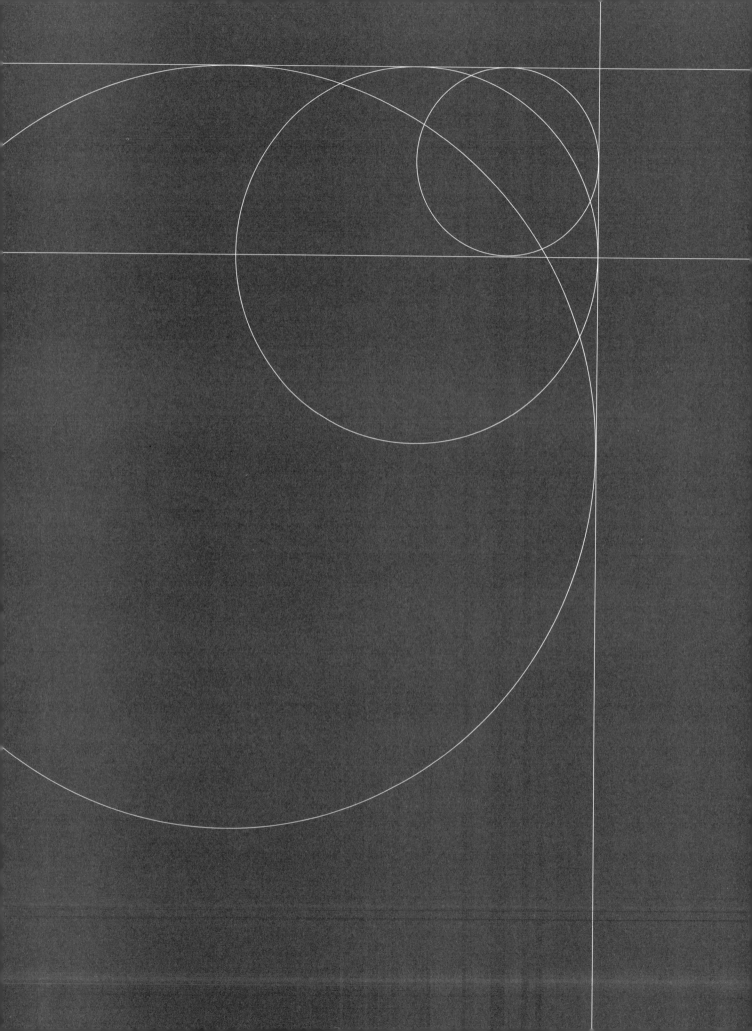

38 OSTEOPOROSIS
A. Epidemiology, Pathology, and Pathogenesis

Osteoporosis is a skeletal disease, marked by low bone mass and microarchitectural deterioration that leads to an increased susceptibility to fracture. Fractures are the single most important clinical consequence of osteoporosis and represent a major health problem in the elderly. Low bone mass, skeletal fragility, and propensity to fall are the primary determinants of fracture risk in older persons. Bone density, a measure of bone mass, can be measured noninvasively using widely available densitometric techniques, and is the main focus of risk assessment and therapy. However, knowledge of other risk factors may be useful in determining fracture risk, understanding the pathophysiology of osteoporosis, and guiding prevention and treatment.

Fractures, Morbidity, and Costs

Fractures affect a substantial proportion of the older population in North America and Europe (Table 38A-1). Older white women are at greatest risk, but all elderly women and elderly men may be affected. Although vertebral and wrist fractures are the most common types of fracture, hip fractures are the most devastating. Adding substantially to the burden of the disease, fractures among the elderly also occur at a variety of other skeletal sites not traditionally considered "osteoporotic."

The risk of most types of fractures in elderly women is related to low bone density (1). Approximately 90% of hip and spine fractures, 70% of wrist fractures, and 50% of all other fractures in white women aged 65–84 years are attributable to osteoporosis. Assuming that 70% of all fractures in the elderly are at least partly due to low bone mass, 1.3 million fractures per year in the United States can be attributed to osteoporosis (2). Because these estimates of attributable risk are higher than that suggested by the relationship between bone mass and fracture risk (3), some component of bone fragility that leads to fractures is independent of bone mass.

Hip fracture risk is strongly related to low bone density, and is more strongly associated with bone density at the hip than at other sites (3). The risk of hip fracture rises exponentially with age, is twice as great in women as it is in men at most ages, and reaches 2% and 3% per year in men and women, respectively, by age 85 (4). Nearly all hip fractures in the elderly (about 90%) occur as a direct result of falls (5).

TABLE 38A-1
Frequency and Impact of Osteoporosis in the United States

Persons with femoral osteoporosis or osteopenia	
White women	17–26 million (59%–84%)
African American women	1.2 million (36%)
Mexican American women	0.5 million (49%)
Men (all races, using male cutoffs)	10 million (37%)
Lifetime risk of hip, wrist, or vertebral fracture	
50-year-old white woman	40%
50-year-old white man	13%
Fractures per year due to osteoporosis	1.3 million
Hip fractures per year	250,000–300,000
Hospitalization per year for osteoporotic fractures	432,000
Outpatient visits per year for osteoporotic fractures	3.4 million
Medical expenditures for osteoporotic fractures in 1995	$13.8 billion

Many other important risk factors, including neuromuscular impairment, poor vision, low body weight, weight loss, a positive family history, sedative use, and a previous vertebral fracture, increase the risk of hip fracture independent of bone density (6). In the first year after a hip fracture, there is a 12%–20% higher mortality rate than that expected in the general population (7), and this increased rate is higher in men and African Americans (8). The mortality risk is greatest during the first six months after a hip fracture, due to acute complications of the fracture and its treatment and to severe coexisting medical conditions. By 12 months after the fracture, 50% or more of hip-fracture survivors show decreased physical function, and 20%–30% of previously noninstitutionalized patients require nursing-home care.

In contrast to hip, wrist, and other long-bone fractures, a majority of vertebral fractures in women are asymptomatic or not diagnosed (9). Severe vertebral fractures usually can be seen on spine radiographs, but the presence of mild fractures can be uncertain. It is important to recognize vertebral fractures, because they are a common hallmark of osteoporosis that requires treatment. They are found on radiographs of 5%–10% of white women at age 55 years, a rate that rises to 30%–40% by age 80 (10,11). The risk of a new vertebral fracture on x-ray in white women is 0.5% per year at age 55 and 2%–3% per year at age 80 years, roughly three times the incidence of clinically diagnosed vertebral fractures (9,11). The risk of vertebral fractures is strongly related to low bone density (3), but few major risk factors other than age have been identified. Recent radiographic surveys have found that vertebral fractures are at least as common in men aged 50–65 years as in women this age, but at older ages, the risk in women exceeds that in men (10). This finding probably reflects the larger role that occupational and sports trauma play in young male vertebral fractures. In the elderly, only about 25% of clinically diagnosed vertebral fractures are due to falls (9).

Vertebral fractures that reach clinical attention usually cause severe back pain and physical disability (12,13). However, even undiagnosed fractures found on radiographs are, on average, associated with increased back pain and disability in such activities as bending, putting on socks, and getting in and out of an automobile (12). Both clinically and radiographically identified vertebral fractures are associated with increased mortality, probably due to an association with comorbid medical conditions (7,14).

Wrist fractures, 90% of which are due to falls, are four times more common in women than in men. Incidence reaches a plateau among women around age 65, increasing

TABLE 38A-2
Types of Fracture in the Elderly Associated with Gender, Age, Bone Density, and Falls

Type of fracture	Fracture risk associated with			% of fractures associated with a fall[b]
	Female gender	Increased age	Low bone density[a]	
Hip	+	+	++	>90
Wrist	+	–	++	>90
Vertebral	+[c]	+[c]	++[d]	<50[c]
Proximal humerus	+	+	++	>90
Pelvis	+	+	++	80–90
Rib	–	+	++	50–79
Clavicle	–	–	++	<50
Femur shaft	+	+	++	50–79
Patella	+	–	++	80–90
Tibia/Fibula	+	–	++	50–79
Ankle	+	–	+	80–90
Heel	NA	–	++	NA
Foot	–	–	+	<50
Toe	NA	–	+	<50
Elbow	NA	–	+	>90
Hand	–	–	++	50–79
Finger	NA	–	+	50–79
Face	–	–	–	50–79

[a] + = relative risk of 1.2–1.7 per standard deviation decrease bone density
  ++ = relative risk of 1.8 or greater per standard deviation decrease in bone density
[b] Fall from standing height or less
[c] Clinical vertebral fractures
[d] Radiographically detected vertebral deformities

TABLE 38A-3
Lifetime Risk of Fracture

	Hip fracture (%)	Distal forearm (%)	Vertebral fracture	
			Clinical (%)	Radiographic (%)
White women	14–17 [a,b,c,d]	14–16 [a,b,c,d]	16 [c,d]	35 [a]
White men	5–6 [a,b,c]	2–3 [a,b,c]	5 [c]	?
Black women	6 [b]	?	?	?
Black men	3 [b]	?	?	?

Lifetime risk of fracture at age 50 years in persons with average risk.
[a] Data from Chrischilles et al (17).
[b] Data from Cummings et al (18).
[c] Data from Melton L, Chrischilles E, Cooper C, Lane A, Riggs B. How many women have osteoporosis? J Bone Miner Res 1992;7:1005–1010.
[d] Data from National Osteoporosis Foundation (11).

only slowly thereafter (2). This seems to be a result of changes in the falling pattern with advancing age; in older persons, for example, slower gait and decreased reflexes make a fall on the hip more likely than one on an outstretched arm (5). The risk of wrist fractures is greater in healthier, more active women with low bone density, and wrist fractures are not associated with increased mortality (2).

Classic osteoporotic fractures (e.g., hip, vertebrae, and wrist) account for considerably less than one-half of all clinical fractures in elderly white women (1) and less than one-third of all fractures in elderly white men (15). Other fractures displaying an age-related increase in incidence and a greater incidence in women than in men include fractures of the pelvis, proximal humerus, and femur shaft (Table 38A-2). The risks of these fractures and fractures of the rib, clavicle, patella, distal tibia/fibula, calcaneus, and hand are all strongly related to low bone density (1,3). Fractures of the ankle, foot, toe, finger, and elbow are more weakly related to low bone density, and face and skull fractures appear to be unrelated to low bone density.

The health care-related costs of osteoporosis are substantial and increasing. Direct U.S. medical expenditures for osteoporotic fractures are estimated at $13.8 billion, with about 60% going for treatment of hip fracture and 30% for fractures other than the hip, spine, or wrist (16). In 1995, an estimated 432,000 U.S. hospital discharges were persons aged 45 years and older with osteoporotic fractures. Of these, 57% (246,600) were hip fractures, 3% (13,400) were forearm fractures, 7% (29,400) were spine fractures, and 33% (142,700) were other fractures. In that same year, there were more than 79,000 nursing-home stays for fractures, 77% of which were for hip fractures. Women accounted for 80% of all hospitalizations for fracture, and 77% of those for hip fracture. Most fractures, however, are treated on an outpatient basis. Overall, osteoporotic fractures were responsible for a total of 3.4 million outpatient physician, hospital, and emergency-room visits, of which nearly two-thirds were for fractures at sites other than hip, spine, or forearm. The cost of treating a hip fracture in the United States averages well over $30,000.

The number of hip fractures and their associated costs could triple by the year 2040, due to aging of the population (2).

Individual Risk of Fracture

The average risk of fracture for an individual is influenced by life expectancy and fracture risk at each age. These factors have been modeled in several studies (11,17,18), producing consistent estimates of the lifetime risks of fracture for an average 50-year-old white woman or man (Table 38A-3). Such estimates are useful for weighing the public health burden of osteoporosis, compared with other conditions. At age 50, the lifetime risk of having a hip, wrist, or clinical vertebral fracture is about 40% in white women and 13% in white men. A 50-year-old white woman has a 30% lifetime risk of having a fracture other than hip, wrist, or spine, and a 70% risk of a fracture at any site. Lifetime risks of hip fracture for blacks have been reported (Table 3), but there are insufficient data for other fractures and for other racial groups. At any given age, fracture risk and mortality correlate strongly with bone density. Incorporating these factors into a model improves estimates of lifetime fracture risk. For example, a 50-year-old white woman has a 19% lifetime risk of hip fracture if her radial bone mass is at the 10th percentile for her age, compared with an 11% lifetime risk if her bone mass is at the 90th percentile (19).

Prevalence of Osteoporosis and Osteopenia

Because the amount of bone mineral per unit volume (bone density) correlates strongly with bone strength (20) and is a major determinant of fracture risk, the proportion of the population with low bone density is a useful estimate of the prevalence of osteoporosis. The World Health Organization has defined low bone mass (osteopenia) in women as a bone mineral density (BMD) between 1.0 and 2.5 standard deviations below the mean for young adult women; it defines osteoporosis as a bone density equal to or greater than 2.5 standard deviations below the young adult mean. Women in the latter group who already have experienced one or more fractures are considered to have "established" osteoporosis.

Using young normal reference values for total femur bone density obtained from the Third National Health and Nutrition Examination Survey (NHANES III), 17% (5 million) of U.S. white women aged 50 and older have osteoporosis, and another 42% (12 million) have osteopenia (21). Using the total femur bone density cutoff values for white women, the same NHANES data suggest that 8% of non-Hispanic African American women (300,000) and 12% of Mexican American women (100,000) have osteoporosis; another 28% (900,000) and 37% (300,000), respectively, have osteopenia. Although the validity of using norms for whites in other racial groups is uncertain, the lower age-adjusted prevalence of osteoporosis in non-Hispanic African American women, compared with white women, is consistent with the lower incidence of fracture among the former (22). Prevalence estimates in women are increased by about 20% when based on bone density of the femoral neck. Higher prevalence estimates in white women are suggested by a combination of bone-density measurements at the hip, spine, and radius (2). Using the lowest value from the three sites, 30% of U.S. postmenopausal white women aged 50 years and older have osteoporosis, and another 54% have low bone mass. The number of older women in the United States with an increased risk of fracture due to low bone density approaches or exceeds the number with hypertension, diabetes, or high blood cholesterol.

For men aged 50 years and older, an adequate sample was available in NHANES III to estimate the prevalence of low bone mass for all races combined. Using a bone density cutoff value derived from young males for the total hip, 4% of all U.S. males over age 50 have osteoporosis and another 33% have low bone mass, for a total of about 10 million men affected. Prevalence estimates for men are 40%–50% higher if bone density of the femoral neck is used in place of the total hip.

These findings underscore several limitations of defining osteoporosis by universal bone density cut-off points derived from means and standard deviations in young normals (commonly called bone density T-scores). Using this approach, the estimated prevalence of osteoporosis in the population varies by the measurement technique or skeletal site used, by the selection of a normal reference population, and by the variability of the measurement in that reference population (11). It also is likely that the young normal reference values should be race- and gender-specific, but gender- and race-specific data on the relationship between bone density and fracture risk is needed before these values can be determined. Although the T-score approach is useful for estimating and comparing the prevalence of osteoporosis among populations, the cut-off points used ultimately are arbitrary. There is little evidence for a threshold of bone density at which fractures occur. The use of universal bone density T-scores as thresholds indicating the need for treatment is controversial, because the risk of fracture is a function of age and risk factors other than bone density (6,11,23).

Pathophysiology

Bone remodeling, or the removal and replacement of old bone, is a normal process needed to maintain the biomechanical integrity of the adult skeleton. Bone resorption and formation are coupled temporally and occur at discrete remodeling sites on the surfaces of cancellous bone and in proximity to the Haversian systems of cortical bone. When these processes are balanced, the quantity of bone replaced at each remodeling site essentially is equal to the quantity removed. In osteoporosis, there is a reduction in the mass of bone during remodeling, but the remaining tissue is normal. Net bone loss due to remodeling occurs when bone resorption exceeds bone formation at each site ("remodeling imbalance") and when there is an increase in bone turnover related to an increase in the number of remodeling sites. In addition, loss of bone mass results when periosteal resorption of cortical bone exceeds endosteal apposition.

Age-related declines in bone strength are caused by a decline in mass, alterations in geometry, and qualitative changes in bone. Bone density is strongly related to the strength of bone, with a correlation of r = 0.6–0.8 between bone density and in vitro fracture loads (20). Bone strength also is affected by geometric, microarchitectural, and qualitative changes that accompany bone loss and aging (24), and as a result, older bones are weaker, independent of their lower mass. Decreases in the thickness and increases in the porosity of cortical bone reduce its strength, although this weakness may be partially compensated for by periosteal bone apposition that increases bone size and strength. Loss of trabecular bone results in thinning, perforation, and reduction in the number and connectivity of the trabecular plates that comprise the internal supporting structure of vertebrae, distal radius, and proximal femur. The accumulation of microfractures impairs the strength of both cortical and trabecular bone. As a result of these qualitative changes, there may be a disproportionately large loss of strength as mass declines. Indeed, bone may become so fragile, particularly in the spine, that loads generated during normal activities can exceed fracture loads (20). At the same time, an increase in falls and a decline in protective responses subject the skeleton to a greater frequency and severity of trauma.

By the fourth to fifth decade of life, both women and men have begun a gradual, age-related process of bone loss that continues into old age (25). By age 80 years, on average, women have lost about 40% of their peak adult bone mass, and men have lost about 25%. A number of age-related changes in mineral metabolism and bone-cell function contribute to bone loss, but the causes are not well-understood. In women, bone loss accelerates after menopause, for a period of five to 15 years, due to a cessation of ovarian function and an estrogen deficiency that trigger increased local production of bone-resorbing cytokines, accelerated turnover, and a remodeling imbalance (26). Low serum estradiol levels also are associated with low bone mass and bone loss in perimenopausal women, and in postmenopausal women up to 25 years after menopause (27). Very low levels of serum estradiol (<5 pg/mL) in elderly women (mean age, 72) are associated with increased risks of hip and vertebral fracture (28). It is not known whether this late effect of estrogen deficiency shares the same biochemical and cellular mechanisms as perimenopausal bone loss (26).

Bone loss in late postmenopausal women and elderly men also has been linked to a constellation of factors that includes age-related decreases in Vitamin D production, changes in Vitamin D metabolism, deficiencies in calcium intake and absorption, secondary hyperparathyroidism (which stimulates bone resorption), and decreased osteoblast function and bone formation. Estrogen deficiency may contribute to this constellation of factors, possibly through extraskeletal effects on calcium homeostasis and down-regulation of bone growth factors that impair bone formation (26). This hypothesis is consistent with the epidemiologic evidence that low estradiol levels increase bone loss and fracture risk in late postmenopausal women (28), and also with a growing body of evidence that low serum estradiol levels are strongly associated with low bone mineral density, high bone turnover, and fracture risk in elderly men (26). No such associations with testosterone deficiency have been observed.

Genetic, Gender, and Racial/Ethnic Differences

Bone mass in women and men at older ages, when fractures are most common, reflects a combination of the peak bone mass achieved as a young adult and subsequent bone loss. Each of these factors accounts for about one-half of the population variance in bone mass at age 70 years. Peak bone mass may be determined largely by genetics. Heritability estimates from twin studies suggest that genetic factors account for about 70%–80% of the interindividual variation in peak bone mass in both genders (29); however, the specific genes involved in determining bone mass, size, geometry, and strength remain undefined. Environmental factors, especially diet and mechanical loading, also play a role in determining peak bone mass. For example, calcium supplementation increases bone accretion in adolescent females, although these gains do not persist after supplements are stopped.

Gender differences in bone size and mass do not appear until the onset of puberty, but by young adulthood, most males have larger and thicker bones than do females (30). The larger bones of men confer a substantial strength advantage that probably underlies at least part of the lower fracture risk among men later in life. Racial differences in bone mass and size are accentuated during the pubertal growth period, and the resulting differences in peak bone mass may contribute to differences in fracture risk later in life. There are few data on racial or gender differences in

age-related bone loss, although limited evidence suggests that bone loss at the hip is greater in women than in men (25).

Hip fracture rates vary substantially by race, ethnicity, and geographic area (31). Age-adjusted hip fracture incidence rates are highest (>six per 1000 per year) in the white populations of Northern Europe and North America. Intermediate rates of four to six per 1000 per year have been observed in Great Britain, New Zealand, and Finland, and rates of two to four per 1000 per year have been found in Hong Kong, China, and Japan, and in Asian, African American, and Hispanic populations in the United States. These patterns are explained only partially by racial differences in bone mass; Asians and Hispanics in the United States have a bone mass similar to whites, but demonstrate a lower fracture risk (22). Large geographic differences in hip fracture rates can be found even within similar racial/ethnic groups, suggesting that lifestyle factors and level of economic development also contribute to the geographic variability in fracture risk.

Risk Factors for Fracture

Bone mass is one of the strongest determinants of fracture risk in both women and men and is a primary focus of risk assessment and treatment. A growing number of pharmacological interventions can reduce bone loss, increase bone density, and lower the risk of fractures in women with osteoporosis. A number of other important risk factors for fracture have been identified, some of which are independent of bone density. Knowledge of even nonmodifiable risk factors can help identify high-risk individuals who may benefit from interventions. Published osteoporosis treatment guidelines for white women include risk factors for fracture in determining recommended bone density treatment thresholds. For example, the U.S. National Osteoporosis Foundation recommends treatment for women with a bone density T-score below −2.5 if no other risk factors are present, and for women with a T-score below −2.0 if the patient has one or more strong risk factors, such as a prior fracture (11).

As discussed above, older age, female gender, and Caucasian race are strong, although nonmodifiable, risk factors for osteoporosis and fractures. Most of our knowledge about other fracture risk factors has been gained from studies of hip fracture in white women (Table 38A-4). The few studies in men and nonwhites indicate that their risk factors for hip fracture are similar to those for white women (22,32,33). Risk factor for hip fracture may not apply to other types of fractures. Different risk factors have been found for fractures of different bones (5), consistent with site-specific differences in the pathophysiology of skeletal fragility and trauma (Table 38A-2).

An existing vertebral fracture found on radiograph signals a fourfold increased risk of having another vertebral fracture, a twofold increased risk of a subsequent hip fracture, and a 50% greater risk of a nonvertebral fracture, compared with the risk for women without a previous vertebral fracture (34). These risks are independent of a

TABLE 38A-4
Risk Factors for Hip Fracture in Women

Established risk factors	**(Relative risk ≥ 2.0)**
Bone mineral density	Per 1 standard deviation decrease
Fall on hip	Versus fall on other body part
Neuromsuscular impairment	Unable to rise from chair without arms
Ethnicity	Caucasians versus African-Americans or Asians
Established risk factors	**(Relative risk ≥ 1.1–1.9)**
Age	Per 5-year increase
Multiple falls in past year	Versus no falls
Estrogen replacement therapy	Nonuse versus current user
Weight	Per 5-kg decrease
Vision impairment	Reduced acuity, depth perception versus no impairment
Physical inactivity	Versus walks for exercise
Likely risk factors	**(Relative risk ≥ 2.0)**
Weight loss since age 25 years	Per 20% loss
Ethnicity	Caucasians versus Hispanics
Poor health status	Versus good/excellent
Likely risk factors	**(Relative risk ≥1.1–1.9)**
History of low trauma fracture	Versus no fracture
Calcium intake < 400 mg/day	Versus ≥ 1000 mg/day
Height	Per 10-cm increase
Hip axis length	Per 1 standard deviation increase
Sedative use	Daily use versus nonuse
Current smoker	Versus never smoked

Adapted from Cumming et al (22)

woman's bone density, suggesting that a vertebral fracture is a marker for general skeletal fragility. A personal history of any nonspine, low-trauma fracture after age 50 years also is associated with an increased risk of subsequent hip, vertebral, and nonspine fractures (6,11).

Consistent with a strong genetic component to bone mass, a familial history also is a risk factor for fracture (29). Daughters of women who have had a vertebral or hip fracture have a lower bone mass in the spine and hip, respectively, than women whose mothers have no such history. Women whose mothers or siblings have had hip fractures have an increased risk of hip fracture. Family predisposition is both site-specific and independent of bone density (35), suggesting a possible genetic influence on fracture risk through variations in bone geometry or some nonskeletal factor.

Body weight is a powerful determinant of bone mass and bone density (36). Women and men who have a low body weight or have lost weight have a high risk of hip fracture, independent of bone density (22). Low body weight may increase hip fracture risk through decreased conversion of androgen precursors to estrone in fat and muscle tissue, bone loss caused by reduced mechanical strain on bone, and reduced soft-tissue padding, especially

overlying the greater trochanter. Muscle size and bone size may share genetic determinants.

Most nonspine fractures in the elderly are the result of a fall (Table 38A-2). A history of previous falls and risk factors for falls (including lower-extremity weakness and impairments of gait and balance) are associated with an increased risk of hip fracture (6,22,32,33). However, only 1%–2% of falls in the elderly result in a hip fracture. Falls to the side, decreased protective neuromuscular responses, reduced soft-tissue padding, and harder landing surfaces are all associated with a greater risk of hip fracture (5). Impaired balance and muscle weakness also increase the risk of nonspine fractures other than hip fracture in both women and men, independent of bone density (15,23). Sedative users have a twofold increased risk of falls and hip fractures (6,22).

Smokers have lower bone mass, faster bone loss, and an increased risk of hip and vertebral fracture compared with nonsmokers (6,22,36). This increased risk is not explained by a lower body weight in smokers, but may be due in part to poorer neuromuscular function.

There is good evidence from randomized trials that calcium supplementation reduces bone loss in postmenopausal women (37). Several randomized trials have found that calcium supplementation plus vitamin D protects against hip and nonspine fractures (38). Observational studies of dietary calcium intake, however, show only a modest and inconsistent protective effect for hip fracture (39). Measurements of dietary calcium intake may be unreliable, and its effect on fractures may be confounded by intake of associated nutrients such as protein from dairy products.

Skeletal loading from weight-bearing and muscle contraction stimulates osteoblast function and bone formation. Conversely, prolonged immobility causes bone loss. It is uncertain whether common forms of moderate exercise, such as walking, are sufficient to prevent bone loss, and at what sites. Randomized trials suggest that vigorous aerobic exercise and strength training preserve or modestly enhance bone mass for as long as the exercise is continued, and such exercise may help prevent falls. Despite the generally modest effects of even strenuous physical activity on bone mass, observational studies find that elderly men and women who maintain some form of regular physical activity have a 50%–70% lower risk of hip fracture (22). Whether this apparent protection is due to effects of exercise on bone mass and neuromuscular function is uncertain; it may reflect better health, superior physical function and nutrition, and increased exposure to sunlight among elderly people who are able to exercise. These findings are consistent with the occurrence of disuse osteoporosis in immobile and sedentary elderly individuals. The risk of peripheral fractures other than those of the hip does not appear to be increased in the inactive elderly, but women who are more active may be more likely to suffer some types of fractures, including fractures of the forearm, foot, and ankle.

Summary

Bone fractures are the primary clinical consequence of osteoporosis. Prevention is particularly important in osteoporosis, because the loss of bone strength may not be completely reversible. White women are the group most frequently affected, but nonwhite women and men also are affected in significant numbers. A large number of pathophysiological processes affecting mineral metabolism, bone cell function, and neuromuscular function play a role in osteoporosis. Low bone mass, bone loss, and a propensity for falling are established causes of osteoporotic fracture in the elderly. Most of the risk factors for fracture are likely to operate through one or more of these pathways. Identifying those at risk by measuring bone mass and assessing risk factors can help target prevention and treatment efforts toward those who will benefit most. There is relatively little epidemiologic data about other potential causes of fracture, including poor bone quality, bone geometry, and trauma biomechanics.

MICHAEL C. NEVITT, PhD, MPH

References

1. Seeley DG, Browner WS, Nevitt MC, Genant HK, Scott JC, Cummings SR. Which fractures are associated with low appendicular bone mass in elderly women? Ann Intern Med 1991;115:837–842.
2. Cooper C, Melton LJ. Magnitude and impact of osteoporosis and fractures. In: Marcus R, Feldman D, Kelsey J (eds). Osteoporosis. San Diego: Academic Press, 1996; pp 419-434.
3. Marshall D, Johnell O, Wedel H. Meta-analysis of how well measures of bone mineral density predict occurrence of osteoporotic fractures. BMJ 1996;312:1254–1259.
4. Jacobsen SJ, Goldberg J, Miles TP, Brody JA, Stiers W, Rimm AA. Hip fracture incidence among the old and very old: a population-based study of 745,435 cases. Am J Public Health 1990;80:871–873.
5. Nevitt MC, Cummings SR. Type of fall and risk of hip and wrist fractures: the study of osteoporotic fractures. J Am Geriatr Soc 1993;41:1226-1234.
6. Cummings SR, Nevitt MC, Browner WS, et al. Risk factors for hip fracture in white women. N Engl J Med 1995;332:767–773.
7. Cooper C, Atkinson EJ, Jacobsen SJ, O'Fallon WM, Melton LJ. Population-based study of survival after osteoporotic fractures. Am J Epidemiol 1993;137:1001–1005.
8. Fisher ES, Baron JA, Malenka DJ, et al. Hip fracture incidence and mortality in New England. Epidemiology 1991;2:116–122.
9. Cooper C, Campion G, Melton LJ. Hip fractures in the elderly: a world-wide projection. Osteoporos Int 1992;2:285–289.
10. O'Neill TW, Felsenberg D, Varlow J, Cooper C, Kanis JA, Silman AJ. The prevalence of vertebral deformity in European men and women: the European Vertebral Osteoporosis Study. J Bone Miner Res 1996;11:1010–1018.
11. National Osteoporosis Foundation. Osteoporosis: review of the evidence for prevention, diagnosis, and treatment and cost-effectiveness analysis: status report. Osteoporos Int 1998;8 (Suppl 4):S1–S88.
12. Nevitt MC, Ettinger B, Black DM, et al. The association of radiographically detected vertebral fractures with back pain and function: a prospective study. Ann Intern Med 1998;128:793–800.
13. Nevitt MC, Thompson DE, Black DM, et al. Effect of alendronate on limited activity days and bed disability days caused by back pain in postmenopausal women with existing vertebral fractures. Fracture Intervention Trial Research Group. Arch Intern Med 2000;160:77–85.
14. Kado DM, Browner WS, Palermo L, Nevitt MC, Genant HK, Cummings SR. Vertebral fractures and mortality in older women: a prospective study. Arch Intern Med 1999;159:1215–1220.
15. Nguyen TV, Eisman JA, Kelly PJ, Sambrook PN. Risk factors for osteoporotic fractures in elderly men. Am J Epidemiol 1996;144:255–263.
16. Ray NF, Chan JK, Thamer M, Melton LJ. Medical expenditures for the treatment of osteoporotic fractures in the United States in 1995: report from the National Osteoporosis Foundation. J Bone Miner Res 1997;12:24–35.

17. Chrischilles EA, Butler CD, Davis CS, Wallace RB. A model of lifetime osteoporosis impact. Arch Intern Med 1991;151: 2026–2032.

18. Cummings SR, Black DM, Rubin SM. Lifetime risks of hip, Colles' or vertebral fracture and coronary heart disease among white postmenopausal women. Arch Intern Med 1989;149: 2445–2448.

19. Black DM, Cummings SR, Melton LJ. Appendicular bone mineral and a woman's lifetime risk of hip fracture. J Bone Miner Res 1992;7:639–646.

20. Bouxsein ML. Applications of biomechanics to the aging human skeleton. In: Rosen CJ, Glowacki J, Bilezikian JP (eds). The Aging Skeleton. San Diego: Academic Press, 1999; pp. 315–331.

21. Looker AC, Orwoll ES, Johnston CC Jr, et al. Prevalence of low femoral bone density in older U.S. adults from NHANES III. J Bone Miner Res 1997;12:1761–1768.

22. Cumming RG, Nevitt MC, Cummings SR. Epidemiology of hip fractures. Epidemiol Rev 1997;19:244–257.

23. Nguyen T, Sambrook P, Kelly P, et al. Prediction of osteoporotic fractures by postural instability and bone density. BMJ 1993;307:1111–1115.

24. Melton LJ, Chao EYS, Lane J. Biomechanical aspects of fractures. In: Riggs BL, Melton LJ (eds). Osteoporosis: Etiology, Diagnosis, and Management. New York: Raven Press, 1988; pp. 111–131.

25. Hannan MT, Felson DT, Anderson JJ. Bone mineral density in elderly men and women: results from the Framingham osteoporosis study. J Bone Miner Res 1992;7:547–553.

26. Riggs BL, Khosla S, Melton LJ. A unitary model for involutional osteoporosis: estrogen deficiency causes both Type I and Type II osteoporosis in postmenopausal women and contributes to bone loss in aging man. J Bone Miner Res 1998; 13:763–773.

27. Slemenda C, Longcope C, Peacock M, Hui S, Johnston CC. Sex steroids, bone mass, and bone loss. A prospective study of pre-, peri-, and postmenopausal women. J Clin Invest 1996; 97:14–21.

28. Cummings SR, Browner WS, Bauer D, et al. Endogenous hormones and the risk of hip and vertebral fractures among older women. Study of Osteoporotic Fractures Research Group. N Engl J Med 1998;339:733–738.

29. Sambrook PN, Kelly PJ, White CP, Morrison NA, Eisman JA. Genetic determinants of bone mass. In: Marcus R, Feldman D, Kelsey J (eds). Osteoporosis. San Diego: Academic Press, 1996; pp. 477–482.

30. Orwoll ES, Klein RF. Osteoporosis in men: Epidemiology, pathophysiology, and clinical characterization. In: Marcus R, Feldman D, Kelsey J (eds). Osteoporosis. San Diego: Academic Press, 1996; pp. 745–784.

31. Maggi S, Kelsey JL, Litvak J, Heyse SP. Incidence of hip fractures in the elderly: a cross-national study. Osteoporos Int 1991;1:232–241.

32. Grisso JA, Chiu GY, Maislin G, Steinmann WC, Portale J. Risk factors for hip fractures in men: a preliminary study. J Bone Miner Res 1991;6:865–868.

33. Grisso JA, Kelsey JL, Strom BL, et al. Risk factors for hip fracture in black women. N Engl J Med, 1994;330:1555–1559.

34. Black DM, Arden NK, Palermo L, Pearson J, Cummings SR. Prevalent vertebral deformities predict hip fractures and new deformities but not wrist fractures. Study of Osteoporotic Fractures Research Group. J Bone Miner Res 1999;14: 821–828.

35. Fox KM, Cummings SR, Powell-Threets K, Stone K. Family history and risk of osteoporotic fracture: the Study of Osteoporotic Fractures Research Group. Osteoporos Int 1998; 8:557–562.

36. Bauer DC, Browner WS, Cauley JA, et al. Factors associated with appendicular bone mass in older women. Ann Intern Med. 1993;118:657–665.

37. Cumming RG. Calcium intake and bone mass: a quantitative review of the evidence. Calcif Tissue Int 1990;47:194–201.

38. Chapuy MC, Arlot ME, Duboeuf F, et al. Vitamin D₃ and calcium to prevent hip fractures in elderly women. N Engl J Med 1992;327:1637–1642.

39. Cumming RG, Nevitt MC. Calcium for prevention of osteoporotic fractures in postmenopausal women. J Bone Miner Res 1997;12:1321–1329.

OSTEOPOROSIS
B. Clinical and Laboratory Features

Osteoporosis, a disease defined by low bone mass and deterioration in bone structure, leads to the occurrence of fractures after relatively low levels of trauma. The most common sites for osteoporotic fractures are the spine, hip, and wrist. However, all fractures that occur from low trauma are considered osteoporotic fractures. The most common osteoporotic fractures occur in the vertebrae. Vertebral fractures can be completely asymptomatic, and fewer than 15% of these fractures ever come to medical attention (1,2). This fact does not lessen the importance of vertebral fractures, as such events are the strongest risk factor for additional fractures (1–4).

Acute symptoms from an osteoporotic vertebral fracture include intense, localized pain and reduced spine motion. Interventions are intended to diminish pain and improve activity, and treatment usually requires a few days of reduced activity or immobilization, with analgesics as needed (5). Acute pain from an osteoporotic fracture generally lasts four to six weeks. If the pain lasts longer, other possible causes of a vertebral fracture, such as metastatic disease, multiple myeloma, and thyroid disease, should be investigated. The development of radicular pain syndromes from osteoporotic vertebral fractures is uncommon, and other diagnoses should be considered in the setting of such symptoms (5).

The anatomy does not return to normal after a vertebral fracture, and refracture of the same vertebrae, with further compression and vertebral deformity, is common (5). All vertebral fractures are associated with losses of height; in the thoracic spine, these losses result in progressive kyphosis. Vertebral fractures in the lumbar spine result in progressive flattening of the lordotic curve, and scoliosis may develop (5,6). When the number and severity of fractured vertebrae increase, kyphosis and loss of the normal lumbar lordosis also increase. In addition, as the number of vertebral fractures increases, loss of truncal shape and protrusion of the abdomen may occur. In severe cases, the lowest thoracic ribs are lowered to the rim of the pelvis and eventually lie within the pelvis (5,6). The height loss results in a progressive shortening of the paraspinal musculature. The muscle-shortening results in prolonged contraction, and patients experience back pain (5).

Physical examination reveals paraspinal muscle pain without much vertebral-body pain. The muscle pain is increased with prolonged standing and may be relieved by walking (5,6). The height loss and abdominal protrusion usually are asymptomatic, but patients may have emotional problems resulting from altered body image (6). Many patients wear abdominal-flattening girdles or go on weight-reduction diets. Both of these measures are of limited benefit and may be harmful. As the deformity progresses, patients may complain of postprandial abdominal pain, which can be prevented by consumption of smaller meals (5).

The long-term care of people with chronic vertebral deformities can be approached in a number of ways (6).

Education is essential, specifically about the nature of the deformity and the need for goal-setting, so that patients will have realistic ideas regarding body image and therapies that reduce pain, restore function, improve quality of life, and prevent additional fractures. Therapy focuses on rehabilitation and appropriate analgesia to reduce chronic back pain (5,6). Caution should be used in prescribing narcotic analgesics, some anti-inflammatory drugs, and generic calcium supplements because they may cause constipation, which can worsen back pain. If constipation develops, a stool softener should be prescribed. Education is required about how to perform such daily activities as bending, lifting, and stooping in ways that do not increase the loads to a brittle skeleton. The inclusion of other health professionals, including physical therapists, occupational therapists, and nurses, is critical in managing the nonpharmacologic treatment of spinal osteoporosis (5,6).

Diagnostic Studies in Osteoporosis

Low bone mass is the strongest predictor of future fracture. The magnitude of the association between low bone mass and the risk of future fracture is greater than that of either elevated cholesterol or hypertension in predicting myocardial infarction and stroke. Historical and lifestyle risk factors are not reliable in identifying individuals with low bone mass (7–9), and bone densitometry is required to identify such individuals (4).

In 1994, the World Health Organization (WHO) provided criteria for the diagnosis of normal bone mass, low bone mass or osteopenia, and osteoporosis (Table 38B-1) (3,7). The WHO criteria for osteoporosis were based on comparisons to peak adult bone mass (PABM) from a pop-

TABLE 38B-1
World Health Organization Criteria for the Diagnosis of Osteoporosis[a]

Normal:	BMC or BMD not more than 1 standard deviation below peak adult bone mass T-score >−1
Osteopenia:	BMC or BMD that lies between 1 and 2.5 standard deviations below peak adult bone mass T-score between −1 and −2.5
Osteoporosis:	BMC or BMD value more than 2.5 standard deviations below peak adult bone mass T-score ≤ −2.5
Severe Osteoporosis:	BMC or BMD value more than 2.5 standard deviations below peak adult bone mass and the presence of one or more fragility fractures T-score ≤ −2.5 plus fragility fracture

[a] World Health Organization criteria for the diagnosis of osteoporosis based on bone mineral content (BMC) or bone mineral density (BMD) measurements. These criteria can be applied to either the central or peripheral skeletal measurement sites.
Adapted from references 3,4,7.

ulation of Caucasian postmenopausal women. Using 2.5 standard deviations below PABM as the definition of osteoporosis (i.e., a T-score of –2.5), a 30% prevalence of osteoporosis was found among older postmenopausal Caucasian women. Although the WHO criteria identify individuals with high fracture risks, the risk of fracture is, in fact, a continuous gradient that increases with decreasing bone mineral density (BMD) levels (3,4,7).

The other WHO criteria for osteopenia (T-score between –1.0 and –2.5) identify individuals who currently are at lower risk of fracture than those with osteoporosis, but who require evaluation and, possibly, treatment. These include individuals who are treated with corticosteroids (in whom vertebral fractures occur at osteopenic BMD levels), have high bone turnover identified by biochemical markers, are at increased risk of falling, or are of advanced age (1,4,9). Because the goal of measuring BMD is to identify individuals at risk for fractures, the paradigm shifts in the setting of osteopenia from the treatment of prevalent fractures to the prevention of incident fractures (1,4).

The WHO criteria, developed from a large population of subjects, assist in determining an individual's risk of an osteoporotic fracture. However, as with most criteria used to diagnose a disease, they have shortcomings (4,5). Because these criteria are based entirely on BMD and do not consider other components of fracture risk, they are imperfect with regard to predicting a given individual's risk (3,4,7). In addition, the WHO criteria do not account for changes in the bone microarchitecture that influence bone strength and fracture risk. Finally, the WHO criteria for the spine, hip, and wrist apply only to Caucasian postmenopausal women. Additional epidemiologic studies are underway in men, younger Caucasian women, and other ethnic groups to make the criteria more useful (1,4).

Despite these limitations, the WHO criteria can help the clinician by providing an objective number for the diagnosis of osteoporosis, similar to a diastolic blood pressure measurement of >90 mm Hg for the diagnosis of hypertension. The criteria also provide objective thresholds for the institution of treatment, regardless of the presence of other risk factors. A T-score of –2 is the number below which the National Osteoporosis Foundation recommends treatment (10). Clinicians should remember that these diagnostic cut-off levels are somewhat arbitrary, and that the gradient for fracture risk correlates with declining levels of BMD and bone microarchitectural changes in an individual (4).

The reference population established by the WHO for osteoporosis of the total hip and femoral neck was the National Health and Examination Survey III (NHANES III) (11). Data derived from this population, which was composed of men and women from many ethnic groups, has proved useful for diagnosing osteoporosis at the hip. Incorporating this reference database, which exists only for the hip, into the software for the three major manufacturers of dual-energy x-ray absorptiometer (DEXA) machines has improved standardized results (12). However, the relationship between BMD and hip-fracture risk has been evaluated only for elderly Caucasian women; low bone mass, regardless of race or gender, is the strongest predictor of future hip fracture (1,4,7).

The WHO criteria use T-scores, the number of standard deviations below PABM, rather than comparing patients to individuals of similar age and gender (3,4,7). This approach is a major strength of the WHO criteria because, although bone mass declines with age, not everyone loses bone as they age. If age-similar standards (Z scores) were used to diagnose osteoporosis, the prevalence of osteoporosis would not increase with age, and osteoporosis would be underestimated (4). Using young, normal BMD as the diagnostic level for subsequent BMD comparisons recognizes the actual prevalence of the problem. However, Z-scores – age-matched BMC/BMD scores – are useful for the growing child or adolescent prior to the acquisition of PABM (2,4).

In clinical practice, the diagnosis of osteopenia or osteoporosis often is made when physicians apply the WHO criteria to premenopausal women (1,2,4). Although these women have low bone mass in the premenopausal state, they do not have an increased risk of fracture, even when compared to age-matched controls with normal bone mass (4). These osteopenic women probably never reached PABM, are generally healthy, have normal rates of bone remodeling, and no increased risk of bone fragility at the time they are evaluated with a BMD measurement. However, when they go through menopause, bone turnover usually increases, remodeling space increases, and these changes may increase their fracture risk. In clinical practice, it is not the standard of care to obtain a bone mass measurement in premenopausal women. However, an exceptionally low bone mass may suggest a secondary cause of osteoporosis and a medical work-up should be initiated.

Bone Mass Measurements

The indications for bone mass measurements are to diagnose osteopenia or osteoporosis, predict fracture risk, and monitor the response of BMD to therapy. Measurement devices are categorized by whether they measure the central skeleton (spine and hip) or the peripheral skeleton (finger, heel, tibia, and wrist/forearm). The DEXA is the central device most commonly used. Peripheral devices include quantitative ultrasound (QUS), peripheral quantitative computed tomography (pQCT), and peripheral DEXA. All of these devices are precise and accurate, but the central DEXA scans have software to measure total body bone mass, body composition, and vertebral morphometry (4). Central and peripheral bone mass measurement devices, the sites they measure, and their precision are listed in Table 38B-2.

The utility of these measurement devices for detecting osteopenia or osteoporosis depends on the age of the patient and the site measured. BMD differs throughout the skeleton, and discrepancies are observed more often in early postmenopausal women (50–55 years) than in women older than 65 years (4,13). However, degenerative changes (osteophytes or facet hypertrophy) in the spine of the elderly

TABLE 38B-2
Characteristics of Bone Densitometry Machines

Technique	Site	Precision error (%CV)[a]	Radiation dose (uSv equivalent)
SEXA	Radius	1–2	< 1
	Calcaneus	1–2	< 1
DEXA	AP-Spine	1–2	1
	Lat-Spine	2–3	3
	Total Hip	1.5–2.5	1
	Total Body	< 1	3
QCT	Lumbar Spine		
	Single Energy	2–4	50
	Dual Energy	4–6	100
QUS	Calcaneus	2–4	0
	Tibia	0.5	0
pDEXA	Forearm	1–1.7	< 1
pQCT	Forearm	1.0	< 5
RA	Phalanges	1.0	< 1

[a] Precision will vary by site of measurement and individual machine use.

% CV, percentage coefficient of variation; SEXA, single-energy x-ray absorptiometry; DEXA, dual-energy x-ray absorptiometry; QCT, quantitative computed tomography; QUS, quantitative ultrasound; pDEXA, peripheral dual-energy x-ray absorptiometry; pQCT, peripheral quantitative computed tomography; RA, radiographic absorptiometry.

that are detected by anteroposterior spine DEXAs can overestimate bone mass. Therefore, a more accurate measurement of true bone mass in these individuals is obtained from the hip.

T-score discrepancies limit the ability of single-site measurements to diagnose osteopenia or osteoporosis, also limiting risk-prediction capabilities. Although differences in bone biology and structure explain some discrepancy, much of this discrepancy is because T-score calculations are based on inconsistent reference population databases. The creation of a consistent database would eliminate much of the confusion surrounding differences in T-scores derived from the 11 FDA-approved peripheral BMD/ultrasound devices. Such a database was created by the National Center for Health Statistics' Third National Health and Nutrition Examination Survey (NHANES III), but only for the hip.

Bone Mass Measurements To Predict Fracture Risk

A diagnosis of osteopenia or osteoporosis made by a BMD measurement is clinically important because it is associated with an increased risk of fracture; as a patient ages, this risk increases at the same BMD level (4,14). In general, as bone mass decreases with age, fracture risk increases. Fracture risk reduction can be expressed as a current fracture risk (within three to five years of the BMD measurement) or a

lifetime fracture risk. The current fracture risk increases 1.5–3.0 times for each standard deviation reduction in BMD (4). In the elderly, BMD correlates at different sites, and the fracture risk prediction is approximately uniform, regardless of the skeletal site measured or device used, except for the hip (4). The prediction of hip fracture risk from the femoral neck bone mass is greater than at any other site. Current fracture risk should not be used for perimenopausal women with or without low BMD, because their fracture risk does not increase in the same way as it does in elderly women (4,15,16). Estimates of lifetime fracture risk are available (see Chapter 38A), but have not been validated in longitudinal studies (7,16). If patients understand that low bone mass at menopause does increase the lifetime risk of fracture, they may more readily accept therapeutic interventions.

When To Repeat Bone Mass Measurements

The ease, precision, and accuracy of BMD measurements make bone densitometry ideal for serial measurements. Central measurement devices typically are used for serial measurements because the areas of the skeleton they measure are rich in trabecular bone. Because trabecular bone has a large surface area and a high turnover rate, responses to therapy can be detected over a short period of time (13). The

TABLE 38B-3
Recommendations for Diagnosis and Treatment of Osteoporosis

1. Urge postmenopausal women to consider their risk of osteoporosis. Osteoporosis is a "silent" risk factor for fracture, just as hypertension is for stroke.

2. Implement a system in your office whereby at-risk women have their skeletal health addressed and recorded at every visit.

3. Evaluate for osteoporosis all postmenopausal women who present with fractures. Use bone mineral density (BMD) testing to confirm the diagnosis and determine disease severity.

4. Recommend BMD testing to postmenopausal women under age 65 who have one or more risk factors, other than menopause, for osteoporotic fractures.

5. Recommend BMD testing for all women aged 65 and older, regardless of additional risk factors.

Adapted from *Physicians Guide to Prevention and Treatment of Osteoporosis*, National Osteoporosis Foundation.

peripheral skeletal sites are not useful for serial measurement because they are composed mainly of cortical bone. When evaluating the effect of a therapeutic intervention, such as estrogen or bisphosphonates, areas of the central skeleton (spine and hip) show the greatest response to therapy in the shortest period of time (17,18). However, if personnel are familiar with a densitometer's in vivo precision error for repeated measurements, changes noted beyond the least significant change represent real BMD changes (4).

In reviews of controlled trials performed to assess the reduction in new vertebral and hip fractures by antiresorptive therapies, the rates of change in BMD differed among study subjects. Although some subjects' BMD improved in the spine and hip in the first year of treatment, other subjects lost BMD in these areas (17,18). Some individuals who gained BMD in the first year actually lost some bone mass during the second year while still on the therapy. This phenomenon, referred to as "regression to the mean," suggests that if a clinician plans to perform serial BMD measurements to assess the response to therapy, scans of the central skeleton probably should not be performed more frequently than every two years (15,17–20). The National Osteoporosis Foundation guidelines for diagnosis and treatment of osteoporosis are shown in Table 38B-3.

Serial BMD measurements obtained on different manufacturers' instruments are difficult to compare. Serial scans performed on a different unit of the same manufacturer's machine also can be difficult to compare, as the precision error of the two devices may be different (4,20). In an attempt

to reduce these technical differences, the Bone Densitometry Standards Committee developed a standardized BMD (sBMD) that has improved comparisons between different manufacturers' instruments. When using the sBMD for the spine or total hip serial measurements, an additional 1% precision error should be included in calculations of the percentage change between measurements performed on instruments from different manufacturers (4,20).

PAUL MILLER, MD
NANCY E. LANE, MD

References

1. NIH Consensus Development Panel. Osteoporosis prevention, diagnosis, and therapy. JAMA 2001;285:785–795.
2. Nevitt MC, Ettinger B, Black DM, et al. The association of radiographically detected vertebral fractures with back pain and function: a prospective study. Ann Intern Med 1998;128:793–800.
3. Assessment of fracture risk and its application to screening for postmenopausal osteoporosis. Report of a WHO Study Group. World Health Organ Techn Rep Ser 1994;843:1–129.
4. Miller PD, Bonnick SL. Clinical application of bone densitometry. In: Fauvus MJ (ed). Primer on the Metabolic Bone Disease and Disorders of Mineral Metabolism, 4th edition. Philadelphia: Lippincott-Raven, 1999; pp 152-159.
5. Kleerekoper M, Avioli L. Evaluation and treatment of postmenopausal osteoporosis. In: Fauvus MJ (ed). Primer on the Metabolic Bone Disease and Disorders of Mineral Metabolism, 3rd Edition. Philadelphia: Lippincott-Raven, 1996; pp 264–268; pp 264–271.
6. Gold DT, Shipp KM, Lyles KW. Managing patients with complications of osteoporosis. Endocrinal Metab Clin North Am 1998;27:485–496.
7. Kanis JA. Diagnosis of osteoporosis. Osteoporos Int 1997;7(Suppl 3):S108–S116.
8. Cummings SR, Nevitt MC, Browner WS, et al. Risk factors for hip fracture in white women. Study of Osteoporotic Fractures Research Group. N Engl J Med 1995;332:767–773.
9. Lane NE, Lukert B. The science and therapy of glucocorticoid-induced bone loss. Endocrinal Metab Clin North Am 1998;27:465–483.
10. National Osteoporosis Foundation. Pocket Guide to Prevention and Treatment of Osteoporosis. Washington DC: National Osteoporosis Foundation, 1999.
11. Looker AC, Wahner HW, Dunn WL, et al. Proximal femur bone mineral levels of US adults. Osteoporos Int 1995;5:389–409.
12. Faulkner KG, Roberts LA, McClung MR. Discrepancies in normative data between Lunar and Hologic DXA systems. Osteoporos Int 1996;6:432–436.
13. Pouilles JM, Tremolliees F, Ribot C. Spine and femur densitometry at the menopause: are both sites necessary in the assessment of the risk of osteoporosis? Calcif Tiss Int 1993;52:344–347.

14. Hui SL, Slemenda CW, Johnston CC Jr. Age and bone mass as predictors of fracture in a prospective study. J Clin Invest 1988;81:1804–1809.
15. Machado A, Hannon R, Eastell R. Monitoring alendronate therapy for osteoporosis. J Bone Miner Res 1999;35:845–852.
16. Huang C, Ross PD, Wasnich RD. Short-term and long-term fracture prediction by bone mass measurements. J Bone Miner Res 1998;13:107–113.
17. Cummings SR, Black DM, Thompson DE, et al. Effect of alendronate on risk of fracture in women with low bone density but without vertebral fractures. JAMA 1998;280:2077–2082.
18. Cummings SR, Palermo L, Browner W, Marcus R, Wallace R. Monitoring osteoporosis therapy with bone densitometry: misleading changes and regression to the mean. Fracture Intervention Trial Research Group. JAMA 2000;283:1318–1321.
19. Yudkin PL, Stratton IM. How to deal with regression to the mean in intervention studies. Lancet 1996;347:241–243.
20. Faulkner KG, McClung MR. Quality control of DXA measurements in multicenter trials. Osteoporos Int 1995;5:218–227.

OSTEOPOROSIS
C. Treatment

The main goal of osteoporosis management is the prevention of fractures. For people who have low bone mass but have not had fractures, the goal is prevention of a first fracture. For the person who already has had one or more fractures, intervention is urgently needed to prevent recurrences.

Agents that treat osteoporosis work by reducing bone resorption. Most of these medications increase bone mineral density (BMD) and reduce biochemical markers of bone turnover. However, recent studies show a reduction in fracture risk even with agents that produce little change in BMD, such as calcitonin and raloxifene. Some of these studies show fracture reduction after one year of treatment, before there has been time to augment BMD substantially. This finding suggests that agents that increase BMD must have some additional effects on bone "quality" to account for the risk reduction. However, it is not clear exactly what aspect of bone quality is improved or how to measure the change.

Lifestyle Issues

Bone health depends on adequate intake of calcium and vitamin D, an active lifestyle that includes regular weight-bearing exercise, and avoidance of cigarette smoking and other factors that impact BMD negatively (Table 38C-1).

The recommended daily intake of calcium is 1200 mg for men and women over the age of 50 (1). The typical postmenopausal woman ingests between 500 mg and 600 mg of calcium daily from dietary sources, and needs a supplement of 600–700 mg of calcium daily. Calcium carbonate is the least expensive form of calcium supplement. For reliable absorption, calcium carbonate should be taken in divided doses of no more than 500 mg per dose, with food. In about 20% of patients, calcium carbonate causes gastrointestinal distress, including upper gastrointestinal gas or constipation. This problem usually does not occur with calcium citrate, which is more expensive.

TABLE 38C-1
Lifestyle Issues Important for Prevention and Treatment of Osteoporosis

Calcium: Recommended intake is 1200 mg daily for adults older than 50 years.
  Most women need a calcium supplement of 500–700 mg daily.
  Calcium carbonate is effective and least expensive.
  Calcium citrate often is tolerated better by patients who have digestive distress.

Vitamin D: Recommended intake is 400–800 IU daily.
  Standard multivitamins contain 400 IU vitamin D.
  Additional vitamin D (total, 800 IU daily) is advisable for persons older than 70 years and can be achieved by taking calcium and vitamin D in combination, in addition to a multivitamin.

Exercise
  Weight-bearing exercise, if possible; recommend walking at least 40 minutes per session, at least four sessions per week.
  Spinal strengthening exercises also are advisable.

Avoid cigarette smoking and other possible negative factors, such as high intake of caffeine, protein, and phosphorus.

Vitamin D is essential for absorption of calcium from the gastrointestinal tract and assimilation into bone. It also has some direct effects on bone remodeling and direct or indirect effects on muscle strength and balance. Although some foods, such as milk and orange juice, are supplemented with vitamin D, and although vitamin D is produced in the skin by ultraviolet light exposure, subclinical vitamin D deficiency does occur. Subclinical vitamin D deficiency was found in 16% of healthy, ambulatory, postmenopausal women in the Southeastern United States and in 50% of hip fracture patients in Boston. Sunblock, although useful for other purposes, filters out the wavelength of light required for vitamin D synthesis. Supplementation with 400–800 IU of vitamin D per day usually is sufficient to assure adequate serum levels of 25-hydroxyvitamin D in most subjects. Standard supplemental multivitamins contain 400 IU of vitamin D; some calcium supplements contain 100 IU or 200 IU of vitamin D.

Calcium and vitamin D may slow, but do not prevent, bone loss in recently menopausal women. In older women, calcium and vitamin D have been shown to prevent bone loss and reduce the risk of spine and nonspine fractures (2).

Weight-bearing exercise, such as walking, is important. Patients should try to walk for 40 minutes or more, four times a week. Carrying light weights (one or two pounds) when walking is desirable. Spinal resistance exercises may be helpful.

TABLE 38C-2
Elements of a Fall-Risk Reduction Program

Hearing and visual impairments corrected as much as possible.

Flooring and carpet in good condition, without uneven surfaces.

No throw rugs.

Lighting bright and without glare.

Night lights present throughout the house.

Telephones readily available.

Electric cords short and not in walkways.

Clutter does not obstruct walkways.

Pets do not lie near feet or bedside.

Railings in tub, shower, and toilet areas.

Nonslip surfaces on floors of tub and shower.

Water drainage in bathroom adequate to prevent slippery floors.

Bedside table for items that might clutter floor.

Kitchen cleaning and cooking supplies within easy reach.

Stairs have railings on both sides, and nonskid surfaces.

No items stored on steps.

All entries maintained in good condition.

Shoes fit well.

Be trained and use a cane if gait is unsteady.

Above all, don't hurry.

Because most osteoporotic fractures involve some element of trauma or falling, patients should be counseled to reduce their risk of falling and avoid activities that produce undesirable forces on the skeleton (e.g., high impact, pushing, pulling, bending, and lifting). Table 38C-2 lists some ways to reduce the risk of falls and injuries.

Pharmacologic Agents

Several pharmacologic agents significantly reduce the risk of osteoporotic fractures in women who already have had a fracture (prevalent fractures) and in women who have low BMD (T-score of –2.5 and below). Some medications also have been shown to prevent bone loss in recently menopausal women. Agents approved by the FDA are shown in Table 38C-3.

Bisphosphonates

Bisphosphonates share a common chemical structure (two phosphonic acids joined to a carbon) that causes them to bind avidly to hydroxyapatite crystals on the surfaces of bone. They resist metabolic degradation, and reduce the ability of individual osteoclasts to resorb bone, reduce the total number of osteoclasts, and accelerate osteoclast apoptosis. Two bisphosphonates (alendronate and risedronate) are approved for the prevention and treatment of postmenopausal osteoporosis. Bisphosphonates are remarkably free from systemic toxicity.

Alendronate

Alendronate was the first bisphosphonate approved by the FDA for treatment of osteoporosis. Results from the Early Postmenopausal Intervention Cohort (EPIC), which involved 2357 recently menopausal women (average age, early 50s) without osteoporosis, showed that 5 mg of daily alendronate was effective in preventing the accelerated bone loss that occurs in the early postmenopausal period (3). In phase III trials involving almost 1000 women in their late 60s who had established osteoporosis, 10 mg of daily alendronate was shown to increase spinal bone density by almost 10% after three years and, to a lesser degree, increase BMD at other sites (4). The average change in BMD at the femoral neck was approximately 4%, with no change noted at the forearm. In the vertebral fracture portion of the Fracture Intervention Trial (FIT), which involved more than 2000 women with low femoral neck BMD and prevalent vertebral fractures, alendronate significantly reduced the frequency of vertebral, hip, and wrist fractures (5).

The FDA-approved dosage of alendronate for treatment of bone loss in recently menopausal women is 5 mg/day or 35 mg, once weekly; the approved dosage for treatment of postmenopausal osteoporosis is 10 mg/day or 70 mg, once weekly. Alendronate also is approved for treatment of corticosteroid-induced osteoporosis (5 mg/day for men and estrogen-replete women, 10 mg daily for estrogen-deficient women, or an equivalent weekly dose).

TABLE 38C-3
FDA-Approved Pharmacologic Agents for Postmenopausal Osteoporosis

Bisphosphonates
  Alendronate (Fosamax)
  Risedronate (Actonel)
Calcitonin (Miacalcin)[a]
Estrogen (several oral and transdermal preparations)[b]
Raloxifene (Evista)

[a] Calcitonin is approved only for treatment of established osteoporosis.
[b] Estrogen is approved only for prevention of bone loss in recently menopausal women.

All bisphosphonates are absorbed poorly when taken by mouth. To ensure absorption, alendronate must be taken on an empty stomach, upon rising in the morning, with nothing but water taken by mouth for at least 30 minutes afterward. Because nitrogen-containing bisphosphonates can be irritating to the esophagus, alendronate should be taken with a glass of water large enough to wash down the tablet; and to avoid reflux, patients should not lie down until they have eaten. Alendronate should not be given to patients who have active upper GI disease, and should be stopped in patients who develop upper GI complaints or who are unable to be upright after taking it.

Risedronate
Risedronate is a nitrogen-containing pyridinyl bisphosphonate. Its effectiveness was shown in two pivotal studies of more than 3600 women with low BMD and prevalent vertebral fractures (6,7). The primary end point in these two trials was new vertebral fractures, which were reduced by 41%–49%. The reduction in the rate of new vertebral fractures was significant after only one year of treatment (8). Nonvertebral fractures, a secondary end point in these studies, were reduced by 33%–39% (6). Risedronate therapy significantly increased BMD at the spine and hip.

In the largest trial of osteoporosis to date, risedronate therapy produced a significant reduction in hip fractures among nearly 9500 postmenopausal women who had low bone mass (9). Of interest, a subset of elderly women who were enrolled in the trial because they had clinical risk factors for fractures, but not necessarily low bone mass, did not show a benefit.

Risedronate was well-tolerated in clinical trials of almost 16,000 subjects, with adverse events no different from those of placebo (6). It appears to have good gastrointestinal tolerability. Risedronate is approved for prevention and treatment of postmenopausal osteoporosis and for prevention and treatment of corticosteroid-induced osteoporosis. The dosage is 5 mg daily for all of these indications. The instructions for dosing of risedronate in the United States are essentially the same as for alendronate. However, a pharmacokinetic study showed similar levels when risedronate was taken two hours before or after a meal, or at least 30 minutes before retiring in the evening, compared with after an overnight fast. Regulatory authorities in Canada and Europe have allowed for this more flexible dosing.

Etidronate and Pamidronate
Etidronate and pamidronate are other bisphosphonates available in the United States. Although neither is approved by the FDA for use in osteoporosis, both are used "off-label."

Etidronate has been shown to increase BMD in two prospective, randomized, controlled trials of women with postmenopausal osteoporosis. When used to treat osteoporosis, etidronate is administered in an intermittent cyclic regimen (400 mg etidronate daily for 14 days every third month) (10). As with all bisphosphonates, etidronate must be taken on an empty stomach to be effective, but it may be taken between meals, at bedtime, or during the night.

Pamidronate can be given by intravenous infusion (11). A typical regimen is an initial dose of 90 mg pamidronate, with subsequent doses of 30 mg every third month. The 30-mg dose can be infused over approximately 60 minutes. Intravenous pamidronate is useful for patients who cannot tolerate oral bisphosphonates.

Calcitonin
Calcitonin is a peptide hormone secreted by specialized cells in the thyroid. Salmon calcitonin is more potent and has a longer duration of action than human calcitonin. Calcitonin acts directly on osteoclasts to reduce bone resorption by binding to specific osteoclast receptors.

Available since 1984, salmon calcitonin (50 to 100 IU daily by subcutaneous injection) results in slight gains in spinal BMD, somewhat less than is achieved with estrogen or bisphosphonates. The effect appears to be greatest in patients who have rapid bone turnover. There has been speculation that the effects of subcutaneous calcitonin would not last because of the development of neutralizing antibodies or down-regulation of receptors. Because of the perception of limited and perhaps only transient effectiveness, the inconvenience and discomfort of injections, the relatively high cost, and limited tolerance (approximately 20% of patients given subcutaneous salmon calcitonin develop nausea or flushing), subcutaneous calcitonin has not been used widely.

Nasal calcitonin, introduced in 1995, is much better tolerated than the subcutaneous form. The recommended dosage of nasal calcitonin is 200 IU (one spray) daily. Relatively small studies with nasal calcitonin showed modest gains in bone mass and suggested a beneficial effect on fracture risk. A recently completed, five-year, multicenter, placebo-controlled, double-blind study of nasal calcitonin in 1255 women with established postmenopausal osteoporosis showed only a modest effect on spinal bone mass, but a 36% reduction in the incidence of new vertebral fractures with 200 IU of nasal calcitonin daily (12). No effect of calcitonin on the incidence of hip fracture or other nonvertebral fracture was shown in this study; however, the study did not have sufficient power to show such an effect.

Nasal calcitonin is extremely well-tolerated. There are no concerns about long-term safety. An important side benefit of calcitonin is a possible analgesic effect, which makes calcitonin a drug to consider for osteoporotic patients for whom acute or chronic pain is a problem, particularly patients with acute painful vertebral fractures.

Estrogen

Estrogen is an effective agent for preventing bone loss in recently menopausal women. Oral conjugated estrogens were shown in a large prospective study to prevent bone loss when begun at menopause. The Postmenopausal Estrogen and Progestin Intervention (PEPI) evaluated 875 recently menopausal women who were randomized to groups receiving estrogen, (with or without progestin) or placebo; women receiving estrogen showed approximately 5% increase in spinal BMD over three years (13). Similar effects on bone loss have been shown for other oral estrogen preparations and for transdermal estradiol in recently menopausal women.

Estrogen increases bone mass by 5%–10% when started after age 65 years. However, once estrogen is stopped, bone mass levels drop fairly quickly. Because of this, estrogen must be continued for the benefits to be maintained. There is one small prospective study of estrogen that suggests a beneficial effect on vertebral fracture risk (14), but no prospective studies are available that show a decrease in hip fractures or other nonspine fractures. However, several large cross-sectional studies suggest that women who take estrogen have approximately 25%–50% fewer spine and hip fractures (15).

Estrogen has a variety of extraskeletal effects. In particular, it relieves such symptoms of estrogen deficiency as hot flashes and vaginal dryness. Symptom relief is the most common reason given by women for starting estrogen.

Although estrogen once was thought to reduce the risk of myocardial infarction, prospective randomized trials have failed to confirm this cardiovascular benefit. Some data suggest that there may be an increased risk of cardiovascular events in women with established coronary disease who begin taking estrogen. Estrogen use is associated with a decreased risk for Alzheimer's disease and colon cancer in cross-sectional studies, but has not been shown to have these benefits in randomized controlled trials. Estrogen also is associated with a small, but significant, increased risk of venous thromboembolic events. Long-term estrogen use may be associated with a slight increase in the risk for breast cancer, an emotionally charged issue that deters many women from starting estrogen or taking it long-term.

The optimal dose, delivery method, and blood level of estrogen for the best bone effects are not clear. For years, it has been thought that 0.625 mg daily of conjugated equine estrogen was the minimally effective and optimal dose. A recent study of esterified estrogens showed a typical dose response, with 0.3 mg daily effective for preventing bone loss, gains in BMD with 0.625 mg daily, and further gains with 1.25 mg daily (16).

Adding a progestin to estrogen protects the endometrium from the effects of unopposed estrogen. Although progestins do not alter the effects of estrogen on the bones, they may increase the risk of breast cancer more than estrogen alone does.

Long-term adherence to estrogen is low. It is estimated that only 15% of women who might benefit actually are taking estrogen. Between 30%–50% of prescriptions for estrogen are never filled, and only 20% of women who begin taking estrogen are still taking it three to five years later. Estrogen should not be used in women who are or might be pregnant, nor in women with undiagnosed genital bleeding, known or suspected cancer of the breast, known or suspected estrogen-dependent neoplasm, or active thrombophlebitis or a thromboembolic disorder.

Selective Estrogen-Receptor Modulator

Raloxifene is a selective estrogen-receptor modulator (SERM). After binding to estrogen receptors, SERMs produce different expression of estrogen-regulated genes in different tissues, activating some and inhibiting others. Raloxifene (60 mg/day) is approved by the FDA for prevention of bone loss in recently menopausal women and for treatment of established osteoporosis. In a study of 607 recently menopausal women, raloxifene prevented bone loss (17) and generally was well-tolerated, but was associated with an increase in leg cramps and a slight increase in hot flashes.

Raloxifene was evaluated for treatment of postmenopausal osteoporosis in the MORE Study (Multiple Outcomes of Raloxifene Evaluation), which involved 7705 women (18). Bone density increased slightly but significantly in the spine and hip, and the risk of new vertebral fractures was reduced by 30%–50%. Although no effect of raloxifene on hip fracture or other nonvertebral fracture was shown in this study, the study was not powered to show such an effect.

Raloxifene produces some favorable changes in lipids, decreasing low-density lipoprotein-cholesterol, and its effect on high-density lipoprotein-cholesterol and triglycerides is neutral. There are no data on the cardiovascular effects of raloxifene, but a large clinical trial is underway to evaluate that aspect. There is a small but significant increased risk of venous thrombosis with raloxifene, similar to that of estrogen. In the osteoporosis trials, raloxifene was associated with approximately 70% fewer cases of breast cancer. This is not surprising in view of raloxifene's known anti-estrogen effect on breast tissue. A large clinical trial is underway to compare raloxifene with tamoxifen for prevention of breast cancer in high-risk patients.

In The Future

New bisphosphonates are in clinical trials. Ibandronate, a third-generation bisphosphonate, was not effective in reducing fractures when given intravenously at 1 mg every three months (19), but is being studied as daily oral therapy. Although more data on the nonskeletal effects of raloxifene are being collected, clinical trials with newer SERMs, such as droloxifene and idoxifene, have been discontinued because of adverse endometrial effects. Trials are beginning on new SERMs, such as lasofoxifene.

All of the agents approved for prevention and treatment of osteoporosis act by reducing bone resorption. There is considerable interest in agents that promote new bone formation. Possible bone-forming agents include parathyroid hormone (20), bone morphogenetic protein, cytokines that stimulate bone formation, and inhibitors of cytokines that reduce bone resorption. HMG-CoA reductase inhibitors (statins), in wide clinical use to treat hypercholesterolemia, are being investigated for possible bone benefits; statins may have antiresorptive effects, anabolic effects, or both. Data from cross-sectional studies suggest that statins may reduce the risk of fractures.

Vertebroplasty and Kyphoplasty

For patients who have painful or deforming vertebral fractures, new procedures – vertebroplasty and kyphoplasty – offer options for relief of pain and possible reversal of deformity (21,22). These procedures, which involve injection of bone cement into an involved vertebra under radiologic guidance, have not been evaluated fully for long-term safety and efficacy. They should be offered only to selected patients and should be performed only by experienced operators.

NELSON B. WATTS, MD

References

1. Institute of Medicine. Dietary reference intakes: calcium, phosphorous, magnesium, vitamin D, and fluoride. Washington, DC: Academy Press, 1997.
2. Dawson-Hughes B, Harris SS, Krall EA, Dallal G. Effects of calcium and vitamin D supplementation on bone density in men and women 65 years of age and older. N Engl J Med 1997; 337:670–676.
3. Ravn P, Weiss S, Rodriguez-Portales JA, et al. Alendronate in early postmenopausal women: effects on bone mass during long-term treatment and after withdrawal. J Clin Endocrinol Metab 2000;85:1492–1497.
4. Liberman UA, Weiss SR, Broll J, et al. Effect of oral alendronate on bone mineral density and the incidence of fractures in postmenopausal osteoporosis. N Engl J Med 1995;333:1437–1443.
5. Black DM, Cummings SR, Karpf DB, et al. Randomised trial of effect of alendronate on risk of fracture in women with existing vertebral fractures. Lancet 1996;348:1535–1541.
6. Harris ST, Watts NB, Genant HK, et al. Effects of risedronate treatment on vertebral and nonvertebral fractures in women with postmenopausal osteoporosis. A randomized controlled trial. JAMA 1999;282:1344–1352.
7. Reginster J, Minne HW, Sorensen OH, et al. Randomized trial of the effects of risedronate on vertebral fractures in women with established postmenopausal osteoporosis. Osteoporos Int 2000;11:83–91.
8. Watts N, Roux C, Genant H, et al. Risedronate reduces vertebral fracture risk after the first year of treatment in postmenopausal women with established osteoporosis. J Bone Miner Res 1999;14(suppl 1):S136.
9. Miller P, Roux C, McClung M, et al. Risedronate reduces hip fractures in patients with low femoral neck bone mineral density. Arthritis Rheum 1999;42(suppl 9):S287.
10. Watts NB, Harris ST, Genant HK, et al. Intermittent cyclical etidronate treatment of postmenopausal osteoporosis. N Engl J Med 1990;323:73–79.
11. Thiebaud D, Burckhardt P, Melchior J, et al. Two years effectiveness of intravenous pamidronate (APD) versus oral fluoride for osteoporosis occurring in the menopause. Osteoporos Int 1994;4:76–83.
12. Chesnut CH, Silverman S, Andriano K, et al. A randomized trial of nasal spray salmon calcitonin in postmenopausal women with established osteoporosis: the prevent recurrence of osteoporotic fractures study. Am J Med 2000;109:267-276.
13. Bush TL, Wells HB, James MK, et al. Effects of hormone therapy on bone mineral density. Results from the postmenopausal estrogen/progestin interventions (PEPI) trial. JAMA 1996;276:1389–1396.
14. Lufkin EG, Wahner HW, O'Fallon WM, et al. Treatment of postmenopausal osteoporosis with transdermal estrogen. Ann Intern Med 1992;117:1–9.
15. Cauley JA, Seeley DG, Browner WS, et al. Estrogen replacement therapy and fractures in older women. Ann Intern Med 1995;122:9–16.
16. Genant HK, Lucas J, Weiss S, et al. Low-dose esterified estrogen therapy: effects on bone, plasma estradiol concentrations, endometrium, and lipid levels. Arch Intern Med 1997;157: 2609–2615.
17. Delmas PD, Bjarnason NH, Mitlak BH, et al. Effects of raloxifene on bone mineral density, serum cholesterol concentrations, and uterine endometrium in postmenopausal women. N Engl J Med 1997;337:1641–1647.
18. Ettinger B, Black DM, Mitlak BH, et al. Reduction of vertebral fracture risk in postmenopausal women with osteoporosis treated with raloxifene. Results from a 3-year randomized clinical trial. JAMA 1999;282:637–645.
19. Recker RR, Stakkestad JA, Felsenberg D, et al. A new treatment paradigm: quarterly injections of ibandronate reduce the risk of fractures in women with postmenopausal osteoporosis (PMO): results of a 3-year trial. Osteoporosis Int 2000;11(suppl 2):S209.
20. Neer RM, Arnaud CD, Zanchetta JR, et al. Recombinant human PTH [rhPTH(1-34)] reduces the risk of spine and nonspine fractures in postmenopausal osteoporosis. Endocrine Society, 82nd Annual Meeting, 2000.
21. Wilson DR, Myers ER, Mathis JM, et al. Effect of augmentation on the mechanics of vertebral wedge fractures. Spine 2000;25:158–165.
22. Deramond H, Depriester C, Galibert P, Le Gars D. Percutaneous vertebroplasty with polymethylmethacrylate. Technique, indications, and results. Radiol Clin North Am 1998;36:533–546.

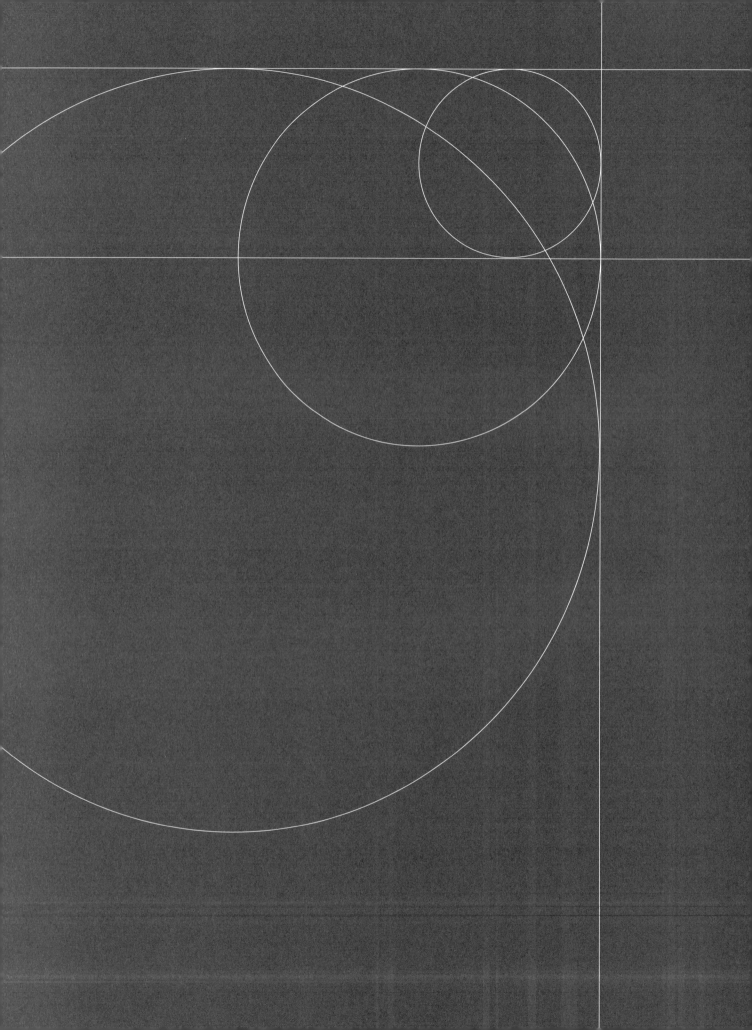

39 PEDIATRIC RHEUMATIC DISEASES
A. Special Considerations

Many rheumatic diseases that occur in adults also affect children, albeit less frequently. Additionally, some diseases, such as systemic-onset or pauciarticular-pattern rheumatoid disease, occur predominantly in children. In all of these diseases, the clinical manifestations are often impacted by the child's growth and development. Four issues that relate to growth and development and contribute to the uniqueness of the child with rheumatic disease will be discussed.

Examination

To perform a valid and complete examination on a child who is ill or in pain can be difficult. Yet an accurate exam is necessary if the correct diagnosis is to be made. Children at different ages and developmental levels respond differently to examination. Rheumatic disease manifestations can also vary with age. It may be helpful to keep certain guidelines in mind. Height and weight should be obtained at each visit, and these growth parameters plotted on an appropriate growth chart. Inadequately controlled disease or medication side-effects can impair normal growth.

Infants and Toddlers

In infants and toddlers, observation skills are particularly important. By looking for movements that cause pain or irritability as well as lack of movement of any joint, you can ascertain much before ever examining the patient. Using toys, talking, and keeping eye contact with the child may help alleviate the child's fear. Having the child sit on a parent's lap or even having the parent assist with the examination may make a more thorough exam possible. Swelling can be subtle in a chubby child and careful attention to range of motion is critical. A single swollen digit may be the only sign of arthritis.

School-Aged Children

Most school-aged children like to actively participate in the examination, particularly if they are in comfortable clothing such as a T-shirt and shorts. It is generally best to examine any painful area last, after completing the general and remainder of the musculoskeletal examination. In addition to joint examination, careful attention should be paid to gait, leg length, and muscle strength. Having a child perform a sit-up or climb a few stairs can be a more helpful screen than specific muscle testing.

Adolescents

In adolescents, the examination itself is not difficult, but relating to the patient can be. It is important that the patient is as comfortable as possible and that rapport is established with the adolescent, not just the parent. In situations where the parent continues to dominate the interactions, it may be helpful to ask to speak to the adolescent alone. The examination should include a scoliosis screen as part of the musculoskeletal exam.

Growth

Juvenile rheumatoid arthritis (JRA) is a chronic disease and has long been known to affect growth of the child. Historically, this clinical effect was noted by Still in 1897 and later described by Kuhns in 1932. JRA's effects on growth are multifactoral and include, not only the disease itself, but medication side effects, nutrition, and mechanical problems. In recent years, the roles of growth hormone and insulin-like growth factors have gradually begun to be elucidated, as described below.

General

It is clear that the onset subtype of JRA is important. In the pauciarticular group, little or no general adverse effect on growth is seen; however, this group may have severe local growth disturbances at the sites of inflammation, particularly leg-length discrepancy and mandibular asymmetries.

A child with polyarticular and systemic disease who has never received corticosteroid therapy may have overall growth retardation, generally related to the severity and duration of disease. In one study, one-fourth of both disease groups lost >1 height Z score* over the 14-year follow-up period (1). Growth impairment generally was not severe, except in a small number of patients with systemic disease. Height velocity during puberty was especially vulnerable. The degree of "catch-up" growth was unpredictable.

In another study involving 64 prepubertal children with primarily mild pauciarticular and polyarticular JRA, growth velocity decreased in the first postdiagnostic year and then increased to normal range with treatment and four-year follow-up. The greatest effect on velocity was seen in children with more severe polyarticular disease. There were only two patients with systemic disease in the study (2). A long-term follow-up study of adults who had JRA and had received corticosteroids showed reduced final height and armspan (3).

---

*Z score = $(X_1-X_2)/SD$ where X_1 = subject's measurement, X_2 = mean of the reference population for age and gender, and SD = standard deviation of the mean for the reference population.

Local

Local growth disturbances occur as a result of inflammation and the accompanying increase in vascularity, which may result in either over- or undergrowth of the affected bone.

The hip frequently is involved in JRA. This occasionally leads to a small femoral head within a larger acetabulum. This was noted in five patients undergoing hip arthroplasty. The small size was thought to be secondary to destruction of the articular cartilage (4). Of note, all patients had disease onset prior to age 3 years.

The knee is the most frequently involved joint in JRA. Persistent synovitis, particularly in an asymmetric fashion, can lead to significant leg-length discrepancy. The distal femoral epiphyses account for approximately 70% of femoral growth, so persistent inflammation leads to overgrowth on the involved side in a child whose epiphyses have not yet closed. Often the medial side predominates, leading to additional knee valgus. Increased use of intra-articular steroids may reduce this risk and appears to have a low level of adverse effects (5).

Micrognathia and malocclusion are known as common sequelae of JRA. Unilateral disease may lead to chin deviation. The temporomandibular joint (TMJ) consists of hyaline cartilage, fibrocartilage, and synovial membrane and constitutes the mandibular cavities and condyles. Computed tomography study revealed TMJ alterations including erosions, cysts, and cavity flattening in 50% of children with JRA, particularly in those with polyarticular and systemic disease. Sixty-nine percent had orthodontic abnormalities (6). Patients with polyarticular disease often have small, short facies with underdeveloped mandibles. These consequences of TMJ arthritis are difficult to treat. MRI may detect early changes. Orthodontic consultation is recommended. Costochondral grafts may be beneficial in those who are severely affected.

Other sites frequently involved include the wrist, with undergrowth of the ulnar head, and the vertebrae, with undergrowth of the cervical spine.

Osteopenia and Osteoporosis

Osteopenia is low bone mass for age, and the child with JRA is at great risk for failure to achieve adequate postpubertal bone mass. The introduction of dual-energy x-ray absorptiometry (DEXA) has enabled osteopenia assessment and has led people to realize the magnitude of the problem. Both the cortical appendicular skeleton and the axial trabecular bone are affected, but the cortical is affected to a greater degree (7). Failure of bone formation results in impaired development of normal bone, and the defect is accentuated at puberty. Osteopenia appears to correlate with disease activity and severity (7). Other contributing factors include decreased physical activity, immobility, decreased sun exposure, and decreased dietary intake of calcium and vitamin D. Peak bone mass is normally reached during adolescence, and this achievement is important to minimize future risk for osteoporosis and fractures. Often in JRA, bone density fails to undergo expected pubertal increase. Significant axial osteopenia of the lumbar spine and femoral neck was found in patients with polyarticular disease (8).

In addition to generalized osteopenia, involved joints often show local juxta-articular demineralization – even on early radiographs. Patients may benefit from DEXA monitoring at selected intervals. Therapy includes weight-bearing exercise, appropriate nutrition, calcium and vitamin D supplementation, and most importantly, adequate disease control with suppression of inflammation.

Endocrine Factors

Low levels of osteocalcin, along with decreased bone mineral content, were found in children with active inflammation, but both parameters were normal in children with inactive disease (9). Osteocalcin levels in patients with heights less than the third percentile were below normal, suggesting decreased osteoblast activity (10). In this study, osteocalcin levels correlated with decreased insulin-like growth factor 1 (IGF-l) levels. However, these patients also were receiving corticosteroid therapy, which can decrease osteocalcin levels.

Children with JRA and short stature may have low human growth hormone (hGH) secretion. Some have inadequate or no response to exogenous hGH administration, suggesting an additional defect in the response pathway or growth hormone insensitivity (11). Other studies have shown levels not significantly different from controls (10).

Insulin-like growth factor 1, a peptide produced in the liver, is the main peripheral mediator of growth hormone. It promotes collagen formation. Serum levels of this peptide have been reduced in most JRA studies, especially in children with systemic disease (12). Levels appear to correlate with the degree of inflammation as measured by acute-phase reactants. Levels returned to normal with recombinant growth hormone (rGH) therapy in one study (10)

Interleukin-6 (IL-6) is markedly elevated in systemic disease and appears to correlate with the degree of inflammation. Studies in transgenic mice show that IL-6 mediates a decrease in IGF-1 production, which might represent a mechanism by which chronic inflammation affects growth (13).

Vascular endothelial growth factor is a mitogen for vascular endothelial cells and a mediator of vascular permeability. Serum levels correlate with disease activity in polyarticular JRA and may play a role in inflammation (14).

Growth Hormone Therapy

In one study, 14 children with JRA on corticosteroid therapy received rGH therapy of 1.4 IU/kg/week with a partial response. The mean height velocity increased from 1.9 to 5.4 cm/year with an accompanying 12% increase in lean body mass. However, at the end of one year the height velocity decreased to pretreatment levels (15).

In another study, rGH increased height velocity during the year of therapy (mean 3.1 cm/year) but the long-term effect was unknown. There was no correlation between growth hormone secretion and rGH therapy response, raising the question of a target-cell defect or peripheral defect regarding growth hormone mediation. Fifty percent of the children in this study had borderline or poor caloric intake (10). Growth hormone therapy may be beneficial in some patients, but the response is unpredictable.

Nutrition

Adequate nutrition, both caloric and protein, is critical for optimizing growth in children with JRA. Up to 30% of children with JRA have some growth abnormality (16). Using anthroprometric measurements, up to 40% have poor nutritional status, and muscle mass is frequently low. Protein stores and specific nutrients such as iron, selenium, vitamin C, and zinc have been reported low (17). Inflammatory cytokines such as IL-1, IL-6, and tumor necrosis factor likely modulate some of the nutritional abnormalities. In addition, some patients have mechanical feeding problems related to jaw or upper-extremity disease.

Monitoring of serial weights during clinic visits should be routine. Dietary logs, nutrient analysis, and consultation with a dietitian is needed for a child with poor weight gain. Nutritional supplementation may be beneficial.

Adherence

Optimal treatment of pediatric rheumatic diseases often requires complex therapeutic strategies that can be both confusing and time-consuming to patients and their families. Strategies often involve a coordinated list of activities, which may include taking regular medication, keeping up with complex exercise regimens, making dietary modifications, making regular clinic visits, undergoing laboratory tests, and, in some children, wearing therapeutic splints. This is complicated by the fact that there is often delayed benefit for good adherence. It is easy to understand why adhering to these regimens is often compromised. In fact, estimates are that only 50%–54% of patients with chronic pediatric disease adhere adequately to their recommended therapy (18). In JRA, medication compliance was found to be of similar frequency, ranging from 38% to 59% (18). In a study of prednisone therapy in children with systemic lupus erythematosus or dermatomyositis, adherence ranged from 33% to 78%, which is similar to that reported in children with cancer (19). Surprisingly in the prednisone study, two-thirds of patients over-medicated themselves, possibly when they felt poorly. Adherence to exercise regimens is likely to be lower than with medication, according to parent report. One must also differentiate between complete non-adherence and periodic nonadherence.

The consequences of not adhering to therapy are multiple, not only for the patient but also for the health care system. The patients' risk for disease complications and long-term sequelae are generally increased with nonadherence. Poor or dishonest communication between patient and physician or health care provider also stresses the relationship and failure to admit nonadherence may lead to needless changes of medication or unnecessary testing. All of these are inefficient and lead to increased health care costs.

Factors Impacting Adherence

Many factors may impede adherence. These factors can generally be grouped into three categories: 1) those related to the disease; 2) those related to the patient; and 3) those related to the regimen itself. There is no typical nonadherent patient and no consistent correlations with obvious demographic factors. However, certain "states" that lead to nonadherence that relate to disease and to the patient and family have been reported (20). They are included in Tables 39A-1 and 39A-2.

Factors Related to Treatment Regimen

The health care provider can increase the likelihood of good therapy adherence by making the treatment regimen as simple as possible and by anticipating some of the known negative factors including bad-tasting medication, frequent dosing, high cost, complexity, delay in therapeutic response, transportation concerns, and the patient's forgetting to take medication or do exercises. Exercise regimens may be especially problematic because the child may experience discomfort and express anger or resentment toward the parent.

The person with chronic disease may be asked to alter his or her lifestyle in a way that restricts sports interests, peer-related social activity, or leisure time. Such changes are especially difficult for active children and adolescents. Parental supervision and appropriate involvement are critical in providing children with needed support.

TABLE 39A-1
Adherence: Factors Relating to Patient and Family

1. Negative reactions from the child, including complaints, refusal, discomfort, embarrassment, or more general oppositional behavior.

2. Lack of understanding of the disease and treatment, especially in younger children.

3. Misunderstanding of the disease and treatment.

4. Lack of patient autonomy and low self-esteem.

5. Dissatisfaction with the provider or the therapeutic intervention.

6. Inadequate family resources.

7. Language barriers.

8. Family instability or disagreement.

9. Other family demands, e.g., parental illness.

10. Parental resentment or anger over the illness.

11. Lack of adequate family coping abilities and strategies.

TABLE 39A-2
Adherence: Factors Related to Disease

1. Disease duration is often prolonged with unpredictable exacerbations. Adherence tends to decrease over time.

2. Age of onset. Younger patients are less adherent.

3. Asymptomatic periods. When a patient is asymptomatic or in remission there is often a temptation to discontinue medication because the patient feels well. This is enhanced by a commonly seen delay in therapeutic response of days to weeks and also by the delay in occurrence of negative effects (recurrence of symptoms) with missed medication.

4. Severity of disease has no clear correlation with adherence.

Assessing Adherence

Adherence can be assessed through direct or indirect means. Indirect means include parental or self-report, medication diary, prescription renewals, and presence of predictable side effects. Direct means include counting pills, measuring laboratory parameters such as drug levels, and using electronic devices that record and store the time and date a pill container is opened (20).

Improving Adherence

Strategies used to improve adherence can be categorized into three types: educational, organizational, and behavioral. These strategies can be used singly or in combination (20).

Educational strategies include providing information, helping prioritize, re-educating, providing written handouts, using reminder systems, referring to community and national resources, providing positive feedback, and using appropriate discipline techniques. Information should be age-, culture-, and language-appropriate and take into account the child's cognitive abilities. It is important not to overwhelm the family early in the process.

Organizational strategies include counseling, increasing supervision, decreasing complexity, decreasing costs, and increasing the palatability of medication. Treatment regimens should fit into the family daily routine as much as possible. Therapeutic exercise and play often can be combined.

Behavioral strategies can include using self-management training to increase self-esteem, training parents to deal with oppositional behavior, monitoring adherence, and using a positive reinforcement or reward system for good adherence. Reinforcement programs are time-consuming and require parental training but can improve adherence (20). Reward systems where tokens are exchanged for privileges can be successful. The child's responsibilities for the treatment regimen should increase as the child gets older, but parents should not completely withdraw supervision.

Regular clinic visits are important for re-educating and re-enforcing adherence strategies and for adapting treatment. They also help build and maintain a cooperative and trusting relationship between clinician and patient. Visits should allow enough time for adherence discussion and re-enforcement. Good documentation is also important to facilitate monitoring of adherence. The clinician must relate to the child, who needs to be an active partner in his or her treatment program. Judgmental attitudes are not helpful. A multidisciplinary team approach is optimal.

Studies are needed to identify children and families at high risk for nonadherence, further define successful family coping mechanisms that can be taught and re-enforced, and to evaluate strategies for improving adherence.

Psychosocial and Educational Issues

Chronic disease has a major impact on the development and daily functioning of children and their families. Unfortunately, there are few and often contradictory studies on the nature of the impact and the contributing factors. Different assessment methods, varying population size, and a mixture of disease subtypes, particularly with JRA, contribute to the different conclusions. Some epidemiologic studies concluded that there is more risk for psychosocial problems in children with JRA (21), others less (22). A recent controlled study (23) used self-report questionnaires combined with personnel interviews to study children (aged seven to 11) and adolescents (aged 12 to 16) with arthritis. Self-esteem, perceived competence, and body image were similar to healthy controls. The arthritis patients did have less energy to participate in social activities, and adolescents received more emotional support from family, peers, and professionals. The amount of support received correlated positively with disease severity. Other studies showed that children with chronic illness do not have a higher incidence of psychiatric disease nor is there any correlation between psychological test scores and disease functional measurements (24).

Family Impact

Long-term psychosocial outcome appears to be favorable overall. Chronic family difficulties predicted psychosocial functioning in people with JRA in a nine-year follow-up study. The study showed no correlation between psychosocial function and disease activity. The most frequent psychiatric disturbance on follow-up was anxiety disorder. No children had depressive disorder and 15% had mild to moderate impairment in psychosocial functioning (25).

Positive family factors may play an important role in the child's ability to cope with chronic illness. In one study, a highly cohesive family structure correlated with a high level of social adjustment in children with JRA (23). An environment with flexibility, individual freedom, and an emphasis on self-mastery appears optimal. Family coping skills can be enhanced by educational programs such as those sponsored by the American Juvenile Arthritis Organization/Arthritis Foundation and by retreats or workshops directed by professionals (26). These also can reduce family stress and improve parent-child relationships.

Pain

Often, inadequate attention is given to pain in children with arthritis. Young children usually do not verbalize discomfort or pain and even the older child may have become accustomed or tolerant to a certain level of pain. Tools are available to help the clinician ascertain the child's perception of pain and can be used as serial measurements. The Pain Coping Questionnaire has been validated in children and adolescents and is good at assessing the child's pain coping strategies. It is simple and applicable over a wide age-range (27). Less coping effectiveness has been related to higher levels of pain. Use of the Visual Analogue Scale of the Pediatric Pain Questionnaire is also a simple tool that can be used during clinic visits to monitor pain levels in patients at risk. Higher patient-perceived pain intensity correlates with higher incidence of depressive and anxiety symptoms (28).

School and Educational Achievement

Many factors affect school attendance, but it is generally high for all but the more severely affected patients. In one study, school absence was associated with decreased adherence to physical therapy and the presence of psychological problems, but not with age or duration of illness (30). School problems for children with arthritis include difficulties with writing, opening doors, participating in physical education, and carrying books, as well as fatigue, absences, inadequate understanding by teachers and peers, and being late to class. School success is critical to the normal development of the child, and school status and educational progress should be assessed regularly at clinic visits. In a study of 44 adults with JRA surveyed 25 years after disease onset, patients and controls showed equivalent levels of educational achievement, income, and insurance coverage; but patients had lower rates of employment, daily energy levels, and exercise tolerance (30).

During the past decade the overall prognosis for children with rheumatic disease has steadily improved. However, for optimal treatment and outcome, attention must be given to their special needs.

CAROL B. LINDSLEY, MD

References

1. Polito C, Strano CG, Olivieri AN, et al. Growth retardation in non-steroid treated juvenile rheumatoid arthritis. Scand J Rheumatol 1997;26:99–103.
2. Saha MT, Verronen P, Liappala P, Lenko HL. Growth of prepubertal children with juvenile chronic arthritis. Acta Paediatr 1999;88:724–728.
3. Zak M, Muller J, Karup-Pedersen F. Final height, armspan, subischial leg length and body proportions in juvenile chronic arthritis. A long-term follow-up study. Horm Res 1999;52: 80–85.
4. Hastings DE, Orsini E, Myers P, Sullivan J. An unusual pattern of growth disturbance of the hip in juvenile rheumatoid arthritis. J Rheumatol 1994;21:744–747.
5. Sherry DD, Stein LD, Reed AM, Schanberg LE, Kredich, DW. Prevention of leg length discrepancy in young children with pauciarticular juvenile rheumatoid arthritis by treatment with intraarticular steroids. Arthritis Rheum 1999;42:2330–2334.
6. Ronchezel MV, Hilario MO, Goldenberg J, et al. Temporomandibular joint and mandibular growth alterations in patients with juvenile rheumatoid arthritis. J Rheumatol 1995; 22:1956–1961.
7. Cassidy JT. Osteopenia and osteoporosis in children. Clin Exp Rheumatol 1999;17:245–250.
8. Kotaniemi A. Growth retardation and bone loss as determinants of axial osteopenia in juvenile chronic arthritis. Scand J Rheumatol 1997;26:14–18.
9. Reed A, Haugen M, Pachman LM. Abnormalities in serum osteocalcin values in children with chronic rheumatic diseases. J Pediatr 1990;116:574–580.
10. Davies UM, Jones J, Reeve J, et al. Juvenile rheumatoid arthritis. Effects of disease activity and recombinant human growth hormone on insulin-like growth factor 1, insulin-like growth factor binding proteins 1 and 3, and osteocalcin. Arthritis Rheum 1997;40:332–340.
11. Hopp RJ, Degan J, Corley K, Lindsley CB, Cassidy JT. Evaluation of growth hormone secretion in children with juvenile rheumatoid arthritis and short stature. Nebr Med J 1995; 80:52–57.
12. Cimaz R, Rusconi R, Cesana B, et al. A multicenter study on insulin-like growth factor-I serum levels in children with chronic inflammatory diseases. Clin and Exp Rheum 1997;15: 691–696.
13. DeBenedetti F, Alonzi T, Moretta A, et al. Interleukin 6 causes growth impairment in transgenic mice through a decrease in insulin-like growth factor-I. A model for stunted growth in children with chronic inflammation. J Clin Invest 1997;99: 643–650.
14. Maeno N, Takei S, Imanaka H, et al. Increased circulating vascular endothelial growth factor is correlated with disease activity in polyarticular juvenile rheumatoid arthritis. J Rheumatol 1999;26:2244–2248.
15. Simon D, Touati G, Prieur AM, Ruiz JC, Czernichow P. Growth hormone treatment of short stature and metabolic dysfunction in juvenile chronic arthritis. Acta Paediatr Suppl 1999;88:100–105.
16. Henderson CT, Lovell DJ. Assessment of protein energy malnutrition in children and adolescents with JRA. Arthritis Care Res 1989;2:108–113.
17. Bacon MC, White PH, Raith DJ, et al. Nutritional status and growth in JRA. Semin Arthritis Rheum 1990;20:97–106.
18. Rapoff MA. Compliance with treatment regimens for pediatric rheumatic diseases. Arthritis Care Res 1989;2(suppl): 40–47.

19. Pieper KB, Rapoff MA, Purviance MR, Lindsley CB. Improving compliance with prednisone therapy in pediatric patients with rheumatic disease. Arthritis Care Res 1989;2:132–135.

20. Rapoff MA. Adherence to Pediatric Medical Regimens. New York: Kluwer Academic/Plenum Publishers, 1999.

21. Gortmaker SL, Walker DK, Weitzman M, Sobol AM. Chronic conditions, socio-economic risks and behavioral problems in children and adolescents. Pediatrics 1990;85:267–276.

22. Vandvik IH. Mental health and psychosocial functioning in children with recent onset of rheumatic disease. J Child Psychol Psychiatry 1990;31:961–971.

23. Huygen ACJ, Kuis W, Sinnema G. Psychological, behavioural, and social adjustment in children and adolescents with juvenile chronic arthritis. Ann Rheum Dis 2000;59:276–282.

24. Frank RG, Hagglund KJ, Schopp LH, et al. Disease and family contributors to adaptation in juvenile rheumatoid arthritis and juvenile diabetes. Arthritis Care Res 1998;11:166–176.

25. Aasland A, Flato B, Vandvik IH. Psychosocial outcome in juvenile chronic arthritis: a nine-year follow-up. Clin Exp Rheumatol 1997;15:561–568.

26. Hagglund KJ, Doyle NM, Clay DL, Frank RG, Johnson JC, Pressly TA. A family retreat as a comprehensive intervention for children with arthritis and their families. Arthritis Care Res 1996;9:35–41.

27. Reid GJ, Gilbert CA, McGrath PJ. The pain coping questionnaire: preliminary validation. Pain 1998;76:83–96.

28. Varni JW, Rapoff MA, Waldron SA, Gragg RA, Bernstein BH, Lindsley CB. Chronic pain and emotional distress in children and adolescents. J Dev Behav Ped 1996;17:154–161.

29. Sturge C, Garralda ME, Boissin M, Dor'e CJ, Woo P. School attendance and juvenile chronic arthritis. Br J Rheumatol 1997;36:1218–1223.

30. Peterson LS, Mason T, Nelson, AM, O'Fallon WM, Gabriel SE. Psychosocial outcomes and health status of adults who have had juvenile rheumatoid arthritis: a controlled, population-based study. Arthritis Rheum 1997;40:2235–2240.

PEDIATRIC RHEUMATIC DISEASES
B. Juvenile Rheumatoid Arthritis and Juvenile Spondyloarthropathies

Juvenile Rheumatoid Arthritis

Juvenile rheumatoid arthritis (JRA) is the most common form of childhood arthritis and one of the more common chronic childhood illnesses. The cause is unknown. Diagnosis requires a combination of data from history, physical examination, and laboratory testing. For the vast majority of patients, the immunogenetic associations, clinical course, and functional outcome are quite different from adult-onset rheumatoid arthritis (RA). However, approximately 5%–10% of people with JRA who have rheumatoid factor-positive polyarticular arthritis beginning during adolescence have a disease that resembles adult-onset RA much more than JRA.

Epidemiology

The prevalence of JRA in the United States has been estimated to be between 57 and 113 per 100,000 children younger than 16 years (1). The overall prevalence rate on January 1, 1980, for this age group in the Mayo Clinic population was estimated to be 113 per 100,000 (95% confidence intervals: 69, 196); the population studied was almost exclusively white and predominately of Northern European ancestry (2). Hochberg et al (3) reported that the prevalence of JRA among urban African Americans was 26 per 100,000 (95% confidence intervals: 7, 66). In a recent population-based study from Sweden, Andersson-Gäre and Fasth estimated the prevalence of JRA to be 86 per 100,000 (4). In addition, they reported that 50% of JRA patients have active disease that persists into adulthood (5). Neither the Mayo Clinic study nor Hochberg et al included adult-age JRA patients, resulting in an underestimation. All prevalence estimates have wide confidence intervals because of the relative rarity of JRA and the small number of actual cases detected in even the largest studies. This leads to enormous differences between the lower and upper estimates of actual JRA cases. The most commonly cited figure is 70,000 to 100,000 cases (active and inactive) of JRA in the US population under age 16 (1). Using Andersson-Gäre and Fasth's report on disease persisting into adulthood, an estimated 35,000 to 50,000 people older than age 16 years have active JRA in the United States (5).

JRA affects a much smaller portion of the U.S. population than adult-onset RA. However, compared to other pediatric-onset chronic illnesses, JRA is relatively common, affecting approximately the same number of children as juvenile diabetes, at least four times as many children as sickle cell anemia or cystic fibrosis, and at least 10 times as many as hemophilia, acute lymphocytic leukemia, chronic renal failure, or muscular dystrophy (6).

Clinical Features

The diagnostic criteria for JRA are disease onset at less than 16 years of age, persistent arthritis in one or more joints for at least six weeks, and exclusion of other types of childhood arthritis (7). Misdiagnosis often results when one or more of four key points are missed: 1) arthritis must be present and is defined as swelling, effusion, or the presence of two or more of the following: limitation of motion, tenderness, pain on motion, or joint warmth; 2) the arthritis must be consistently present for at least six weeks (Many European criteria require at least 12 weeks of persistent arthritis); 3) more than 100 other causes of chronic arthritis in children must be excluded; and 4) no specific laboratory or other test can establish the diagnosis of JRA.

JRA is subdivided into three types: systemic, polyarticular, and pauciarticular. These subtypes demonstrate unique clinical presentations, immunogenetic associations, and clinical courses (Table 39B-1). Within the polyarticular and pauciarticular subtypes, further clinical grouping can be done, supporting the concept that JRA represents different forms of chronic arthritis.

Recognizing that chronic arthritis in childhood is a heterogeneous group of diseases, the International League Against Rheumatism (ILAR) has developed an alternative classification system that is being used increasingly in many parts of the world, especially Europe. The idiopathic arthritidies of childhood (IAC) are separated into eight separate categories, with each category defined by specific inclusion and exclusion criteria (8). The current IAC classification scheme is currently being validated by both clinical and immunogenetic methods to assess the homogeneity and stability of the diagnostic categories (9). For the next several years, both classification systems (JRA and IAC) will continue to appear in the literature. For a more complete description of the IAC classification system see Table 39B-2.

Systemic Onset JRA (sJRA)
Approximately 10% of children with JRA have systemic onset characterized by daily or twice-daily intermittent fever spikes of >101°F and the presence of a rash that is pale pink, blanching, transient (lasting minutes to a few hours), nonpuritic in 95% of cases, and characterized by small macules or maculopapules. Children with sJRA often have growth delay, osteopenia, diffuse lymphadenopathy, hepatosplenomegaly, pericarditis, pleuritis, anemia, leukocytosis, thrombocytosis, and elevated acute-phase reactants. Positive rheumatoid factor (RF) and uveitis are rare. The extra-articular features are mild to moderate in severity and almost always self-limited. Most symptoms resolve when the fevers resolve; however, sJRA patients can develop pericardial tamponade, severe vasculitis with secondary consumptive coagulopathy, and macrophage activation syndrome – all of which require intense corticosteroid therapy.

The long-term prognosis for systemic-onset JRA is determined by the severity of the arthritis, which usually develops concurrently with the fever and rash, but in some patients does not develop for weeks or months after the onset of the fever. sJRA may develop at any age younger than 16 years, but the peak age of onset is 1–6 years old. Boys and girls are equally affected.

Polyarticular Onset (poJRA)
To be characterized as having poJRA a child must have arthritis in five or more joints (Table 39B-1). Approximately 40% of children with JRA have polyarticular involvement. At least two distinct disease groups comprise poJRA and are most easily distinguished by the presence or absence of RF. Rheumatoid factor-positive patients are almost always girls with later disease onset (at least 8 years old) who are usually HLA-DR4 positive, have symmetric small-joint arthritis,

TABLE 39B-1
JRA Subtype Characteristics

Characteristic	Systemic	Polyarticular	Pauciarticular
Frequency of cases	10%	40%	50%
Number of joints with arthritis at onset	Variable	≥5	≤4
Sex ratio (F:M)	1:1	3:1	5:1
Frequency of uveitis	1%	5%	20%
Frequency of rheumatoid factor positivity	<2%	5%–10%	<2%
Frequency of ANA positivity	5%–10%	40%–50%	75%–85%
Frequency of ≥5 joints involved any time during course of JRA	50%–60%	100%	50%
Frequency of active disease >10 years follow-up	42%	45%	41%
Frequency of erosions or joint space narrowing on radiographs	45%	54%	28%
Median time to develop erosions or joint space narrowing on radiographs (years after disease onset)	2.2	2.4	5.4
Frequency of adult height <5th percentile	50%	16%	11%

JRA, juvenile rheumatoid arthritis; ANA, antinuclear antibody.

TABLE 39B-2
Proposed Classification Criteria for the Idiopathic Arthritidies of Childhood

Diagnostic subcatagory	Description	Percentage of childhood onset arthritis patients seen in pediatric rheumatology clinic
Systemic	Arthritis with or preceded by daily fever of at least 2 weeks duration, documented to be quotidian for at least 3 days, and accompanied by at least one of the following: rheumatoid rash, generalized lymphadenopathy, hepato- or splenomegaly and serositis.	4%
Oligoarthritis – persistent	Arthritis in ≤ 4 joints at any time during the onset or course of the disease	20%
Oligoarthritis – extended	Arthritis in ≤ 4 joints in first 6 months of disease but affecting a cumulative total of ≥5 joints after the first 6 months	13%
	Exclusion criteria for *both* the oligoarthritis categories: Definite psoriasis in first- or second-degree relative confirmed by dermatologist Family history of HLA-B27 associated disease Positive test for rheumatoid factor Patient is an HLA-B27 positive male with onset of arthritis after 8 years old Presence at any time of diagnosis of "systemic arthritis" (see above)	
Polyarthritis – rheumatoid factor negative	Arthritis affecting ≥5 joints during first 6 months Exclusion criteria: Positive test for rheumatoid factor Presence at any time of diagnosis of "systemic arthritis" (see above)	22%
Polyarthritis – rheumatoid factor positive	Arthritis affecting ≥5 joints during first 6 months and positive test for rheumatoid factor at least twice at least 3 months apart Exclusion criteria: Rheumatoid factor test positive <2 times Presence at any time of diagnosis of "systemic arthritis" (see above)	6%

Adapted from Petty et al. (8) with permission. HLA, human leukocyte antigen.

and are at greater risk for developing erosions, nodules, and poor functional outcome compared with RF-negative patients. RF-positive polyarticular JRA resembles adult-onset RA more than any other JRA subset. Clinical manifestations and outcome are highly variable, and include fatigue, anorexia, protein-caloric malnutrition, anemia, growth retardation, delay in sexual maturation, and osteopenia. Polyarticular-onset JRA may develop at any age younger than 16 years, and girls with poJRA outnumber boys with this form three to one.

Pauciarticular JRA (paJRA)
To be characterized as having paJRA a child must have arthritis in four or fewer joints. Patients are subdivided into at least two distinct clinical groups: early onset and late onset.

Early-onset paJRA patients are typically very young (1–5 years old), are more likely to be girls (girls outnumber boys four to one), are often antinuclear antibody (ANA)-positive, have the greatest risk for developing chronic eye inflammation, and have the best overall articular outcome. Eye involvement occurs in 30%–50% of early-onset paJRA patients. The inflammatory process primarily involves the anterior chamber of the eye and is associated with minimal, if any, symptoms in more than 80% of affected children. Because severe, irreversible eye changes, including corneal clouding, cataracts, glaucoma, and partial or total visual loss, can occur, patients should be screened at regular intervals and treated by experienced eye specialists (Table 39B-3; 10).

Late-onset paJRA is more common in boys; 50% are HLA-B27 positive. Patients are more likely to have enthesitis

Diagnostic subcatagory	Description	Percentage of childhood onset arthritis patients seen in pediatric rheumatology clinic

Enthesitis-related arthritis	Arthritis and enthesitis or arthritis plus any 2 of the following:
	    Sacroiliac joint tenderness
	    Inflammatory spinal pain
	    Positive HLA-B27
	    Physician-diagnosed HLA-B27–associated disease in first- or
	        second-degree relative
	    Symptomatic anterior uvieits
	    Male >8 years old at onset of arthritis or enthesitis
	
	Exclusions:
	    Definite psoriasis in first- or second-degree relative confirmed
	        by dermatologist
	    Presence at any time of diagnosis of "systemic arthritis"
	        (see above)
		12%

Psoriatic arthritis	Arthritis and psoriasis or arthritis and all of the following:
	    Physician-diagnosed psoriasis in parents or siblings
	    Dactylitis
	    Nail abnormalities (pitting or onycholysis)
	
	Exclusions:
	    Positive rheumatoid factor
	    Presence at any time of diagnosis of "systemic arthritis"
	        (see above)
		12%

Other	Arthritis for ≥6 months and does not fit into any of the above categories or fits into more than 1 category	11%

or tendinitis, with the arthritis often affecting large joints (shoulders, hips, and knees) or the spine. Eye involvement, if it occurs, is usually of sudden onset; chronic eye complications are less likely to occur than in early-onset paJRA.

Treatment

The standard of care for JRA incorporates the comprehensive, coordinated efforts of an interdisciplinary team of health care professionals and the family to address all facets of life that may be affected by a chronic illness. These include education, peer relations, self-esteem, social adjustment, family dynamics, vocational planning, and financial concerns. In clinical settings that have used this approach, young adults with JRA have been shown to surpass community standards and even their own siblings in

levels of post-secondary schooling and professional degree attainment (11).

The treatment of JRA begins during the diagnostic process. The patient, parents, influential extended family members (for example, grandparents), and the health care team must be convinced and convincing that the patient really does have JRA and that other diseases have been considered and eliminated. The family shoulders the largest responsibility for the child's ongoing treatment, such as giving medications, putting on splints, assisting with prescribed exercises and maintaining the family schedule to facilitate regular school attendance. The therapeutic goals for children with JRA are relieving symptoms, maintaining joint motion and muscle strength, preventing or minimizing anatomic joint damage, maximizing functional status, promoting

TABLE 39B-3
American Academy of Pediatrics Guidelines for Screening Eye Exams in JRA

JRA onset subtype	Age at onset	
	<7 years	>7 years
Systemic	Annual	Annual
Polyarticular		
ANA positive	Every 3–4 months for 4 years, then every 6 months for 3 years, then annually	Every 6 months for 4 years, then annually
ANA negative	Every 6 months for 4 years, then annually	Every 6 months for 4 years, then annually
Pauciarticular		
ANA positive	Every 3–4 months for 4 years, then every 6 months for 3 years, then annually	Every 6 months for 4 years, then annually
ANA negative	Every 6 months for 4 years, then annually	Every 6 months for 4 years, then annually

JRA, juvenile rheumatoid arthritis; ANA, antinuclear antibody. Adapted with permission from Yancey and Gross (10).

positive self-image, and encouraging productive family dynamics. Studies have shown that the negative psychologic impact of JRA is greater on patients' siblings than on the patients themselves (11).

The treatment program can be divided into physical, social, and pharmacologic components. Physical and occupational therapists oversee the physical component, which consists of performing range-of-motion exercises for the involved joints two or three times per day; fabricating splints to minimize joint deformity of mechanical stress or to correct contractures; and teaching joint-protection techniques to minimize joint trauma while the young person participates in activities of daily living. The physical and occupational therapists often consult with school personnel about physical education and classroom adaptations.

The social program relates to psychosocial adjustments, school adaptations, and vocational issues. The patient's social worker and rheumatology nurse are deeply involved in this area. Patients and families often feel quite isolated and benefit from introduction to other families with children with JRA. The Arthritis Foundation sponsors national and regional activities of the American Juvenile Arthritis Organization (AJAO). The AJAO is a membership organization for children with juvenile-onset rheumatic diseases and their families. Early involvement of families with the AJAO can greatly facilitate productive adjustment to the challenges of a rheumatic disease.

Juvenile rheumatoid arthritis does not affect intellectual capacity but can significantly impair educational achievement. However, most roadblocks to educational progress can be avoided or corrected with minor adaptations in the school environment. The AJAO has developed written materials and training workshops to aid health care profes-

sionals and parents in working with their child's school and teachers. In addition, a number of federal laws support the rights of children with chronic illness (including JRA) to receive education in the "least restrictive environment."

The pharmacologic management encompasses treatment of articular, ocular, and other manifestations of JRA. Pediatric rheumatologists have become more aggressive in the use of anti-inflammatory medications because of the frequent chronicity and risk of irreversible damage to joints or eyes in children with JRA whose chronic arthritis or uveitis is only partially controlled. The overall goal of treatment for either arthritis or uveitis should be prompt, consistent, complete (or very nearly complete) suppression of the inflammation while avoiding chronic corticosteroid therapy (including topical opthalmic use for uveitis). This goal can be accomplished in almost all JRA patients, but requires aggressive use of, oftentimes, several anti-inflammatory medications with the early introduction of one or more second-line medications such as methotrexate, etanercept, and sulfasalazine (see below).

In patients with very mild arthritis, the articular manifestations can be treated with nonsteroidal anti-inflammatory drugs (NSAIDs) alone. NSAIDs are the first-line treatment for JRA. Achieving an anti-inflammatory effect requires larger doses than are needed for pain control (up to twice the analgesic dose) and consistent ingestion over a longer period of time. The average time to demonstrate clinical response to a particular NSAID in JRA patients is one month (12). Approximately one-half of children with JRA who will respond to a particular NSAID have done so by two weeks of regular therapy, but up to 25% do not demonstrate clinical response until eight to 12 weeks of continued therapy. Many NSAIDs have been prospectively evaluated in patients with JRA, and overall efficacy rates are similar. However, individual patient response is idiosyncratic. A favorable response to the first NSAID used occurs in 50%–60% of children with JRA. About 50% of those demonstrating inadequate clinical response to the first NSAID improve with the next NSAID tried (13). In general, the selection of NSAID is driven more by logistics than scientific concerns. Liquid NSAIDs are often necessary in young patients and four-times-a-day preparations are avoided in school-aged children if at all possible.

Most children tolerate NSAID therapy well. The most frequent side effects are abdominal pain and anorexia. H2 blockers, misoprostol, or antacids are often given to minimize these complaints. The actual prevalence of gastritis or gastrointestinal ulceration with NSAID use in JRA patients is unknown, but it seems to be less common in children than in adults (13). NSAIDs should be taken with food.

NSAIDs also may adversely affect coagulation, the liver, or renal function, or may cause central nervous system (CNS) symptoms. Increased bruising associated with daily activities is common, but significantly increased bleeding with trauma or surgery is rare. However, with most elective surgeries, especially those involving the mouth or throat, surgeons recommend temporary termination of NSAID therapy. Although elevated liver enzymes occur in 3%–5% of children with JRA treated with nonsalicylate NSAIDs and 15%–30% treated with salicylates, very few patients demonstrate clinical or laboratory evidence of functional liver impairment. Fewer than 5% demonstrate proteinuria or hematuria. CNS symptoms generally develop soon after starting treatment and are primarily mood changes (drowsiness or irritability), headaches, and tinnitus. Mood changes occur in 3%–5%. Headaches are much more common with indomethacin, and tinnitus occurs primarily but not exclusively with salicylate use. A unique skin toxicity seen in children taking naproxen is the development of small pinhead-size blisters that heal leaving a hypopigmented scar. These lesions usually are minimally symptomatic and the scars resolve very slowly, often taking several years to fade. The skin also can become fragile and scars can develop in even the smallest scratch or abrasion. These skin findings are very seldom seen in adults taking naprosyn and are seldom seen in children taking other NSAIDs. If observed, naproxen therapy should be discontinued permanently. The general practice is to perform complete blood cell count, serum glutamic-oxaloacetic transaminase, serum glutamate pyruvate transaminase, blood urea nitrogen, creatinine, and routine urinalysis every three to six months in JRA patients taking NSAIDS regularly.

At least two-thirds of children with JRA are inadequately treated with NSAIDs alone (13). In a prospective blinded trial, oral methotrexate given once weekly at 10 mg/m² body surface area (BSA) was well tolerated and significantly more effective than either placebo or oral methotrexate at 5 mg/m² BSA (14). Methotrexate is used primarily for sJRA or poJRA patients. Overall, approximately 70% of JRA patients demonstrate clinical improve-

ment on methotrexate therapy, although the rate of response is lower in sJRA patients still demonstrating systemic features (14). In patients with significant arthritis despite methotrexate therapy at 10 mg/m² BSA, higher doses (up to 1 mg/kg/week, maximum of 50 mg/week) have been shown to be beneficial and generally well tolerated in short-term uncontrolled trials (13,15). At doses greater than 20 mg/m² BSA per week, oral absorption is unpredictable, and parenteral administration results in more reliable dosing and fewer gastrointestinal side effects. The pharmacokinetic profiles of subcutaneous and intramuscular administration are similar, with the former causing less patient discomfort. Therapeutic benefits of methotrexate do not usually become evident for at least three to four weeks, and maximal response is not reached until three to six months. Methotrexate not uncommonly causes oral ulcers, nausea, decreased appetite, and abdominal pain, but these side effects are generally mild and do not require alteration in dosage. Pulmonary complications from methotrexate are very rare in JRA patients, and reports of liver biopsies have been reassuring (16,17). Folic acid (1 mg orally daily) is often given to decrease the frequency and severity of side effects. At the current time, most pediatric rheumatologists follow the American College of Rheumatology monitoring guidelines for methotrexate toxicity developed for adult RA patients (18) (see Appendix II), even though the guidelines have not been evaluated or validated in patients with JRA.

In a randomized, prospective, placebo-controlled trial in children with severe methotrexate-resistant poJRA, etanercept demonstrated a clinically significant, rapid onset, comprehensive improvement in JRA-related symptoms, functional ability, joint exam, erythrocyte sedimentation rate, and C-reactive protein. The median improvements in clinical and laboratory outcome measures from baseline after three months of etanercept therapy ranged from 40%–95%. The drug was well tolerated and not associated with any treatment-related laboratory abnormalities in this study of up to seven months of etanercept treatment (19), leading to FDA approval of etanercept for poJRA. Longer-term safety studies are ongoing. Etanercept and very likely other tumor necrosis factor (TNF)-blocking agents, once they have been tested in children, should be utilized in children achieving less than optimal disease control with methotrexate. Studies in adults with RA have shown that the TNF-blocking agents etanercept and infliximab are safe and synergistic when given with methotrexate, and are able to arrest or significantly slow the development of radiologic evidence of joint damage (20). TNF blockade has great potential to significantly improve the long-term outcome of people with severe poJRA.

Sulfasalazine demonstrated superiority to placebo in a prospective, double-blind trial (21). A phase I study of intravenous gamma globulin (IVIgG) has shown promising results in patients with poJRA (13). However, given the expense of IVIgG therapy, clear-cut efficacy should first be established in controlled trials. Prospective controlled trials of oral gold (22), D-penicillamine, and hydroxychloroquine (23) in children with JRA documented no greater efficacy than placebo, and, accordingly, these drugs are infrequently used. Injectable gold has never been evaluated in JRA patients in a controlled trial, but significant clinical improvement is seen in 50%–60% of patients on injectable gold therapy (13). Injectable gold therapy requires painful intramuscular injections, is associated with a high frequency of side effects, and has been almost entirely replaced by methotrexate in the treatment of JRA.

Systemic corticosteroids have been and will continue to be used for severe life-threatening complications of sJRA. The high frequency of significant side effects and lack of evidence that these drugs alter the natural history of articular manifestations strongly weigh against routine use in JRA.

Intra-articular corticosteroids are indicated for patients with limited joint involvement. In people with active paJRA in the knees, intra-articular triamcinolone resulted in suppression of the arthritis for longer than six months in 70% of patients in one study and longer than 12 months in 50% of patients in another study (13). Recently, magnetic resonance imaging demonstrated that intra-articular steroid therapy resulted in significant long-lasting suppression of inflammation and pannus formation without evidence of toxic effects on cartilage (24).

Treatment of ocular inflammation in JRA should be directed by an ophthalmologist experienced in treating inflammatory eye disorders. Early detection, topical corticosteroids, dilating agents, and frequent follow-up are critical in the management of JRA-associated uveitis. If these measures are not effective, then systemic or subtenons injections of corticosteroids are used. An open trial suggested that NSAIDs are beneficial in decreasing the severity of ocular inflammation in JRA-associated uveitis (7). Increasingly, systemic treatment with methotrexate is used to control chronic steroid-dependent uveitis. In severe cases, chlorambucil and cyclophosphamide have been used (7).

A significant number of children with JRA demonstrate generalized retardation of linear growth. Growth retardation is discussed in more detail in Chapter 39A.

Outcome

In a summary of published outcome studies, more than 30% of people with JRA had significant functional limitations after 10 or more years of follow-up (25). Twelve percent of people with JRA were in Steinbrocker classes III (limited self-care) or IV (bed or wheelchair bound) three to seven years after disease onset, but 48% were classified in class III or IV 16 or more years after disease onset (7). Active synovitis can be detected in 30%–55% of JRA patients 10 years after disease onset (25). In a longitudinal study of JRA patients referred to a pediatric rheumatologist within the first six months of disease onset, 28% of the paJRA, 54% of the poJRA, and 45% of the sJRA patients demonstrated either erosions or joint-space narrowing on standard radiographs (25).

Mortality rate estimates in JRA have ranged from 0.29 to 1.1 per 100 patients. These estimates represent a mortality rate three to 14 times greater than the standardized mortality rate for a similarly aged US population (25).

The outcome for JRA patients with uveitis has significantly improved over the past several decades but still is associated with an unacceptably high rate of ocular complications. In the most recent study of ocular outcomes, at a mean follow-up of 9.4 years since onset of eye disease, 85% of patients had normal visual acuity but 15% had significant visual loss, including 10% who were blind in at least one eye (7).

Juvenile Spondyloarthropathies

The spondyloarthropathies in childhood encompass four discrete clinical entities: juvenile ankylosing spondylitis, reactive arthritis, psoriatic arthritis, and arthropathies associated with inflammatory bowel disease. However, since these diseases often take many years to fully evolve and satisfy existing diagnostic criteria, it is not uncommon for children to have symptoms suggestive of spondyloarthropathy but not satisfy full criteria for diagnosis. For that reason, it has been suggested that spondyloarthropathies in children include another syndrome – seronegative enthesopathy and arthropathy (SEA syndrome). The SEA syndrome is applied to people who are negative for RF, negative for ANA, and have enthesitis and either arthritis or arthralgia (7). SEA syndrome is designed to distinguish those children who may have symptoms consistent with other rheumatic diseases, such as JRA, but actually are more likely to develop spondyloarthropathy over time. In one series, 69% of children characterized as having SEA syndrome developed probable or definite spondyloarthropathy at a mean follow-up of 11 years. Children with a much higher risk for developing definite spondyloarthropathy were HLA-B27 positive, had a family history of spondyloarthropathy, or had definite arthritis and not just arthralgia (26). The IAC categories of enthesitis-related arthritis and psoriatic arthritis (see Table 39B-2) represent these cases as well (8).

Epidemiology

The incidence and prevalence of the spondyloarthropathies in childhood are much less well-studied than the epidemiology of JRA. In general, spondyloarthropathies are less common in children than JRA. Juvenile ankylosing spondylitis is reported to have a prevalence of two to 10 per 100,000 individuals and an incidence of 0.3 to 0.4 per 100,000. The prevalence for psoriatic arthritis is two to 12 per 100,000 and for the arthritis associated with inflammatory bowel disease, 0.5 to 1 per 100,000 (26).

Juvenile Ankylosing Spondylitis

Most published reports of juvenile ankylosing spondylitis use the same diagnostic criteria as for diagnosing ankylosing spondylitis in adults. However, to have juvenile ankylosing spondylitis, the patient's disease onset must occur at age 16 years or younger. The adult criteria for ankylosing spondylitis require plain radiographic evidence of sacroiliitis. Because radiographic changes are known to occur years after the onset of clinical symptoms in many cases, establishing a definite diagnosis of juvenile ankylosing spondylitis may be delayed for many years. Of the patients who satisfy the diagnostic criteria, there is a male:female ratio of 6:1, and 82%–95% are HLA-B27 positive (27). The arthritis is usually episodic rather than chronic, and large joints of the lower extremities and the tarsal bones are much more commonly affected than the upper extremities or small joints of the hands. Enthesitis is common, as is lower back or buttock pain. When following patients with probable juvenile ankylosing spondylitis, it is important to monitor the lumbar spine motion and chest expansion very closely.

The primary extra-articular manifestation of juvenile ankylosing spondylitis is acute iritis, which occurs in 5%–10% of patients. Tests for ANA and RF are characteristically negative, and plain radiographs often do not show the characteristic changes in the sacroiliac or lumbosacral spine for many years. Bone scans seldom are helpful because radioisotope uptake is typically increased in the sacroiliac joints and the lumbar spine as a consequence of skeletal growth. Computed tomography and magnetic resonance imaging scans are difficult to interpret because experience with normal findings in sacroiliac joints in children is limited. There are no pathognomonic laboratory tests.

Treatment for juvenile ankylosing spondylitis is primarily NSAIDs; methotrexate and sulfasalazine have been shown to be potentially useful in a few open studies. Patients with severe enthesis unresponsive to NSAIDs may benefit from low-dose prednisone (27).

Reactive Arthritis

Reactive arthritis follows genitourinary or gastrointestinal infection and most commonly is in association with conjunctivitis and urethritis. The vast majority of cases are associated with dysenteric infection. Genitourinary infection as an initiating event is seen primarily in adolescents but also in sexually abused children. Large weight-bearing joints are usually involved. These patients often have enthesitis, and the onset of the musculoskeletal symptoms can be quite acute. Urethritis is frequently asymptomatic and detected only as sterile pyuria, while conjunctivitis is almost always acute in onset. The patient may have oral ulcers and a characteristic (but relatively uncommon) skin rash, keratoderma blennorrhagicum, which starts as a papular eruption on the soles or palms that becomes pustular within a matter of days and then later becomes scaly. Often the clinical manifestations appear asynchronously. The arthritis and conjunctivitis, although sometimes acute, are usually self-limited and associated with excellent clinical outcomes. Treatment with NSAIDs is usually sufficient for musculoskeletal symptoms.

Arthritis Associated with Inflammatory Bowel Disease

Significant peripheral or axial arthritis may occur with either Crohn's disease or ulcerative colitis. Overall, 7%–20% of people with inflammatory bowel disease develop arthritis, which, in the vast majority of instances, will involve primarily the large joints of the lower extremities. The male-to-female ratio is essentially equal, and there is no obvious association with HLA-B27. A small subset of people with inflammatory bowel disease develop axial arthritis; the male-to-female ratio is four to one in these patients, and HLA-B27 is positive in approximately 80%. In most instances, the arthritis is episodic and occurs with worsening of the bowel symptoms.

In some cases, arthritis precedes the onset of gastrointestinal symptoms by months or, rarely, years. The association with underlying bowel disease may be suspected in these patients by the presence of frequent subclinical gastrointestinal symptoms and intermittent nocturnal diarrhea, as well as in patients who have severe systemic symptoms and signs (such as fatigue, weight loss, or fever) that seem excessive relative to the severity of the arthritis. In addition, the presence of erythema nodosum, frequent oral ulcers, pyoderma gangrenosum, digital clubbing, significant anemia, or significant hypoalbuminemia suggest the presence of inflammatory bowel disease.

In most instances, the arthritis improves dramatically with treatment of the underlying bowel disease. The musculoskeletal manifestations are frequently episodic and last for one to two months.

Psoriatic Arthritis

Patients manifesting chronic arthritis in association with psoriasis with an onset at or before the age of 16 years are said to have juvenile psoriatic arthritis. However, the classic psoriatic rash may not appear for many years. According to diagnostic criteria for childhood psoriatic arthritis developed in Vancouver, patients with "definite psoriatic arthritis" have arthritis and psoriasis or arthritis in association with any three of the following clinical characteristics: 1) dactylitis, 2) nail pitting or onycholysis, 3) history of psoriasis in first- or second-degree relatives, or 4) an atypical psoriatic rash. Patients are said to have "probable psoriatic arthritis" if arthritis and two of these four clinical characteristics are present (9). The IAC criteria for psoriatic arthritis are shown in Table 39B-2.

In the vast majority of cases, the arthritis is peripheral, and it may be associated with asymptomatic chronic uveitis in some patients. In studies of pediatric psoriatic arthritis, the association with HLA-B27 positivity is mixed in patients who have axial arthritis. About 50% of children have arthritis before the psoriatic rash appears. Flexor tenosynovitis in fingers or toes (sausage digits) is not uncommon in psoriatic arthritis.

The treatment for psoriatic arthritis is essentially the same as for JRA. A comprehensive physical program should be instituted. NSAIDs are the first line of treatment, but patients with more severe disease may require methotrexate (7,27). Monitoring for asymptomatic uveitis by slit-lamp examination should be done at the same frequency as for children with JRA (Table 39B-3).

DANIEL J. LOVELL, MD, MPH

References

1. Singsen BH. Rheumatic diseases of childhood. Rheum Dis Clin North Am 1990;16:581–599.

2. Towner SR, Michet CJJ, O'Fallen WM, Nelson AM. The epidemiology of juvenile arthritis in Rochester, Minnesota. Arthritis Rheum 1983;26:1208–1213.

3. Hochberg MC, Linet MS, Sills EM. The prevalence and incidence of juvenile rheumatoid arthritis in an urban black population. Am J Public Health 1983;73:1202–1203.

4. Andersson-Gäre BA, Fasth A. Epidemiology of juvenile chronic arthritis in Southwestern Sweden – 5-year prospective population study. Pediatrics 1992;90:950–958.

5. Andersson-Gäre BA, Fasth A. The natural history of juvenile chronic arthritis: a population based cohort study. II. Outcome. J Rheumatol 1995;22:308–319.

6. Gortmaker S. Chronic childhood disorders. Prevalence and impact. Ped Clin North Am 1984;31:3–18.

7. Cassidy JT, Petty RE. Textbook of Pediatric Rheumatology, 3rd ed. Philadelphia: WB Saunders, 1995.

8. Petty RE, Southwood TR, Baum J. Revision of the proposed classification criteria for juvenile idiopathic arthritis. Durban, 1997. J Rheumatol 1997;25:1991–1994.

9. Ramsey SE, Bolaria RK, Cabral DA, Malleson PN, Petty RE. Comparison of criteria for the classification of childhood arthritis. J Rheumatol 2000;27:1283–1286.

10. Yancey C, Gross R. Guidelines for ophthalmologic examinations in children with juvenile rheumatoid arthritis. Peds 1993;92:295–296.

11. White PH, Shear ES. Transition/job readiness for adolescents with juvenile arthritis and other chronic illness. J Rheumatol 1992;19:28–31.

12. Lovell DJ, Giannini EH, Brewer EJ. Time course of response to nonsteroidal anti-inflammatory drugs in juvenile rheumatoid arthritis. Arthritis Rheum 1984;27:1433–1437.

13. Giannini EH, Cawkwell GD. Drug treatment in children with juvenile rheumatoid arthritis past, present and future. Ped Clin North Am 1995;42:1099–1125.

14. Giannini EH, Brewer EJ, Kuzmina N. Methotrexate in resistant juvenile rheumatoid arthritis: results of the U.S.A.-U.S.S.R. double-blind, placebo-controlled trial. N Engl J Med 1991; 326:1043–1049.

15. Wallace CA, Sherry DD. Preliminary report of higher dose methotrexate and treatment in juvenile rheumatoid arthritis. J Rheumatol 1992;19:1604–1607.

16. Kugathasan S, Newman AJ, Dahms BB, Boyle JT. Liver biopsy findings in patients with juvenile rheumatoid arthritis receiving long-term, weekly methotrexate therapy. J Pediatr 1996;128:149–151.

17. Hashkes PJ, Balistreri WF, Bove KE, Ballard ET, Passo MH. The long-term effect of methotrexate therapy on the liver in patients with juvenile rheumatoid arthritis. Arthritis Rheum 1997;40:2226–2234.

18. Kremer JM, Alarcón GS, Lightfoot RW, et al. Methotrexate for rheumatoid arthritis: suggested guidelines for monitoring liver toxicity. Arthritis Rheum 1994;37:316–328.

19. Lovell DJ, Giannini EH, Reiff A, et al. for The Pediatric Rheumatology Collaborative Study Group. Etanercept in children with polyarticular juvenile rheumatoid arthritis. N Engl J Med 2000;342:763–769.

20. Pisetsky DS. Tumor necrosis factor blockers in rheumatoid arthritis. N Engl J Med 2000;342:810–811.

21. Van Rossum M, Fiselier TJW, Franssen M, et al. Sufasalazine in the treatment of juvenile chronic arthritis – a randomized, double-blind, placebo-controlled, multicenter study. Arthritis Rheum 1998;41:808–816.

22. Giannini EH, Brewer EJ, Kuzmina N. Auranofin in the treatment of juvenile rheumatoid arthritis. Results of the USA-USSR double-blind, placebo-controlled cooperative trial. Arthritis Rheum 1990;33:466–476.

23. Brewer EJ, Giannini EH, Kuzmina N. D-penicillamine and hydroxychloroquine in the treatment of severe juvenile rheumatoid arthritis. Results of the U.S.A.-U.S.S.R. double-blind, placebo-controlled trial. N Engl J Med 1986;314:1269–1276.

24. Huppertz H-I, Tschammler A, Horwitz A, Schwab O. Intra-articular corticosteroids for chronic arthritis in children: efficacy and effects on cartilage and growth. J Pediatr 1995;127:317–321.

25. Levinson JE, Wallace CA. Dismantling the pyramid. J Rheumatol 1992;19:6–10.

26. Cabral DA, Malleson PN, Petty RE. Spondyloarthropathies of childhood. Ped Clin North Am 1995;42:1051–1070.

27. Burgos-Vargas R, Petty RE. Juvenile ankylosing spondylitis. Rheum Clin North Am 1992;18:123–142.

PEDIATRIC RHEUMATIC DISEASES
C. Connective-Tissue Diseases

The connective-tissue diseases occur infrequently in childhood (Table 39C-1). However, the diversity of their manifestations makes them integral to the differential diagnosis of every child or adolescent who appears systemically ill. Each disease may initially present with diffuse aches and pains, prolonged fever of unknown origin, chronic anemia, recurrent infections, or unexplained fatigue and weight loss.

Children and adolescents with nonarticular rheumatism also present with fatigue, aches, pains, or stiffness. However, in contrast to the children with connective-tissue diseases, they often appear well and lack systemic inflammatory changes. Nonarticular rheumatism includes both benign entities (e.g., "growing pains") and disabling illnesses such as fibromyalgia and reflex sympathetic dystrophy, which produce significant morbidity. It is essential that all children with suspected nonarticular rheumatism be carefully evaluated. Many children initially diagnosed with nonarticular rheumatism are determined to have true connective-tissue diseases over time.

Systemic Lupus Erythematosus

Systemic lupus erythematosus (SLE) is the most common major connective tissue disease of childhood, with an estimated prevalence five to 10 per 100,000 (1). SLE predominantly affects adolescent females but may affect males and younger children. It is more common in African Americans, Asians, and Hispanics, but it may affect children of any age, race, and gender. Antinuclear antibodies (ANA) are found in virtually all cases of SLE, but this alone does not establish the diagnosis. ANA testing has high sensitivity (virtually all children with SLE are ANA-positive) but low specificity (many children who are ANA-positive do not have SLE). Hypocomplementemia and antibodies to Sm in children with ANA are important findings that greatly increase the probability of SLE.

The American College of Rheumatology criteria for the classification of definite SLE apply to children (2). However, it is important to recognize that the disease may evolve over time in childhood. Children may initially be diagnosed with idiopathic thrombocytopenic purpura because they do not fulfill four or more of the recognized criteria, only to develop renal involvement and hypocomplementemia typical of SLE months or even years later.

The onset of SLE in children is often gradual, and the malar rash seen in textbooks is not reliably present. In children and adolescents with fatigue and malaise, evidence of multisystem involvement should be actively sought. Pleural effusions, synovitis affecting the small joints of the hands or feet, hemolytic anemia, proteinuria, and hematuria are common manifestations of SLE that may not be detected during a routine office evaluation.

Less frequently, the onset is dramatic. Fever and rash may be accompanied by polyserositis (abdominal pain, pleural effusions), neurologic manifestations (seizures, hallucinations, depression, coma), renal involvement (hematuria, proteinuria, hypertension, nephrotic syndrome), or pulmonary disease (effusions, hemorrhage, respiratory failure) occurring in any combination. Sudden overwhelming sepsis (resulting from neutropenia, functional asplenia, or hypocomplementemia) may also be present. Frequently, both antibiotics and corticosteroids are required in this setting because active SLE and infection may present simultaneously.

Renal involvement is common, occurring in up to two-thirds of children with SLE (3). There may be only mild glomerulitis, but many children suffer from diffuse proliferative glomerulonephritis or membranous nephritis that may ultimately lead to renal failure. Central nervous system involvement also is a common cause of morbidity. Dramatic manifestations such as transverse myelitis, seizures, coma, and psychosis are less common than subtle findings such as chronic depression, poor judgment, and impaired short-term memory. These changes result in poor

TABLE 39C-1
Rheumatic Disease Diagnoses in a Large Tertiary Referral Center[a]

Juvenile rheumatoid arthritis	189
Spondyloarthropathies	161
Nonarticular rheumatism (e.g., fibromyalgia)	160
Systemic lupus erythematosus	53
Mechanical syndromes	49
Vasculitic diseases	37
Lyme disease	25
Rheumatic manifestations of endocrine disease	11
Scleroderma	10
Skeletal dysplasias	7
Disorders of collagen metabolism (e.g., Marfan's, Ehlers–Danlos)	6
Acute rheumatic fever	5
Infections of bones and joints	2
Malignancies (leukemia, neuroblastoma)	2
Other	5

[a] 722 individual patients seen in a single calendar year for new or follow-up appointments; all initially referred for rheumatic disease evaluation by other physicians.

school performance and family disruptions that contribute significantly to the morbidity of SLE. It is extremely important that the treating physician recognize that nonadherence with medications frequently accompanies "acting out" by children and adolescents with SLE. In such circumstances, it is important to make certain the child is taking the prescribed medications.

Corticosteroids are extremely effective in reducing the inflammatory manifestations of SLE, but in children and adolescents the use of these drugs is associated with substantial morbidity. Cushingoid facies, short stature, acne, osteonecrosis, cataracts, pancreatitis, and accelerated atherosclerosis are well-recognized complications. For patients with severe disease, immunosuppressive drug regimens (such as periodic intravenous cyclophosphamide) have been associated with a dramatic reduction in both disease and steroid-related morbidity without excessive toxicity (4,5). The key to high-quality survival for children with SLE is early recognition and comprehensive management of both their medical and psychosocial needs.

Mixed Connective Tissue Disease

Mixed connective tissue disease (MCTD) is a variant of SLE with a greater frequency of Raynaud's phenomenon and hypergammaglobulinemia but a lower frequency of hypocomplementemia. Children with MCTD are also less likely to develop severe nephritis or require immunosuppressive therapy (6). A significant proportion of children with MCTD ultimately develops scleroderma (7). Childhood MCTD should be suspected when both ANA and rheumatoid factor are found in a child with what appears to be SLE or dermatomyositis. Antibodies to Sm are typically absent, whereas those to U_1 ribonucleoprotein are typically present; however, some patients with characteristic clinical features lack the expected serologic findings. Interestingly, MCTD shares with scleroderma and juvenile dermatomyositis the frequent occurrence of nail-fold capillary changes and Gottren's papules, suggesting an etiopathogenic association. The treatment of childhood MCTD is identical to that for SLE with similar manifestations.

Antiphospholipid Antibody Syndromes

Antiphospholipid antibodies (APL) occur in children and adolescents with SLE, but also in many children with a positive ANA without SLE. In addition, APL are found in a high percentage of children with unexplained strokes, and have also been reported in children with multiple pulmonary emboli and chorea (8–11). Proper therapy is uncertain. The risks of anticoagulation with warfarin seem greater than the risk of thrombosis in unselected APL-positive children and adolescents. Some physicians observe conservatively; others treat with a small daily dose of aspirin. Children with a history of stroke or embolic phenomena should be appropriately anticoagulated.

Juvenile Dermatomyositis

Juvenile dermatomyositis (JDMS) affects both genders with a slight female predominance. Most often, the onset is slow and the initial symptoms are not recognized. Parents of small children usually first notice a reluctance to go up or down stairs and an increased desire to be carried. With time, the child becomes "clumsy." Ultimately, medical intervention is sought because of rash, progressive weakness, or constitutional symptoms such as fever or weight loss.

There are several distinct subsets of JDMS. The most common subset consists of proximal muscle weakness and mild heliotropic rash in children who have no evidence of vasculitis. The illness often resolves over a six-month period with corticosteroid therapy alone. Children with a vasculitic rash or nail-fold capillary abnormalities are more likely to have a chronic course and internal organ involvement. This subset includes those with Gottren's papules. Children with severe rash and markedly elevated muscle enzymes but only moderate weakness are in another, less common, subset that may represent a distinct illness.

Clinical and Laboratory Features

The rash of JDMS is an erythematous discoloration most prominent on the face and the extensor surfaces of the elbows and knees. It is often ascribed by parents to the child's frequent falling. The heliotropic rash characteristic of this condition is a violaceous discoloration over the eyelids. Gottren's papules are inflammatory vasculitic lesions overlying the interphalangeal joints. They may be an early clue to the diagnosis but are not always present. Proximal muscle weakness may be overlooked if testing for weakness is limited to evaluating grip strength, which tests only distal muscle function. Frequently the diagnosis of JDMS is first considered when laboratory evaluation demonstrates muscle enzyme abnormalities [creatinine phosphokinase (CPK), aspartate aminotransferase (AST), or aldolase (ALD)]. All of these enzymes may be abnormal, but in some children, only the aldolase is elevated. The diagnosis is confirmed by characteristic electromyographic abnormalities, muscle biopsy, or the typical clinical picture. Arthritis may be present, but it usually resolves promptly after therapy is initiated.

Special care must be taken to evaluate swallowing function and the gag reflex of children with dermatomyositis. A more nasal voice or frequent coughing when eating should be regarded with extreme concern. Aspiration due to weakness of the voluntary muscles that initiate swallowing is a prominent hazard. Chronic abdominal pain also must be regarded with concern. Although it may be benign, it sometimes results from small-vessel vasculitis. Small areas of bowel involvement may initially produce nonspecific abdominal pain, but progressive involvement may lead to perforation with catastrophic consequences. Cerebritis, which may be associated with hallucinations and dementia, or retinal vasculitis is also sometimes present. Other major internal organ complications include pulmonary fibrosis and cardiac damage with scarring, poor contractility, and possible conduction abnormalities.

Diffuse calcification of subcutaneous tissues or muscle groups may be a debilitating complication of JDMS. Small areas of discrete calcification do not warrant surgical intervention unless they are causing discomfort. Rarely a patient will develop severe, diffuse calcification (calcinosis universalis) following the acute phase of illness. No satisfactory treatment exists. Regimens that interfere with calcification appear to have greater effects on normal bone than on ectopic bone. However, there is speculation that newer agents may be beneficial. Secondary infection of calcium deposits is a constant concern. Fortunately, severe complications are infrequent in children who are promptly diagnosed and appropriately treated.

Differential Diagnosis
MCTD should be considered in children with persistent arthritis and muscle inflammation.

Chronic weakness in childhood may also be the result of genetic conditions such as muscular dystrophy or metabolic conditions such as hyperthyroidism. Although some of these conditions are accompanied by elevated muscle enzyme levels, they lack the characteristic rash and other evidence of vasculitis that commonly accompany JDMS. Isolated polymyositis is very rare in childhood.

Treatment
The majority of children with JDMS recover completely with corticosteroids alone. However, some have persistent active disease or develop unacceptable corticosteroid side effects (12). Low-dose oral methotrexate is often effective for mild disease. There are reported experiences with larger doses of methotrexate administered intramuscularly or intravenously, cyclophosphamide, intravenous gamma globulin, and cyclosporine (13–15).

Scleroderma

In children, scleroderma is often present for a prolonged period before clinicians recognize the progressive thickening and hardening of the skin. Children suffer from the focal forms (morphea and linear scleroderma) more often than the systemic forms of progressive systemic sclerosis (PSS) and CREST syndrome (calcinosis, Raynaud's phenomenon, esophageal dysmotility, sclerodactyly, telangiectasia).

Clinical Features
Linear scleroderma (LS) in childhood is a tight band-like constriction of the skin over the extremities or trunk. If involvement is limited and does not cross a joint, the condition is benign. However, thickening of the skin may be associated with atrophy of the underlying muscle and bone, as well as synovitis. LS crossing a joint or involving a large proportion of a limb in childhood often produces contractures and stunted growth. These cases may warrant therapy.

Some children develop lesions of both morphea and LS. There are also cases in which the skin lesions are associated with an inflammatory myopathy (sclerodermatomyositis) or other inflammatory lesions including uveitis. LS *en coup de sabre* is a special case involving the scalp and face. Typically, there is an area of thickening of the scalp that may extend down onto to the face. This condition is often confused with Parry-Romberg syndrome of progressive facial hemiatrophy. Parry-Romberg syndrome is associated with inflammation and atrophy of the deeper underlying tissues and often involves the central nervous system and tongue. Although typical cases of linear scleroderma *en coup de sabre* and Parry-Romberg syndrome are easily distinguished, there are cases that do not clearly fall into either category. The two diseases may be related (16). Mild cases of LS that do not produce contractures do not require therapy. Methotrexate has been effective for more severe cases (17).

In contrast to LS, PSS in childhood may be life-threatening. Diffuse tightening of the skin is accompanied by inflammation and fibrosis of the internal organs (heart, lungs, and kidneys). The onset of PSS is usually gradual. Often, patients first seek care because of worsening Raynaud's phenomenon. On careful inspection, skin tightening is evident proximal to the forearm. Facial skin tightening results in a characteristic appearance with a sharp nose, almond-shaped eyes, and difficulty opening the mouth fully. Distal fingertip lesions, nail-fold capillary abnormalities, or Gottren's papules also suggest progessive systemic sclerosis in a child with Raynaud's phenomenon. In rare instances, the first indications of illness may be swallowing difficulties, malabsorption, or restrictive pulmonary disease (18).

The diagnosis of CREST syndrome in childhood is usually first suggested by the prominent telangiectasias. Induration and skin thickening are much less striking than in PSS. Both PSS and CREST may have life-threatening pulmonary involvement with fibrosis and decreased diffusion capacity. Swallowing dysfunction and widespread internal organ involvement resulting in malabsorption, cardiorespiratory failure, or renal disease are common late in the disease course in both conditions. Catastrophic hypertension secondary to renal involvement (scleroderma renal crisis) is described but is infrequent in childhood.

Gottren's papules and nail-fold capillary abnormalities are found in JDMS, PSS, and MCTD but in no other conditions. This suggests that despite their highly varied clinical expression and prognosis, there is a fundamental relationship between these diseases. The explanation for this association and its etiopathogenic basis are not yet clear.

Laboratory Features
The laboratory abnormalities associated with both PSS and CREST syndrome are primarily those of chronic inflammation and those appropriate to the internal organ involvement. Most patients have ANA, and antibodies to Scl-70 are found in some but not all children with PSS. Similarly, anticentromere antibodies are considered characteristic of CREST syndrome, but they are not always present.

Treatment

There is no uniformly satisfactory treatment for childhood scleroderma. Localized forms that are only cosmetically disturbing are best treated topically. The systemic forms of scleroderma are traditionally treated with D-penicillamine, but although this drug has been beneficial for some patients, it has been ineffective for others. Trials involving methotrexate, cyclosporine, and a variety of biologic agents are underway (19,20). The long-term prognosis for children with PSS or CREST is highly variable. In some, the disease relentlessly progresses, but others survive well into adulthood despite internal organ involvement.

Henoch–Schönlein Purpura

Henoch–Schönlein purpura (HSP) is a common form of small-vessel vasculitis seen almost exclusively in childhood. The typical child with HSP presents with abdominal pain following an upper-respiratory infection. This is followed by petechiae that are predominantly present over dependent areas such as the lower extremities, the buttocks, and the extensor surface of the upper extremities (Fig. 39C-1). Widespread immune complex deposition results in arthritis, abdominal pain, and nephritis in some patients. These manifestations may be severe, with varying degrees of skin rash and edema in dependent areas. Intestinal inflammation may lead to edema and bleeding with potential complications of intussusception, infarction, or perforation. Renal involvement may be chronic but rarely leads to renal failure (21).

There are no distinguishing laboratory abnormalities in HSP. The diagnosis is established by the characteristic clinical picture. Most children recover without therapy as the immune complexes are cleared from their sites of deposition. Typically, the illness is resolved within two weeks. Occasionally, recurrent immune complex deposition causes the illness to be prolonged or episodic. A development of great concern is the development of nephritis, which may be severe. For children with severe abdominal pain or possible intussusception, corticosteroids may be helpful. There is no clear evidence that corticosteroids are beneficial for renal involvement (21). The arthritis associated with HSP is typically transient, but if it persists, nonsteroidal anti-inflammatory drugs usually provide relief. If a child appears to have unusually chronic or severe HSP, polyarteritis nodosa should be excluded.

Medium- and Large-Vessel Vasculitis

The presenting manifestations of polyarteritis nodosa (PAN) in childhood are highly variable. PAN often involves the renal vessels, producing hematuria and hypertension; it may affect the mesenteric vessels, causing abdominal pain. If it affects more superficial vessels, rash or unexplained extremity pain can result. PAN may begin as a fever of unknown origin. It should be suspected in children with chronic fever and abdominal pain if infec-

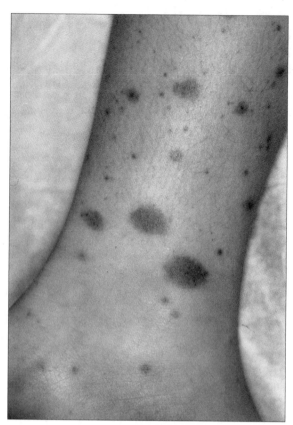

Fig. 39C-1. Evolving rash of Henoch–Schönlein purpura on the lower extremity.

tions, neoplasia, and inflammatory bowel disease have been excluded. When PAN presents with fever, rash, and joint pains, it may be confused with systemic-onset juvenile rheumatoid arthritis. In other instances, the renal involvement and abdominal pain can be confused with HSP. PAN is distinguished by the presence of arterial inflammation that may be demonstrated by biopsy of involved tissues or angiographic studies. In patients with hematuria or hypertension, renal angiography is useful to rapidly establish the correct diagnosis (Fig. 39C-2).

Like Kawasaki disease, PAN may produce coronary artery lesions. Nonspecific thickening of the coronary arteries is found in many inflammatory conditions. Whenever children with suspected Kawasaki disease fail to respond rapidly to the administration of intravenous gamma globulin (IVIgG), alternative diagnoses such as PAN must be carefully considered. Corticosteroids are the treatment of choice for children with PAN and for children with IVIgG-resistant Kawasaki disease (22).

Cutaneous PAN in childhood presents with tender subcutaneous nodules associated with markedly elevated erythrocyte sedimentation rate and, in some cases, fever or malaise. All children should be investigated for evidence of internal organ involvement. Similar lesions may be seen in erythema nodosum, in the panniculitis of Weber–Christian disease, and in patients abusing intravenous drugs, but each has a different pathologic appearance.

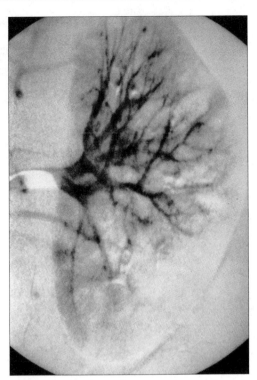

Fig. 39C-2. Renal angiogram demonstrating small aneurysms of polyarteritis nodosa.

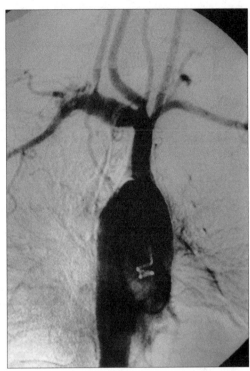

Fig. 39C-3. Angiogram of the aortic arch demonstrating both aneurysmal dilation and stenosis of proximal vessels in a patient with Takayasu's arteritis.

Other forms of medium- and large-vessel vasculitis are rare in children and adolescents. Takayasu's arteritis frequently has its onset in adolescence (Fig. 39C-3) and is more common in females. The presenting complaints are fever, anemia, and elevated acute-phase reactants without apparent explanation. Involvement of the abdominal branches of the aorta may produce abdominal pain. The diagnosis is made only if it is actively sought. Most often, the left radial pulse is reduced or absent, but carotid, femoral, and renal arteries may be selectively involved. The diagnosis is suggested by the presence of asymmetric pulses, widening of the aortic arch on chest radiograph, or arterial bruits.

Wegener's granulomatosis and lymphomatoid granulomatosis are uncommon in adolescents. Their manifestations in childhood do not differ significantly from the findings in adults (see Chapter 21).

THOMAS J. A. LEHMAN, MD

References

1. Lehman TJA. Systemic lupus erythematosus in childhood and adolescence. In: Wallace DJ, Hahn BH (eds). Dubois' Lupus Erythematosus, 4th ed. Philadelphia: Lea and Febiger, 1993.
2. Tan EM, Cohen AS, Fries JF, et al. The 1982 revised criteria for the classification of systemic lupus erythematosus. Arthritis Rheum 1982;25:1271–1277.
3. Lehman TJA, Mouradian JA. Systemic lupus erythematosus. In: Barratt TM, Avner ED, Harmon WE (eds). Pediatric Nephrology 4th ed. Baltimore: Lippincott Williams and Wilkins, 1999.
4. Lehman TJ, Sherry DD, Wagner-Weiner L, et al. Intermittent intravenous cyclophosphamide therapy for lupus nephritis. J Pediatr 1989;114:1055–1060.
5. Lehman TJA, Onel KB. Intermittent intravenous cyclophosphamide arrests progression of the renal chronicity index in childhood systemic lupus erythematosus. J Pediatr 2000;136:243–247.
6. Singsen BH, Bernstein BH, Kornreich HK, King KK, Hanson V, Tan EM. Mixed connective tissue disease in childhood. J Pediatr 1977;90:893–900.
7. Nimelstein SH, Brody S. McShane D, Holman HR. Mixed connective tissue disease: a subsequent evaluation of the original 25 patients. Medicine 1980;59:239–248.
8. Kenet G, Sadetzki S, Murad H, et al. Factor V Leiden and antiphospholipid antibodies are significant risk factors for ischemic stroke in children. Stroke 2000;31:1283–1284.
9. Nordal EB, Nielsen J, Marhaug G. Chorea in juvenile primary antiphospholipid syndrome. Scand J Rheumatol 1999;28:324–327.
10. Toren A, Toren P, Many A, et al. Spectrum of clinical manifestations of antiphospholipid antibodies in childhood and adolescence. Pediatr Hematol Oncol 1993;10:311–315.
11. Tucker LB. Antiphospholipid syndrome in childhood the great unknown. Lupus 1994;3:367–369.
12. Spencer CH, Hanson V, Singsen BH, Bernstein BH, Kornreich HK, King KK. Course of treated juvenile dermatomyositis. J Pediatr 1984;105:399–408.
13. Ansell BM. Management of polymyositis and dermatomyositis. Clin Rheum Dis 1984;10:205–213.

14. Lang BA, Laxer RM, Murphy G, Silverman ED, Roifman CM. Treatment of dermatomyositis with intravenous gamma-globulin. Am J Med 1991;91:169–172.

15. Girardin E, Dayer JM, Paunier L. Cyclosporine for juvenile dermatomyositis. J Pediatr 1988;112:165–166.

16. Lehman TJA. The Parry Romberg syndrome of progressive facial hemiatrophy and linear scleroderma en coup de sabre: mistaken diagnosis or overlapping conditions? J Rheumatol 1992;19:844–845.

17. Uziel Y, Feldman BM, Krafchik BR, Yeung RS, Laxer RM. Methotrexate and corticosteroid therapy for pediatric localized scleroderma. J Pediatr 2000;136:91–95.

18. Garty BZ, Athreya BH, Wilmott RR, Scarpa N, Doughty R, Douglas SD. Pulmonary functions in children with progressive systemic sclerosis. Pediatrics 1991;88:1161–1167.

19. Lehman TJA. Systemic and localized scleroderma in children. Cur Opin in Rheumatol 1996;8:576–579.

20. Foldevari I, Lehman TJA. Is methotrexate a new perspective in the treatment of juvenile progressive systemic scleroderma? Arthritis Rheum 1993;36:S218.

21. Steward M, Savage JM, Bell B, McCord B. Long term renal prognosis of Henoch-Schoenlien purpura in an unselected childhood population. Eur J Pediatr 1988;147:113–115.

22. Wright DA, Newburger JW, Baker A, Sundel RP. Treatment of immune globulin-resistant Kawasaki disease with pulsed doses of corticosteroids. J Pediatr 1996;128:146–149.

23. Cabral DA, Tucker LB. Malignancies in children who initially present with rheumatic complaints. J Pediatr 1999;134:53–57.

24. Cassidy J, Petty R. Musculoskeletal manifestations of systemic disease. In: Textbook of Pediatric Rheumatology, 3rd ed. Philadelphia: W.B. Saunders, 1995.

PEDIATRIC RHEUMATIC DISEASES
D. Pain Syndromes

Pain is an unpleasant sensory and emotional experience associated with actual or potential tissue damage or described in such terms (1). All children experience pain with the notable exception of children with congenital indifference to pain. Most pain is of short duration and directly due to noxious stimuli. Chronic or recurrent musculoskeletal pain, however, can arise from a variety of conditions including those of an inflammatory, traumatic, or psychologic nature. The amount of pain, especially chronic pain, is not directly proportional to the amount of noxious stimuli. Because pain is subjective, the amount of pain is what the child reports. This makes the evaluation and treatment of children with chronic pain challenging.

There are a variety of presentations of childhood chronic musculoskeletal pain. An individual child may have more than one subtype of musculoskeletal pain. Hypermobility, both generalized and localized, growing pains, and then the amplified musculoskeletal pain syndromes will be discussed.

Generalized Hypermobility

Many children are flexible; however, hypermobility is defined by either the Beighton criteria (2) or modified criteria of Carter and Wilkinson (3). These criteria are summarized in Table 39D-1. Estimates of the prevalence of hypermobility are between 10% and 20% for Caucasians, with a higher prevalence in those of Chinese and East African decent. Girls are approximately twice as likely to be hypermobile as boys. Various syndromes are associated with hypermobility, the best known are Marfan's and Ehlers-Danlos (see Chapter 33) syndromes. These syndromes are not benign and require specialist care to monitor for ocular, cardiac, and vascular complications.

Hypermobility syndrome generally occurs in children between the ages of 3 and 10 years (4). It is characterized by intermittent nocturnal leg pain. The pain, which is frequently in the leg muscles or behind the knee, can awaken the child and cause him or her to cry with pain. There is a notable absence of morning stiffness or limping even after a particularly severe attack. Certain activities, such as playing soccer or climbing on the monkey bars, may precipitate an attack of pain. The pain is generally short-lived (lasting 30–60 minutes), but more severe and prolonged episodes may occur. On examination, there is no suggestion of inflammation such as guarding, muscular atrophy, or bony enlargement, although a small bland joint effusion is rarely present.

Reassurance is the primary treatment of hypermobility; however, supportive footwear may be helpful. An evening dose of acetaminophen or a nonsteroidal anti-inflammatory drug (NSAID) may abort the attack. Very rarely is a change of activity indicated, but if so, alternative activities should be encouraged so that the child is not discouraged from participating in sports and physical education. Older children with severe hypermobility pains may be helped by formal physical therapy to strengthen the supportive muscles and to learn joint protection techniques.

There are some less benign associations with hypermobility. Delayed motor development in infants may lead to parental anxiety and unnecessary physiotherapy. In older children and adults hypermobility has been associated with soft tissue rheumatism including fibromyalgia. Hypermobility is also associated with temporomandibular joint dysfunction, chondromalacia patellae, back pain, osteoarthritis, and increased joint injuries, especially to the knee. Hypermobility, by itself, is not associated with aortic dilatation or mitral value prolapse.

TABLE 39D-1
Criteria for Hypermobility

Beighton criteria
  Six points or more of possible nine is considered hypermobile. One point for each motion:
  Touching each thumb to volar forearm
  Extending each 5th metacarpophalangeal joint to 90°
  Greater than 10° hyperextension of each elbow
  Greater than 10° hyperextension of each knee
  Able to touch palms to floor with knees straight

Carter and Wilkinson criteria
  Three points or more of possible five is considered hypermobile. One point for each:
  Touching either thumb to volar forearm
  Hyperextending the metacarpophalangeal joints of one hand so that the fingers parallel the forearm
  Greater than 10° of hyperextension of either elbow
  Greater than 10° of hyperextension of either knee
  Able to touch palms to floor with knees straight

Other non-criteria signs include excessive internal rotation to hip, excessive ankle dorsiflexion, excessive eversion of the foot, and the ability to place one's heel behind one's head or to have one's elbows passively touch behind one's back.

Localized Hypermobility

Any joint can suffer from hypermobility and present as unstable or painful. The three most common areas to raise questions or problems are pes planus, genu recurvatum, and recurrent patella dislocation.

The flexible flat foot is normal and present in infants. The arch forms as part of normal growth. Persistence of a flexible flat foot is not usually a cause of significant discomfort. A rare adolescent with a short Achilles tendon and hypermobile flat foot may have pain from excessive weight bearing on the talar head. Treatment is controversial, but conservative management would include aggressive heel cord stretching, adjusting the shoes, and, if that fails, soft foot orthoses (5). Surgery is rarely indicated even in the most extreme cases and then, only once skeletal maturity has been reached.

Genu recurvatum, like pes planus, may be part of a generalized hypermobility syndrome or may occur in isolation. Adolescent girls are prone to develop symptomatic genu recurvatum manifested by popliteal pain and an increased incidence of anterior cruciate ligament injury (6). Symptoms are worse when standing or walking and improve with rest. Treatment involves physical therapy with special attention to biomechanics, orthotics, strengthening, and improving knee proprioception.

Recurrent patellar dislocation causes a sudden giving way of the knee with pain and inability to straighten the knee (approximately 25° flexed) (7). The patella dislocates laterally. On examination, femoral anteversion, patella alta, and an increased Q angle are common. There is involuntary contraction of the quadriceps muscle if the examiner tries to displace the patella laterally. The Q angle is the angle formed by a line from the anterior-superior iliac spine through the center of the patella and a line from the center of the tibial tubercle to the center of the patella. A normal Q angle is 10°–20°. If chronic, premature degeneration of the articular cartilage of the patella-femoral joint may ensue. Treatment is physical therapy to strengthen the vastus. It that is unsuccessful, surgical realignment of the extensor system may be indicated.

Growing Pains

Growing pains occur in 10%–20% of school-aged children. They are most frequent in children of elementary or preschool age. The pains occur in the early evening or nighttime and may awaken the child. The pain is crampy, usually located deep in the thigh, shin, or calf, and is frequently relieved by massage. There is no residual pain, stiffness, or limping in the morning. Laboratory studies and radiographs, if done, are normal. The term growing pain is a misnomer because the rate of growth is not associated with these pains; however, using the term may reassure the family that the pains are benign. Usually, other family members have experienced growing pains. Only children with typical symptoms and a normal examination, including the absence of hypermobility, should be diagnosed with growing pains.

The etiology is unknown but experience has proved that growing pains do not portend serious illness. Successful management includes reassurance, decreasing excessive secondary gain, and gentle massage. An evening dose of either acetaminophen or an NSAID may be preventive in children with frequent attacks of pain. Passive stretching may also help (8).

Amplified Musculoskeletal Pain Syndromes

There are a variety of distinct pain amplification syndromes in children with differing presentations; however, each is characterized by marked pain and disability beyond what one would expect given the history and physical examination (9). These syndromes are on a continuum and frequently overlap, so the established nomenclature, which divides these conditions into separate groups, leads to oversimplification. A way of looking at the various syndrome subsets is shown in Table 39D-2, along with some of the synonyms. Most children will present with a single subset but there are many in whom these subsets coexist (such as a painful foot with autonomic signs and a painful hand without) or who present with a different subset during a subsequent relapse. Still, there are consistent features to the presentation, physical examination, and treatment.

The etiology of amplified musculoskeletal pain in children is unknown; most authors relate the onset to injury, illness, or psychologic distress. Other factors such as age, sex, hormonal, and genetic factors may play a role. Psychologic distress, in both patient and family, is usually significant either as a cause of or effect of the pain and dysfunction; however, high-quality controlled studies are lacking. Minor trauma is also present as an initial step in many children. Major trauma usually precedes the development of complex regional pain syndrome type I (CRPSI) in adults, but prior fracture is relatively rare in children. Illness, especially arthritis, can serve as the initiating event.

Pain amplification syndromes are not entirely diagnoses of exclusion; characteristic historical and physical examination features emerge to form a typical pattern that will help positively make the diagnosis (Table 39D-3). The typical patient is a 12-year-old girl from an upper-middle class family who has leg pain without overt autonomic dysfunction. One needs to be very circumspect in making this diagnosis in children under the age of 8 years. Boys with amplified musculoskeletal pain present in very similar fashion to girls.

Historical features include minor trauma that may not even be remembered (e.g., "I must have hit my foot."), allodynia, and symptoms of autonomic dysfunction – especially color and temperature changes. In children, these are almost always cold and blue (very rarely will children have the warm, red phase seen in adult CRPSI). There is marked dysfunction with inability to attend school, carry out activities of daily living, or ambulate (if the lower extremity is involved). The examiner is frequently struck by a remarkable interdependency, or enmeshment, between the patient and mother. This interdependency usually manifests itself through body language, and by the mother answering all questions, even when the child is addressed directly. Also striking is the incongruent affect of the child who is cheerful and perfectly calm when reporting severe pain. Most children have a distinct *la belle indifference* about both the pain and the dysfunction it causes. Typically these children are overly mature, seemingly bright (but may have average intelligence), are accomplished in school and extracurricular activities, and are described by their parents as perfectionistic, empathetic, pleasers who will sacrifice their own needs to help others.

Concurrent conversion symptoms and other somatic complaints are common. Conversion, by definition, is not painful, and the more common symptoms are numbness, dizziness, and paralysis. Conversion symptoms are more common in children without overt autonomic dysfunction compared to those with CRPSI. Frequent somatic complaints include headache, abdominal pain, dysmenorrhea, and hyperventilation. Other helpful historical information includes the presence of a role model for chronic pain in the family, the failure of prior medications and treatments, and recent major life events such as divorce, moving, school changes, school stress, siblings moving away, or an illness or death of a family member or friend.

The physical examination is notable for absence of underlying disease; normal neurological examination, especially sensory tests; and allodynia. Allodynia is present if the child reports pain when lightly touched or when a fold of skin is gently pinched; the border of the allodynia can vary greatly on repeat testing. Most children will be

TABLE 39D-2
Names for the Musculoskeletal Pain Syndromes

Intermittent pain without overt autonomic dysfunction
Psychosomatic musculoskeletal pain
Growing pains

Continuous pain without signs of autonomic dysfunction
Psychosomatic musculoskeletal pain
Pseudodystrophy
Diffuse idiopathic pain syndrome
Localized idiopathic pain syndrome

Pain with signs of autonomic dysfunction
Complex regional pain syndrome, types I and II
Reflex sympathetic dystrophy
Reflex neurovascular dystrophy
Algodystrophy
Sudeck's atrophy
Shoulder-hand syndrome
Causalgia, major or minor
Localized idiopathic pain syndrome

Pain with painful points
Fibromyalgia
Fibrositis
Diffuse idiopathic pain syndrome

Hypervigilance
Psychosomatic musculoskeletal pain
Growing pains

TABLE 39D-3
Clues to Childhood Amplified Pain From the History and Physical Examination

Preadolescent to adolescent age (mean age 12 years)
Female (80%)
Increasing pain after minor or no trauma
Marked disability
Crawls around house or up stairs
Allodynia (unable to bear light touch, clothing, or
  bedcovers)
May have symptoms of autonomic changes (any)
  Cold
  Color changes: purple, blue, or gray
  Clammy
  Edema
Worse or no better with splint or cast
Unsuccessful prior therapies
High-level athlete, dancer
Typical personality
  Mature beyond years
  Excels at school and extracurricular activities
  Perfectionist
  Pleaser (meets the needs of others at her own expense)
Role model for chronic pain or a similar pain in family
  or friends
Recent major life event (may be multiple)
  Moving
  Change of school, friends
  Divorce
  Change in nuclear family
Mother acts as spokesperson
Incongruent affect for amount of pain reported
La belle indifference about pain and disability
Compliant when requested to use limb
Autonomic signs, especially after use
Allodynia with a variable border
Pain is not restricted to a dermatome or peripheral nerve
Otherwise a normal neurologic examination

extremely compliant; children who are nonambulatory due to foot pain will stand and even walk upon request. Signs of autonomic dysfunction, if not initially present, may appear after the child uses the limb. Painful points are tested by direct digital pressure of 3–4 kg in a perpendicular direction to the skin (10, 11). In addition to the 18 criteria points for fibromyalgia (see Chapter 8E), control points such as the forehead, mid-radius, shin, clavicle, and thumbnail should be tested. Many children with widespread pain report that nearly every point on their body is painful; these children should not be classified as having the fibromyalgic subset of pain amplification (10,12).

There are some differences between the various subsets of amplified pain. Children with overt autonomic dysfunc-

tion, categorized as having a CRPSI subset syndrome, have continuous pain in a limb (more commonly the lower extremity) and usually can recall the exact time of onset. Although most have an incongruent affect, some display marked pain behavior such as crying or screaming when touched. Children without overt autonomic dysfunction, categorized as having a psychosomatic pain subset syndrome, are less sure of the exact onset, and are more likely to have multiple sites involved (including centrally located sites such as the back, chest, and jaw), concurrent conversion symptoms, and a longer duration of pain. They can have intermittent pain and dysfunction that usually follows strenuous physical activities. Children with painful points, categorized as having a fibromyalgia-subset syndrome, are more likely to be depressed and fatigued, have non-restorative sleep, and have multiple somatic complaints. Approximately 50% of those in the fibromyalgic subset are depressed, whereas 10% of those in the CRPSI subset are depressed. Children with marked anxiety about normal body sensations, categorized as having a hypervigilant subset syndrome, are truly concerned that the sensations they interpret as painful are a sign of major illness. The pain is usually quite short-lived, lasting only a few seconds at times, or it may be prolonged at sites of injury ("slow healing"). Children with any form of amplified pain may also be hypervigilant.

Blood tests, if done, are normal unless there is a concurrent illness. Radiographs are normal or show osteoporosis. Technetium bone scans may be normal or reveal decreased blood flow and decreased uptake in the involved limb (13,14). In adults with CRPSI, the technetium bone scans typically show spotty increased uptake, but this is rare in children.

After the diagnosis is clear, the first step is establishing trust and convincing the child and family that this is the diagnosis. All medical investigations and drug treatments should stop. The nature of the condition should be fully explained, stressing that although the etiology is unknown, there should be a psychological evaluation because psychological factors need attention in most, but not all, children (15).

Treatment
The treatments proposed for amplified musculoskeletal pain syndromes are legion, bespeaking the lack of controlled trials. The most common treatments reported to be beneficial for children with the CRPSI subset are exercise therapy, transcutaneous electrical stimulation, and sympathetic blocks (9,16–18). The majority of these patients were successfully treated with aggressive physical therapy alone (see below). Treatments used in a few children with variable results include corticosteroids, tricyclic antidepressants, opioids, anticonvulsants, sympathectomy, immobilization, biofeedback, behavioral treatment, and a coping approach. NSAIDs are not helpful.

Treatment of the nonautonomic subset has been less studied, but aggressive exercise therapy has been very successful in one large series (14).

TABLE 39D-4
Aggressive Exercise Therapy for Childhood Amplified Pain – Typical Day

Morning

1 hour occupational therapy:

Functional activities to simulate normal chores such as sweeping, carrying, and upper extremity strengthening (especially in those with upper extremity pain). Timed activities include weight bearing on the painful body part. Desensitize regions of allodynia with contrast baths, towel rubs, and massage (children learn to do the desensitization on themselves). Intermittent upper extremity stretching before and after exercise.

1 hour physical therapy:

Endurance and strengthening exercises including bicycling, walking and jogging, mini-trampoline jumping, and jumping rope. Sport-specific activities are simulated such as soccer drills. Intermittent lower extremity stretching before and after exercise.

1 hour pool therapy:

Water aerobics and weight-bearing activities.

Afternoon

1 hour occupational therapy:

As in the morning, reevaluate the child's function and timed activities and quality of movement. Goals advanced as appropriate.

1 hour physical therapy:

As in the morning, reevaluate the child's function and timed activities and quality of movement. Goals advanced as appropriate.

1 hour family swim (not therapy supervised) for play and relaxation in the therapy pool.

Evening

An evening home exercise program consisting of 30–40 minutes of activities to be done independently with compliance being checked by the therapist. If the child has an increase in pain during the night, he or she is to repeat this program. Recreational activities are encouraged.

Schoolwork is usually suspended and make-up work is done once the child returns to school.

Again, there is no consensus about treating children in the fibromyalgic subset, but most authors suggest treating with a tricyclic antidepressant, more to improve the sleeping pattern than for depression, and some form of exercise therapy, either daily aerobic or more intense exercise therapy (9,19,20). Some advocate low-dose NSAIDs (19). Patients with the best long-term outcome are those who have continued an exercise program. There is a host of other therapies, but these involve such small numbers that they cannot be recommended at present. The outcome of children with fibromyalgia is reported as better than is the outcome of adults with fibromyalgia, but this is controversial (21–24).

Children with hypervigilance alone are usually anxious. Reassurance that there is not an ominous underlying disease is all that is needed. A few will benefit from a home exercise program that gives them something to do to treat the pain without medication.

Aggressive exercise therapy, when used for any of the pain amplification syndromes, is one-on-one, functionally focused, intense aerobic exercise (generally five to six hours a day, daily; see Table 39D-4). All aids are discontinued as soon as possible. The therapist modifies the exercises continually to gain maximum function, because restoration of function is the primary goal of therapy. Allodynia is directly treated with desensitization such as towel rubs and massage.

The average duration of therapy is two to three weeks, during which time the child must work through the initial muscle aches and build cardiovascular endurance. Most children are treated as outpatients; however, inpatient therapy is indicated if outpatient therapy fails, if the child has uncontrollable pain at night after exercising, or if the amount of dysfunction interferes with the child's ability to carry out routine activities of daily living. The pain may change location as the exercise therapy progresses. After the intensive program has ended, the child does a daily home exercise program. This takes 40–60 minutes to complete and, over a month or two, the home program is replaced by normal activities. Some children can be treated exclusively with a home program.

The goal of the exercise therapy is restoration of full function, which usually is obtained in the first week or two. Pain diminishes in most children over the following few weeks. In our clinic, 80% are free of pain within one to two months, and an additional 15% are fully functional but report mild to moderate pain. Older children with less pain at onset may fare more poorly. There is little difference in the treatment and outcome in those with and without overt autonomic dysfunction.

The long-term outcome of each subset is not fully defined and there are no natural history studies. However, after five years, approximately 90% of children, with or without autonomic dysfunction, treated with an intense exercise program are without symptoms or limitations. Approximately 30% of children thus treated will have a relapse, but half of these will be able to resolve their symptoms with reinstitution of their home exercise program and will not require formal exercise therapy. Children with the fibromyalgic subset may do somewhat more poorly, with 50% reporting some pain after five years, but 90% are not disabled.

Psychotherapy is indicated in about 80% of the children we see. Recommendations may be for individual therapy, family therapy, and/or marital therapy, depending on the evaluation. Some children require specific educational help or counseling for appropriate academic expectations.

Although pain amplification syndromes are challenging, most children do well and the outcome is extremely gratifying.

Musculoskeletal Pain as a Manifestation of Other Diseases

Many childhood malignancies that affect the bones or bone marrow may present with musculoskeletal pain (25). A child with excessive bone pain should always be evaluated for leukemia, even if definite synovitis is present. Leukemia, lymphoma, rhabdomyosarcoma, and neuroblastoma all may initially present with musculoskeletal pain or synovitis. With the exception of systemic lupus erythematosus, arthritis in childhood is commonly associated with an elevation of the platelet count. Musculoskeletal pain, a decreased platelet count, and arthritis suggest bone marrow infiltration and can be seen with both malignancies and storage diseases such as histiocytosis X.

Endocrine disorders including hypo- or hyperthyroidism, diabetes mellitus, hypo- and hyperparathyroidism, and pituitary tumors producing excessive amounts of growth hormone all may be complicated by musculoskeletal complaints. Musculoskeletal problems are also a major component of many genetic disorders of collagen metabolism including Marfan's syndrome, Ehlers–Danlos syndrome, and the epiphyseal dysplasias.

It is also important to note that gout does not occur in children except as a complication of malignancy, other causes of accelerated cell lysis, or renal compromise. Even under these circumstances, gouty arthritis in childhood is extremely rare (26).

DAVID D. SHERRY, MD

References

1. Merskey DM, Bogduk N (eds). Classification of Chronic Pain. Descriptions of Chronic Pain Syndromes and Definitions of Pain Terms. 2nd ed. Seattle: IASP Press, 1994.

2. Beighton P, Solomon L, Soskolne C. Articular mobility in an African population. Ann Rheum Dis 1973;32:413–418.

3. Carter C, Wilkinson J. Persistent joint laxity and congenital dislocation of the hip. J Bone Joint Surg 1964;46B:40–45.

4. Everman DB, Robin NH. Hypermobility syndrome. Pediatr Rev 1998;19:111–117.

5. Mosca VS. Flexible flatfoot and skewfoot. Instr Course Lect 1996;45:347–354.

6. Loudon JK, Goist HL, Loudon KL. Genu recurvatum syndrome. J Orthop Sports Phys Ther 1998;27:361–367.

7. Thabit Gd, Micheli LJ. Patellofemoral pain in the pediatric patient. Orthop Clin North Am 1992;23:567–585.

8. Baxter MP, Dulberg C. "Growing pains" in childhood — a proposal for treatment. J Pediatr Orthop 1988;8:402–406.

9. Sherry DD. Pain syndromes. In: Isenberg DA, Miller JJI (eds). Adolescent Rheumatology. London: Marin Duntz LTD, 1998; pp 197–227.

10. Buskila D, Press J, Gedalia A, et al. Assessment of nonarticular tenderness and prevalence of fibromyalgia in children. J Rheumatol 1993;20:368–370.

11. Okifuji A, Turk DC, Sinclair JD, Starz TW, Marcus DA. A standardized manual tender point survey. I. Development and determination of a threshold point for the identification of positive tender points in fibromyalgia syndrome. J Rheumatol 1997;24:377–383.

12. Croft P, Burt J, Schollum J, Thomas E, Macfarlane G, Silman A. More pain, more tender points: is fibromyalgia just one end of a continuous spectrum? Ann Rheum Dis 1996;55:482–485.

13. Laxer RM, Allen RC, Malleson PN, Morrison RT, Petty RE. Technetium 99m-methylene diphosphonate bone scans in children with reflex neurovascular dystrophy. J Pediatr 1985;106:437–440.

14. Sherry DD, McGuire T, Mellins E, Salmonson K, Wallace CA, Nepom B. Psychosomatic musculoskeletal pain in childhood: clinical and psychological analyses of 100 children. Pediatrics 1991;88:1093–1099.

15. Sherry DD, Weisman R. Psychologic aspects of childhood reflex neurovascular dystrophy. Pediatrics 1988;81:572–578.

16. Bernstein BH, Singsen BH, Kent JT, et al. Reflex neurovascular dystrophy in childhood. J Pediatr 1978;93:211–215.

17. Wilder RT, Berde CB, Wolohan M, Vieyra MA, Masek BJ, Micheli LJ. Reflex sympathetic dystrophy in children. Clinical characteristics and follow-up of seventy patients. J Bone Joint Surg N Am 1992;74:910–919.

18. Sherry DD, Wallace CA, Kelley C, Kidder M, Sapp L. Short- and long-term outcomes of children with complex regional pain syndrome type I treated with exercise therapy. Clin J Pain 1999;15:218–223.

19. Russell IJ. Fibromyalgia syndrome: approaches to management. Bull Rheum Dis 1996;45:1–4.

20. Wigers SH, Stiles TC, Vogel PA. Effects of aerobic exercise versus stress management treatment in fibromyalgia. A 4.5 year prospective study. Scand J Rheumatol 1996;25:77–86.

21. Buskila D, Neumann L, Hershman E, Gedalia A, Press J, Sukenik S. Fibromyalgia syndrome in children — an outcome study. J Rheumatol 1995;22:525–528.

22. Rabinovich CE, Schanberg LE, Stein LD, Kredich DW. A follow up study of pediatric fibromyalgia patients (abstract). Arthritis Rheum 1990;33(suppl):S146.

23. Mikkelsson M. One year outcome of preadolescents with fibromyalgia. J Rheumatol 1999;26:674–682.

24. Siegel DM, Janeway D, Baum J. Fibromyalgia syndrome in children and adolescents: clinical features at presentation and status at follow-up. Pediatrics 1998;101:377–382.

25. Cabral DA, Tucker LB. Malignancies in children who initially present with rheumatic complaints. J Pediatr 1999;134:53–57.

26. Cassidy J, Petty R. Musculoskeletal manifestation of systemic disease. In: Textbook of Pediatric Rheumatology, 3rd edition. Philadelphia: WB Saunders, 1995.

40 REHABILITATION

The primary factors addressed in rehabilitating people with rheumatic diseases are activity and mobility limitation. Rehabilitation uses all healing disciplines and technologies, with an emphasis on preservation and restoration of function. The rheumatologist is the leader and coordinator of an interdisciplinary team that uses medical, surgical, psychological, and physical treatments. Such a program can provide functional success even when the disease process is not controlled.

WHO Classification of Impairment, Activities, and Participation

To provide standards for classification of disabilities, the World Health Organization (WHO) published The International Classification of Impairments, Disabilities, and Handicaps (ICIDH) in 1980 (1). This report was an attempt to understand and categorize the experiences of people living with chronic illnesses. The basis of the classification is that a health condition (i.e., disease or disorder) may result in an impairment, disability, or handicap, and these three states interrelate. In this context, impairment is the loss or abnormality of a physiological or psychological function. Disability, the result of impairment, limits performance of an activity in a manner considered normal for a person. Handicap, the consequence or disadvantage resulting from an impairment or disability, affects an individuals' ability to participate or perform a societal role considered normal for that individual (1). This classification scheme has been criticized because of its dependence on the medical model of disease and its inattention to societal impact upon disability, particularly handicap. Much of current health care delivery and education continues to consider disability a disease-related deficit that prevents an individual's normal function, without considering the role of society and the interaction of the disabled individual in that society over a life span.

In 1998, the WHO presented ICIDH-2 (The International Classification of Impairments, Activities and Participation) (2). The intent was to use neutral terminology, include environmental factors, and provide a societal model orientation. *Impairment* remains, but *disability* has been replaced by *activity*, and *handicap* is replaced by *participation*. By the revised statement, a disease may result in *impairment* that affects activity and participation, and these three factors may interrelate. *Activity* is defined as a person's functional level and may be limited in nature, duration, and quality. *Participation* is involvement in life situations in relation to impairments, activities, health conditions, and contextual factors, and it may be restricted in nature, duration, and quality (2). In this new classification, activity limitation equates with disability, and participation restriction equates with handicap. Impairment occurs at the body level, activity at the whole person level, and participation at the societal level. Examples of rheumatic disease disablements are illustrated in Table 40-1. In the ICIDH-2 model, medical treatment is directed toward impairment, and rehabilitation therapies are directed toward activity limitation. Public education, legislation, and universal architectural design would improve limited participation by the disabled community.

Rehabilitation Team and Setting

A holistic health approach that fosters optimal function should focus on the remission or absence of the underlying rheumatic disease, yet promote consideration of the individual as a whole, functioning person. Patient involvement with the physical, psychological, social, and societal aspects of health and well-being is central to this approach.

Access to multidisciplinary expertise can help achieve optimal outcomes. In the hospital, the multidisciplinary team may consist of a rheumatologist as team leader, occupational and physical therapists, psychologists and social workers, rehabilitation nurses, and orthopedic surgeons. Integral to this rehabilitation team is the patient, who must accept responsibility for selecting and implementing realistic goals. In early disease and in the outpatient setting, it may be unnecessary to include all disciplines in the rehabilitation process. However, the expertise of a team is required for complicated, advanced disease, when the patient may face disease elements, mobility problems, impaired activities of daily living, depression, job loss, and insurance loss. The team leader selects the appropriate consultations as problems arise, assures communication between team members, and guides the patient toward realistic goals.

Rehabilitation should start with the first doctor visit and extend throughout the course of the disease. During early disease, the physician can address most functional problems with attention to the medical regimen. Rehabilitation can occur in a physician's office and by referral to the appropriate practitioner. For example, mobility problems are referred to physical therapists; activities of daily living problems, to occupational therapists; and psychological problems, to psychologists. For more advanced disease, short-term inpatient rehabilitation can provide more intense, daily treatment. Daily observation of the patient will permit adjustment of medical and therapy programs.

TABLE 40-1
Rheumatic Disease Disablement Examples

Disease	Impairment	Activity limitation	Participation restriction
Rheumatoid arthritis	Knee pain and contracture	Unable to walk long distances	Unable to participate in recreation (golf, walking, etc.)
DLE	Hair loss and skin depigmentation	None	Social activity restrictions (self-conscious, shy)
Scleroderma	Raynaud's phenomenon	None	Unable to participate in winter sports
Polymyositis	Proximal muscle weakness	Limited on stairs	Unable to enter houses, public buildings, climb curbs
SLE	Photosensitivity	None	Unable to participate in outdoor activities
Ankylosing spondylitis	Back pain and stiffness	Limited ability to lift and bend	Unable to do medium and heavy jobs or engage in recreation

DLE, discoid lupus erythematosis; SLE, systemic lupus erythematosus

In the United States, diagnostic related groups (DRGs) govern the current medical care system and reimbursement for inpatient stays. This system was designed to reduce the total cost of health care in the United States and has been successful in doing so. For acute illnesses, both inpatient stays and health care costs have been reduced. Inpatient rehabilitation is not defined by the DRG system, but it reflects the trend of reduced inpatient days. Currently, inpatient care is reserved for patients who have the most advanced rheumatic disease with the most functional impairment.

Medicare rules dictate the requirements for inpatient hospitalization, and Medicare requires that patients with rheumatic disease have reductions in activities of daily living and mobility that have not responded to outpatient treatment. The illness must be sufficiently severe to require daily monitoring by a physician and other health professionals. Three hours of multidisciplinary inpatient treatment must be provided daily from two major rehabilitative disciplines, such as physical therapy, occupational therapy, or speech therapy. Social services and psychological rehabilitation can be provided during the hospitalization and may contribute to required daily treatment, but not as major treatment modalities.

A transitional inpatient care unit or skilled nursing facility can be used for people who have significant functional problems and require at least one modality for one hour per day, but who do not need three hours of daily treatment. This option should be considered for patients who have less disability but require skilled nursing and functional training (e.g., postoperative total joint arthroplasty strengthening and gait training). The goal for inpatient and outpatient programs is maintenance of the rehabilitative program by patients in the home environment.

Clinical trials have shown beneficial response to multidisciplinary team care when compared with regular outpatient care. For people with active rheumatoid arthritis (RA), improvement from inpatient rehabilitation was maintained for up to two years (3). The greatest changes were observed two weeks after discharge, when there was statistical improvement in the Ritchie articular index, number of swollen joints, disease activity by visual analogue scale (VAS), pain by VAS, and physician global assessment. At four weeks, 18% of people who had received inpatient rehabilitation achieved American College of Rheumatology (ACR)-20 status (see Appendix I) or better; none who had received outpatient treatment showed such improvement. One year after treatment, disease activity by VAS still was significantly lower for the inpatient group, and the percentage of patients achieving an ACR-20 was 46% in the inpatient group and 23% in the outpatient group.

Multidisciplinary rehabilitation treatment also is efficacious in ankylosing spondylitis (4). Considering the similar inflammatory, multiarticular nature of many other rheumatic diseases, rehabilitative medical therapies probably would be beneficial and should be made available to all patients.

Patient Assessment

In addition to the usual history and physical examination, an assessment of the patient's function is needed. This information is best obtained by indirect questions, such as, "How does your arthritis effect your life?" or "Describe to me what you do on a usual day." Such questions give patients an opportunity to relate the functional impact of their disease to activities that are important to them. The patient and health care team can use this information to establish goals. All team members should obtain discipline-specific information. Patients should be asked about activities of daily living, including personal grooming, toileting, eating, transfers, and ambulation; vocational activities, such as jobs and homemaking; and avocational activities, such as hobbies. Patient abilities regarding activities of daily living usually are described as independent, supervised, assisted, or unable. Dressing is subdivided further into ability to dress upper body and lower body.

The occupational therapist records specific hand and upper-extremity function, including power grip, power and precision pinch, pill handling, and cylindrical grasp. The physical therapist records activities stressing trunk and lower-extremity functions and mobility, such as the ability to lie prone or on one's side, roll from side to side, go from a supine position to sitting, move from sitting to standing, ambulate, and climb stairs. Ambulation can be divided into household and community, and with and without aids or wheelchair assistance.

Because rheumatic diseases cause problems related primarily to mobility, muscular strength, and joint range of motion, the physical examination is functionally oriented. Manual muscle testing is a common way of measuring strength (Table 40-2). This ability is graded from zero to five, encompassing a range from no motor activity to normal strength. Assessment of normal strength varies, depending on gender, size, and training status. Because individuals with normal strength can lose considerable motor function before it is detectable by an examiner, range of motion is measured by a goniometer. Particular attention should be given to alignment, noting flexion contractures, joint instabilities, and deformities.

There are multiple ways to record longitudinal function. The method most commonly used in the rheumatologic community is the ACR Functional Classification, groups I–IV (see Appendix I). This classification groups individuals into broad categories that indicate functional ranges from

TABLE 40-2
Grades of Muscle Strength in Manual Muscle Testing

Grade	Description
5 (Normal)	Full ROM against gravity, strong resistance
4 (Good)	Full ROM against gravity, some- but not full-resistance
3 (Fair)	Full ROM against gravity, no resistance
2 (Poor)	Full ROM, gravity eliminated
1 (Trace)	Slight contracture, no ROM
0 (Zero)	No muscle activity demonstrable

ROM, range of motion

normal to incapacitated (i.e., where assistance is needed in ambulation and activities of daily living). The ACR classification, a widely applicable, time-tested tool, is insensitive to small changes in function. Other useful functional assessment tools are the Arthritis Impact Measurement Scale (AIMS), the Stanford Health Assessment Questionnaire (HAQ), and the Functional Impact Measure (see Chapter 7B). Each of these scales relies on self-administered reports or professional observation of functional activities.

Pain Control

Pain is a common chief complaint and a cause of inactivity and functional losses for people with rheumatic disease. Cooperation and success with rehabilitation cannot be achieved if patients are in pain. Disease control through standard medical regimens sometimes is the most efficient way of controlling pain and improving activities. Supplemental use of intra-articular corticosteroids in resistant joints can control inflammation and pain, prevent flexion contractures, and improve range of motion and function. The use of topically applied medications (e.g., capsaicin and salicylic acid creams) may be helpful, particularly as an adjunct to physical therapy and occupational therapy. Oral analgesics, including low-dose nonsteroidal anti-inflammatory drugs and narcotics, are useful adjuncts to physical therapy when given 20–30 minutes before beginning a session. They can be used on an intermittent basis to permit normal exercise or work periods.

Physical Modalities
Heat and Cold

Of the physical modalities commonly prescribed for musculoskeletal illnesses, heat and cold have the largest body of literature to support their use. Heat and cold have been used for centuries in musculoskeletal impairments, especially in acute injuries. There is no evidence that any harm is done when these modalities are applied properly, and there is substantial anecdotal evidence of beneficial effects, including reduced pain and muscle spasms, increased circulation, and improved range of motion (5). Temperature changes occur in the skin, deeper tissues, and on occasion, joint cavities. In addition to beneficial effects reported in clinical conditions, there is experimental evidence for diminished pain response to both heat and cold in animal models of joint inflammation. Heat or cold treatment did not change joint inflammation, but secondary pain response and behavior were improved (6).

A systematic review of the medical literature for clinical benefit from heat and cold treatment showed few controlled studies of acceptable quality, particularly with regard to randomization and masking. However, of those studies that did meet such criteria, heat and cold had no effect on the objective measures of disease activity, including inflammation (7). All patients reported that they preferred heat or cold therapy to no treatment, but there was no preference for either modality. Because there are no harmful effects from heat or cold, it should be prescribed as a home treatment as needed for pain relief.

Heat therapy usually is administered as a superficial application of hot packs, electric heating pads, water baths, paraffin wax, or thermal packs. The use of water or whirlpool baths can be combined with active or passive motion to improve joint range of motion. Thermal packs contain chemical agents that produce heat by exothermic reactions when activated. They have no advantages over electrical heating pads or moist heat, and have the disadvantages of one time usage and increased cost. Heat therapy is contraindicated when there is loss of normal sensation and diminished or faulty blood supply.

With thermal therapy, deeper heating of tissues can be achieved by the use of therapeutic ultrasound. There are no controlled trials to indicate its utility in rheumatic disease, but the disadvantage of ultrasound therapy is that it must be performed in a specialist's office, with the associated inconvenience and cost.

Cold reduces pain and muscle spasm and leads to vasospasm with a consequent decrease in tissue metabolism, inflammation, and edema. Because of these effects, it is standard treatment for immediate care after musculoskeletal injury. Applied locally for up to 30 minutes, cold produces a cooling of the skin and subcutaneous tissues. Deep cooling does occur and is dependent on application time and soft-tissue depth.

Cold typically is prescribed as ice packs, reusable gel packs, chemical packs, or ice massage directly over the painful area. Chemical packs, which produce cold by endothermic reactions, have little utility except on an infrequent basis because of their expense and one-time use. Cooling sprays, such as ethyl chloride, are used commonly in rheumatology in a "spray and stretch" technique, especially for painful syndromes of the neck and back. The skin is cooled superficially by the spray, resulting in pain relief and relief of muscle spasm. Active or passive stretching then can be achieved.

Electrical Stimulation

Transcutaneous electrical nerve stimulation (TENS) may be used for outpatient treatment of pain. A low-voltage electrical stimulus is delivered to the skin either intermittently or continuously by activation of a battery-operated device worn at the waist. The patient can activate and control intensity as needed. TENS is administered for noninflammatory conditions, particularly chronic back pain from osteoarthritis (OA), knee pain, chronic shoulder pain, or pain in other major joints of the body. TENS usually is prescribed for patients who are resistant to heat, cold, stretching, exercise, and other modalities. Although commonly used, there are no controlled studies validating its efficacy.

Hydrotherapy

Hydrotherapy combines exercise therapy and warm-water immersion. It may be prescribed intermittently on an outpa-

tient basis or as part of a sustained regimen in the form of spa therapy. There are few controlled trials of this treatment. However, there is some indication that people who received hydrotherapy on a regular, outpatient basis had greater benefit than did those who were treated by seated immersion in water, land exercises, or relaxation therapy (8). This improvement was physical and emotional, as reflected by the AIMS-2 questionnaire. A more extensive systematic review of the published literature for spa therapy showed many flaws in the designs of the treatments, with little use of important outcome measures, such as quality-of-life instruments. The conclusion was that spa therapy could not be supported as an efficacious treatment (9).

Rest

Local or systemic rest reduces acute inflammation and pain, and promotes normal joint position. Local rest is achieved by use of splints or braces; systemic rest, by bed rest. Short periods of rest as part of a comprehensive program enables patients to participate in exercise programs and work activities. However, prolonged rest, whether local or systemic, should be avoided because it is associated with significant muscle loss. Just a few weeks of local immobilization can reduce muscle mass by 21% (10), and evidence suggests that prolonged bed rest as a primary treatment is not helpful and should not be prescribed routinely. Some medical conditions, including acute back pain, may worsen with bed rest (11).

Exercise Therapy

Exercise therapy must take into consideration the underlying disease activity, including degree of inflammation, joint stability, muscle atrophy, and anticipated short- and long-term functional goals. Prescribed exercise may be active or passive, assisted, resistive, or aerobic.

Passive exercises, including stretching and gentle range-of-motion exercises, are administered by a physical therapist with the goal of maintaining joint flexibility and reducing contractures. Passive exercises are used for conditions associated with severe pain and weakness, such as acute joint inflammation, inflammatory myositis, and postoperative periods. Isometric exercise, in which there is active muscle contracture without muscle shortening or joint motion, helps maintain muscle strength and is prescribed as initial therapy for people unable to tolerate range-of-motion exercises due to pain, such as people who recently have undergone joint arthroplasty.

Most people with a rheumatic disease benefit from resistive and aerobic exercise programs. Resistive exercises should be tailored to the individual, the area of weakness, and the underlying disorder, with a goal of increasing strength and endurance.

Walking and resistive exercises, administered for one hour three times per week, are associated with less pain, less disability, and greater flexion strength in people with OA of the knee (12). Similar effects are seen with hip OA. Results include mild to moderate improvements in pain, disability outcome measures, and greater benefit on patients' global assessments (13).

Exercise therapy for people with RA improves aerobic capacity and motor strength, without worsening pain or disease activity (14).

In ankylosing spondylitis, pain and stiffness are improved with recreational exercise of at least 30 minutes daily (15). Back exercises, prescribed five days a week, improved health status as measured by the HAQ Disability Index. The greatest benefit was seen in people with early disease.

In patients with systemic lupus erythematosus, aerobic and strengthening exercises did not worsen disease activity and were associated with decreased fatigue and improvement in functional status, strength, and cardiovascular fitness (16).

Ambulatory Aids

Canes, crutches, and walkers are prescribed to improve gait and ease weakness, pain, and instability in lower-extremity joints. The most useful canes are those made of wood or aluminum. They should be inexpensive, lightweight, easily adjusted for height, and have a comfortable grip and wide rubber tip. Cane length should be fitted so that the elbow is flexed to 30°. By the use of a single cane or crutch, at least 25% of normal weight-bearing can be shifted from a weak or painful joint to the opposite limb. With bilateral support, up to 100% of weight-bearing can be unloaded from a painful lower extremity to the upper extremities. Some patients who choose to carry a cane do not use it for support, but only as a signal that they have ambulatory problems.

Patients need instruction on the proper use of an ambulatory aid. Single support is carried contralateral to the painful leg. It is advanced and used to bear weight during stance on the opposite (painful) leg. Multiple tips (e.g., the quad cane) provide increased security for those with impaired proprioception or balance problems. For people who can not bear weight on the wrist or who have significant hand deformities, ambulatory aids can be modified to accommodate these problems with forearm troughs, hand grips, and Velcro straps. To avoid wrist and hand stress, these devices are fitted with the elbow at 90° flexion.

Crutches are prescribed for more severe problems, and provide increased support when used bilaterally. They are most useful in the postoperative period and for acute injuries and illnesses, as they allow people to put little or no weight on a painful or weak leg. They should be adjusted so that no pressure occurs on the axilla. Patients need to be instructed about proper weight-bearing on the upper extremities, with the wrist and elbow in extension. Platform crutches should be prescribed for people with significant hand and wrist arthritis who have discomfort using conventional crutches.

For those in need of greater ambulatory stability, walkers provide a wider support base than do canes or crutches. Walkers also are useful in the postoperative period, for the elderly, frail, and those who need maximum support for balance. They must be lightweight so that they can be picked up and advanced. Wheels, brakes, and seats can be attached for comfort and safety.

Wheelchairs can promote increased independence and interaction when ambulation is restricted to the household level. A manual wheelchair is advised for people with normal upper-extremity function and sufficient strength and endurance to propel the chair. Manual wheelchairs to be propelled by family can be prescribed for the postoperative period and for the frail and elderly who do not wish to travel alone. Electric wheelchairs and carts should be prescribed for those with poor upper-extremity function.

Upper-Extremity Aids

A large variety of commercially available assistive devices can improve activities of daily living for people with impaired upper-extremity function. Pinch and grasp can be improved by building up handles on tools, cookware, and eating utensils. Power equipment, such as electric knives and tools, can substitute for decreased power grip and poor upper-extremity strength. Reachers can be used to retrieve objects from floors and shelves. Long handled brushes, combs, and sponges can help with upper-extremity grooming and perineal care.

Buttonhooks, zippers with tabs, clothing and shoes with Velcro closures, elastic-waist trousers, and V-neck pullovers can facilitate dressing. Sock cones and long-handled shoehorns ease the donning and doffing of socks and shoes, and dressing sticks assist those with impaired shoulder mobility.

Home safety and accessibility can be evaluated during home visits by physical and occupational therapists. People with impaired mobility can be aided by the installation of half steps, ramps, and handrails in entryways. Doorways should be wide enough to permit easy access for walkers and wheelchairs. Furniture placement and room size should be sufficient for easy mobility with walking aids and wheelchairs. Throw rugs and loose electrical cords should be removed. For those with knee and hip problems, chair height can be increased by adding blocks under the chair legs or supplementing chair seats with four-inch thick, high-density foam cushions. Elevated seats facilitate transfer on and off the toilet. In the bathroom, rubber mats should be placed on tub and shower floors to improve traction and prevent falls. Grab-bars and tub and shower benches should be used for those with balance problems. Handheld shower nozzles facilitate bathing.

Orthotic Devices

Splints and braces can improve stability and reduce pain and inflammation. However, because effective orthoses restrict motion, only short-term use is recommended to preserve muscle strength. Splints for the upper extremity are used commonly and have general patient and physician acceptance (Table 40-3). Although splints reduce pain and inflammation, no studies indicate that they prevent deformities. Wrist orthoses may decrease hand function (as measured by grip strength), finger dexterity, and hand dexterity, at least in the short term (17). People with severe deformities may need to consult an orthotist or occupational therapist for a custom-made device.

Orthoses that immobilize the wrist in a neutral position, with 20°–30° extension of the hand at the wrist, are used in carpal tunnel syndrome. For flexible swan-neck deformities of the digits, ring splints can improve pinch strength and precision by putting the proximal interphalangeal joint in a slightly flexed and more functional position. Ring splints are not effective for fixed deformities, and there are no studies to support their prolonged use to prevent the development of such deformities. Ring splints may be made of silver to enhance cosmesis and promote compliance.

The carpometacarpal (CMC) immobilization splint (thumb post splint) reduces pain when patients with degenerative CMC joint disease have flares at the base of the thumb. However, these patients should avoid activities that increase forces across the CMC joints, such as power pinch. Strategies to reduce such forces include increasing the size of pens and pencils by using a rubber or foam grip and using a light touch with writing instruments.

Plaster or lightweight fiberglass casts can be used for trial immobilization. If cast immobilization results in pain relief, a more expensive, rigid orthosis or surgical arthrodesis also will decrease pain and improve function, and these options should be considered.

Lower-Extremity Orthoses

The simplest orthoses for restricting range of motion and decreasing pain in lower extremities are elastic bandages, elastic or neoprene sleeves, and taping. Many patients with osteoarthritis (OA) of the knee relieve pain and improve function by using sleeves to reduce range of motion. For people with patellofemoral joint arthritis and abnormal tracking, taping the knee to promote normal patellar tracking reduced knee pain by 25%, compared with a control group (18). For people who have marked weakness and deformities, consultation with an orthotist or an orthopedic surgeon skilled in biomechanics can provide more extensive bracing. Disadvantages to more extensive bracing include high cost and a low rate of compliance.

Footwear

Foot pain and deformities are common in RA and OA. Many of these problems can be addressed adequately by careful attention to footwear (Table 40-4). The upper portion of the shoe should be soft, and the toe box deep and wide enough to accommodate deformities. These measures will prevent rubbing, blisters, and skin breakdown.

Many people with RA have pain on the soles of their feet, particularly at the metatarsal areas. Cock-up deformities of the toes and prominent metatarsal heads, with anterior displacement of the fat pad, are common. These deformities can cause painful metatarsalgia, with calluses and skin breakdown. These problems can be avoided by using inserts, metatarsal pads placed proximal to the metatarsal heads on the insole of the shoe, or external metatarsal bars placed proximal to the metatarsal heads. Commercially available inserts of high-density polypropylene may be satisfactory treatment for metatarsalgia and painful bony prominences. For persistent symptoms, patients may be referred to an orthotist for a custom-made polypropylene insert or a molded insert. The use of sandals and footwear custom-made from molded impressions may provide pain-free ambulation.

Vocational Rehabilitation and Disability

Musculoskeletal diseases are the leading cause of disability and absence from work in the United States (19). Rheumatoid

TABLE 40-3
Shoe Specifics

Disease	Deformity	Problem	Solutions
RA/OA	Hallux valgus with bunion formation	Pain, inflammation	Wide, soft, deep toebox; stretch medial leather
RA	Cock-up toes	Pain, redness, ulcers on dorsum of toes	Deep toebox, soft leather upper; stretch upper; donut pads; sandals
RA	Valgus hindfoot	Hindfoot pain	Medial wedge; lace-up canvas ankle support; ankle-hindfoot orthosis
RA	MTP subluxation with callosities	Metatarsalgia	Metatarsal bar; metatarsal pad; sole inserts
OA	Hallux rigidus	MTP pain	Metatarsal bar; rigid sole; rocker-bottom sole

RA, rheumatoid arthritis; OA, osteoarthritis; MTP, metatarsophalangeal

TABLE 4
Common Upper-Extremity Orthotics

Disorder	Deformity	Problem	Solution
RA	Flexible swan-neck digits	None; clicking; cosmetic appearance	Ring splints (stabilizes PIP in flexion)
Carpal tunnel syndrome	None	Night pain, dysesthesias	Wrist splint, 20°–30° extension
OA of first CMC	None	CMC pain with pinch	Thumb post splint, thumb spica
RA	None	Pain and inflammation of wrist, MCPs and PIPs	Hand-resting splint (resting posture from wrist to DIPs)
Mallet finger	Flexion of DIP	None	Rigid DIP splint, 20° hyperextension

RA, rheumatoid arthritis; OA, osteoarthritis; PIP, proximal interphalangeal; DIP, distal interphalangeal; CMC, carpal metacarpal

arthritis is associated with a high rate of disability; more than one-third of working persons who develop RA are unable to work after five years (20). Three years after diagnosis with systemic lupus erythematosus, 40% of patients no longer are working (21). One of the goals of rehabilitation is to maintain employment, and achieving this goal may require job modification, retraining, and vocational rehabilitation. Among people with arthritis and musculoskeletal disorders, 71% of those accepted for vocational rehabilitation return to work (22).

Disability insurance payments are the main impediment to successful vocational rehabilitation. Among people with RA, high pain level, older age, and lower educational status are barriers to re-employment. For people with systemic lupus erythematosus, low education level, receipt of Medicaid, absence of medical insurance, engagement in physically demanding jobs, poverty level, and greater disease activity are predictors of early work disability. Race, gender, cumulative organ damage, and disease duration do not predict work disability (21).

The Social Security Administration administers the uniform disability program throughout the United States. There are two programs for which patients are eligible: Social Security Disability Insurance (SSDI) and Social Security Insurance (SSI). For SSDI, patients must meet the requirements of being disabled and having paid into the Social Security system for the required amount of time, usually 40 quarters. For SSI eligibility, patients must be disabled and have reduced income, but there is no work requirement. Under the Social Security system, disability is defined by law, and essentially means an inability to do any type of work, regardless of previous job or experience. The definition of disability is, "inability to engage in any substantial gainful activity by reason of a medically determinable physical or mental impairment(s) which can be expected to result in death or which has lasted or can be expected to last for a continuous period of not less than 12 months" (23).

Once the decision to apply for disability is made, longitudinal evidence-based information that demonstrates the impact of the illness on function and ability to work must be provided to the Social Security office. To apply for disability under the Social Security system, patients complete applications at their local district offices. The application is reviewed to see whether the patient is eligible for disability. If patients do not meet eligibility requirements, additional medical information is requested from the patient and the physician. A consultative examination by a medical or psychological expert may be requested and paid for by the Social Security Administration. If disability is not allowed, appeal by the patient is permitted, and a court hearing is held before an administrative law judge. At that meeting, patients are queried about how their rheumatic diseases affect their lives and ability to work. Patients can present additional medical information, call witnesses, and retain a lawyer as their advocate to interpret the legal aspects of disability. When disability is granted, the amount of payment made is determined by law. In addition to monthly payments, people receiving SSI are eligible for Medicaid immediately. Those receiving SSDI are eligible for Medicare after two years.

THOMAS BEARDMORE, MD

References

1. World Health Organization. *International Classification of Impairments, Disabilities and Handicaps (ICIDH). Geneva: World Health Organization, 1980.*

2. World Health Organization. *International Classification of Impairments, Activities and Participation (ICIDH-2). Geneva: World Health Organization, 1998.*

3. Vliet Vlieland TP, Breedveld FC, Hazes JM. *The two year follow-up of a randomized comparison of in-patient multidisciplinary team care and routine out-patient care for active rheumatoid arthritis. Br J Rheumatol 1997;36:82–85.*

4. Band DA, Jones SD, Kennedy LG, et al. Which patients with ankylosing spondylitis benefit from an inpatient management program? J Rheumatol 1997;24:2381–2384.

5. Oosterveld FG, Rasker JJ. Treating arthritis with locally applied heat or cold. Semin Arthritis Rheum 1994;24:82–90.

6. Sluka KA, Christy MR, Peterson WL, Rudd SL, Troy SM. Reduction of pain-related behaviors with either cold or heat treatment in an animal model of acute arthritis. Arch Phys Med Rehabil 1999;80:313–317.

7. Welch V, Broseau L, Shea B, McGowan J, Wells G, Tugwell P. Thermotherapy for treating rheumatoid arthritis (Cochrane review). Cochrane Database Syst Rev 2000;4:CD002826.

8. Hall J, Skevington SM, Maddison PJ, Chapman K. A randomized trial of hydrotherapy in rheumatoid arthritis. Arthritis Care Res 1996;9:206–215.

9. Verhagen AP, de Vet HC, de Bie RA, Kessels AG, Boers M, Knipschild PG. Taking baths: the efficacy of balneotherapy in patients with arthritis. A systematic review. J Rheumatology 1997;24:1964–1971.

10. Veldhuizen JW, Verstappen FT, Vroemen JP, Kuipers H, Greep JM. Functional and morphological adaptations following four weeks of knee immobilization. Int J Sports Med 1993;14:283–287.

11. Allen C, Glasziou P, Del Mar C. Bed rest: a potentially harmful treatment needing more careful evaluation. Lancet 1999;354:1229–1233.

12. Ettinger WH Jr, Burns R, Messier SP, et al. A randomized trial comparing aerobic exercise and resistance exercise with a health education program in older adults with knee osteoarthritis. The Fitness Arthritis and Seniors Trial. JAMA 1997;277:25–31.

13. Van Baar ME, Assendelft WJ, Dekker J, Oostendorp RA, Bijlsma JW. Effectiveness of exercise therapy in patients with osteoarthritis of the hip or knee: a systematic review of randomized clinical trials. Arthritis Rheum 1999;42:1361–1369.

14. Van den Ende CH, Vliet Vlieland TP, Munneke M, Hayes JM. Dynamic exercise therapy in rheumatoid arthritis: a systematic review. Br J Rheumatol 1998;37:677–687.

15. Uhrin Z, Kuzis S, Ward MM. Exercise and changes in health status in patients with ankylosing spondylitis. Arch Intern Med 2000;160:2969–2975.

16. Ramsey-Goldman R, Schilling EM, Dunlop D, et al. A pilot study on the effects of exercise in patients with systemic lupus erythematosus. Arthritis Care Res 2000;13:262–269.

17. Stern EB, Ytterberg SR, Krug HE, Mullin GT, Mahowald ML. Immediate and short-term effects of three commercial wrist extensor orthoses on grip strength and function in patients with rheumatoid arthritis. Arthritis Care Res 1996;9:42–50.

18. Cushnaghan J, McCarthy C, Dieppe P. Taping the patella medially: a new treatment for osteoarthritis of the knee joint? BMJ 1994;308:753–755.

19. Colvez A, Blanchet M. Disability trends in the United States population 1966-76: analysis of reported causes. Am J Public Health 1981;71:464–471.

20. Yelin E, Meenan R, Nevitt M, Epstein W. Work disability in rheumatoid arthritis: effects of disease, social, and work factors. Ann Intern Med 1980;93:551–556.

21. Partridge AJ, Karlson EW, Daltroy LH, et al. Risk factors for early work disability in systemic lupus erythematosus: results from a multicenter study. Arthritis Rheum 1997;40:2199–2206.

22. Straaton KV, Maisiak R, Wrigley JM, Fine PR. Musculoskeletal disability, employment, and rehabilitation. J Rheumatol 1995;22:505–513.

23. Disability Evaluation Under Social Security. SSA Publication No. 64-039. ICN No. 486600, U.S. Department of Health and Human Services, Social Security Administration, Office of Disability, Washington, DC, 1998.

41 PSYCHOSOCIAL FACTORS

A variety of psychosocial factors may influence the health status and behavior of people with arthritis. Although most studies of the psychosocial dimensions of arthritis have focused on patients with rheumatoid arthritis (RA), psychosocial factors are important in all rheumatic conditions and disorders of the musculoskeletal system. For example, stress and depression are two important psychosocial factors that influence patients' symptom reports and their abilities to cope effectively with their illnesses.

Stress

Stress is defined as any event that an individual perceives as a threat to his or her well-being and which exceeds his or her resources for managing the threat (1). Arthritis and related musculoskeletal disorders (ARMD) are important stressors because they are a source of multiple threats to well-being, such as chronic health problems, restricted activities, long-term disabilities, and direct (e.g., loss of employment) and indirect (e.g., health care costs) economic losses. In addition, ARMD may contribute to the development of other stressors, such as psychological disorders, that pose additional threats to the well-being of vulnerable individuals.

Assessments of individual patients should examine stress associated both with *major life events*, such as the death of a spouse or other family member, and common, *persistent negative events*, such as conflicts with neighbors or one's employer. These two forms of stress may impact patients differently, although there is conflicting evidence about which type of stressor is more influential (2,3). For example, evidence indicates that major life events are associated with short-term decreases in symptoms of RA (4), although they tend to make patients more vulnerable to the deleterious effects of common, persistent negative events (5). These common negative events, or "daily hassles," are associated with altered immune function and symptom severity. It has been shown, for example, that increases in interpersonal stress tend to produce increases in physicians' global ratings of RA disease activity, measures of total T-cell activation, and interleukin 2 receptor expression, as well as a higher ratio of circulating B cells to T cells (6). The severity of daily hassles is associated with measures of physical health in people with systemic lupus erythematosus (SLE) and with psychological distress in people with SLE and fibromyalgia (2). High levels of daily stressors also are associated with increased symptom reports in children with juvenile rheumatic disease (7). These findings are consistent with patient beliefs about an association between stress and symptom flares, and suggest that stress management or other interventions designed to enhance coping may be helpful adjuncts to the medical management of ARMD.

Depression

Depression is common among people with ARMD. The U.S. National Health and Nutrition epidemiologic study showed that 16% of persons with chronic musculoskeletal pain had scores indicative of depression on the Center for Epidemiologic Studies Depression Scale (8). Similarly, a 12-year study of 6153 patients found that the frequency of probable depression was 37% in people with RA, 33% in people with osteoarthritis (OA) of the knee or hip, and 49% in people with fibromyalgia (9).

The relationships between depression and health status variables in people with ARMD are complex. In general, the relationships between depression and pain, disability, and loss of valued activities are independent of disease activity. The US National Health and Nutrition survey suggested that depression amplifies pain and is influenced by pain (10). Among people with RA, the most important predictors of patients' reports of depression are their ratings of pain intensity and scores on the Health Assessment Questionnaire (HAQ) Disability Index (11). Among women with RA, however, loss of valued activities may be a better predictor of depression than is increased disability. Younger patients with RA appear to be at particularly high risk for developing depressive symptoms. The inverse relationship between age and depression in RA may be mediated by the relatively high levels of stress and pain reported by younger patients. Finally, depressive disorders may produce negative consequences for people with RA, even after the depression is successfully treated or resolved. One study indicates that a history of depression in these patients makes them vulnerable to higher levels of pain, fatigue, and disability when they are experiencing dysphoric mood, even if they are not currently depressed (12).

Most studies of the relationship between affect and symptoms in people with ARMD have focused solely on such negative states as depression. Although there is no consensus as to whether negative and positive emotional states are polar opposites or whether they are independent states, it generally is accepted that evaluations of patients with ARMD should take into account both positive and negative affect. For example, HAQ measures of activity limitation in people with RA are associated with frequent use of maladaptive pain-coping strategies and relatively infrequent use of adaptive strategies (13). There are important differences in the determinants of these coping strategies. Maladaptive coping is associated with low positive affect and high negative affect, whereas adaptive coping is associated only with high positive affect. Thus, both positive and negative affect contribute to the relationships between pain-coping strategies and activity limitations. This work suggests that affective states may influence patient beliefs about ARMD and strategies for coping with the stressors produced by illness.

Cognitive Beliefs and Coping Strategies

Cognitive Beliefs

Health-related beliefs and coping strategies used by people with ARMD are reliably associated with their health status. Two important beliefs involve perceptions of learned helplessness and self-efficacy.

Learned helplessness is a stable belief that no viable solutions are available to eliminate or reduce the source of stressful events. Learned helplessness is associated with emotional, motivational, and cognitive deficits in adaptive coping with stress, and may contribute to psychological distress and functional disability in people with ARMD. For example, helplessness beliefs regarding multiple illness-related stressors may cause individuals to experience anxiety and depression. These emotional deficits, in turn, may lead to increased pain and reduced attempts to engage in activities of daily living (motivational deficits) or to develop new means of adapting to disabilities and distress (cognitive deficits).

These relationships between helplessness and adaptation to ARMD have been confirmed in many studies. Most of these investigations have used the Arthritis Helplessness Index to measure helplessness. High levels of helplessness in people with RA are associated with low self-esteem, the use of maladaptive coping strategies, and high levels of pain, depression, and functional impairment. Helplessness also correlates with poorer physical health in people with SLE (14). Because helplessness beliefs also mediate the relationship between low formal education level and greater mortality among persons with RA (15), improving perceptions of control over arthritis symptoms may be desirable. However, the belief that one can manage symptoms of ARMD may not always be helpful. Patients who believe they can control their symptoms tend to suffer psychological distress in response to increased pain unless they find a way to cognitively restructure their pain experiences, such as adopting the belief that pain has made life more precious.

Another cognitive factor closely related to perceptions of symptom control is *self-efficacy*. In contrast to perceptions of control over multiple stressors or symptoms, self-efficacy represents a belief that one can perform specific actions in particular situations to achieve specific health-related goals. An individual may exhibit great variation in self-efficacy for different actions. For example, an individual may have high self-efficacy for pacing daily activities with scheduled rest periods in her home environment, but low self-efficacy for performing exercises prescribed in physical therapy.

Self-efficacy is associated with multiple dimensions of health status across several rheumatic disorders. High baseline levels of self-efficacy for pain and functional ability among people with RA and OA correlate strongly with low levels of pain, disability, and depression at initial assessment, and at a four-month follow-up evaluation (16). High self-efficacy for pain is correlated with low frequencies of observable pain behaviors among persons with RA and fibromyalgia, even after controlling for demographic factors and measures of disease severity (17,18). Among SLE patients, self-efficacy for disease management is related to physical and mental health status and to disease activity (19). The two measures of self-efficacy are an instrument for people with arthritis (16) and a questionnaire for people with various chronic pain syndromes (20).

Coping Strategies

The coping process comprises several stages that include appraising the threat associated with a particular stressor; performing motor and cognitive actions (coping strategies) that may control the impact of the stressor; and evaluating the outcomes produced by these actions and, if necessary, performing alternative coping responses.

Studies of coping among people with ARMD primarily have used three instruments: the Ways of Coping Scale, the Coping Strategies Questionnaire, and the Vanderbilt Pain Management Inventory. Passive coping strategies, such as catastrophizing (believing that no coping strategy will effectively control symptoms), are associated with high levels of pain, disability, and poor adaptation to illness. Indeed, recent evidence suggests that the higher levels of pain and disability found in women with OA, compared with those found in men with OA, may be due to greater use of catastrophizing among the women (21). Conversely, psychological adjustment and relatively low levels of pain and functional impairment in persons with RA, OA, and fibromyalgia are related to positive strategies, such as focusing on positive thoughts during pain episodes and infrequent use of catastrophizing (22). However, there are no data concerning whether the positive effects of psychosocial interventions are mediated in part by reductions in catastrophizing.

Psychosocial Interventions

Given the relationships between health status and psychosocial factors, great effort has been devoted to testing psychosocial interventions that may improve patients' pain, affect, and function. Investigations also have assessed the extent to which these interventions help patients reduce health care utilization and costs. There is no single, standard psychosocial treatment protocol for ARMD, but most interventions share common treatment components, such as education, acquisition and home practice of new coping skills, and relapse prevention.

Several investigators have examined the effects of group psychologic therapies on symptom control and health status. For example, a biofeedback-assisted group therapy intervention trained RA patients and their family members in relaxation and behavioral problem-solving skills. This intervention, relative to attention-placebo and no adjunct treatment conditions, significantly reduced pain behavior and disease activity after treatment ended, although it did not influence patient perceptions of helplessness (23). A one-year follow-up showed that patients who received the psychologic intervention reported lower levels of pain and depression than were reported by those who received no adjunct treatment. This intervention, compared with no adjunct treatment and attention-placebo conditions, was associated with significantly lower use of health care resources and lower medical service costs (24). Similar interventions have produced reductions in pain and psychologic distress in people with RA for periods ranging from 15 to 30 months (25).

Several investigations have shown that psychosocial interventions may reliably increase self-efficacy beliefs and health status in people with ARMD. For example, a stress-management training program that focused specifically on increasing self-efficacy produced significant improvements in ratings of depression, pain, and walking speed among people with RA at 15-month follow-up (26). The Arthritis Self-Management Program (ASMP), developed by Lorig and colleagues at Stanford and adopted by the Arthritis Foundation, produces reliable increases in self-efficacy and exercise time, as well as significant reductions in pain, health distress, and health care system utilization among people with RA and OA; these improvements persist for four years after treatment initiation (27). Although the ASMP has not been shown to significantly alter functional ability, certain psychosocial interventions may increase function in patients with specific disorders. For example, it has been found that, among people with knee OA, coping-skills training, relative to arthritis education and standard care, produced significant reductions in ratings of pain and psychologic disability that generally were maintained at six-month follow-up (28). In addition, patients who received coping-skills training reported significant reductions in physical disability from post-treatment to follow-up.

Similar psychosocial interventions have been developed for people with fibromyalgia and SLE. However, few evaluations of these protocols have had adequate experimental controls for the effects of special attention given to participants in treatment trials or adequate follow-up evaluation. Although several uncontrolled trials have suggested that coping skills training for fibromyalgia patients may produce improvements in pain and function, none of the three attention-placebo–controlled trials performed to date have shown that psychosocial interventions are superior to placebo (29,30). Indeed, the efficacy of psychosocial interventions using the criteria for efficacy established by the American Psychological Association indicates that the ASMP and several similar interventions meet the criteria for well-established treatments for people with RA and OA (30). However, the efficacy of psychosocial interventions for people with fibromyalgia has not been established.

Innovations in Psychosocial Interventions

Several investigators have tested novel methods for delivering psychosocial interventions to patients outside of the clinic setting. For example, several investigators have examined the efficacy of telephone-based interventions for people with ARMD. These interventions, which are delivered by trained lay personnel, produce significant improvements in pain and disability among patients with OA (31), as well as significant improvements in psychological status among patients with SLE (32).

Fries and colleagues (33) evaluated the outcomes produced by an ASMP-based intervention delivered by booklets, audiotapes, and videotapes that were mailed to people with OA and RA. This intervention produced significant improvements in physical function, pain, joint count, global vitality, exercise, self-efficacy, and number of physician visits. All outcomes, with the exception of increased exercise, were maintained at six-month follow-up.

Another promising approach is the identification of patient subgroups that may show optimal response to psychosocial interventions. One uncontrolled trial of cognitive-behavioral therapy for people with fibromyalgia suggests that patients characterized by high levels of affective distress and pain are most likely to respond to this intervention (34). Another recent study indicates that people with RA and OA may be reliably differentiated from one another with respect to their readiness to adopt the self-management strategies emphasized by most psychosocial interventions (35). This suggests that it may be possible to enhance the outcomes produced by these interventions by tailoring treatment to individuals' specific stage of readiness for self-management.

Relatively few preventive interventions have been evaluated in the United States. However, Linton and colleagues (36) in Sweden have documented the efficacy of brief self-management interventions for reducing work absenteeism in persons with either initial episodes of musculoskeletal pain or recurrent back pain over a two-year period. Indeed, it was found that the intervention for persons with initial episodes of back pain produced an eight-fold reduction in the risk of developing a chronic pain syndrome. Felson and Zhang (37) have reviewed the risk factors that may serve as targets for primary, secondary, and tertiary prevention programs for persons with OA.

LAURENCE A. BRADLEY, PhD
NANCY L. McKENDREE-SMITH, PhD

References

1. Lazarus RL, Folkman S. Stress, Appraisal, and Coping. New York: Springer Publishing, 1998.

2. DaCosta D, Dobkin PL, Pinard L, et al. The role of stress in functional disability among women with systemic lupus erythematosus: A prospective study. Arthritis Care Res 1999;12: 112-119.

3. Adams SG Jr, Dammers PM, Saia TL, Brantley PJ, Gaydos G. Stress, depression, and anxiety predict average symptom severity and daily symptom fluctuation in systemic lupus erythematosus. J Behav Med 1994;17:459-477.

4. Potter PT, Zautra AJ. Stressful life events' effects on rheumatoid arthritis disease activity. J Consult Clin Psychol 1997;65: 319-323.

5. Affleck G, Tennen H, Urrows S, Higgins P. Person and contextual features of daily stress reactivity: Individual differences in relations of undesirable daily events with mood disturbance and chronic pain intensity. J Pers Soc Psychol 1994;66:329-340.

6. Harrington L, Affleck G, Urrows S, et al. Temporal covariation of soluble interleukin-2 receptor levels, daily stress, and disease activity in rheumatoid arthritis. Arthritis Rheum 1993; 36:199-203.

7. Schanberg LE, Sandstrom MJ, Starr K, et al. The relationship of daily mood and stressful events to symptoms in juvenile rheumatic disease. Arthritis Care Res 2000;13:33-41.

8. Magni G, Marchetti M, Moreschi C, Merskey H, Luchini SR. Chronic musculoskeletal pain and depressive symptoms in the National Health and Nutrition Examination. I. Epidemiologic follow-up study. Pain 1993;53:163-168.

9. Hawley DJ, Wolfe F. Depression is not more common in rheumatoid arthritis: A 10-year longitudinal study of 6,153 patients with rheumatic disease. J Rheumatol 1993;20:2025-2031.

10. Magni G, Moreschi C, Rigatti-Luchini S, Merskey H. Prospective study on the relationship between depressive symptoms and chronic musculoskeletal pain. Pain 1994;56: 289-297.

11. Wolfe F, Hawley DJ. The relationship between clinical activity and depression in rheumatoid arthritis. J Rheumatol 1993;20: 2032-2037.

12. Fifield J, Tennen H, Reisine S, McQuillan J. Depression and the long-term risk of pain, fatigue, and disability in patients with rheumatoid arthritis. Arthritis Rheum 1998;41:1851-57.

13. Zautra AJ, Burleson MH, Smith CA, et al. Arthritis and perceptions of quality of life: An examination of positive and negative affect in rheumatoid arthritis patients. Health Psychol 1995;14:399-408.

14. Thumboo J, Fong KY, Chan SP, et al. A prospective study of factors affecting quality of life in systemic lupus erythematosus. J Rheumatol 2000;27:1414-20.

15. Callahan LF, Cordray DS, Wells G, Pincus T. Formal education and five-year mortality in rheumatoid arthritis: Mediation by helplessness scale score. Arthritis Care Res 1996;9:463-72.

16. Lorig K, Chastain RL, Ung E, Shoor S, Holman HR. Development and evaluation of a scale to measure perceived self-efficacy in people with arthritis. Arthritis Rheum 1989;31:37-44.

17. Buckelew SP, Parker JC, Keefe FJ, et al. Self-efficacy and pain behavior among subjects with fibromyalgia. Pain 1994;59: 377-384.

18. LeFebvre JC, Keefe FJ, Affleck G, et al. The relationship of arthritis self-efficacy to daily pain, daily mood, and daily pain coping in rheumatoid arthritis patients. Pain 1999;80:425-435.

19. Karlson EW, Daltroy LH, Lew RA, et al. The relationship of socioeconomic status, race, and modifiable risk factors to outcomes in patients with systemic lupus erythematosus. Arthritis Rheum 1997;40:47-56.

20. Anderson KO, Dowds BN, Pelletz RE, Edwards WT, Peeters-Asdourian C. Development and initial validation of a scale to measure self-efficacy beliefs in patients with chronic pain. Pain 1995;63:77-84.

21. Keefe FJ, Lefebvre JC, Egert JR, Affleck G, Sullivan MJ, Caldwell DS. The relationship of gender to pain, pain behavior, and disability in osteoarthritis patients: The role of catastrophizing. Pain 2000;87:325-334.

22. Blalock SJ, DeVellis BM, Giorgino KB. The relationship between coping and psychological well-being among people with osteoarthritis: A problem-specific approach. Ann Behav Med 1995;17:107-115.

23. Bradley LA, Young LD, Anderson KO, et al. Effects of psychological therapy on pain behavior of rheumatoid arthritis patients: Treatment outcome and six-month follow-up. Arthritis Rheum 1987;30:1105-1114.

24. Young LD, Bradley LA, Turner RA. Decreases in health care resource utilization in patients with rheumatoid arthritis following a cognitive behavioral intervention. Biofeedback Self Regul 1995;20:259-268.

25. Keefe FJ, Van Horn Y. Cognitive-behavioral treatment of rheumatoid arthritis pain: Maintaining treatment gains. Arthritis Care Res 1993;6:213-222.

26. Smarr KL, Parker JC, Wright GE, et al. The importance of enhancing self-efficacy in rheumatoid arthritis. Arthritis Care Res 1997;10:18-26.

27. Lorig KR, Mazonson PD, Holman HR. Evidence suggesting that health education for self-management in patients with chronic arthritis has sustained health benefits while reducing health care costs. Arthritis Rheum 1993;36:439-446.

28. Keefe FJ, Caldwell DS, Williams DA, et al. Pain coping skills training in the management of osteoarthritic knee pain. II: Follow-up results. Behav Ther 1990;21:49-62.

29. Sandstrom MJ, Keefe FJ. Self-management of fibromyalgia: The role of formal coping skills training and physical exercise training programs. Arthritis Care Res 1998;11:432-447.

30. Bradley LA, Alberts KR. Psychological and behavioral approaches to pain management for patients with rheumatic disease. Rheum Dis Clin North Am 1999;25:215-232.

31. Weinberger M, Tierney WM, Cowper PA, Katz BP, Booher PA. Cost-effectiveness of increased telephone contact for patients with osteoarthritis: A randomized, controlled trial. Arthritis Rheum 1996;36:243-246.

32. Maisiak R, Austin JS, West SG, Heck L. The effect of person-centered counseling on the psychological status of persons with systemic lupus erythematosus or rheumatoid arthritis: a randomized, controlled trial. Arthritis Care Res 1996;9:60-66.

33. Fries JF, Carey C, McShane DJ. Patient education in arthritis: randomized controlled trial of a mail-delivered program. J Rheumatol 1997;24:1378-1383.

34. Turk DC, Okifuji A, Sinclair JD, Starz TW. Interdisciplinary treatment for fibromyalgia syndrome: Clinical and statistical significance. Arthritis Care Res 1998;11:186-195.

35. Keefe FJ, Lefebvre JC, Kerns RD, et al. Understanding the adoption of arthritis self-management: Stages of change profiles among arthritis patients. Pain 2000;87:303-313.

36. Linton SJ, Hellsing AL, Andersson D. A controlled study of the effects of an early intervention on acute musculoskeletal pain problems. Pain 1993;54:353-359.

37. Felson DT, Zhang Y. An update on the epidemiology of knee and hip osteoarthritis with a view to prevention. Arthritis Rheum 1998;41:1343-1355.

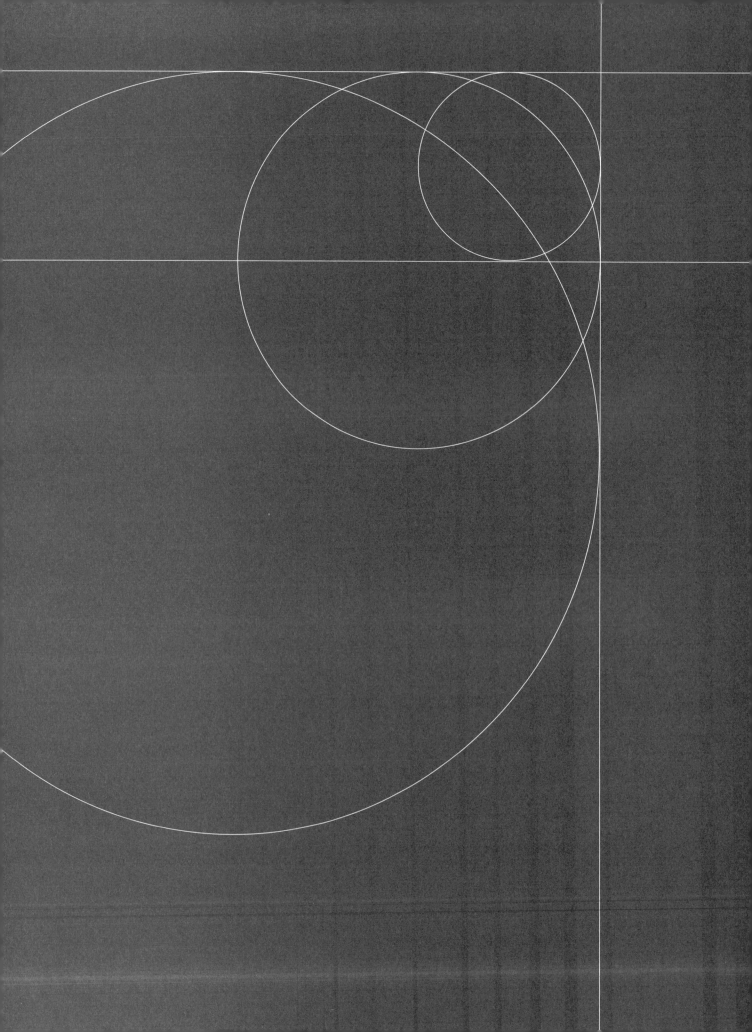

42 PATIENT EDUCATION AND SELF-MANAGEMENT

In an era of exploding information due to the World Wide Web and rapidly expanding use of the Internet, the field of patient education is on the brink of major expansion and growth. This, along with increasing consumer demand for information and an emphasis on disease self-management, has created an opportunity for patients and health-care providers alike.

Over the past few decades, the community of rheumatology health professionals has developed a strong theoretical foundation and research portfolio focused on patient education. This foundation has led to the current emphasis on the efficacy of programs, how they work and for whom, and the application of these programs to a broad base of patient populations. Direct consumer marketing by private industries has resulted in higher consumer demand for immediate information on new medications and state-of-the-art treatments. The promise of future therapies evolving from the mapping of the human genome is creating uncharted territory in all fields, including education. Moreover, as we begin to understand, accept, and research the effectiveness of complimentary medicines used by consumers, patient education becomes an even more essential component of the comprehensive clinical care of people living with rheumatic diseases (1).

Another first in the field of rheumatology is the emphasis on prevention. As prevention becomes part of practice and research, the need for new and effective patient-education programs is unprecedented. The National Arthritis Action Plan: A Public Health Strategy is the blueprint to address the causes of chronic pain and disability for the country (2). A major component of that plan is an emphasis on developing strategies for education of the public, people with arthritis and their families, and health professionals. The rheumatology community is poised to meet this challenge. Development of and research on education programs have contributed to the development of health-education theories. There is a vast information base on effecting knowledge change, understanding the impact of psychological factors on coping and disease management, and quantifying the effect of self-management education programs on health status (3,4).

What Is Patient Education?

Patient education is defined as "planned, organized learning experiences designed to facilitate voluntary adaptation of behaviors or beliefs conducive to health" (5). The "voluntary adaptation" is key to successful patient education programs and relates to issues of motivation and adherence. Education programs are most effective when they are planned and designed with well-defined goals and learning objectives targeted toward specific groups of people with similar forms of arthritis. Successful programs are designed to provide information that helps patients initiate behavior change and maintain healthy behaviors.

Patient education is interpreted to cover a broad spectrum of human factors. Although the focus is primarily on behaviors and beliefs, the scope of patient education also incorporates additional elements that motivate people to change health behaviors. These factors include knowledge, communication abilities, and sense of control, all of which affect health outcomes. A challenge to health educators is the fact that people all learn differently, making it more difficult to develop educational programs that meet individuals' needs. Proponents of distance learning, that is providing a broad base of education programs via the Internet, contend that the vast array of communication technology will enable educators to more easily design individual programs that achieve similar goals (6). If proven true, this very well may be the future direction in patient education.

Goals of Patient Education

A wide range of patient-education programs now exist, from structured traditional classes to on-line tutorials. However, the underlying goals of patient education follow basic learning principles. The goals of education programs for rheumatology patients are as varied as the theoretical framework that shape them. Daltroy and Liang (7) have emphasized that patient education goals are similar to those of traditional medical care: to improve function, relieve pain, enhance psychological well being, maintain satisfactory social interaction and employment, and control disease activity. Lorig has demonstrated that additional aims of patient education are to maintain or improve health and to slow deterioration. Research has effectively demonstrated the value of planned, goal-oriented programs. Patient education programs should always be evaluated to be certain the desired goals are achieved. Evaluation tools developed to measure educational outcomes, psychologic function, social function, and quality of life should be used when developing and implementing programs. Table 42-1 summarizes the variety of goals that can be achieved in developing these and other patient-education programs. With these goals as the foundation, one can develop successful patient-education programs. There are three key components to developing

TABLE 42-1
Goals of Patient-Education Programs

Understand disease and treatment(s)
Control or relieve pain and other symptoms
Enable psychosocial well being
Control or alter disease activity and its consequences
Prevent or minimize disability
Decrease inappropriate use of health services
Increase/foster independence
Enhance functional health status
Enhance social functioning
Improve communication skills

Modified from Allegrante JP. Patient education. In: Paget SA, Gibofsky A, Beary JF III (eds). Manual of Rheumatology and Outpatient Orthopedic Disorders. Philadelphia: Lippincott Williams & Wilkins, 2000.

patient-education programs. First, know your target population. Assess what the patients already know, the source of this information, perceptions about the cause of and treatments for the disease, and in what way they will best receive the information. Second, pilot test the program to evaluate if the goals have been met, and if not, why. Third, modify the program based on feedback from patients and the results of your evaluations.

Role of Self-Management

In the late 1970s, the self-help movement centered on individuals with common physical and/or emotional concerns who met on a regular basis to offer mutual support, information, education, and advocacy. Although the movement continues today, the emphasis in rheumatology patient education has been on self-management programs, the development of programs by health professionals in partnership with the patient community. These programs incorporate the reported experiences and invaluable advice from patients who live with rheumatic diseases. For example, programs such as the Arthritis Self-Management Program (8) and telephone education and support programs (9,10) include patients who use their experiences after having completed professionally led training. These types of collaborations allow for the patients, as well as the health educators, to maximize their expertise. Patient-education programs utilize the expertise of many different groups of people, including physicians, nurses, and social workers, as well as what are traditionally called *lay persons* – patients or volunteers that have familiarity with or relationship to a specific disease. Rheumatology patient education programs are based on a multitude of methods. These range from formal, didactic education sessions led by a health professional to information groups that are facilitated by people who have a specific rheumatic disease.

Theoretical Frameworks

The contributions of health educators, behavioral psychologists, and social psychologists have resulted in numerous modifications in the types of arthritis education programs available. The capacious definition of patient education has resulted in the concentration of programs designed to increase or change knowledge, behavior and beliefs, psychosocial function, and health status. Traditionally, health-education programs have emphasized increased knowledge about disease as the main outcome. In studies developed to enhance knowledge, 94% were successful in reaching their desired goals (11). This is not surprising because people diagnosed with chronic disease often seek information of various sorts during the course of their illness. Transfer of knowledge is essential in any learning process. However, many variables can interfere with a patient's quest for information. Culturally determined health beliefs and behaviors (12), as well as generation gaps, may prohibit some patients from seeking information about their disease. Physicians also may not have effective communication skills or teaching capabilities. Moreover, acquisition of knowledge alone does not result in changing health beliefs or health behaviors.

The focus over recent years has not been whether there should be patient-education programs but rather *which* programs to offer, to *whom,* and through *what* educational modality. Most recently this focus has included an emphasis on documenting the relationship of education interventions to expected health outcomes. The traditional education programs that have been successful include patient-education classes, peer telephone information and counseling lines, videoconferences, and educational support groups. Through the use of the Internet, distance learning is opening up a whole new way of delivering information on disease management that will not only achieve educational goals but has the potential to affect communication between patient and physician, and ultimately to enhance patient care and treatment (13).

The current focus of educational planning is on identifying the specific factors that cause patients to learn new information and subsequently alter their behavior. Perhaps the greatest contribution to the field of patient education has been the research findings that have influenced education programs towards effecting positive health outcomes.

Self-efficacy, an extension of social learning theory, refers to an individual's belief in his or her capability to mobilize the motivation, cognitive resources, and courses of action needed to meet situation demands (14). Lorig and colleagues have used the concept of self-efficacy to help patients live their lives with the chronic symptoms of their illness. The emphasis is on behavior and one's belief that a behavior can be carried out in a specific situation. Work in this area has led to further research demonstrating that a sense of control over one's illness is a precursor to resulting behaviors. In arthritis-education programs, the aim is to develop interventions that increase self-efficacy and self-confidence to enable patients to meet the physical and emotional challenges posed by their illness. Examples of the types of interventions used to enhance a patient's self-efficacy are mastery of skills, role modeling, reinterpreting symptoms, and persuasion. In recent years, social support has emerged as a concept vital to the success of patient-education programs. Patient-education programs have also been shown to have a significant effect on patients' health status. Bradley et al (15) demonstrated reduced pain behavior using a psychologic intervention, and Parker et al (16) have shown that a cognitive-behavioral pain management program can increase coping behaviors and one's confidence in the ability to control pain. These studies on educational interventions address the most common concerns reported by patients: pain, depression, and disability.

Challenges in Patient Education

Perhaps the major challenge for patient educators is to develop programs that effectively reach diverse patient populations. Some forms of rheumatic disease are disproportionately prevalent in the Latino, African American, and Asian communities. To date, education programs have been found effective in the population for which they were developed – that is white, middle-class patients. Little is known about the adaptability of current programs for people from various cultural backgrounds who adhere to culture-specific health beliefs and behaviors, and for whom English is not the primary spoken and written language. Robbins and colleagues (17) piloted a culturally sensitive Spanish version of the Systemic Lupus Erythematosus Self-Help Course, but there was no evidence of pre- and post-test change in depression, self-efficacy, or functional status. These findings raise questions about programs and the reliability of outcome measures for culturally diverse populations. There is a need to further understand how culturally determined health beliefs and behaviors affect health status.

As more people use on-line technology, the opportunities for patient education programs via the Internet are virtually unlimited. Programs are already available that can be accessed by patients from their homes and have similar effects on health status as the more traditional face-to-face program formats. Horton's LupusLine (18), a peer-counseling telephone service, and its Spanish counterpart, Charle de Lupus, are examples. These programs have been developed to enhance coping ability, increase knowledge about lupus, and reduce isolation. Maisiak's arthritis information telephone line also allows patients access to information via telephone (19). Building on interventions such as these will open an untapped source for new programs targeted to specific patient populations.

Practical Applications

Patient education is a mutual responsibility of the patient and the physician. Physicians must recognize that educational information is a vital component of the treatment plan that empowers patients to manage their disease and

ultimately alter their functional and social status. Through education, patients who become experts about their disease contribute to the treatment plan and enhance their own quality of life.

With the changing role of physicians in the current health care environment, it is unrealistic for the primary health care provider also to be the health educator. The physician's role is to recognize the patient's educational needs and, as part of the treatment plan, make a referral to the appropriate health care provider. The office practice nurse, physical therapist, and other health care providers are excellent sources of information on education programs. The most comprehensive references for education programs are available from the Arthritis Foundation, the American College of Rheumatology (ACR), and the Association of Rheumatology Health Professionals, a division of ACR composed of nurses, physical and occupational therapists, psychologists, social workers, and health educators. Practitioners today can also refer patients to information sources on the Web; however, the accuracy and effectiveness of Internet sources to date have not been validated.

Current Patient-Education Programs

The Arthritis Foundation offers a variety of programs disseminated through its regional and statewide chapters. The Arthritis Self-Management Program (ASMP), developed by Lorig and colleagues, has become the gold standard in self-management education programs for people with chronic illness. The six-week program is offered to lay persons who are taught, and in turn teach the course to other arthritis patients. The original goals of ASMP were to provide knowledge about chronic illness and teach skills to assist patients in coping with their illness. The theoretical assumption is that enhanced knowledge and adoption of self-management behaviors will result in improved functional outcomes (20). Many of the program activities teach people new behaviors that lead to increased function. Randomized research trials of the program have found that participants improve health behaviors, self-efficacy, and health status (8).

The Arthritis Foundation also has a plethora of educational literature, ranging from information for the newly diagnosed patient to more extensive information for the patient who has been living with arthritis for an extended period of time. Two recent Arthritis Foundation publications, *Good Living with Rheumatoid Arthritis* (21) and *Alternative Therapies* (22) are excellent examples of user-friendly guides that provide state-of-the-art information to the general public as well as patients. These and additional education materials can be found on the Arthritis Foundation's Web site at www.arthritis.org.

Other sources of patient education programs are available to both patients and professionals. Disease-specific organizations such as the Lupus Foundation of America, the Scleroderma Society, and the National Fibromyalgia

Partnership offer programs for patients and their families. These organizations have national offices with regional or statewide local chapters. In addition, hospitals often offer programs through departments of public health and patient education, nursing, or social services. Due to the National Arthritis Action Plan and collaborations with the Centers for Disease Control and Prevention, statewide education programs are now being designed to raise public awareness about the seriousness of arthritis as well as to assist patients and their families through education programs (23). Academic institutions with rheumatology research centers have education programs that are part of the overall services offered. Most are Musculoskeletal Disease Centers funded by the National Institutes of Health and are located throughout the country. These centers are engaged in arthritis studies, some of which include education programs that are available to the patient population.

The opportunities for people with arthritis to learn about their disease are numerous. The expansion of technology has set the stage for tremendous growth over the next decade, which will build upon that knowledge base and ultimately lead to enhancing the quality of life for the millions of people living with arthritis.

LAURA ROBBINS, DSW

References

1. Allegrante JP. Patient Education. In: Paget SA, Gibofsky A, Beary JF III (eds). Manual of Rheumatology and Outpatient Orthopedic Disorders. Philadelphia: Lippincott Williams & Wilkins, 2000.

2. Arthritis Foundation, Association of State and Territorial Officials, Centers for Disease Control. National Arthritis Action Plan: A Public Health Strategy. 1999.

3. Daltroy LH, Liang MH. Arthritis education: opportunities and state of the art. Health Education Quarterly 1993;20(1): 3–16.

4. Parker JC, Frank RG, et al. Pain management in rheumatoid arthritis patients – a cognitive-behavioral approach. Arthritis Rheum 1988;31:593–601.

5. Burckhardt C. Arthritis and musculoskeletal patient education standards. Arthritis Care Res 1994;7:1–4.

6. Moore M, Kearsley G. Distance Education: A Systems View. Stamford, Conn: Wadsworth Publishing, 1996.

7. Daltroy L, Liang M. Advances in patient education in rheumatic disease. Ann Rheum Dis 1991;50:415–417.

8. Lorig K, Holman H. Arthritis self-management studies: a twelve-year review. Health Education Quarterly 1993;20:17–28.

9. Maisiak RS, Austin JS, Heck L. A controlled comparison of the effects of two interventions on the health status of rheumatoid arthritis or osteoarthritis patients (abstract). Arthritis Rheum 1995;38:9 S383.

10. Horton R, Peterson MG, Powell S, Engelhard E, Paget SA. Users evaluate LupusLine, a telephone peer counseling service. Arthritis Care Res 1997;10:257–263.

11. Lorig K, Konkol L, Gonzalez V. Arthritis patient education: a review of the literature. Patient Education Counsel 1987; 10:207–252.

12. Robbins L. Social and cultural assessment. In: Robbins L, Burckhardt C, Hannan M, DeHoratius R (eds). Clinical Care in the Rheumatic Diseases 2nd Edition. Atlanta: American College of Rheumatology, in press.

13. Shore D. Harvard Review. April, 1999.

14. Gonzalez V, Goeppinger J, Lorig K. Four psychosocial theories and their application to patient education and clinical practice. Arthritis Care Res 1990;3:132–143.

15. Bradley LA, Young LD, Anderson KO, et al. Effects of psychosocial therapy on pain behavior of rheumatoid arthritis patients: treatment outcome and six-month follow up. Arthritis Rheum 1987;30:1105–1114.

16. Parker J, Frank RG, Beck NC, et al. Pain management in rheumatoid arthritis patients: a cognitive-behavioral approach. Arthritis Rheum 1988;31:593–601.

17. Robbins L, Allegrante JP, Paget SA. Adapting the systemic lupus erythematosus self-help (SLESH) for Latino SLE patients. Arthritis Care Res 1993;6:97–103.

18. Horton R, Steiner-Grossman P. LupusLine Leader's Manual: A Step-By-Step Guide to Starting a Peer Counseling Service. New York: Hospital for Special Surgery, 1993.

19. Maisiak R, Koplon S, Heck L. User evaluation of an arthritis information telephone service. Arthritis Care Res 1989;2:75–79.

20. Lorig K, Seieznick M, Lubeck D, Ung E, Chastain R, Holman H. The beneficial outcomes of the arthritis self-management course are not adequately explained by behavior change. Arthritis Rheum 1989;32:91–95.

21. Arthritis Foundation. The Arthritis Foundation's Guide to Good Living with Rheumatoid Arthritis. Atlanta: Arthritis Foundation, 2000.

22. Horstman J. The Arthritis Foundation's Guide to Alternative Therapies. Arnold W, Berman B, Hollister JR, Liang M (eds). Atlanta: Arthritis Foundation, 1999.

23. Centers for Disease Control and Prevention, National Center for Chronic Disease Prevention and Health Promotion, http://www.cdc.gov/nccdphp.

43 PAIN MANAGEMENT

All too often in office-based practice, treatment of pain is of less concern than diagnosis and treatment of the disease. Patients with chronic diffuse pain frequently are dismissed as not having "real" pain, which only perpetuates their illness. Presence of pain should be specifically sought in all patients. Pain relief should always be a primary focus of the physician's efforts.

Nature of Pain

A useful definition adopted by the International Association for the Study of Pain (1) defines pain as "an unpleasant sensory and emotional experience associated with actual or potential tissue damage, or described in terms of such damage." Neurophysiologically, pain is a complex sensation-perception interaction that involves simultaneous parallel processing of nociceptive signals from the spinal cord that activate a central network encompassing the pain experience (Fig. 43-1).

In addition to strictly sensory-discriminative elements of nociception and afferent input from somatic reflexes, there are major contributions from pathways and regions of the brain concerned with emotional, motivational, and cognitive aspects of pain. These factors determine the subjective intensity of pain. The two principal effectors of the stress response, the hypothalamic–pituitary–adrenal axis and the sympathetic nervous system, are also activated. The stress response may become maladaptive in chronic pain syndromes such as fibromyalgia. Negative emotions (depression and anxiety), other negative psychological factors (loss of control, unpredictability in one's environment), and certain cognitive aspects (negative beliefs and attributions, catastrophizing) all can function as stressors with actions in these systems.

Pain Categories

There are four principal categories of pain: nociceptive pain, neuropathic pain, chronic pain of complex etiology, and psychogenic pain.

Nociceptive Pain

Nociceptive pain is due to stimulation of peripheral pain receptors on thinly myelinated $A\delta$ and/or unmyelinated (C) afferent nerves during inflammation, injury, or tissue destruction. The pain experienced generally "matches" the noxious stimulus. However, both peripheral sensitization (reduction in the threshold of nociceptor endings) and central sensitiza-

tion (amplification of pain in the CNS) with input into the CNS via thickly myelinated $A\beta$ touch afferent nerves can occur in "normal" nociceptive pain. These inputs may result in primary allodynia (pain felt with non-noxious stimuli, such as gentle touching) and primary hyperalgesia (more pain than normal felt with noxious stimuli). In addition to systemic inflammatory or degenerative rheumatic diseases, nociceptive pain occurs as regional musculoskeletal pain in tenosynovitis, compressive neuropathies, nerve entrapment syndromes, bursitis, and various localized forms of arthritis (e.g., acromioclavicular osteoarthritis). Usually self-limited with conventional treatment strategies, regional musculoskeletal pain may become chronic and disabling.

Neuropathic Pain

Both peripheral and central nervous system processes play a role in neuropathic pain, which may follow injuries and diseases that directly affect the nervous system. Examples include trigeminal neuralgia, postherpetic neuralgia, radiculopathic pain due to injury to spinal nerve roots, sympathetic-related pain conditions (e.g., reflex sympathetic dystrophy), and central pain following strokes. Here the pain may be paroxysmal with electric shock-like, shooting, or burning characteristics. It may be associated with hyperpathia (persistence after the stimulus has ended, spreading or worsening in crescendo-fashion with repeated touching). Central sensitization and ectopic firing of peripheral neu-

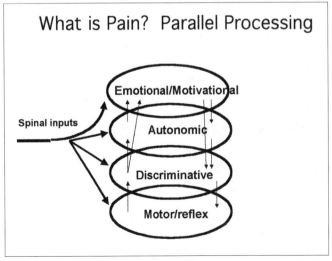

Fig. 43-1. A neurophysiologist's view of pain. Courtesy of Alan R. Light, PhD.

rons, either spontaneously or through mechanical forces developed during movement, contribute to this peculiar type of pain. Management may require special pharmacologic approaches, as discussed below.

Chronic Pain of Complex Etiology

Chronic pain of complex etiology occurs in fibromyalgia and a large number of regional pain syndromes, such as migraine headache, temporomandibular disorders (TMD), irritable bowel syndrome, atypical chest pain, myofascial pain, and chronic low-back pain. The bases for this type of pain are complex and poorly understood. There is question whether some (e.g., myofascial pain syndrome) even exist as distinct entities (2). Indeed, there is growing evidence that many or even most overlap, with very close relationships etiologically and pathophysiologically. The diagnostic label applied to an illness in a given patient often depends on which medical specialist evaluates the patient first.

Collectively, these chronic pain syndromes constitute huge personal and societal burdens. All too frequently, the problem is not approached effectively by traditional medicine. In fibromyalgia, which can be taken as a prototype for this category, pain diffusely radiates from the axial skeleton over large areas of the body, predominately involving muscles. The patient describes the symptoms as "exhausting," "miserable," or "unbearable." Altered central nociceptive processing results in a decrease in the pain-perception threshold and in the threshold for pain tolerance. The hallmarks of fibromyalgia – chronic widespread pain, fatigue, and multiple somatic symptoms – have both psychologic and biologic bases that derive, at least in part, from chronic stress and distress. Female gender, adverse experiences during childhood, psychological vulnerability to stress, and a stressful, often frightening environment and culture are important antecedents. Thus, fibromyalgia and related syndromes should be viewed from a biopsychosocial perspective (3).

More purely *psychogenic pain* is seen in somatoform and somatization disorders and hysteria.

Management

The first element in pain management is accurate assessment and diagnosis of the cause of the pain. Assessment should include attention to possible psychological and sociocultural factors that could be contributing to the pain experience. Diagnostic "waffling," the ordering of frightening tests, excessive use of physical therapy modalities after minor trauma, excessive activity limitation, and overly liberal work-release are among the important factors that can convert what should be a self-limited acute pain condition into a chronic pain syndrome. It also is important to be aware of confounders to recovery, such as pending litigation or compensation claims. On the other hand, patients become frustrated with comments such as, "It's all in your mind." To the patient, the pain is real.

For acute nociceptive pain (less than 30 days duration), pharmacological interventions should follow a step-wise approach using nonopioid and opioid analgesics either singly or in combination, as indicated by pain intensity. Depending on the specific musculoskeletal disorder, initially conservative combinations of corticosteroid injections, activity modification, splints, counterforce bracing, local heat or cold, and in some cases, surgical procedures may be indicated for pain relief and/or to preserve function. Education about the nature of the underlying problem, limitations, and prognosis should err on the side of optimism. Whenever possible, rapid return to full activity and work is best.

If there is a significant nociceptive pain element, chronic pain (longer than six months duration) may be managed pharmacologically with analgesics using the same step-wise approach outlined for acute pain. Especially important is a multifaceted treatment plan that incorporates various adjuvant medicines, exercise, and psychological and behavioral approaches to reduce distress and promote self-efficacy and self-management. For many regional chronic pain syndromes, e.g., TMD (4), referral to an experienced specialist who advocates holistic, nonsurgical approaches is recommended.

Assessment

Assessment of pain in the physician's office should be based on a biopsychosocial perspective, i.e., identifying biological variables that contribute to pain and recognizing that psychological and sociocultural factors potentially amplify or perpetuate the pain experience (5). Pain intensity should be measured with either a verbal or numerical rating scale or a visual analog scale. It can be useful to determine pain-detection threshold (normal = 4 kg/cm^2) at four convenient fibromyalgia tender-point sites by pressure algometry in all patients, regardless of diagnosis. Note pain behaviors, such as guarding, rubbing, grimacing, and sighing, which may vary inversely with patients' self-efficacy for control of chronic pain.

A simple self-report form that incorporates validated scales for physical and psychological health status (Modified Health Assessment Questionnaire), visual analog scales for pain, fatigue, patient global self-assessment, a checklist of current symptoms, and scales for helplessness and cognitive performance can be completed in just a few minutes (6). Easily adaptable to a busy practice, such information is invaluable for the psychosocial assessment of pain, both diagnostically and in monitoring response to therapy. Marital adjustment, perceived levels of social support, and current stressors in the patient's life are important topics for evaluation. The simple inquiry "How was your childhood?" often reveals adverse childhood experiences such as abuse that have increased the patient's vulnerability to chronic pain (7).

In multidisciplinary settings, information obtained from the Minnesota Multiphasic Personality Inventory (MMPI), the Social Support Questionnaire (SSQ), the Sickness Impact Profile (SIP), and the Multidimensional Pain Inventory (MPI) is useful for more comprehensive assessments. For example, subgroups of patients with chronic pain have been identified from MPI responses that appear to predict response to interdisciplinary therapeutic interventions (8).

Pharmacologic Management

A useful step-wise approach for pharmacologic interventions based on pain intensity is illustrated in Fig. 43-2. Addition of tramadol, propoxyphene, codeine, or timed-release oxycodone (9) for people with osteoarthritis who do not find relief with acetaminophen plus nonsteroidal anti-inflammatory drugs (NSAIDs) or cyclooxygenase-2 (COX)-2 inhibitors is effective. Glucosamine, chondroitin, and intra-articular hyaluronate sodium or hylan G-F 20 may be helpful adjuncts in OA. Reasonable guidelines for use of opioids in more severe chronic musculoskeletal pain include exclusion of substance abusers, concomitant attention to psychological and social perpetuators of pain, use of an "opioid treatment contract," "one physician, one dispensing pharmacy," and close monitoring. Drug-seeking behavior (pseudoaddiction) often indicates that pain is not being controlled adequately.

Opioid Analgesic Drugs

Opioids bind to μ, κ, or δ opioid receptors (predominately μ for analgesic effects) in regions of the brain involved in integrating pain and to pre- and postsynaptic terminals of peripheral sensory fibers, where they inhibit release of substance P and other mediators. Tramadol also inhibits reuptake of norepinehrine and serotonin. Table 43-1 lists opioids commonly in use. The side effects of opioids include constipation, nausea and vomiting, sedation, cognitive impairment, miosis, myoclonus, urinary retention, and respiratory depression. Older persons are more sensitive to opioids with respect to both efficacy for pain relief and vulnerability to side effects; starting doses should be reduced 25%–50% in this population. In the great majority of patients with well-defined chronic rheumatic disease pain, opioids are effective, safe, and well-tolerated (10,11). Several weeks or months are required to titrate opioid therapy in the out-patient setting. During opiod tapers, which require two to three weeks, clonidine (0.2–0.4 mg/day) is helpful in controlling withdrawal symptoms. Monitoring of patients taking analgesic medications requires frequent re-evaluation for efficacy and side effects during initiation, titration, dose changes, and maintenance therapy.

Muscle Relaxants

Centrally acting skeletal muscle relaxants (carisprodol, cyclobenzaprine, chlorzoxazone, metaxolone, methocarbamol, and orphenedrine citrate) have had a modest benefit as adjunctive therapy for nociceptive pain associated with muscle strains. Used intermittently, they also have limited effectiveness for certain regional and diffuse chronic pain syndromes. Sedation and other CNS side effects occur frequently. Abuse may occur, particularly with carisprodol, and abrupt cessation may be associated with withdrawal symptoms.

Antidepressants

Tricyclic antidepressants (TCAs) clearly are effective in neuropathic pain and in diffuse and regional chronic pain syndromes, but side effects (dry mouth, drowsiness, and weight gain) limit patient acceptance. Selective serotonin reuptake inhibitors, and the large number of other antidepressants with different mechanisms of action, are not effective substitutes for TCAs as analgesic agents, but should be used for the frequently concomitant depression that amplifies pain.

Antiepileptic drugs (AEDs)

Carbamazepine and a series of other new AEDs, some of which potentiate γ-amino butyric acid (GABA) in the CNS, have become first-line agents for neuropathic pain (12). Gabapentin, a 3-alkylated GABA analog originally introduced as an anticonvulsant, is useful in chronic pain states including fibromyalgia, related syndromes, and various types of neuropathic pain (reviewed in 13). Gabapentin may ameliorate associated depressed mood and anxiety as well. Doses as high as 3600 mg/day in divided doses may be used with few side effects. Pregabalin, another GABA analog, also is promising.

Capsaicin

Obtained from red chili peppers, topical capsaicin binds to vanilloid receptors on peripheral terminals of nociceptive neurons, thereby inhibiting activation of the pain pathway by noxious stimuli. Essentially free of toxicity other than mild burning at the site of application, capsaicin is useful as adjunctive therapy in diffuse and regional musculoskeletal pain syndromes, joint pain in arthritis, and in neuropathic pain disorders.

Other Pharmacologic Agents

Neuroleptics (phenothiazines, thioxanthenes, butyrophenones, clozapine, risperidone) and anxiolytics (clonazepam, lorazepam, temazepam, alprazolam, and buspirone) have antinociceptive effects in chronic pain and are often used in combination with antidepressants and AEDs. Benzodiazepines (temazepam, zolpidem, and triazolam) are widely used for the poor sleep associated with fibromyalgia and related chronic pain syndromes, but are no substitute for the maintenance of common-sense sleeping practices (e.g., avoidance of excessive caffeine intake, moderation of alcohol use). Dextromethorphan, an n-methyl-D-aspartate

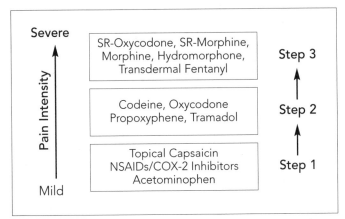

Fig. 43-2. Step-wise approach to pharmacologic management of pain.

TABLE 43-1
Opioid Analgesic Drugs

Drug	Oral equivalent	Starting dose	Comment
Short-Acting			For all, start low and titrate; begin bowel program early; most of these opiods are available in combination with acetaminophen or aspirin (do not exceed maximum dose). For all, short-acting opioid often is needed for break-through pain.
Morphine sulfate (*Roxanol*)	30 mg	15-30 mg every 4 h	
Codeine (*Fiornal*)	120 mg	30-60 mg every 4-6 h	
Hydrocodone (*Lortab*)	30 mg	5-10 mg every 3-4 h	
Oxycodone (*Percodan*)	20-30 mg	5-10 mg every 3-4 h	
Hydromorphone (*Dilaudid*)	7.5 mg	1.5 mg every 3-4 h	
Propoxyphene (*Darvon*)	100 mg	100 mg every 4 h	
Tramadol (*Ultram*)	120 mg	50-100 mg every 6 h	
Methadone (*Dolophine*)		15-60 mg every 8 h	
Long-acting			
SR-Morphine (*MS Contin*)	30 mg	5-10 mg every 3-4 h	
SR-Oxycodone (*Oxycontin*)	20-30 mg	10-20 mg every 12 h	
Transdermal fentanyl (*Duragesic*)	NA	see pkg insert	

(NMDA) receptor antagonist available as an over-the-counter antitussive or as specially compounded capsules, can be used ~1:1 with morphine for neuropathic pain. Anecdotally, the combination is of benefit as adjunctive therapy in diffuse and regional chronic pain syndromes. Mexilitine (a sodium channel blocker), baclofen (which activates GABA β-receptors), clonidine (a centrally acting antiadrenergic), and tizanidine (an α_2-adrenergic agonist), all have special uses in neuropathic and other pain states. Tropisetron is one of several highly selective, competitive antagonists of 5-HT$_3$, a serotonin receptor located exclusively on peripheral and central neurons. Very effective as an antiemitic in patients undergoing cancer chemotherapy, preliminary data suggest that tropisetron improves self-reported pain, anxiety, and depression in fibromyalgia, as well as pain due to inflammatory and degenerative rheumatic diseases (14).

Pharmacologic Management of Chronic Pain of Complex Etiology
Amitriptyline at bedtime (10–50 mg) is a well-established therapy for fibromyalgia and related chronic pain syndromes. Although not effective as single agents for pain control, non-TCA antidepressants may be useful in combination with TCAs. The skeletal muscle relaxant cyclobenzaprine improves sleep and reduces pain (15). Corticosteroids and NSAIDs are useful only as treatment for coexisting inflammatory processes. Pharmacologic and nonpharmacologic treatment of poor sleep is crucial for improving the patient's overall sense of well-being. Some experts advocate opioid analgesics as therapy for patients with severe allodynia and hyperalgesia. If used, opioids should be combined with multidisciplinary approaches, psychotherapeutic interventions, and the cautions mentioned above. Gabapentin is one of a number of promising novel approaches. Growth hormone and cytokine therapies are still experimental.

Psychological and Behavioral Approaches
The importance of strategies in this area has been emphasized recently by Keefe and Bonk (5) and Bradley and Alberts (16). Depression, anxiety, stress, sleep disturbance, pain beliefs and coping strategies, and self-efficacy all are central to the pain experience in many patients, and frequently determine the outcome of chronic pain. Unless psychosocial and behavioral variables are recognized and approached, strictly pharmacologic interventions to reduce nociceptive pain from inflammation or the diffuse pain in fibromyalgia and related syndromes are of limited benefit. Showing special promise is cognitive–behavioral therapy (CBT), which includes components for education, training in relaxation and coping skills, rehearsals of the skills learned, and relapse prevention. Well-established behavioral treatments in rheumatoid arthritis and osteoarthritis that improve ratings of pain or pain behavior include CBT and the Arthritis Self-Management Program (17). Self-care education and telephone counseling are probably efficacious in osteoarthritis, but have not been studied in rheumatoid arthritis. CBT for the diffuse pain of fibromyalgia and related regional pain syndromes has garnered mixed results (16)

Physical Therapy and Physical Modalities
The objectives here are to diminish pain, improve function, minimize disability, and promote self-efficacy. Although certain strategies and modalities are clearly beneficial, this area needs properly designed trials to establish efficacy.

Exercise
In addition to the positive effects on underlying pathologic processes in bones, joints, and muscles, exercise to improve

cardiovascular fitness, muscle tone, and strength is essential to the treatment of fibromyalgia and related chronic pain syndromes. The benefits of exercise include improvements in subjective and objective measures of pain and in overall sense of well-being. Many people with chronic pain have the negative belief (fear) that activity will harm them and they perceive their muscles to be weak and easily fatigued. Consequently, exercise is avoided and their muscles become deconditioned. Normal activities become challenging. Excessive activity "on a good day" induces a major flare of pain and fatigue, possibly due in part to the peripheral and central effects of proinflammatory cytokines (TNF, IL-1, IL-6) released in response to exercise-damaged myofibers. Ideally, exercise should be low impact (walking, water aerobics, or stationary bicycling rather than running), begin very gently, and progress gradually to endurance and strength training. Encouragement and positive reinforcement can reduce the virtually universal problem of poor compliance. Obesity, poor posture, and overloading activities at work and home also contribute to muscle pain and fatigue and should be addressed. Daily stretching exercises after hot showers are very helpful.

Heat and Cold
Heat (hot packs, paraffin, hydrotherapy in its many forms) is of proven benefit in nociceptive pain, especially when combined with exercise (range of motion, stretching, strengthening). Diffuse and regional pain is improved by such strategies as sauna, hot baths and showers, and hot mud. While not superior to superficial heat, cold (cold packs, immersion, or vapocoolant sprays) may provide more immediate analgesic benefit, particularly when applied soon after an injury.

Other Physical Modalities
Gentle massage is well received by people with diffuse pain syndromes, but it is a totally passive modality that fails to promote self-efficacy for control of pain. Trigger-point injections are of short-term benefit only and should generally be avoided. Neurophysiologic effects of acupuncture and electroacupuncture include release of opioids and other mediators in the nervous system. Several randomized controlled trails have shown acupuncture to improve subjective pain and to raise pain thresholds, but its long-term benefit in chronic pain syndromes remains unclear. Although transcutaneous electrical nerve stimulation (TENS) is widely used for localized musculoskeletal pain, its mechanisms of action remain unclear. An advantage of TENS is that the patient can apply this modality at home.

Complementary and Alternative Medicine (CAM)
The immense popularity of CAM today contrasts with the current paucity of data regarding the biochemical nature and mechanism of action of most alternative remedies and the lack of rigorous studies addressing efficacy, safety, and cost-effectiveness of these strategies. Many physicians lack knowledge about CAM, and patients are reluctant to inform their physicians about CAM approaches. This can be dangerous because of unsuspected drug interactions. Despite these concerns, patients with chronic pain and fatigue are the largest group using CAM. Until neuroscience, behavioral science, and health care systems evolve to such a point that effective biopsychosocial treatment strategies are applied in most people with chronic pain, CAM approaches will continue to proliferate. In the meantime, a practical approach is to inquire about CAM usage, refrain from expression of negative opinions if a particular CAM treatment is relatively inexpensive and appears to be safe, and to encourage "whatever works" in the context of the power of the placebo effect and promotion of self-efficacy for control of pain. See Chapter 50 for more on CAM.

Procedure-Based Pain Management
Injection of local anaesthetics, epidural techniques, and root and ganglion surgery may have a place in certain cases, but risk-benefit ratios and long-term efficacy in chronic pain have not been fully established.

Pain in Children

Except for children younger than 1 year, the approach to the management of pain in children is similar to that in adults. Issues meriting particular attention include the young child's inability to self-report pain, fear (e.g., of doctors and needles), age-related pharmacologic factors, and psychosocial variables that differ from those in adults (e.g., school absenteeism). Although clinically significant pain often is not fully recognized and treated, recurrent complaints of pain all over the body are common in otherwise healthy children. In such cases, the physician must be sensitive and wise, avoid unnecessary testing, and emphasize lifestyle interventions, reduction of school stressors, and aerobic exercise (18).

Pain in Older Persons

Pain, particularly musculoskeletal pain, is very common in older persons and is neither part of normal aging nor better tolerated than in younger persons. Those misconceptions contribute importantly to the unfortunate undertreatment (or no treatment) of chronic pain in the elderly in both community and institutional settings. Indeed, in a study of nursing home residents, 71% had at least one pain complaint, and for 34% of those, pain was constant. Yet only 15% had received analgesic medication in the previous 24 hours (19). The experience of pain in older persons differs somewhat from that in young or middle-aged individuals: less frequent self-report of pain, atypical presentation of pain (e.g., as confusion, restlessness, or other behavioral change), less prominent anxiety associated with the pain, and frequent coexisting depression. Older persons exhibit lower self-efficacy and tend to use passive coping strategies (e.g., praying and hoping) rather than cognitive coping methods. Their susceptibility to associated impairments is greater.

The American Geriatrics Society has published clinical practice guidelines for the management of chronic pain in older persons (20). Special barriers to accurate pain assessment in this population include reluctance to report pain, use of atypical descriptors of pain, fear of diagnostic tests and medications, and communication difficulties due to sensory and cognitive impairments. With respect to pharmacologic therapy in the elderly, goals, hopes, and tradeoffs should be discussed openly. Dosing of medications should follow the "start low, go slow" maxim, particularly with opioids. Nevertheless, the use of opioids for moderate or severe pain is appropriate. COX-2 inhibitors are preferred to traditional NSAIDs in the elderly. The health care provider also must be aware of economic barriers that some elderly patients confront in obtaining medications. Nonpharmacologic treatment of pain in older persons should be an integral part of care plans.

JOHN B. WINFIELD, MD

References

1. Merskey H. Classification of Chronic Pain. Description of Chronic Pain Syndromes and Definitions of Pain Terms. International Association for the Study of Pain. New York: Elsevier, 1994.
2. Wolfe F, Simons DG, Fricton J, et al. The fibromyalgia and myofascial pain syndromes: a preliminary study of tender points and trigger points in persons with fibromyalgia, myofascial pain syndrome and no disease. J Rheumatol 1992; 9:944–951.
3. Winfield JB. Pain in fibromyalgia. Rheum Dis Clinics North Am 1999;25:55–79.
4. Differential diagnosis and management considerations of temporomandibular disorders. In: Okeson JP (ed). Orafacial Pain: Guidelines of Assessment, Diagnosis, and Management. Carol Stream, Illinois: Quintessence, 1996; pp 113–184.
5. Keefe FJ, Bonk V. Psychosocial assessment of pain in patients having rheumatic diseases. Rheum Dis Clin North Am 1999; 25:81–103.
6. Pincus T. Documenting quality management in rheumatic disease: are patient questionnaires the best (and only) method? Arthritis Care Res 1996;9:339–348.
7. Winfield JB. Psychological determinants of fibromyalgia. Current Reviews in Pain 2000;4:276–286.
8. Turk DC, Rudy TE, Kubinski JA, et al. Dysfunctional patients with temporomandibular disorders: evaluating the efficacy of a tailored treatment protocol. J Consult Clin Psychol 1996;64: 139–146.
9. Caldwell JR, Hale ME, Boyd RE, et al. Treatment of osteoarthritis pain with controlled release oxycodone or fixed combination oxycodone plus acetaminophen added to nonsteroidal antiinflammatory drugs: a double blind, randomized, multicenter, placebo controlled trial. J Rheumatol 1999;26:862–869.
10. Ytterberg SR, Mahowald ML, Woods SR. Codeine and oxycodone use in patients with chronic rheumatic disease pain. Arthritis Rheum 1998;41:16.
11. Pappagallo M. Aggressive pharmacologic treatment of pain. Rheum Dis Clin North Am 1999;25:193–213.
12. Sindrup SH, Jensen TS. Efficacy of pharmacological treatments of neuropathic pain: an update and effect related to mechanism of drug action. Pain 1999;83:389–400.
13. Bryans JS, Wustrow DJ. 3-substituted GABA analogs with central nervous system activity: a review. Med Res Rev 1999;19: 149–177.
14. Färber L, Stratz T, Brückle M, et al. Efficacy and tolerability of troisetron in primary fibromyalgia – a highly selective and competitive 5-HT$_3$ receptor antagonist. Scand J Rheumatol 2000;29(Suppl 113):49–54.
15. Bennett RM, Gatter RA, Campbell SM, et al. A comparison of cyclobenzaprine and placebo in the management of fibrositis. A double-blind controlled study. Arthritis Rheum 1988;31: 1535–1542.
16. Bradley LA, Alberts KR. Psychological and behavioral approaches to pain management for patients with rheumatic disease. Rheum Dis Clin North Am 1999;25:215–232.
17. Lorig KR, Mazonson PD, Holman HR. Evidence suggesting that health education for self-management in patients with chronic arthritis has sustained health benefits while reducing health care costs. Arthritis Rheum 1993;36:439–446.
18. Zempsky WT, Schechter NL. Office-based pain management. The 15-minute consultation. Ped Clin North Am 2000;47: 601–615.
19. Ferrell BA, Ferrell BR, Osterweil D. Pain in the nursing home. J Am Geriatr Soc 1990;38:409–414.
20. AGS panel on Chronic Pain in Older Persons. The management of chronic pain in older persons. J Am Geriatrics Soc 1998;46:635–651.

44 THERAPEUTIC INJECTION OF JOINTS AND SOFT TISSUES

Treatment of joint inflammation by local injection has been an important facet of arthritis care ever since Hollander demonstrated that hydrocortisone salts could be effective when used this way (1). Of the many other compounds that have been injected with therapeutic intent (2), only corticosteroids and hyaluronates for knee osteoarthritis are widely used for injection. The major objectives of local injection are to enter a painful structure, remove any excess fluid, and instill the corticosteroid suspension likely to provide the longest duration of relief. Salutary results may ensue from temporary relief of pain by a local anesthetic that often is admixed with the corticosteroid, relief of distention of a contracted joint space, and systemic effects of corticosteroids. Local injection minimizes the hazards inherent in systemic corticosteroid therapy, while assuring the direct application of potent medication to the active site of disease.

The indications for local injection are listed in Table 44-1. Injections should never be the sole intervention, even for isolated regional disorders, and other aspects of a treatment program should be respected and continued. Joint injection is relatively contraindicated when the process causing the regional problem is obscure, especially if infection enters the differential diagnosis. Established infections, either regional (cellulitis) or systemic (bacteremia), constitute absolute contraindication to therapeutic injections, although swollen joints or bursae definitely should be entered if these sites are suspected to be the source or seed of infection.

TABLE 44-1
Indications for Therapeutic Injection of Musculoskeletal Structures

1. When only one or a few joints are inflamed, provided infection has been excluded.

2. In systemic polyarthritis syndromes (e.g., rheumatoid arthritis, psoriatic arthritis, others), as an adjunct to systemic drug therapy.

3. To assist in rehabilitation and prevent deformity.

4. To relieve pain in osteoarthritis exhibiting local inflammatory signs.

5. Soft-tissue regional disorders (e.g., bursitis, tenosynovitis, periarthritis, nodules, epicondylitis, ganglia).

Previous failure to respond to local injection should preclude a repeat attempt, unless technical features of the last treatment (including strict adherence to a postinjection rest regimen) were suboptimal. Bleeding diatheses dictate caution when induction of hemarthrosis seems possible, but should not avert decompression of established joint swelling that might be due to bleeding. Joint or soft-tissue injections and aspirations in people taking warfarin are associated with low risk, provided the most recent international normalized ratio (INR) is <4.5 (4).

The most common complication following a single injection is a transient increase in pain, often accompanied by local inflammatory signs. This effect, most likely from a local reaction to corticosteroid crystals, was seen following 6% of injections in a large series of people with rheumatoid arthritis (RA) (5). The reaction generally subsided within four to 24 hours, and was managed with rest, analgesia, and cold packs. Because such flares tend to be provoked by the less-soluble corticosteroid preparations, one of the more soluble corticosteroids should be used when injecting patients with a history of postinjection flare. Rarely, skin and subcutaneous tissue atrophy at the site of injection; darker-skinned patients should be forewarned about potential loss of pigmented cells, which can be distressing. Systemic effects from single injections are common, but usually mild and transient, and include flushing, slight agitation, and exacerbation of diabetic tendencies. People who have received repeated injections can show signs of exogenous hypercortisolism. Adrenal suppression is possible when injections are given more than once or twice per month; hence, frequently injected patients facing major physiologic stress (e.g., abdominal surgery) should have their adrenal reserve tested to determine if supplemental corticosteroids should be given.

Concerns that cartilage and supporting structures might be weakened by repeated corticosteroid injections, with accelerated demise of a joint as a consequence, have not been supported by clinical observations or studies of primate models (6). The commonly stated limit of three to four injections per year for large, weight-bearing joints should be observed for the nearly normal joint, but patients with established arthritis for which few therapeutic alternatives exist can be injected more frequently. Tendons, ligaments, and their attachments to bone can be disrupted by corticosteroids when injected directly, and care must be taken to confine injections to adjacent synovial sheaths and bursae. Chances for directly inducing infection are extremely slim, with incidence rates from 1:1000 to 1:16,000 in experienced hands; however, in several series that examined risk factors for septic arthritis, up to 20% of infected joints had been injected within the previous three months (7).

Injection Technique

Successful therapeutic injection depends on familiarity with the regional anatomy of the structure to be entered. Before other preparations take place, the injector should form a clear mental image of the site to be entered, which can be marked by penpoint or fingernail indentation, and the path to be taken by the needle. The patient should be positioned so that structures on either side of the injection target are relaxed. Skin-cleansing and hand-washing provide sufficient asepsis (8); sterile gloves are advised when extensive palpation is anticipated; and sterile draping is reserved for the immunocompromised patient or a probable lengthy or difficult procedure. Patients generally appreciate measures to reduce the sensation of needle puncture, such as spraying the site with ethyl chloride solution or infiltrating the skin and subcutaneous tissues with lidocaine delivered through an ultrathin needle. When lidocaine is used, the track to the structure of interest can be found with certainty and marked by leaving the needle in place, pending puncture of the same site with a larger needle. Even when delivery of medication is the sole purpose, success in obtaining fluid assures that the needle has indeed entered a synovial space (9). Evacuating all obtainable synovial fluid removes phlogistic material, minimizes dilution of the injected compound, and has been shown in a prospective controlled trial to prolong relief (compared with no aspiration) in RA patients injected with triamcinolone for knee synovitis (10).

Of the several corticosteroid preparations available (Table 44-2), the less-soluble compounds tend to be preferred for joint-space injections, although some physicians avoid the fluorinated compounds for peritendon and bursal injections because of their propensity to cause soft-tissue atrophy (5). The optimal dose and volume to be injected into any specific structure has not been determined, but most clinicians deliver 1–2 cc of corticosteroid preparation to large joints (knees, hips, shoulders), half that amount to medium joints (wrists, elbows, ankles), and half-again as much (or less) to small joints and soft-tissue sites. Dilution with lidocaine provides some immediate temporary relief to the patient, assures the clinician that the desired structure was entered, and provides a vehicle to deliver corticosteroid to all reaches of the joint space. To promote this latter effect, some clinicians inject a 10-cc steroid–lidocaine admixture into larger joints (11), although most use less. Moving an injected joint through its physiologic range and gently massaging an injected soft-tissue structure also promote drug delivery. Some limitation on joint use following injection can prolong therapeutic benefit, but optimum duration of joint rest has not been determined; mandated rest (enforced with a sling, splint, or crutches) as long as three weeks for upper-extremity joints and six weeks for lower-extremity joints has been described. The only con-

TABLE 44-2
Corticosteroid Preparations for Therapeutic Injection

Compound (in order of relative solubility)	Concentration (mg/mL)	Glucocorticoid potency (hydrocortisone equivalents/mg)
Triamcinolone hexacetonide[a]	20	5
Triamcinolone acetonide[a]	40	5
Prednisolone tebutate	20	4
Methylprednisolone acetate	20, 40, 80	5
Dexamethasone acetate[a]	8	25
Hydrocortisone acetate	25, 50	1
Triamcinolone diacetate[a]	40	5
Betamethasone sodium phosphate and acetate[a]	6	25
Dexamethasone sodium phosphate[a]	4	25
Prednisolone sodium phosphate	20	4

[a] Fluorinated compounds.

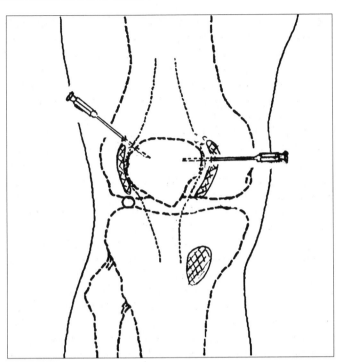

Fig. 44-1. Aspiration and injection sites for the painful knee. The circle lateral to the patellar tendon at the joint line can be entered to deliver corticosteroids into a flexed knee. Hatched areas on either side of the patella correspond to soft-tissue injection sites. The hatched area medial and inferior to the joint line represents the region of pes anserine bursa.

trolled trial published to date found that triamcinolone-injected knees that received 24 hours of rest after injection fared significantly better six months later, compared with injected knees that had not been rested (12).

Injections in Specific Disorders

Rheumatoid Arthritis

The often-dramatic effects of corticosteroid injections in RA can sometimes lead to an unfortunate overdependence on this modality and a neglect of other forms of therapy. For the person with RA who receives more than an occasional injection, a dedicated log in the outpatient record that tracks such injections can show overreliance on intra-articular therapy. Certain extra-articular features of RA respond well to local injections, particularly entrapment neuropathies due to synovial proliferation at the volar aspect of the wrist (carpal tunnel), medial aspect of the elbow (cubital tunnel), and medial aspect of the ankle (tarsal tunnel). Rheumatoid nodules usually shrink in response to corticosteroid delivered nearby (13).

Osteoarthritis

The role of local corticosteroids in OA remains relatively controversial. An older study of knee OA showing no additional benefit from cortisone, when compared with injections of inert compounds or placebo puncture (14), has not stemmed

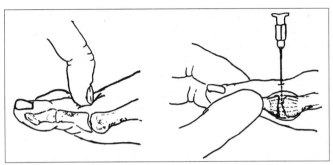

Fig. 44-2. Arthrocentesis/injection of the first metatarsophalangeal joint. Joint line is palpated, then marked with imprint of thumbnail (left panel). Gentle distraction of the phalanx widens joint space, easing entry into capsule by needle oriented perpendicularly to phalanx, penetrating skin at marked joint line just medial to extensor tendon (right panel).

the popularity of intra-articular corticosteroids for painful knee OA, and has been partly contraverted by subsequent studies (6,15). Although inflammation in OA is considered a secondary phenomenon, features of local inflammation often are present and predict response to injection (15). However, pain often arises from structures that are exterior to the joint capsule. Experienced clinicians seek and inject the irritated pes anserine bursa in people with knee pain and OA (Fig. 44-1) (16). A study that compared periarticular delivery of corticosteroids to the traditional intra-articular route found OA pain relief to be greater and longer lasting in patients given soft-tissue injection (17).

Crystalline Arthropathy

Joint entry is important for diagnosis of crystalline arthropathy and can be used for treatment, often at the same time.

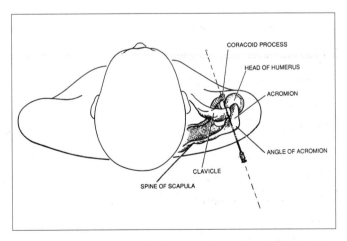

Fig. 44-3. Posterior approach for entry of glenohumeral joint. Line drawn from point 1 cm medial to angle of acromion through tip of coracoid process passes directly through glenohumeral joint. Optimal site for entry located 1 cm inferior and 1 cm medial to bend of acromial angle, found by palpating spine of scapula. Keeping index finger of opposite hand on coracoid process during procedure provides mental "target" for the aspirating/injecting needle.

Intra-articular injection avoids the potential toxicities of systemic nonsteroidal anti-inflammatories, colchicine, or corticosteroids, and is safe, provided infection is unlikely. Because concomitant gout and infection is a negligible possibility when a typical joint flares without systemic features (18), local injection immediately after obtaining synovial fluid may be the treatment modality of choice (Fig. 44-2).

Others

Several regional disorders respond to local injection. Certain common entities, such as trochanteric bursitis, require only that the tender site be pinpointed before being entered. Injections for tendinitis and entrapment neuropathies require additional skill and should not be attempted without an experienced guide (19). Only a few entities affect the true shoulder (glenohumeral) joint in isolation, including primary OA, infection, and adhesive capsulitis. The latter process can be treated by injecting a large volume of diluted corticosteroid–anesthetic mixture (20), but requires definite joint entry (Fig. 44-3).

ROBERT W. IKE, MD

References

1. Hollander JL, Brown EM, Jessar RA, Brown CY. Hydrocortisone and cortisone injected into arthritic joints. Comparative effects of and use of hydrocortisone as a local antiarthritic agent. JAMA 1951;147:1629–1635.

2. Hunter JA, Blyth TH. A risk-benefit assessment of intra-articular corticosteroids in rheumatic disorders. Drug Saf 1999;21: 353–365.

3. Brandt KD, Smith GN Jr, Simon LS. Intraarticular injection of hyaluronan as treatment for knee osteoarthritis: what is the evidence? Arthritis Rheum 2000;43:1192–1203.

4. Thumboo J, O'Duffy JD. A prospective study of the safety of joint and soft tissue aspirations in patients taking warfarin sodium. Arthritis Rheum 1998;41:736–739.

5. McCarty DJ, Harman JG, Grassanovich JL, Qian C. Treatment of rheumatoid joint inflammation with intrasynovial triamcinolone hexacetonide. J Rheumatol 1995;22:1631–1635.

6. Creamer P. Intra-articular corticosteroid treatment in osteoarthritis. Curr Opin Rheumatol 1999;11:417–421.

7. von Essen R, Savolainen HA. Bacterial infection following intra-articular injection. Scand J Rheumatol 1989;18:7–12.

8. Cawley PJ, Morris IM. A study to compare the efficacy of two methods of skin preparation prior to joint injection. Br J Rheumatol 1992;31:847–848.

9. Jones A, Regan M, Ledingham J, Pattrick M, Manhire A, Doherty M. Importance of placement of intra-articular steroid injections. Br Med J 1993;307:1329–1330.

10. Weitoft T, Uddenfeldt P. Importance of synovial fluid aspiration when injecting intra-articular corticosteroids. Ann Rheum Dis 2000;59:233–235.

11. Schaffer TC. Joint and soft-tissue arthrocentesis. Primary Care 1993;20:757–770.

12. Chakravarty K, Pharoah PD, Scott DG. A randomized controlled study of post-injection rest following intra-articular steroid therapy for knee synovitis. Br J Rheumatol 1994;33: 464–468.

13. Ching DW, Petrie JP, Klemp P, Jones JG. Injection therapy of superficial rheumatoid nodules. Br J Rheumatol 1992;31: 775–777.

14. Miller JH, White J, Norton TH. The value of intra-articular injections in osteoarthritis of the knee. J Bone Joint Surg [Br] 1958;40B:636–643.

15. Gaffney K, Ledingham J, Perry JD. Intra-articular triamcinolone hexacetonide on knee osteoarthritis: factors influencing the clinical response. Ann Rheum Dis 1995;54:379–381.

16. Larsson LG, Baum J. The syndrome of anserina bursitis: an overlooked diagnosis. Arthritis Rheum 1985;28:1062–1065.

17. Sambrook PN, Champion GD, Browne CD, et al. Corticosteroid injection for osteoarthritis of the knee: peripatellar compared to intra-articular route. Clin Exp Rheum 1989;7:609–613.

18. Ike RW. Bacterial arthritis. In: Koopman WJ (ed). Arthritis and Allied Conditions, 13th edition. Baltimore: Lippincott Williams & Wilkins, 2001; pp 2570–2599.

19. Doherty M, Hazleman BL, Hutton CW, Maddison PJ, Perry JD (eds). Rheumatology Examination and Injection Techniques. London: WB Saunders, 1992.

20. Gam AN, Schydlowsky P, Rossel I, Remvig L, Jensen EM. Treatment of "frozen shoulder" with distension and glucocorticoid compared with glucocorticoid alone. Scand J Rheumatol 1998;27:425–430.

45 NONSTEROIDAL ANTI-INFLAMMATORY DRUGS

Nonsteroidal anti-inflammatory drugs (NSAIDs) are anti-inflammatory, analgesic, and antipyretic agents used to reduce pain, decrease gelling, and improve function in people with many different forms of arthritis. However, these drugs have never been shown to alter the natural history of any disease. There are at least 20 different NSAIDs currently available in the United States (Table 45-1). In addition, cyclooxygenase-2 (COX-2)-specific inhibitors are available with similar efficacy but significantly decreased gastrointestinal (GI) and platelet effects.

NSAIDs represent one of the most commonly used classes of drugs in the world. Approximately 60 million NSAID prescriptions are written each year in the United States; the number for elderly patients exceeds that for younger patients by approximately 3.6-fold. Aspirin (ASA), ibuprofen, naproxen, and ketoprofen are available over the counter. At equipotent doses, the clinical efficacy and tolerability of the various NSAIDs are similar; however, individual responses are highly variable. Although it is believed that if a patient does not respond to an NSAID of one class, it is reasonable to try an NSAID from a different class, this theory has not been studied in a prospective, controlled manner (1,2).

Sodium salicylic acid was discovered in 1763. Impure forms of salicylates had been used as analgesics and antipyretics throughout the previous century. Once purified and synthesized, the acetyl derivative of salicylate (acetylsalicylic acid, or ASA) was found to provide more anti-inflammatory activity than salicylate alone. Due to the toxicity of ASA, particularly related to the potential for upper gastrointestinal (GI) intolerance, phenylbutazone, an indoleacetic acid derivative, was introduced in the early 1950s. This agent was the first nonsalicylate NSAID developed for use in people with painful and inflammatory conditions. However, due to concerns related to bone-marrow toxicity, particularly in women over the age of 60, this compound now is rarely prescribed. Indomethacin, another indoleacetic acid derivative, was developed in the 1960s to substitute for phenylbutazone.

Mechanisms of Action

The primary mechanism of action of the NSAIDs is the inhibition of prostaglandin (PG) synthesis (3,4). Some NSAIDs are potent inhibitors of prostaglandin synthesis, but others more prominently affect biologic events not mediated by prostaglandins. Differential effects have been attributed to variations in the enantiomeric state of the agent, and to its pharmacokinetics, pharmacodynamics, and metabolism. Although variability can be explained in part by absorption, distribution, and metabolism, potential differences in mechanism of action must be considered (5).

Inhibition of Prostaglandin Synthesis

By decreasing the production of prostaglandins of the E series, NSAIDs produce anti-inflammatory and analgesic effects. These prostanoic acids are proinflammatory, increase vascular permeability, and increase sensitivity to the release of bradykinins. NSAIDs also inhibit the formation of prostacyclin and thromboxane, resulting in complex effects on vascular permeability and platelet aggregation (6).

NSAIDs specifically inhibit COX, and thereby reduce the conversion of arachidonic acid to PGs. ASA acetylates the COX enzyme, but all of the nonsalicylate NSAIDs are reversible inhibitors, maintaining an effect based on serum half-life (7).

There are at least two isoforms of the COX enzymes (6,8), and they differ most importantly in their regulation and expression. COX-1 is expressed constitutively in most tissues, and is inhibited by all NSAIDs to varying degrees, depending on the system used to measure drug effects. COX-1 helps maintain the integrity of the gastric and duodenal mucosa; many of the toxic effects of the NSAIDs on the GI tract are attributed to its inhibition. It is important in modulating renal plasma flow, particularly in patients who are relatively dehydrated, or who have clinically significant congestive heart failure, cirrhosis with or without ascites, or such intrinsic kidney disease as systemic lupus erythematosus (SLE) or diabetes.

The other isoform, COX-2, is an inducible enzyme and is usually undetectable in most tissues. Its expression is increased during states of inflammation or, experimentally, in response to mitogenic stimuli. The expression of COX-2 is inhibited by corticosteroids (9,10). COX-2 activity is important for modulating glomerular blood flow and renal electrolyte and water balance.

The activity of both COX-1 and COX-2 is inhibited, to some degree, by all of the currently available NSAIDs. The clinical effectiveness of these drugs is believed to be due to their effects on COX-2, whereas many of the mechanism-based toxic effects are secondary to inhibition of COX-1.

Evidence has accumulated that several NSAIDs are more selective for COX-2 than for COX-1. For example, in vitro effects of low-dose etodolac and meloxicam demonstrate approximately a 10-fold inhibition of COX-2 compared to COX-1 (6). At higher, anti-inflammatory doses, this specificity is mitigated. Specific COX-2 inhibitors (or COX-1–sparing agents) are at least 300 times more effective

TABLE 45-1
Nonsteroidal Anti-Inflammatory Drugs

NSAID	Trade name	Usual dosage[a]	Approved use[b]
Carboxylic Acids			
Aspirin (acetylsalicylic acid)	Multiple	2.4–6 g/24 h in 4–5 divided doses	RA, OA, AS, JCA, ST
Buffered aspirin	Multiple	Same	Same
Enteric-coated salicylates	Multiple	Same	Same
Salsalate	Disalcid	1.5–3.0 g/24 h bid	Same
Diflunisal	Dolobid	0.5–1.5 g/24 h bid	Same
Choline magnesium trisalicylate	Trilisate	1.5–3 g/24 h bid–tid	RA, OA, pain, JCA
Propionic Acids			
Ibuprofen	Motrin, Rufen, OTC	OTC: 200–400 mg qid Rx: 400, 600, 800 max: 3200 mg/24 h	RA, OA,JCA
Naproxen	Naprelan, Anaprox	250, 375, 500 mg bid	RA, OA, JCA, ST
Fenoprofen	Nalfon	300-600 mg qid	RA, OA
Ketoprofen	Orudis	75 mg tid	RA, OA
Flurbiprofen	Ansaid	100 mg bid–tid	RA, OA
Tolmetin	Tolectin	400, 600, 800 mg; 800–2400 mg/24 h	RA, OA, JCA
Acetic Acid Derivatives			
Indomethacin	Indocin, Indocin	SR 25, 50 mg tid–qid SR:75 mg bid; rarely >150 mg/24 h	RA, OA,G, AS
Tolmetin	see above		
Sulindac	Clinoril	150, 200 mg bid (some increase to tid)	RA, OA, AS, ST, G
Diclofenac	Voltaren, Arthrotec	50 tid, 75 mg bid	RA, OA, AS
Etodolac	Lodine	200, 300 mg b-t-qid. max: 1200 mg/24 h	OA, pain
Fenamates			
Meclofenamate	Meclomen	50–100 mg tid–qid	RA, OA
Mefenamic acid	Ponstel	250 mg qid	RA, OA
Enolic Acids			
Piroxicam	Feldene	10, 20 mg qd	RA, OA
Phenylbutazone	Butazolidin	100 mg tid up to 600 mg/24 h	AS, gout
Meloxicam	Mobic	7.5 mg qd USA	OA
		15 mg qd elsewhere	OA, RA
Naphthylkanones			
Nabumetone	Relafen	500 mg bid up to 1500 mg/24 h	RA, OA
COX-2 Inhibitors			
Celecoxib	Celebrex	100, 200 mg bid,	RA, OA
		200 mg qd	OA
Rofecoxib	Vioxx	12.5, 25 mg qd	RA, OA
		50 mg qd	acute pain
Valdecoxib	Bextra	25 mg qd	RA, OA

[a] bid, twice per day; tid, three times per day; qid, four times per day; qd, per day

[b] FDA approved: RA, rheumatoid arthritis; OA, osteoarthritis; AS, ankylosing spondylitis; G, gout; JCA, juvenile chronic polyarthritis; ST, soft tissue injury.

at inhibiting COX-2 activity than COX-1, and have no measurable effect on COX-1–mediated events at therapeutic dose (8). Both celecoxib and rofecoxib are as effective at inhibiting OA pain, dental pain, and the pain and inflammation associated with RA as is naproxen at 500 mg twice per day, ibuprofen at 800 mg three times per day, and diclofenac at 75 mg twice per day, without endoscopic evidence of gastroduodenal damage and without affecting platelet aggregation (11). Large GI outcome trials have demonstrated that celecoxib and rofecoxib, at two to four times the normal treatment dosages for RA and OA (respectively), have a twofold to threefold decreased incidence of important GI bleeding, perforation, or obstruction, as compared with ibuprofen or naproxen at normal treatment dosages (12,13). Unfortunately, due to the design of the randomized, controlled trials, many of the important questions regarding the renal effects of the specific COX-2 inhibitors remain unanswered.

It has been described that PGs inhibit apoptosis and that NSAIDs, via inhibition of PG synthesis, may reestablish more normal cell-cycle responses. Evidence also suggests that some NSAIDs may reduce PGH synthase gene expression, supporting the clinical evidence of differences in activity in NSAIDs in sites of active inflammation (10).

Other Potential Mechanisms

NSAIDs are lipophilic and become incorporated in the lipid bilayer of cell membranes, and thereby may interrupt protein-protein interactions important for signal transduction. For example, stimulus-response coupling, which is critical for recruitment of phagocytic cells to sites of inflammation, has been demonstrated in vitro to be inhibited by some NSAIDs. NSAIDs inhibit activation and chemotaxis of neutrophils and reduce toxic oxygen radical production in stimulated neutrophils. NSAIDs scavenge superoxide radicals (14,15).

Salicylates inhibit phospholipase C activity in macrophages, inhibiting the arachidonic cascade earlier than do the COX enzymes. Some NSAIDs affect T-lymphocyte function experimentally by inhibiting rheumatoid factor production in vitro. Neutrophil endothelial cell adherence, which is critical to migration of granulocytes to sites of inflammation, is disrupted, and expression of L-selectins is decreased (14,15,16). NSAIDs have been demonstrated in vitro to inhibit NF-κB (nitric oxide transcription factor)-dependent transcription, thereby inhibiting inducible nitric-oxide synthetase (17). Anti-inflammatory levels of ASA inhibit expression of inducible nitric-oxide synthetase and subsequent production of nitrite in vitro. At pharmacologic dosages, sodium salicylate, indomethacin, and acetaminophen were studied and had no effect, but at suprapharmacologic dosages, sodium salicylate inhibited nitrite production. Although nonacetylated salicylates have been shown in vitro to inhibit neutrophil function and to have equal efficacy in patients with RA (18), clinically, there is no evidence to suggest that biologic effects other than PG synthase inhibition are more important.

Pharmacology

Bioavailability

All NSAIDs are absorbed completely after oral administration. Absorption rates may vary in patients with altered GI blood flow or motility and, with certain NSAIDs, when taken with food. Enteric coating may reduce direct effects of NSAIDs on the gastric mucosa, but also may reduce the rate of absorption.

Most NSAIDs are weak organic acids; once absorbed, they are >95% bound to serum albumin. Clinically significant decreases in serum albumin levels or institution of other highly protein-bound medications may lead to an increase in the free component of NSAID in serum. This process may be important in people who are elderly or chronically ill with associated hypoalbuminemic states. Due to increased vascular permeability in localized sites of inflammation, this high degree of protein binding may result in delivery of higher levels of NSAIDs.

Metabolism

NSAIDs are metabolized predominantly in the liver and excreted in the urine. This process must be considered when prescribing NSAIDs for people with hepatic or renal dysfunction. Some NSAIDs, such as oxaprozin, have two metabolic pathways, through which some portion is secreted directly into the bile and another part is further metabolized and excreted in the urine. Other NSAIDs (e.g., indomethacin, sulindac, and piroxicam) have prominent enterohepatic circulation, resulting in a prolonged half-life, and should be used with caution in the elderly. In patients with renal insufficiency, some inactive metabolites may be resynthesized in vivo to the active compound. Diclofenac, flurbiprofen, celecoxib, and rofecoxib are metabolized in the liver, and should be used with care and at lowest possible doses in patients with clinically significant liver disease, including cirrhosis with or without ascites, prolonged prothrombin times, falling serum albumin levels, or important elevations in liver transaminases in blood. Most of the NSAIDs and celecoxib are metabolized through the P450 CYP2C9 isoenzyme; however, rofecoxib is not. The exact metabolic pathways for rofecoxib remain unknown.

Salicylates are the least highly protein-bound NSAID: approximately 68%. Zero-order kinetics are dominant in salicylate metabolism, and increasing the dose of salicylates is effective over a narrow range, but once the metabolism is saturated, incremental dose increases may lead to very high serum salicylate levels. Changes in salicylate doses need to be considered carefully at chronic steady-state levels, particularly in patients with altered renal or hepatic function.

Plasma Half-Life

Significant differences in plasma half-lives of the NSAIDs may be important in explaining their diverse clinical effects. Those with long half-lives typically do not attain maximum plasma concentrations quickly, and clinical responses may be delayed. Piroxicam has the longest serum half-life of currently marketed NSAIDs: 57 ± 22 hours, and diclofenac has one of the shortest: 1.1 ± 0.2 hours. Although drugs have been developed with very long half-lives to improve patient adherence, it sometimes is preferable to use drugs of shorter half-life so that when the drug is discontinued, the unwanted effects disappear more rapidly.

Sulindac and nabumetone are "prodrugs" in which the active compound is produced after first-pass metabolism through the liver. Prodrugs were developed to decrease the exposure of the GI mucosa to the local effects of the NSAIDs. Unfortunately, the patient is placed at substantial risk of an NSAID-induced upper GI event as long as COX-1 activity is inhibited systemically.

Once plasma steady-state has been achieved, synovial-fluid concentrations of NSAIDs do not vary greatly. Choice of a specific NSAID is based largely on issues of safety and convenience.

Other pharmacologic properties may be important clinically. NSAIDs that are highly lipid-soluble in serum will penetrate the central nervous system more effectively and occasionally produce striking changes in mentation, perception, and mood. Indomethacin has been associated with many of these side effects, even after a single dose, particularly in the elderly.

Adverse Effects

The NSAIDs may produce toxic effects in any organ system. Some effects are mediated by PG synthesis inhibition, and other effects are mediated by unknown mechanisms. Table 45-2 lists important effects, many of which will be discussed in this section.

Hepatotoxicity

Elevation in hepatic transaminase levels is not uncommon, although it occurs more often in patients with juvenile rheumatoid arthritis or SLE. Although many reports indicate that elevated serum transaminases are common in people taking NSAIDs, unless elevations exceed two to three times the upper limits of normal (19), or serum albumin or prothrombin times are altered, these effects usually are not considered clinically significant. However, overt liver failure has been reported following use of many NSAIDs, including diclofenac, flurbiprofen, and sulindac. Of all NSAIDs, sulindac has been associated with the highest incidence of cholestasis (19). When NSAID treatment is initiated, patients should be evaluated within eight to 12 weeks and blood analysis for serum transaminase changes should be considered.

Prostaglandin-Related Adverse Effects

Many adverse reactions attributed to NSAIDs are due to inhibition of PG synthesis in local tissues. For example, people with allergic rhinitis, nasal polyposis, or a history of asthma, in whom NSAIDs effectively inhibit PG synthetase, are at increased risk for anaphylaxis. Although the exact mechanism for this effect remains unclear, it is known that

TABLE 45-2
Adverse Reactions to the NSAIDs

Gastrointestinal
Nausea, vomiting, dyspepsia, diarrhea, constipation

Gastric mucosal irritation, superficial erosions, peptic ulceration, increased fecal blood wasting

Major gastrointestinal hemorrhage, penetrating ulcers, small-bowel erosions, induce "diaphragm" development in small bowel

Liver
Hepatotoxicity, hepatitis, fulminant hepatic failure

Renal
Glomerulopathy, interstitial nephritis, alterations in renal plasma flow leading to fall in glomerular filtration rates, interfere with naturesis induced by diuretics, inhibit renin release, induce edema

Alterations in tubular functions

Central Nervous System
Headaches, confusion, hallucinations, depersonalization reactions, depression, tremor

Aseptic meningitis, tinnitus, vertigo, neuropathy, toxic amblyopia, transient transparent corneal deposits

Hematologic
Anemia, marrow depression, Coomb's-positive anemia, decrease platelet aggregation

Hypersensitivity
Asthma, asthma/urticaria syndrome, urticaria, rashes, photosensitivity, Stevens-Johnson syndrome

Other
Drug interactions such as displacement of oral hypo-glycemics and warfarin from protein-binding sites and from sites of metabolism

Interference with the actions of β blockers and some diuretics

E prostaglandins serve as bronchodilators. When COX activity is inhibited in people at risk, a decrease in synthesis of PGs that contribute to bronchodilation results. Another explanation implicates the alternate pathway of arachidonate metabolism, whereby shunting of arachidonate into the leukotriene pathway occurs when COX is inhibited. This explanation implies that large stores of arachidonate released in certain inflammatory situations lead to excess substrate for leukotriene metabolism. This process results in release of products that are highly reactive, such as the "SRSA" pathway that stimulates anaphylaxis.

Platelet Effects

Platelet aggregation is induced primarily by stimulating thromboxane production with activation of platelet COX-1. There is no COX-2 in platelets. NSAIDs and ASA inhibit the activity of COX-1, but the COX-2–specific inhibitors have no effect on COX-1 at therapeutic doses.

The effect of the nonsalicylate NSAIDs on platelet function is reversible and related to the half-life of the drug; however, ASA acetylates the COX-1 enzyme, serving to permanently inactivate it. The individual platelet cannot make new COX enzyme, so after exposure to ASA, the platelet does not function appropriately. Only with repopulation of platelets not exposed to ASA will normal platelet aggregation return. Therefore, people awaiting surgery should discontinue NSAIDs at a time determined by four to five times their serum half-life. Aspirin needs to be discontinued one to two weeks before the planned procedure to allow a normal platelet population to re-establish.

ASA decreases the risk of recurrent thromboembolic disease in patients with a history of cerebrovascular or cardiovascular disease. It is useful partly because it decreases platelet aggregation through inhibition of COX-1. Because the COX-2–specific inhibitors do not affect platelets, patients at risk for a thromboembolic event who are to be treated with a COX-2–specific inhibitor must be treated with concomitant low-dose ASA. Furthermore, it is not known whether the long-acting, nonselective NSAIDs are as effective as low-dose ASA in preventing further thromboembolic events in people at risk. Only ASA has been studied prospectively, and low-dose aspirin should be given concomitantly with either nonselective NSAIDs or specific COX-2 inhibitors in patients at risk for thrombosis.

Gastrointestinal Effects

The most clinically significant adverse effects following use of NSAIDs occur in the GI tract. NSAIDs cause a wide range of GI problems, including abdominal pain, dyspepsia, nausea, and vomiting, as well as esophagitis, esophageal stricture, gastritis, mucosal erosions, hemorrhage, peptic ulceration and perforation, obstruction, and death (20). The cause of such NSAID-induced GI symptoms as abdominal pain, dyspepsia, and diarrhea remains unknown. The structural changes beginning with ulcers are due to systemic inhibition of PG synthesis. In addition to the known effects on gastric and duodenal mucosa, there is increasing evidence that the mucosa of the large and small bowel are affected. These agents also may induce stricture formation. These strictures may manifest as diaphragms that precipitate small- or large-bowel obstruction, and may be very hard to detect on contrast radiographic studies. There also is evidence to suggest that NSAIDs induce dysfunction in GI mucosal permeability (20,21).

NSAIDs rapidly penetrate the GI mucosa in the presence of stomach acid, leading to oxidative uncoupling of cellular metabolism that leads to local tissue injury and cell death. This damage consists of local erosions and hemorrhages that can, with further damage, lead to formation of clinically significant ulcers (21).

The magnitude of risk for clinically important adverse GI events is controversial. The FDA reports an overall risk of 2%–4% per year for NSAID-induced gastric ulcer development and its complications (20,22). In general, the relative risk as summarized in multiple clinical trials ranges from 4.0 to 5.0 for the development of gastric ulcer, from 1.1 to 1.6 for the development of duodenal ulcer, and from 4.5 to 5.0 for the development of clinically significant gastric ulcer with hemorrhage, perforation, or death. Some data suggest that the risk of hospitalization for adverse GI effects may be sevenfold to 10-fold greater in people with RA treated with NSAIDs, compared with those who are not receiving these agents.

Epidemiologic studies suggest that the safest NSAIDs are nonacetylated salicylates. However, there are controversial data about their efficacy at safe doses. Those NSAIDs with prominent enterohepatic circulation and significantly prolonged half-lives, such as sulindac and piroxicam, have been linked to increased gastrointestinal toxicity due to re-exposure of gastric and duodenal mucosa to bile reflux, and thus the active moiety of the drug. Other sites in the GI tract, including the esophagus and small and large bowel, also may be affected. Exposure to NSAIDs probably is a major factor in the development of esophagitis and subsequent stricture formation.

Endoscopic studies have demonstrated that NSAID administration results in shallow erosions or submucosal hemorrhages that, although they can occur at any site in the GI tract, are observed more commonly in the stomach, near the prepyloric area and the antrum. Typically, these lesions are asymptomatic, making prevalence data difficult to determine. There are data demonstrating that NSAID-induced ulcers >3 mm in diameter, with obvious depth, are found in 15%–31% of patients so treated. It is unknown how many lesions spontaneously heal or progress to ulceration, frank perforation, gastric or duodenal obstruction, serious GI hemorrhage, and subsequent death. Risk factors for developing GI toxicity in people receiving NSAIDs include age >60 years, history of peptic ulcer disease, prior use of anti-ulcer therapies for any reason, concomitant use of corticosteroids (particularly in people with RA), such comorbidities as significant cardiovascular disease, and severe RA. Other risk factors include increased doses of specific and singular NSAIDs (Table 45-3).

Endoscopic data from large numbers of people treated with COX-2–specific inhibitors demonstrate that induction of ulcers occurs at the same rate as in patients who received placebo (4–8%). After one week of treatment, the active comparators induced ulcers >3 mm in diameter, with obvious depth, in 15% of healthy volunteers taking diclofenac (75 mg twice per day) or ibuprofen (800 mg three times per day) and in 19% of healthy volunteers taking naproxen (500 mg twice per day). After 12 weeks of treatment, ulcers

TABLE 45-3
Risk Factors for NSAID-Induced Gastroduodenal Toxic Effects

Increasing patient age (>60 years)
Extent of current and past disease
History of peptic ulcer disease
History of gastrointestinal bleeding
Concomitant use of NSAIDs with corticosteroid therapy
Dose of the NSAID
Combinations of NSAIDs
History of GI intolerance to NSAIDs

were induced in 26% of patients with OA and RA taking naproxen (500 mg twice per day) or ibuprofen (800 mg three times per day) (23,24). In addition, ulcer complications, such as obstruction, perforation, or bleeds, are two to three times less with the COX-2–specific inhibitors than with the active comparators (12,13). It is possible that patients with ulcers secondary to low-dose aspirin administration for cardiovascular prophylaxis and patients infected with *Helicobacter pylori* may demonstrate delay in healing of those ulcers when treated with COX-2–specific inhibitors, but this association was not observed in the long-term outcome trials of the COX-2–specific inhibitors.

Approach to the Patient at Risk for GI Events
The approach to the patient who requires chronic NSAID treatment and has developed or is at risk for an NSAID-induced GI event is controversial (Table 45-4). Many patients who have dyspepsia or upper-GI distress while being treated with nonselective NSAIDs typically manifest superficial erosions by endoscopy, which often heal spontaneously without change in therapy. Even more difficult to evaluate is whether agents documented as cytoprotective actually alter NSAID-induced symptoms, which may or may not predict significant GI events. Clinical studies have demonstrated that more than 80% of patients who develop significant NSAID-induced endoscopic abnormalities are asymptomatic (25). However, prospective observational trials have demonstrated that patients are more symptomatic when they develop NSAID-induced toxicities than was previously believed.

If a patient develops a gastric or duodenal ulcer while taking NSAIDs, treatment should be discontinued and therapy for ulcer disease instituted with H_2-antagonist or proton-pump inhibitors (PPIs). If NSAIDs must be continued, the patient will need anti-ulcer therapy for longer periods of time. Diagnostic tests to determine if the patient is *H. pylori*-positive should be performed; if the patient has measurable antibodies, specific antibiotic therapy to eradicate the infection should be administered.

Preventing NSAID-induced gastric and duodenal ulcers is more complicated. There is no evidence that agents other than

misoprostol will prevent NSAID-induced gastric ulceration and its complications. Although H_2-antagonists and PPIs have been demonstrated to prevent NSAID-induced duodenal ulcers, prevention of gastric ulcerations has not been clearly shown. An endoscopy study has shown that famotidine at twice the approved dose (40 mg twice per day) significantly decreased the incidence of both gastric and duodenal ulcers. Similarly, an endoscopy study demonstrated that treatment with omeprazole decreased gastroduodenal ulcers. Although H_2-antagonists and PPIs effectively decrease NSAID-induced dyspeptic symptoms, neither has been studied to determine if they decrease the incidence of ulcer complications.

Misoprostol is a PG analog that locally replaces the PGs normally synthesized in the gastric mucosa, but its synthesis is inhibited by NSAIDs. Misoprostol has been shown to successfully inhibit by 40% the development of such ulcer complications as bleeding, perforation, and obstruction, compared to placebo. Further analysis of these data demonstrate that patients with health assessment questionnaire (HAQ) scores >1.5 (worse disease) had an 87% reduction in risk for an NSAID-induced toxic event if concomitantly treated with misoprostol, 200 µg four times per day.

These data suggest that high-risk patients may benefit from concomitant misoprostol therapy if NSAID treatment

TABLE 45-4
Prophylaxis and Treatment of NSAID-Induced GI Disease

Antacids
 No data demonstrates usefulness

Sulcrafate
 No data demonstrates prevention or improvement of
  gastric ulcers

H_2-antagonists
 Heal duodenal lesions
 Prevent duodenal lesions
 High dosages prevent gastric lesions and heal
 NSAID-induced lesions
 Improves symptoms

Omeprazole
 Demonstrates prophylaxis and heals both
  gastroduodenal lesions
 Improves symptoms

Misoprostol
 Heals NSAID-induced gastroduodenal erosive disease
 200 mg qid prevents NSAID-induced gastric and
  duodenal disease
 200 mg bid, tid, qid prevents NSAID-induced erosive
  disease
 Does not improve symptoms

bid, twice per day; tid, three times per day; qid, four times per day is indicated. The pharmacoeconomic utility of such therapy in the high-risk patient has been proved. Unfortunately, 30% of patients complained of diarrhea, the most common adverse event, and diarrhea caused withdrawal of approximately 10% of patients.

The COX-2–specific inhibitors are a choice with less risk for important GI damage and associated complications. These drugs also induce less nonspecific GI complaints than do the nonselective NSAIDs; however, more events are observed than with placebo in randomized, controlled trials.

Renal Adverse Effects

The effects of NSAIDs on renal function include sodium retention, changes in tubular function, interstitial nephritis, and reversible renal failure due to alterations in filtration rate and renal plasma flow (26). Prostaglandins and prostacyclins are important for maintaining intrarenal blood flow and tubular transport of electrolytes and water. All NSAIDs (including the COX-2–specific inhibitors), except nonacetylated salicylates, have the potential to induce reversible impairment of glomerular filtration rate. This effect occurs more frequently in people with congestive heart failure; established renal disease with altered intrarenal plasma flow, including diabetes, hypertension, or atherosclerosis; and induced hypovolemia, due to salt depletion or significant hypoalbuminemia (Table 45-5). Triamterene-containing diuretics, which increase plasma renin levels, may predispose patients receiving NSAIDs to precipitously develop acute renal failure.

NSAID-associated interstitial nephritis typically is manifested as nephrotic syndrome, characterized by edema or anasarca, proteinuria, hematuria, and pyuria. The usual stigmata of drug-induced allergic nephritis, such as eosinophilia, eosinophiluria, and fever, typically are absent. Interstitial infiltrates of mononuclear cells are seen histologically, with relative sparing of the glomeruli. Phenylpropionic acid derivatives, such as fenoprofen, naproxen, and tolmetin, along with the indoleacetic acid derivative indomethacin, most commonly are associated with the development of interstitial nephritis.

Inhibition of PG synthesis intrarenally by NSAIDs decreases renin release, producing a state of hyporeninemic hypoaldosteronism, with resulting hyperkalemia. Physiologically, this effect may be amplified in patients taking potassium-sparing diuretics. Salt retention precipitated by some NSAIDs, which may lead to peripheral edema, likely is due to inhibition of intrarenal prostaglandin production (which decreases renal medullary blood flow), increases in tubular reabsorption of sodium chloride, and direct tubular effects. The frequency of such peripheral edema with standard doses of both the nonselective NSAIDs and the COX-2–specific inhibitors is about 2%–3% in most patients, but in patients at risk, the rate may increase. With increasing dosages of several of the NSAIDs, there is an increased incidence of peripheral edema. NSAIDs also have been reported to increase the effect of antidiuretic hormone, reducing excretion of free water and resulting in hyponatremia. Thiazide diuretics may produce an added effect on

the NSAID-induced hyponatremia. All NSAIDs have been demonstrated to interfere with medical management of hypertension and heart failure by inhibiting the clinical effects of angiotensin-converting enzyme (ACE) inhibitors, β-blockers, and diuretics. All NSAIDs, with the exception of the nonacetylated salicylates, have been associated with increases in mean blood pressure. Patients receiving antihypertensive agents must be checked regularly when initiating therapy with a new NSAID to insure no significant, continued, and sustained rises in blood pressure.

The mechanism of acute renal failure induced in the at-risk patient treated with NSAIDs is believed to be PG-mediated. However, the role of COX-2 in maintenance of renal homeostasis in humans remains unclear. COX-2 activity is notably present in the macula densa and tubules in animals and man, and is up-regulated in salt-depleted animals. In humans, COX-1 is an important enzyme for controlling intrarenal blood flow. There is sufficient evidence to indicate that the COX-2–specific inhibitors will not be safer than traditional NSAIDs in terms of renal function. Until further appropriate clinical trials are conducted, any patient at high risk for renal complications should be monitored carefully. No patient with a creatinine clearance of <30 cc/min should be treated with an NSAID or a COX-2–specific inhibitor.

Other Adverse Effects

Typical nonspecific reactions associated with NSAIDs include skin rash and photosensitivity. The phenylpropionic acid derivatives may induce aseptic meningitis, especially in patients with SLE. The underlying mechanism of action remains unknown. This class of NSAIDs also has been associated with a reversible toxic amblyopia.

TABLE 45-5
Risk Factors for Renal Failure Associated With NSAIDs

High risk
   Volume depletion such as hemodynamically significant bleed, or a patient with hemodynamic compromise such as septic shock
   Severe congestive heart failure
   Hepatic cirrhosis with or without ascites
   Clinically significant dehydration

Low to moderate risk
   Intrinsic renal disease
      Diabetic nephropathy
      Nephrotic syndrome
      Hypertensive nephropathy
   Induction of anesthesia

Questionable risk
   Advanced age

Tinnitus is a common problem with higher doses of salicylates and the nonsalicylate NSAIDs. The mechanism is unknown. The very young and the elderly may not complain of tinnitus, but only of hearing loss. Decreasing the dose usually alleviates the effect. In all circumstances, tinnitus is reversible with discontinuation of medication.

Due to the antiplatelet effects of nonselective NSAIDs (except the nonacetylated salicylates), concomitant therapy with warfarin puts patients at great risk for bleeding. As concomitant NSAID therapy would displace warfarin from its albumin-binding sites, the prothrombin time may be prolonged. In addition, given the increased relative risk for NSAID-induced gastroduodenal ulcers and bleeding, there is an increased risk for bleeding when the NSAIDs are used concomitantly with warfarin. In that the COX-2–specific inhibitors do not cause ulcers of the GI tract nor do they alter platelet function, the patient on warfarin would have less risk for a significant GI bleed when treated with these drugs. Competitive binding effects such as these also may be seen with phenytoin or other highly protein-bound drugs, such as antibiotics. The NSAIDs inhibit the renal excretion of lithium and should be used with caution in patients taking this drug. Cholystyramine, an anion-exchange resin, reduces the rate of NSAID absorption and its bioavailability.

The central nervous system side effects of NSAIDs include aseptic meningitis, psychosis, and cognitive dysfunction (27). The latter changes are seen more commonly in elderly patients treated with indomethacin, and the phenylpropionic acid derivatives are associated more commonly with the development of aseptic meningitis and toxic amblyopia.

Although there are case reports of reversible infertility associated with the use of NSAIDs, given the large numbers of patients who regularly use NSAIDs, there does not appear to be a generalized epidemic of infertility. In addition, there is ample evidence that traditional use of NSAIDs does not lead to osteoporosis. Although inflammation in the joint leads to juxta-articular osteopenia, this development is the result of increased PG synthesis in the inflamed joint, which likely is directly related to increased COX-2 activity.

Some of the early NSAIDs, particularly phenylbutazone and indomethacin, have been associated with an increased risk for bone marrow failure (28). In a case-controlled study using Medicaid claims data, the adjusted odds ratio for neutropenia for patients treated with an NSAID is 4.2 (confidence interval, 2.0–8.7). When patients treated with either phenylbutazone or indomethacin were excluded, the odds ratio for the development of neutropenia still was quite robust, at 3.5 (CI 1.6–7.6). There were no specific risks associated with specific NSAIDs. In general, the NSAIDs are commonly used drugs, yet the incidence of neutropenia is quite small.

There are few data documenting the effects of the NSAIDs on pregnancy or the fetus. In animal models, the NSAIDs have been shown to increase the incidence of dystocia, postimplantation loss, and delay of parturition. The effect of prostaglandin inhibition may result in premature closure of the ductus arteriosus. ASA has been associated with smaller babies and neonatal bruising; however, it has been used for many years in the treatment of people who require NSAIDs while pregnant. In animals, there is no evidence that ASA is a teratogen. The NSAIDs are excreted in breast milk, and it is believed that salicylates in normally recommended doses are not dangerous to nursing infants (29).

A potential pulmonary toxic reaction is the development of pulmonary infiltrates with eosinophilia. Patients with the reaction presented with pneumonia-like symptoms, including shortness of breath and, at times, high fever. Peripheral blood eosinophilia was noted. Corticosteroids and discontinuance of the drug were required to reverse the process. It is unknown whether this reaction is associated with specific NSAIDs or the general class (30).

Summary and Conclusions

Although NSAIDs are known to relieve pain, decrease inflammation, and be antipyretic, they have not been shown to decrease erosions in RA, retard osteophyte formation in OA, or protect cartilage from mechanical or inflammatory injury. However, pretreatment with NSAIDs repeatedly has been demonstrated to decrease heterotopic bone formation after joint replacement. Specific NSAIDs have been shown in vitro to inhibit chondrocyte proteoglycan synthesis. There are a few case reports that suggest the chronic use of some NSAIDs accelerated cartilage damage in OA, and some investigators believe the data to be compelling enough to preclude the use of NSAIDs as standard therapy for OA. Although this effect may have profound implications clinically, only inferential evidence suggests that long-term use of NSAIDs damages cartilage in humans and worsens the clinical course of OA.

The choice of NSAID typically is based on physician-prescribing behaviors. Historically, aspirin congeners, including enteric-coated aspirin, were the first choice for treating inflammatory and degenerative arthritic conditions. Although low in cost, problems included GI intolerance and the need for multiple regular doses throughout the day to maintain adequate anti-inflammatory blood levels. Depending upon body mass, concomitant drug use, serum albumin levels, and other physiologic factors, 10 to 20 plain aspirin tablets daily, taken no more than eight hours apart, usually are required to achieve anti-inflammatory salicylate blood levels. Doses may need to be increased if enteric-coated aspirin is chosen, due to variable absorption within the bowel. The nonsalicylate NSAIDs continue to be important therapeutic choices to alleviate pain and edema associated with chronic joint disease. With the advent of the COX-2–specific inhibitors, there are drugs available that are safer for the GI tract. The important use of these drugs for palliative therapy to reduce pain, edema, and other evidence of inflammation will continue. The choice of the safest possible therapies, which preserve efficacy during long-term use, should be paramount.

LEE S. SIMON, MD

References

1. Baum C, Kennedy DL, Forbes MB. Utilization of nonsteroidal anti-inflammatory drugs Arthritis Rheum 1985;28:686–692.

2. Phillips AC, Polisson RP, Simon LS. NSAIDs and the elderly: toxicity and the economic implications. Drugs Aging 1997;10: 119–130.

3. Brooks PM, Day RO. Nonsteroidal antiinflammatory drugs: differences and similarities. N Engl J Med 1991;324:1716–1725.

4. Furst DE. Are there differences among nonsteroidal antiinflammatory drugs? Comparing acetylated salicylates, nonacetylated salicylates, and nonacetylated nonsteroidal antiinflammatory drugs. Arthritis Rheum 1994;37:1–9.

5. Simon LS, Strand V. Clinical response to nonsteroidal antiinflammatory drugs. Arthritis Rheum 1997;40:1940–1943.

6. Vane JR, Bakhle YS, Botting RM. Cyclooxygenase 1 and 2. Annu Rev Pharmacol Toxicol 1998;38:97–120.

7. Smith WL. Prostanoid biosynthesis and mechanisms of action. Am J Physiol 1992; 263:F181–F196.

8. Lipsky LP, Abramson SB, Crofford L, DuBois RN, Simon L, van de Putte LB. The classification of cyclooxygenase inhibitors. J Rheumatol 1998;25:2298–2303.

9. DuBois RN, Abramson SB, Crofford L, et al. Cyclooxygenase in biology and disease. FASEB J 1998;12:1063–1073.

10. Crofford LJ, Lipsky PE, Brooks P, Abramson SB, Simon LS, Van de Putte LB. Basic biology and clinical application of specific Cyclooxygenase-2 inhibitors. Arthritis Rheum 2000;43: 4–13.

11. Simon LS. Are the biologic and clinical effects of the COX-2-specific inhibitors an advance compared with the effects of traditional NSAIDs? Curr Opin Rheum 2000;12:163–170.

12. Silverstein FE, Faich G, Goldstein JL, et al. Gastrointestinal toxicity with celecoxib vs nonsteroidal anti-inflammatory drugs for osteoarthritis and rheumatoid arthritis. JAMA 2000;284: 1247–1255.

13. Bombardier C, Laine L, Reicin A, et al. Comparison of upper gastrointestinal toxicity of rofecoxib and naproxen in patients with rheumatoid arthritis. N Engl J Med 2000;343:1520–1528.

14. Simon LS. Nonsteroidal anti-inflammatory drugs and their effects: the importance of COX selectivity. J Clin Rheum 1996; 2:135–140.

15. Abramson SB, Leszczynska-Piziak J, Clancy RM, Philips M, Weissmann G. Inhibition of neutrophil function by aspirin-like drugs (NSAIDs): requirement for assembly of heterotrimeric G proteins in bilayer phospholipid. Biochem Pharmacol 1994;47: 563–572.

16. Díaz-González F, González-Alvero I, Companero MR, et al. Prevention of in vitro neutrophil-endothelial attachment through shedding of L-selectin by nonsteroidal antiinflammatory drugs. J Clin Invest 1995;95:1756–1765.

17. Amin AR, Vyas P, Attur M, et al. The mode of action of aspirin-like drugs: effect on inducible nitric oxide synthase. Proc Natl Acad Sci USA 1995;92:7926–7930.

18. Bombardier C, Peloso PM, Goldsmith CH. Salsalate, a nonacetylated salicylate, is as efficacious as diclofenac in patients with rheumatoid arthritis. Salsalate-Diclofenac Study Group. J Rheumatol 1995;22:617–624.

19. Garcia Rodriguez LA, Williams R, Derby LE, Dean AD, Jick H. Acute liver injury associated with nonsteroidal anti-inflammatory drugs and the role of risk factors. Arch Intern Med 1994;154:311–316.

20. Wolfe MM, Lichtenstein DR, Singh G. Gastrointestinal toxicity of the nonsteroidal antiinflammatory drugs. N Engl J Med 1999;340:1888–1899.

21. Mahmud T, Rafi SS, Scott DL, Wrigglesworth JM, Bjarnason I. Nonsteroidal antiinflammatory drugs and uncoupling of mitochondrial oxidative phosphorylation. Arthritis Rheum 1996;39:1998–2003.

22. Fries J. NSAID gastropathy: the second most deadly rheumatic disease? Epidemiology and risk appraisal. J Rheumatol Suppl 1991;28:6–10.

23. Simon LS, Weaver AL, Graham DY, et al. The Anti-inflammatory and upper gastrointestinal effects of celecoxib in rheumatoid arthritis: a randomized, controlled trial. JAMA 1999;282:1921–1928.

24. Laine L, Harper S, Simon T, et al. A randomized trial comparing the effect of rofecoxib, a cyclooxygenase 2-specific inhibitor, with that of ibuprofen on gastroduodenal mucosa of patients with osteoarthritis. Gastroenterology 1999;117:776–783.

25. Singh G, Ramey DR, Morfeld D, Shi H, Hatoum HT, Fries JF. Gastrointestinal tract complications of nonsteroidal antiinflammaotry drug treatment in rheumatoid arthritis. A prospective observational study. Arch Intern Med 1996;156:1530-1536.

26. Whelton A. Nephrotoxicity of nonsteroidal anti-inflammatory drugs: physiologic foundations and clinical implications. Am J Med 1999;106:13S–24S.

27. Hoppmann RA, Peden JG, Ober SK. Central nervous system side effects of nonsteroidal anti-inflammatory drugs. Aseptic meningitis, psychosis, and cognitive dysfunction. Arch Intern Med 1991;151:1309–1313.

28. Strom BL, Carson JL, Schinnar R, Snyder ES, Shaw M, Lundin FE Jr. Nonsteroidal anti-inflammatory drugs and neutropenia. Arch Intern Med 1993;153:2119–2124.

29. Ostensen M, Ostensen H. Safety of nonsteroidal anti-inflammatory drugs in pregnant patients with rheumatic disease. J Rheumatol 1996;23:1045–1049.

30. Goodwin SD, Glenny RW. Nonsteroidal anti-inflammatory drug-associated pulmonary infiltrates with eosinophilia. Arch Intern Med 1992;152:1521–1524.

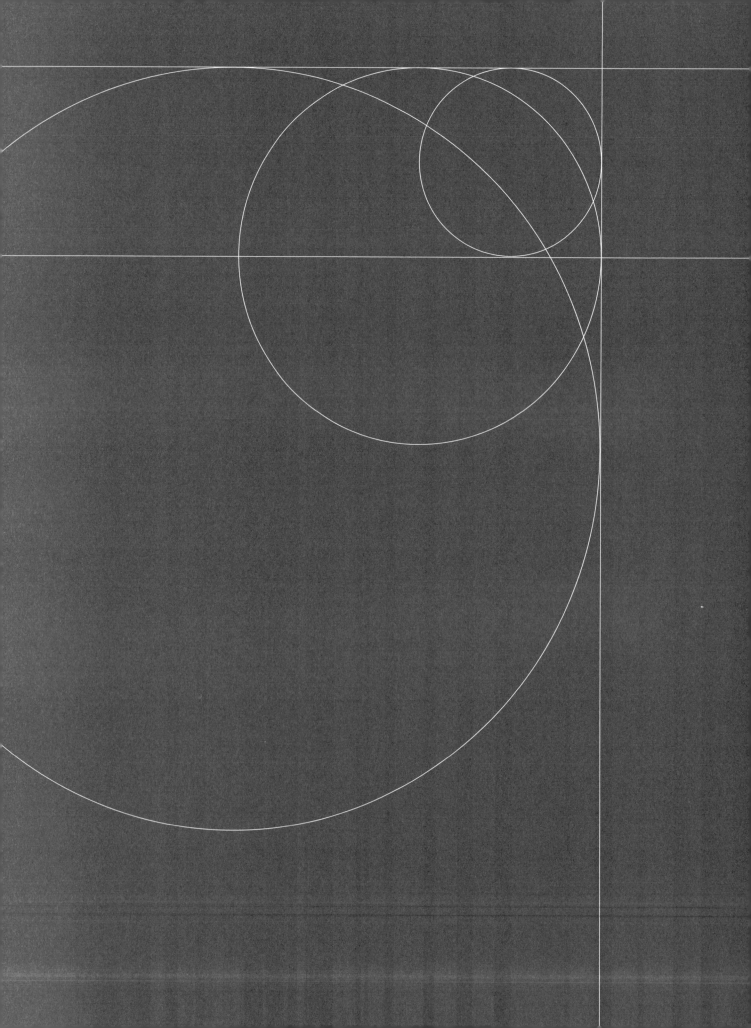

46 CORTICOSTEROIDS

Corticosteroid use is one of the most important and controversial subjects in rheumatology. The dramatic anti-inflammatory effects of corticosteroids were first described in the setting of treating rheumatoid arthritis (RA). This unexpected discovery resulted in a Nobel Prize in 1950 (1,2). The subsequent realization, however, that long-term supraphysiologic therapy produced devastating side effects led to polarized views of the role of corticosteroids in the therapy of rheumatic diseases. Many of the issues remain unresolved, and the controversies continue today (3–7). Nevertheless, corticosteroid therapy remains a prominent component of rheumatologic practice because the short-term efficacy of these powerful hormones remains unsurpassed.

Corticosteroid Physiology

Corticosteroid hormones are essential for normal development and homeostasis maintenance during both basal and stress conditions. They represent one of the most important products of the hypothalamic–pituitary–adrenal (HPA) axis and the central stress response system. In addition to their powerful anti-inflammatory actions, they regulate a broad array of metabolic and central nervous system (CNS) functions (Table 46-1). Under basal conditions, corticosteroid levels fluctuate with a circadian rhythm that follows the light–dark cycle. Under stressful conditions, however, the central stress response ("fight or flight") is stimulated and markedly enhances the production and secretion of adrenal corticosteroids. Inflammatory stress is associated with production of cytokines such as tumor necrosis factor α (TNF-α) and interleukins 1 and 6 (IL-1 and IL-6). These cytokines normally stimulate the HPA axis and corticosteroid production, which results in feedback suppression of cytokine production and the inflammatory response. Inadequate corticosteroid production facilitates unchecked amplification of inflammatory mechanisms and concomitant tissue injury (3,8,9). Defects in this bidirectional feedback loop between the CNS and peripheral inflammatory pathways are suspected to contribute to several rheumatic diseases, including RA (8–10). Tissue resistance to the actions of corticosteroids (Table 46-1) has also been postulated to play a role in the pathogenesis of several rheumatic diseases. It is these pathogenetic hypotheses that, in the context of the potentially serious side effects of corticosteroid therapy, drive the continuing interest in and controversies over corticosteroids (3–6). Although corticosteroids are not a "cure" for any rheumatic disease, their involvement in the pathogenesis of many diseases, particularly RA, appears highly probable (8).

Cellular and Molecular Effects of Corticosteroids

All of the effects of corticosteroids are mediated by receptors designated as type 1, or mineralocorticoid, receptors and type 2, or corticosteroid, receptors. Type 1 receptors are located mainly in the kidneys and various parts of the CNS and are believed to be critical in the basal regulation of circadian adrenocortical activity. Type 2 receptors are present in virtually all cells of the body and mediate the anti-inflammatory and metabolic actions of corticosteroids. In the absence of corticosteroid ligands, type 2 receptors normally exist in association with several classes of heat-shock proteins. Upon corticosteroid binding, the heat-shock proteins disassociate from the receptor, and the corticosteroid–receptor complex then migrates to the nucleus to regulate gene expression and other cellular activities. Major intracellular activities of the corticosteroid–receptor complex include competitive inactivation of c-fos:c-jun complexes and nuclear factor (NF)-κB activity. Inhibition of NF-κB is mediated through the induction of an inhibitory factor, IκB (11,12). c-fos:c-jun and NF-κB are important transcriptional activating factors and have prominent roles in driving the cellular production of most proinflammatory cytokines, as well as other inflammatory mediators. Corticosteroids also alter gene transcription by hindering nearby gene promoter-enhancer sequences that reside near corticosteroid receptor binding sites (13). Moreover, they enhance production of cyclic AMP and destabilize several classes of messenger RNA, including cytokine mRNA. Type 2 receptors are produced in two alternatively spliced forms: alpha and beta. The alpha form mediates the classic anti-inflammatory activities of the corticosteroid receptor. The beta form, interestingly, inhibits corticosteroid action and competes with the alpha form (14). Thus, the ratio of alpha to beta type 2 receptors in a cell is hypothesized to modulate the cellular actions of corticosteroids. If beta forms predominate in a cell, they confer "resistance" to corticosteroid action in that cell (14).

The primary outcome of corticosteroid action at the cellular level is inhibition of the cascade of inflammatory and immune mechanisms at virtually all levels (Table 46-1). Neutrophil and monocyte migration into the inflammatory site, antigen processing and presentation to lymphocytes, and cellular activation and differentiation are all suppressed. Corticosteroids are particularly active on immature T lymphocytes, activated T-effector lymphocytes, natural killer cells, and immature B cells, but they have minimal suppres-

TABLE 46-1
Major Physiologic, Cellular, and Molecular Effects of Corticosteroids Relevant to the Rheumatic Diseases

Physiologic effects
Enhance behavioral arousal and euphoria.
Increase blood glucose and liver glycogen.
Promote insulin resistance.
Depress thyroid function.
Depress reproductive function and reproductive hormone synthesis.
Increase muscle catabolic activity.
Enhance activity of detoxifying enzymes.
Impair wound healing.
Suppress acute inflammation.
Suppress type 1 (cell-mediated/delayed hypersensitivity type) immune responsiveness relative to type 2 (humoral).

Cellular effects
Alter neuronal activities in many parts of the brain, resulting in changes in neuropeptide and neurotransmitter synthesis, release, and actions (particularly catecholamines, γ-aminobutyric acid, and prostaglandins).
Suppress synthesis and release of corticotropin- and gonadotropin-releasing hormones from the hypothalamus.
Suppress synthesis and release of adrenocorticotropic, thyroid-stimulating, and growth hormone by the pituitary.
Suppress synthesis and release of cortisol and androgens by the adrenal gland.
Suppress estrogen synthesis by ovary and testosterone synthesis by testes, and decrease the action of these hormones on target cells.
Suppress osteoblast growth and osteoprotegerin production.
Promote type IIb skeletal muscle fiber atrophy.
Alter adipocyte activity resulting in changes in adipose tissue distribution.
Decrease fibroblast proliferation, DNA, and collagen synthesis.
Decrease fibroblast production of phospholipase A_2, cyclooxygenase-2, prostaglandins, and metalloproteinases.
Depress endothelial cell functions including expression of adhesion molecules involved in inflammatory cell recruitment to inflammatory sites.
Suppress neutrophil, eosinophil, monocyte migration.
Inhibit macrophage antigen presentation to lymphocytes.
Suppress immune/inflammatory effector cell activation and differentiation (macrophages, T cells, mast cells, natural killer cells, and immature B cells).
Increase apoptosis of immature and activated T lymphocytes.
Suppress proinflammatory mediator production (e.g., tumor necrosis factor α, interleukin 1, interleukin 12, interferon γ, prostaglandins, leukotrienes).

Molecular effects
Bind plasma cortisol-binding globulin and cellular type 1 or type 2 corticosteroid receptors.
Stimulate disassociation of corticosteroid receptor from heat-shock protein-90, 70, 56, and 26, translocation to nucleus, and binding to glucocorticoid-responsive genes.
Enhance transcriptional activity of genes to which cortisol-receptor complexes bind, although the overall effect may be inhibitory.
Inactivate c-jun:c-fos transcriptional activator proteins.
Enhance IκB production and suppress NF-κB activity.
Destabilize mRNA for many proinflammatory cytokine genes.
Enhance β-adrenergic receptor expression.
Enhance cyclic-adenosine monophosphate production.

sive effects on mature antibody-producing B cells. Normally, they potently suppress production of proinflammatory cytokines such as TNF-α, IL-1, IL-12, and related mediators such as gamma interferon, prostaglandin E$_2$, and leukotrienes. Importantly, suppressive effects are minimal on the production of anti-inflammatory cytokines such as IL-4 and IL-10. As a consequence, corticosteroids tend to skew or bias immune responses toward humoral immunity (or type 2 immune responses) and suppress macrophage activation and cellular immunity (or type 1 immune responses). These differential immunologic effects may play a role in determining the therapeutic response to corticosteroids, or lack thereof, in various rheumatic diseases. Diseases mediated primarily by macrophages and type 1 cellular immunity, such as RA, tend to respond dramatically to corticosteroid therapy; Diseases that probably involve type 2 humoral-immune mechanisms, such as lupus glomerulonephritis, require therapy with supraphysiologic levels of corticosteroids for disease suppression.

Corticosteroid Pharmacology

Corticosteroids are 17-hydroxy-21-carbon steroid molecules, the principal, naturally occurring form of which is cortisol (hydrocortisone). Numerous synthetic derivatives have been produced for systemic therapy (Table 46-2), but prednisone, prednisolone, and methylprednisolone are the most widely used. One of the most potent synthetic corticosteroids is dexamethasone, but it is not commonly used for anti-inflammatory therapy because of its long half-life. The biologic effects of these preparations are influenced by multiple factors including dose, scheduling, route of administration, and patient, disease, and tissue variables. For example, corticosteroid availability is influenced by its binding to cortisol-binding globulin (transcortin), which is not only present in plasma but is also expressed at different levels in various tissues.

Corticosteroid therapy is not rigorously standardized. Therapeutic dosing regimens are usually individualized in a manner that attempts to maximize therapeutic effects and minimize side effects. To achieve these goals, a variety of approaches have evolved. In general, increasing doses and

frequency of administration enhance anti-inflammatory activity and increase side effects, and high-dose schedules tend to be used when urgent control of the disease process is required. For example, intermittent high-dose supraphysiologic intravenous bolus treatment (e.g., 1000 mg of methylprednisolone daily for three days) may be used to treat acute glomerulonephritis in systemic lupus erythematosus (SLE) or vasculitis in RA. Although this regimen has pronounced effects on lymphocyte function and numbers, it often produces sustained clinical effects for weeks or even months. Daily or alternate-day high-dose oral treatment (e.g., 60 mg of prednisone daily for up to one month, followed by tapering to the lowest possible dose that maintains disease control) is often employed in the setting of acute, severe, but less threatening disease such as thrombocytopenia or pleurisy in SLE. Intermittent low oral doses in the physiologic range (e.g., <7 mg of prednisone daily on an as-needed basis) can be used for symptomatic control in RA. With this regimen, rapid development of side effects is unlikely, and it gives the patient control over withdrawing from corticosteroid therapy. Alternate-day therapy is usually preferred to minimize side effects, but in many conditions such as RA, patients cannot tolerate alternate-day schedules.

Local injections or topical therapy are also very useful for many conditions and are preferred when possible because they target the area specifically involved. Toxicity is also minimized. Several corticosteroid formulations are available for these indications (e.g., triamcinolone acetonide, or hexacetonide) (3).

Side Effects of Corticosteroid Therapy

The pharmacologic side effects of corticosteroids are not distinct from their normal physiologic effects, but reflect the same underlying biologic actions. The likelihood of developing side effects depends on the type of corticosteroid, dose, duration of exposure, and a multitude of host, tissue, and cell variables. It needs to be emphasized that corticosteroids are not merely powerful anti-inflammatory drugs, but rather are essential hormones involved in maintaining homeostasis of numerous physiologic func-

TABLE 46-2
Corticosteroid Formulations Used for Systemic Therapy

Form	Relative anti-inflammatory potency	Equivalent dose (mg)	Biologic half-life (hours)
Hydrocortisone	1	20	8–12
Cortisone	0.8	25	8–12
Prednisone	4	5	12–36
Methylprednisolone	5	4	12–36
Prednisolone	5	4	12–36
Dexamethasone	20–30	0.75	36–54

tions. Not surprisingly, both corticosteroid deficiency and excess have pathophysiologic consequences. Therapeutic administration that supplements an endogenous deficiency is less likely to produce side effects. In contrast, therapy that exceeds physiologic need will produce a syndrome that resembles Cushing syndrome, except that adrenal production of corticosteroids and androgens is suppressed in iatrogenic Cushing syndrome (Table 46-3). Several side effects that deserve particular emphasis are osteoporosis, infection, adrenal insufficiency, and corticosteroid withdrawal syndromes (3).

Osteoporosis

All corticosteroid preparations currently in use inhibit bone formation and promote the development of osteoporosis. As a consequence, vertebral compression fractures are a frequent and devastating complication, and active prevention measures should be employed. The likelihood of developing osteoporosis is closely linked to the maximum dose and cumulative duration of therapy, but it should always be anticipated with any extended period of therapy regardless of dose (15). Men and postmenopausal women are most sensitive, and people in whom the disease process itself causes bone loss (such as RA) are at high risk. Corticosteroids induce osteoporosis by inhibiting ovarian and testicular sex steroid hormones, as well as adrenal androgens. They also inhibit intestinal calcium absorption and promote secondary hyperparathyroidism, which leads to osteoclast activation and osteoblast inhibition. Thus, therapeutic and preventive measures should emphasize adequate intake of calcium (1500 mg/day) and vitamin D (400–800 IU/day). Estrogen replacement therapy should be considered for postmenopausal women, and androgen replacement therapy should possibly be considered for men. Bisphosphonate therapy should also be considered in high-risk patients (3,16–18). Recent surveys indicate that many patients receive inadequate treatment to prevent this complication. Intensive efforts are required to educate both patients and health-care professionals in the standards of care for this preventable complication (19).

Infections

Corticosteroid deficiency renders patients susceptible to severe, even life-threatening, tissue injury in response to infection because of the unrestrained inflammatory response. Conversely, corticosteroid excess leads to impaired inflammatory and immune responses and an increased incidence and severity of infections (i.e., impaired host defense). As expected, the likelihood of developing infection in the course of corticosteroid treatment depends on the maximum dose and cumulative duration of therapy. Prednisone dosages of about 2–10 mg/day are rarely associated with infectious complications, whereas prednisone dosages in the range of 20–60 mg/day have pronounced suppressive effects on host defense mechanisms and lead to a progressive increase in infection risk after 14 days of treatment. Cumulative doses greater than 700 mg are associated with progressively increased risk of infection.

TABLE 46-3
Side Effects of Long-Term Corticosteroid Therapy[a]

Common
Hypertension
Negative balance of calcium and secondary hyperparathyroidism
Negative balance of nitrogen
Truncal obesity; moon facies; supraclavicular fat deposition; posterior cervical fat deposition (buffalo hump); mediastinal widening (lipomatosis); weight gain
Impaired wound healing; facial erythema; thin, fragile skin; violaceous striae; petechiae and ecchymoses
Acne
Suppression of growth in children
Adrenal insufficiency secondary to hypothalamic-pituitary-adrenal axis suppression
Hyperglycemia; diabetes mellitus
Hyperlipoproteinemia; atherosclerosis
Sodium retention, hypokalemia
Increased risk of infection; neutrophilia; monocytopenia; lymphopenia; suppressed delayed-type hypersensitivity reactions
Myopathy
Osteoporosis; vertebral compression fractures
Osteonecrosis
Alterations in mood or behavior, such as euphoria, emotional lability, insomnia, depression; increased appetite
Posterior subcapsular cataracts

Uncommon
Metabolic alkalosis
Diabetic ketoacidosis; hyperosmolar, nonketotic diabetic coma
Peptic ulcer disease (usually gastric); gastric hemorrhage
"Silent" intestinal perforation
Increased intraocular pressure and glaucoma
Benign intracranial hypertension or pseudotumor cerebri
Spontaneous fractures
Psychosis

Rare
Sudden death with rapid administration of high-dose, pulse therapy
Cardiac valvular lesions in patients with systemic lupus erythematosus
Congestive heart failure in predisposed patients
Panniculitis (following withdrawal)
Hirsutism or virilism; impotence; secondary amenorrhea
Hepatomegaly due to fatty liver
Pancreatitis
Convulsions
Epidural lipomatosis
Exophthalmos
Allergy to synthetic corticosteroids resulting in urticaria, angioedema

[a] Reprinted with permission from Wilder (3).

The primary risk is for infections with facultative intracellular microbes such as mycobacteria, *Pneumocystis carinii*, and fungi. Patients also develop more severe cases of acute pyogenic infections. It is important to note that high-dose corticosteroids can mask the symptoms of infectious diseases such as abscesses and bowel perforation. Thus, unusual degrees of suspicion are required to make these diagnoses. Except for herpes, viral infections are generally not a major problem during corticosteroid treatment (3,4).

Adrenal Insufficiency

Administration of corticosteroids suppresses endogenous HPA axis function and may produce secondary adrenal deficiency. The development of this side effect can occur with as little as five days of prednisone treatment at 20–30 mg/day, although in this setting, pituitary-adrenal function normally returns rapidly after stopping corticosteroids. In contrast, patients treated for more prolonged periods of time (weeks to months) may require up to 12 months for HPA axis function to return to normal, and it should be assumed that all patients treated with more than 20 mg of prednisone per day for one month have some degree of HPA axis deficiency.

The risk to the patient is during periods of corticosteroid taper and warrants close follow-up and attention to symptoms of deficiency. The major concern is the development of acute adrenal insufficiency during general anesthesia, surgery, trauma, or an acute infectious disease. Patients may require supplemental corticosteroid therapy in these settings. If doubt exists about the existence of adrenal insufficiency, an adrenocorticotropic hormone (ACTH) stimulation test may be indicated (3).

Withdrawal Syndromes

Corticosteroid deficiency classically presents in Addisonian crisis with fever, nausea, vomiting, hypotension, hypoglycemia, hyperkalemia, and hyponatremia, but other syndromes are also noted. Most often, patients develop an exacerbation of their underlying inflammatory disease. Some patients develop a symptom complex consisting of diffuse muscle and joint pain, weight loss, fever, and headache. In this setting, plasma cortisol levels do not correlate with symptoms and are frequently higher than "normal." Withdrawal syndromes require increased dosages of corticosteroid administration and careful slow taper over a period of weeks to months. In general, at doses greater than 40 mg/day, prednisone can be tapered at a rate of about 10 mg/week. At doses between 20 and 40 mg/day, one can usually taper about 5 mg/week. Below 20 mg/day, and especially less than 5 mg/day, withdrawal symptoms are common, because the dosage changes are occurring within the normal physiologic range of corticosteroids. For example, a rapid reduction of prednisone from 5 to 2.5 mg/day represents a 50% reduction in available corticosteroid and, not surprisingly, is often associated with severe withdrawal symptoms. Reductions in these situations can often be best managed by a patient-dictated schedule. Close follow-up is indicated in all cases. Occasionally, a switch to an alternate-day schedule is done as the first step before reducing the average daily dose. This therapeutic strategy frequently works well in conditions such as SLE, but it is rarely tolerated by patients with RA, who report marked worsening of symptoms on the "off" day of therapy.

In general, considering the broad spectrum of rheumatic diseases and patient variables, corticosteroid therapy must be individualized with attention directed at avoiding or preventing the side effects associated with both corticosteroid excess and deficiency.

RONALD L. WILDER, MD, PhD

References

1. Hench PS, Kendall EC, Slocumb CH, Polley HF. *The effect of a hormone of the adrenal cortex (17-hydroxy-11-dehydrocorticosterone: compound E) and of pituitary adrenocorticotropic hormone on rheumatoid arthritis. Proc Staff Meet Mayo Clin* 1949;24:181–197.
2. Hench PS, Kendall EC, Slocumb CH, Polley HF. *Effects of cortisone acetate and pituitary ACTH on rheumatoid arthritis, rheumatic fever and certain other conditions. Arch Intern Med* 1950;85:545–666.
3. Wilder RL. Corticosteroids. In: McCarty DJ, Koopman WJ (eds). *Arthritis and Allied Conditions: A Textbook of Rheumatology*, 13th ed. Philadelphia: Williams & Wilkins, 1996; pp 731–750.
4. Boumpas DT, Chrousos GP, Wilder RL, Cupps TR, Balow JE. *Glucocorticoid therapy for immune-mediated diseases: basic and clinical correlates. Ann Intern Med* 1993;119:1198–1208.
5. Kirwan JR. *The effect of glucocorticoids on joint destruction in rheumatoid arthritis. The Arthritis and Rheumatism Council Low-Dose Glucocorticoid Study Group. N Engl J Med* 1995; 333:142–146.
6. Saag KG. *Low-dose corticosteroid therapy in rheumatoid arthritis: balancing the evidence. Am J Med* 1997;103:31S–39S.
7. Strand V. *Steroid withdrawal favours joint erosion in rheumatoid arthritis. Clin Exp Rheumatol* 1999;17:519–520.
8. Wilder RL. *Neuroendocrine-immune system interactions and autoimmunity. Annu Rev Immunol* 1995;13:307–338.
9. Chrousos GP. *The hypothalamic-pituitary-adrenal axis and immune-mediated inflammation. N Engl J Med* 1995;332: 1351–1362.
10. Kanik KS, Chrousos GP, Schumacher HR, Crane ML, Yarboro CH, Wilder RL. *Adrenocorticotropin, glucocorticoid, and androgen secretion in patients with new onset synovitis/rheumatoid arthritis: relations with indices of inflammation. J Clin Endocrinol Metab* 2000;85:1461–1466.
11. Auphan N, DiDonato JA, Rosette C, Helmberg A, Karin M. *Immunosuppression by glucocorticoids: inhibition of NF-kappa B activity through induction of I kappa B synthesis. Science* 1995;270:286–290.
12. Scheinman RI, Cogswell PC, Lofquist AK, Baldwin AS, Jr. *Role of transcriptional activation of I kappa B alpha in mediation of immunosuppression by glucocorticoids. Science* 1995;270:283–286.

13. Akerblom IE, Slater EP, Beato M, Baxter JD, Mellon PL. Negative regulation by glucocorticoids through interference with a cAMP responsive enhancer. Science 1988;241:350–353.

14. Bamberger CM, Bamberger AM, de Castro M, Chrousos GP. Glucocorticoid receptor beta, a potential endogenous inhibitor of glucocorticoid action in humans. J Clin Invest 1995;95: 2435–2441.

15. Van Staa TP, Leufkens HG, Abenhaim L, Zhang B, Cooper C. Use of oral corticosteroids and risk of fractures. J Bone Miner Res 2000;15:993–1000.

16. Saag KG, Emkey R, Schnitzer TJ, et al. Alendronate for the prevention and treatment of glucocorticoid-induced osteoporosis. Glucocorticoid-Induced Osteoporosis Intervention Study Group. N Engl J Med 1998;339:292–299.

17. Reid DM, Hughes RA, Laan RF, et al. Efficacy and safety of daily risedronate in the treatment of corticosteroid-induced osteoporosis in men and women: a randomized trial. European Corticosteroid-Induced Osteoporosis Treatment Study. J Bone Miner Res 2000;15:1006–1013.

18. Eastell R, Devogelaer JP, Peel NF, et al. Prevention of bone loss with risedronate in glucocorticoid-treated rheumatoid arthritis patients. Osteoporos Int 2000;11:331–337.

19. Buckley LM, Marquez M, Feezor R, Ruffin DM, Benson LL. Prevention of corticosteroid-induced osteoporosis: results of a patient survey. Arthritis Rheum 1999;42:1736–1739.

47 DISEASE-MODIFYING ANTIRHEUMATIC DRUGS

Disease-modifying antirheumatic drugs (DMARDs) are a diverse group of agents that reduce the signs and symptoms of rheumatoid arthritis (RA) and other arthritides such as psoriatic arthritis. These drugs are called disease-modifying because of their ability to prevent radiologic joint damage. This terminology may be imprecise because hydroxychloroquine (HCQ) and auranofin, though conventionally classified as DMARDs, have not been shown to retard radiologic damage. The newly approved biologic agents are considered DMARDs because of their favorable impact on structural damage. For completeness, minocycline, which is not considered to be a traditional DMARD, and the staphyloccal protein A column, a medical device, are also included within this chapter.

Although the older DMARDs are distinguished by their delayed onset of action, the current group includes agents that range from rapid to slow-acting in onset. For example, the new anti-tumor necrosis factor (TNF) drugs suppress disease manifestations relatively quickly. Also, loading dose strategies (e.g., leflunomide) and rapid dose escalation (e.g., methotrexate) have been utilized successfully with certain agents to compensate for otherwise delayed effects. The recognition that joint damage may occur within the first three to 12 months of RA has led to earlier introduction of DMARDs and more aggressive treatment with combination DMARD therapy. Rheumatologists typically initiate DMARD therapy within the first three to six months to control persistently active disease and prevent irreversible joint damage. Although disease remission is the primary goal, this endpoint is often not achieved with standard DMARD monotherapy. Residual disease activity, if sufficiently pronounced, may warrant treatment modification. If one agent produces intolerable side effects or lacks evidence of clinical efficacy, another DMARD may be substituted. Alternatively, the existing DMARD may be maintained and other DMARDs added to improve the clinical response. When to change DMARD therapy and the selection of particular agents is a matter of clinical judgement, depending on the degree of joint inflammation determined by rheumatologic examination.

Each of the DMARDs is summarized below, with emphasis on the pharmacology, mechanisms, clinical efficacy, and possible side effects of each agent. The accompanying tables are meant to offer practical information for clinicians. Table 47-1 reviews dosing guidelines and clinically important toxicities for each of the DMARDs. The procedures for monitoring possible toxicities are detailed in Table 47-2.

Methotrexate

Methotrexate (MTX) is commonly employed as the initial DMARD for the treatment of moderate to severe RA. MTX, a folate analogue, inhibits dihydrofolate reductase, thereby reducing tetrahydrofolate formation and blocking DNA synthesis (tetrahydrofolate is a single-carbon donor that is essential for purine and pyrimidine synthesis). Because MTX inhibits DNA synthesis, its therapeutic efficacy has been attributed to the suppression of lymphocyte proliferation. However, studies have shown that the antirheumatic properties of MTX are more likely related to its anti-inflammatory effects.

Inside cells, MTX forms polyglutamates that inhibit the enzyme 5-aminoimidazole-4-carboxamidoribonucleotide (AICAR) transformylase. This enzymatic block leads to the intracellular accumulation of AICAR and in turn, extracellular adenosine release (1). Adenosine binds to specific receptors on the surface of lymphocytes, monocytes, and neutrophils, and down-regulates inflammatory pathways. MTX also has been reported to inhibit neovascularization, neutrophil activity and adherence, interleukin (IL)-1 and IL-8 production by stimulated peripheral blood mononuclear cells, and TNF production by stimulated peripheral T cells.

The clinical efficacy and safety of MTX therapy in RA has been firmly established by prospective, controlled trials. Uncontrolled observations have also shown that MTX therapy produces long-term benefits for up to 11 years (2). In addition, nearly 50% of patients remain on MTX therapy for at least five years (3). The long-term efficacy and tolerability of this agent is a major reason for the preference of MTX over other DMARDs. MTX treatment favorably impacts RA in its early stages. In a recent one-year study of people with RA of less than three years' duration, MTX therapy was associated with an ACR-20 (see Table 47-4) response rate of nearly 60%, a rate not significantly different from that of the comparison group receiving etanercept (4).

Methotrexate therapy is generally well-tolerated, but some patients experience side effects. The dose-related side effects of MTX are nausea, stomatitis, and bone-marrow suppression. Concurrent treatment with folic or folinic acid lowers the frequency and severity of these side effects (5). Fatigue, flu-like symptoms, and headache may also occur following MTX administration. Pulmonary (pneumonitis) and hepatic (fibrosis and cirrhosis) toxicities appear to be idiosyncratic and may depend on other risk factors. MTX

TABLE 47-1
Disease-Modifying Antirheumatic Drugs for Treating Rheumatoid Arthritis

Drug	Route	Usual dosage	Side effects
Methotrexate	Oral, SQ, IM	Initial: 7.5–10 mg/wk; maintenance: 7.5–25 mg/wk	Fatigue, flu-like symptoms, nausea, stomatitis, bone marrow suppression, pneumonitis, hepatic fibrosis
Hydroxychloroquine	Oral	400 mg/day	Nausea, abdominal pain, headache, rash, retinal toxicity, blurred vision
Sulfasalazine	Oral	Initial: 500 mg bid; maintenance: 1–1.5 g bid	Nausea, diarrhea, rash, bone marrow suppression, severe allergic reactions, hepatitis
Gold sodium malate	IM	Initial: 10, 25, 50 mg/wk x 15-20 wks, maintenance: 50 mg/wk+ 50 mg every 4 wks	Rash, stomatitis, bone marrow suppression, proteinuria, hematuria
Auranofin	Oral	3 mg bid	Nausea, diarrhea, abdominal pain rash, stomatitis, bone marrow suppression
Minocycline	Oral	100 mg bid	Dizziness, dyspepsia, skin rash, skin discoloration, headaches
Azathioprine	Oral	2–2.5 mg/kg/day	Nausea, vomiting, diarrhea, bone marrow suppression, hepatitis
Cyclosporine	Oral	2.5–5 mg/kg/day	Hypertension, renal toxicity, hirsutism, tremor, gingival hyperplasia
Leflunomide	Oral	Loading: 100 mg/day x 3 days; maintenance: 10–20 mg/day	Diarrhea, nausea, vomiting, abdominal pain, alopecia, rash, mouth ulcers, allergic reactions, liver enzymes
D-Penicillamine	Oral	Loading: 125–250 mg/day; maintenance: 750 mg/day	Rashes, proteinurea, hematuria, neutropenia, thrombocytopenia, SLE-like reactions
Etanercept	SQ	25 mg twice weekly	Injection-site reactions, infections, SLE-like reactions
Infliximab	IV	Induction: 3 mg/kg on wk 0, 2, 6; maintenance: 3 mg/kg every 8 wk[a]	Infusion reactions, infections, SLE-like reactions

SQ, subcutaneous; IM, intramuscular; IV, intravenous; bid, twice daily; SLE, systemic lupus erythematosus

therapy also increases the risk of infections and, in rare instances, leads to B-cell lymphoma.

Methotrexate therapy is contraindicated in the setting of significant renal insufficiency because its major clearance is by the kidney. Thus, the drug is contraindicated in patients with serum creatinine levels >2.0–2.5 mg/dL, or if substantial renal insufficiency is suspected despite a lower creatinine. MTX should also not be given to people with significant liver disease. Patients who routinely drink alcohol (more than two drinks per week) should not receive MTX because of the increased risk for liver damage.

The starting dose of MTX is usually 7.5–10 mg/week. The MTX dose can be advanced to 15–25 mg/week to achieve maximum clinical efficacy, depending on the limits of tolerability. The oral route is most convenient for MTX administration. For more predictable absorption, however,

TABLE 47-2
DMARD Monitoring for Possible Toxicity[a]

DMARD	Toxicities requiring monitoring	Baseline evaluation	Monitoring
Hydroxychloroquine	Macular damage	Eye exam age > 40 years or prior eye disease	Annual eye exam
Sulfasalazine	Myelosuppression	CBC, ALT, G6PD levels	CBC every 2–4 wks for first 3 mo, then every 3 mo
Methotrexate	Myelosuppression, liver fibrosis, pneumonitis	CBC, ALT, AST, albumin, creatinine, chest x-ray[b], screen for HBV and HCV[c]	CBC, ALT, AST, and serum albumin every 8 wks
Parenteral gold	Myelosuppression, proteinuria	CBC, creatinine, urinalysis	CBC and urinalysis every 1–2 wks for first 20 wks, then at time of each injection
Azathioprine	Myelosuppression, hepatotoxicity	CBC, creatinine, AST, ALT	CBC every 1–2 wks for first 2 mo or with dosage changes, then every 1–3 mo
Cyclosporin A	Renal insufficiency, hypertension	CBC, urinalysis, creatinine	Creatinine and BP every 2 wks for the first 3 mo, and then monthly, if stable[d]
Minocycline	None	None	None
Leflunomide	Thrombocytopenia, hepatotoxicity	CBC, ALT, AST	CBC, ALT, and AST every 8 wks
D-Penicillamine	Myelosuppression, proteinuria	CBC, creatinine, urinalysis	CBC, urinalysis every 2 wks until stable dosage, then every 1–3 mo
Infliximab	Clinically important infections	CBC	None
Etanercept	Clinically important infections	CBC	None

[a] See Appendix II for American College of Rheumatology guidelines for monitoring drug therapy.
[b] If medical history of respiratory symptoms, known lung disease, or cigarette smoking (some authorities recommend a chest x-ray for every patient before starting MTX).
[c] If at risk for acquiring HBV or HCV.
[d] If serum creatinine increases to 30% of baseline on two occasions, then the daily dose of CsA should be decreased by 0.5 to 1.0 mg/kg; if the diastolic BP rises above 95 mm Hg, then the hypertension should be treated with medications that do not significantly interfere with the metabolism of cyclosporine (e.g., verapamil, diltiazem); most authorities recommend in order the use of a β-blocker, diuretic, angiotensin converting enzyme inhibitor, and amlodipine; if the serum creatinine or BP is elevated above normal values, then consideration should also be given to discontinuing any nonsteroidal anti-inflammatory drugs, or lowering their dosage.

CBC, complete blood count; ALT, alanine aminotransferase; AST, aspartate aminotransferase; G6PD, glucose 6-phosphate dehydrogenase; HBV, hepatitis B virus; HCV, hepatitis C virus; BP, blood pressure

MTX may be administered parenterally. The drug's bioavailability is similar via subcutaneous (SQ) and intramuscular (IM) routes. Because the SQ route is easier and less painful, it is preferred to IM administration. The clinical efficacy of MTX can sometimes be enhanced by switching from oral to parenteral administration.

Sulfasalazine

Sulfasalazine (SSZ) was synthesized in 1942 to link an antibiotic, sulfapyridine, with an anti-inflammatory agent, 5-aminosalicylic acid (5-ASA). Approximately 30% of SSZ is absorbed from the gastrointestinal (GI) tract. The remainder is degraded in the gut to sulfapyridine and 5-ASA. Whereas the bulk of the sulfapyridine is absorbed from the gut, most 5-ASA is excreted in the feces. SSZ suppresses various lymphocyte and leukocyte functions and, like MTX, inhibits AICAR transformylase, resulting in extracellular adenosine release (6). In addition, SSZ reduces the activation of nuclear factor κB (NF-κB), a transcriptional factor that promotes the expression of certain genes associated with inflammation (7).

Sulfasalazine is effective for the treatment of mild to moderate RA. In a randomized, double-blind, placebo-controlled trial that lasted 24 weeks, treatment with SSZ produced an ACR-20 response rate of 56%, compared with a 29% rate for placebo-treated subjects (8). The same study also revealed that patients treated with SSZ had less radiographic progression of joint damage than the placebo group. SSZ is generally well-tolerated and does not increase the risk for infection. The most common side effects are nausea, diarrhea, abdominal pain, dyspepsia, and rash. Rarely, SSZ may cause severe agranulocytosis. SSZ should not be used in patients with sulfa allergies or glucose 6-phosphate dehydrogenase deficiency. Three months of treatment are usually required to achieve maximum clinical effect.

Antimalarials

Hydroxychloroquine and chloroquine are prescribed widely for the treatment of RA. These medications are absorbed efficiently from the GI tract and show extended serum half-lives due to tissue depot effects. The antimalarials are concentrated inside cells, principally within acidic cytoplasmic vesicles. In lysosomes, accumulation of antimalarials raises the intravesical pH, and may thereby interfere with the processing of autoantigenic peptides (9).

Hydroxychloroquine is indicated primarily for the treatment of mild RA. Its treatment superiority over placebo has been shown in a randomized, controlled trial involving 126 patients with relatively mild disease of less than five years' duration (10). Six to 12 months of HCQ therapy at the usual doses (e.g., 400 mg/day) are generally required to achieve a clinical effect.

The most common side effects from HCQ are nausea, abdominal pain, and headache. HCQ is rarely associated with retinal toxicity, mostly when it has been used for longer than 10 years and at doses exceeding 400 mg/day. Physicians have questioned the value of screening eye examinations for patients who have been treated with HCQ for relatively short periods of time and with standard doses. However, annual eye exams are a common practice and highly advisable for patients with long-term use (>10 years) or high daily dosage (>6.5 mg/kg/day).

Minocycyline

Oral minocycline is used principally for the treatment of mild RA. Rationale for its use in RA stems from an old (and still unsubstantiated) theory that infection is a triggering event for this disease. Despite the lack of any conclusive evidence to support this theory, oral minocycline has been shown to decrease the signs and symptoms of RA in several placebo-controlled trials (11). The mechanisms by which minocycline controls joint inflammation are unknown. Minocycline has several biologic activities that may confer antirheumatic properties; it inhibits collagenase activity and the expression of nitric oxide synthase type 2, and up-regulates the synthesis of IL-10, an anti-inflammatory cytokine.

The most frequently observed side effects from oral minocycline therapy are dizziness, gastrointestinal symptoms, and skin rash. Skin hyperpigmentation, which reverses after stopping the drug, is a potential problem with long-term therapy. This antibiotic also has been rarely associated with the development of systemic lupus erythematosus-like symptoms.

Gold Compounds

The past decade has witnessed a steady decline in the use of gold compounds for the treatment of RA. There are two parenteral gold formulations, gold sodium malate and myochrysine, and an oral compound, auranofin. The efficacy of gold injections for the treatment of RA has been documented in several prospective clinical trials. Although injectable gold and MTX therapy produce similar rates of clinical response in trials, gold has a higher incidence of toxicity requiring drug discontinuation.

Auranofin (oral gold) has fewer side effects than gold injections. Although auranofin has been shown to improve the clinical manifestations of RA in controlled studies, it has seen limited use in clinical practice owing to a lack of sustained clinical efficacy, slow onset of action, and poor GI tolerability.

Leflunomide

Leflunomide (LEF), a newly approved oral therapy for RA, is indicated for the treatment of moderate to severe RA. LEF selectively inhibits dihydroorotate dehydrogenase, a key enzyme in the de novo pyrimidine synthesis pathway. In trials, LEF has shown superior clinical efficacy to placebo, and benefits comparable to those of MTX or SSZ (8,12). Treatment with LEF also retards radiologic progression of joint disease (13) and improves quality of life (14).

Leflunomide is a pro-drug rapidly converted to its active metabolite, A77 1726, which is extensively bound to plasma proteins. A77 1726 has a long plasma half-life: 15–18 days. Common side effects from LEF therapy are diarrhea, nausea, skin rash, alopecia, and elevated serum transaminases. Lowering the maintenance dose of LEF from 20 mg/day to 10 mg/day may resolve mild toxic reactions. LEF should be discontinued in the event of moderate or serious toxicity. Depending on the severity of the adverse reaction, cholestyramine may be given 8 mg three times daily to facilitate clearance of A77 1726 from the body.

Azathioprine

Azathioprine (AZA) is used primarily for treating people with RA whose disease has not been managed with other DMARD therapy. There is evidence from small controlled studies that AZA is more effective than placebo for the treatment of RA. In larger trials, AZA shows less efficacy than MTX and similar efficacy as D-penicillamine and cyclosporine for reducing the signs and symptoms of RA. Treatment with AZA has also been associated with greater radiologic progression of joint damage than MTX therapy after four years of follow-up.

Azathioprine is an orally administered purine analogue, which is converted in the liver to 6-mercaptopurine, its active metabolite. Patients with RA are more frequently intolerant of AZA than MTX. In one study, more than 25% of patients discontinued AZA because of GI distress and other side effects. AZA also may cause hepatitis, pancreatitis, or myelosuppression, and increases the risk for lymphoproliferative disorders.

Cyclosporine

Evidence from controlled trials shows that treatment with cyclosporine (CsA) reduces the signs and symptoms of RA and slows the development of joint erosions. CsA inhibits IL-2 production and the proliferation of activated T cells, which may explain its efficacy in RA. CsA, initially studied in RA at doses of 5–10 mg/kg/day, caused unacceptable renal toxicity. More recent trials have shown that CsA treatment in doses of 2.5–5.0 mg/kg/day affords similar clinical benefits as the higher doses, with a lower incidence of renal toxicity (15).

Toxicity has been a limiting factor in the use of CsA. In particular, nephrotoxicity commonly leads to hypertension and a rise in the serum creatinine. For this reason, CsA is contraindicated for people with uncontrolled hypertension or renal insufficiency. Other CsA side effects include GI distress, hypertrichosis, tremor, paresthesias, and gum hyperplasia. There is also an increased risk for infection. Although CsA has been associated with the development of cancer, a retrospective case-controlled study has recently found that its use in RA does not increase the risk of lymphoproliferative disease or skin cancer (16). CsA is associ-

TABLE 47-4
American College of Rheumatology Preliminary Definition of Improvement in Rheumatoid Arthritis

≥ 20 % improvement in the tender joint count
≥ 20 % improvement in the swollen joint count

and

≥ 20 % improvement in at least three of these five measures:

- Patient pain
- Patient global assessment of disease severity
- Physician global assessment of disease severity
- Physical function
- Acute-phase-reactant level (CRP or ESR)

To achieve an ACR-20 response, the patient must meet criteria for improvement in tender and swollen joint counts plus three of the five other measures of disease activity. Clinical responses are often assessed using ACR-50 and ACR-70 responses, which require ≥50% or ≥70% improvement, respectively, in the same measures (27).

ated with numerous clinically important drug interactions. For example, CsA levels are increased by concomitant administration of ketoconazole, calcium antagonists, and H2 antagonists, and decreased by the addition of anticonvulsants and rifampicin.

The conventional oil-based CsA formulation shows considerable individual variability in pharmacokinetic properties. The mean oral bioavailability of the oil-based CsA formulation is 30%. A newer, microemulsion-based formulation of CsA (Neoral) has higher oral bioavailability and more predictable absorption. For people with RA, these two formulations appear to be equivalent in clinical efficacy and toxicity. The microemulsion-based product often can be dosed at lower levels than the oil-based formulation to achieve the same blood concentration and therapeutic effect.

The recommended starting dose of CsA is 2.5–3.5 mg/kg/day as a twice-daily regimen, with a maximum dose of 5 mg/kg/day. CsA therapy requires close monitoring (Table 47-2). In practice, some authorities use only two doses of CsA: 75 mg twice daily for patients less than 60 kg and 100 mg twice daily for patients greater than 60 kg. If patients do not respond to CsA after three months of treatment, then the physician may check a serum-trough level. If patients are not absorbing CsA adequately, then the serum trough level should be below 100 mg/mL. In general, a 1:1 dose-conversion is recommended when changing from the conventional to the microemulsion formulation. A serum-trough level should be obtained for patients receiving CsA >4 mg/kg/day before switching from the oil-based to microemulsion-based formula. If the serum-trough level is >100mg/mL, then the initial dose of Neoral should be no higher than 4/mg/kg/day.

D-Penicillamine

D-Penicillamine is rarely used today for the treatment of RA because of its high incidence of toxicity. However, it is an approved DMARD for this indication. The mode of action of D-penicillamine is uncertain. Penicillamine is effective in RA in doses of 600–1500 mg daily, although the higher dose is associated with a significant increase in side effects. There are conflicting data as to whether penicillamine prevents joint erosions in RA.

More than 25% of patients taking penicillamine have to discontinue the drug because of side effects within the first 12 months. The major adverse reactions are skin rashes, proteinuria, hematuria, neutropenia, thrombocytopenia, and a variety of autoimmune phenomena including the induction of antinuclear antibodies and drug-induced lupus, Goodpasture's syndrome, and myasthenia gravis. Some of these adverse reactions occur more frequently in patients who demonstrate slow sulfoxidation, and there may also be an association with HLA-DR3 and B8. Penicillamine should be started in doses between 125 and 250 mg/day and increased to a maximum of 750 mg/day over a period of a few months. When disease is controlled the dose can be reduced, but most patients suffer an exacerbation of their symptoms if the drug is stopped. While taking penicillamine patients need to have regular blood and urine tests, as outlined in Table 47-2.

Biologic Agents

Two TNF inhibitors have been approved for the treatment of RA: etanercept and infliximab. Etanercept, a soluble p75TNF receptor fusion protein (sTNFR-Ig), binds to TNF and neutralizes its biologic activities. Etanercept also reacts with lymphotoxin α, but the role of this cytokine in amplifying joint inflammation is unknown. Results from two placebo-controlled trials have shown that etanercept, 25 mg SQ twice daily, is effective for the treatment of RA, producing ACR-20 response rates in the range of 60% to 75% (17,18). A six-month clinical trial has also shown that etanercept affords incremental clinical benefits when added to background MTX therapy (19). For people with early RA, etanercept has proven to be similar to MTX in clinical efficacy, although numerical trends suggest that etanercept may be slightly more effective than MTX for preventing joint damage (4).

Infliximab is a chimeric antibody composed of a human IgG1κ Fc region linked to an Fv domain of a murine anti-TNF monoclonal antibody. Infliximab is formulated for intravenous administration. In a large clinical trial, 428 patients with active RA despite MTX therapy were maintained on a constant dose of MTX and randomly treated with placebo or 3 mg/kg or 10 mg/kg of intravenous infliximab at week zero, two, and six, and then every four or eight weeks. After 30 weeks, infliximab-treated patients achieved ACR-20 response rates of 50%–58% compared to 20% for the placebo group (20). Importantly, treatment with infliximab and MTX significantly reduced radiologic progression of joint damage compared to MTX alone (21).

Side effects may occur with TNF blockade therapy. Injection-site reactions have been noted with etanercept administration, but they are usually mild. Infliximab infusions may produce mild reactions consisting of headache, nausea, rash, hypertension, or hypotension. Rarely, infliximab may provoke a severe allergic reaction. Neither etanercept nor infliximab has been associated with an increased rate of serious bacterial infections in trials, but concerns linger about the possibility that chronic TNF inhibition may predispose to infectious complications, especially tuberculosis. Approximately 10% of infliximab- and etanercept-treated patients with RA develop antibodies to double-stranded DNA. Rarely, the induction of these autoantibodies has been associated with systemic lupus erythematous (SLE)-like reactions. These reactions have not been life-threatening and resolve after stopping the anti-TNF agent and treating with a brief course of corticosteroids. In isolated cases, etanercept therapy has been associated with pancytopenia and a demyelinating process resembling multiple sclerosis.

Protein A Column

A staphylococcal protein A (Prosorba) column recently has been approved as a medical device for the treatment of moderate to severe RA. The device is used in conjunction with plasmapheresis, which takes the separated plasma and passes it through the column. Studies have shown that 12 weekly treatments with the Prosorba column afford modest benefits over a sham treatment (22). Prosorba is reserved for treatment of the most refractory cases.

Combination DMARD Therapy

Methotrexate has emerged as the anchor drug for most combination regimens. Many patients who are treated with MTX are only partial responders and require further DMARD therapy. Rheumatologists often add one or two DMARDs to background MTX therapy ("step-up" approach) in an attempt to improve the clinical response. A growing number of studies support the clinical efficacy and safety of this strategy.

The most commonly used DMARD combinations are "triple therapy" (MTX + SSZ + HCQ), MTX plus CsA, and MTX plus a TNF inhibitor (23,24). DMARD combinations have proven efficacious for treating patients with both advanced and early RA. The relative benefits and risks of simultaneously initiating therapy with multiple DMARDs versus the step-up approach described above are unknown. The potential advantages of an aggressive multidrug approach is shown by the results of a 56-week clinical trial comparing treatment with 2 g/day SSZ alone to a regimen of SSZ 2 g/day, prednisolone 60 mg/day, and MTX 7.5 mg/week (25). At the trial's conclusion, patients taking the combination regimen had significantly less joint damage than those receiving SSZ alone. In contrast, an open randomized trial enrolling 82 people with active RA of less than 12 months' duration found that standard monotherapy with SSZ produced similar levels of clinical improvement as initial therapy with MTX plus CsA and intra-articular corticosteroid injections (26). Further studies are needed to clarify the best treatment strategy.

Conclusions

The treatment of RA evolves as new evidence-based therapies reach the clinic. Once a DMARD becomes established in clinical practice, additional data comes to light regarding the drug's long-term efficacy and tolerability in diverse patient populations with varying levels of disease severity. Experience has taught that results from short-term trials do not extrapolate readily to the clinical situation. For example, auranofin was indistinguishable in clinical efficacy from MTX in a trial setting, but it has shown poor efficacy and tolerability in practice. On the other hand, MTX has grown in clinical utility due to its excellent long-term efficacy and tolerability. This hierarchy of effectiveness may be best reflected in the length of time patients take a DMARD, which is significantly longer for MTX than other agents, such as SSZ, HCQ, and gold (3).

The current DMARDs are a group of agents with varied biologic activities. In the past, DMARDs have been primarily adopted for the treatment of RA on empirical grounds. However, recent insights into the pathogenesis of RA have allowed the development of novel agents that specifically target pathogenic mechanisms. Etanercept and infliximab are examples of such agents. The newer DMARDs have expanded the treatment options for RA and enable greater flexibility in decision-making. The observed clinical benefits of these newer agents provide optimism that prevention of joint destruction and physical disability are attainable goals. Current efforts are directed towards the discovery of combination DMARD regimens that more effectively suppress joint inflammation and damage.

E. WILLIAM St. CLAIR, MD

References

1. Cronstein BN. *The mechanism of action of methotrexate. Rheum Dis Clin North Am* 1997;23:739–755.
2. Weinblatt ME, Maier AL, Fraser PA, Coblyn JS. *Longterm prospective study of methotrexate in rheumatoid arthritis: conclusion after 132 months of therapy. J Rheumatol* 1998;25: 238–242.
3. Pincus T, Marcum SB, Callahan LF. *Longterm drug therapy for rheumatoid arthritis in seven rheumatology private practices: Second line drugs and prednisone. J Rheumatol* 1992;19: 1885–1894.
4. Bathon JM, Martin RW, Fleischmann RM, et al. *A comparison of etanercept and methotrexate in patients with early rheumatoid arthritis. N Engl J Med* 2000;343:1586–1593.
5. Morgan SL, Baggott JE, Vaughn WH, et al. *Supplementation with folic acid during methotrexate therapy for rheumatoid arthritis. A double-blind, placebo-controlled trial. Ann Intern Med* 1994;121:833–841.
6. Gadangi P, Longaker M, Naime D, et al. *The anti-inflammatory mechanism of sulafasalazine is related to adenosine release at inflamed sites. J Immunol* 1996;156:1937–1941.
7. Wahl C, Liptay S, Guido A, Schmid RM. *Sulfasalazine: a potent and specific inhibitor of nuclear factor kappa B. J Clin Invest* 1998;101:1163–1174.
8. Smolen JS, Kalden JR, Scott DL, et al. *Efficacy and safety of leflunomide compared with placebo and sulphasalazine in active rheumatoid arthritis: a double-blind, randomised, multicentre trial. Lancet* 1999;353:259–266.
9. Fox RI. *Mechanism of action of hydroxychloroquine as an antirheumatic drug. Semin Arthritis Rheum* 1993;23:82–91.
10. Clark P, Casas E, Tugwell P, et al. *Hydroxychloroquine compared with placebo in rheumatoid arthritis. A randomized controlled trial. Ann Intern Med* 1993;119:1067–1071.
11. Alarcon GS. *Minocycline for the treatment of rheumatoid arthritis. Rheum Dis Clin North Am* 1998;24:489–499.
12. Strand V, Cohen S, Schiff M, et al. *Treatment of active rheumatoid arthritis with leflunomide compared with placebo and methotrexate. Arch Intern Med* 1999;159:2542–50.
13. Sharp JT, Strand V, Leung H, Hurley, Loew-Friedrich I on behalf of the Leflunomide Rheumatoid Arthritis Investigators Group. *Treatment with leflunomide slows radiographic progression of rheumatoid arthritis. Arthritis Rheum* 2000;43:495–505.
14. Strand V, Tugwell P, Bombardier C, et al. *Function and health-related quality of life. Results from a randomized controlled trial of leflunomide versus methotrexate or placebo in patients with active rheumatoid arthritis. Arthritis Rheum* 1999;42: 1870–1878.
15. Cranney A, Tugwell P. *The use of Neoral in rheumatoid arthritis. Rheum Dis Clin North Am* 1998;24:479–488.
16. van den Borne BEEM, Landewe RBM, Houkes I, et al. *No increased risk of malignancies and mortality in cyclosporin A-treated patients with rheumatoid arthritis. Arthritis Rheum* 1998;41:1930–1937.
17. Moreland LW, Baumgartner SW, Schiff MH, et al. *Treatment of rheumatoid arthritis with a recombinant human tumor necrosis factor receptor (p75)-Fc fusion protein. N Engl J Med* 1997;337:141–147.
18. Moreland LW, Schiff MH, Baumgartner SW, et al. *Etanercept therapy in rheumatoid arthritis. A randomized, controlled trial. Ann Intern Med* 1999;130:478–486.
19. Weinblatt ME, Kremer JM, Bankhurst AD, et al. *A trial of etanercept, a recombinant tumor necrosis factor receptor:Fc fusion protein, in patients with rheumatoid arthritis receiving methotrexate. N Engl J Med* 1999;340:253–259.

20. Maini RN, St.Clair EW, Breedveld F, et al. Infliximab (chimeric anti-tumor necrosis factor a monoclonal antibody) versus placebo in rheumatoid arthritis patients receiving concomitant methorexate: a randomised phase III trial. Lancet 1999;354: 1932–1939.

21. Lipsky PE, van der Meijde DMFM, St.Clair EW, et al. Infliximab and methotrexate in the treatment of rheumatoid arthritis. N Engl J Med 2000;343:1594–1602.

22. Felson DT, LaValley MP, Baldassare AR, et al. The Prosorba column for treatment of refractory rheumatoid arthritis. A randomized, double-blind, sham-controlled trial. Arthritis Rheum 1999;42:2153–2159.

23. O'Dell JR, Haire CE, Erikson N, et al. Treatment of rheumatoid arthritis with methotrexate alone, sulfasalazine and hydroxy-chloroquine, or a combination of all three medications. N Engl J Med 1996;334:1287–1291.

24. Tugwell P, Pincus T, Yocum D, et al. Combination therapy with cyclosporine and methotrexate in severe rheumatoid arthritis. N Engl J Med 1995;333:137–141.

25. Boers M, Verhoeven AC, Markusse HM, et al. Randomised comparison of combined step-down prednisolone, methotrexate and sulphasalazine with sulfasalazine alone in early rheumatoid arthritis. Lancet 1997;350:309–318.

26. Proudman SM, Conaghan PG, Richardson C, et al. Treatment of poor-prognosis early rheumatoid arthritis. A randomized study of treatment with methotrexate, cyclosporine A, and intraarticular corticosteroids compared with sulfasalazine alone. Arthritis Rheum 2000;43:1809–1819.

27. Felson DT, Anderson JJ, Boers M, et al. American College of Rheumatology preliminary definition of improvement in rheumatoid arthritis. Arthritis Rheum 1995;38:727–735.

28. American College of Rheumatology Ad Hoc Committee on Clinical Guidelines. Guidelines for monitoring drug therapy in rheumatoid arthritis. Arthritis Rheum 1996;39:713–732.

48 BIOLOGIC AGENTS

Remarkable progress has been made in the development of immunomodulatory interventions collectively referred to as biologic agents. These therapies are distinct from the majority of traditional antirheumatic drugs in that they: 1) are often large molecules; 2) are derived from or resemble naturally occurring effector molecules such as antibodies or soluble cell-surface receptors; and 3) target specific components of the immune response. Several biologic agents, including inhibitors of the proinflammatory cytokine tumor necrosis factor (TNF), are now available for the treatment of rheumatoid arthritis (RA). The development of additional agents for RA and the testing of biologic therapies in other conditions are proceeding swiftly.

Several factors encouraged the development of biologic agents. From a clinical standpoint, there has been a growing appreciation of the impact of rheumatic diseases. In years past, RA was considered to be a relatively benign disease, but it is now recognized as a chronic, progressive condition that exacts a tremendous toll on patients. There has also been growing dissatisfaction with the currently available medications for rheumatic diseases. Many drugs, including the so-called disease-modifying agents employed in RA and other conditions, often cannot be used long-term because of toxicities or ineffectiveness. Central to the development of biologic agents has been the tremendous progress in delineating the dysregulations in the immune response underlying the initiation and propagation of rheumatic diseases. Accompanying this greater understanding of immunopathogenesis has been the expectation that specific components of the immune response are tenable therapeutic targets. Finally, the ability to target specific cell-surface and soluble molecules was created by the remarkable advances made in the last decade in biotechnology, molecular biology, and pharmaceutical development.

Approaches to Therapy

Because rheumatic diseases are driven by the immune system, the goals of therapy with biologic agents are the induction of immunologic tolerance and disease remission. The choices of targets for immunomodulatory therapy are based on understanding both physiologic and pathologic immune responses. In the generation of productive immune responses, antigens are processed by antigen-presenting cells (APCs) and presented in the context of appropriate major histocompatibility complex (MHC) molecules (e.g., MHC class II) to subsets of T lymphocytes that bear antigen-specific T-cell receptors (TCRs).

When this first signal is accompanied by additional stimulation, provided by interaction of the T cell with costimulatory cell-surface molecules and cytokines, an immune response is generated. If the first signal is inhibited, no response will occur. If the second signal is inhibited, the result will be ignorance (i.e., no immune reaction to the antigen) or tolerance (specific anergy to the antigen). After an immune reaction has begun, the propagation and shaping of the response (e.g., T-helper 1 versus T-helper 2 predominance) depend on the overall activity of mediators such as cytokines and chemokines present in the local milieu. Various cells function in complex interactive networks to amplify and sustain the inflammation characteristic of rheumatic disease. Using biologic agents to interfere with this cascade might interrupt the ongoing immune response, and allow the re-establishment of normal immune homeostasis.

The approach to immunomodulatory therapy may be conceptualized as consisting of specific, semispecific, and nonspecific approaches. The ability to target components of the immune response in a more specific fashion is one of the major advantages of biologic agents over traditional therapies.

Ag/TCR/MHC-Specific Therapies

Therapy specific for the agents causing the disease, or for the clones of T or B cells programmed to respond to the etiologic antigens, has the greatest theoretical appeal. Not only might such specific therapy obviate many of the adverse effects observed with nonspecific immunosuppressive agents, it could also prevent further reactivity to the etiologic antigen, thereby inducing remission of disease (1,2).

A number of biologic agents that target the trimolecular complex (Ag/TCR/MHC) have been used successfully in animal models of autoimmune disease. Although these therapies can induce tolerance and completely abrogate disease in animals, at present, several considerations preclude the use of such an approach in human rheumatic diseases. The greatest of these is the fact that, in contrast to the situation in animal models, the specific antigens causing rheumatic disease in humans remain largely undefined. Even without knowledge of the inciting antigen, however, specific inhibition could be achieved if the particular TCR/MHC interactions driving the immune response were known. Yet these also remain largely unidentified. Moreover, in animal models of autoimmune disease, Ag/TCR/MHC-specific therapies are most successful when administered before or soon after disease initiation. Such timely institution of therapy is rarely possible in humans, who present for treatment only long after the disease has begun. Another potentially con-

TABLE 48-1
Targets of Biologic Therapy in Rheumatic Diseases

Specific
  Ag/TCR/MHC-directed
  Other relevant antigens

Semispecific
  Cell subsets
    CD4⁺ T cells
      Memory T cells
      Th1 versus Th2 T cells
    Others (dendritic cells, B cells, mast cells,
      macrophages, etc)
  Costimulatory molecules
    CD80/CD86 – CD28/CTLA-4
    CD40 – CD40L (CD154)
    Others
  Adhesion molecules
    LFA-1 (CD11a/CD18)/ICAM-1 (CD54)
    VLA-4 / VCAM-1
    Others (E-selectin, CD44, etc)
  Cytokines
    Proinflammatory cytokines
      TNF
      IL-1
      Others (IL-6, IL-17, etc)
    Immunoregulatory cytokines
      IL-4, IL-10 (Th2)
      IL-12, IL-18, IFN-γ (Th1)
      Others (TGF-β, IL-2, IL-15, Interferons [γ, β, α], etc)
  Other inflammatory mediators
    Chemokines (IL-8, MCP-1, RANTES, MIP-1α, etc)
    Complement proteins
    Others (PAF, substance P, NO, etc)

Nonspecific
  Pan-T cell
  Pan-lymphocyte

TCR, T-cell receptor; MHC, major histocompatibility complex; TNF, tumor necrosis factor; IL, interleukin; IFN, interferon; TGF, transforming growth factor; PAF, platelet activating factor; NO, nitric oxide.

founding factor is the "antigenic drift" seen in chronic immune reactions.

Nevertheless, several interventions targeting the Ag/TCR/MHC complex have been tested in human disease. These include vaccinations with TCR-derived peptides; vaccination with MHC fragments or with relevant peptides linked to MHC fragments (e.g., cartilage protein gp39/DR4 in RA); and administration of antibodies to MHC molecules (2,3). Although these interventions appear to be tolerated well, the demonstration of efficacy awaits further testing.

Other potential approaches are based in the induction of bystander tolerance, using antigens distinct from the etiologic agent but relevant to the disease. An example of this is oral ingestion of type II collagen in RA (4). Although theoretically appealing, there has not yet been conclusive proof of the efficacy of oral tolerance in human disease.

Semispecific Therapy
The majority of biologic approaches to rheumatic diseases are considered semispecific (Table 48-1). Although not specific for etiologic antigens, they target important components of the dysregulated immune response that are central to the propagation of disease. These same molecules are involved in normal immunity but are upregulated at sites of active disease. Importantly, some semispecific approaches are also capable of inducing immunologic tolerance.

T-Cell–Directed Therapies
One of the earliest targets chosen for study of biologic agents in human rheumatic disease was CD4. The CD4⁺ subset of T lymphocytes serves a key role in the inflammation of RA and other rheumatic diseases. Biologic therapy targeting CD4 achieved remarkable success in animal models of autoimmune disease, inducing specific immunologic tolerance and long-term clinical benefit. Moreover, anti-CD4 therapy with foreign antibodies induced tolerance to the treating agent as well. Early uncontrolled studies in people with RA showed biologic effects (i.e., decreases in the numbers of circulating CD4⁺ cells) and suggested clinical benefit. However, in more rigorous, double-blind placebo-controlled trials, the clinical efficacy of anti-CD4⁺ therapy was no greater than that of placebo, despite the induction of long-term decreases in CD4⁺ T cells (5). Moreover, the antibodies used elicited an immune response.

Despite the failure of anti-CD4 antibodies in RA, a number of important lessons have come from these trials. First, determination of clinical efficacy of prospective therapies for rheumatic diseases must come from rigorously controlled clinical trials. Second, it is possible that rheumatic diseases such as RA are heterogeneous, and that the efficacy of particular biologic therapies may vary with particular patient subsets or stages of disease. Finally, the characteristics of the biologic agent are crucial. For example, some anti-CD4 antibodies preferentially target naive CD4 T cells rather than the populations of memory Th1 CD4 T cells presumably of greatest relevance to rheumatic disease (6). In the future, CD4-targeted therapies may be tenable options, for example, with non-depleting antibodies.

Inhibition of Costimulatory Molecules
Potentially one of the most exciting avenues for biologic therapy focuses on costimulatory molecules, the cell-surface molecules that provide the second signal governing immune responses. Among the most important pairs of costimulatory molecules are 1) CD28 and CTLA-4, which bind B7-1 (CD80) and B7-2 (CD86); and 2) CD40 ligand (CD40L; CD154), which binds CD40 (7–9).

The interactions of T-cell surface molecules CD28 and CTLA-4 with B7-1 and B7-2 (present on APCs) are essential to the initiation, sustenance, and regulation of T-cell driven immune responses. Interactions between CD40L (present on T cells) and CD40 (on APCs) are essential for the formation of lymph node germinal centers and the production of antibodies. CD28 and CD40 interactions also affect Th1/Th2 balance (9). Inhibition of these molecules is effective in several animal models of diseases such as RA and systemic lupus erythematosus (SLE) (7–9). In some cases, e.g., solid organ allograft transplant, antigen-specific immune tolerance has been achieved using biologic agents that inhibit CD28 and CD40. A number of clinical studies using these approaches in RA, SLE, and other autoimmune diseases have begun (10).

Inhibition of Adhesion Molecules

Adhesion molecules serve several roles relevant to the generation of autoimmune responses in rheumatic diseases. These include regulation of the recruitment, retention, and activation of inflammatory cells at sites of active disease (11). Several adhesion molecules also provide costimulatory signals to T cells and mediate functions such as angiogenesis. Among adhesion molecules, the interaction of LFA-1 (CD11a/CD18) with ICAM-1 (CD54) and that of VLA-4 (CD49d/CD29) with VCAM-1 (CD106) may be the most important, making these molecules attractive targets for biologic therapies. Inhibition of these molecules has led to clinical improvement in numerous animal models of autoimmune disease and, in some cases, to immunologic tolerance. Anti-adhesion therapy with an anti-ICAM-1 antibody has been tested in humans. Although therapy appeared to be effective and capable of modulating immune responsiveness, repeated use of the agent was precluded by the immunogenicity of the murine antibody. This highlights the concept that for biologic agents to be viable in the clinic, the characteristics of the agent are as important as those of the target. Trials of anti-adhesion therapy are currently ongoing in several immune-mediated conditions including psoriasis, ulcerative colitis, and multiple sclerosis (10).

Inhibition of Cytokines

To date, the greatest success with biologic agents has been achieved by inhibitors of proinflammatory cytokines. Two biologic agents, both inhibitors of TNF, are currently approved for the treatment of RA: etanercept, a soluble p75-TNF-receptor/Fc fusion protein; and infliximab, a chimeric anti-TNF monoclonal antibody. In addition, a recombinant version of the naturally occuring IL-1 inhibitor (IL-1Ra) is being evaluated in advanced-phase clinical trials, as is the human anti-TNF monoclonal antibody known as D2E7.

The success of anti-TNF strategies in RA raises several questions not only about TNF inhibitors, but also about future biologic agents (12). For example, although some patients achieve complete suppression of disease activity with long-term use of TNF inhibitors, others show minimal clinical effect. Identification of factors that might explain this variability, such as heterogeneity in synovial TNF expression or genetic polymorphisms encoding TNF, would be of tremendous value. Deeper understanding of the mechanisms of these agents would allow further treatment paradigms to be assessed rationally, including combinations of therapies. Interestingly, although the currently available TNF-blocking agents are all capable of inhibiting TNF, there are differences among them in terms of target specificity and binding avidity; the implications of these differences remain to be determined.

Modification of Th1/Th2 Balance

An important advance in the understanding of the pathogenesis of autoimmune diseases has been the elucidation of T-cell subsets, identified by the patterns of cytokines they secrete. The Th1 subset of cells, which functions primarily in cell-mediated immunity, seems to play a dominant role in RA and several other rheumatic conditions (13). Therefore, alteration of the Th1/Th2 balance may be a valuable therapeutic approach in RA. As the generation of these cells is regulated largely by specific cytokines (i.e., IL-12, IL-18, and IFN-γ drive Th1 development; IL-10 and IL-4 drive Th2 development and inhibit Th1 cells), therapeutic administration or targeting of these cytokines may be a practical approach to this goal. IL-10 exerts additional anti-inflammatory effects that could impact rheumatic diseases. Both IL-4 and IL-10 have been assessed in preliminary studies in people with RA. Of note, a number of other factors can modulate Th1/Th2 balance, including the relative strength or timing of costimulation, the presence of specific chemokines or other mediators in the local milieu (e.g., TNF, substance P) (7,9,13). These factors provide additional potential therapeutic avenues for Th1/Th2 regulation.

Inhibition of Other Inflammatory Mediators

A variety of inflammatory mediators contribute to immune responses and could therefore serve as targets for biologic interventions. Recently, there has been an explosion in knowledge about chemokines. These small molecules direct the trafficking of specific populations of leukocytes to inflammatory sites and regulate their activation (14). Driven in part by their potential utility in allergic and infectious diseases, there has been substantial interest in developing chemokine inhibitors. Other immune-system components that have attracted renewed interest are the interferons and components of the complement cascade. Specific inhibitors of complement proteins, including antibodies to C5, are under evaluation (10).

Types of Biologic Agents

The current types of biologic agents are shown in Fig. 48-1. The development of monoclonal antibodies (mAbs), which allowed targets such as cell-surface molecules and cytokines to be bound and inhibited with unprecedented specificity, ushered in the era of therapeutic biologic agents (15). Initially developed in mice, refinements in genetic engineering and biotechnology have allowed the development of progressively less foreign constructs. Chimeric antibodies (e.g., infliximab) are about 70% human (the Fc fragment and constant regions) and 30% murine (the antigen-binding variable regions). Humanized mAbs are approximately 95% human (only the complementarity-determining regions are murine). Monoclonal antibodies derived entirely from human sequences (e.g., D2E7) can now also be produced, for example, by repertoire cloning of phage libraries. Technological advances have enabled the development of additional types of immunomodulatory biologic agents, such as recombinant forms or homologues of naturally occurring inhibitors. Examples include the recombinant IL-1Ra anakinra, which binds to the IL-1 receptor but

transduces no signal, and soluble forms of the p75 cell-surface receptor for TNF. Modifications of these compounds, such as coupling soluble tumor necrosis factor receptor (sTNF-R) with the Fc piece of IgG (e.g., etanercept) have improved pharmacokinetic characteristics.

Although extraordinary additions to the therapeutic armamentarium, mAbs, soluble receptors, and other such constructs are less than ideal drugs. First, the production of these macromolecules is exacting and expensive. Emerging genetic technologies may enable large-scale production of pharmaceutical proteins (including mAbs) in transgenic plants or in the milk or urine of transgenic animals (16), decreasing the cost. Other developments may improve the pharmacokinetic and pharmacodynamic characteristics of

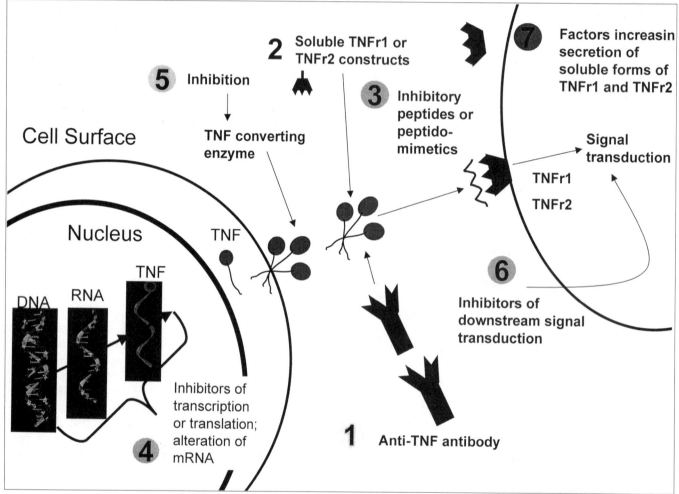

Fig. 48-1. Potential approaches for biologic therapy. A given immunologic target, in this case the binding of tumor necrosis factor (TNF) to its specific cell-surface receptors [TNFRI (CD120a), TNFRII (CD120b)] can be inhibited through multiple approaches. After a stimulatory signal, genes encoding TNF are transcribed, and subsequently the mRNA translated into protein. The mRNA for TNF is assembled into an active trimer at the cell surface. The TNF homotrimer is cleaved from the cell surface by a specific protease (TNF concerting enzyme, or TACE); subsequently it binds to its specific cell-surface receptors, and transduces a signal. Inhibitory approaches include: 1) monoclonal antibodies specifically bind TNF, preventing it from binding to its receptors; 2) soluble forms of the TNF receptors bind TNF and lymphtoxin α (LT-α), preventing their binding to the cell-surface receptors; 3) small peptide or peptidomimetic inhibitors block the TNF/TNFR interactions; 4) transcription, translation, and mRNA stability can be modulated by gene therapy, kinase inhibitors, and other factors; 5) inhibition of TACE prevents TNF from being secreted; 6) various factors can affect signal transduction post-receptor; and 7) the secretion of TNFR can be increased by various means (e.g., gene therapy, cytokines).

such compounds. Techniques such as the use of liposomes, gelatin microspheres, or bispecific antibodies may allow greater precision in drug delivery to specific inflammatory sites (17–19). This could conceivably reduce the price and diminish the risk of untoward effects.

Because mAbs and soluble receptors are large protein molecules, these agents may be immunogenic, which potentially decreases the half lives and clinical utility of these agents and also leads to adverse effects. Factors that affect whether an agent will elicit an immune response include: 1) route of administration (e.g., subcutaneous is generally more immunogenic than intravenous, and oral doses tend to be the least immunogenic); 2) immunosuppressive effects of the agent or concomitant medications (this can minimize immune responses); 3) dose and dosing frequency (regular administration of larger doses tends to minimize immune responses); and 4) modifications to the compound (e.g., polyethylene glycol treatment or glycosylation of proteins can reduce immunogenicity). The more foreign a protein is, the more likely it is to induce an immune response. However, even fully human compounds can be immunogenic.

Considerations such as these, along with the success of the TNF inhibitors, have spawned intense efforts to develop other approaches to modulate the immune response (Fig. 48-1). For example, small molecule peptides or peptidomimetics that could inhibit TNF/TNF-R interactions have been tested in vitro (20). Much attention has also focused on gene-based strategies. Many of the key cell-surface molecules and cytokines involved in the immunopathogenesis of rheumatic diseases are upregulated through the action of factors controlling transduction and translation (21). With further understanding of the molecular mechanisms and their role in disease, interventions such as anti-sense oligonucleotides, gene transfer of regulatory factors, ribozyme treatment, and specific protease inhibitors (e.g., p38 MAP kinase inhibitor) may have entered clinical studies (22,23). Potential therapies such as protease inhibitors and peptidomimetic inhibitors could be small, orally bioavailable molecules that would be cheaper to produce than macromolecules.

Future Directions

The future for biologic agents in rheumatic diseases is promising. Greater understanding of the immune responses that underlie rheumatic diseases should continue to yield novel and viable targets for specific therapies. Advances in biopharmaceuticals should generate agents that possess desirable characteristics in terms of pharmacokinetics, immunogenicity, adverse effects, ease of administration, and cost. Research defining the populations of patients expected to derive the greatest benefit from particular types of therapy should optimize efficacy and minimize toxicity. Combinations of biologic agents for synergy (e.g., the combination of TNF and IL-1 inhibitors) (24) and the combined use of biologic agents and traditional therapies are

being assessed. These developments may allow clinicians to maximize their use of these novel therapies and achieve clinical benefits previously considered unattainable.

ARTHUR KAVANAUGH, MD

References

1. Cush JJ, Kavanaugh AF. Biologic interventions in rheumatoid arthritis. Rheum Dis Clin N Am 1995;23:797–816.
2. Adorini L, Guery J-C, Rodriguez-Tarduchy G, Trembleau S. Selective immunosuppression. Immunol Today 1993;14:285–289.
3. Moreland L, Morgan E, Adamson T, et al. T cell receptor peptide vaccination in rheumatoid arthritis: a placebo-controlled trial using a combination of Vβ3, Vβ14, and Vβ17 peptides. Arthritis Rheum 1998;41:1919–1929.
4. Kalden JR, Sieper J. Oral collagen in the treatment of rheumatoid arthritis. Arthritis Rheum 1998;41:191–194.
5. van der Lubbe PA, Dijkmans BAC, Markusse HM, Nässander U, Breedveld FC. A randomized, double-blind, placebo-controlled study of CD4 monoclonal antibody therapy in early rheumatoid arthritis. Arthritis Rheum 1995;38:1097–1106.
6. Rep M, van Oosten B, Roos M, Ader H, Polman C, van Lier R. Treatment with depleting CD4 monoclonal antibody results in a preferential loss of circulating naive T cells but does not affect IFN-γ secreting Th1 cells in human. J Clin Invest 1997;99:2225–2231.
7. Reiser H, Stadecke M. Costimulatory B7 molecules in the pathogenesis of infectious and autoimmune diseases. N Engl J Med 1996;335:1369–1377.
8. Datta S, Kalled S. CD40-CD40 ligand interaction in autoimmune disease. Arthritis Rheum 1997;40:1735–1745.
9. Daikh D, Finck B, Linsley P, Hollenbough D, Wofsy D. Long-term inhibition of murine lupus by brief simultaneous blockade of the B7/CD28 and CD40/gp39 costimulation pathways. Immunol Today 1997;159:3104–3108.
10. Glennie M, Johnson P. Clinical trials of antibody therapy. Immunol Today 2000;21:403–410.
11. Kavanaugh A. Antiadhesion therapy in rheumatoid arthritis: a review of recent progress. BioDrugs; Clin Immunotherapeutics 1997;7:119–133.
12. Kavanaugh A, Cohen S, Cush J. Inhibitors of tumor necrosis factor in rheumatoid arthritis. Will that dog hunt? J Rheum 1998;25:2049–2053.
13. Miossec P, van den Berg W. Th1/Th2 cytokine balance in arthritis. Arthritis Rheum 1997;40:2105–2115.
14. Nickel R, Beck L, Stellato C, Schleimer R. Chemokines and allergic disease. J Allergy Clin Immunol 1999;104:723–742.
15. Breedveld F. Therapeutic monoclonal antibodies. Lancet 2000;355:735–740.
16. Kerr D, Liang F, Bondioli K, et al. The bladder as a bioreactor: urothelium production and secretion of growth hormone into urine. Nature Biotechnology 1998;16:75–79.
17. Spragg D, Alford D, Greferath R, et al. Immunotargeting of liposomes to activated vascular endothelial cells: a strategy for site-selective delivery in the cardiovascular system. Proc Natl Acad Sci USA. 1997;94:8795–8800.

18. *van Spriel A, van Ojik, van de Winkel J. Immunotherapeutic perspective for bispecific antibodies. Immunol Today 2000; 21:391–397.*

19. *Brown K, Leong K, Huang C-H, et al. Gelatin/chondroitin 6-sulfate microspheres for the delivery of therapeutic proteins to the joint. Arthritis Rheum 1998;41:2185–2195.*

20. *Takasaki W, Kajino Y, Kajino K, Murali R, Greene M. Structure-based design and characterization of exocyclic peptidomimetics that inhibit TNFα binding to its receptor. Nature Biotechnology 1997;15:1266–1270.*

21. *Firestein G, Manning A. Signal transduction and transcription factors in rheumatic disease. Arthritis Rheum 1999;42:609–621.*

22. *Wrighton C, Hofer-Warbinek R, Moll T, Eytner R, Bach F, de Martin R. Inhibition of endothelial cell activation by adenovirus-mediated expression of IκBα, an inhibitor of the transcription factor NF-κB. J Exp Med 1996;183:1013–1022.*

23. *Evans C, Ghivizzani S, Kang R, et al. Gene therapy for rheumatic diseases. Arthritis Rheum 1999;42:1–16.*

24. *Bendele A, Chilpala E, Scherrer J, et al. Combination benefit of treatment with the cytokine inhibitors interleukin-1 receptor antagonist and soluble tumor necrosis factor type I in animal models of rheumatoid arthritis. Arthritis Rheum 2000;43:2648-2659.*

49 OPERATIVE TREATMENT OF ARTHRITIS

Pain not relieved by other treatments is the most common indication for operative treatment of arthritis. Loss of joint function is a less common indication for surgical treatment because function restoration is usually less predictable than pain relief. Operative treatments include joint debridement, synovectomy, osteotomy, soft-tissue arthroplasty, resection arthroplasty, fusion, and joint replacement. In addition, people with rheumatoid arthritis (RA) may benefit from tenosynovectomy and repair or reconstruction of ruptured tendons.

Although operative treatments can produce excellent results, they also expose patients to serious risks. Potential operative and perioperative complications include extensive blood loss, cardiac arrhythmia and arrest, nerve and blood vessel injury, infection, venous thrombosis, and pulmonary embolism. Late postoperative complications include delayed infection and loosening and wear of implants. Even in the absence of complications, the results of surgical procedures such as joint debridements, synovectomies, and osteotomies may deteriorate with time. For these reasons, the potential risks and expected short-term and long-term outcomes of operative treatment must be carefully considered for each patient. Nonetheless, individuals who fail to gain satisfactory results from nonsurgical therapy or who have progressive disease should be evaluated by a surgeon before they develop deformity, joint instability, contractures, or advanced muscle atrophy. Delaying surgery until these problems develop can compromise the results and increase the risk of complications.

Preoperative Evaluation

With the exception of people in whom arthritic disorders have caused or may cause spinal instability and neurologic damage, operative treatment is elective. Patients should have an extensive preoperative evaluation and should understand the full range of therapeutic options. The physician needs a thorough understanding of the degree of pain and functional limitation and an understanding of the patient's social and occupational needs and expectations. Before planning surgery, patients should understand the potential benefits and risks. In general, the patients most likely to notice significant lasting benefit from operative treatment are those with joint pain unrelieved by nonsurgical treatment. Patient age, overall health status, and capacity to adhere to postoperative rehabilitation and precautions also help determine the outcome.

Even in people with obvious joint disease, pain, and loss of function, failure to carefully evaluate the cause of the symptoms can lead to disappointing results. Common diagnostic dilemmas include differentiating hip joint pain from lumbar radicular pain and shoulder joint pain from cervical radicular pain. Rheumatoid arthritis and other types of inflammatory arthritis may cause such severe joint deformity that detecting neurologic involvement becomes difficult. Patients may develop joint sepsis that is not readily apparent because of the inflammatory nature of their underlying disease and the use of medications that suppress the inflammatory response to infection. A careful history, physical examination, and plain radiographs are sufficient to define the cause of symptoms for most, but in some cases, joint aspiration, electrodiagnostic studies, and additional imaging studies are needed to clarify the cause of pain and loss of function.

Before considering surgical intervention, patients should first be treated with nonoperative interventions including medications, ambulatory aides, activity modification, physical therapy, and orthoses. Braces may control instability and decrease pain in the spine, knee, ankle, wrist, or thumb. A cane may be considered for patients with lower-extremity arthritis. In addition to reducing the body-weight load to the joints of the lower extremity, a cane reduces the hip abductor forces required to keep the pelvis level during gait, thereby reducing hip-joint reactive forces by up to 20% in the contralateral hip.

Weight reduction for obese patients can decrease symptoms and increase the probability of successful operative treatment. There is some evidence of an increased incidence of infection in obese patients following total joint arthroplasty (1), as well as increased intraoperative blood loss (2). Obesity does not appear to increase the risk of implant loosening, but this may be because heavier patients are less active. For some overweight patients, the pain and loss of mobility caused by arthritis makes it more difficult to reduce their weight or avoid gaining weight. In these individuals, surgeons may recommend proceeding with operative treatment despite the increased risks associated with obesity.

The importance of a thorough preoperative history and physical examination, as well as careful perioperative medical management, cannot be overemphasized. Many patients who could benefit from surgical treatment, especially people with osteoarthritis (OA), are elderly and may have decreased cardiac, pulmonary, renal, or peripheral vascular function. These conditions require evaluation and, in some cases, treatment before surgery. Carious teeth, pharyngitis, cystitis, and other potential sources of infection should be treated prior to surgery. Men with symptoms of prostatic hypertrophy need a urologic evaluation before surgery and women should be evaluated for asymptomatic urinary tract infections. Preoperative laboratory evaluation should include a measure of hemoglobin and hematocrit, urinalysis, and other diagnostic tests as indicated by the individual's medical history.

Preparation for Operative Treatment

All patients should receive instruction concerning the planned procedure, the risks and common complications, the type and extent of postoperative rehabilitation, and expectations for postoperative pain relief and function. To reduce the risks of operative and postoperative complications, including excessive bleeding and compromised healing, doses of nonsteroidal anti-inflammatory drugs (NSAIDs) and corticosteroids should be decreased before surgery when possible. Preoperative evaluation and instruction by physical and occupational therapists facilitate rehabilitation for some patients. In selected patients, delaying surgery will make it possible to achieve optimal management of cardiovascular or other systemic disorders, allow them to improve their nutritional status and muscle strength, or reduce their weight.

Disease-Related Factors

Options and indications for surgical treatment vary considerably among the arthritic diseases. Thus, the physician must consider the unique features of each disease in making decisions or advising patients concerning operative treatment.

Osteoarthritis

A number of surgical procedures have the intent of decreasing symptoms for people with OA while preserving or restoring a cartilaginous articular surface. These include arthroscopic joint debridement, resection or perforation of subchondral bone to stimulate formation of cartilaginous tissue, and use of grafts to replace degenerated articular cartilage. By removing loose fragments of cartilage, bone, and meniscus (and in some instances osteophytes), joint debridement may improve joint mechanical function and may decrease pain. Penetration of subchondral bone in regions of advanced cartilage degeneration stimulates formation of cartilaginous repair tissue, but because it lacks the properties of normal articular cartilage, this tissue frequently degenerates. Replacing localized regions of degenerated cartilage with osteochondral, perichondral, periosteal, and chondrocyte grafts has produced promising short-term results in small series of patients. Overall, current procedures performed with the intent of preserving or restoring a cartilaginous articular surface and decreasing symptoms are not likely to be beneficial in people with advanced joint degeneration, but they may be helpful in selected people with less severe disease.

Osteotomies correct malalignment and shift loads from severely degenerated regions of the articular surface to regions that have remaining articular cartilage. In selected patients with OA, osteotomies of the hip and knee decrease pain, but in general the results are less predictable than joint replacement. For these reasons, surgeons most commonly recommend osteotomies for young active people who have a stable joint with a functional range of motion, good muscle function, and some remaining articular cartilage.

Joint fusion (i.e., arthrodesis) can relieve pain and restore skeletal stability and alignment in people with advanced OA. Because this procedure eliminates joint motion, it has limited application. Furthermore, fusion of one joint increases the loading and motion of other joints, perhaps accelerating degeneration. For example, fusion of the hip increases the probability of developing degenerative disease in the lumbar spine and ipsilateral knee joints. Currently, surgeons most commonly perform fusions for treating degeneration of cervical and lumbar spine, hand interphalangeal, first metatarsophalangeal, wrist, and ankle joints.

For selected joints, resection of degenerated articular surfaces and replacement with implants fabricated from polyethylene, metal, or other synthetic materials can relieve pain and allow the patient to maintain joint mobility (Fig. 49-1). Over the past several decades, replacing the hip and knee have proven to be effective methods of relieving pain and maintaining or improving function. Recent advances have led to better methods and implants for replacement of the hip, knee, shoulder, and elbow. Unfortunately, joint replacements have limitations, primarily because the new surface lacks the mechanical properties and durability of articular cartilage and because the prostheses must be fixed to the patients' bones. None of the currently available synthetic materials duplicates the ability of articular cartilage to provide a painless, low-friction gliding surface and to distribute loads across the synovial joint, nor can current implants achieve the stability and durability of the bond between articular cartilage and bone. Thus, wear of implants limits their life span, and loosening can lead to failure. For these reasons, current joint replacements cannot be expected to provide a lifetime of normal function for young active patients.

Rheumatoid Arthritis

People with RA require careful evaluation to prevent operative and perioperative neurologic injury, establish the sequence and timing of joints to be treated surgically, and reduce the risks of infection and other complications.

People with RA commonly have cervical spine involvement that can lead to spinal instability and increased risk of neurologic deficits. Neurologic changes may be difficult to recognize due to limited joint motion and associated disuse muscle atrophy. To evaluate the risk of neurologic injury, people with RA should have active flexion and extension lateral cervical radiographs within one year before surgery. In a retrospective review of 113 patients with RA who underwent total hip or knee arthroplasty, Collins et al (3) reported significant atlantoaxial subluxation, atlantoaxial impaction, and/or subaxial subluxation in 69 patients (61%). Thirty-five

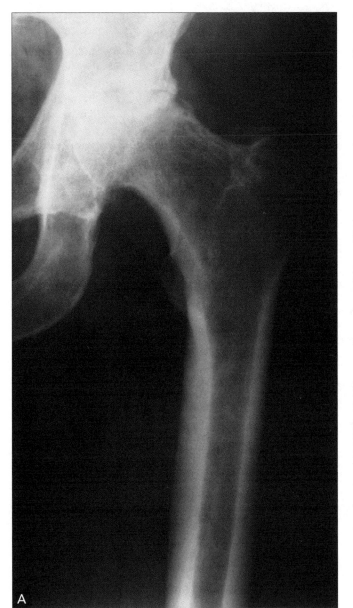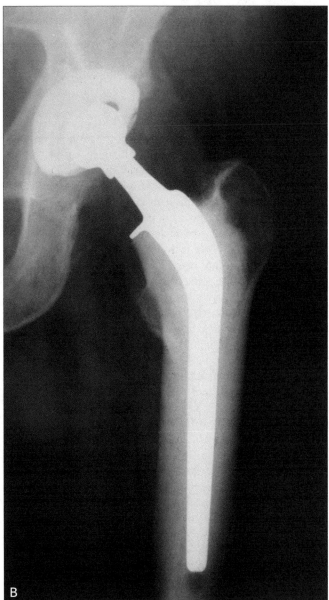

Fig. 49-1. Radiographs showing a hip replacement. **A:** The left hip of a 52-year-old man with avascular necrosis and advanced osteoarthritis. Loss of articular cartilage has reduced the radiographic joint space to a thin line. The patient has severe hip pain and minimal hip motion. **B:** The joint has been resected and replaced with a metal femoral component fixed with methylmethacrylate (cement) and an uncemented metal acetabular component containing a polyethylene liner. The patient no longer has hip pain and lacks only a few degrees of normal hip motion.

of these 69 patients (50%) had no clinical signs or symptoms of instability at the time of admission for joint replacement arthroplasty. Instability of greater than 7–10 mm at the atlantoaxial joint or greater than 4 mm at subaxial levels on flexion and extension lateral radiographs generally requires stabilization prior to other elective surgery. Patients with lesser degrees of atlantoaxial and subaxial involvement should be evaluated by the anesthesiologist preoperatively and consideration given to an awake intubation.

Patients with multiple-joint involvement require careful planning and timing of various joint procedures to allow optimal rehabilitation. Patients undergoing lower-extremity surgery may require surgical stabilization of the upper extremity first to allow crutch ambulation and use of the upper extremities to assist with transfers, rising from a chair, and stair climbing. For example, a person with severe wrist involvement as well as hip involvement may benefit from wrist arthrodesis prior to total hip arthroplasty. The patient with multiple lower-extremity joint involvement may benefit from treating joints either sequentially or simultaneously, depending on the joints involved and the severity of the disease. The patient with severe disease and contractures of both knees, for example, may benefit from having both knees replaced at the same time. In that situation, if only one knee is replaced, a flexion contracture in the untreated knee will cause the patient to keep the operatively treated knee flexed when standing and thereby compromise rehabilitation following surgery. Foot and ankle disease are generally addressed prior to hip and knee arthroplasty to provide the patient a stable lower extremity on which to stand and rehabilitate the hip and knee.

Long-term use of corticosteroids increases the complexity of surgical treatment of people with RA. In general, these patients will require "stress dose" steroids perioperatively due to inhibition of their adrenal function. Long-term corticosteroid use combined with the effects of the disease can cause connective tissue changes that make the skin and superficial blood vessels friable. Extreme caution must be used in physically handling such a patient. For example, in severely affected patients, mild pressure can cause a hematoma or skin ulceration and adhesive tape can tear the skin. In addition, chronic low-dose corticosteroid use in patients with RA has been correlated with an increased incidence of fracture, infection, and gastrointestinal hemorrhage or ulcer. People with RA treated with total joint arthroplasties demonstrated a higher incidence of infection than patients with OA treated with total joint arthroplasties (1). Patients with RA frequently have more than one joint arthroplasty, and infection of one arthroplasty is associated with an increased incidence of subsequent infection of another replaced joint (4).

Many people with RA are treated with NSAIDs and/or methotrexate preoperatively. A review of 165 patients undergoing total hip arthroplasty found a higher incidence of gastrointestinal bleeding and/or hypotension in patients receiving NSAIDs at the time of hospital admission (5). Several studies have demonstrated that there is no increase in wound or other postoperative complications in patients who continue methotrexate therapy perioperatively. Perhala et al (6) compared 60 patients with RA who underwent a total of 92 joint arthroplasties without interruption of methotrexate therapy to a group of 61 patients not receiving methotrexate who underwent a total of 110 joint arthroplasties. Eight patients on methotrexate had a total of eight wound complications (8.7%) versus five patients with a total of six wound complications in the nonmethotrexate group (5.5%, $P = 0.366$). In a randomized, nonblinded prospective study of 64 patients with RA on methotrexate therapy, Sany et al (7) reported no infections and no difference in wound healing between patients whose therapy was discontinued seven days before an orthopaedic procedure and those whose therapy was continued perioperatively.

Juvenile Rheumatoid Arthritis

Joint replacement arthroplasty in children with juvenile rheumatoid arthritis (JRA) is reserved for patients who are debilitated by pain and/or decreased function, and is generally delayed until patients are skeletally mature. Joint replacement is also delayed because the life expectancy of the young patient is greater than that of current prostheses. Moreover, each subsequent revision surgery necessarily involves greater periprosthetic bone loss and less predictable long-term results. People with JRA are often candidates for tendon lengthening to correct contractures, and prophylactic procedures, such as synovectomy, to alleviate symptoms and possibly delay articular destruction.

Patients with JRA present important anesthetic risks. Although they do not develop cervical spine involvement and accompanying neurologic deficits as commonly as adults with RA, these problems do occur in association with JRA. Therefore, people with JRA require preoperative screening radiographs as described for patients with RA. Unilateral collapse of the lateral mass of the atlas, with or without axis involvement, may result in a fixed rotational head tilt deformity that makes it difficult to establish an airway for general anesthesia. Micrognathia associated with temporomandibular joint involvement can also make endotracheal intubation difficult. Restricted motion of the axial and appendicular skeleton can make regional anesthesia difficult as well.

Osteonecrosis

Treatment of osteonecrosis remains controversial, partially because the natural history of the disorder remains unknown. Nonsteroidal anti-inflammatory agents and decreased joint loading are commonly employed for temporary symptomatic relief, though neither has been shown to affect the long-term results. Electromagnetic stimulation has also been employed on an experimental basis. Most surgical treatments of osteonecrosis have been developed for treatment of the hip. Core decompression (i.e., drilling a channel from the lateral surface of the femur into the necrotic region of the femoral head) with or without bone grafting, has been advocated for patients who have femoral osteonecrosis without collapse or acetabular changes. In most series, these procedures have decreased pain in a high percentage of the patients. This treatment is generally considered ineffective in people whose femoral head shows any signs of collapse; however, for these patients, various other surgical options exist. These options include femoral osteotomies, designed to place an intact segment of the femoral head in a weight-bearing position, and hip arthrodesis. Replacement of the femoral head or total hip have met with excellent results in this population, but prosthesis durability is a concern, particularly in young patients.

Ankylosing Spondylitis

Joint replacements decrease pain and improve function for people with advanced joint disease due to ankylosing spondylitis (AS). Osteotomies that correct spinal deformities can also be of benefit for some. Spinal involvement can lead to extensive ligamentous calcification and heterotopic ossification that make regional anesthesia difficult, if not impossible. Patients with prolonged disease also develop severe kyphotic deformities of the cervical, thoracic, and lumbar spine that impede endotracheal intubation. Restricted chest excursion may further complicate intraoperative and postoperative care. Patients with AS tend to bleed more during and after surgery than similar, otherwise-healthy individuals. The explanation for this bleeding tendency appears to be that compared with normal tissues, the ossified soft tissues are less capable of contracting to assist in hemostasis. There does not appear to be an associated defect in blood coagulation or platelet function.

People with AS, diffuse idiopathic skeletal hyperostosis, or post-traumatic osteoarthrosis are at increased risk for postoperative heterotopic ossification. Although patients with AS have excellent pain relief after total hip arthroplasty, gains in total range of motion are often limited due to periarticular heterotopic ossification, as well as long-standing soft tissue contractures and muscle atrophy. Various regimens have been tried to prevent postoperative soft tissue ossification, but radiation therapy delivered locally appears to be the most effective means of preventing heteotopic bone formation after surgery. Fractionated and single low-dose radiation therapy to the hip and abductor musculature have been effective when begun early in the postoperative period.

Psoriatic Arthritis

The perioperative concerns with NSAIDs and methotrexate discussed with RA apply to psoriatic arthritis as well. A unique perioperative risk in people with psoriatic arthritis is the development of a flare of psoriasis at the operative site due to the physiologic and/or psychologic stress of surgery. Also known as isomorphic or Koebner's phenomenon, this process may predispose the patient to a generalized flare of psoriasis as well. People with psoriatic arthritis may have an increased incidence of postoperative infections. Menon and Wroblewski (8) reported superficial wound infection in 9.1% and deep wound infections in 5.5% of their 38 patients with psoriasis treated with total hip arthroplasty.

Hemophilic Arthropathy

Despite the risk of excessive bleeding, operative treatment can produce good results in people with hemophilic arthropathy. Synovectomy is commonly performed in the knee and elbow, and gives improved range of motion and decreased pain to the majority of patients. Total knee and total hip replacements can improve function and relieve pain in hemophilic patients with advanced joint degeneration (9).

Hemophilic arthropathy may be particularly difficult to manage perioperatively. Factor replacement has important risks and must be carefully monitored. A thrombotic event may be precipitated by repeated factor infusions, and resultant disseminated intravascular coagulation after elective surgery has been reported. The subgroup of patients with high levels of factor antibody are generally contraindicated for major elective surgery.

Whether or not people with well-controlled hemophilia without aquired immunodeficiency syndrome (AIDS) are at increased risk for non-transfusion–related infection is unclear. Septic arthritis has been reported as a rare complication of hemophilia, but one that must be promptly diagnosed and definitively treated. Human immunodeficiency virus (HIV)-1-infected hemophilia patients who have not developed AIDS do not appear to have an increased incidence of infection after surgery when compared with patients who are seronegative for HIV-1.

Pigmented Villonodular Synovitis

Pigmented villonodular synovitis most commonly involves the knee and has been reported in patients ranging in age from the second to the ninth decade. It also occurs in the ankle and shoulder, as well as in other joints where it may be more difficult to detect. Arthroscopy may allow for early diagnosis. Synovectomy, by arthrotomy or arthroscopy, usually provides symptomatic relief, and may be curative in patients with the localized form of the disease. The diffuse form of the disease responds less favorably to synovectomy, with recurrences in more than one-third of patients. Radiation does not appear to decrease the recurrence rate, and may lead to local soft-tissue complications.

Synovial Chondromatosis

Synovial chondromatosis is a rare condition that results in the formation of cartilaginous fragments that may lie in synovial joint cavities, the synovium, or, in some instances, in the periarticular soft tissues. The condition causes pain, catching, and locking of the joint as well as loss of joint motion and possible degeneration of the articular surfaces. Removal of intra-articular loose bodies and, in some instances, synovectomy can relieve symptoms and improve motion in patients who have not developed degenerative joint disease. However, the cartilage fragments reaccumulate in many joints. In patients with degenerative joint disease, joint replacement combined with synovectomy can cure the disease.

Sites of Surgical Intervention

The operative treatments that provide the best results vary not only among the different types of arthritis, but also among anatomic sites. Thus, the most appropriate procedure should be chosen based on the joint involved, the type of arthritis, the patient's age, and other social and medical factors.

Hip

The most commonly employed operative treatments for arthritis of the hip are cemented (i.e., anchored with polymethymethacrylate cement) and uncemented total hip arthroplasty. More than 120,000 hip prostheses are implanted in the United States each year (10) (Fig. 49-1). Osteotomies and fusions are performed less frequently than hip replacements, but can produce good results in certain patients.

Nearly 30 years of clinical studies now document the success of total hip replacement for the treatment of disabling pain and impairment due to chronic hip diseases. Recent long-term follow-up studies show that total hip replacements will provide excellent function for more than 20 years in appropriately selected patients (11). Initially, surgeons limited hip replacement to patients between the ages of 60 and 75 years, but over the last decade studies have shown that younger and more elderly patients also can benefit from this procedure. Although most patients who have a hip replacement increase their level of physical function, patients with limited expectation for improved function also can benefit from the procedure.

The risk of postoperative venous thrombosis and infection in people treated who have undergone hip replacements has significantly decreased in the past two decades. Early series of hip replacements reported a high rate of failure due to infection, but modern aseptic techniques and prophylactic antibiotics have reduced the incidence of infection to less than 1% (12). Loosening remains the predominant cause of long-term failure of hip replacements, but recent research has clarified the causes of this problem. Particulate debris, the majority of which appears to be generated from wear of polyethylene surfaces, stimulates osteoclastic bone lysis at the bone–cement interface in prostheses fixed with methylmethacrylate and at the prosthesis–bone interface in uncemented implants. The osteolysis can lead to loosening of the prostheses, bone loss, and bone fractures (Fig. 49-2). Improvements in cement techniques have decreased the incidence of aseptic femoral loosening from as high as 40% to less than 5% 10 years after the procedure for many groups of patients. Even in a group of patients who were younger than 50 years at the time of cemented hip arthroplasty, only 8% had evidence of femoral component loosening 16–20 years after the procedure (13). In contrast, cemented acetabular components continue to have a high rate of loosening despite improved cement techniques. Preliminary reviews of the results with uncemented acetabular components (Fig. 49-1B) suggest that they may have better results. Uncemented femoral components have been associated with postoperative thigh pain, yet some surgeons use them in young patients in an effort to give these patients increased prosthetic durability. Uncemented femoral components also may have a potential advantage in revision surgery where there is hope of regaining lost bone stock with bone growth into and around the prosthesis. In September 1994, a National Institute of Health Consensus Development Conference Panel convened to evaluate the available scientific information concerning total hip replacement, and concluded that total hip replacement is a highly successful method of treating pain and disability and that the vast majority of the patients have an excellent prognosis for long-term improvement in symptoms and function (10). The panel noted that implant loosening remains a problem and recommended regular follow-up to detect impending failure early and allow treatment before significant bone loss or fracture occur (Fig. 49-2).

Despite its great success, total hip arthroplasty has important limitations, particularly for young patients who are likely to outlive the prosthesis. Alternatives to arthroplasty include osteotomy, arthrodesis, and resection arthroplasty. Femoral and pelvic osteotomy have been shown to be effective in relieving pain in young patients with acetabular dysplasia and minimal or no radiographic degenerative change. Whether or not they alter the natural history of hip dysplasia is unclear. Results are less favorable in adults older

than 40 years and in patients with significant degenerative change. Arthrodesis of the hip offers young patients with hip arthritis a dependable, durable, pain-free hip. Once fusion is obtained, the patient may return to vigorous activity without the limitations imposed on arthroplasty patients. However, some patients find the prospect of a stiff hip unacceptable. At long-term follow-up, patients complain of some difficulty sitting in a chair and using public transportation, but otherwise perform activities of daily living very well with excellent pain relief. Patients who develop associated lumbosacral pain later in life may be considered for conversion of the arthrodesis to a total hip arthroplasty.

Resection arthroplasty, originally described for treatment of tuberculous arthritis of the hip and osteomyelitis, is seldom employed as a primary procedure today. It remains an option for people with recalcitrant infection involving a total hip arthroplasty and for low-demand patients who are not candidates for more extensive reconstruction. After resection arthroplasty, the proximal femur is allowed to articulate with the acetabulum or the ilium.

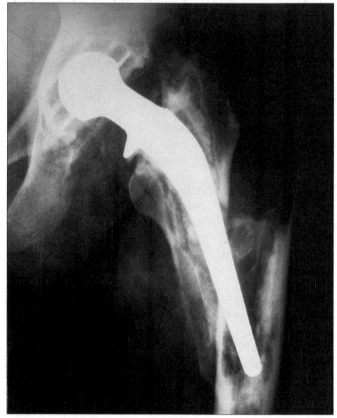

Fig. 49-2. Radiograph showing a left hip replacement with bone resorption around the femoral bone cement, loosening of the prosthesis, and a fracture through the proximal femur. This 67-year-old man had a hip replacement 14 years ago. He was not evaluated for the last seven years. Despite the development of severe periprosthetic osteolysis, he did not notice any problems with his hip until he tripped on an electrical cord and sustained the fracture. Earlier detection of the asymptomatic osteolysis followed by surgical revision would have prevented the fracture and extensive loss of bone.

Surprisingly, the majority of otherwise healthy patients are pain-free and ambulatory, but generally require one or two crutches and a substantial heel lift to walk. Today, resection arthroplasty is generally reserved for salvage of a failed hip arthroplasty that is not amenable to revision.

Knee

A variety of operative procedures have been described for treatment of arthritis of the knee, including arthroscopy, osteotomy, and replacement arthroplasty. The indications for these procedures differ significantly.

Arthroscopy has advanced the diagnosis and treatment of many forms of knee arthritis. It is particularly useful for people whose symptoms may be attributed to a specific mechanical etiology, such as a meniscus tear or loose body. Arthroscopic synovectomy can decrease pain and swelling for patients with hemophilia, pigmented villonodular synovitis, synovial chondromatosis, and early RA without significant cartilage erosion. Whether or not it alters the long-term course of these diseases is unclear. Arthroscopic debridement or chondroplasty for degenerative knee arthritis, except in cases of degenerative meniscal tears or intra-articular loose bodies, does not appear to affect the natural history of the disease. It may, however, provide short-term relief of symptoms for some patients.

Osteotomy about the knee is intended to redirect the weight-bearing axis away from a degenerative portion of the tibiofemoral joint, and may also stimulate development of fibrocartilage in the unloaded degenerative compartment. The majority of knee osteotomies are valgus osteotomies of the proximal tibia, performed to redirect weight-bearing forces from a degenerative medial tibiofemoral articulation through a better-preserved lateral compartment. Femoral osteotomies are preferred for valgus and excessive varus deformities of the knee. Osteotomies generally are chosen over total knee arthroplasties for young, heavy, active patients, and should be reserved for patients with noninflammatory disease. Appropriate candidates have <5° of flexion contracture, >90° of flexion, and isolated medial or lateral tibiofemoral arthritis without significant patellofemoral involvement. Good results have been reported in 80%–90% of patients for six to nine years postosteotomy, with 60%–70% good results at 10 to 15 years follow-up (14). It is difficult to compare these results with those of total knee arthroplasty, where the patients are generally older and less active.

Total knee arthroplasty, similar to total hip arthroplasty, may be performed with cement or bone ingrowth as the means of fixation. Several large series reveal that tibial and femoral results are excellent regardless of the type of fixation, with 97% survivorship of prostheses at 10- and 12-year analyses (15). Despite excellent results with cement fixation, some surgeons reserve cemented tibial and femoral components for patients older than 50 or 60, or patients with poor bone stock, based on the assumption that uncemented components will last longer for young patients and preserve their bone stock. Patellar problems are the leading cause of failure

after total knee arthroplasty. Unlike tibial and femoral results, results of uncemented patellar components, which require a metal-backing for bone ingrowth, are substantially inferior to results of cemented all-polyethylene patellar components, and have thus fallen out of favor in recent years.

Knee arthrodesis is an option for patients with recalcitrant infection or failed total knee arthroplasty that cannot be revised effectively. Despite loss of knee motion, a functional lower extremity that permits painless weight bearing can be expected using current techniques. Resection arthroplasty has also been used for patients with failed total knee arthroplasty.

Foot and Ankle

Surgical options for arthritis of the foot and ankle include cheilectomy (resection of an osteophyte), arthroscopic debridement, osteotomy, arthrodesis, and replacement arthroplasty.

Osteophytes may develop at the periphery of a joint and cause symptoms related to impingement during normal walking. These are not uncommon on the dorsum of the first metatarsophalangeal joint and the anterior aspect of the tibiotalar joint. Although it does not cure the underlying disease, cheilectomy often provides relief of mechanical symptoms and associated pain. Loose bodies may also be a source of mechanical symptoms and are amenable to arthroscopic removal.

Supramalleolar tibial osteotomy allows realignment of the weight-bearing axis through the tibiotalar joint. This can help to preserve the joint in various congenital and post-traumatic degenerative conditions of the ankle. Low tibial osteotomy has been shown to be particularly effective in long-term relief of symptoms with intermediate-stage primary OA. Osteotomy is generally reserved for noninflammatory arthritides, but it may also provide relief of pain and decreased frequency of intra-articular bleeding in patients with haemophilic arthropathy.

Arthrodeses of the foot and ankle offer pain relief and stability to people with severe arthritis. Fusions of these joints are well tolerated, even by children, despite some restriction of stressful activities such as hill climbing and running. Although the vast majority of patients with ankle and/or peritalar arthrodeses obtain excellent relief of pain and increased function, initial nonunion of the arthrodesis occurs in 5%–30% of cases. Infection and delayed wound healing have been reported in 25%–40% of patients with RA who undergo tibiotalar arthrodesis, yet the majority have an excellent long-term result.

Unlike total replacement arthroplasty of the hip and knee, ankle replacement arthroplasties have not produced predictable results. By five to 10 years after surgery, 60%–90% of these prostheses have failed. Most surgeons now limit the use of this procedure to treatment of inflammatory arthritis in minimally active elderly patients who have multiple joint involvement.

Hand and Wrist

The distal interphalangeal joints and thumb carpometacarpal joints are the most commonly involved joints in OA of the hand, while proximal interphalangeal, metacarpophalangeal, carpometacarpal, radiocarpal, and distal radioulnar joints are more commonly involved in inflammatory arthropathy. Surgeons use a variety of joint and soft-tissue procedures to treat these disorders.

When evaluating the wrist and hand in people with RA, it is imperative to obtain a history of the patient's functional abilities, carefully noting any recent changes. Inability to actively flex or extend interphalangeal and/or metacarpophalangeal joints with preservation of passive motion usually signals a ruptured tendon. Flexor and extensor tendons in patients with rheumatoid disease are more susceptible to rupture than normal tendons. Underlying ultrastructural changes associated with the inflammatory process weaken the tendons, and abnormal bony prominences, particularly at the distal radioulnar joint, abrade the weakened tendons, making them prone to rupture. Tenosynovectomy not only provides decreased pain with increased range of motion and grip strength, but also appears to protect the tendons, particularly when combined with resection of abnormal bony prominences. Acute tendon ruptures should be evaluated early by a surgeon for consideration of reconstruction prior to the development of fibrosis and contractures. In the rheumatoid hand, the metacarpophalangeal joints of the fingers are generally reconstructed with silicone implants that function as flexible spacers. Ulnar drift of the digits with resultant ulnar subluxation of the extensor tendons may be at least partially corrected by surgical centralization of the extensor tendons and transfer of the intrinsic hand muscle insertions from one digit to the adjacent digit on the ulnar side.

Arthrodesis is commonly employed in the interphalangeal joints, carpus, and wrist for end-stage joint degeneration due to most arthritic disorders. Interphalangeal joints are best managed with arthrodesis in a partially flexed position. Solid fusion can be reliably obtained in more than 95% of cases using various techniques. Arthrodesis may also be performed at the radiocarpal joint or selectively at diseased intercarpal joints. Although some reduction in wrist motion and grip strength are commonly noted with limited intercarpal arthrodeses, long-term pain relief and stability are excellent.

Surgeons rarely recommend arthrodesis of arthritic thumb carpometacarpal joints, because motion of these joints is particularly important for overall hand function. The degenerative thumb carpometacarpal joint is amenable to interposition arthroplasty (resection of the joint surfaces and interposition of soft tissue, usually a portion of the abductor pollicis longus or flexor carpi radialis tendons), which yields excellent pain relief and increased grip strength.

Experience with arthroplasty of the wrist is limited, partially due to the predictable results obtained with wrist fusion. Intermediate-term results have been mixed. Silicone spacer implants yielded a high incidence of failure with poor pain relief in approximately 50% of patients an average of five to six years after the procedure. Wrist arthroplasty designs have yielded improved clinical outcome, but component failure remains a problem. In selected patients with degenerative disease of the radiocarpal joint, resection of the proximal row of carpal bones (i.e., proximal row carpectomy) can reduce pain.

Elbow

Routine activities of daily living require a wide range of elbow flexion and extension as well as pronation and supination. Although elbow fusion can be reliably obtained with internal fixation, this results in substantial impairment because shoulder and wrist motion cannot adequately compensate for loss of elbow motion. Fortunately, radial head excision, synovectomy, arthroscopy, and arthroplasty are alternatives that have yielded good results.

Arthritis involving primarily the radiohumeral articulation is not uncommon with rheumatoid and post-traumatic joint disease. Radial-head resection offers increased range of motion and decreased pain in appropriately selected patients. Resultant proximal migration of the radius is minimal after this procedure, and elbow instability is seldom a concern if the medial collateral ligament complex is intact. Patients generally have good intermediate-term relief of pain with increased range of motion. In one series, 84% of people with RA reported good pain relief six months after the procedure (16). Synovectomy may be performed alone or in conjunction with other procedures, such as radial-head resection. Patients with hemophilia likewise have decreased pain and swelling following synovectomy, as well as a decreased incidence of hemarthrosis. Arthroscopy has been used effectively to perform synovectomies as well as remove loose bodies and osteophytes from arthritic elbows.

Elbow joint replacement arthroplasty, while newer than hip and knee arthroplasty, has developed rapidly. The rate of loosening in young active patients with post-traumatic arthropathy approaches 50% at five- to eight-year follow-up. However, intermediate-term results in low-demand patients with inflammatory disease are promising, with survival of the components and good or excellent results reported in more than 90% of RA patients at three- to eight-year follow-up (17). Motion was reportedly improved to a functional range and pain relief was substantial for >90% of these patients.

Shoulder

The high degree of compensatory movement in the scapulothoracic articulation, as well as elsewhere throughout the upper extremity, may be responsible for the relatively low incidence of patients requiring operative treatment of arthritic glenohumeral joints. Nonetheless, some patients will be debilitated by an arthritic shoulder, fail nonoperative treatment, and present for consideration of surgical intervention.

Shoulder arthrodesis yields excellent pain relief and provides a stable upper extremity with long-term durability for young patients with severe glenohumeral arthritis. Fusion is reliably obtained in the majority of patients with relatively few complications. Despite rigid fusion of the glenohumeral joint, abduction of 50° and flexion of 40° in the shoulder girdle is possible via scapulothoracic motion.

The majority of total shoulder arthroplasties are performed for RA of the glenohumeral joint. Pain relief and improved general functions of daily living are reported in the majority of patients; the most common long-term complication reported is glenoid component loosening (18). To this end, recent efforts have explored the use of hemiarthroplasty, which is the replacement of the humeral head without resurfacing the glenoid. This method has proven effective in selected patients including those with cuff-tear arthropathy — chronic, massive rotator cuff tears with secondary superior migration of the humeral head and resultant erosive changes of the glenohumeral joint and inferior surface of the acromion.

Cervical Spine

The clinical problems caused by arthritis of the cervical spine are pain, compromised neurologic function, and mechanical instability that causes or has the potential to cause pain and neurologic deficits. Spinal fusions can decrease pain, restore stability, and, in some instances, prevent development of neurologic deficits. Surgical decompression of the spinal cord and nerve roots can relieve pain and improve neurologic function in selected patients.

Generally accepted indications for surgical intervention in people with RA with cervical spine involvement are pain refractory to nonoperative modalities, neurologic deterioration, and radiographic evidence of impending spinal cord compression. Whereas the anterior atlantodental interval has been traditionally used to determine the degree of atlantoaxial instability, the posterior atlantodental interval has been shown to be an important predictor of the potential for postoperative neurologic improvement (19). The available evidence also suggests that patients who undergo cervical arthrodesis earlier in the course of their disease have more satisfactory results than those in whom arthrodesis is delayed. Some authors have recommended that patients with atlantoaxial subluxation and a posterior atlanto-odontoid interval of 14 mm or less, patients who have atlantoaxial subluxation and at least 5 mm of basilar invagination, and patients who have subaxial subluxation and a sagittal spinal canal diameter of 14 mm or less, even in the absence of neurologic findings, undergo posterior surgical fusion at the involved levels. Pain is relieved in the majority of patients, but neurologic improvement is variable and closely related to preoperative radiographic instability and neurologic status.

Radiographic evidence of OA in the cervical spine occurs in about 50% of people older than 50 years and 75% of people older than 65. In contrast to people with RA, these patients rarely have instability. However, they may develop pain and neurologic signs as a result of degenerative stenosis. Posterior decompression may be accomplished via laminectomy or laminaplasty. Laminectomy, or removal of part or all of one or more cervical laminae, allows excellent visualization and decompression at the expense of potentially destabilizing the spine with resultant kyphosis. Laminaplasty may be performed by one of many techniques, but in general involves cutting through the lam-

inae completely on one side at the involved levels of the spine and cutting 80% of the way through the contralateral laminae at those same levels. The cervical spinal canal may then be opened on the hinge of the partially cut laminae. This allows excellent multi-level decompression at the expense of decreased cervical motion. The choice between these two procedures remains controversial.

Perioperative Management

The goals of perioperative management include restoration of motion and function, relief of pain, and prevention of complications. To obtain optimal surgical results, joint replacement patients must participate in a physical therapy regimen directed at improving range of motion and restoring function. Physical therapy typically starts within 24 hours after a joint replacement and is generally continued for six or more weeks through a combination of inpatient rehabilitation, home health care, and outpatient services. Continuous passive motion (CPM) machines are frequently used in the early stages of rehabilitation after a total knee replacement, and have more recently been utilized in certain situations for hip and shoulder patients as well.

Narcotic analgesics are generally required in the acute postoperative period, and are tapered off during the ensuing weeks. Patient-controlled analgesia (PCA) pumps provide effective and efficient delivery of narcotics through a combination of basal infusion rate and intermittent dosing, which the patient dictates as needed by pressing a button. The maximum dose per hour is preset by the physician. As an alternative, spinal and epidural infusions have become increasingly popular for total hip and knee arthroplasty patients. Each not only may be used for surgical anesthesia, but also can provide postoperative analgesia. An indwelling epidural catheter can be left in place for two to three days postoperatively and titrated to provide pain relief while sparing motor control for ambulation and other exercises. As an added benefit, the vasodilation associated with epidural anesthesia may further decrease the risk of thromboembolus.

Thromboembolic disease is a potential complication after any spine or lower extremity procedure. This complication is particularly common among unprophylaxed hip arthroplasty patients. In the absence of prophylaxis, the incidence of deep venous thrombosis has been reported as high as 74% and the incidence of symptomatic pulmonary embolism as high as 3.4% (20). A recent meta-analysis of thromboembolic prophylactic agents has shown a significantly lower risk of deep venous thrombosis and symptomatic pulmonary embolism with warfarin, pneumatic compression, and low-molecular-weight heparins (20). Of these, warfarin was thought to be the safest and most effective. Low-molecular-weight heparins were associated with a risk of postoperative bleeding.

Patients undergoing major joint reconstruction commonly require perioperative blood transfusion. Concern regarding the associated risks of blood-borne disease, anaphylaxis, and transfusion reaction has given rise to improved techniques for postoperative blood management. For many years, preoperative autologous donation has provided a relatively safe, albeit expensive and time-consuming, alternative to allogeneic transfusion. More recent advances have seen the advent of perioperative blood salvage and erythropoietin analogs. Blood-salvage devices that reinfuse blood from the operative site are an effective means of reducing allogenic transfusion after arthroplasty (21). Erythropoietin analogs may further reduce the risk by stimulating the patient's marrow to increase erythrocyte production prior to elective surgery.

Postoperative Complications

The majority of serious postoperative complications, including infection, nerve and blood vessel injury, pulmonary embolus, and joint dislocation, occur within the first postoperative weeks; however, complications may occur at any time after surgery. Arthroplasty patients in particular must be monitored indefinitely for subtle radiographic evidence of periprosthetic osteolysis, which, when treated early, may halt progression to massive bone loss and catastrophic failure (Fig. 49-2) (10). The vast majority of failures among lower-extremity total joint prostheses occur after the first decade postoperatively, and most patients remain asymptomatic until substantial bone loss, subsidence, and even fracture have occurred. It is therefore imperative that routine follow-up, including careful standardized clinical and comparative radiographic evaluation, be obtained on a regular basis throughout the patient's life.

In addition, patients must be carefully monitored for early signs of infection. Early detection of infection in a prosthetic joint may make it possible to save the implants. However, successful treatment of chronic joint infections without removal of the implants occurs rarely. Patients with multiple joint arthroplasties who develop sepsis in one prosthetic joint should be treated aggressively and observed closely, because they have a substantial risk of developing a metachronous infection in another artificial joint.

The relationship between bacteremias caused by diagnostic and surgical procedures and subsequent infection of a total joint arthroplasty remain uncertain. However, several reports suggest that bacteremias associated with dental procedures can seed total joint arthroplasties. For this reason, 2 g of penicillin one hour prior to dental manipulation and 1 g six hours after the first dose have been recommended for patients with total joint arthroplasties (22). One gram of erythromycin one hour prior to dental manipulation and 500 mg six hours after the first dose may be utilized for penicillin-sensitive patients. Oral antibiotic prophylaxis appropriate for the regional flora has also been recommended prior to and following urologic, gastrointestinal, and other bacteremia-evoking manipulations.

New Operative Treatments

Replacements of the hip and knee predictably relieve pain and provide stability and motion for large numbers of patients. Unfortunately, wear and loosening can cause failure of these implants. Other current operative treatments also relieve or reduce pain for many patients with arthritis: however, they are generally less successful in restoring joint function. Joint fusions and even joint replacements place important limits on function and other current treatments do not reliably arrest or reverse joint degeneration. Thus, there is a clear need for new therapeutic approaches. Advances in surgical techniques, implant materials and methods of fixing implants to bone may decrease the frequency and severity of long-term wear and loosening of joint replacements, making it possible to provide more patients with joint replacements that last a lifetime. Improved results of wrist and ankle joint replacement may be possible with new implant designs. Although they have not yet been shown to be effective in arthritic joints, operative approaches intended to preserve or restore cartilaginous articular surfaces that include surgical debridement of degenerated tissue and correction of mechanical abnormalities combined with implantation of artificial matrices, growth factors, and transplanted chondrocytes or mesenchymal stem cells have the potential to restore a joint surface.

JOSEPH A. BUCKWALTER, MD
W. TIMOTHY BALLARD, MD

References

1. Wymenga AB, Horn JRV, Theeuwes A, Muytjens HL, Slooff TJ. Perioperative factors associated with septic arthritis after arthroplasty. Prospective multicenter study of 362 knee and 2,651 hip operations. Acta Orthop Scand 1992;63:665–671.
2. Lehman DE, Capello WN, Feinberg JR. Total hip arthroplasty without cement in obese patients. J Bone Joint Surg 1994; 76A:854–862.
3. Collins DN, Barnes CL, FitzRandolph RL. Cervical spine instability in rheumatoid patients having total hip or knee arthroplasty. Clin Orthop Rel Res 1991;272:127–135.
4. Murray RP, Bourne MH, Fitzgerald RH. Metachronous infections in patients who have had more than one total joint arthroplasty. J Bone Joint Surg 1991;73A:1469–1474.
5. Connelly CS, Panush RS. Should nonsteroidal anti-inflammatory drugs be stopped before elective surgery? Arch Intern Med 1991;151:1963–1966.
6. Perhala RS, Wilke WS, Clough JD, Segal AM. Local infectious complications following large joint replacement in rheumatoid arthritis patients treated with methotrexate versus those not treated with methotrexate. Arthritis Rheum 1991;34:146–152.
7. Sany J, Anaya JM, Canovas F, et al. Influence of methotrexate on the frequency of postoperative infectious complications in patients with rheumatoid arthritis. J Rheumatol 1993;20:1129–1132.
8. Menon TJ, Wroblewski BM. Charnley low-friction arthroplasty in patients with psoriasis. Clin Orthop Rel Res 1983;300:127–128.
9. Kelly SS, Lachiewicz PF, Gilbert MS, Bolander ME, Jankiewicz JJ. Hip arthroplasty in hemophilic arthropathy. J Bone Joint Surg 1995;67A:828–834.

10. Total Hip Replacement. NIH Concensus Statement 1994;12 (5):1–31.
11. Callagham JJ, Albright JC, Goetz DD, Olejniczak JP, Johnston RC. Charnley total hip arthroplasty. Minimum twenty-five-year follow-up. J Bone Joint Surg 2000;82A: 487–497.
12. Fitzgerald RH. Total hip arthroplasty sepsis. Prevention and diagnosis. Orthop Clin North Am 1992;23:259–264.
13. Sullivan PM, MacKenzie JR, Callaghan JJ, Johnston RC. Total hip arthroplasty with cement in patients who are less than fifty years old. J Bone Joint Surg 1994;76A:863–869.
14. Insall JN, Joseph DM, Msika C. High tibial osteotomy for varus gonarthrosis. A long-term follow-up study. J Bone Joint Surg 1984;66A:1040–1048.
15. Rand JA, Ilstrup DM. Survivorship analysis of total knee arthroplasty. Cumulative rates of survival of 9200 total knee arthroplasties. J Bone Joint Surg 1991;73A:397–409.
16. Summers GD, Talor AR, Webley M. Elbow synovectomy and excision of the radial head in rheumatoid arthritis: a short term palliative procedure. J Rheumatol 1988;15:566–569.
17. Kraay MJ, Figgie MP, Inglis AE, Wolfe SW, Ranawat CS. Primary semiconstrained total elbow arthroplasty. Survival analysis of 113 consecutive cases. J Bone Joint Surg 1994;76B: 636–640.
18. Brostrom LA, Wallensten R, Olsson E, Anderson D. The Kessel prosthesis in total shoulder arthroplasty. A five-year experience. Clin Orthop Rel Res 1992;277:155–160.
19. Boden SD, Dodge LD, Bohlman HH, Rechtine GR. Rheumatoid arthritis of the cervical spine. J Bone Joint Surg 1993;75A:1282–1297.
20. Freedman KB, Brookenthal KR, Fitzgerald RH, Williams S, Lonner JH. A meta-analysis of thromboembolic prophylaxis following elective total hip arthroplasty. J Bone Joint Surg 2000;82A:929–938.
21. Grosvenor D, Goyal V, Goodman S. Efficacy of postoperative blood salvage following total hip arthroplasty in patients with and without deposited autologous units. J Bone Joint Surg 2000;82A:951–954.
22. Nelson JP, Fitzgerald RH, Jaspers MT, Little JW. Prophylactic antimicrobial coverage in arthroplasty patients. J Bone Joint Surg 1990;72A:1–2.

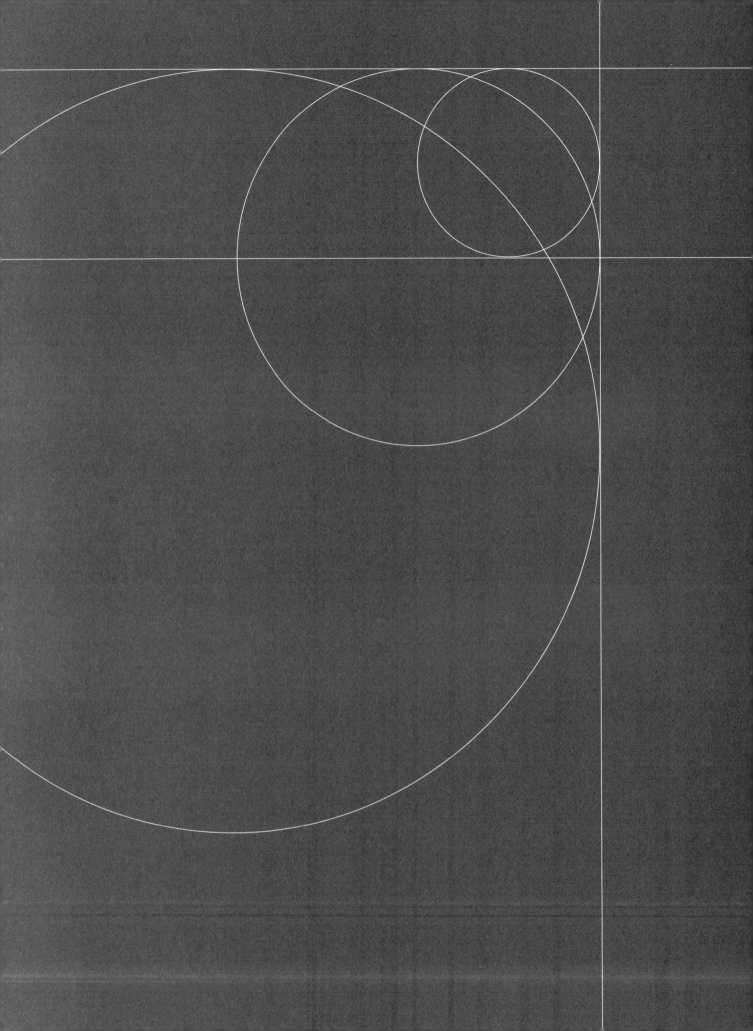

50 COMPLEMENTARY AND ALTERNATIVE THERAPIES

More and more people are employing complementary and alternative medicine (CAM) to treat their illnesses. In 1997, a survey of English-speaking patients found that 42.1% used at least one of 16 specific CAM therapies during a 12-month period (1). More than 50% of these patients had a musculoskeletal disease (arthritis, back, or neck pain). In this study population, visits to CAM practitioners exceeded total visits to primary care physicians. Total out-of-pocket expenditures for CAM treatments were approximately $27 billion, similar to out-of-pocket expenditures for all US physician services.The study found that these patients were most likely to use CAM therapies in conjunction with, rather than in place of, conventional therapies.

Many rheumatic conditions – e.g., osteoarthritis (OA), rheumatoid arthritis (RA), and fibromyalgia – have no known etiology or cure, are characterized by chronic pain and an unpredictable disease course, and often are without a complete or satisfactory therapy. As a consequence, patients often seek out CAM therapies in addition to the conventional treatment their doctors recommend (2).

Although physician and patient ideally are motivated by the same desired outcome (relief of symptoms and, when possible, disease modification), their acceptance of available CAM therapies differs greatly. Between 38.5% and 55% of patients do not disclose use of CAM therapies to their physicians (1,2) simply because their physicians do not ask. The fear of physician disapproval of CAM therapies accounts for only 15% of patient nondisclosure (2). As the medical community awaits more rigorous assessment of CAM therapies, physicians should be motivated by existing evidence (1–3) to ask patients about their use of CAM therapies. To protect patients from dangerous drug interactions and treatment modalities known to be harmful, use of CAM therapies must be elicited as a part of the comprehensive history and physical examination (3).

Meditation, Biofeedback, and Stress Reduction

Meditation, biofeedback, and stress reduction are used widely for the treatment of pain, depression, and anxiety. These therapeutic modalities are especially popular with people who have fibromyalgia.

Meditation teaches the patient to develop concentration, calmness, and insight as a way of treating symptoms (5). A prospective, observational, case-control study found that people with fibromyalgia were more likely than control patients in a rheumatology practice ($P < 0.01$) to use CAM (4). Study participants with fibromyalgia reported the use of spiritual practices (meditation, relaxation, self-help groups, prayer) more commonly than did control patients. People with fibromyalgia also perceived spiritual practices as the most successful interventions, compared with over-the-counter products, use of other health care practitioners, and dietary modifications. In an uncontrolled study of 225 patients with chronic pain enrolled in a meditation program, 60% showed continued improvement of pain at four years follow-up (5).

Biofeedback, with the assistance of electronic monitors, teaches people how to use their mind to affect body functions (e.g., circulation and pain sensation). In people with RA, biofeedback has been shown to decrease clinic visits, hospitalization days, and medical costs (6). In a review of 23 people with Raynaud's phenomenon participating in biofeedback therapy, Yocum and colleagues (7) found that at 18 months, patients continued to be able to raise baseline finger temperatures and that the greatest temperature increase was observed in patients with connective-tissue disorders, including lupus and scleroderma.

Relaxation techniques focus on the reduction of stress by using such tactics as breathing exercises to help provide relief. In a randomized, controlled trial of people with RA, relaxation techniques were shown to significantly reduce pain, disease activity, and anxiety (8).

Prayer and Spirituality

A majority of Americans believe in the healing power of prayer. Seven percent of patients surveyed by Eisenberg et al (1) reported using some form of spiritual healing in conjunction with conventional therapies, and 35% reported using prayer to address health-related problems. Patients with chronic illnesses seek treatment that includes attention to the mind and spirit as well as the body.

A number of studies have shown an association between spiritual involvement and positive health outcomes. A recent systematic review of randomized trials examined the efficacy of distant healing (9). Distant healing is considered to be a conscious, dedicated act directed at benefiting another person's physical or emotional well-being at a distance. It includes prayer, therapeutic touch, Reiki, and LeShane healing. Astin et al (9) found that 13 of 23 studies (57%) that met inclusion criteria yielded statistically significant, positive treatment effects of distant healing. Nine of the 23 studies showed no effect and one showed a negative effect, making it difficult to draw definitive conclusions about efficacy, but also difficult to simply dismiss the power of distant healing.

Exercise

Strengthening, stretching, general conditioning exercises, and yoga have been shown to provide symptomatic relief for various forms of arthritis, including OA of the hip and knee (10) and carpal tunnel syndrome (11). Tai chi exercise has been shown to significantly decrease the risk of falling in the elderly (12). In a randomized, controlled trial, people with OA of the knee who were enrolled in a program of physical therapy combined with supervised and unsupervised exercise were found to have clinically and statistically significant improvement (10). The benefits attained in the treatment group continued to be apparent at one year, with fewer patients requiring knee surgery than did patients in the control group. In a separate study, patients with carpal tunnel syndrome experienced a statistically significant improvement in grip strength and pain reduction with a yoga program based on upper body postures; flexibility exercises; correct alignment of hands, wrists, arms, and shoulders; stretching; and increased awareness of optimal joint position (11).

Acupuncture

Based on the belief that there are patterns of energy flow (Qi) that are essential for health, acupuncture is a procedure that treats illness by correcting Qi imbalances. Solid, sterile metal needles are used to penetrate the skin and manually or electrically stimulate known flow patterns. Acupuncture frequently is used to treat pain and is considered a useful therapy for such conditions as OA, Raynaud's phenomenon, fibromyalgia, and low back pain (13). A meta-analysis of randomized, controlled trials of acupuncture for the treatment of back pain found that acupuncture was superior to other control interventions (14). A randomized, controlled trial of acupuncture in people with OA of the knee found statistically significant reductions of pain in patients treated with acupuncture (15).

Massage

Massage is one of the CAM interventions used most frequently (1) and is, in general, risk-free. Various massage techniques can be used (Table 50-1), and patients need to be encouraged to discuss their medical conditions with the massage therapist. With this information, therapists can devise a plan for massage that will achieve the desired outcome and avoid negative experiences. For example, people at risk for fracture because of known osteoporosis or chronic corticosteroid use should avoid deep pressure. In a randomized, placebo-controlled trial comparing Swedish massage, transcutaneous electrical nerve stimulation (TENS), and sham TENS therapy in people with fibromyalgia, patients in the massage group showed decreases in insomnia, pain, fatigue, anxiety, and depression as well as decreased cortisol production (16).

Herbs, Supplements, and Vitamins

Herbal remedies are the fastest-growing form of CAM therapy in the United States. Viewed as "natural," and therefore safe, herbs actually are potent medications. Potential benefits of herbal therapy must be balanced against the possible harmful side effects from interactions with other prescription medications or the presence of illicit constituents or contaminants. Because most herbs used to relieve pain affect eicosanoid metabolism, the side effects may be similar to those of nonsteroidal anti-inflammatory drugs (NSAIDs).

TABLE 50-1
Massage and Bodywork

Western massage
  Swedish massage: full-body stroking and kneading of superficial muscle layers, using oil or lotion.
  Deep-tissue massage: strong pressure on deep muscles or tissue layers.
  Trigger-point therapy: deep finger pressure on trigger points.
  Myofascial release: steady pressure to stretch fascia.

Oriental bodywork and massage
  Acupressure (i.e., Shiatsu): finger and hand pressure used at acupuncture points.

Structural integration bodywork
  Chiropractic adjustment: short-level, high-velocity thrust directed specifically at a "manipulable lesion."
  Osteopathic manipulation: thrust, muscle energy, counterstrain, articulation, and myofascial release directed at a specific lesion.
  Rolfing: release of muscles and tissue layers from surrounding fascia using deep pressure and fascia release techniques.
  Reflexology: stimulation of massage points in the feet, hands, and ears that correspond to organs and body parts.
  CranioSacral therapy: gentle manipulation of the skull bones to balance the fluids in the craniosacral system.

TABLE 50-2
Resources Available on the Internet

Alternative medicine
Altmednet.com: http://www.altmednet.com – many CAM links
Arthritis Foundation: http://www.arthritis.org
Cochrane Collaboration: http://www.cochrane.org – systematic reviews
National Center for Complementary and Alternative Medicine: http://nccam.nih.gov – affiliated with NIH, conducts and
  supports research as well as providing information about CAM

Healing systems
Ayurvedic medicine: http://ayurvedahc.com
Chinese medicine: http://acupuncture.com
Naturopathic medicine: The American Association of Naturopathic Physicians: http://www.naturopathic.org
Homeopathic medicine: National Center for Homeopathy: http://www.homeopathic.org
Chiropractic medicine: American Chiropractic Association: http://www.amerchiro.org
Osteopathic medicine: American Osteopathic Association: http://www.aoa-net.org

Meditation, Biofeedback, Stress Reduction
The Mind-Body Medical Institute: http://www.mindbody.harvard.edu – information and referrals
Insight Meditation Society: http://www.dharma.org – information and links

Prayer and Spirituality
National Institute for Healthcare Research: http://www.nihr.org

Yoga
The American Yoga Association: http://americanyogaassociation.
Yoga Research Center : http://yrec.org

Massage
The National Certification Board for Therapeutic Massage and Body work: http://www.ncbtmb.com – referral list
The American Massage Therapy Association: http://www.amtamassage.org – information about massage as well as
  locator service for therapists

Herbs, supplements, vitamins
US Food and Drug Administration: http://www.fda.gov – access to MEDWATCH as well as warnings on herbal products
American Botanical Council: http://www.herbs.org – factual information about herbs
HerbMed: http://www.amfoundation.org/ – herbal database
NIH Office of Dietary Supplements: http://dietary-supplements.info.nih.gov
American Dietetic Association: http://www.eatright.org – referrals to registered dietitians
American Herbalists Guild: http://www.americanherbalistsguild.com – referrals to herbal practitioners

Many commonly used herbs and supplements affect the clotting system, and preoperative assessments must include questions concerning herbal intake.

Neither herbal nor supplement preparations undergo strict production inspection or quality control under the 1994 Dietary Supplement Health Education Act. Contaminants, such as lead and arsenic, as well as NSAIDs and steroids have been found in herbal preparations. Supplement preparations may or may not contain specified amounts or even any of the advertised supplement. Besides presenting a patient safety issue, this variability also makes any studies of these supplements difficult to interpret.

The best-studied nutritional supplements are glucosamine sulfate and chondroitin sulfate. A comprehensive meta-analysis concluded that there is sufficient evidence to suggest a moderate but definite reduction in pain for patients with OA of the knee who are treated with glucosamine and chondroitin (17). Since neither of these supplements have significant side effects, most clinicians have accepted or even encouraged their use in people with OA of the knee.

Evidence from studies in an animal model of inflammatory arthritis suggests a protective effect of polyphenols contained in green tea (Camelia senensis) (18). The equivalent of three to four daily cups of green tea prevented or ameliorated the development of arthritis. Other supplements that are commonly used by patients with arthritis include dimethyl sulfone (MSM) and S-adenosylmethionine (SAM-e), but the evidence for their effectiveness is not as compelling.

Vitamins C and D have been hypothesized to benefit patients with OA. Low levels of Vitamin D have been found in people with OA of the hip and knee (19). Patients with higher levels of Vitamin C intake appear to have a lower incidence of OA. Theoretically, antioxidant supplements could help to prevent the progression of OA of the knee (20).

Diet and Arthritis

Except for prevention and treatment of gout, there is no definitive scientific evidence that what an individual eats can cause or cure arthritis. Although an increasing amount of literature suggests that a change in diet may relieve some symptoms and even impact the progression of disease, the lack of consistency among findings limits the ability to make specific dietary recommendations for the prevention or treatment of arthritis. However, encouraging patients to modify their diets may result in beneficial weight loss as well as an overall improvement in health. A weight loss of as little as 5 kg may reduce the incidence of OA of the knees by 50% in women, particularly women who are more than 10% over their ideal body weight (21).

Red meat and certain vegetable oils (corn, sunflower, and safflower) contain omega-6 fatty acids, which are synthesized into arachidonic acid, the building blocks for prostaglandins and leukotrienes. Eliminating or reducing the amount of omega-6, while substituting omega-3 oils, may help reduce pain and inflammation. Omega-3 fatty acids are eicosapentaenoic acid (EPA) and docosahexaenoic acid (DHA), fatty acids that compete with omega-6 fatty acids to form arachidonic acid. Good sources for omega-3 fatty acids are fresh cold-water fish, sardines in their own oil, flaxseed, green soybeans and tofu, and canola and olive oils. Patients also can take food supplements to get more omega-3 fatty acids.

Miscellaneous Therapies

Wearing copper bracelets is believed to ease arthritis pain. In a placebo-controlled trial, Walker and Keats reported that a significant number of patients assigned to wear copper bracelets experienced arthritis pain relief, compared with little relief reported by individuals assigned to wear bracelets that were painted to look like copper (22). These investigators also reported that the copper bracelets were lighter at the end of the study period and suggested that copper was absorbed by the skin. While the concept of absorbing copper through the skin is controversial, it is worthwhile to recommend that patients who are interested in trying this alternative therapy buy a bracelet that has not been treated to prevent tarnishing.

Static magnet therapy, as opposed to pulsed electromagnetic therapy (the use of pulsed electric current in combination with a permanent magnet, a medically accepted therapy), is believed to relieve pain by increasing circulation, suppressing inflammation, affecting C-fibers, and changing the polarization of cells. Two scientific trials (23,24) have suggested that static magnetic therapy may relieve arthritis symptoms. However, the short follow-up periods and the small sample sizes limit the results' applicability and emphasize the need for more studies.

Bee stings or injections are believed by some to reduce arthritis symptoms. Applied at painful areas or trigger points, the known anti-inflammatory chemicals in bee venom are thought to relieve inflammation. Animal studies have shown that bee venom reduces inflammation (5) and prevents rats from getting an induced form of arthritis (25). However, no human studies have been done, and it is felt that the risk of an anaphylactic reaction outweighs the unproven benefit of symptom relief.

Available Resources

Internet sites to help physicians assist their patients in making educated decisions about the use of CAM therapies can be found in Table 50-2 and Appendix IV.

ERIN L. ARNOLD, MD
WILLIAM J. ARNOLD, MD

References

1. Eisenberg DM, Davis RB, Ettner SL, et al. Trends in alternative medicine use in the United States. 1990-1997. JAMA 1998;280:1569–1575.
2. Rao JK, Mihaliak K, Kroenke K, Bradley J, Tierney WM, Weinberger M. Use of complementary therapies for arthritis among patients of rheumatologists. Ann Intern Med 1999; 131:409–416.
3. Sugarman J, Burk L. Physicians' ethical obligations regarding alternative medicine. JAMA 1998;280:1623–1625.
4. Pioro-Boisset M, Esdaile JM, Fitzcharles MA. Alternative medicine use in fibromyalgia syndrome. Arthritis Care Res 1996;9:13–17.
5. Kabat-Zinn J, Lipworth L, Burney R, Sellers W. Four year follow-up of a meditation-based program for the self-regulation of chronic pain: treatment outcomes and compliance. Clin J Pain 1986;2:159–173.
6. Young LD, Bradley LA, Turner RA. Decreases in health care resource utilization in patients with rheumatoid arthritis following a cognitive behavioral intervention. Biofeedback Self Regul 1995;20:259–268.
7. Yocum DE, Hodes R, Sundstrom WR, Cleeland CS. Use of biofeedback training in treatment of Raynaud's disease and phenomenon. J Rheumatol 1985;12:90–93.
8. Bradley LA, Young LD, Anderson KO, et al. Effects of psychological therapy on pain behavior of rheumatoid arthritis patients. Treatment outcome and six-month followup. Arthritis Rheum 1987;30:1105–1114.
9. Astin JA, Harkness E, Ernst E. The efficacy of "distant healing": a systematic review of randomized trials. Ann Intern Med 2000; 132:903–910.

10. Deyle D, Henderson NE, Matekel RL, Ryder MG, Garber MB, Allison SC. *Effectiveness of manual physical therapy and exercise in osteoarthritis of the knee. Ann Intern Med 2000; 132:173–181.*

11. Garfinkel MS, Singhal A, Katz WA, Allan DA, Reshetar R, Schumacher HR. *Yoga-based intervention for carpal tunnel syndrome: a randomized trial. JAMA 1998;280:1601–1603.*

12. Wolf SL, Barnhart H, Kutner NG, et al. *Reducing frailty and falls in older persons: an investigation of tai chi and computerized balancing training. J Am Geriatr Soc 1996;44:489–497.*

13. NIH Consensus Development Panel on Acupuncture. *Acupuncture. JAMA 1998;280:1518–1524.*

14. Ernst E, White AR. *Acupuncture for back pain: a meta-analysis of randomized controlled trials. Arch Intern Med 1998;158: 2235–2241.*

15. Berman BM, Singh EB, Lao L, Langenberg P, Li H, Hochberg M. *A Randomized trial of acupuncture as an adjunctive therapy in osteoarthritis of the knee. Rheumatology 1999;38:346–354.*

16. Sunshine W, Field TM, Quintino O, et al. *Fibromyalgia benefits from massage therapy and transcutaneous electrical stimulation. J Clin Rheumatol 1996;2:18–22.*

17. McAlindonTE. *Glucosamine and chondroitin for treatment of osteoarthritis. A systematic quality assessment and metaanalysis. JAMA 2000;283:1469–1475.*

18. Haqqui TM, Anthony DD, Gupta S, et al. *Prevention of collagen-induced arthritis in mice by a polyphenolic fraction from green tea. Proc Natl Acad Sci USA 1999;96:4524–4529.*

19. McAlindon TE. *Influence of vitamin D status on the incidence of progression of knee osteoarthritis. Annals Intern Med 1996;125:353–361.*

20. McAlindon TE, Jacques P, Zhang Y, et al. *Do antioxidant micronutrients protect against the development of knee osteoarthritis? Arthritis Rheum. 1996;39:648-656.*

21. Felson DT. *Weight loss reduces the risk for symptomatic knee OA in women: the Framingham study. Annals Intern Med 1992;116:535–542.*

22. Walker WR, Keats DM. *An investigation of the therapeutic value of the "copper bracelet" – dermal assimilation of copper in arthritic/rheumatoid conditions. Agents Actions 1976;6: 454–459.*

23. Valbona C, Hazlewood CF, Jurida G. *Response of pain to static magnetic fields in postpolio patients: a double-blind pilot study. Arch Phys Med Rheab 1997;78:1200–1203.*

24. Weintraub MI. *Magnetic biostimulation in painful diabetic peripheral neuropathy: a novel intervention. Am J Pain Management 1999;9:9–18.*

25. Chang YH, Bliven ML. *Anti-arthritic effect of bee venom. Agents Actions 1979;9:205–211.*

26. Eiseman JL, vonBredow J, Alvares AP. *Effect of honeybee (Apis mellifera) venom on the course of adjuvant-induced arthrits and depression of drug metabolism in the rat. Biochem Pharmacol 1982;31:1139–1146.*

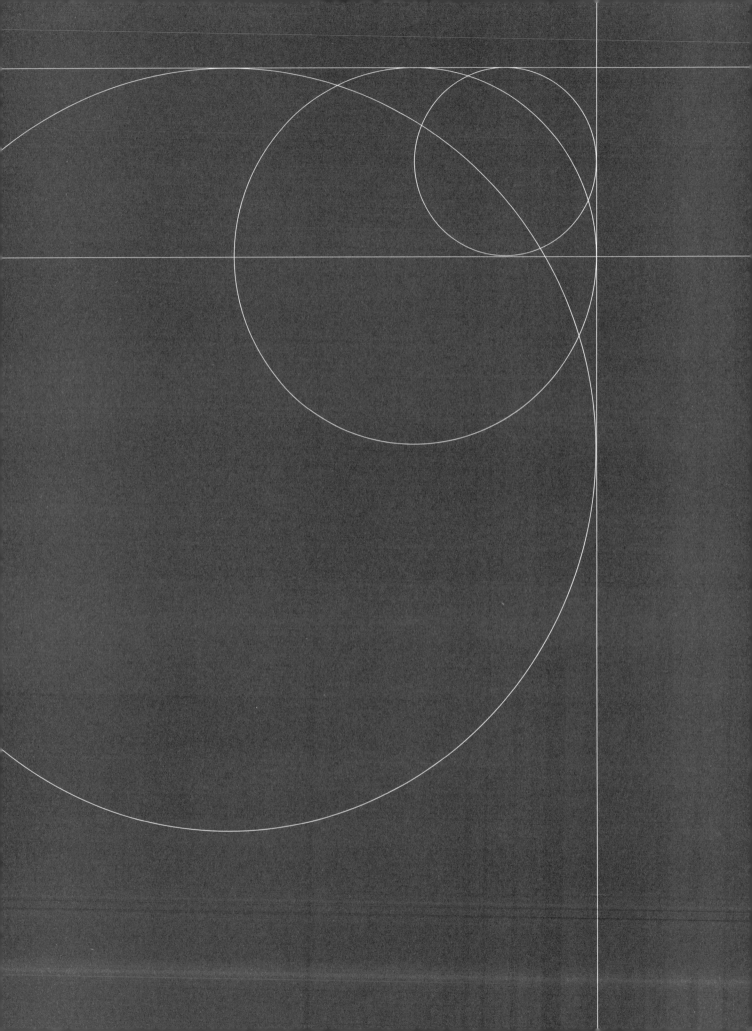

APPENDIX I
CRITERIA FOR THE CLASSIFICATION AND DIAGNOSIS OF THE RHEUMATIC DISEASES

The criteria presented in the following section have been developed with several different purposes in mind. For a given disorder, one may have criteria for: 1) classification of groups of patients (e.g., for population surveys, selection of patients for therapeutic trials, or analysis of results on interinstitutional patient comparisons); 2) diagnosis of individual patients; and 3) estimations of disease frequency, severity, and outcome.

The original intention was to propose criteria as guidelines for classification of disease syndromes for the purpose of assuring correctness of diagnosis in patients taking part in clinical investigation rather than for individual patient diagnosis. However, the proposed criteria have in fact been used as guidelines for patient diagnosis as well as for research classification. One must be cautious in such application because the various criteria are derived from the use of analytic techniques that allow the minimum number of variables to achieve the best group discrimination, rather than to attempt to arrive at a diagnosis in an individual patient.

The proposed criteria are empiric and not intended to include or exclude a particular diagnosis in any individual patient. They are valuable in offering a standard to permit comparison of groups of patients from different centers that take part in various clinical investigations, including therapeutic trials.

The ideal criterion is absolutely sensitive (i.e., all patients with the disorder show this physical finding or the positive laboratory test) and absolutely specific (i.e., the positive finding or test is never present in any other disease). Unfortunately, few such criteria or sets of criteria exist. Usually, the greater the sensitivity of a finding, the lower its specificity, and vice versa. When criteria are established attempts are made to select reasonable combinations of sensitivity and specificity.

Criteria for the Classification of Fibromyalgia[a]

1. History of widespread pain
   Definition. Pain is considered widespread when all of the following are present: pain in the left side of the body, pain in the right side of the body, pain above the waist, and pain below the waist. In addition, axial skeletal pain (cervical spine or anterior chest or thoracic spine or low back) must be present. In this definition, shoulder and buttock pain is considered as pain for each involved side. "Low back" pain is considered lower segment pain.

2. Pain in 11 of 18 tender point sites on digital palpation.[†]
   Definition. Pain, on digital palpation, must be present in at least 11 of the following 18 tender point sites:
   Occiput: bilateral, at the suboccipital muscle insertions.
   Low cervical: bilateral, at the anterior aspects of the intertransverse spaces at C5-C7.
   Trapezius: bilateral, at the midpoint of the upper border.
   Supraspinatus: bilateral, at origins, above the scapula spine near the medial border.
   Second rib: bilateral, at the second costochondral junctions, just lateral to the junctions on upper surfaces.
   Lateral epicondyle: bilateral, 2 cm distal to the epicondyles.
   Gluteal: bilateral, in upper outer quadrants of buttocks in anterior fold of muscle.
   Greater trochanter: bilateral, posterior to the trochanteric prominence.
   Knee: bilateral, at the medial fat pad proximal to the joint line.

---

[a] For classification purposes, patients will be said to have fibromyalgia if both criteria are satisfied. Widespread pain must have been present at least 3 months. The presence of a second clinical disorder does not exclude the diagnosis of fibromyalgia. [†] Digital palpation should be performed with an approximate force of 4 kg. For a tender point to be considered "positive" the subject must state that the palpation was painful. "Tender" is not to be considered "painful."

Adapted from Wolfe F, Smythe HA, Yunus MB, et al. The American College of Rheumatology 1990 criteria for the classification of fibromyalgia. Report of the multicenter criteria committee. Arthritis Rheum 1990;33:160–172, with permission of the American College of Rheumatology.

Criteria for the Classification of Rheumatoid Arthritis[a]

Criterion	Definition
1. Morning stiffness	Morning stiffness in and around the joints, lasting at least 1 hour before maximal improvement
2. Arthritis of three or more joint areas	At least three joint areas simultaneously have had soft tissue swelling or fluid (not bony overgrowth alone) observed by a physician. The 14 possible areas are right or left PIP, MCP, wrist, elbow, knee, ankle, and MTP joints
3. Arthritis of hand joints	At least one area swollen (as defined above) in a wrist, MCP, or PIP joint
4. Symmetric arthritis	Simultaneous involvement of the same joint areas (as defined in 2) on both sides of the body (bilateral involvement of PIPs, MCPs, or MTPs is acceptable without absolute symmetry)
5. Rheumatoid nodules	Subcutaneous nodules, over bony prominences, or extensor surfaces, or in juxtaarticular regions, observed by a physician
6. Serum rheumatoid factor	Demonstration of abnormal amounts of serum rheumatoid factor by any method for which the result has been positive in <5% of normal control subjects
7. Radiographic changes	Radiographic changes typical of rheumatoid arthritis on posteroanterior hand and wrist radiographs, which must include erosions or unequivocal bony decalcification localized in or most marked adjacent to the involved joints (osteoarthritis changes alone do not qualify)

[a] For classification purposes, a patient shall be said to have rheumatoid arthritis if he/she has satisfied at least four of these seven criteria. Criteria 1 through 4 must have been present for at least 6 weeks. Patients with two clinical diagnoses are not excluded. Designation as classic, definite, or probable rheumatoid arthritis is *not* to be made.

Reprinted from Arnett FC, Edworthy SM, Bloch DA, et al. The American Rheumatism Association 1987 revised criteria for the classification of rheumatoid arthritis. Arthritis Rheum 1988;31:315–324, with permission of the American College of Rheumatology.

Classification of Progression of Rheumatoid Arthritis

Stage I, Early
* 1. No destructive changes on roentgenographic examination
  2. Radiographic evidence of osteoporosis may be present

Stage II, Moderate
* 1. Radiographic evidence of osteoporosis, with or without slight subchondral bone destruction; slight cartilage destruction may be present
* 2. No joint deformities, although limitation of joint mobility may be present
  3. Adjacent muscle atrophy
  4. Extraarticular soft tissue lesions, such as nodules and tenosynovitis may be present

Stage III, Severe
* 1. Radiographic evidence of cartilage and bone destruction, in addition to osteoporosis
* 2. Joint deformity, such as subluxation, ulnar deviation, or hyperextension, without fibrous or bony ankylosis
  3. Extensive muscle atrophy
  4. Extra-articular soft tissue lesions, such as nodules and tenosynovitis may be present

Stage IV, Terminal
* 1. Fibrous or bony ankylosis
  2. Criteria of stage III

* The criteria prefaced by an asterisk are those that must be present to permit classification of a patient in any particular stage or grade.

Reprinted from Steinbrocker O, Traeger CH, Batterman RC. Therapeutic criteria in rheumatoid arthritis. JAMA 1949;140:659–662, with permission.

Criteria for Clinical Remission in Rheumatoid Arthritis[a]

Five or more of the following requirements must be fulfilled for at least two consecutive months:
1. Duration of morning stiffness not exceeding 15 minutes
2. No fatigue
3. No joint pain (by history)
4. No joint tenderness or pain on motion
5. No soft tissue swelling in joints or tendon sheaths
6. Erythrocyte sedimentation rate (Westergren method) less than 30 mm/hour for a female or 20 mm/hour for a male

[a] These criteria are intended to describe either spontaneous remission or a state of drug-induced disease suppression, which simulates spontaneous remission.

No alternative explanation may be invoked to account for the failure to meet a particular requirement. For instance, in the presence of knee pain, which might be related to degenerative arthritis, a point for "no joint pain" may not be awarded. Exclusions: Clinical manifestations of active vasculitis, pericarditis, pleuritis or myositis, and unexplained recent weight loss or fever attributable to rheumatoid arthritis will prohibit a designation of complete clinical remission.

Reprinted from Pinals RS, Masi AT, Larsen RA, et al. Preliminary criteria for clinical remission in rheumatoid arthritis. Arthritis Rheum 1981;24:1308–1315, with permission of the American College of Rheumatology.

Criteria for Classification of Functional Status in Rheumatoid Arthritis[a]

Class I: Completely able to perform usual activities of daily living (self-care, vocational, and avocational)
Class II: Able to perform usual self-care and vocational activities, but limited in avocational activities
Class III: Able to perform usual self-care activities, but limited in vocational and avocational activities
Class IV: Limited in ability to perform usual self-care, vocational, and avocational activities

[a] Usual self-care activities include dressing, feeding, bathing, grooming, and toileting. Avocational (recreational and/or leisure) and vocational (work, school, homemaking) activities are patient-desired and age- and sex-specific.

Reprinted from Hochberg MC, Chang RW, Dwosh I, et al. The American College of Rheumatology 1991 revised criteria for the classification of global functional status in rheumatoid arthritis. Arthritis Rheum 1992;35:498–502, with permission of the American College of Rheumatology.

American College of Rheumatology Preliminary Definition of Improvement in Rheumatoid Arthritis (ACR-20)

Required $\left\{\begin{array}{l}\geq 20\% \text{ improvement in tender joint count} \\ \geq 20\% \text{ improvement in swollen joint count}\end{array}\right.$

+

≥20% improvement in three of the following five
    Patient pain assessment
    Patient global assessment
    Physician global assessment
    Patient self-assessed disability
    Acute-phase reactant (ESR or CRP)

Disease activity measure	Method of assessment
1. Tender joint count	ACR tender joint count, an assessment of 28 or more joints. The joint count should be done by scoring several different aspects of tenderness, as assessed by pressure and joint manipulation on physical examination. The information on various types of tenderness should then be collapsed into a single tender-versus-nontender dichotomy.
2. Swollen joint count	ACR swollen joint count, an assessment of 28 or more joints. Joints are classified as either swollen or not swollen.
3. Patient's assessment of pain	A horizontal visual analog scale (usually 10 cm) or Likert scale assessment of the patient's current level of pain.
4. Patient's global assessment of disease activity	The patient's overall assessment of how the arthritis is doing. One acceptable method for determining this is the question from the AIMS instrument: "Considering all the ways your arthritis affects you, mark 'X' on the scale for how well you are doing." An anchored, horizontal, visual analog scale (usually 10 cm) should be provided. A Likert scale response is also acceptable.
5. Physician's global assessment of disease activity	A horizontal visual analog scale (usually 10 cm) or Likert scale measure of the physician's assessment of the patient's current disease activity.
6. Patient's assessment of physical function	Any patient self-assessment instrument which has been validated, has reliability, has been proven in RA trials to be sensitive to change, and which measures physical function in RA patients is acceptable. Instruments which have been demonstrated to be sensitive in RA trials include the AIMS, the HAQ, the Quality (or Index) of Well Being, the MHIQ, and the MACTAR.
7. Acute-phase reactant value	A Westergren ESR or a CRP level.

ACR, American College of Rheumatology; ESR, erythrocyte sedimentation rate; CRP, C-reactive protein; AIMS, Arthritis Impact Measurement Scales; RA, rheumatoid arthritis; HAQ, Health Assessment Questionnaire; MHIQ, McMaster Health Index Questionnaire; MACTAR, McMaster Toronto Arthritis Patient Preference Disability Questionnaire.

Reprinted from Felson DT, Anderson JJ, Boers M, et al. American College of Rheumatology preliminary definition of improvement in rheumatoid arthritis. Arthritis Rheum 1995;38:727–35, with permission of the American College of Rheumatology.

Criteria for the Classification of Spondyloarthropathy[a]

    Inflammatory spinal pain
      or
    Synovitis
        Asymmetric or
        Predominantly in the lower limbs
      and one or more of the following
        Positive family history
        Psoriasis
        Inflammatory bowel disease
        Urethritis, cervicitis, or acute diarrhea within 1 month before arthritis
        Buttock pain alternating between right and left gluteal areas
        Enthesopathy
        Sacroiliitis

[a] This classification method yields a sensitivity of 78.4% and a specificity of 89.6%. When radiographic evidence of sacroiliitis was included, the sensitivity improved to 87.0% with a minor decrease in specificity to 86.7%. Definition of the variables used in classification criteria follow.

Varible	Definition
Inflammatory spinal pain	History or present symptoms of spinal pain in back, dorsal, or cervical region, with at least four of the following: (a) onset before age 45, (b) insidious onset, (c) improved by exercise, (d) associated with morning stiffness, (e) at least 3 months' duration
Synovitis	Past or present asymmetric arthritis or arthritis predominantly in the lower limbs
Family history	Presence in first-degree or second-degree relatives of any of the following: (a) ankylosing spondylitis, (b) psoriasis, (c) acute uveitis, (d) reactive arthritis, (e) inflammatory bowel disease
Psoriasis	Past or present psoriasis diagnosed by a physician
Inflammatory bowel disease	Past or present Crohn's disease or ulcerative colitis diagnosed by a physician and confirmed by radiographic examination or endoscopy
Alternating buttock pain	Past or present pain alternating between the right and left gluteal regions
Enthesopathy	Past or present spontaneous pain or tenderness at examination of the site of the insertion of the Achilles tendon or plantar fascia
Acute diarrhea	Episode of diarrhea occurring within one month before arthritis
Urethritis	Nongonococcal urethritis or cervicitis occurring within one month before arthritis
Sacroiliitis	Bilateral grade 2–4 or unilateral grade 3–4, according to the following radiographic grading system: 0 = normal, 1 = possible, 2 = minimal, 3 = moderate, and 4 = ankylosis

Reprinted from Dougados M, Van Der Linden S, Juhlin R, et al. The European Spondylarthropathy Study Group preliminary criteria for the classification of spondylarthropathy. Arthritis Rheum 1991;34:1218–1227, with permission of the American College of Rheumatology.

Criteria for the Diagnosis of Rheumatic Fever[a]

Major manifestations	Minor manifestations	Supporting evidence of preceding streptococcal infection

Carditis
Polyarthritis
Chorea
Erythema marginatum
Subcutaneous nodules
	Clinical findings
	Arthralgia
	  Fever
	Laboratory findings
	  Elevated acute phase reactants
	    Erythrocyte
	      sedimentation rate
	    C-reactive protein
	  Prolonged PR interval
		Positive throat culture or rapid streptococcal antigen test
		Elevated or rising streptococcal antibody titer

[a] If supported by evidence of preceding group A streptococcal infection, the presence of two major manifestations, or of one major and two minor manifestations indicates a high probability of acute rheumatic fever.

Reprinted from Special Writing Group of the Committee on Rheumatic Fever, Endocarditis, and Kawasaki Disease of the Council on Cardiovascular Disease in the Young, American Heart Association: Guidelines for the diagnosis of rheumatic fever: Jones criteria, updated 1992. JAMA 1992;268:2069–2073, with permission.

Criteria for the Classification and Reporting of Osteoarthritis of the Hand, Hip, and Knee

Classification criteria for osteoarthritis of the hand, traditional format[a]

Hand pain, aching, or stiffness
  and
Three or four of the following features:
  Hard tissue enlargement of two or more of 10 selected joints
  Hard tissue enlargement of two or more DIP joints
  Fewer than three swollen MCP joints
  Deformity of at least one of 10 selected joints

[a] The 10 selected joints are the second and third distal interphalangeal (DIP), the second and third proximal interphalangeal, and the first carpometacarpal joints of both hands. This classification method yields a sensitivity of 94% and a specificity of 87%. MCP = metacarpophalangeal.

Reprinted from Altman R, Alarcón G, Appelrouth D, et al: The American College of Rheumatology criteria for the classification and reporting of osteoarthritis of the hand. Arthritis Rheum 1990;33: 1601–1610, with permission of the American College of Rheumatology.

Classification criteria for osteoarthritis of the hip, traditional format[a]

Hip pain
  and
At least two of the following three features:
  ESR <20 mm/hour
  Radiographic femoral or acetabular osteophytes
  Radiographic joint space narrowing (superior, axial, and/or medial)

[a] This classification method yields a sensitivity of 89% and a specificity of 91%. ESR = erythrocyte sedimentation rate (Westergren).

Reprinted from Altman R, Alarcón G, Appelrouth D, et al: The American College of Rheumatology criteria for the classification and reporting of osteoarthritis of the hip. Arthritis Rheum 1991; 34:505–514, with permission of the American College of Rheumatology.

Criteria for classification of idiopathic osteoarthritis (OA) of the knee[a]

Clinical and laboratory	Clinical and radiographic	Clinical[b]

Knee pain plus at least five of nine:
  Age >50 years
  Stiffness <30 minutes
  Crepitus
  Bony tenderness
  Bony enlargement
  No palpable warmth
  ESR <40 mm/hr
  RF <1:40
  SF OA
	Knee pain plus at least one of three:
	  Age >50 years
	  Stiffness <30 minutes
	  Crepitus
	    +
	  Osteophytes
		Knee pain plus at least three of six:
		  Age >50 years
		  Stiffness <30 minutes
		  Crepitus
		  Bony tenderness
		  Bony enlargement
		  No palpable warmth

92% sensitive 75% specific	91% sensitive 86% specific	95% sensitive 69% specific

[a] ESR, erythrocyte sedimentation rate (Westergren); RF, rheumatoid factor; SF OA, synovial fluid signs of OA (clear, viscous, or white blood cell count <2,000/mm^3).

[b] Alternative for the clinical category would be four of six, which is 84% sensitive and 89% specific.

Reprinted from Altman R, Asch E, Bloch G, et al. Development of criteria for the classification and reporting of osteoarthritis: classification of osteoarthritis of the knee. Arthritis Rheum 1986;29:1039–1049, with permission of the American College of Rheumatology.

Criteria for the Classification of Acute Gouty Arthritis

A. The presence of characteristic urate crystals in the joint fluid, or
B. A tophus proved to contain urate crystals by chemical means or polarized light microscopy, or
C. The presence of six of the following 12 clinical, laboratory, and x-ray phenomena listed below:
   1. More than one attack of acute arthritis
   2. Maximal inflammation developed within 1 day
   3. Attack of monarticular arthritis
   4. Joint redness observed
   5. First metatarsophalangeal joint painful or swollen
   6. Unilateral attack involving first metatarsophalangeal joint
   7. Unilateral attack involving tarsal joint
   8. Suspected tophus
   9. Hyperuricemia
  10. Asymmetric swelling within a joint (radiograph)
  11. Subcortical cysts without erosions (radiograph)
  12. Negative culture of joint fluid for microorganisms during attack of joint inflammation

Adapted from Wallace SL, Robinson H, Masi AT, et al: Preliminary criteria for the classification of the acute arthritis of primary gout. Arthritis Rheum 1977;20:895–900, with permission of the American College of Rheumatology.

Criteria for the Classification of Systemic Lupus Erythematosus[a]

Criterion	Definition
1. Malar rash	Fixed erythema, flat or raised, over the malar eminences, tending to spare the nasolabial folds
2. Discoid rash	Erythematous raised patches with adherent keratotic scaling and follicular plugging; atrophic scarring may occur in older lesions
3. Photosensitivity	Skin rash as a result of unusual reaction to sunlight, by patient history or physician observation
4. Oral ulcers	Oral or nasopharyngeal ulceration, usually painless, observed by a physician
5. Arthritis	Nonerosive arthritis involving two or more peripheral joints, characterized by tenderness, swelling, or effusion
6. Serositis	a) Pleuritis—convincing history of pleuritic pain or rub heard by a physician or evidence of pleural effusion OR b) Pericarditis—documented by ECG or rub or evidence of pericardial effusion
7. Renal disorder	a) Persistent proteinuria greater than 0.5 grams per day or greater than 3+ if quantitation not performed OR b) Cellular casts—may be red cell, hemoglobin, granular, tubular, or mixed
8. Neurologic disorder	a) Seizures—in the absence of offending drugs or known metabolic derangements; eg, uremia, ketoacidosis, or electrolyte imbalance OR b) Psychosis—in the absence of offending drugs or known metabolic derangements; eg, uremia, ketoacidosis, or electrolyte imbalance
9. Hematologic disorder	a) Hemolytic anemia—with reticulocytosis OR b) Leukopenia—less than 4000/mm^3 total on two or more occasions OR c) Lymphopenia—less than 1500/mm^3 on two or more occasions OR d) Thrombocytopenia—less than 100,000/mm^3 in the absence of offending drugs
10. Immunologic disorder[b]	a) Anti-DNA: antibody to native DNA in abnormal titer OR b) Anti-SM: presence of antibody to SM nuclear antigen OR c) Positive finding of antiphospholipid antibodies based on (1) an abnormal serum level of IgG or IgM anti-cardiolipin antibodies, (2) a positive test result for lupus anticoagulant using a standard method, or (3) a false positive serologic test for syphilis known to be positive for at least 6 months and confirmed by *Treponema pallidum* immobilization or fluorescent treponemal antibody absorption test
11. Antinuclear antibody	An abnormal titer of antinuclear antibody by immunofluorescence or an equivalent assay at any point in time and in the absence of drugs known to be associated with "drug-induced lupus" syndrome

[a] This classification is based on 11 criteria. For the purpose of identifying patients in clinical studies, a person must have SLE if any four or more of the 11 criteria are present, serially or simultaneously, during any interval of observation.

[b] The modifications to criterion number 10 were made in 1997.

Adapted from Tan EM, Cohen AS, Fries JF, et al. The 1982 revised criteria for the classification of systemic lupus erythematosus (SLE). Arthritis Rheum 1982;25:1271–7, with permission of the American College of Rheumatology.

Adapted from Hochberg MC. Updating the American College of Rheumatology revised criteria for the classification of systemic lupus erythematosus [letter]. Arthritis Rheum 1997;40:1725, with permission of the American College of Rheumatology.

Criteria for the Classification of Systemic Sclerosis (Scleroderma)[a]

A. Major criterion

Proximal scleroderma: Symmetric thickening, tightening, and induration of the skin of the fingers and the skin proximal to the metacarpophalangeal or metatarsophalangeal joints. The changes may affect the entire extremity, face, neck, and trunk (thorax and abdomen).

B. Minor criteria

1. *Sclerodactyly:* Above-indicated skin changes limited to the fingers

2. *Digital pitting scars or loss of substance from the finger pad:* Depressed areas at tips of fingers or loss of digital pad tissue as a result of ischemia

3. *Bibasilar pulmonary fibrosis:* Bilateral reticular pattern of linear or lineonodular densities most pronounced in basilar portions of the lungs on standard chest roentgenogram; may assume appearance of diffuse mottling or "honeycomb lung." These changes should not be attributable to primary lung disease.

---

[a] For the purposes of classifying patients in clinical trials, population surveys, and other studies, a person shall be said to have systemic sclerosis (scleroderma) if the one major or two or more minor criteria are present. Localized forms of scleroderma, eosinophilic fasciitis, and the various forms of pseudoscleroderma are excluded from these criteria.

Adapted from Subcommittee for Scleroderma Criteria of the American Rheumatism Association Diagnostic and Therapeutic Criteria Committee. Preliminary criteria for the classification of systemic sclerosis (scleroderma). Arthritis Rheum 1980;23:581–590, with permission of the American College of Rheumatology.

Criteria for the Diagnosis of Polymyositis and Dermatomyositis[a]

Criterion	Definition
1. Symmetrical weakness	Weakness of limb-girdle muscles and anterior neck flexors, progressing over weeks to months, with or without dysphagia or respiratory muscle involvement
2. Muscle biopsy evidence	Evidence of necrosis of Type I and II fibers, phagocytosis, regeneration with basophilia, large vesicular sarcolemmal nuclei and prominent nucleoli, atrophy in a perifascicular distribution, variation in fiber size, and an inflammatory exudate, often perivascular
3. Elevation of muscle enzymes	Elevation in serum of skeletal muscle enzymes, particularly creatine phosphokinase and often aldolase, serum glutamate oxaloacetate, and pyruvate transaminases, and lactate dehydrogenase
4. Electromyographic evidence	Electromyographic triad of short, small, polyphasic motor units, fibrillations, positive sharp waves, and insertional irritability, and bizarre, high-frequency repetitive discharges
5. Dermatologic features	A lilac discoloration of the eyelids (heliotrope) with periorbital edema, a scaly, erythematous dermatitis over the dorsum of the hands (especially the metacarpophalangeal and proximal interphalangeal joints, Gottron's sign), and involvement of the knees, elbows, and medial malleoli, as well as the face, neck, and upper torso

[a] Confidence limits can be defined as follows. For a definite diagnosis of dermatomyositis, three of four criteria plus the rash must be present; for a definite diagnosis of polymyositis, four criteria must be present without the rash. For a probable diagnosis of dermatomyositis, two criteria plus the rash must be present; for a probable diagnosis of polymyositis, three criteria must be present without the rash. For a possible diagnosis of dermatomyositis, one criterion plus the rash must be present; for a possible diagnosis of polymyositis, two criteria must be present without the rash.

The following findings exclude a diagnosis of dermatomyositis or polymyositis.

- Evidence of central or peripheral neurologic disease, including motor-neuron disorders with fasciculations or long-tract signs, sensory changes, decreased nerve conduction times, and fiber-type atrophy and grouping on muscle biopsy.
- Muscle weakness with a slowly progressive, unremitting course and a positive family history or calf enlargement to suggest a muscular dystrophy.
- Biopsy evidence of granulomatous myositis such as with sarcoidosis.
- Infections, including trichinosis, schistosomiasis, trypanosomiasis, staphylococcosis, and toxoplasmosis.
- Recent use of various drugs and toxins, such as clofibrate and alcohol.
- Rhabdomyolysis as manifested by gross myoglobinuria related to strenuous exercise, infections, crush injuries, occlusions of major limb arteries, prolonged coma or convulsions, high-voltage accidents, heat stroke, the malignant-hyperpyrexia syndrome, and envenomation by certain sea snakes.
- Metabolic disorders such as McArdle's syndrome.
- Endocrinopathies such as thyrotoxicosis, myxedema, hyperparathyroidism, hypoparathyroidism, diabetes mellitus, or Cushing's syndrome.
- Myasthenia gravis with response to cholinergics, sensitivity to d-tubocurarine, and decremental response to repetitive nerve stimulation.

Data from Bohan A, Peter JB. Polymyositis and dermatomyositis (first of two parts). N Engl J Med 1975;292:344–347, with permission.

Criteria for the Classification of Sjögren's Syndrome[a]

1. Ocular symptoms
    Definition. A positive response to at least one of the following three questions:
    (a) Have you had daily, persistent, troublesome dry eyes for more than 3 months?
    (b) Do you have a recurrent sensation of sand or gravel in the eyes?
    (c) Do you use tear substitutes more than three times a day?
2. Oral symptoms
    Definition. A positive response to at least one of the following three questions:
    (a) Have you had a daily feeling of dry mouth for more than 3 months?
    (b) Have you had recurrent or persistently swollen salivary glands as an adult?
    (c) Do you frequently drink liquids to aid in swallowing dry foods?
3. Ocular signs
    Definition. Objective evidence of ocular involvement, determined on the basis of a positive result on at least one of
        the following two tests:
    (a) Schirmer-I test (≤ 5 mm in 5 minutes)
    (b) Rose bengal score (≥ 4, according to the van Bijsterveld scoring system)
4. Histopathologic features
    Definition. Focus score ≥ 1 on minor salivary gland biopsy (focus defined as an agglomeration of at least 50 mononuclear
        cells; focus score defined as the number of foci per 4 mm^2 of glandular tissue)
5. Salivary gland involvement
    Definition. Objective evidence of salivary gland involvement, determined on the basis of a positive result on at least
        one of the following three tests:
    (a) Salivary scintigraphy
    (b) Parotid sialography
    (c) Unstimulated salivary flow (≤ 1.5 ml in 15 minutes)
6. Autoantibodies
    Definition. Presence of at least one of the following serum autoantibodies:
    (a) Antibodies to Ro/SS-A or La/SS-B antigens
    (b) Antinuclear antibodies
    (c) Rheumatoid factor
Exclusion criteria: preexisting lymphoma, acquired immunodeficiency syndrome, sarcoidosis, or graft-versus-host disease

---

[a] For primary Sjögren's syndrome, the presence of three of six items showed a very high sensitivity (99.1%), but insufficient specificity (57.8%). Thus, this combination could be accepted as the basis for a diagnosis of probable primary Sjögren's syndrome. However, the presence of four of six items (accepting as serologic parameters only positive anti-Ro/SS-A and anti-La/SS-B antibodies) had a good sensitivity (93.5%) and specificity (94.0%), and therefore may be used to establish a definitive diagnosis of primary Sjögren's syndrome.

Reprinted from Vitali C, Bombardieri S, Moutsopoulos HM, et al. Preliminary criteria for the classification of Sjögren's syndrome. Arthritis Rheum 1993;36:340–347, with permission of the American College of Rheumatology.

Criteria for the Classification of Polyarteritis Nodosa[a]

Criterion	Definition
1. Weight loss ≥4 kg	Loss of 4 kg or more of body weight since illness began, not due to dieting or other factors
2. Livedo reticularis	Mottled reticular pattern over the skin of portions of the extremities or torso
3. Testicular pain or tenderness	Pain or tenderness of the testicles, not due to infection, trauma, or other causes
4. Myalgias, weakness, or leg tenderness	Diffuse myalgias (excluding shoulder and hip girdle) or weakness of muscles or tenderness of leg muscles
5. Mononeuropathy or polyneuropathy	Development of mononeuropathy, multiple mononeuropathies, or polyneuropathy
6. Diastolic BP >90 mm Hg	Development of hypertension with the diastolic BP higher than 90 mm Hg
7. Elevated BUN or creatinine	Elevation of BUN >40 mg/dL or creatinine >1.5 mg/dL, not due to dehydration or obstruction
8. Hepatitis B virus	Presence of hepatitis B surface antigen or antibody in serum
9. Arteriographic abnormality	Arteriogram showing aneurysms or occlusions of the visceral arteries, not due to arteriosclerosis, fibromuscular dysplasia, or other noninflammatory causes
10. Biopsy of small or medium-sized artery containing PMN	Histologic changes showing the presence of granulocytes or granulocytes and mononuclear leukocytes in the artery wall

[a] For classification purposes, a patient shall be said to have polyarteritis nodosa if at least three of these 10 criteria are present. The presence of any three or more criteria yields a sensitivity of 82.2% and a specificity of 86.6%. BP, blood pressure; BUN, blood urea nitrogen; PMN, polymorphonuclear neutrophils.

Reprinted from Lightfoot RW Jr, Michel BA, Bloch DA, et al. The American College of Rheumatology 1990 criteria for the classification of polyarteritis nodosa. Arthritis Rheum 1990;33:1088–1093, with permission of the American College of Rheumatology.

Criteria for the Classification of Henoch-Schönlein Purpura[a]

Criterion	Definition
1. Palpable purpura	Slightly raised "palpable" hemorrhagic skin lesions, not related to thrombocytopenia
2. Age ≤20 at disease onset	Patient 20 years or younger at onset of first symptoms
3. Bowel angina	Diffuse abdominal pain, worse after meals, or the diagnosis of bowel ischemia, usually including bloody diarrhea
4. Wall granulocytes on biopsy	Histologic changes showing granulocytes in the walls of arterioles or venules

[a] For purposes of classification, a patient shall be said to have Henoch-Schönlein purpura if at least two of these four criteria are present. The presence of any two or more criteria yields a sensitivity of 87.1% and a specificity of 87.7%.

Reprinted from Mills JA, Michel BA, Bloch DA, et al. The American College of Rheumatology 1990 criteria for the classification of Henoch-Schönlein purpura. Arthritis Rheum 1990;33:1114–1121, with permission of the American College of Rheumatology.

Criteria for the Classification of Churg-Strauss Syndrome[a]

Criterion	Definition
1. Asthma	History of wheezing or diffuse high-pitched rales on expiration
2. Eosinophilia	Eosinophilia >10% on white blood cell differential count
3. Mononeuropathy or polyneuropathy	Development of mononeuropathy, multiple mononeuropathies, or polyneuropathy (ie, glove/stocking distribution) attributable to a systemic vasculitis
4. Pulmonary infiltrates, non-fixed	Migratory or transitory pulmonary infiltrates on radiographs (not including fixed infiltrates), attributable to a systemic vasculitis
5. Paranasal sinus abnormality	History of acute or chronic paranasal sinus pain or tenderness or radiographic opacification of the paranasal sinuses
6. Extravascular eosinophils	Biopsy including artery, arteriole, or venule, showing accumulations of eosinophils in extravascular areas

[a] For classification purposes, a patient shall be said to have Churg-Strauss syndrome if at least four of these six criteria are positive. The presence of any four or more of the six criteria yields a sensitivity of 85% and a specificity of 99.7%.

Adapted from Masi AT, Hunder GG, Lie JT, et al. The American College of Rheumatology 1990 criteria for the classification of Churg-Strauss syndrome (allergic granulomatosis and angiitis). Arthritis Rheum 1990;33:1094–1100, with permission of the American College of Rheumatology.

Criteria for the Classification of Wegener's Granulomatosis[a]

Criterion	Definition
1. Nasal or oral inflammation	Development of painful or painless oral ulcers or purulent or bloody nasal discharge
2. Abnormal chest radiograph	Chest radiograph showing the presence of nodules, fixed infiltrates, or cavities
3. Urinary sediment	Microhematuria (>5 red blood cells per high power field) or red cell casts in urine sediment
4. Granulomatous inflammation on biopsy	Histologic changes showing granulomatous inflammation within the wall of an artery or in the perivascular or extravascular area (artery or arteriole)

[a] For purposes of classification, a patient shall be said to have Wegener's granulomatosis if at least two of these four criteria are present. The presence of any two or more criteria yields a sensitivity of 88.2% and a specificity of 92.0%.

Reprinted from Leavitt RY, Fauci AS, Bloch DA, et al. The American College of Rheumatology 1990 criteria for the classification of Wegener's granulomatosis. Arthritis Rheum 1990;33:1101–1107, with permission of the American College of Rheumatology.

Criteria for the Classification of Giant Cell Arteritis[a]

Criterion	Definition
1. Age at disease onset ≥50 years	Development of symptoms or findings beginning at age 50 or older
2. New headache	New onset of or new type of localized pain in the head
3. Temporal artery abnormality	Temporal artery tenderness to palpation or decreased pulsation, unrelated to arteriosclerosis of cervical arteries
4. Elevated erythrocyte sedimentation rate	Erythrocyte sedimentation rate ≥50 mm/hour by the Westergren method
5. Abnormal artery biopsy	Biopsy specimen with artery showing vasculitis characterized by a predominance of mononuclear cell infiltration or granulomatous inflammation, usually with multinucleated giant cells

[a] For purposes of classification, a patient shall be said to have giant cell (temporal) arteritis if at least three of these five criteria are present. The presence of any three or more criteria yields a sensitivity of 93.5% and a specificity of 91.2%.

Reprinted from Hunder GG, Bloch DA, Michel BA, et al. The American College of Rheumatology 1990 criteria for the classification of giant cell arteritis. Arthritis Rheum 1990;33:1122–1128, with permission of the American College of Rheumatology.

Criteria for the Classification of Takayasu Arteritis[a]

Criterion	Definition
1. Age at disease onset ≤40 years	Development of symptoms or findings related to Takayasu arteritis at age ≤40 years
2. Claudication of extremities	Development and worsening of fatigue and discomfort in muscles of one or more extremity while in use, especially the upper extremities
3. Decreased brachial artery pulse	Decreased pulsation of one or both brachial arteries
4. BP difference >10 mm Hg	Difference of >10 mm Hg in systolic blood pressure between arms
5. Bruit over subclavian arteries or aorta	Bruit audible on auscultation over one or both subclavian arteries or abdominal aorta
6. Arteriogram abnormality	Arteriographic narrowing or occlusion of the entire aorta, its primary branches, or large arteries in the proximal upper or lower extremities, not due to arteriosclerosis, fibromuscular dysplasia, or similar causes; changes usually focal or segmental

[a] For purposes of classification, a patient shall be said to have Takayasu arteritis if at least three of these six criteria are present. The presence of any three or more criteria yields a sensitivity of 90.5% and a specificity of 97.8%. BP = blood pressure (systolic; difference between arms).

Reprinted from Arend WP, Michel BA, Bloch DA, et al. The American College of Rheumatology 1990 criteria for the classification of Takayasu arteritis. Arthritis Rheum 1990;33:1129–1132, with permission of the American College of Rheumatology.

Criteria for the Classification of Hypersensitivity Vasculitis[a]

Criterion	Definition
1. Age at disease onset >16 years	Development of symptoms after age 16
2. Medication at disease onset	Medication was taken at the onset of symptoms that may have been a precipitating factor
3. Palpable purpura	Slightly elevated purpuric rash over one or more areas of the skin; does not blanch with pressure and is not related to thrombocytopenia
4. Maculopapular rash	Flat and raised lesions of various sizes over one or more areas of the skin
5. Biopsy including arteriole and venule	Histologic changes showing granulocytes in a perivascular or extravascular location

[a] For purposes of classification, a patient shall be said to have hypersensitivity vasculitis if at least three of these five criteria are present. The presence of any three or more criteria yields a sensitivity of 71.0% and a specificity of 83.9%.

Reprinted from Calabrese LH, Michel BA, Bloch DA, et al. The American College of Rheumatology 1990 criteria for the classification of hypersensitivity vasculitis. Arthritis Rheum 1990;33:1108–1113, with permission of the American College of Rheumatology.

Diagnostic Guidelines for Kawasaki Syndrome[a]

Fever lasting >5 days plus four of the following criteria
1. Polymorphous rash
2. Bilateral conjunctival injection
3. One or more of the following mucous membrane changes:
    Diffuse injection of oral and pharyngeal mucosa
    Erythema or fissuring of the lips
    Strawberry tongue
4. Acute, nonpurulent cervical lymphadenopathy (one lymph node must be >1.5 cm)
5. One or more of the following extremity changes:
    Erythema of palms and/or soles
    Indurative edema of hands and/or feet
    Membranous desquamation of the fingertips

[a] Other illnesses with similar clinical signs must be excluded.

Reprinted from Kawasaki T, Kosaki T, Okawa S, et al. A new infantile acute febrile mucocutaneous lymph node syndrome (MLNS) prevailing in Japan. Pediatrics 1974;54:271–276, with permission.

Criteria for the Diagnosis of Behçet's Disease[a]

Criterion	Definition
1. Recurrent oral ulceration	Minor aphthous, major aphthous, or herpetiform ulceration observed by physician or patient, which recurred at least three times in one 12-month period
Plus two of	
2. Recurrent genital ulceration	Aphthous ulceration or scarring, observed by physician or patient
3. Eye lesions	Anterior uveitis, posterior uveitis, or cells in vitreous on slit lamp examination; or retinal vasculitis observed by ophthalmologist
4. Skin lesions	Erythema nodosum observed by physician or patient, pseudofolliculitis, or papulopustular lesions; or acneiform nodules observed by physician in postadolescent patients not on corticosteroid treatment
5. Positive pathergy test	Read by physician at 24–48 hours

[a] Findings applicable only in the absence of other clinical explanations. The presence of recurrent oral ulceration and any two of the remaining criteria yields a sensitivity of 91% and a specificity of 96%.

Reprinted from International Study Group for Behçet's Disease. Criteria for diagnosis of Behçet's disease. Lancet 1990;335:1078–1080, with permission.

Preliminary Classification Criteria for Antiphospholipid Syndrome[a]

Vascular thrombosis
   a) One or more clinical episodes of arterial, venous or small-vessel thrombosis in any tissue or organ *and*
   b) Thrombosis confirmed by imaging or Doppler studies or histopathology, with the exception of superficial venous thrombosis *and*
   c) For histopathologic confirmation, thrombosis present without significant evidence of inflammation in the vessel wall.

Pregnancy morbidity
   a) One or more unexplained deaths of a morphologically normal fetus at or beyond the 10th week of gestation, with normal fetal morphology documented by ultrasound or by direct examination of the fetus *or*
   b) One or more premature births of a morphologically normal neonate at or before the 34th week of gestation because of severe preeclampsia or severe placental insufficiency *or*
   c) Three or more unexplained consecutive spontaneous abortions before the 10th week of gestation, with maternal anatomic or hormonal abnormalities and paternal and maternal chromosomal causes excluded.

Laboratory criteria
   a) Anticardiolipin antibody of IgG and/or IgM isotype in blood, present in medium or high titer on two or more occasions at least six weeks apart, measured by standard enzyme linked immunosorbent assay for β_2 glycoprotein-1 dependent anticardiolipin antibodies *or*
   b) Lupus anticoagulant present in plasma on two or more occasions at least six weeks apart, detected according to the guidelines of the International Society on Thrombosis and Hemostasis.

[a] Definite APS is considered to be present if at least one of the clinical and one of the laboratory criteria are met.

Adapted from Wilson WA, Gharavi AE, Koike T, et al. International consensus statement on preliminary classification criteria for definite antiphospholipid syndrome. Report of an International Workshop. Arthritis Rheum 1999;42:1309–1311 with permission of the American College of Rheumatology.

World Health Organization Criteria for the Diagnosis of Osteoporosis[a]

Normal: BMC or BMD not more than 1 standard deviation below peak adult bone mass
T-score >–1

Osteopenia: BMC or BMD that lies between 1 and 2.5 standard deviations below peak adult bone mass
T-score between –1 and –2.5

Osteoporosis: BMC or BMD value more than 2.5 standard deviations below peak adult bone mass
T-score ≤ –2.5

Severe
Osteoporosis: BMC or BMD value more than 2.5 standard deviations below peak adult bone mass and the presence of one or more fragility fractures
T-score ≤ –2.5 plus fragility fracture

[a] World Health Organization criteria for the diagnosis of osteoporosis based on bone mineral content (BMC) or bone mineral density (BMD) measurements. These criteria can be applied to either the central or peripheral skeletal measurement sites.

Adapted from Assessment of fracture risk and its application to screening for postmenopausal osteoporosis. Report of a WHO study group. World Health Organ Techn Rep Ser 1994;843:1–129.

Criteria for the Diagnosis of Juvenile Rheumatoid Arthritis

I. General

The JRA Criteria Subcommittee in 1982 reviewed the 1977 Criteria (1) and recommended that *juvenile rheumatoid arthritis* be the name for the principal form of chronic arthritic disease in children and that this general class should be classified into three onset subtypes: systemic, polyarticular, and pauciarticular. The onset subtypes may be further subclassified into subsets as indicated below. The following classification enumerates the requirements for the diagnosis of JRA and the three clinical onset subtypes and lists subsets of each subtype that may be useful in further classification.

II. General criteria for the diagnosis of juvenile rheumatoid arthritis:
   A. Persistent arthritis of at least six weeks duration in one or more joints
   B. Exclusion of other causes of arthritis (see list of exclusions)

III. JRA onset subtypes

The onset subtype is determined by manifestations during the first six months of disease and remains the principal classification, although manifestations more closely resembling another subtype may appear later.
   A. Systemic onset JRA: This subtype is defined as JRA with persistent intermittent fever (daily intermittent temperatures to 103°F or more) with or without rheumatoid rash or other organ involvement. Typical fever and rash will be considered probable systemic onset JRA if not associated with arthritis. Before a definite diagnosis can be made, arthritis, as defined, must be present.
   B. Pauciarticular onset JRA: This subtype is defined as JRA with arthritis in four or fewer joints during the first six months of disease. Patients with systemic onset JRA are excluded from this onset subtype.
   C. Polyarticular JRA: This subtype is defined as JRA with arthritis in five or more joints during the first six months of disease. Patients with systemic JRA onset are excluded from this subtype.
   D. The onset subtypes may include the following subsets:
      1. Systemic onset
         a. Polyarthritis
         b. Oligoarthritis
      2. Oligoarthritis (Pauciarticular onset)
         a. Antinuclear antibody (ANA) positive-chronic uveitis

         b. Rheumatoid factor (RF) positive
         c. Seronegative, B27 positive
         d. Not otherwise classified
      3. Polyarthritis
         a. RF positivity
         b. Not otherwise classified

IV. Exclusions
   A. Other rheumatic diseases
      1. Rheumatic fever
      2. Systemic lupus erythematosus
      3. Ankylosing spondylitis
      4. Polymyositis or dermatomyositis
      5. Vasculitic syndromes
      6. Scleroderma
      7. Psoriatic arthritis
      8. Reiter's syndrome
      9. Sjögren's syndrome
      10. Mixed connective tissue disease
      11. Behçet's syndrome
   B. Infectious arthritis
   C. Inflammatory bowel disease
   D. Neoplastic diseases including leukemia
   E. Nonrheumatic conditions of bones and joints
   F. Hematologic diseases
   G. Psychogenic arthralgia
   H. Miscellaneous
      1. Sarcoidosis
      2. Hypertrophic osteoarthropathy
      3. Villonodular synovitis
      4. Chronic active hepatitis
      5. Familial Mediterranean fever

V. Other proposed terminology

Juvenile chronic arthritis (JCA) and juvenile arthritis (JA) are new diagnostic terms currently in use in some places for the arthritides of childhood. The diagnoses of JCA and JA are not equivalent to each other, nor to the older diagnosis of juvenile rheumatoid arthritis or Still's disease. Hence reports of studies of JCA or JA cannot be directly compared with one another nor to reports of JRA or Still's disease. Juvenile chronic arthritis is described in more detail in a report of the European Conference on the Rheumatic Diseases of Children (2) and juvenile arthritis in the report of the Ross Conference (3).

1. JRA Criteria Subcommittee of the Diagnostic and Therapeutic Criteria Committee of the American Rheumatism Association: Current proposed revisions of the JRA criteria. Arthritis Rheum 1977;20(Suppl)195–199.
2. Ansell BW: Chronic arthritis in childhood. Ann Rheum 1978;Dis 37:107–120.
3. Fink CW: Keynote address: Arthritis in childhood, Report of the 80th Ross Conference in Pediatric Research. Columbus, Ross Laboratories, 1979, pp 1-2.

APPENDIX II
GUIDELINES FOR THE MANAGEMENT OF RHEUMATIC DISEASES

Practice guidelines represent a recent and important development in rheumatology. Guidelines, which are developed by a panel of experts, address a broad range of clinical issues from the approach to diagnosis of musculoskeletal signs and symptoms to patient management. Guidelines provide a framework for clinical practice and serve a valuable educational function for students of the rheumatic diseases. Moreover, because in very few instances have guidelines been tested in clinical settings, they present an opportunity to study whether they result in efficiencies or improvements in diagnosis and patient management.

Initial Evaluation of the Adult Patient With Acute Musculoskeletal Symptoms

"Red flags" suggesting the need for urgent evaluation and management of the patient with musculoskeletal symptoms

Feature	Differential diagnosis
History of significant trauma	Soft tissue injury, internal derangement, or fracture
Hot, swollen joint	Infection, systemic rheumatic disease, gout, pseudogout
Constitutional signs and symptoms (e.g., fever, weight loss, malaise)	Infection, sepsis, systemic rheumatic disease
Weakness	
Focal	Focal nerve lesion (compartment syndrome, entrapment neuropathy, mononeuritis multiplex, motor neuron disease, radiculopathy[a])
Diffuse	Myositis, metabolic myopathy, paraneoplastic syndrome, degenerative neuromuscular disorder, toxin, myelopathy,[a] transverse myelitis
Neurogenic pain (burning, numbness, paresthesia)	
Asymmetric	Radiculopathy,[a] reflex sympathetic dystrophy, entrapment neuropathy
Symmetric	Myelopathy,[a] peripheral neuropathy
Claudication pain pattern	Peripheral vascular disease, giant cell arteritis (jaw pain), lumbar spinal stenosis

[a] Radiculopathy and myelopathy may be due to infectious, neoplastic, or mechanical processes.

Reprinted from American College of Rheumatology Ad Hoc Committee on Clinical Guidelines: Guidelines for the initial evaluation of the adult patient with acute musculoskeletal symptoms. Arthritis Rheum 1996;39:1–8, with permission of the American College of Rheumatology.

Monitoring Drug Therapy in Rheumatoid Arthritis

Recommended monitoring strategies for drug treatment of rheumatoid arthritis[a]

Drugs	Toxicities requiring monitoring[b]	Baseline evaluation	Monitoring	
			System review/examination	Laboratory
Salicylates, nonsteroidal anti-inflammatory drugs	Gastrointestinal ulceration and bleeding	CBC, creatinine, AST, ALT	Dark/black stool, dyspepsia, nausea or vomiting, abdominal pain, edema, shortness of breath	CBC yearly, LFTs, creatinine testing may be required[c]
Hydroxychloroquine	Macular damage	None unless patient is over age 40 or has previous eye disease	Visual changes, funduscopic and visual fields every 6–12 months	–
Sulfasalazine	Myelosuppression	CBC, and AST or ALT in patients at risk, G6PD	Symptoms of myelosuppression[d], photosensitivity, rash	CBC every 2–4 weeks for first 3 months, then every 3 months
Methotrexate	Myelosuppression, hepatic fibrosis, cirrhosis, pulmonary infiltrates or fibrosis	CBC, chest radiography within past year, hepatitis B and C serology in high-risk patients, AST or ALT, albumin, alkaline phosphatase, and creatinine	Symptoms of myelosuppression[d], shortness of breath, nausea/vomiting, lymph node swelling	CBC, platelet count, AST, albumin, creatinine every 4–8 weeks
Gold, intramuscular	Myelosuppression, proteinuria	CBC, platelet count, creatinine, urine dipstick for protein	Symptoms of myelosuppression[d], edema, rash, oral ulcers, diarrhea	CBC, platelet count, urine dipstick every 1–2 weeks for first 20 weeks, then at the time of each (or every other) injection
Gold, oral	Myelosuppression, proteinuria	CBC, platelet count, urine dipstick for protein	Symptoms of myelosuppression[d], edema, rash, diarrhea	CBC platelet count, urine dipstick for protein every 4–12 weeks
D-penicillamine	Myelosuppression, proteinuria	CBC, platelet count, creatinine, urine dipstick for protein	Symptoms of myelosuppression[d], edema, rash	CBC, urine dipstick for protein every 2 weeks until dosage stable, then every 1–3 months
Azathioprine	Myelosuppression, hepatotoxicity, lymphoproliferative disorders	CBC, platelet count, creatinine, AST or ALT	Symptoms of myelosuppression[d]	CBC and platelet count every 1–2 weeks with changes in dosage, and every 1–3 months thereafter
Corticosteroids (oral ≤ 10 mg of prednisone or equivalent)	Hypertension, hyperglycemia	BP, chemistry panel, bone densitometry in high-risk patients	BP at each visit, polyuria, polydipsia, edema, shortness of breath, visual changes, weight gain	Urinalysis for glucose yearly
Agents for refractory RA or severe extraarticular complications				
Cyclophosphamide	Myelosuppression, myeloproliferative disorders, malignancy, hemorrhagic cystitis	CBC, platelet count, urinalysis, creatinine, AST or ALT	Symptoms of myelosuppression[d], hematuria	CBC and platelet count every 1–2 weeks with changes in dosage, and every 1–3 months thereafter, urinalysis and urine cytology every 6–12 months after cessation
Chlorambucil	Myelosuppression, myeloproliferative disorders, malignancy	CBC, urinalysis, creatinine, AST or ALT	Symptoms of myelosuppression[d]	CBC and platelet count every 1–2 weeks with changes in dosage, and every 1–3 months thereafter
Cyclosporin A	Renal insufficiency, anemia, hypertension	CBC, creatinine, uric acid, LFTs, BP	Edema, BP every 2 weeks until dosage stable, then monthly	Creatinine every 2 weeks until dose is stable, then monthly; periodic CBC, potassium, and LFTs

[a] CBC = complete blood cell count (hematocrit, hemoglobin, white blood cell count) including differential cell and platelet counts; ALT = alanine aminotransferase; AST = aspartate aminotransferase; LFTs = liver function tests; BP = blood pressure.

[b] Potential serious toxicities that may be detected by monitoring before they have become clinically apparent or harmful to the patient. This list mentions toxicities that occur frequently enough to justify monitoring. Patients with comorbidity, concurrent medications, and other specific risk factors may need further studies to monitor for specific toxicity.

[c] Package insert for diclofenac (Voltaren) recommends that AST and ALT be monitored within the first 8 weeks of treatment and periodically thereafter. Monitoring of serum creatinine should be performed weekly for at least 3 weeks in patients receiving concomitant angiotensin-converting enzyme inhibitors or diuretics.

[d] Symptoms of myelosuppression include fever, symptoms of infection, easily bruisability, and bleeding.

Reprinted from American College of Rheumatology Ad Hoc Committee on Clinical Guidelines: Guidelines for monitoring drug therapy in rheumatoid arthritis. Arthritis Rheum 1996;39:723–731, with permission of the American College of Rheumatology.

Antirheumatic drug therapy in pregnancy and lactation, and effects on fertility[a]

Drug	FDA use-in-pregnancy rating†	Crosses placenta	Major maternal toxicities	Fetal toxicities	Lactation	Fertility
Aspirin	C; D in third trimester	Yes	Anemia, peripartum hemorrhage, prolonged labor	Premature closure of ductus, pulmonary hypertension, ICH	Use cautiously; excreted at low concentration; doses > 1 tablet (325 mg) result in high concentration in infant plasma	No data
NSAIDs	B; D in third trimester	Yes	As for aspirin	As for aspirin	Compatible according to AAP	No data
Corticosteroids						
Prednisone	B	Dexamethasone and betamethasone	Exacerbation of diabetes and hypertension, PROM	IUGR	5–20% of maternal dose excreted in breast milk; compatible, but wait 4 hours if dose > 20 mg	No data
Dexamethasone	C					No data
Hydroxychloroquine	C	Yes: fetal concentration 50% of maternal	Few	Few	Contraindicated (slow elimination rate, potential for accumulation)	No data
Gold	C	Yes	No data	1 report of cleft palate and severe CNS abnormalities	Excreted into breast milk (20% of maternal dose); rash, hepatitis, and hematologic abnormalities reported, but AAP considers it compatible	No data
D-penicillamine	D	Yes	No data	Cutis laxa connective tissue abnormalities	No data	No data
Sulfasalazine	B; D if near term	Yes	No data	No increase in congenital malformations, kernicterus if administered near term	Excreted into breast milk (40–60% maternal dose); bloody diarrhea in 1 infant; AAP recommends caution	Females: no effect; males: significant oligospermia (2 months to return to normal)
Azathioprine	D	Yes	No data	IUGR (rate up to 40%) and prematurity; transient immunosuppression in neonate, possible effect on germlines of offspring	No data; hypothetical risk of immunosuppression outweighs benefit	Not studied; can interfere with effectiveness of IUD
Chlorambucil	D	Teratogenic effects potentiated by caffeine	No data	Renal angiogenesis	Contraindicated	No data
Methotrexate	X	No data	Spontaneous abortion	Fetal abnormalities (including cleft palate and hydrocephalus)	Contraindicated; small amounts excreted with potential to accumulate in fetal tissues	Females: infrequent long-term effect; males: reversible oligospermia
Cyclophosphamide	D	Yes: 25% of maternal level	No data	Severe abnormalities; case report: male twin developed thyroid papillary cancer at 11 years and neuroblastoma at 14 years	Contraindicated; has caused bone marrow depression	Females: age > 25 years, concurrent radiation, and prolonged exposure increase risk of infertility; males: dose-dependent oligospermia and azoospermia regardless of age or exposure
Cyclosporin A	C	Yes	No data	IUGR and prematurity; 1 case report: hypoplasia of right leg; not an animal teratogen and unlikely to be a human one	Contraindicated due to potential for immunosuppression	No data

* ICH = intracranial hemorrhage; AAP = American Academy of Pediatrics; PROM = premature rupture of membranes; IUGR = intrauterine growth retardation; CNS = central nervous system; IUD = intrauterine device.

† Food and Drug Administration (FDA) use-in-pregnancy ratings are as follows: A = Controlled studies show no risk. Adequate, well-controlled studies in pregnant women have failed to demonstrate risk to the fetus. B = No evidence of risk in humans. Either animal findings show risk but human findings do not, or, if no adequate human studies have been performed, animal findings are negative. C = Risk cannot be ruled out. Human studies are lacking and results of animal studies are either positive for fetal risk or lacking as well. However, potential benefits may justify the potential risk. D = Positive evidence of risk. Investigational or post-marketing data show risk to the fetus. Nevertheless, potential benefits may outweigh the potential risk. X = Contraindicated in pregnancy. Studies in animals or humans, or investigational or post-marketing reports, have shown fetal risk which clearly outweighs any possible benefit to the patient.

Reprinted from American College of Rheumatology Ad Hoc Committee on Clinical Guidelines. Guidelines for monitoring drug therapy in rheumatoid arthritis. Arthritis Rheum 1996;39:723–731, with permission of the American College of Rheumatology.

Monitoring Drug Therapy in Systemic Lupus Erythematosus

Drug	Toxicities requiring monitoring	Baseline evaluation
Salicylates, NSAIDs	Gastrointestinal bleeding, hepatic toxicity, renal toxicity, hypertension	CBC, creatinine, urinalysis, AST, ALT
Glucocorticoids	Hypertension, hyperglycemia, hyperlipidemia, hypokalemia, osteoporosis, avascular necrosis, cataract, weight gain, infections, fluid retention	BP, bone densitometry, glucose, potassium, cholesterol, triglycerides (HDL, LDL)
Hydroxychloroquine	Macular damage	None unless patient is over 40 years of age or has previous eye disease
Azathioprine	Myelosuppression, hepatotoxicity, lymphoproliferative disorders	CBC, platelet count, creatinine, AST or ALT
Cyclophosphamide	Myelosuppression, myeloproliferative disorders, malignancy, immunosuppression, hemorrhagic cystitis, secondary infertility	CBC and differential and platelet count, urinalysis
Methotrexate	Myelosuppression, hepatic fibrosis, cirrhosis, pulmonary infiltrates, fibrosis	CBC, chest radiograph within past year, hepatitis B and C serology in high-risk patients, AST, albumin, bilirubin, creatinine

Reproduced from Guidelines for referral and management of systemic lupus erythematosus in adults. Arthritis Rheum 1999;42:1785–1796, with permission of the American College of Rheumatology.
CBC, complete blood cell count; AST, aspartate transaminase; ALT, alanine transaminase; BP, blood pressure; HDL, high-density lipoprotein; LDL, low-density lipoprotein; Pap, Papanicolaou

Monitoring	
System review	Laboratory
Dark/black stool, dyspepsia, nausea/vomiting, abdominal pain, shortness of breath, edema	CBC yearly, creatinine yearly
Polyuria, polydipsia, edema, shortness of breath, BP at each visit, visual changes, bone pain	Urinary dipstick for glucose every 3–6 months, total cholesterol yearly, bone densitometry yearly to assess osteoporosis
Visual changes	Fundoscopic and visual fields every 6–12 months
Symptoms of myelosuppression	CBC and platelet count every 1–2 weeks with changes in dose (every 1–3 months thereafter), AST yearly, Pap test at regular intervals
Symptoms of myelosuppression, hematuria, infertility	CBC and urinalysis monthly, urine cytology and Pap test yearly for life
Symptoms of myelosuppression, shortness of breath, nausea/vomiting, oral ulcer	CBC and platelet count, AST or ALT, and albumin every 4–8 weeks, serum creatinine, urinalysis

Guidelines for Clinical Use of the Antinuclear Antibody Test

Conditions Associated with Positive IF-ANA Test Results[a]

Disease	Frequency of Positive ANA Result, %
Diseases for which an ANA test is very useful for diagnosis	
SLE	95–100
Systemic sclerosis (scleroderma)	60–80
Diseases for which an ANA test is somewhat useful for diagnosis	
Sjögren's syndrome	40–70
Idiopathic inflammatory myositis (dermatomyositis or polymyositis)	30–80
Disease for which an ANA test is useful for monitoring or prognosis	
Juvenile chronic oligoarticular arthritis with uveitis	20–50
Raynaud phenomenon	20–60
Conditions in which a positive ANA test result is an intrinsic part of the diagnostic criteria	
Drug-induced SLE	~100
Autoimmune hepatic disease	~100
MCTD	~100
Diseases for which an ANA test is not useful in diagnosis	
Rheumatoid arthritis	30–50
Multiple sclerosis	25
Idiopathic thrombocytopenic purpura	10–30
Thyroid disease	30–50
Discoid lupus	5–25
Infectious diseases	Varies widely
Malignancies	Varies widely
Patients with silicone breast implants	15–25
Fibromyalgia	15–25
Relatives of patients with autoimmune diseases (SLE or scleroderma)	5–25
Normal persons[b]	
≥1:40	20–30
≥1:80	10–12
≥1:160	5
≥1:320	3

[a] IF indicates immunofluorescent; ANA, antinuclear antibody; SLE, systemic lupus erythematosus; MCTD, mixed connective tissue disease.

[b] Values are titers. Prevalence of positive ANA test result varies with titer. Female sex and increasing age tend to be more commonly associated with positive ANA.

Flow chart for clinical antinuclear antibody testing

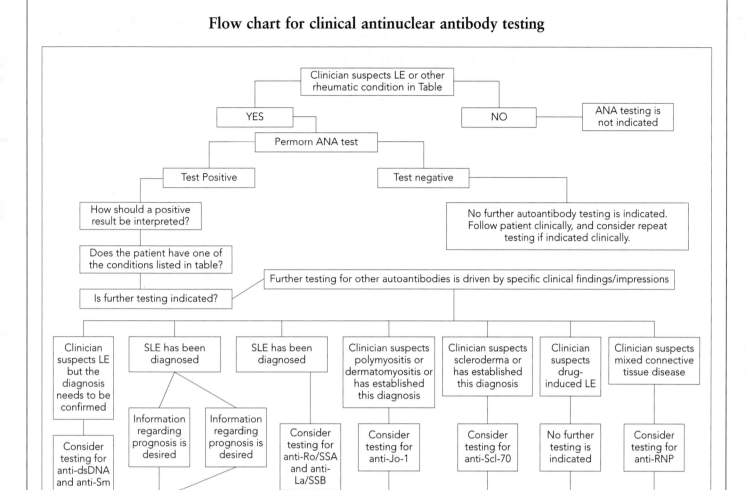

LE, lupus erythematosus; RNP, ribonucleoprotein

Reprinted from Kavanaugh A, Tomar R, Reveille J, Solomon DH, Homburger HA. Guidelines for clinical use of the antinuclear antibody test and tests for specific autoantibodies to nuclear antigens. Arch Pathol Lab Med 2000;124:71–81, with permission of the College of American Pathologists.

Recommendations for the Medical Management of Osteoarthritis of the Hip and Knee

Nonpharmacologic Therapy for Patients With Osteoarthritis

Patient education
Self-management programs (e.g., Arthritis Foundation Self-Management Program)
Personalized social support through telephone contact
Weight loss (if overweight)
Aerobic exercise programs
Physical therapy
Range-of-motion exercises
Muscle-strengthening exercises
Assistive devices for ambulation
Patellar taping
Appropriate footwear
Lateral-wedged insoles (for genu varum)
Bracing
Occupational therapy
Joint protection and energy conservation
Assistive devices for activities of daily living

Pharmacologic Therapy for Patients With Osteoarthritis[a]

Oral
    Acetaminophen
    COX-2-specific inhibitor
    Nonselective NSAID plus misoprostol or a proton pump inhibitor[b]
    Nonacetylated salicylate
    Other pure analgesics
        Tramadol
        Opioids
Intraarticular
    Glucocorticoids
    Hyaluronan
Topical
    Capsaicin
    Methylsalicylate

[a] The choice of agent(s) should be individualized for each patient. COX-2, cyclooxygenase 2; NSAID, nonsteroidal anti-inflammatory drug.
[b] Misoprostol and proton pump inhibitors are recommended in patients who are at increased risk for upper gastrointestinal adverse events.

Reprinted from American College of Rheumatology Subcommittee on Osteoarthritis Guidelines. Recommendations for the medical management of osteoarthritis of the hip and knee. Arthritis Rheum 2000;43:1905–1915, with permission of the American College of Rheumatology.

Recommendations for the Prevention and Treatment of Glucocorticoid-Induced Osteoporosis

Patient Beginning Therapy With Glucocortocoid (Prednisone Equivalents of ≥5 mg/day) With Plans for Treatment Duration of ≥3 Months

Modify lifestyle risk factors for osteoporosis.
    Smoking cessation or avoidance
    Reduction of alcohol consumption if excessive
Instruct in weight-bearing physical exercise.
Initiate calcium supplementation.
Initiate supplementation with vitamin D (plain or activated form).
Prescribe bisphosphonate (use with caution in premenopausal women).

Patient Receiving Long-Term Glucocorticoid Therapy (Prednisone Equivalent of ≥5 mg/day)

Modify lifestyle risk factors for osteoporosis.
    Smoking cessation or avoidance
    Reduction of alcohol consumption if excessive
Instruct in weight-bearing physical exercise.
Initiate calcium supplementation.
Initiate supplementation with vitamin D (plain or activated form).
Prescribe treatment to replace gonadal sex hormones if deficient or otherwise clinically indicated.
Measure bone mineral density (BMD) at lumbar spine and/or hip.
If BMD is not normal (i.e., T-score below −1), then
    Prescribe bisphosphonate (use with caution in premenopausal women).
    Consider calcitonin as second-line agent if patient has contraindication to or does not tolerate bisphosphonate therapy.
If BMD is normal, follow-up and repeat BMD measurement either annually or biannually.

Reprinted from American College of Rheumatology Ad Hoc Committee on Glucocorticoid-Induced Osteoporosis. Recommendations for the prevention and treatment of glucocorticoid-induced osteoporosis. 2001 update. Arthritis Rheum 2001;44:1496–1503, with permission of the American College of Rheumatology.

APPENDIX III
DRUGS USED IN TREATING RHEUMATIC DISEASES

This appendix provides practical information on the drugs most commonly used to treat people with rheumatic disorders. The drugs are listed alphabetically by the clinical category that best describes their pharmacologic class or action or primary indication in rheumatology. It is not intended to be all inclusive nor to provide comparative information helpful for the selection of individual drugs. Chapters within the *Primer* provide more detailed descrip-

tions of the drugs, and the prescribing physician is strongly encouraged to consult these chapters or other similar text reference material for drug indications and comparisons of drug efficacy or toxicity. In addition, it is recommended that before prescribing these drugs, the prescribing physician be familiar with the package insert provided by the manufacturer and available in the *Physician's Desk Reference* (PDR) or similar publication.

Nonsteroidal Anti-inflammatory Drugs

Drug	Brand Name(s)	Dosage
Diclofenac potassium	Cataflam	For OA: 100 to 150 mg per day in 2 or 3 doses. For RA: 100 to 200 mg per day in 3 or 4 doses
Diclofenac sodium	Voltaren	For OA: 100 to 200 mg per day in 2 or 3 doses. For RA: 150 to 200 mg per day in 3 or 4 doses
	Voltaren XR	100 mg per day in a single dose
Diclofenac sodium with misoprostol	Arthrotec	For OA: 150 mg per day in 3 doses. For RA: 150 to 200 mg per day in 2 to 4 doses*
Diflunisal	Dolobid	For RA or OA: 500 to 1,500 mg per day in 2 doses
Etodolac	Lodine	800 to 1,200 mg per day in 2 to 4 doses
	Lodine XL	400 to 1,000 mg per day in a single dose
Fenoprofen calcium	Nalfon	900 to 2,400 mg per day in 3 or 4 doses; never more than 3,200 mg per day
Flurbiprofen	Ansaid	200 to 300 mg per day in 2 to 4 doses
Ibuprofen	Prescription: Motrin	1,200 to 3,200 mg per day in 3 or 4 doses
	Non-prescription: Advil, Motrin IB, Nuprin	200 to 400 mg every 4 to 6 hours as needed, no more than 1,200 mg per day
Indomethacin	Indocin	50 to 200 mg per day in 2 to 4 doses
	Indocin SR	75 mg per day in a single dose or 150 mg per day in 2 doses
Ketoprofen	Prescription: Orudis Oruvail	200 to 225 mg per day in 3 or 4 doses 200 mg per day in a single dose
	Non-prescription: Actron, Orudis KT	12.5 mg every 4 to 6 hours as needed
Meclofenamate sodium	Meclomen	200 to 400 mg per day in 4 doses
Mefenamic acid	Ponstel	250 mg every 6 hours as needed, for up to 7 days
Meloxicam	Mobic	For OA: 7.5 to 15 mg per day in a single dose
Nabumetone	Relafen	1,000 mg per day in 1 or 2 doses; 2,000 mg per day in 2 doses.
Naproxen	Naprosyn	500 to 1,500 mg per day in 2 doses
	Naprelan	750 mg or 1,000 mg per day in a single dose

*These doses are for diclofenac portion of tablet. Misoprostol dosage varies based on pill strength.
+NSAID dosages are for "arthritis" unless otherwise noted.

Special Instructions	Possible Side Effects	Be Aware	Cautions
For all traditional NSAIDs: Do not take with other prescription or OTC NSAIDs. Take in morning or evening at the same time every day. Take with food, a glass of milk or an antacid. **For OTC NSAIDs:** Do not take for more than 10 days for pain or more than 3 days for fever unless directed by a doctor.	**For all traditional NSAIDs:** abdominal pain, dizziness, drowsiness, fluid retention, gastric ulcers and bleeding, greater susceptibility to bruising or bleeding from cuts, heartburn, indigestion, lightheadedness, nausea, nightmares, rash, ringing in ears, reduction in kidney function, increase in liver enzymes **For indomethacin only:** depression, headache, "spaced-out" feeling **For diclofenac sodium with misoprostol only:** Same as other NSAIDs except risk of gastric ulcers is decreased; risk of abdominal pain and diarrhea is increased. **For meloxicam only:** Same as other NSAIDs, except some studies have shown it is less likely to cause gastric ulcers and susceptibility to bruising and bleeding.	**For all traditional NSAIDs:** Because ulcers or internal bleeding can occur without warning, regular checkups are important. If you consume more than 3 alcoholic drinks daily, check with your doctor before using these products. Side effects may be more pronounced for people with pre-existing heart or kidney disease. May cause confusion in elderly people with kidney impairment. **For mefenamic acid only:** This medication is for short-term relief of pain and should not be used for more than 7 days. **For meloxicam only:** There is no evidence this drug will provide aspirin's protection against heart attack or stroke. Meloxicam may be used with low-dose aspirin, but doing so may slightly increase risk of gastric bleeding.	**For all traditional NSAIDs:** sensitivity or allergy to aspirin or similar drugs, kidney or liver disease, heart disease, high blood pressure, asthma, peptic ulcers, use of blood thinners **For meloxicam only:** sensitivity or allergy to meloxicam; sensitivity or allergy to aspirin or other NSAIDs; advanced kidney disease; liver disease; hypertension; heart failure; use of ACE inhibitors, lithium, warfarin or furosemide

(Continued on next page)

Nonsteroidal Anti-inflammatory Drugs (continued)

Drug	Brand Name(s)	Dosage
Naproxen sodium	Prescription: Anaprox	550 to 1,650 mg per day in 2 doses
	Non-prescription: Aleve	220 mg every 8 to 12 hours as needed
Oxaprozin	Daypro	1,200 mg per day in 1 or 2 doses or 1,800 mg per day in 2 or 3 doses
Piroxicam	Feldene	20 mg per day in 1 or 2 doses
Sulindac	Clinoril	300 to 400 mg per day in 2 doses
Tolmetin sodium	Tolectin	1,200 to 1,800 mg per day in 3 doses
COX-2 INHIBITORS		
Celecoxib	Celebrex	For OA: 200 mg per day in 1 or 2 doses. For RA: 200 to 400 mg per day in 2 doses
Rofecoxib	Vioxx	For OA: 12.5 mg or 25 mg per day in a single dose For RA: 25 mg per day in a single dose
Valdecoxib	Bextra	10 mg per day in a single dose
SALICYLATES		
ACETYLATED SALICYLATES		
Aspirin	Non-prescription: Anacin, Ascriptin, Bayer, Bufferin, Ecotrin, Excedrin tablets	3,600 to 5,400 mg per day in several doses
NONACETYLATED SALICYLATES		
Choline and magnesium salicylates	CMT, Tricosal, Trilisate	2,000 to 3,000 mg per day in 2 or 3 doses
Choline salicylate	Arthropan	3,480 to 6,960 mg per day in several doses
Magnesium salicylate	Prescription: Magan, Mobidin, Mobogesic Non-prescription: Bayer Select, Doan's Pills, Arthritab	2,600 to 4,800 mg per day in 3 to 6 doses
Salsalate	Amigesic, Anaflex 750, Disalcid, Marthritic, Mono-Gesic, Salflex, Salsitab	1,000 to 3,000 mg per day in 2 or 3 doses
Sodium salicylate	(Available as generic only)	3,600 to 5,400 mg per day in several doses

Special Instructions	Possible Side Effects	Be Aware	Cautions
For all traditional NSAIDs: Take in morning or evening at the same time every day. Take with food, a glass of milk or an antacid. **For traditional OTC NSAIDs:** Do not take for more than 10 days for pain or more than 3 days for fever unless directed by a doctor.	**For all traditional NSAIDs:** abdominal pain, dizziness, drowsiness, fluid retention, gastric ulcers and bleeding, greater susceptibility to bruising or bleeding from cuts, heartburn, indigestion, lightheadedness, nausea, nightmares, rash, ringing in ears, reduction in kidney function, increase in liver enzymes	**For all traditional NSAIDs:** Because ulcers or internal bleeding can occur without warning, regular checkups are important. If you consume more than 3 alcoholic drinks daily, check with your doctor before using these products. Side effects may be more pronounced for people with pre-existing heart or kidney disease. May cause confusion in elderly people with kidney impairment.	**For all traditional NSAIDs:** sensitivity or allergy to aspirin or similar drugs, kidney or liver disease, heart disease, high blood pressure, asthma, peptic ulcers, use of blood thinners
For COX-2s: Do not take with prescription or OTC NSAIDs.	**For COX-2s:** Same as traditional NSAIDs, except less likely to cause gastric ulcers and susceptibility to bruising or bleeding.	**For COX-2s:** There is no evidence these drugs will provide aspirin's protection against heart attack or stroke. (Use of celecoxib with low-dose aspirin [325 mg per day] is permitted, but will increase ulcer risk.)	Hypersensitivity to celecoxib, sensitivity to sulfonamides or allergy to aspirin or other NSAIDs Sensitivity or allergy to rofecoxib, aspirin or other NSAIDs Sensitivity or allergy to valdecoxib, aspirin or other NSAIDs
Take with food. Do not chew tablets; do not crush enteric-coated or time-release forms and mix with water. Do not combine with other NSAIDs.	Abdominal cramps and pain, deafness, gastric ulcers, heartburn or indigestion, increased bleeding tendency, nausea or vomiting, ringing in ears	Ulcers or internal bleeding can occur without warning, so regular checkups are important. Confusion, deafness, dizziness, or ringing in the ears indicate you are taking too much. If you consume more than 3 alcoholic drinks daily, see your doctor before using these drugs.	Sensitivity or allergy to aspirin or similar drugs, kidney or liver disease, heart disease, high blood pressure, asthma, peptic ulcers, use of blood thinners

For all nonacetylated salicylates: Take with food. Do not chew tablets; do not crush enteric-coated or time-release forms and mix with water. Do not combine with other NSAIDs.	**For all nonacetylated salicylates:** Bloating, confusion, deafness, diarrhea, dizziness, heartburn, stomach distress, rash, ringing in ears (associated with fewer side effects than other NSAIDs)	**For all nonacetylated salicylates:** Dizziness, deafness, or ringing in the ears indicate that you are taking too much. Taking this drug along with other NSAIDs may increase the side effects of both medications.
		    Use of alcohol may increase your risk of gastric irritation and bleeding, as well as liver damage.
		    Side effects may be more pronounced for people with pre-existing heart or kidney disease. May cause confusion in elderly people with kidney impairment.
			For all nonacetylated salicylates: Previous allergy to a nonacetylated medicine

Analgesics

Drug	Brand Name(s)	Dosage
Acetaminophen	Non-prescription: Anacin (aspirin-free), Excedrin caplets, Panadol, Tylenol	325 to 1,000 mg every 4 to 6 hours as needed, no more than 4,000 mg per day
Acetaminophen with codeine	Fioricet, Phenaphen with Codeine, Tylenol with Codeine	15 to 60 mg codeine every 4 hours as needed
Oxycodone	OxyContin	20 to 30 mg every 12 hours (New users should start at 10 mg every 12 hours and work up to an effective dosage)
	Roxicodone	5 mg every 3 to 6 hours or 10 mg 3 or 4 times a day as needed
Hydrocodone with acetaminophen	Dolacet, Hydrocet, Lorcet, Lortab, Vicodin	2.5 to 10 mg hydrocodone every 4 to 6 hours as needed
Propoxyphene hydrochloride	Darvon, PP-Cap	65 mg every 4 hours as needed, no more than 390 mg per day
Tramadol	Ultram	50 to 100 mg every 6 hours as needed

Special Instructions	Possible Side Effects	Be Aware	Cautions
Do not use with any other product containing acetaminophen. Do not use for more than 10 days for pain — unless directed by a doctor.	When taken as prescribed, acetaminophen is usually not associated with side effects.	In case of an accidental overdose, contact a physician or poison control center immediately. If you consume more than 3 alcoholic drinks daily, check with your doctor before using one of these products.	A history of alcohol abuse
Take with food or milk. Do not drive or operate heavy machinery while on this medication. Do not take more than 60 mg of codeine in a single dose.	Constipation, dizziness or lightheadedness, drowsiness, nausea, unusual tiredness or weakness, vomiting	**For all narcotic analgesics:** Long-term treatment can cause tolerance, the need to increase the dose over time to maintain pain relief, and physical dependence, meaning withdrawal symptoms will appear if the drug is stopped abruptly.	A history of drug or alcohol abuse; head injury; sensitivities to acetaminophen, codeine or sulfites
Do not increase dose on your own because side effects increase and tolerance develops as dosage increases; do not stop abruptly unless advised to do so by your doctor; do not drive or operate heavy machinery until you know how your body reacts to this medication.	Dizziness, drowsiness, lightheadedness or feeling faint, nausea or vomiting, unusual tiredness or weakness		Use of central nervous system depressants; drinking 3 or more alcoholic drinks daily
Do not increase dose on your own because tolerance develops as dosage increases.	Dizziness or lightheadedness, drowsiness, nausea, vomiting		Current or previous serious depression, use of tranquilizers or antidepressants
	Dizziness, nausea, constipation, headache, sleepiness		Liver disease, asthma, kidney disease, history of drug or alcohol abuse, use of central nervous system depressants

Biologic Response Modifiers

Drug Brand	Brand Name(s)	Dosage
Anakinra	Kineret	100 mg per day in a single dose adminstered via subcutaneous (beneath the skin) injection
Etanercept +	Enbrel	25 mg twice per week, given by subcutaneous (beneath the skin) injection
Infliximab ++	Remicade	Range based on body weight, initial dose repeated at 2 and 6 weeks and once every 8 weeks thereafter

Corticosteroids

Drug*	Brand Name(s)	Dosage**
Cortisone	Cortone Acetate	5 to 150 mg per day in a single dose
Dexamethasone	Decadron, Hexadrol	0.5 to 9 mg per day in a single dose
Hydrocortisone	Cortef, Hydrocortone	20 to 240 mg per day in a single dose or divided into several doses
Methylprednisolone	Medrol	4 to 160 mg per day in a single dose or divided into several doses
Prednisolone	Prelone	5 to 200 mg per day in a single dose or divided into several doses
Prednisolone sodium phosphate (liquid only)	Pediapred	5 to 60 mL per day in 1 to 3 doses
Prednisone	Deltasone, Orasone, Prednicen-M, Sterapred	1 to 60 mg per day in a single dose or divided into several doses
Triamcinolone	Aristocort	4 to 60 mg per day in a single dose or divided into several doses

* Only oral corticosteroids are listed in this chart.
** Dosages of corticosteroids are highly variable and based on the disease being treated.
+ Etanercept was approved in 2002 for the treatment of psoriatic arthritis in addition to rheumatoid arthritis.
++ Infliximab, in combination with methotrexate, is indicated for reducing signs and symptoms, inhibiting the progression of structural damage, and improving physical function in patients with severely active rheumatoid arthritis who have had an inadequate response to methotrexate.

Special Instructions	Possible Side Effects	Be Aware	Cautions
Drug is supplied in single-use, 1mL prefilled glass syringes with a 27-gauge needle. Each prefilled glass syringe contains 0.67 mL (100 mg) of anakinra.	Mild and transient local injection site that typically lasts 14-28 days	Administration of these drugs should be discontinued if you develop a serious infection. Live vaccines should not be given concurrently with these drugs. Supplies of Enbrel may be temporarily limited in 2001. Register with manufacturer to help ensure access. Call 888/4ENBREL.

Anakinra may be used alone or in combination with DMARDs other than tumor necrosis factor (TNF) blocking agents. | Active infection, central nervous system disorders, including demyelinating disorders such as multiple sclerosis, myelitis, and optic neuritis |
| Drug must be refrigerated prior to use. Mix prior to injection. Do not shake. May be injected into the thigh, abdomen or upper arm. | Redness and/or itching, pain or swelling at injection site | | |
| Drug is infused intravenously (IV) during a 2-hour procedure. It is administered in conjunction with methotrexate. | Upper respiratory infections, headache, cough, sinusitis | | |

Special Instructions	Possible Side Effects	Be Aware	Cautions
Take with food. A single daily dose should be taken with breakfast. Don't stop medication abruptly; dosage must be tapered or reduced gradually.	With high-dosage and long-term use: Cushing's syndrome (weight gain, moonface, thin skin, muscle weakness, brittle bones), cataracts, hypertension, increased appetite, elevated blood sugar, indigestion, insomnia, mood changes, nervousness or restlessness	These drugs reduce resistance to and mask symptoms of infection, so alert your doctor if you develop fever or other signs of infection or if you just don't feel well.	Fungal infection, inactive tuberculosis, underactive thyroid, herpes simplex of the eye, high blood pressure, osteoporosis, stomach ulcer, allergy to FD&C Yellow No. 5 (applies only to 24 mg tablet of Medrol)

Disease-Modifying Antirheumatic Drugs

Drug	Brand Name(s)	Dosage	Special Instructions
Auranofin (oral gold)	Ridaura	6 to 9 mg per day in 1 or 2 doses	Take with a glass of milk or water. If stomach upset occurs, take with food.
Azathioprine	Imuran	50 to 150 mg per day in 1 to 3 doses, based on body weight	Take with food.
Cyclophosphamide	Cytoxan	50 to 150 mg per day in a single dose; may also be given intravenously	Take oral medication with breakfast. Drink lots of fluids throughout the day and empty bladder before bedtime.
Cyclosporine	Neoral, Sandimmune	100 to 400 mg per day in 2 doses, based on body weight	Be consistent: Take at the same time every day, either with a meal or between meals.
Hydroxychloroquine sulfate	Plaquenil	200 to 600 mg per day in 1 or 2 doses, based on body weight	Take with food or a glass of milk or water.
Leflunomide	Arava	10 to 20 mg per day in a single dose	Treatment starts with a loading dose of 100 mg per day for 3 days.
Methotrexate	Rheumatrex, Trexall	7.5 to 15 mg per week in 3 doses, or 10 mg per week in a single dose; may also be given by injection	Take with food or a glass of milk or water.
Minocycline	Minocin	200 mg per day in 2 doses	Take on an empty stomach with water.
Penicillamine	Cuprimine, Depen	125 to 250 mg per day in a single dose to start, increased to not more than 1,500 mg per day in 3 doses	Take on an empty stomach, at least 1 hour before or 2 hours after any food, milk or medicine.
Sulfasalazine	Azulfidine, Azulfidine EN-Tabs	500 mg to 3 grams per day in 2 to 4 doses	Take with food or a glass of milk or water.
Gold sodium thiomalate	Myochrysine	10 mg in a single dose the first week, 25 mg the following week, then 25 to 50 mg per week thereafter. Frequency may be reduced after several months.	
Aurothioglucose (both injectable)	Solganal		

Possible Side Effects	Be Aware	Cautions
Abdominal or stomach cramps or pain, bloated feeling, decrease in or loss of appetite, diarrhea or loose stools, gas or indigestion, mouth sores, nausea or vomiting, skin rash or itching	This drug can cause sun sensitivity, so minimize exposure to sunlamps and sunlight and wear a sunscreen when outdoors. Your doctor may order periodic blood and urine tests to check for effects on blood and kidneys.	Adverse reaction to a gold-containing medication in the past, a history of blood-cell abnormality, inflammatory bowel disease, kidney or liver disease
Cough, fever and chills, loss of appetite, nausea or vomiting, skin rash, unusual bleeding or bruising, unusual tiredness or weakness	This drug can reduce your ability to fight infection, so call your doctor immediately if you develop chills, fever or a cough.	Kidney or liver disease, use of allopurinol
Blood in urine or burning on urination, confusion or agitation, cough, dizziness, fever and chills, infertility in men and women, loss of appetite, missed menstrual periods, nausea or vomiting, unusual bleeding or bruising, unusual tiredness or weakness	This drug can reduce your ability to fight infection, so call your doctor immediately if you develop chills, fever or a cough, or if you have burning on urination or blood in urine.	Kidney or liver disease, any active infection
Tender or enlarged gums, high blood pressure, increase in hair growth, kidney problems, loss of appetite, tremors	Because this drug's rate of absorption is unpredictable, your doctor will monitor it through blood tests. Use of this drug may make you more susceptible to infection and certain cancers. Do not get live vaccines while on this drug. Stop taking cyclosporine for a few days before and after having non-live vaccines.	Sensitivity to castor oil (if receiving drug by injection), liver or kidney disease, active infection, high blood pressure
Black spots in visual field, diarrhea, loss of appetite, nausea, rash	Because vision may be damaged with long-term therapy (given over several years), have an eye exam before starting drug and every 12 months thereafter to detect retinal changes.	Allergy to any antimalarial drug, retinal abnormality
Diarrhea, skin rash, liver toxicity, hair loss	Either member of a couple who is taking leflunomide and would like to have a child should not take leflunomide or should discontinue leflunomide and go through an 11-day drug elimination process using the cholesterol-lowering drug cholestyramine.	Active infection, liver disease, known immune deficiency, renal insufficiency, underlying malignancy
Cough, diarrhea, hair loss, loss of appetite, unusual bleeding or bruising	Chest X-rays, liver tests and blood counts are advised before starting this drug and throughout treatment to monitor side effects. Alert doctor immediately if you have a dry cough, fever or difficulty breathing. May temporarily reduce fertility in men and women. Causes birth defects if taken during pregnancy.	Abnormal blood count, liver and lung disease, alcoholism, immune-system deficiency, active infection
Dizziness, vaginal infections, nausea, headache, skin rash	This drug is not yet FDA-approved for arthritis. It is an antibiotic.	Sensitivity to tetracycline medications
Diarrhea, joint pain, lessening or loss of sense of taste, loss of appetite, fever, hives or itching, mouth sores, nausea or vomiting, skin rash, stomach pain, swollen glands, unusual bleeding or bruising, weakness	Because this drug can cause blood abnormalities and kidney damage, your doctor will order periodic blood and urine tests to check for unwanted effects. Take consistently; stopping and starting can worsen side effects.	Penicillin allergy, blood disease, kidney disease, lupus
Stomach upset, diarrhea, dizziness, headache, light sensitivity, itching, appetite loss, liver abnormalities, lowered blood count, nausea or vomiting, rash	Failure to drink adequate fluids while on this medication can lead to the formation of urine crystals. Azulfidine EN-Tabs have a special coating that prevents the tablets from disintegrating in your stomach and irritating the stomach lining.	Allergy to sulfa drugs or aspirin, kidney or liver disease, blood disease
Irritation or soreness of tongue, metallic taste, skin rash or itching, soreness, swelling or bleeding of gums, unusual bleeding or bruising	Increased joint pain may occur for one or two days after injection, but it usually disappears after the first few injections. Your doctor will order periodic urine and blood tests to check for side effects.	Penicillamine use, lupus, skin disease, kidney disease, blood disease, colitis

Osteoporosis Medications

Drug	Brand Name(s)	Dosage
Alendronate	Fosamax	For osteoporosis treatment: 10 mg per day in a single dose For osteoporosis prevention: 5 mg per day in a single dose
Calcitonin (injectable)	Calcimar, Miacalcin	100 IUs per day in a single dose
Calcitonin (nasal spray)	Miacalcin	200 IUs per day in a single dose
Conjugated estrogens	With progesterone: Premphase, Prempro Without progesterone: Premarin	0.625 mg per day continuously in 28-day cycles (progesterone component of drug varies depending on day of cycle) Taken daily or in 4-week cycles of 0.625 mg per day for 3 weeks followed by 1 week of rest from drug
Esterified estrogen	Estratab Menest	0.3 mg to 0.6 mg per day in a single dose
Raloxifene hydrochloride	Evista	60 mg per day in a single dose
Risedronate sodium	Actonel	For osteoporosis treatment: 5 mg per day in a single dose For osteoporosis prevention: 5 mg per day in a single dose

Special Instructions	Possible Side Effects	Be Aware	Cautions
Take with a full glass (6 to 8 ounces) of water first thing in the morning. Do not eat or drink anything else or take any other medication or supplements for at least 30 minutes. Stay upright (sitting or standing) for at least 30 minutes after taking the drug.	Abdominal pain	Calcium can prevent absorption of this drug when taken at the same time. Make sure your doctor is aware if you are taking supplements or antacids containing calcium, aluminum, magnesium, or iron.	Allergy to alendronate; problems with one or more of the following: digestion, esophagus, intestines, stomach or kidneys; pregnancy; inability to sit or stand for 30 minutes
To gain the full benefits of this drug, you should follow a diet rich in calcium and vitamin D. Store medication in refrigerator prior to opening. Store at room temperature after opening. Do not use if solution has changed colors or has particles floating in it.	Diarrhea, flushing of skin, inflamed skin at injection site, loss of appetite, nausea, stomach pain, vomiting	Allergic skin reaction or infection may occur at injection site.	Protein allergy
Alternate nostrils daily. Store medication in refrigerator prior to opening. Store at room temperature after opening.	Nasal irritation, diarrhea, flushing of the skin, loss of appetite, nausea, stomach pain, vomiting	Allergic reaction could occur in nasal tissues.	Protein allergy
To gain the full benefits of these drugs, you should follow a diet rich in calcium and vitamin D.	Breast tenderness and enlargement, enlargement of benign tumors of the uterus, irregular bleeding or spotting, change in amount of cervical secretion, vaginal yeast infections, fluid retention, skin rashes, hair loss or abnormal hairiness, weight changes, changes in sex drive	Women who have not had a hysterectomy should take this drug in conjunction with progesterone. Consult with your doctor regarding the possible risk of cancer of the uterus or breast, gallbladder disease, inflammation of the pancreas, abnormal blood clotting.	Liver dysfunction or disease; hypersensitivity to ingredients
	Abdominal cramps, breast swelling and tenderness, change in vaginal bleeding, loss of appetite, contact lens intolerance, nausea, rapid weight gain, stomach bloating, swelling of feet and lower legs	You should have your blood pressure monitored while on this drug. Women who have not had a hysterectomy should take this drug in conjunction with progesterone.	Undiagnosed vaginal bleeding; breast cancer or other estrogen-dependent cancer, a family history of breast cancer, problems related to circulation or blood clotting
	Hot flashes and abdominal pain	This drug should not be used prior to menopause.	Pregnancy or potential pregnancy; history of blood clots
Take with a full glass (6 to 8 ounces) of water first thing in the morning. Do not eat or drink anything else or take any other medication or supplements for at least 30 minutes. Stay upright (sitting or standing) for at least 30 minutes after taking the drug.	Abdominal or stomach pain, diarrhea, headache, joint pain, skin rash	Calcium can prevent absorption of this drug when taken at the same time. Make sure your doctor is aware if you are taking supplements or antacids containing calcium, aluminum, magnesium, or iron.	Allergy to risedronate sodium; digestive problems, including trouble swallowing, inflammation of the esophagus, or ulcer; kidney problems; pregnancy; inability to sit or stand for 30 minutes

Fibromyalgia Medications

Drug	Brand Name(s)	Dosage	Special Instructions
ANTIDEPRESSANTS | TRICYCLICS			
Amitriptyline hydrochloride	Elavil, Endep	10 to 50 mg per day in a single dose	Take at bedtime. Avoid alcohol, which may increase drowsiness.
Doxepin	Adapin, Sinequan	10 to 100 mg per day in a single dose	Take in the morning with or without food.
Nortriptyline	Aventyl, Pamelor	10 to 100 mg per day in a single dose	Take in the morning with or without food.
ANTIDEPRESSANTS | SSRIs			
Fluoxetine	Prozac	20 mg per day in a single dose	**For all SSRIs:** Always take at the same time in relation to meals and snacks to make sure that it is absorbed in the same way.
Paroxetine	Paxil	10 mg per day in a single dose	
Sertraline	Zoloft	25 to 50 mg per day in a single dose	
BENZODIAZEPINES			
Temazepam	Restoril	15 mg per day in a single dose	Take at bedtime.
BENZODIAZEPINES			
Cyclobenzaprine	Cycloflex, Flexeril	10 to 30 mg per day in 1 to 3 doses	

Possible Side Effects	Be Aware	Cautions
For all tricyclic antidepressants: Difficulty concentrating, dizziness, drowsiness, dry mouth, headache, increased appetite (including craving for sweets), nausea, sleep disturbances, unpleasant taste, urinary retention, weakness or tiredness, weight gain	**For all tricyclic antidepressants:** Adverse side effects can occur if you stop using these drugs abruptly; discontinue gradually to avoid withdrawal symptoms. Driving and operating heavy machinery while on this drug are not recommended.	**For all tricyclic antidepressants:** a history of seizures, urinary retention, heart problems, glaucoma or other chronic eye conditions, use of another antidepressant
Anxiety and nervousness, diarrhea, dry mouth, headache, increased sweating, nausea, trouble sleeping		**For all SSRIs:** use of alcohol or other central nervous system depressants, including antihistamines, narcotic medications and some dental anesthetics
Constipation, decreased sexual ability, dizziness, dry mouth, headaches, nausea, difficulty urinating, tremors, trouble sleeping, unusual tiredness or weakness, vomiting		
Decreased appetite or weight loss; decreased sexual drive or ability; diarrhea; drowsiness; dryness of the mouth; headaches; stomach or abdominal cramps; gas or pain; tremors; trouble sleeping; clumsiness or unsteadiness; dizziness or lightheadedness; drowsiness; slurred speech		
	Monoamine oxidase (MAO) inhibitors may increase risk of harmful side effects.	Use of alcohol or other central nervous system depressants, including antihistamines, narcotic medications, or anesthetics, including some dental anesthetics
Dizziness or lightheadedness, drowsiness, dry mouth, confusion		Use of alcohol or other central nervous system depressants, glaucoma, problems with urination, heart or blood vessel disease, overactive thyroid

Fibromyalgia Medications (continued)

Drug	Brand Name(s)	Dosage	Special Instructions
OTHER			
Maprotiline	Ludiomil	25 to 150 mg per day in 1 to 3 doses	Take this drug only for the length of time your doctor recommends.
Trazodone	Desyrel, Trazon, Trialodine	50 to 150 mg per day in 2 or 3 doses	Take only before bed, when you are ready to go to sleep.
Zolpidem	Ambien	5–10 mg per day in a single dose	

Gout Medications

Drug	Brand Name(s)	Dosage	Special Instructions
Allopurinol	Lopurin, Zyloprim	100 to 300 mg per day in a single dose	Take immediately after a meal. Stop taking medication at the first sign of a rash, which may indicate an allergic reaction.
Colchicine	Only available as generic	0.6 to 1.2 mg per day in 1 or 2 doses for prevention. 0.5 or 0.6 mg every 1 or 2 hours (no more than 8 doses per day) to stop acute attacks	Take with food if stomach upset occurs. Drink plenty of fluids.
Probenecid	Benemid, Probalan	500 to 1,000 mg per day in 2 doses	Take with food or an antacid. Do not take with aspirin or other NSAIDs. Avoid alcohol.
Probenecid and colchicine	ColBenemid, Col-Probenecid, Proben-C	1 tablet (500 mg probenicid and 0.5 mg colchicine) 1 or 2 times per day	Take with food or an antacid. Drink plenty of fluids. Do not take with aspirin or other NSAIDs. Avoid alcohol.
Sulfinpyrazone	Anturane	100 to 800 mg per day in 1 or 2 doses	Take with food, milk or antacids. Avoid aspirin and aspirin-containing products or other NSAIDs since they may decrease the effect of sulfinpyrazone.

Possible Side Effects	Be Aware	Cautions
Blurred vision, decreased sexual ability, dizziness or lightheadedness, drowsiness, dry mouth, headaches, increased or decreased sexual drive, tiredness or weakness	Side effects are more likely to occur in older adults.	Alcohol use, seizure disorders, glaucoma, asthma, enlarged prostate, heart or blood vessel disease, overactive thyroid, liver disease, use of MAO inhibitors
Dizziness or lightheadedness, drowsiness, dry mouth, headaches, nausea and vomiting, unpleasant taste in mouth	Do not stop taking abruptly; your doctor may gradually reduce the dosage before stopping medication altogether.	History of alcohol abuse or heart, liver, or kidney disease
Side effects are uncommon at prescribed dosage.	Because this medication can cause short-term loss of memory (for several hours), take only on nights when you don't have to be active again for 7 or 8 hours.	History of alcohol abuse, drug abuse or dependence, sleep apnea, kidney or liver disease

Possible Side Effects	Be Aware	Cautions
Hives, itching, liver-function abnormalities, nausea, skin rash or sores	Acute gout attacks are common when this drug is started, but attacks will gradually decrease and eventually stop after several weeks and can be minimized by taking lower doses and by taking along with colchicine.	Kidney disease, use of azathioprine or mercaptopurine
Diarrhea, nausea and vomiting, stomach pain		Intestinal disease, kidney or liver disease
Headache, joint pain and swelling, loss of appetite, nausea, skin rash, vomiting	This drug may interfere with the copper sulfate urine sugar tests taken by people with diabetes.	Blood disease, kidney disease, kidney stones, use of antineoplastics, heparin, nitrofurantoin, or zidovudine
Diarrhea, nausea and vomiting, stomach pain, headache, joint pain and swelling, loss of appetite, skin rash		Intestinal disease, kidney or liver disease, blood disease, use of antineoplastics, heparin, NSAIDs, nitrofurantoin or zidovudine
Lowered blood count, rash, stomach pain	In rare cases, this medication may lower blood cell counts; therefore, you may need to have periodic blood tests.	Stomach ulcers, anemia, low white blood cell count, use of other sulfa drugs or blood thinners

Reprinted from Dunkin MA. 2001 Drug guide. Get smart about the drugs you take. Arthritis Today 2001;15(1):39–60, with permission of the Arthritis Foundation.

APPENDIX IV
SUPPLEMENT GUIDE

This appendix lists dietary supplements commonly used by people with arthritis and related diseases and are listed alphabetically under Herbs and Other Remedies and Vitamins and Minerals. Knowledge for many of these products is incomplete, but attempts have been made to list the most common source of the product, claims by manu-factures and available evidence to support the claim, dose recommended by the manufacturer, known side effects or interactions, and comments on select products. More detailed information on dietary supplements, including other sources of information, can be found in *The Arthritis Foundation's Guide to Alternative Therapies* (1999).

Herbs and Other Remedies

Boswellia serrata
Indian olibanum, salai guggul; an Ayurvedic remedy
Source: Resin from the bark of boswellia trees.
Claims: Reduces inflammation. In human studies, some evidence of efficacy for effects on pain in rheumatoid arthritis (RA) and osteoarthritis (OA), when combined with ginger and aswagandha. Contains boswellian acid, known to have anti-inflammatory actions.
How It's Used: Taken in pills or capsules.
Cautions/Side Effects/Interactions: None known.

Bovine cartilage
Source: Ground cattle cartilage, usually from the trachea.
Claims: Psoriasis, OA, and RA. No good human studies for arthritis.
How It's Used: As an ointment for psoriasis; internally for OA and RA.
Cautions/Side Effects/Interactions: May cause allergic reaction, diarrhea, and nausea.

Bromelain
Ananas comosus, pineapple
Source: A protein-digesting enzyme from the juice of pineapples.
Claims: OA and RA. A combination enzyme product with trypsin and rutin has been shown to relieve OA pain as well as nonsteroidal anti-inflammatory drugs (NSAIDs). One promising animal study for arthritis, but no scientific evidence that bromelain alone is effective in humans.
How It's Used: Comes in capsules. To relieve inflammation, typical dose is 80 mg to 320 mg in two or three doses per day for eight to 10 days, and as needed after 10 days.
Cautions/Side Effects/Interactions: Avoid if allergic to pineapple. Can increase the effect of blood-thinning drugs. Large doses can cause upset stomach and cramps.

Cartilage
Shark cartilage, chicken cartilage, collagen
Source: Shark or chicken cartilage.
Claims: Pain and stiffness of OA, gout, RA, and juvenile RA (JRA). No evidence that it affects OA or other kinds of arthritis. Note: In clinical studies, a specific Type II chicken collagen given in 20 µg to 2,300 µg daily doses appeared to reduce RA symptoms through a presumed oral tolerance mechanism.
How It's Used: Internally, taken as capsules or in a drink, in doses of up to 2000 mg per day for chicken cartilage and 4500 mg per day for shark cartilage. Collagen and cartilage appear in many combination products.
Cautions/Side Effects/Interactions: Safety and effectiveness of commercially available substances unknown. People with chicken or egg allergies should not use chicken collagen; can cause nausea in high doses. Shark cartilage may be contaminated with heavy metals and may cause nausea, vomiting, fatigue, and symptoms of acute hepatitis.

Cat's claw
Uncaria tomentosa
Source: Roots and bark of a vine that grows wild in the Peruvian Amazon.
Claims: Pain and inflammation in RA. No human studies. One animal study suggested that it may have anti-inflammatory properties.
How It's Used: Comes in tablets, capsules, and tea bags. Usual dosage is 500 mg to 1000 mg three times a day. The level of active ingredients varies greatly, depending on when the plant is harvested.
Cautions/Side Effects/Interactions: May increase the risk of bleeding if taken with other blood thinners. Side effects can include diarrhea, hypotension, unusual bruising, and bleeding gums.

Chondroitin sulfate
Source: Cattle trachea.
Claims: Pain and stiffness associated with OA; repairs cartilage. Clinical studies from Europe show internal use relieves OA symptoms and has few or no side effects. Several studies have shown that chondroitin sulfate added to conventional analgesics or NSAIDs is significantly better than analgesics or NSAIDs alone for reducing pain. In one Belgian study, long-term use of chondroitin appeared to prevent cartilage loss in fingers.
How It's Used: Recommended dosage is 1200 mg per day, divided into two doses. Taken in pill, capsule, or drink.

Chondroitin sulfate is slow-acting, so it can take two months or longer for effects to show. Often sold in combination products with glucosamine. No studies show that glucosamine and chondroitin taken together are more effective than either taken alone. Available in creams and lotions. No evidence that external use has any effect.

Cautions/Side Effects/Interactions: Occasional mild side effects include nausea and indigestion. Theoretically, may increase chances of bleeding if taken with a blood thinner.

CMO
Cetyl myristoleate, cerasomal-cis-9-cetylmyristoleate
Source: A waxy substance that comes from beef tallow.
Claims: Symptomatic relief in RA, OA, fibromyalgia, Sjögren's syndrome, and ankylosing spondylitis. No human studies.
How It's Used: Comes in capsules. No typical dosage. Also available in creams.
Cautions/Side Effects/Interactions: Not known.

Collagen hydrolysate
Gelatin, gelatine
Source: Hides and bones of cattle, pigs, and sheep.
Claims: Relieves pain and inflammation of OA; repairs cartilage. Results in European studies vary for effects on pain in OA. No studies to show if it repairs cartilage.
How It's Used: Internally, in capsules or as a powder dissolved in fluids and taken as a drink. Considered safe in daily doses up to 10 grams.
Cautions/Side Effects/Interactions: May cause gastrointestinal upset.

Curcumin
see Turmeric

Devil's claw
Harpagophytum procumbens
Source: The root of an African plant named for the bumpy hooks that cover its fruit.
Claims: Pain and inflammation of OA and gout. No clinical studies for arthritis. In one human study, relieved low back pain better than placebo.
How It's Used: Internally as tea, tincture, or capsules, in doses as high as 2000 mg to 10,000 mg per day for RA.
Cautions/Side Effects/Interactions: Devil's claw is used to stimulate stomach acids. May cause diarrhea; may interfere with antacids; may interfere with cardiac and diabetes medications.

DHEA
Dehydroepiandrosterone
Source: Derived from chemically treated wild yam.
Claims: Relieves pain, inflammation, and fatigue; used for lupus. In clinical studies, a prescription grade of DHEA was shown to lower glucocorticoid doses and increase bone density in patients with mild to moderate SLE.
How It's Used: Internally, in pill form.

Cautions/Side Effects/Interactions: Possible side effects include acne, hair growth, changes in menstrual pattern, abdominal pain, and hypertension.. DHEA can increase insulin resistance or sensitivity. Possibility of liver damage when combined with azathioprine or methotrexate.

DMSO
Dimethyl sulfoxide (*see also* MSM)
Source: Chemical byproduct of wood processing.
Claims: Eases pain, inflammation, and stiffness associated with RA, OA, and scleroderma. No U.S. human studies for arthritis. Some animal studies show it is effective for inflammation. US animal studies were halted in the mid-1960s after high doses of DMSO damaged the eye lenses in animals.
How It's Used: Given orally or intravenously or applied externally. A 70% solution of DMSO for treating scleroderma is available in Canada. A new drug, Pennsaid, which uses DMSO to carry NSAIDs through the skin into painful areas, is available in the UK and expected to be marketed in Canada and the United States.
Cautions/Side Effects/Interactions: DMSO can cause drowsiness, headache, dizziness, nausea, vomiting, diarrhea, and constipation. Can worsen asthma and cardiac conditions. Can cause a garlic-like smell in those who use it. Non-pharmaceutical products may be contaminated.

Eleuthero
Eleutherococcus senticosus
see Ginseng

Evening primrose oil
see GLA

Feverfew
Tanacetum parthenium
Source: Dried leaves of the plant.
Claims: Relieves pain and inflammation. No clinical studies in arthritis.
How It's Used: Taken internally as whole fresh leaves, dried leaves, and in capsules.
Cautions/Side Effects/Interactions: May increase the effects of blood thinners and NSAIDs. Can provoke allergies and cause mouth sores, nausea, and vomiting. May stimulate uterine contractions and cause abortion.

Fish oil
Source: Oils from cold-water fish, such as salmon and mackerel.
Claims: Pain, stiffness, inflammation, fatigue, and depression; eases symptoms of RA, Raynaud's phenomenon, systemic lupus. Several human studies have shown that the omega-3 fatty acids EPA and DHA in fish oil reduce inflammation and pain of RA; may ease symptoms of Raynaud's and may relieve depression.
How It's Used: Internally, in capsules; usual dose is about 3 grams of the active ingredients EPA and DHA. Side

effects can be minimized by taking the supplements with meals and starting with low doses, increasing gradually.

Cautions/Side Effects/Interactions: Can multiply the effects of other blood thinners; may cause belching, bad breath, heartburn, and nosebleeds. High doses can cause nausea and diarrhea.

Flaxseed

Linum usitatissimum

Source: Meal or oil from the flax plant.

Claims: Relieves pain, stiffness, and inflammation from RA; possibly eases symptoms of lupus and Raynaud's phenomenon. No good clinical studies to show flaxseed relieves arthritis symptoms, but it is a source of omega-3 fatty acids, which have anti-inflammatory properties.

How It's Used: Available in capsules and as meal, flour, seeds, or oil. Some sources recommend taking 1 to 3 tablespoons per day of flaxseed oil or about 30 grams of the meal.

Cautions/Side Effects/Interactions: Flaxseed is a natural laxative and may cause gas or loose bowels. The fiber in flaxseed can impair absorption of some drugs; women with hormone-sensitive conditions, such as breast or uterine cancer, should avoid it.

Frankincense

see Boswellia

GLA

Gamma linolenic acid

Source: Black currant oil, borage oil, and evening primrose oil.

Claims: Eases pain, inflammation, and stiffness of RA; eases symptoms of Raynaud's phenomenon and Sjögren's syndrome. Several human studies show GLA taken internally can ease RA pain and inflammation.

How It's Used: Internally, in capsules and oil. Usual dosage is about 1800 mg per day. Externally, as oil. There is no evidence to support using the oil topically on aching joints.

Cautions/Side Effects/ Interactions: Can increase the effects of blood thinners; evening primrose oil can lead to indigestion, nausea, diarrhea, and abdominal pain.

Gelatin, gelatine

see Collagen hydrolysate

Ginger

Zingiber officinale

Source: The root of a lily.

Claims: Relieves pain and inflammation of RA and OA. Studies show ginger inhibits production of substances that contribute to pain and swelling, and one uncontrolled human study showed some pain relief. Clinical studies of a combination product that included boswellia and turmeric suggest some improvement in RA and OA symptoms.

How It's Used: Internally as tea, tablets, capsules, or tinctures. Dose varies; as a tea, use 1 teaspoon fresh, grated ginger steeped in a cup of water.

Cautions/Side Effects/Interactions: Ginger is a mild blood thinner. Ginger can cause skin irritation, and large overdoses can cause central nervous system damage and irregular heartbeat. Should not be used if the patient has gallstones.

Ginkgo

Ginkgo biloba

Source: An extract of the leaves of the gingko, the world's oldest living species of trees.

Claims: Increases circulation in Raynaud's phenomenon. No clinical studies in patients with Raynaud's, but German study showed increased blood flow in finger capillaries of subjects without Raynaud's.

How It's Used: Capsules; usual dosage is 120 mg to 240 mg per day. Choose a product that is standardized to 6% terpene lactones and 24% flavone glycosides.

Cautions/Side Effects/Interactions: Low risk of side effects, but mild headache and upset stomach are possible. Ginkgo may increase the risk of bleeding, especially in patients taking other blood thinners.

Ginseng

American ginseng: *Panax quinquefolius*

Asian ginseng: *Panax ginseng*

Siberian ginseng: *Eleutherococcus senticosus*

Source: The roots of two different but related plant types.

Claims: Reduces fatigue; eases fibromyalgia symptoms. No evidence it helps any kind of arthritis, including fibromyalgia.

How It's Used: Usually taken in capsules or tablets; also available as a tea; dosage varies, but usually about 100 mg standardized extract twice a day; powdered root dosage usually 500 mg to 1000 mg daily.

Cautions/Side Effects/Interactions: Can act as a mild stimulant. Women with hormone-sensitive conditions and people with hypertension should avoid ginseng. Panax ginseng may amplify effects of corticosteroids. Can change blood glucose level. May increase effects of estrogen drugs. Should not be used with monoamine oxidase (MAO) inhibitors.

Glucosamine

Glucosamine hydrochloride, glucosamine sulfate

Source: Supplements are made from chitin in the shells of crab, lobster, and shrimp.

Claims: Eases pain and stiffness of OA; contributes to cartilage repair. Many European studies show glucosamine sulfate taken internally eases OA pain as well as NSAIDs; one long-term Belgian study has suggested glucosamine sulfate may reduce cartilage loss in OA of the knee. Studies of a combination product that includes glucosamine HCL, chondroitin, and manganese showed it eased OA symptoms for some. However, two studies suggest it has little or no effect on those with severe OA or those who are overweight.

How It's Used: Internally, as capsules, tablets, and a drink. Usual dosage is 1500 mg per day taken in two doses; 2000 mg for those who weigh 200 pounds or more. Often combined with chondroitin. No studies show glucosamine and chondroitin taken together are any more effective than either taken alone. Applied externally in creams and ointments, often in combination products. No evidence it works when applied externally.

Cautions/Side Effects/Interactions: Side effects include indigestion and nausea, but a different brand might alleviate the side effects. Possible reaction if allergic to shellfish. Avoid glucosamine N-acetyl version.

Gotu kola
Centella asiatica, Centella coriacea

Source: Above-ground part of a low-growing plant from Asia and Africa.

Claims: Taken internally, increases circulation, eases symptoms of "rheumatism" and lupus; externally, relieves psoriasis and scleroderma. No human studies or evidence for arthritis.

How It's Used: As an extract, taken internally or applied externally; as dried leaves, in capsules, tea, or tinctures.

Cautions/Side Effects/Interactions: Taken internally, may cause nausea, abortion, allergic reactions, and sun sensitivity. External use may result in allergic reactions. High doses may increase cholesterol, blood glucose levels, and the sedative effects of other drugs and supplements.

Green Tea
Camellia sinensis

Source: A tea that is steamed and dried, rather than fermented like black teas.

Claims: Relieves pain and inflammation. No human studies or evidence that green tea is effective for RA or any other kind of arthritis. Some evidence of efficacy in animal models of arthritis. Green tea contains polyphenols, antioxidant compounds believed to reduce inflammation.

How It's Used: As a beverage, or as an extract in capsules, tablets, and tinctures. Available loose and in bags for brewing. Suggested dosage is three or four cups of tea per day or the equivalent in green tea extract.

Cautions/Side Effects/Interactions: Green tea may cause an allergic reaction. Contains caffeine; can cause stomach upset and constipation; can amplify the effects of such drugs as aspirin and acetaminophen.

Guggul
Commiphora mukul

Source: A gum resin from the guggul tree, which grows throughout India.

Claims: Arthritis. No human studies for arthritis.

How It's Used: Taken in pills or capsules. Dosage recommendations vary widely.

Cautions/Side Effects/Interactions: Can stimulate uterus and menstrual flow. May cause stomach and intestinal upsets, and interfere with drugs for thyroid conditions and some hypertension drugs.

Indian frankincense
see Boswellia

Kava kava
Piper methysticum

Source: The root of the kava plant.

Claims: Pain, anxiety, depression relief. No clinical studies in arthritis.

How It's Used: Usual daily dosage 140 mg to 210 mg of an ingredient called kava lactones in capsules; as a drink, 1 mL to 3 mL of fresh kava.

Cautions/Side Effects/Interactions: Can cause nausea, headache, and dizziness. Heavy use of kava may impair thinking and activities that require concentration, such as driving; do not mix with tranquilizers, sleeping medications, or alcohol.

Melatonin
N-acetyl-5-methoxytryptamine

Source: Supplements usually synthetic, but some come from animal pineal tissue.

Claims: Boosts the immune system; cures sleep problems; prevents osteoporosis. Studies show melatonin appears to boost the immune system and help regulate sleep. One study showed that women with fibromyalgia slept better after a 2 mg dose.

How It's Used: Usual dose is 0.3 mg to 3 mg taken a few hours before bedtime.

Cautions/Side Effects/Interactions: Since melatonin is a hormone, it can have far-reaching and unpredictable effects. Should not be used in patients with lupus or other, related autoimmune diseases. Because some melatonin comes from cattle organs, bovine spongiform encephalopathy contamination is possible.

MSM
Methylsulfonylmethane

Source: A sulfur compound formed by the breakdown of DMSO (dimethyl sulfoxide).

Claims: Pain and inflammation in arthritis. No human studies. In animal studies, some evidence of effects on animal models of arthritis and lupus.

How It's Used: Internally, in capsules; typical dose is 1000 mg to 3000 mg daily with meals; some people take 250 mg to 500 mg per day as a dietary supplement. Externally as a lotion; no typical topical dosage.

Cautions/Side Effects/Interactions: Can cause nausea, diarrhea, and headache.

New Zealand green-lipped mussels
Perna canaliculus
Source: Mussels from New Zealand.

Claims: Eases symptoms associated with OA and RA. Reported to be effective in one clinical study, but results were not confirmed by later study.

How It's Used: Available freeze-dried or ground. Taken internally in capsules of 300 mg to 350 mg three times per day.

Cautions/Side Effects/Interactions: Should be avoided by those with seafood or shellfish allergies. May cause nausea, diarrhea, and gas. One case of hepatitis from New Zealand green-lipped mussels has been reported.

SAM-e
S-adenosylmethionine

Source: Naturally occurring compound produced from methionine, a sulfur-containing amino acid, and adenosine triphosphate (ATP); supplements are made from fermented yeast or are synthesized.

Claims: Relieves symptoms of OA and fibromyalgia. Several human studies have shown SAM-e relieves OA pain and other symptoms as well as NSAIDs do, without side effects. Some studies show it relieved pain and other fibromyalgia symptoms. Other studies show it is as effective as tricyclic antidepressants, without the side effects.

How It's Used: Internally, in tablets. In OA studies, SAM-e was taken in doses of 200 mg to 400 mg three times per day. For fibromyalgia, 800 mg per day is typical, increasing dosage gradually from 200 mg per day. For depression, 1600 mg per day is recommended. SAM-e is a prescription drug in Europe.

Cautions/Side Effects/Interactions: May cause nausea or upset stomach; side effects more common with higher doses; might interact with certain antidepressants; SAM-e should not be taken by people who are seriously depressed or have bipolar disorder; may contribute to a manic state.

St. John's wort
Hypericum perforatum

Source: A small yellow flower that grows wild throughout Europe and the United States, primarily in northern California and Oregon.

Claims: Acts as "natural Prozac" for depression; may have anti-inflammatory effects. St. John's wort contains hypericin and hyperforin, chemicals that raise the levels of serotonin in the brain. Studies have shown St. John's wort can relieve mild depression about as well as tricyclic and SSRI antidepressants. However, a large recent study found it ineffective for serious depression.

How It's Used: Internally, in pills, teas, and tinctures. Dose in some clinical trials is 300 mg three times daily of an extract standardized to 0.3 percent hypericin. One cup of the tea usually is taken one to three times per day. Oily topical solution used for muscle pain to relieve inflammation.

Cautions/Side Effects/Interactions: May increase sensitivity to sunlight and risk of sunburn in fair-skinned people. Can block the effects of drugs, including oral contraceptives, human immunodeficiency virus (HIV) medications, tricyclic antidepressants, cyclosporin, several heart drugs, and warfarin. Can amplify the effects of many herbs and drugs, such as MAO inhibitors, SSRI antidepressants, tranquilizers, and alcohol. Should not be taken by people who are severely depressed or have bipolar disorder. Side effects may include insomnia (which can be avoided by taking St. John's wort in the morning or by decreasing the dose), restlessness, anxiety, irritability, stomach pain, fatigue, dry mouth, dizziness, and headache.

Siberian ginseng
see Ginseng

Stinging nettle
Urtica dioica

Source: A common weed with tiny stingers that cause painful irritation.

Claims: Reduces pain and swelling of stiff joints associated with OA and RA. No human studies for arthritis. Some human studies show eating stewed nettle leaves might reduce the amount of anti-inflammatory drugs needed for pain relief.

How It's Used: Commonly taken internally as an extract or by eating the cooked leaves. Nettle extract is sold in capsules. In urtication, one area of skin at a time is "stung" by grasping the nettles with a gloved hand and applying to sore area. To eat, the fresh leaves are steamed and served as a vegetable.

Cautions/Side Effects/Interactions: Cooked nettle has no known side effects, but could cause an allergic reaction. When taken orally, stinging nettle juice may cause diarrhea. It can decrease effects of some cardiac and diabetes drugs and may increase effects of sedatives and tranquilizers. Fresh nettle applied topically can cause skin irritation at the source; can enhance the effects of other herbal sedatives.

Thunder god vine
Tripterygium wilfordii (T2 Hook)

Source: Roots of a vine-like plant from Asia.

Claims: Eases pain and inflammation; treats RA and autoimmune diseases. Some in vitro and animal studies have shown it can interfere with the production of chemical mediators of immunity and inflammation. In one Chinese study, it improved symptoms of RA in people taking it with conventional drugs.

How It's Used: The active ingredient is found in the plant's root, and extracts have been used in the studies. No standard dose for humans has been established. In one study for RA, 30 mg of extract per day was used.

Cautions/Side Effects/Interactions: Leaves and flowers are highly toxic and can cause death. Side effects include dry mouth, loss of appetite, nausea, rash, stomach upset, infertility, and skin reactions. Can enhance the effect of immunosuppressive drugs.

Turmeric

Curcuma longa, Curcuma domestica

Source: A root related to ginger.

Claims: Eases pain, stiffness, and inflammation associated with RA and OA; treats bursitis. In human studies, some evidence of efficacy in RA and OA when combined with boswellia, ginger, and aswagandha.

How It's Used: Internally, as a powdered root in capsules or tablets; the usual dose is 400 mg to 1000 mg three times daily.

Cautions/Side Effects/Interactions: Turmeric is a food spice with no known side effects. Should not be used as a supplement by those with gallstones or during pregnancy. Can cause nausea and may increase risk of bleeding if taken with other blood thinners.

Valerian

Valeriana officinalis

Source: The root of a pink flower that grows wild throughout the Americas, Europe, and Asia.

Claims: Sleep disturbances, muscle and joint pain. Several studies show it's an effective alternative to sleep drugs. No evidence it eases other arthritis-related symptoms.

How It's Used: Internally, usually taken as an herbal extract in capsules or tea about an hour before bedtime. Also comes in a tincture or in combination with other hops and herbs. The tea is prepared by steeping 2 grams to 3 grams of the root in boiling water. Typical dose is one cup of the tea taken one to several times per day; maximum dose is 15 grams of the root per day. Externally, can be used in a bath for restlessness and sleep disorders.

Cautions/Side Effects/Interactions: No known serious side effects. Should not be used with other sleep aids, tranquilizers or alcohol, as it increases the effects. May cause morning drowsiness; after extended use, reduce dose gradually.

White willow bark, willow bark

Salix alba

Source: White willow trees.

Claims: Reduces inflammation and pain; eases gout, OA, and RA symptoms.

How It's Used: The bark is made into a tea, tincture, or extract. The amount of salicin in bark varies considerably among willow species. Possibly safe when used appropriately, and possibly effective for joint and muscle aches.

Cautions/Side Effects/Interactions: Contains salicin, the chemical from which aspirin is derived, so it has many of the same potential adverse effects. May cause nausea, upset stomach, and intestinal bleeding. Could have the same drug interactions as aspirin. May increase effects of blood-thinning drugs or supplements. Could increase any kidney and liver problems. Should not be used in people with known aspirin allergies, or in children because of the possibility of Reye's syndrome.

Wild yam

Dioscorea villosa

Source: The root of a plant that is the source of chemicals used to make many synthetic hormones.

Claims: A "natural" source of DHEA (*see* DHEA). No evidence it helps with any arthritis-related symptoms. Does not contain DHEA. Contains diosgenin, the raw ingredient to make DHEA, not the product itself. Possibly safe, but ineffective.

How It's Used: Varying doses internally, and in creams externally.

Cautions/Side Effects/Interactions: None known.

Vitamins and Minerals

Vitamin A

Use: As an antioxidant; protects cells.

Scientific Evidence: In one clinical study, reduced risk of OA progression when used with vitamin E; in another study, associated with an increased risk of knee OA.

Dosage: Usual supplement dose is 1000 µg (3000 IU to 4000 IU) per day. Recommended dietary allowance (RDA) is 700 µg for women, 900 µg for men.

Cautions/Comments: Supplementation over RDA not recommended for those with OA. Good food sources include dairy products, eggs, meat, salmon, and green and yellow vegetables. Eating one sweet potato a day supplies 10,000 IU of natural beta carotene, a form of vitamin A. Risk of toxicity with high doses.

Vitamin B3

Niacin

Use: For various arthritis symptoms, including pain, stiffness, and RA and OA symptoms.

Scientific Evidence: A clinical study in OA found that NSAID dosage could be lowered by 13% if a patient took B3 vitamins.

Dosage: Usual dose is 10 mg to 25 mg per day. RDA is 14 mg for women, 16 mg for men.

Cautions/Comments: B3 can interfere with diabetes drugs. Food sources include lean meat, fish, peanuts, brewer's yeast, and soy.

Vitamin B5

Pantothenic acid

Use: May help with RA pain and stiffness.

Scientific Evidence: Some research shows that B5 can help with morning stiffness and pain of RA.

Dosage: Usual dose is 250 mg per day, but some people with RA may take up to 2000 mg per day. RDA not established, but an estimated adequate dose for adults is 5 mg per day.

Cautions/Comments: Large amounts of B5 can cause diarrhea. Good food sources are soybeans, lentils, meats, eggs, and grains.

Vitamin B6
Pyridoxine

Use: To lower homocysteine levels in people with lupus (*see* Folic acid).

Scientific Evidence: B vitamins and folic acid decrease blood levels of homocysteine, an amino acid associated with stroke and heart disease, which is high in many people with lupus.

Dosage: Usual dose is 5 mg of B6, with 1 mg of B12 and 1 mg of folic acid. The RDA is 1.3 mg to 1.7 mg per day.

Cautions/Comments: Side effects include nausea, vomiting, abdominal pain, loss of appetite, and headache. Good food sources include soybeans, meats, fish, poultry, whole grains, and bananas.

Vitamin B12

Use: To help lower homocysteine levels.

Scientific Evidence: No evidence it helps arthritis. May lower homocysteine levels, known to be high in those with lupus, when 1 mg is taken daily with 1 mg folic acid and 5 mg B6.

Dosage: RDA is 2.4 µg. A multivitamin should provide enough B12.

Cautions/Comments: Food sources include meat, fish, dairy products; vegetarians may need supplements.

Boron

Use: To relieve pain and inflammation of RA and OA; for osteoporosis; promotes bone health.

Scientific Evidence: Some human and animal studies found boron to ease arthritis symptoms.

Dosage: The RDA for boron is not established. Estimated adequate intake is 1 mg per day.

Cautions/Comments: Could raise estrogen levels in dosages higher than 3 mg; women with hormone-sensitive conditions should avoid. People with kidney problems also should avoid. Food sources include fruits, vegetables, nuts, dried beans, wine, cider, and beer.

Copper

Use: For pain and inflammation of RA.

Scientific Evidence: European studies found copper complexes given by injection or intravenously helped some people with RA, ankylosing spondylitis, gout, and Reiter's syndrome. However, not everyone benefited, and many had unacceptable side effects.

Dosage: Usual dosage is 1 mg to 3 mg per day taken internally. RDA is 800 mg. However, many multi-vitamins contain copper, and drinking water from copper plumbing also may contain it.

Cautions/Comments: Can cause nausea, vomiting, diarrhea, and anemia. People with Wilson's disease should never take copper supplements. Copper deficiency is rare, and there is no evidence to suggest that copper supplements are needed if the diet is balanced.

Food sources include chocolate, lobster, nuts, seeds and dried beans.

Vitamin C
Ascorbic acid

Use: For OA symptoms; necessary for collagen formation and tissue repair.

Scientific Evidence: A Framingham study found a high dietary intake of vitamin C was associated with a three-fold decrease in risk of OA pain and progression. Animal studies offer conflicting results.

Dosage: Usual dose is 100 mg to 1000 mg per day. RDA is 75 mg for women, 90 mg for men. Many people take much more.

Cautions/Comments: Large amounts of supplements can cause upset stomach and diarrhea; may increase iron absorption and worsen hemochromatosis. Good sources include citrus fruits, bell peppers, strawberries, and broccoli.

Calcium

Use: Along with vitamin D, protects bones and joints, prevents osteoporosis; offsets bone effects of glucocorticoids; essential for healthy teeth, blood-clotting, and muscle contractions.

Scientific Evidence: Supplements are recommended for all women past menopause, especially those with arthritis.

Dosage: Usual dose and estimated adequate dose is 1000 mg to 1200 mg per day.

Cautions/Comments: Avoid if there is a history of kidney stones. Calcium from oyster shells or dolomite may be contaminated with heavy metals; taking with vitamin D or estrogen supplements increases calcium absorption. Good food sources include dairy products, salmon, sardines, green leafy vegetables, and soy.

Vitamin D

Use: To build bone mass, prevent bone loss and muscle weakness, slow OA progression, and aid in calcium absorption.

Scientific Evidence: A large study found OA progressed three times faster in people who consumed low amounts of vitamin D. Studies show it decreased incidence and progression of hip OA.

Dosage: Usual dose is 400 IU to 800 IU per day. No RDA; estimated adequate amount is 10 mg to 15 mg.

Cautions/Comments: Vitamin D can be made in the body with exposure to sunlight. Many elderly people in northern climates need supplements because they don't get enough sun. Sunblocks will block vitamin D absorption through the skin. People with a history of kidney stones should use with caution. Risk of toxicity in high doses. Good food sources are fortified milk and fatty cold-water fish, such as salmon and sardines.

Vitamin E

Use: To relieve OA and RA symptoms.

Scientific Evidence: Human studies showed vitamin E eased OA and RA pain better than a placebo and one study found that it was better than NSAIDs for OA. One study showed it may not give identical results in different ethnic groups.

Dosage: Dose for pain was 400 IU to 600 IU per day. Use the natural alpha-tocopherol form. RDA is 15 mg.

Cautions/Comments: High doses of vitamin E could increase risk of bleeding in people taking anti-bleeding medications. Whole grains, nuts, and oils are good food sources.

Folic acid

Use: To lower homocysteine levels associated with stroke and heart disease; to offset side effects of methotrexate.

Scientific Evidence: A study shows folic acid taken with B vitamins lowers homocysteine levels, which are high in people with lupus.

Dosage: Usual dose is 1 mg per day for methotrexate side effects. To lower homocysteine levels, 1 mg per day is taken with 5 mg B6 and 1 mg B12. RDA is 400 µg.

Cautions/Comments: High doses can cause many side effects, such as mood changes. Good food sources are spinach, broccoli, fruits, and dried beans.

Magnesium

Use: To relieve pain and inflammation; to ease fibromyalgia and chronic fatigue symptoms.

Scientific Evidence: A placebo-controlled study of a magnesium and malic acid combination product found it eased pain and boosted energy in 24 women with fibromyalgia.

Dosage: Comes in many forms, and usually is combined with malic acid for treatment of fibromyalgia. Suggested daily dose: malic acid, 1200 mg to 2400 mg; magnesium, 300 mg to 600 mg, divided into several doses. Magnesium RDA is 320 mg for women, 420 mg for men.

Cautions/Comments: Chronic fatigue symptoms are connected to low magnesium levels, and supplements have been shown to improve those symptoms. Can interact with blood pressure medication; may cause loose stools; can cause kidney failure in people with kidney disease; may cause nausea, vomiting, diarrhea, and stomach irritation. Food sources include nuts, grains, and whole foods.

Manganese

Use: For osteoporosis; relieves OA symptoms in a combination product with glucosamine hydrochloride and chondroitin sulfate.

Scientific Evidence: Studies show it's effective for osteoporosis when taken with calcium, zinc, and copper. A glucosamine-chondroitin-manganese combination has been shown effective for OA pain, but it's not known if manganese contributes to these results.

Dosage: For osteoporosis, 5 mg a day usually is combined with elemental calcium, zinc, and copper. The glucosamine combination remedy has a much higher amount. No RDA established. Estimated adequate intake is 1.8 mg to 2.3 mg per day. Dose should not exceed 11 mg per day.

Cautions/Comments: High doses might lead to manganese accumulation and symptoms similar to Parkinson's disease, including psychosis. Those with chronic liver disease should use cautiously. Manganese is found in leafy green vegetables, nuts, seeds, tea, and whole grains.

Selenium

Use: To ease pain, stiffness, and inflammation; for RA symptoms.

Scientific Evidence: One human study for RA showed fewer tender joints, less stiffness, and less swelling after six months; however, the study group also was taking fish oil supplements. No human studies show selenium supplements alone can improve RA symptoms.

Dosage: A usual dose is 50 µg to 200 µg. RDA is 55 µg.

Cautions/Comments: Selenium levels are low in people with RA and other inflammatory conditions, but the human body requires a very small amount of selenium. Some multi-vitamins contain selenium, and care should be taken to avoid overdose. Can cause nausea, vomiting, nail changes, fatigue, and irritability. Good food sources are crab, liver, fish, poultry, and wheat.

Zinc sulfate

Use: To ease pain, stiffness, and inflammation of RA; to ease psoriasis.

Scientific Evidence: A small study showed zinc sulfate improved RA; in another study, it eased psoriatic symptoms. An FDA-approved treatment for Wilson's disease.

Dosage: RDA is 12 mg for women, 15 mg for men. Appears safe when taken in doses less than 50 mg per day.

Cautions/Comments: May interfere with corticosteroids and other immunosuppressive drugs. Can cause nausea, vomiting, diarrhea; taking zinc regularly may impair copper absorption; drinking coffee may decrease zinc absorption up to 50%. Food sources include meat, seafood, egg yolk, dairy, soy, and wheat products.

Resources

The Arthritis Foundation's Guide to Alternative Therapies by Judith Horstman, a comprehensive resource for nearly 90 different forms of alternative treatments. 800/207-8633 or www.arthritis.org. **Natural Medicines Comprehensive Database** is an online resource for evidence-based clinical information on natural medicines. Also in book form. The site is designed for health professionals. Access by subscription only. www.naturaldatabase.com. **HerbMed** is a free online database that provides access to scientific data behind the use of herbs for health. www.herbmed.org. **The US Food & Drug Administration Center for Food Safety & Applied Nutrition** offers online dietary supplement information from the government. www.cfsan.fda.gov/~dms/supplmnt.html.

Adapted from Horstman J. Arthritis Today's supplement guide: herbs, vitamins and other natural remedies. Arthritis Today 2001;15 (July/Aug):34–49, with permission of the Arthritis Foundation.

INDEX

Page numbers followed by "t"
refer to information found in tables.

Notes

Notes

Notes

Notes

Notes

Notes